M
W9-AHM-193

Clinical
Anesthesiology

Fourth edition

G. Edward Morgan, Jr., MD
President and Chief Executive Officer
Excellence in Medicine, LLC
OrthoSource Medical Clinics, Inc.
Pasadena, California

Maged S. Mikhail, MD
San Fernando Valley Heart Institute
Encino-Tarzana Regional Medical Center
Los Angeles, California

Michael J. Murray, MD, PhD
Colonel, Medical Corps, US Army Reserves
Professor of Anesthesiology, Mayo Clinic College of Medicine
Chair, Department of Anesthesiology
Mayo Clinic Jacksonville
Jacksonville, Florida

Lange Medical Books/McGraw-Hill
Medical Publishing Division
New York   Chicago   San Francisco   Lisbon
London   Madrid   Mexico City   Milan   New Delhi
San Juan   Seoul   Singapore   Sydney   Toronto

The McGraw·Hill Companies

Clinical Anesthesiology, Fourth Edition

Copyright © 2006, 2002 by the McGraw-Hill Companies, Inc. All rights reserved. Printed in the United States of America. Except as permitted under the United States Copyright Act of 1976, no part of this publication may be reproduced or distributed in any form or by any means, or stored in a database or retrieval system, without the prior written permission of the publisher.

Previous editions copyright © 1996, 1992 by Appleton & Lange

4 5 6 7 8 9 0 DOCDOC 0 9 8 7

ISBN 0-07-142358-3

Notice

Medicine is an ever-changing science. As new research and clinical experience broaden our knowledge, changes in treatment and drug therapy are required. The editors and the publisher of this work have checked with sources believed to be reliable in their efforts to provide information that is complete and generally in accord with the standards accepted at the time of publication. However, in view of the possibility of human error or changes in medical sciences, neither the editors nor the publisher nor any other party who has been involved in the preparation or publication of this work warrants that the information contained herein is in every respect accurate or complete, and they disclaim all responsibility for any errors or omissions or for the results obtained from use of the information contained in this work. Readers are encouraged to confirm the information contained herein with other sources. For example and in particular, readers are advised to check the product information sheet included in the package of each drug they plan to administer to be certain that the information contained in this work is accurate and that changes have not been made in the recommended dose or in the contraindications for administration. This recommendation is of particular importance in connection with new or infrequently used drugs.

This book was set in Adobe Garamond by Silverchair Science + Communications, Inc..
The editors were Marc Strauss, Harriet Lebowitz, and Peter J. Boyle.
The production supervisor was Philip Galea.
The art manager was Charissa Baker; the illustration coordinator was Maria T. Magtoto.
The text was designed by Eve Siegel.
The index was prepared by Kathrin Unger.
RR Donnelley was printer and binder.

This book is printed on acid-free paper.

INTERNATIONAL EDITION ISBN 0-07-110515-8

To my sister, Jane Morgan, and my mother, Iva Morgan

Edward Morgan

To my entire family, especially my son Daniel Mikhail,
who was born after the last edition

Maged Mikhail

To the men and women in the Armed Forces, and especially
to those who provide health care

Michael Murray

Contents

IV. PHYSIOLOGY, PATHOPHYSIOLOGY, & ANESTHETIC MANAGEMENT

V. SPECIAL PROBLEMS

Contents: Profiles in Anesthetic Practice

Contributors

Contributing Authors

Wayne Kleinman, MD
Director of Obstetrical Anesthesia
Encino-Tarzana Regional Medical Center
Tarzana, California

Gary J. Nitti, MD
Chairman, Department of Anesthesiology
Director, Cardiac Anesthesia Services
Encino-Tarzana Regional Medical Center
Los Angeles, California

Joseph T. Nitti, MD
Staff Anesthesiologist
Encino-Tarzana Regional Medical Center
Los Angeles, California

Julio Raya, MD
Arthritis Institute
Centinela Hospital
Los Angeles, California

Contributors to Profiles in Anesthetic Practice

Robert F. Bedford, MD
Professor, Department of Anesthesiology
University of Virginia School of Medicine
Charlottesville, Virginia

Julian F. Bion, FRCP, FRCA, MD
Reader in Intensive Care Medicine
Birmingham University
Honorary Consultant in Intensive Care Medicine
University Hospital Birmingham NHS Trust
Birmingham, United Kingdom

John Butterworth, MD
Professor and Robert K. Stoelting Chair
Department of Anesthesia
Indiana University School of Medicine
Indianapolis, Indiana

Neal H. Cohen, MD, MPH, MS
Professor, Anesthesia and Perioperative Care
and Medicine
Vice Dean, School of Medicine
University of California, San Francisco
San Francisco, California

Jerry A. Dorsch, MD
Associate Professor Emeritus
Mayo Clinic College of Medicine
Jacksonville, Florida

Roy A. Greengrass, MD
Associate Professor of Anesthesiology
Mayo Clinic College of Medicine
Jacksonville, Florida

Gerald A. Gronert, MD
Professor Emeritus, Department of Anesthesiology
University of California, Davis
Davis, California
Adjunct Professor, Department of Anesthesiology
University of New Mexico
Albuquerque, New Mexico

Carl C. Hug, Jr., MD, PhD
Professor of Anesthesiology Emeritus
Emory University School of Medicine
Attending Physician in Surgical Intensive Care
Emory University Hospital
Atlanta, Georgia

Jennifer M. Hunter, MD
Professor, University Department of Anesthesia
University of Liverpool
Liverpool, United Kingdom

Shauna Irgin, FRCA
Specialist Registrar Anesthesia and Intensive
Care Medicine
University Hospital NHS Trust
Birmingham, United Kingdom

Patricia Kapur, MD
Professor and Chair, Department of
Anesthesiology
David Geffen School of Medicine at UCLA
Los Angeles, California

C. Philip Larson, Jr., MD, CM
Professor Emeritus, Anesthesia and
Neurosurgery
Stanford University
Palo Alto, California
Professor of Clinical Anesthesiology
David Geffen School of Medicine at UCLA
Los Angeles, California

John R. Moyers, MD
Professor, Department of Anesthesia
University of Iowa College of Medicine
Iowa City, Iowa

J. G. Reves, MD
Professor of Anesthesiology
Professor of Pharmacology
Dean, College of Medicine
Vice-President of Medical Affairs
Medical University of South Carolina
Charleston, South Carolina

Takefumi Sakabe, MD
Professor and Chairman
Department of Anesthesiology-Resuscitology
Yamaguchi University School of Medicine
Minami-Kogushi, Ube, Yamaguchi
Japan

John J. Savarese, MD
Professor and Chair, Department of Anesthesiology
Weill Medical College of Cornell University
New York, New York

Peter Slinger, MD, FRCPC
Professor of Anesthesia
University of Toronto
Toronto, Ontario
Canada

Daniel M. Thys, MD
Professor, Department of Anesthesiology
College of Physicians & Surgeons,
   Columbia University
Chair, Department of Anesthesiology
St. Luke's-Roosevelt Hospital Center
New York, New York

Preface

This new edition of *Clinical Anesthesiology* contains several important improvements and refinements of the three highly successful prior editions. For the first time, we have sought the expertise of non-anesthesiologist authorities in specific fields to review the content of selected chapters. The purpose of this plan was to put commonly accepted anesthetic tenets under the spotlight of the scientific literature of related, yet distinct, specialties. For example, those chapters dealing with the anesthetic management of surgical cases were typically reviewed by a surgeon specializing in that field, the pharmacology chapters by pharmacologists, and the equipment chapters by engineers. We hope the results of this endeavor provide the reader with as educational an exercise as was experienced by the authors.

For their review of specific chapters, the authors wish to express their gratitude to Nelson Koe, MD; Duraiyah Thangathurai, MD; Diana Wong, MD; Nabil Rashad, MD; Karen Morgan, MD; Rafael Llerena; Jodi Wabiszewski; Douglas Bacon, MD; C. George Merridew, MBBS; Barry Harrison, MBBS; Jerry Dorsch, MD; Stephen Grinton, MD; Octavio Pajaro, MD, PhD; John Odell, MD; Javier Aduen, MD; Patrick Kamath, MD; Wolf Stapelfeldt, MD; and Robert Hale, DDS.

 Profiles in Anesthetic Practice are exciting, unique features introduced in the third edition, but expanded in the fourth edition. These brief essays, written by eighteen internationally recognized leaders in anesthesiology (five of whom practice anesthesiology outside the United States) present editorialized counterpoints to the usual textbook dogma. They involve the reader in the dynamics of thinking through anesthetic problems and controversies. Thus each essay is a profile in the sense that it represents more of a side perspective as opposed to a straight-on view. The Profiles in Anesthetic Practice are easily identified by the use of color, icons, and a line drawing of each author's profile.

 Key Concepts are listed in the front of each chapter and a corresponding numbered icon identifies the section(s) within the chapter in which each concept is discussed. These should help the reader focus on truly important themes that constitute the core of understanding anesthesiology.

 Case Discussions deal with clinical problems of current interest and provide a methodology and framework to approach oral examinations.

Key Terms and Topics are identified with color type. These highlighted words, the number of which has been significantly expanded in this edition, provide the reader with a quick guide to the subject matter, on which many written exam questions are based.

- All chapters have been thoroughly updated and revised. Chapters 4, 5, 6, and 17 underwent particularly extensive rewriting. The chapter on "Outpatient Anesthesia" was deleted in this edition, ironically because the outpatient setting has become so ubiquitous that it is an integral part of every chapter.
- The suggested reading has been expanded and updated to include pertinent Web addresses.
- Several new illustrations have been added.

Nonetheless, the goal of *Clinical Anesthesiology* remains unchanged from the first edition: "to provide a concise, consistent presentation of the basic principles essential to the modern practice of anesthesia." To this end, the authors strove to minimize redundancies, eliminate contradictions, and write in a highly readable style. The case discussions that conclude each chapter continue to address the whys of clinical medicine, serve as a self-examination tool for the reader, and instill a logical approach to clinical situations. The suggested reading includes relevant texts, chapters, and review articles, emphasizing material published since 2000.

We wish to acknowledge Martin L. DeRuyter, MD, who helped with the extensive revision of Chapter 17 on Peripheral Nerve Blocks. We are also grateful to individuals who offered their expertise in addressing specific questions in selected chapters. They include Douglas Coursin, MD; Jeffrey Vender, MD; Roy Greengrass, MD; Udaya Prakash, MD; Roy Cucchiara, MD; Eric Bloomfield, MD; Jasper Daube, MD; John Noseworthy, MD; Gregory Cascino, MD; W. Andrew Oldenburg, MD; James Meschia, MD; Thomas Brott, MD; Thomas Bower, MD; Richard Prielipp, MD; Daniel Hurley, MD; John Miles, MD; Roger White, MD; Andrea Gabrielli, MD; Gale Van Norman, MD; Lance Oyen, PharmD; Jeffrey Ward, RRT; Steve Holets, RRT; and Frances Kennedy.

Other individuals who offered insights include Alex Aidinoff, MD; Beverly Philip, MD; John Maydak, MD; and Sarah Tierney, CRNA. Also gratefully acknowledged is the assistance of Robin Williams. We would also like to thank Marc Strauss, Harriet Lebowitz, Marsha Loeb, and Arline Keithe for their invaluable assistance.

G. Edward Morgan, Jr., MD
Maged S. Mikhail, MD
Michael J. Murray, MD, PhD
May 2005

The Practice of Anesthesiology

KEY CONCEPTS

 An anesthetic plan should be formulated that will optimally accommodate the patient's baseline physiological state, including any medical conditions, previous operations, the planned procedure, drug sensitivities, previous anesthetic experiences, and psychological makeup.

 Inadequate preoperative planning and errors in patient preparation are the most common causes of anesthetic complications.

 Anesthesia and elective operations should not proceed until the patient is in optimal medical condition.

 To be valuable, performing a preoperative test implies that an increased perioperative risk exists when the results are abnormal and a reduced risk exists when the abnormality is corrected.

 The usefulness of a screening test depends on its sensitivity and specificity. Sensitive tests have a low rate of false-negative results, whereas specific tests have a low rate of false-positive results.

 If any procedure is performed without the patient's consent, the physician may be liable for assault and battery.

 The intraoperative anesthesia record serves many purposes. It functions as a useful intraoperative monitor, a reference for future anesthetics for that patient, and a tool for quality assurance.

The Greek philosopher Dioscorides first used the term *anesthesia* in the first century AD to describe the narcotic-like effects of the plant mandragora. The term subsequently was defined in Bailey's *An Universal Etymological English Dictionary* (1721) as "a defect of sensation" and again in the *Encyclopedia Britannica* (1771) as "privation of the senses." The present use of the term to denote the sleeplike state that makes painless surgery possible is credited to Oliver Wendell Holmes in 1846. In the United States, use of the term *anesthesiology* to denote the practice or study of anesthesia was first proposed in the second decade of the twentieth century to emphasize the growing scientific basis of the specialty. Although the specialty now rests on a scientific foundation that rivals any other, anesthesia remains very much a mixture of both science and art. Moreover, the practice of anesthesiology has

expanded well beyond rendering patients insensible to pain during surgery or obstetric delivery (Table 1–1). The specialty is unique in that it requires a working familiarity with most other specialties, including surgery and its subspecialties, internal medicine, pediatrics, and obstetrics as well as clinical pharmacology, applied physiology, and biomedical technology. The application of recent advances in biomedical technology in clinical anesthesia continues to make anesthesia an exciting and rapidly evolving specialty. A significant number of physicians applying for residency positions in anesthesiology already have training and certification in other specialties.

This chapter reviews the history of anesthesia, its British and American roots, and the current scope of the specialty and presents the general approach to the preoperative evaluation of patients and documentation

Table 1–1. Definition of the practice of anesthesiology, which is the practice of medicine.[1]

Assessment of, consultation for, and preparation of, patients for anesthesia.

Relief and prevention of pain during and following surgical, obstetric, therapeutic, and diagnostic procedures.

Monitoring and maintenance of normal physiology during the perioperative period.

Management of critically ill patients.

Diagnosis and treatment of acute, chronic, and cancer-related pain.

Clinical management and teaching of cardiac and pulmonary resuscitation.

Evaluation of respiratory function and application of respiratory therapy.

Conduct of clinical, translational, and basic science research.

Supervision, teaching, and evaluation of the performance of both medical and paramedical personnel involved in perioperative care.

Administrative involvement in health care facilities, organizations, and medical schools necessary to implement these responsibilities.

[1]From the American Board of Anesthesiology Booklet of Information, January 2003.

of the patient's anesthetic experience. The Case Discussion at the end of the chapter considers medicolegal aspects of the specialty.

■ THE HISTORY OF ANESTHESIA

Anesthetic practices date from ancient times, yet the evolution of the specialty began in the mid-nineteenth century and only became firmly established less than six decades ago. Ancient civilizations had used opium poppy, coca leaves, mandrake root, alcohol, and even phlebotomy (to the point of unconsciousness) to allow surgeons to operate. It is interesting that the ancient Egyptians used the combination of opium poppy (morphine) and hyoscyamus (hyoscyamine and scopolamine); a similar combination, morphine and scopolamine, is still used parenterally for premedication. Regional anesthesia in ancient times consisted of compression of nerve trunks (nerve ischemia) or the application of cold (cryoanalgesia). The Incas may have practiced local anesthesia as their surgeons chewed coca leaves and spat saliva (presumably containing cocaine) into the operative wound. Surgical procedures were for the most part limited to caring for fractures, traumatic

wounds, amputations, and the removal of bladder calculi. Amazingly, some civilizations were also able to perform trephination of the skull. A major qualification for a successful surgeon was speed.

The evolution of modern surgery was hampered not only by a poor understanding of disease processes, anatomy, and surgical asepsis but also by the lack of reliable and safe anesthetic techniques. These techniques evolved first with inhalation anesthesia, followed by local and regional anesthesia, and finally intravenous anesthesia. The development of surgical anesthesia is considered one of the most important discoveries in human history.

INHALATION ANESTHESIA

Because the invention of the hypodermic needle did not occur until 1855, the first general anesthetics were destined to be inhalation agents. Ether (really diethyl ether, known at the time as "sulfuric ether" because it was produced by a simple chemical reaction between ethyl alcohol and sulfuric acid) was originally prepared in 1540 by Valerius Cordus, a 25-year-old Prussian botanist. Ether was used by the medical community for frivolous purposes ("ether frolics") and was not used as an anesthetic agent in humans until 1842, when Crawford W. Long and William E. Clark used it independently on patients. However, they did not publicize this discovery. Four years later, in Boston, on October 16, 1846, William T.G. Morton conducted the first publicized demonstration of general anesthesia using ether. The dramatic success of that exhibition led the operating surgeon to exclaim to a skeptical audience: "Gentlemen, this is no humbug!"

Chloroform was independently prepared by von Leibig, Guthrie, and Soubeiran in 1831. Although first used by Holmes Coote in 1847, chloroform was introduced into clinical practice by the Scottish obstetrician Sir James Simpson, who administered it to his patients to relieve the pain of labor. Ironically, Simpson had almost abandoned his medical practice after witnessing the terrible despair and agony of patients undergoing operations without anesthesia.

Joseph Priestley produced nitrous oxide in 1772, but Humphry Davy first noted its analgesic properties in 1800. Gardner Colton and Horace Wells are credited with having first used nitrous oxide as an anesthetic in humans in 1844. Nitrous oxide's lack of potency (an 80% nitrous oxide concentration results in analgesia but not surgical anesthesia) led to clinical demonstrations that were less convincing than those with ether.

Nitrous oxide was the least popular of the three early inhalation anesthetics because of its low potency and its tendency to cause asphyxia when used alone (see Chapter 7). Interest in nitrous oxide was revived in 1868 when Edmund Andrews administered it in 20% oxygen; its use was, however, overshadowed by the popularity of ether and chloroform. It is ironic that nitrous oxide is the only one of these agents still in common use today. Chloroform initially superseded ether in popularity in many areas (particularly in the United Kingdom), but reports of chloroform-related cardiac arrhythmias, respiratory depression, and hepatotoxicity eventually caused more and more practitioners to abandon it in favor of ether.

Even after the introduction of other inhalation anesthetics (ethyl chloride, ethylene, divinyl ether, cyclopropane, trichloroethylene, and fluroxene), ether remained the standard general anesthetic until the early 1960s. The only inhalation agent that rivaled ether's safety and popularity was cyclopropane (introduced in 1934). However, both are highly combustible and have since been replaced by the nonflammable potent fluorinated hydrocarbons: halothane (developed in 1951; released in 1956), methoxyflurane (developed in 1958; released in 1960), enflurane (developed in 1963; released in 1973), and isoflurane (developed in 1965; released in 1981).

New agents continue to be developed. One such agent, desflurane (released in 1992), has many of the desirable properties of isoflurane as well as the rapid uptake and elimination characteristics of nitrous oxide. Sevoflurane, another agent, also has low blood solubility, but concerns about potentially toxic degradation products delayed its release in the United States until 1994 (see Chapter 7).

LOCAL & REGIONAL ANESTHESIA

The origin of modern local anesthesia is credited to Carl Koller, an ophthalmologist, who demonstrated the use of topical cocaine for surgical anesthesia of the eye in 1884. Cocaine had been isolated from the coca plant in 1855 by Gaedicke and later purified in 1860 by Albert Neimann. In 1884 the surgeon William Halsted demonstrated the use of cocaine for intradermal infiltration and nerve blocks (including the facial nerve, the brachial plexus, the pudendal nerve, and the posterior tibial nerve). August Bier is credited with administering the first spinal anesthetic in 1898; he used 3 mL of 0.5% cocaine intrathecally. He was also the first to describe intravenous regional anesthesia (Bier block) in 1908. Procaine was synthesized in 1904 by Alfred Einhorn and within a year was used clinically as a local anesthetic by Heinrich Braun. Braun was also the first to add epinephrine to prolong the action of local anesthetics. Ferdinand Cathelin and Jean Sicard introduced caudal epidural anesthesia in 1901. Lumbar epidural anesthesia was described first in 1921 by Fidel Pages and again in 1931 by Achille Dogliotti. Additional local anesthetics subsequently introduced clinically include dibucaine (1930), tetracaine (1932), lidocaine (1947),

chloroprocaine (1955), mepivacaine (1957), prilocaine (1960), bupivacaine (1963), and etidocaine (1972). Ropivacaine and levobupivacaine, an isomer of bupivacaine, are newer agents with the same duration of action as bupivacaine but less cardiac toxicity (see Chapter 14).

INTRAVENOUS ANESTHESIA

Induction Agents

Intravenous anesthesia followed the invention of the hypodermic syringe and needle by Alexander Wood in 1855. Early attempts at intravenous anesthesia included the use of chloral hydrate (by Oré in 1872), chloroform and ether (Burkhardt in 1909), and the combination of morphine and scopolamine (Bredenfeld in 1916). Barbiturates were synthesized in 1903 by Fischer and von Mering. The first barbiturate used for induction of anesthesia was diethylbarbituric acid (barbital), but it was not until the introduction of hexobarbital in 1927 that barbiturate induction became a popular technique. Thiopental, synthesized in 1932 by Volwiler and Tabern, was first used clinically by John Lundy and Ralph Waters in 1934, and remains the most common induction agent for anesthesia. Methohexital was first used clinically in 1957 by V.K. Stoelting and is the only other barbiturate currently used for induction. Since the synthesis of chlordiazepoxide in 1957, the benzodiazepines—diazepam (1959), lorazepam (1971), and midazolam (1976)—have been extensively used for premedication, induction, supplementation of anesthesia, and intravenous sedation. Ketamine was synthesized in 1962 by Stevens and first used clinically in 1965 by Corssen and Domino; it was released in 1970. Ketamine was the first intravenous agent associated with minimal cardiac and respiratory depression. Etomidate was synthesized in 1964 and released in 1972; initial enthusiasm over its relative lack of circulatory and respiratory effects was tempered by reports of adrenal suppression after even a single dose. The release of propofol, diisopropylphenol, in 1989 was a major advance in outpatient anesthesia because of its short duration of action (see Chapter 8).

Neuromuscular Blocking Agents

The use of curare by Harold Griffith and Enid Johnson in 1942 was a milestone in anesthesia. Curare greatly facilitated tracheal intubation and provided excellent abdominal relaxation for surgery. For the first time, operations could be performed on patients without having to administer relatively large doses of anesthetic to produce muscle relaxation. These large doses of anesthetic often resulted in excessive circulatory and respiratory depression as well as prolonged emergence; moreover, they were often not tolerated by frail patients.

Other neuromuscular blocking agents (NMBAs) (see Chapter 9)—gallamine, decamethonium, metocurine, alcuronium, and pancuronium—were soon introduced clinically. Because the use of these agents was often associated with significant side effects (see Chapter 9), the search for the ideal NMBA continued. Recently introduced agents that come close to this goal include vecuronium, atracurium, pipecuronium, doxacurium, rocuronium, and cis-atracurium. Succinylcholine was synthesized by Bovet in 1949 and released in 1951; it has become a standard agent for facilitating tracheal intubation. Until recently, succinylcholine remained unparalleled in its rapid onset of profound muscle relaxation, but its occasional side effects continued to fuel the search for a comparable substitute. Mivacurium, a newer short-acting nondepolarizing NMBA, has minimal side effects, but it still has a slower onset and longer duration of action than succinylcholine. Rocuronium is an intermediate-acting relaxant with a rapid onset approaching that of succinylcholine. Rapacuronium, the most recently released NMBA, finally combined succinylcholine's rapid onset and short duration of action with an improved safety profile. However, the manufacturer of rapacuronium voluntarily withdrew it from the market due to several reports of serious bronchospasm.

Opioids

Morphine was isolated from opium in 1805 by Sertürner and subsequently tried as an intravenous anesthetic (see above). The morbidity and mortality initially associated with high doses of opioids in early reports caused many anesthetists to avoid opioids and favor pure inhalation anesthesia. Interest in opioids in anesthesia returned following the synthesis of meperidine in 1939. The concept of balanced anesthesia was introduced in 1926 by Lundy and others and evolved to consist of thiopental for induction, nitrous oxide for amnesia, meperidine (or any opioid) for analgesia, and curare for muscle relaxation. In 1969, Lowenstein rekindled interest in opioid anesthesia by reintroducing the concept of high doses of opioids as complete anesthetics. Morphine was initially employed, but fentanyl, sufentanil, and alfentanil were all subsequently used as sole agents. As experience grew with this technique, its limitations in reliably preventing patient awareness and suppressing autonomic responses during surgery were realized. Remifentanil is a new rapidly metabolized opioid that is broken down by nonspecific plasma and tissue esterases.

EVOLUTION OF THE SPECIALTY

British Origins

Following its first public demonstration in the United States, the use of ether quickly spread to England. John Snow, generally considered the father of anesthesia, became the first physician to take a full-time interest in this new anesthetic, for which he invented an inhaler. He was the first to scientifically investigate ether and the physiology of general anesthesia. (Snow was also a pioneer in epidemiology who helped stop a cholera epidemic in London by proving that the causative agent was transmitted by ingestion rather than inhalation.) In 1847, Snow published the first book on general anesthesia, *On the Inhalation of Ether.* When the anesthetic properties of chloroform were made known (see above), he quickly investigated and developed an inhaler for that agent as well. He believed that an inhaler should be used in administering these agents to control the dose of the anesthetic. His second book, *On Chloroform and Other Anaesthetics,* was published posthumously in 1858.

After Snow's death, Joseph T. Clover took his place as England's leading physician anesthetist. Clover emphasized continuously monitoring the patient's pulse during anesthesia, a practice that was not widely accepted at the time. He was the first to use the jaw-thrust maneuver for relieving airway obstruction, the first to have resuscitation equipment always available during anesthesia, and the first to use a cricothyroid cannula (to save a patient with an oral tumor who developed complete airway obstruction). Sir Frederick Hewitt became England's foremost anesthetist at the turn of the century. He was responsible for many inventions, including the oral airway. Hewitt also wrote what many consider to be the first true textbook of anesthesia, which went through five editions. Snow, Clover, and Hewitt established a tradition of physician anesthetists that still exists in England. In 1893, the first organization of physician specialists in anesthesia, the London Society of Anaesthetists, was formed in England by J.F. Silk.

American Origins

In the United States, few physicians had specialized in anesthesia by the turn of the century. The task of giving anesthesia was usually delegated to junior surgical house officers or medical students, who tended to be more interested in the surgical procedure than in monitoring the patient. Because of the shortage of physicians interested in the specialty in the United States and the relative safety of ether anesthesia, surgeons at both the Mayo Clinic and Cleveland Clinic trained and employed nurses as anesthetists. The first organization of physician anesthetists in the United States was the Long Island Society of Anesthetists formed in 1905, which, as it grew, was renamed the New York Society of Anesthetists in 1911. In 1936, it became the American Society of Anesthetists, and later, in 1945, the American Society of Anesthesiologists (ASA).

Three physicians stand out in the early development of anesthesia in the United States after the turn of the century: Arthur E. Guedel, Ralph M. Waters, and John S. Lundy. Guedel was the first to elaborate on the signs of general anesthesia after Snow's original description. He advocated cuffed tracheal tubes and introduced artificial ventilation during ether anesthesia (later called *controlled respiration* by Waters). Ralph Waters added a long list of contributions to the specialty in the United States; probably the most important of these was his insistence on the proper training of specialists in anesthesia. Waters developed the first academic department of anesthesiology at the University of Wisconsin in Madison. Lundy was instrumental in the formation of the American Board of Anesthesiology, chaired the American Medical Association's Section on Anesthesiology for 17 years, and established the first advanced degree in the United States, a Master of Science in Anesthesiology.

The first elective tracheal intubations during anesthesia were performed in the late nineteenth century by surgeons: Sir William MacEwen in Scotland, Joseph O'Dwyer in the United States, and Franz Kuhn in Germany. Tracheal intubation during anesthesia was popularized in England by Sir Ivan Magill and Stanley Rowbotham in the 1920s.

Official Recognition

Thomas D. Buchanan was appointed the first Professor of Anesthesiology at the New York Medical College in 1904. The American Board of Anesthesiology was established in 1938 with Buchanan as its first president. In England, the first examination for the Diploma in Anaesthetics took place in 1935, and the first Chair in Anaesthetics was awarded to Sir Robert Macintosh in 1937 at Oxford University. Anesthesia became an officially recognized specialty in England only in 1947, when the Faculty of Anaesthetists of the Royal College of Surgeons was established.

THE SCOPE OF ANESTHESIA

The practice of anesthesia has changed dramatically since the days of John Snow. The modern anesthesiologist is now both a consultant and a primary care provider. The consultant role is appropriate because the primary goal of the anesthetist—to see the patient safely and comfortably through an operation—generally takes only a short time (minutes to hours). However, because anesthesiologists manage all "noncutting" aspects of the patient's care in the immediate perioperative period, they are also primary care providers. The "captain of the ship" doctrine, which held the surgeon responsible for every aspect of the patient's perioperative care (including anesthesia), is no longer valid. The surgeon and anesthesiologist must function together effectively, but both are ultimately answerable to the patient rather than to each other. Patients can select their own anesthesiologists, but their choices are usually limited by who is on the medical staff at a particular hospital, the surgeon's preference (if any), or the on-call schedule for anesthesiologists on a given day.

The practice of anesthesia is no longer limited to the operating room nor even confined to rendering patients insensible to pain (Table 1–1). Anesthesiologists are now routinely asked to monitor, sedate, and provide general or regional anesthesia outside the operating room—for lithotripsy, magnetic resonance imaging, computed tomography, fluoroscopy, endoscopy, electroconvulsive therapy, and cardiac catheterization. Anesthesiologists have traditionally been pioneers in cardiopulmonary resuscitation and continue to be integral members of resuscitation teams. An increasing number of practitioners have subspecialized in cardiac anesthesia (see Chapter 21), critical care (see Chapter 49), neuroanesthesia (see Chapter 26), obstetric anesthesia (see Chapter 43), pediatric anesthesia (see Chapter 44), and pain medicine (see Chapter 18). Certification requirements for special competence in critical care and pain medicine already exist in the United States. Anesthesiologists are actively involved in the administration and medical direction of many operating rooms, intensive care units, and respiratory therapy departments. They have also assumed administrative and leadership positions on the medical staffs of many hospitals and ambulatory care facilities.

PREOPERATIVE EVALUATION OF PATIENTS

As will become clear in later chapters, no one standard anesthetic meets the needs of all patients. Rather, an anesthetic plan (Table 1–2) should be formulated that will optimally accommodate the patient's baseline physiological state, including any medical conditions, previous operations, the planned procedure, drug sensitivities, previous anesthetic experiences, and psychological makeup. Inadequate preoperative planning and errors in patient preparation are the most common causes of anesthetic complications. To help formulate the anesthetic plan, a general outline for assessing patients preoperatively is an important starting

Shauna Irgin, FRCA

Julian Bion, FRCP, FRCA, MD

THE ROLE OF THE ANESTHETIST IN MANAGING THE ACUTELY ILL HOSPITALIZED PATIENT

Hospitals have changed markedly over recent years, with increasing throughput, fewer acute beds, more emergency admissions involving acutely ill patients, and a greater proportion of elderly patients undergoing complex interventional procedures. These changes have occurred in an environment of cost containment, constrained working hours and reduced training times for junior doctors, diminution in the authority of doctors and greater involvement of managers in the health care system, a growing demand for outcomes-based monitoring of health care, and increased public expectations. At the same time we have learned that health care is not quite as good as we thought: somewhere between 3% and 16% of patients suffer avoidable adverse events through system errors in health care processes, with clinical staff in the front line taking the blame.[1–3]

Safe care of the acutely ill or high-risk hospitalized patient presents special difficulties in this environment.[4] Outside the confines of single-organ disease such as myocardial infarction or acute asthma, there are few standardized care pathways of the type developed for trauma management. Unpredictability and rapid changes in the patient's condition, multiple therapies, gaps and discontinuities in clinical care, and the difficulty of providing quality care out of "normal" working hours all contribute to the risk of adverse outcomes. Taken together, these changes may explain some of the current phenomenon of "getting better but feeling worse."[5,6] They certainly present clinicians with some important challenges. Responding to these challenges in innovative ways is an important element in professionalism, and is essential for maintaining—or restoring—a sense of ownership, empowerment, and self-respect.

Three countries have developed innovative approaches to acute hospital care: Australia, the United Kingdom, and the United States. Australia has created the concept of the intensive care unit-based Medical Emergency Team (MET) to replace the traditional cardiac arrest team,[7] responding to calls for assistance from staff in other wards and departments using calling criteria based on abnormal vital signs. The United Kingdom has developed nurse-led Outreach care, in which intensive care-trained medical and nursing staff form a link between ward and critical care areas, supporting ward staff and pro-

point (Table 1–3). This assessment includes a pertinent history (including a review of medical records), a physical examination, and any indicated laboratory tests. (This book will present detailed discussions about evaluating patients with specific disorders and those undergoing unusual procedures.) Classifying the patient's physical status according to the ASA scale completes the assessment. Anesthesia and elective operations should not proceed viding continuity of care for acutely ill patients throughout the patient journey.[8] The approach in the United States has been to develop a new medical speciality—the hospitalist, a generalist physician located in the hospital.[9,10] The skill sets required of these different practitioners have not been properly defined, but they all share a need for transdisciplinary team-based working that should appeal to anesthetists.[11]

Anesthetists have an essential role in making hospitals safer places for acutely ill patients. They possess unique skill sets, combined with an impressive track record in safe practice. From the early days of intraoperative administration of anesthesia and airway support during surgery, the anesthetist may now be involved in perioperative care, intensive care medicine, physiological manipulation, monitoring, pharmacology, and acute and chronic pain management, as well as clinical and laboratory research. In parallel with this expansion in role, the discipline has also made major contributions to patient safety in the operating theater, at a level that has been likened to that of aviation.[12] Part of this achievement must be attributable to attitudinal competencies— a mindset that favors teamwork and facilitation of good outcomes over personal aggrandizement. This places anesthetists in the center of developments for managing the acutely ill patient—if they wish to take that opportunity.

The best mechanism for consolidating a role for anesthetists in acute care is through education and training. Training in anesthesia provides many essential skills of value to other acute care disciplines. Similarly, anesthetists could enhance their skills by additional exposure to training in acute medicine. Modular competency-based training programs are the key to this, but they require greater flexibility and collaboration between different disciplines. Multidisciplinary critical care provides a very good model in this respect. In Europe the majority of intensive care training programs are now multidisciplinary, and this year sees the launch of CoBaTrICE—competency-based training in intensive care in Europe. This 3-year project, funded by the European Union and directed by the European Society of Intensive Care Medicine, is using consensus techniques to de-

velop an internationally acceptable set of competencies for intensivists, with appraisal methods and educational resources available via the internet. Anesthetists will have an essential role in helping to provide the education required to support the acquisition of these competencies. They will also access this multidisciplinary training themselves, not only as part of their continuing contribution to intensive care but also to develop new skills in managing acutely ill patients as they travel through the hospital system. As health care becomes increasingly team-based, anesthetists are in a prime position to develop a new role as acute physicians.

1. Wilson RM, Runciman WB, Gibberd RW, et al: The Quality in Australian Health Care Study. Med J Aust 1995;163(9):458.

2. Vincent C, Neale G, Woloshyrowych M: Adverse events in British hospitals: a preliminary retrospective record review. BMJ 2001;322:517.

3. To Err Is Human: Building a Safer Health System: Institute of Medicine, November 1999.

4. Bion JF, Heffner J: Improving hospital safety for acutely ill patients: a Lancet quintet. I: Current challenges in the care of the acutely ill patient. Lancet 2004;363:970.

5. Smith R: Is the NHS getting better or worse? BMJ 2003;327:1239.

6. Zuger A: Dissatisfaction with medical practice. N Engl J Med 2004;350:69.

7. Bellomo R, Goldsmith D, Russell S, et al: Post-operative serious adverse events in a teaching hospital: a prospective study. Med J Aust 2002;176(5):216.

8. Department of Health. Comprehensive Critical Care: Critical care without walls. London, May 2000.

9. Auerbach AD, Nelson EA, Lindenauer PK, et al: Physician attitudes toward and prevalence of the hospitalist model of care: results of a national survey. Am J Med 2000; 109:648.

10. Hilman K: The hospitalist: a US model ripe for importing? Med J Aust 2003;178(2):54.

11. Risser DT, Rice MM, Salisbury ML, et al: The potential for improved teamwork to reduce medical errors in the emergency department. Ann Emerg Med 1999;34(3):373.

12. Morey JC, Simon R, Jay GD, et al: Error reduction and performance improvement in the emergency department through teamwork training: evaluation results of the MedTeams project. Health Serv Res 2002;37(6):1553.

until the patient is in optimal medical condition. Assessing patients with complications may require consultation with other specialists to help determine whether the patient is in optimal medical condi-

tion for the procedure and to have the specialist's assistance, if necessary, in perioperative care. Following the assessment, the anesthesiologist must discuss with the patient realistic options available for anesthetic manage-

Table 1–2. The anesthetic plan.

Premedication
Type of anesthesia
General
Airway management
Induction
Maintenance
Muscle relaxation
Regional
Technique
Agents
Monitored anesthesia care
Supplemental oxygen
Sedation
Intraoperative management
Monitoring
Positioning
Fluid management
Special techniques
Postoperative management
Pain control
Intensive care
Postoperative ventilation
Hemodynamic monitoring

ment. The final anesthetic plan is based on that discussion and the patient's wishes (reflected in the informed consent; see below).

The Preoperative History

The preoperative history should clearly establish the patient's problems as well as the planned surgical, therapeutic, or diagnostic procedure. The presence and severity of known underlying medical problems must also be investigated as well as any prior or current treatments. Because of the potential for drug interactions with anesthesia, a complete medication history including use of any **herbal therapeutics (Table 1–4)** should be elicited from every patient. This should include the use of tobacco and alcohol as well as illicit drugs such as marijuana, cocaine, and heroin. An attempt must also be made to distinguish between true drug allergies (often manifested as dyspnea or skin rashes) and drug intolerances (usually gastrointestinal upset). Detailed questioning about previous operations and anesthetics may uncover prior anesthetic complications. A family history of anesthetic problems may suggest a familial problem such as malignant hyperthermia (see Case Discussion in Chapter 44). A general review of organ systems is important in identifying undiagnosed medical problems. Questions should emphasize cardiovascular, pulmonary, endocrine, hepatic, renal, and neurological function. A positive response to any of these questions should prompt more detailed inquiries to determine the extent of any organ impairment.

Physical Examination

The history and physical examination complement one another: The examination helps detect abnormalities not apparent from the history and the history helps focus the examination on the organ systems that should be examined closely. Examination of healthy asymptomatic patients should minimally consist of measurement of vital signs (blood pressure, heart rate, respiratory rate, and temperature) and examination of the airway, heart, lungs, and musculoskeletal system using standard techniques of inspec-

Table 1–3. Routine preoperative anesthetic evaluation.

I. History
1. Current problem
2. Other known problems
3. Medication history
Allergies
Drug intolerances
Present therapy
Prescription
Nonprescription
Nontherapeutic
Alcohol
Tobacco
Illicit
4. Previous anesthetics, operations, and, if applicable, obstetric history and pain history
5. Family history
6. Review of organ systems
General (including activity level)
Respiratory
Cardiovascular
Renal
Gastrointestinal
Hematological
Neurological
Endocrine
Psychiatric
Orthopedic
Musculoskeletal
Dermatological
7. Last oral intake
II. Physical examination
1. Vital signs
2. Airway
3. Heart
4. Lungs
5. Extremities
6. Neurological examination
III. Laboratory evaluation
IV. ASA[1] classification: see Table 1–5.

[1]ASA, American Society of Anesthesiologists.

Table 1–4. Perioperative effects of common herbal medicines.[1]

Name (Other Names)	Alleged Benefits	Perioperative Effects	Recommendations
Echinacea	Stimulates immune system	Allergic reactions; hepatotoxicity; interference with immune suppressive therapy (eg, organ transplants)	Discontinue as far in advance of surgery as possible
Ephedra (ma huang)	Promotes weight loss; increases energy	Ephedrine-like sympathetic stimulation with increased heart rate and blood pressure, arrhythmias, myocardial infarction, stroke	Discontinue at least 24 h prior to surgery; avoid monoamine oxidase inhibitors
Garlic (ajo)	Reduces blood pressure and cholesterol levels	Inhibition of platelet aggregation (irreversible)	Discontinue at least 7 days prior to surgery
Ginkgo (duck foot, maidenhair, silver apricot)	Improves cognitive performance (eg, dementia), increases peripheral perfusion (eg, impotence, macular degeneration)	Inhibition of platelet-activating factor	Discontinue at least 36 h prior to surgery
Ginseng	Protects against "stress" and maintains "homeostasis"	Hypoglycemia; inhibition of platelet aggregation and coagulation cascade	Discontinue at least 7 days prior to surgery
Kava (kawa, awa, intoxicating pepper)	Decreases anxiety	GABA-mediated hypnotic effects may decrease MAC (see Chapter 7); possible risk of acute withdrawal	Discontinue at least 24 h prior to surgery
St. John's wort (amber, goatweed, *Hypericum perforatum*, klamathe-weed)	Reverses mild to moderate depression	Inhibits serotonin, norepinephrine, and dopamine reuptake by neurons; increases drug metabolism by induction of cytochrome P-450	Discontinue at least 5 days prior to surgery
Valerian	Decreases anxiety	GABA-mediated hypnotic effects may decrease MAC; benzodiazepinelike withdrawal syndrome	Taper dose weeks before surgery if possible; treat withdrawal syndrome with benzodiazepines

[1]For more details, see Ang-Lee MK, Moss J, Yuan C: Herbal medicines and perioperative care. JAMA 2001;286:208. GABA, γ-aminobutyric acid; MAC, minimum alveolar concentration.

tion, eg, auscultation, palpation, and percussion. An abbreviated neurological examination is important when regional anesthesia is being considered and serves to document any subtle preexisting neurological deficits. The patient's anatomy should be specifically evaluated when procedures such as a nerve block, regional anesthesia, or invasive monitoring are planned; evidence of infection over or close to the site or significant anatomic abnormalities may contraindicate such procedures (see Chapters 6, 16, and 17).

The importance of examining the airway cannot be overemphasized. The patient's dentition should be inspected for loose or chipped teeth and the presence of caps, bridges, or dentures. A poor anesthesia mask fit should be expected in some edentulous patients and those with significant facial abnormalities. Micrognathia (a short distance between the chin and the hyoid bone), prominent upper incisors, a large tongue, limited range of motion of the temporomandibular joint or cervical spine, or a short neck suggests

Table 1–5. Preoperative physical status classification of patients according to the American Society of Anesthesiologists.[1]

Class	Definition
P1	A normal healthy patient
P2	A patient with mild systemic disease (no functional limitations)
P3	A patient with severe systemic disease (some functional limitations)
P4	A patient with severe systemic disease that is a constant threat to life (functionality incapacitated)
P5	A moribund patient who is not expected to survive without the operation
P6	A brain-dead patient whose organs are being removed for donor purposes
E	If the procedure is an emergency, the physical status is followed by "E" (for example, "2E")

[1]Modified from the American Society of Anesthesiologists, last amended October 1984.

that difficulty may be encountered in tracheal intubation (see Chapter 5).

Laboratory Evaluation

Routine laboratory testing for healthy asymptomatic patients is not recommended when the history and physical examination fail to detect any abnormalities. Such routine testing is expensive and rarely alters perioperative management; moreover, abnormalities often are ignored—or result in unnecessary delays. Nonetheless, because of the current litigious environment in the United States, many physicians continue to order a hematocrit or hemoglobin concentration, urinalysis, serum electrolyte measurements, coagulation studies, an electrocardiogram, and a chest radiograph for all patients.

 To be valuable, performing a preoperative test implies that an increased perioperative risk exists when the results are abnormal and a reduced risk exists when the abnormality is corrected. The usefulness of a screening test for disease depends on its sensitivity and specificity as well as the prevalence of the disease. Sensitive tests have a low rate of false-negative results, whereas specific tests have a low rate of false-positive results. The prevalence of a disease varies with the population tested and often depends on sex, age, genetic background, and lifestyle practices. Testing is therefore most effective when sensitive and specific tests are used in patients in whom the abnormality might be expected. Accordingly, laboratory testing should be based on the presence or absence of underlying diseases and drug therapy as suggested by the history and physical examination. The nature of the procedure should also be taken into consideration. Thus, a baseline hematocrit is desirable in any patient about to undergo a procedure that may result in extensive blood loss and require transfusion.

Testing fertile women for an undiagnosed early pregnancy may be justified by the potentially teratogenic effects of anesthetic agents on the fetus; pregnancy testing involves detection of chorionic gonadotropin in urine or serum. Routine testing for AIDS (detection of the HIV antibody) is highly controversial. Routine coagulation studies and urinalysis are not cost effective in asymptomatic healthy patients.

ASA Physical Status Classification

In 1940, the ASA established a committee to develop a "tool" to collect and tabulate statistical data that would be used to predict operative risk. The committee was unable to develop such a predictive tool, but instead focused on classifying the patient's physical status, which led the ASA to adopt a five-category physical status classification system (Table 1–5) for use in assessing a patient preoperatively. A sixth category was later added to address the brain-dead organ donor. Although this system was not intended to be used as such, the ASA physical status generally correlates with the perioperative mortality rate (Figure 1–1). Because underlying disease is only one of many factors contributing to perioperative complications (see Chapter 46), it is not surprising that this correlation is not perfect. Nonetheless, the ASA physical status classification remains useful in planning anesthetic management, particularly monitoring techniques (see Chapter 6).

Informed Consent

The preoperative assessment culminates in giving the patient a reasonable explanation of the options available for anesthetic management: general, regional, local, or topical anesthesia; intravenous sedation; or a combination thereof. The term *monitored anesthesia care* (previously referred to as *local standby*) is now commonly used and refers to monitoring the patient during a procedure performed with intravenous sedation or local anesthesia administered by the surgeon. Regardless of the technique chosen, consent must always be obtained for general anesthesia in case other techniques prove inadequate.

If any procedure is performed without the patient's consent, the physician may be liable for assault and battery. When the patient is a minor or otherwise not competent to consent, the consent must be obtained from someone legally authorized to give it, such as a parent, guardian, or close relative. Although

Figure 1-1. American Society of Anesthesiologists' (ASA) physical status classification and correlation with mortality. Trends in two separate retrospective studies suggest that information on surgical mortality rates with respect to ASA physical status is similar, although coming from disparate practices. (Reproduced from ASA Newsletter 2002;66(9) [Mark J. Lema, editor]. http://www.asahq.org/ Newsletters/2002/9_02/vent_0902.htm. Reprinted with permission of the American Society of Anesthesiologists.)

oral consent may be sufficient, written consent is usually advisable for medicolegal purposes. Moreover, consent must be informed to ensure that the patient (or guardian) has sufficient information about the procedures and their risks to make a reasonable and prudent decision whether to consent. It is generally accepted that not all risks need be detailed—only risks that are realistic and have resulted in complications in similar patients with similar problems. It is generally advisable to inform the patient that some complications may be life-threatening.

The purpose of the preoperative visit is not only to gather important information and obtain informed consent, but also to help establish a healthy doctor–patient relationship. Moreover, an empathically conducted interview that answers important questions and lets the patient know what to expect has been shown to be at least as effective in relieving anxiety as some premedication drug regimens (see Case Discussion in Chapter 8).

■ DOCUMENTATION

Documentation is important for both quality assurance and medicolegal purposes. Adequate documentation is essential for the defense of a malpractice action (see Case Discussion below).

The Preoperative Note

The preoperative note should be written in the patient's chart and should describe all aspects of the preoperative assessment, including the medical history, anesthetic history, medication history, physical examination, laboratory results, ASA classification, and recommendations of any consultants. It also describes the anesthetic plan and includes the informed consent. The plan should be as detailed as possible and should include the use of specific procedures such as tracheal intubation, invasive monitoring, and regional or hypotensive techniques. Documentation of informed consent usually takes the form of a narrative in the chart indicating that the plan, alternative plans, and their advantages and disadvantages (including the risk of complications) were presented, understood, and agreed to by the patient. Alternatively, the patient signs a special anesthesia consent form that contains the same information. A sample preanesthetic report form is illustrated in Figure 1–2. Although a completely handwritten note in the chart is acceptable, the use of a printed form decreases the likelihood of omitting important information.

The Intraoperative Anesthesia Record

The intraoperative anesthesia record (Figure 1–3) serves many purposes. It functions as a useful intraoperative monitor, a reference for future anesthetics for that patient, and a tool for quality assurance. This record should be as pertinent and accurate as possible. It should document all aspects of anesthetic care in the operating room, including the following:

- A preoperative check of the anesthesia machine and other equipment.
- A review or reevaluation of the patient immediately prior to induction of anesthesia.
- A review of the chart for new laboratory results or consultations.

ANESTHESIOLOGY PREOPERATIVE NOTE

DATE: TIME: HT.   PREOP DIAGNOSIS:

AGE: SEX: M F   WT.   PROPOSED OPERATION:

MEDICAL HISTORY   **MEDICATIONS:**
ALLERGIES:
INTOLERANCES:
DRUG USE: TOBACCO: ETOH:

PRESENT PROBLEM:

CARDIOVASCULAR

RESPIRATORY

DIABETES

NEUROLOGIC   RENAL

ARTHRITIS/MUSCULO-SKELETAL   HEPATIC

        OTHER

PREVIOUS ANESTHETICS:

FAMILY HISTORY

LAST ORAL INTAKE

PHYSICAL EXAMINATION   BP   P   R   T

  HEART   EXTREMITIES

  LUNGS   NEUROLOGIC

  AIRWAY   OTHER

  TEETH

LABORATORY

  Hct/Hgb   ECG   CHEST X-RAY
  URINE
  LYTES: Na   Cl
        K   GLUCOSE   OTHER
        CO_2 BUN: CREATININE

PLAN ☐ GENERAL   INVASIVE MONITORS
        ☐ REGIONAL
        ☐ MONITORED ANESTHESIA CARE   SPECIAL TECHNIQUES

ASA CLASS   SIGNATURE _____ M.D.
        (RESIDENT)   (STAFF)

PATIENT CONSENT
ANESTHETIC ALTERNATIVES AND RISKS RANGING FROM TOOTH DAMAGE
TO LIFE-THREATENING EVENTS HAVE BEEN EXPLAINED AND ACCEPTED.

PATIENT
NAME

PATIENT'S SIGNATURE

#

Figure 1–2. The preoperative note.

ANESTHESIA RECORD

AGE:_____ SEX: M F PRE MED: S U _____ ASA _____

DENTITION _____ NPO _____ PROPOSED SURGERY _____

☐ PT. IDED ☐ CONSENT ✓ED ☐ CHART REVIEWED SURGEON _____

OPERATION PERFORMED _____

PRE OP: BP_____ P_____ R_____ T_____ Hct_____ ALLERGIES _____

TIME		TOTALS
OXYGEN		
NITROUS OXIDE		
HALO/ENFL/ISOFL/DES/SEVO		
TEMP		
URINE		
FLUIDS/BLOOD		

IV # _____ 240

BP ∨ SYS ECG
   ∧ DIA   FiO₂ 220
PULSE •   EtCO₂ 200
             SaO₂ 180
RESP. ⊘ ASSISTED EtA
      ○ SPONT.
      ● CONTROLLED Temp 160

MONITORS: 140
☐ MACHINE ✓ED ☐ RAPID TRANSFER 120
☐ OXIMETER ☐ FORCED AIR WARMER
☐ BP. SITE ☐ FiO₂ 100
☐ EKG ☐ EtCO₂ 80
☐ FLUID WARMER ☐ ESOPH 60
☐ PRECORDIAL ☐ NERVE STIM
☐ TEMP ☐ CVP 40
☐ HUMIDIFIER ☐ A-LINE 20
☐ BLANKET WARM/COOL ☐ PA CATHETER 0

VENT. | VT/RR | |
      | AIRWAY | P |
BLOOD LOSS
POSITION

REMARKS: _____

☐ MONITORED ANESTHESIA CARE
☐ REGIONAL
☐ GENERAL
BLADE _____
ETT# _____
BBS _____
CUFF _____ cc.
☐ ATRAUMATIC
☐ CO₂
COMMENTS:

EYE PROTECTION:

ANESTH. START _____
ANESTH. INDUC _____
SURG. START _____
SURG. END _____
ANESTH. END _____
ANESTH. NET _____

RECOVERY ROOM B.P. _____ P. _____ R.R. _____ TIME _____ O₂ SAT. _____

CONDITION _____

_____ M.D.
SIGNED (RESIDENT)

_____ M.D.
SIGNED (STAFF)

DATE _____

PAGE _____ OF _____

PATIENT NAME

#

Figure 1–3. The intraoperative anesthesia record.

- A review of the anesthesia and surgical consents.
- The time of administration, dosage, and route of intraoperative drugs.
- All intraoperative monitoring (including laboratory measurements, blood loss, and urinary output).
- Intravenous fluid administration and blood product transfusions.
- All procedures (such as intubation, placement of a nasogastric tube, or placement of invasive monitors).
- Routine and special techniques such as mechanical ventilation, hypotensive anesthesia, one-lung ventilation, high-frequency jet ventilation, or cardiopulmonary bypass.
- The timing and course of important events such as induction, positioning, surgical incision, and extubation.
- Unusual events or complications.
- The condition of the patient at the end of the procedure.

Vital signs are recorded graphically at least every 5 min. Other monitoring data are also usually entered graphically, whereas descriptions of techniques or complications are handwritten. Automated recordkeeping systems are available, but their use is still not widespread. Unfortunately, the intraoperative anesthetic record is often inadequate for documenting critical incidents, such as a cardiac arrest. In such cases, a separate note in the patient's chart may be necessary. Careful recording of the course of events, actions taken, and their timing is necessary to avoid discrepancies between multiple simultaneous records (anesthesia record, nurses' notes, cardiopulmonary resuscitation record, and other physicians' entries in the medical record). Such discrepancies are frequently targeted as evidence of incompetence or dissembling by malpractice attorneys. Incomplete, inaccurate, or illegible records may subject physicians to otherwise unjustified legal liability.

The Postoperative Notes

The anesthesiologist's immediate responsibility to the patient does not end until the patient has completely recovered from the effects of the anesthetic. After accompanying the patient to the postanesthesia care unit (PACU), the anesthesiologist should remain with the patient until normal vital signs have been established and the patient's condition is deemed stable (see Chapter 48). Prior to discharge from the PACU, a discharge note should be written by the anesthesiologist to document the patient's recovery from anesthesia, any apparent anesthesia-related complications, the immediate postoperative condition of the patient, and the patient's disposition (discharge to an outpatient area, an inpatient ward, an intensive care unit, or home). Inpatients should be seen again at least once within 48 h after discharge from the PACU. Postop-

erative notes should document the general condition of the patient, the presence or absence of any anesthesia-related complications, and any measures undertaken to treat such complications (Figure 1–4).

CASE DISCUSSION: MEDICAL MALPRACTICE

A healthy 45-year-old man has a cardiac arrest during an elective inguinal hernia repair. Although cardiopulmonary resuscitation is successful, the patient is left with permanent changes in mental status that preclude his return to work. One year later, the patient files a complaint against the anesthesiologist, surgeon, and hospital.

What four elements must be proved by the plaintiff (patient) to establish negligence on the part of the defendant (physician or hospital)?

1. Standard of Care: *Once a physician establishes a professional relationship with a patient, the physician owes that patient certain obligations, such as adhering to the "standard of care."*

2. Breach of Duty: *If these obligations are not fulfilled, the physician has breached his duties to the patient.*

3. Causation: *The plaintiff must demonstrate that the breach of duty was causally related to the injury. This proximate cause does not have to be the most important or immediate cause of the injury.*

4. Damages: *An injury must result. The injury may result in general damages (eg, pain and suffering) or special damages (eg, loss of income).*

How is the standard of care defined and established?

Individual physicians are expected to perform as any prudent and reasonable physician would in light of the surrounding circumstances. As a specialist, the anesthesiologist is held to a higher standard of knowledge and skill with respect to the subject matter of that specialty than would a general practitioner or a physician in another specialty. Expert witnesses usually establish the standard of care. Although most jurisdictions have extended the "locality rule" to encompass a national standard of care, the specific circumstances pertaining to each individual case are taken into account. The law recognizes that there are differences of opinion and varying schools of thought within the medical profession.

ANESTHESIA POSTOP NOTES

IMMEDIATE POSTOP NOTE (BEFORE DISCHARGE FROM RECOVERY ROOM):

_____ NO COMPLICATIONS OF ANESTHESIA IMMEDIATELY APPARENT;
PATIENT HAS RECOVERED FROM IMMEDIATE EFFECTS OF
ANESTHESIA AND MAY BE TRANSFERRED TO WARD OR
OUTPATIENT DEPARTMENT.

_____ OTHER:

_____ M.D. _____
　　　　　　　SIGNED　　　　　　　　　　　　　　　　DATE　　　　　　　　　TIME

FOLLOW-UP POSTOP NOTE (AFTER DISCHARGE FROM RECOVERY ROOM, BEFORE DISCHARGE
FROM HOSPITAL):

_____ NO APPARENT POSTANESTHETIC COMPLICATIONS.

_____ PATIENT DISCHARGED FROM HOSPITAL BY SURGEON PRIOR TO
POSTANESTHETIC VISIT.

_____ OTHER:

_____ M.D. _____
　　　　　　　SIGNED　　　　　　　　　　　　　　　　DATE　　　　　　　　　TIME

PATIENT
NAME

\#

CHART COPY

Figure 1–4. The postoperative note.

How is causation determined?

It is usually the plaintiff who bears the burden of proving that the injury would not have occurred "but for" the negligence of the physician, or that the physician's action was a "substantial factor" in causing the injury. An exception is the doctrine of res ipsa loquitur ("the thing speaks for itself"), which permits a finding of negligence based solely on circumstantial evidence. For res ipsa to apply in this case, the plaintiff would have to establish that cardiac arrest does not ordinarily occur in the absence of negligence and that it could not have been due to something outside the control of the anesthesiologist. An important concept is that causation in civil cases need only be established by a preponderance of the evidence ("more likely than not")—as opposed to criminal cases, in which all elements of a charged offense must be proved "beyond a reasonable doubt."

What factors influence the likelihood of a malpractice suit?

1. The Physician–Patient Relationship: *This is particularly important for the anesthesiologist, who usually does not meet the patient until the night before or the morning of the operation. Another problem is that the patient is unconscious while under the anesthesiologist's care. Thus, the preoperative and postoperative visits with the patient assume vital importance. Although anesthesiologists have less long-term contact with patients than other medical specialists, it is possible and desirable to make this contact meaningful. Family members should also be included during these meetings, particularly during the postoperative visit if there has been an intraoperative complication.*

2. Adequacy of Informed Consent: *Rendering care to a competent patient who does not consent constitutes assault and battery. Consent is not enough, however. The patient should be informed of the contemplated procedure, including its reasonably anticipated risks, its possible benefits, and the therapeutic alternatives. The physician may be liable for a complication— even if it is not due to the negligent performance of a procedure—if a jury is convinced that a reasonable person would have refused treatment if properly informed of the possibility of the complication. This does not mean, of course, that a documented consent relieves from liability physicians who violate the standard of care.*

3. Quality of Documentation: *Careful documentation of the perioperative visits, informed consent, consultation with other specialists, intra-*

operative events, and postoperative care is absolutely essential. The viewpoint of many courts and juries is that "if it isn't written, it wasn't done." It goes without saying that medical records should never be intentionally destroyed or altered.

SUGGESTED READING

Abenstein JP, Warner MA: Anesthesia providers, patient outcomes, and costs. Anesth Analg 1996;82:1273. An interesting look at the relative safety of the anesthesia team concept.

Ang-Lee MK, Moss J, Yuan C: Herbal medicines and perioperative care. JAMA 2001;286:208. Herbal medications can negatively impact anesthetic management.

Byrne AJ, Sellen AJ, Jones JG: Errors on anaesthetic record charts as a measure of anaesthetic performance during simulated critical incidents. Br J Anaesth 1998;80:58. There is a high error rate in the charting of critical incidents.

Dzankic S, Pastor D, Gonzalez C, Leung JM: The prevalence and predictive value of abnormal preoperative laboratory tests in elderly surgical patients. Anesth Analg 2001;93:301. This is an excellent review of how to evaluate the utility of preoperative laboratory tests in elderly patients.

Kam PCA: Occupational stress in anaesthesia. Anaesth Intensive Care 1997;25:686. Highly recommended reading for anyone considering a career in anesthesia!

Little DM Jr: *Classical Anesthesia Files.* Wood Library—Museum of Anesthesiology, 1985. Writings of historical interest.

Malviya S, D'Errico C, Reynolds P, et al: Preoperative pregnancy testing in adolescent patients: a survey of current practice. Am J Anesthesiol 1997;24:23. Most clinicians ask about the possibility of pregnancy but proceed with a pregnancy test only if indicated by history.

Overdyk FJ, Harvey SC, Fishman RL: Successful strategies for improving operating room efficiency at academic institutions. Anesth Analg 1998;86:896.

Posner KL, Caplan RA, Cheney FW: Variation in expert opinion in medical malpractice review. Anesthesiology 1996;85:1049. This article points out one of the major injustices inherent in the current medical malpractice system in the United States.

Practice Advisory for Preanesthesia Evaluation (approved by the ASA House of Delegates on October 17, 2001). Anesthesiology 2002;96:485. Excellent evidence-based medicine review of the preanesthetic evaluation of patients.

Waisel DB, Truog RD: The benefits of the explanation of the risks of anesthesia in the day surgery patient. J Clin Anesth 1995;7:200. Most parents want to be made aware of the risks of anesthesia.

Waisel DB, Truog RD: An introduction to ethics. Anesthesiology 1997;87:411.

Waisel DB, Truog RD: Informed consent. Anesthesiology 1997;87:968.

Warner MA, Caplan RA, Epstein BS, et al: Practice guidelines for preoperative fasting and the use of pharmacologic agents to reduce the risk of pulmonary aspiration: application to healthy patients undergoing elective procedures. Anesthesiology 1999;90:896. A review by the ASA Task Force on Preoperative Fasting that suggests these fasting guidelines for infants and adults: 2 hours for clear liquids, 4 hours for breast milk, 6 hours for infant formula or light solids.

SECTION I
Anesthetic Equipment & Monitors

The Operating Room: Medical Gas Systems, Environmental Factors, & Electrical Safety

2

KEY CONCEPTS

 Liquid oxygen must be stored well below its critical temperature of –119°C because gases can be liquefied by pressure only if stored below their critical temperature.

 The only reliable way to determine residual volume of nitrous oxide is to weigh the cylinder.

 Because the critical temperature of air is –140.6°C, it exists as a gas in cylinders whose pressures fall in proportion to their content.

 A pin index safety system has been adopted by cylinder manufacturers to discourage incorrect cylinder attachments.

 Body contact with two conductive materials at different voltage potentials may complete a circuit and result in an electrical shock.

 The magnitude of a leakage current is normally imperceptible to touch (less than 1 mA and well below the fibrillation threshold of 100 mA). If the current bypasses the high resistance offered by skin, however, and is applied directly to the heart (microshock), a current as low as 100 μA (microamperes) may be fatal. The maximum leakage allowed in operating room equipment is 10 μA.

 Unlike the utility company's pole-top transformer, the secondary wiring of an isolation transformer is not grounded and provides two live ungrounded voltage lines for operating room equipment.

 Malfunction of the return electrode may result from disconnection from the electrosurgical unit, inadequate patient contact, or insufficient conductive gel. In these situations, the current will find another place to exit (eg, electrocardiogram pads or metal parts of the operating table), which may result in a burn.

 Because pacemaker and electrocardiogram interference is possible, pulse or heart sounds should be closely monitored when any electrosurgical unit is used.

Figure 2–1. A bank of oxygen H-cylinders connected by a manifold.

Anesthesiologists, who spend more time in operating rooms than any other group of physicians, are responsible for protecting unconscious patients from a multitude of possible dangers during surgery. Some of these threats are unique to the operating room. As a result, the anesthesiologist is primarily responsible for ensuring the proper functioning of the operating room's medical gases, environmental factors (eg, temperature, humidity, ventilation, and noise), and electrical safety. This chapter describes the major features of operating rooms that are of special interest to anesthesiologists and the potential hazards associated with these systems. A case summary organizes some of this information into a protocol for testing a new operating room's medical gas pipeline system.

■ MEDICAL GAS SYSTEMS

The medical gases commonly used in operating rooms are oxygen, nitrous oxide, air, and nitrogen. Although technically not a gas, vacuum exhaust for waste anesthetic gas disposal (WAGD or scavenging)

and surgical suction must also be provided and is considered an integral part of the medical gas system. Patients are endangered if medical gas systems, particularly oxygen, malfunction. The main features of such systems are the sources of the gases and the means of their delivery to the operating room. The anesthesiologist must understand both these elements to prevent and detect medical gas depletion or supply line misconnection. Estimates of a particular hospital's peak demand determine the type of medical gas supply system required. Design and standards follow National Fire Protection Association (NFPA) 99 in the United States and HTM 2022 in the United Kingdom.

SOURCES OF MEDICAL GASES

Oxygen

A reliable supply of oxygen is a critical requirement in any surgical area. Medical grade oxygen (99% or 99.5% pure) is manufactured by fractional distillation of liquefied air. Oxygen is stored as a compressed gas at room temperature or refrigerated as a liquid. Most small hospitals store oxygen in two sep-

NITROUS OXIDE

OXYGEN

LIQUID OXYGEN
HIGHLY FLAMMABLE AREA

HAZARDOUS AREA
No Smoking within 25 ft.

Figure 2–2. A liquid storage tank with reserve oxygen tanks in background.

arate banks of high-pressure cylinders (H-cylinders) connected by a manifold (Figure 2–1). Only one bank is utilized at one time. The number of cylinders in each bank depends on anticipated daily demand. The manifold contains valves that reduce the cylinder pressure (approximately 2000 pounds per square inch [psig]) to line pressure (55 ± 5 psig) and automatically switch banks when one group of cylinders is exhausted.

A liquid oxygen storage system (Figure 2–2) is more economical for large hospitals. Liquid oxygen must be stored well below its critical temperature of –119°C because gases can be liquefied by pressure *only* if stored below their critical temperature. A large hospital may have a smaller liquid oxygen supply or a bank of compressed gas cylinders that can provide one day's oxygen requirements as a reserve. To guard against a hospital gas-system failure, the anesthesiologist must always have an emergency (E-cylinder) supply of oxygen available in the operating room.

Most anesthesia machines accommodate one or two E-cylinders of oxygen (Table 2–1). **As oxygen is expended, the cylinder's pressure falls in proportion to its content.** A pressure of 1000 psig indicates an E-cylinder that is approximately half full and represents 330 L of oxygen at atmospheric pressure and a tem-

perature of 20°C. If the oxygen is exhausted at a rate of 3 L/min, a cylinder that is half full will be empty in 110 min. Oxygen cylinder pressure should be monitored before use and periodically during use.

Nitrous Oxide

Nitrous oxide, a most commonly used anesthetic gas, is manufactured by heating ammonium nitrate (thermal decomposition). It is almost always stored by hospitals in large H-cylinders connected by a manifold with an automatic crossover feature. Bulk liquid storage of nitrous oxide is economical only in very large institutions.

Because the critical temperature of nitrous oxide (36.5°C) is above room temperature, it can be kept liquefied without an elaborate refrigeration system. If the liquefied nitrous oxide rises above its critical temperature, it will revert to its gaseous phase. Because nitrous oxide is not an ideal gas and is easily compressible, this transformation into a gaseous phase is not accompanied by a great rise in tank pressure. Nonetheless, all gas cylinders are equipped with an emergency pressure relief valve (rupture disk) to prevent explosion under conditions of unexpectedly high gas pressure (eg, unintentional overfilling). The pressure-relief valve is designed to rupture at 3300 psig, well below the pres-

Table 2–1. Characteristics of medical gas cylinders.

Gas	E-Cylinder Capacity[1] (L)	H-Cylinder Capacity[1] (L)	Pressure[1] (psig at 20°C)	Color (USA)	Color (international)	Form
O_2	625–700	6000–8000	1800–2200	Green	White	Gas
Air	625–700	6000–8000	1800–2200	Yellow	White and black	Gas
N_2O	1590	15,900	745	Blue	Blue	Liquid
N_2	625–700	6000–8000	1800–2200	Black	Black	Gas

[1]Depending on the manufacturer.

sure E-cylinder walls should be able to withstand (more than 5000 psig).

Although a disruption in supply is usually not catastrophic, most anesthesia machines have reserve nitrous oxide E-cylinders. Because these smaller cylinders also contain nitrous oxide in its liquid state, the volume remaining in a cylinder is *not* proportional to cylinder pressure. By the time the liquid nitrous oxide is expended and the tank pressure begins to fall, only about 400 L of nitrous oxide remains. **If liquid nitrous oxide is kept at a constant temperature (20°C), it will vaporize at the same rate at which it is consumed and will maintain a constant pressure (745 psig) until the liquid is exhausted.**

 The only reliable way to determine residual volume of nitrous oxide is to weigh the cylinder. For this reason, the tare weight (TW), or empty weight, of cylinders containing a liquefied compressed gas (eg, nitrous oxide) is often stamped on the shoulder of the cylinder. The pressure gauge of a nitrous oxide cylinder should not exceed 745 psig at 20°C. A higher reading implies gauge malfunction, tank overfill (liquid fill), or a cylinder containing a gas other than nitrous oxide.

Because energy is consumed in the conversion of a liquid to a gas (the latent heat of vaporization), the liquid nitrous oxide cools. The drop in temperature results in a lower vapor pressure and lower cylinder pressure. The cooling is so pronounced at high flow rates that pressure regulators may freeze.

Air

The use of air is becoming more frequent in anesthesiology as the potential hazards of nitrous oxide and high concentrations of oxygen receive increasing attention. Cylinder air is medical grade and is obtained by blending oxygen and nitrogen. Dehumidified but unsterile air is provided to the hospital pipeline system by compression pumps. The inlets of these pumps must be distant from vacuum exhaust vents to minimize contamination. Because the critical temperature of air is –140.6°C, it exists as a gas in cylinders whose pressures fall in proportion to their content.

Nitrogen

Although compressed nitrogen is not administered to patients, it may be used to provide power to some operating room equipment, such as saws and drills. Increasingly much of this equipment is battery operated. Nitrogen is most commonly stored in H-cylinders connected by a manifold.

Vacuum

A central hospital vacuum system usually consists of two independent suction pumps, each capable of handling peak requirements. Traps at every user location prevent contamination of the system with foreign matter. The medical-surgical vacuum may be used for WAGD providing it does not affect the performance of the system. A dedicated WAGD vacuum system is generally preferable.

DELIVERY OF MEDICAL GASES

Medical gases are delivered from their central supply source to the operating room through a piping network. Pipes are sized such that the pressure drop across the whole system never exceeds 5 psig. Gas pipes are usually constructed of seamless copper tubing using a special welding technique. Internal contamination of the pipelines with dust, grease, or water must be avoided. The hospital's gas delivery system appears in the operating room as hose drops, gas columns, or elaborate articulating arms (Figure 2–3). Operating room equipment, including the anesthesia machine, interfaces with these pipeline system outlets by color-coded hoses. Quick-coupler

Figure 2–3. Typical examples of (**A**) gas columns, (**B**) ceiling hose drops, and (**C**) articulating arms. One end of a color-coded hose connects to the hospital medical gas supply system by way of a quick-coupler mechanism. The other end connects to the anesthesia machine through the diameter index safety system.

mechanisms, which vary in design with different manufacturers, connect one end of the hose to the appropriate gas outlet. The other end connects to the anesthesia machine through a noninterchangeable diameter index safety system fitting that prevents incorrect hose attachment.

E-cylinders of oxygen, nitrous oxide, and air attach directly to the anesthesia machine. To discourage incorrect cylinder attachments, a pin index safety system has been adopted by cylinder manufacturers. Each gas cylinder sizes A–E) has two holes in its cylinder valve that mate with corresponding pins in the yoke of the anesthesia machine (Figure 2–4). The relative positioning of the pins and holes is unique for each gas. This system has been unintentionally defeated by multiple washers placed between the cylinder and yoke, which prevents proper engagement of the pins and holes. The pin index safety system is also ineffective if yoke pins are damaged or the cylinder is filled with the wrong gas.

The functioning of medical gas supply sources and pipeline systems is constantly monitored by central and area alarm systems. Indicator lights and audible signals warn of changeover to secondary gas sources and abnormally high (eg, pressure regulator malfunction) or low (eg, supply depletion) pipeline pressures (Figure 2–5).

Despite a multitude of safety devices, alarms, and detailed regulations (established by NFPA, the Compressed Gas Association, and the Department of Transportation), anesthetic catastrophes continue to result from malfunctioning medical gas systems. Mandatory periodic inspections of hospital gas delivery systems by independent agencies and increased involvement by anesthesiologists in gas-system design could ameliorate this problem.

◼ ENVIRONMENTAL FACTORS IN THE OPERATING ROOM

TEMPERATURE

The temperature in most operating rooms seems uncomfortably cold to many conscious patients and, at times, to

Figure 2–4. Pin index safety system interlink between the anesthesia machine and gas cylinder.

anesthesiologists. However, scrub nurses and surgeons stand in surgical garb for hours under hot operating room lights. As a general principle, the comfort of operating room personnel must be reconciled with patient needs. For example, for small children and patients with large exposed surfaces (eg, those with thermal burns) the operating room temperature should be 24°C or higher, since these patients lose heat rapidly and have a limited ability to compensate. Hypothermia has been associated with an increased incidence of wound infection, greater intraoperative blood loss (impaired coagulation assessed by thromboelastography), and prolonged hospitalization (see Chapter 6). On the other hand, intraoperative hypothermia may offer a degree of neurological protection during some intracranial or cardiopulmonary bypass surgeries.

HUMIDITY

In past decades, static discharges were a feared source of ignition in an operating room filled with flammable anesthetic vapors. Because increased humidity decreases the likelihood of static discharges, a relative humidity of at least 50% was recommended. Routine compliance with this requirement is no longer important in the modern era of nonflammable anesthetic agents. However, static sparks can still damage sensitive electrical equipment or lead to microshock (see the section below on The Risk of Electrocution).

VENTILATION

A high rate of operating room airflow decreases contamination of the surgical site. These flow rates are usu-

Figure 2–5. An example of a master alarm panel that monitors gasline pressure.

ally achieved by blending recirculated air with fresh air. Although recirculation conserves energy costs associated with heating and air conditioning, it is unsuitable for WAGD. Therefore, a separate anesthetic gas scavenging system must always supplement operating room ventilation. Extreme rates of flow, such as those produced by a laminar air system, have been proposed for procedures with particularly high risks of infection (eg, total hip replacement).

NOISE

Multiple studies have demonstrated that exposure to noise can have a detrimental effect on multiple human cognitive functions. Operating room noise has been measured at 70–80 dB(A) with frequent sound peaks exceeding 80 dB, depending on which ventilation system (eg, laminar flow) and surgical instruments (eg, power drills and saws) were being used. One study demonstrated a reduction in mental efficiency and short-term memory in anesthesia residents exposed to operating room noise.

■ ELECTRICAL SAFETY

THE RISK OF ELECTROCUTION

The use of electronic medical equipment subjects patients and hospital personnel to the risk of electrocution. Anesthesiologists must have at least a basic understanding of electrical hazards and their prevention.

Body contact with two conductive materials at different voltage potentials may complete a circuit and result in an electrical shock. Usually, one point of exposure is a live 110-V or 240-V conductor, with the circuit completed through a ground contact. For example, a grounded person need contact only one live conductor to complete a circuit and receive a shock. The live conductor could be the frame of a patient monitor that has developed a fault to the hot side of the power line. A circuit is now complete between the power line (which is earth grounded at the utility company's pole-top transformer) through the victim and back to the ground (Figure 2–6). The physiological effect of electrical current depends on the location, duration, frequency, and magnitude (more accurately, current density) of the shock.

Leakage current is present in all electrical equipment as a result of capacitive coupling, induction between internal electrical components, or defective insulation. Current can flow as a result of capacitive coupling between two conductive bodies (eg, a circuit board and its casing) even though they are not physically connected. Some monitors are doubly insulated to decrease the effect of capacitive coupling. Other monitors are designed to be connected to a low-impedance ground (the safety ground wire) that should divert the current away from a person touching the instrument's case. The magnitude of such leaks is normally imperceptible to touch (less than 1 mA and well below the fibrillation threshold of 100 mA). If the current bypasses the high resistance offered by skin, however, and is applied directly to the heart (microshock), current as low as 100 µA may be fatal. The maximum leakage allowed in operating room equipment is 10 µA.

Cardiac pacing wires and invasive monitoring catheters provide a conductive pathway to the myocardial endothelium. In fact, blood and normal saline can serve as electrical conductors. The exact amount of current required to produce fibrillation depends on the timing of the shock relative to the vulnerable period of heart repolarization (the T wave on the electrocardiogram). Even small differences in potential between the earth connections of two electrical outlets in the same operating room might place a patient at risk for microelectrocution.

PROTECTION FROM ELECTRICAL SHOCK

Most patient electrocutions are caused by current flow from the live conductor of a grounded circuit through the body and back to a ground (Figure 2–6). This would be prevented if everything in the operating room were grounded except the patient. Although direct patient grounds should be avoided, complete patient isolation is not feasible during surgery. Instead, the operating room power supply can be isolated from grounds by an isolation transformer (Figure 2–7).

Unlike the utility company's pole-top transformer, the secondary wiring of an isolation transformer is not grounded and provides two live ungrounded voltage lines for operating room equipment. Equipment casing—but not the electrical circuits—is grounded through the longest blade of a three-pronged plug (the safety ground). If a live wire is then unintentionally contacted by a grounded patient, current will not flow through the patient since no circuit back to the secondary coil has been completed (Figure 2–8).

Of course, if both power lines are contacted, a circuit is completed and a shock is possible. In addition, if either power line comes into contact with a

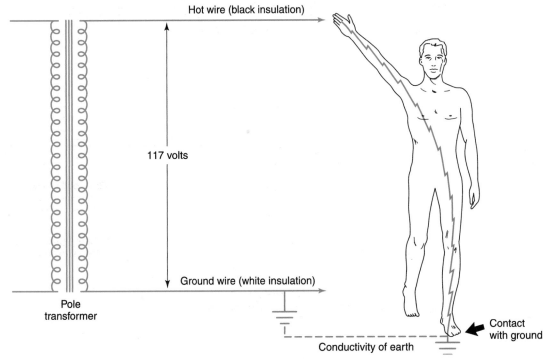

Figure 2–6. The setting for the great majority of electric shocks. An accidentally grounded person simultaneously contacts the hot wire of the electric service, usually via defective equipment that provides a pathway linking the hot wire to an exposed conductive surface. The complete electrical loop originates with the secondary of the pole transformer (the voltage source) and extends through the hot wire, the victim and the victim's contact with a ground, the earth itself, the neutral ground rod at the service entrance, and back to the transformer via the neutral (or ground) wire. (Modified and reproduced, with permission, from Bruner J, Leonard PF: *Electricity, Safety, and the Patient.* Mosby Year Book, 1989.)

ground through a fault, contact with the other power line will complete a circuit through a grounded patient. To reduce the chance of two coexisting faults, a **line isolation monitor** measures the potential for current flow from the isolated power supply to the ground (Figure 2–9). Basically, the line isolation monitor determines the degree of isolation between the two power wires and the ground and predicts the amount of current that *could* flow if a second shortcircuit were to develop. An alarm is activated if an unacceptably high current flow to the ground becomes possible (usually 2 mA or 5 mA), but power is not interrupted unless a ground-leakage circuit breaker (also called a ground-fault circuit interrupter) is also activated. The latter is usually not installed in locations such as operating rooms, where discontinuation of life support systems is more haz-

ardous than the risk of electrical shock. The alarm of the line isolation monitor merely indicates that the power supply has partially reverted to a grounded system. In other words, while the line isolation monitor warns of the existence of a single fault (between a power line and a ground), two faults are required for a shock to occur. If an alarm is activated, the last piece of equipment that was plugged in is suspect and should be removed from service until it is repaired.

Even isolated power circuits do not provide complete protection from the small currents capable of causing microshock fibrillation. Furthermore, the line isolation monitor cannot detect all faults, such as a broken safety ground wire within a piece of equipment. Despite the overall utility of isolated power systems, their requirement in operating rooms was deleted from the National

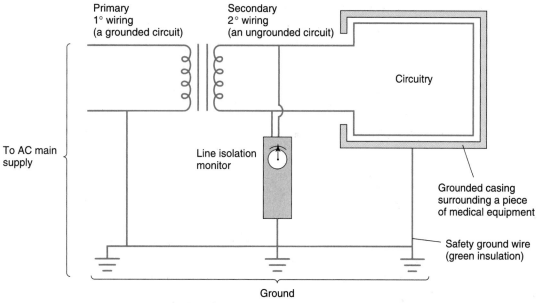

Figure 2–7. A circuit diagram of an isolation transformer and monitor.

Electrical Code in 1984, and newer or remodeled operating rooms may not offer this protection.

There are, however, modern equipment designs that decrease the possibility of microelectrocution. These include double insulation of the chassis and casing, ungrounded battery power supplies, and patient isolation from equipment-connected grounds by using optical coupling or transformers.

SURGICAL DIATHERMY

Electrosurgical units (ESUs) generate an ultrahigh-frequency electrical current that passes from a small active electrode (the cautery tip) through the patient and exits by way of a large plate electrode (the grounding pad, or return electrode). The high current density at the cautery tip is capable of tissue coagulation or cutting, depending on the electrical waveform. Ventricular fibrillation is prevented by the use of ultrahigh electrical frequencies (0.1–3 MHz) compared with line power (50–60 Hz). The large surface area of the low-impedance return electrode avoids burns at the current's point of exit by providing a low current density (the concept of *exit* is technically incorrect, as the current is alternating rather than direct). The high power levels of ESUs (up to 400 W) can cause inductive coupling with monitor cables, leading to electrical interference.

Malfunction of the return electrode may result from disconnection from the ESU, inadequate patient contact, or insufficient conductive gel. In these situations, the current will find another place to exit (eg, electrocardiogram pads or metal parts of the operating table), which may result in a burn (Figure 2–10). Precautions to prevent diathermy burns include proper return electrode placement, avoiding bony protuberances, and elimination of patient-to-ground contacts. Current flow through the heart may lead to pacemaker dysfunction. This can be minimized by placing the return electrode as close to the surgical field and as far from the heart as practical.

Newer ESUs are isolated from grounds using the same principles as the isolated power supply (isolated output versus ground-referenced units). Because this second layer of protection provides ESUs with their own isolated power supply, the operating room's line isolation monitor may not detect an electrical fault. Although some ESUs are capable of detecting poor contact between the return electrode and the patient by monitoring impedance, many older units trigger the alarm only if the return electrode is unplugged from the machine. Bipolar electrodes confine current propagation to a few millimeters, eliminating the need for a return electrode. Because pacemaker and electrocardiogram interfer-

Figure 2–8. Even though a person is grounded, no shock results from contact with one wire of an isolated circuit. The individual is in simultaneous contact with two separate voltage sources but does not close a loop including either source. (Modified and reproduced, with permission, from Bruner J, Leonard PF: *Electricity, Safety, and the Patient.* Mosby Year Book, 1989.)

ence is possible, pulse or heart sounds should be closely monitred when any ESU is used.

◼ OPERATING ROOM FIRES, EXPLOSIONS, & BURNS

FIRES & EXPLOSIONS

Operating room fires and explosions are uncommon (about 100 per year in the United States) but the outcome can be tragic. There are three requisites for a fire or explosion: a flammable agent (fuel), a gas that supports combustion, and a source of ignition (Table 2–2). Although flammable anesthetic agents (diethyl ether,

divinyl ether, ethyl chloride, ethylene, and cyclopropane) are no longer used, the risk of fires or explosions has not been eliminated.

Both oxygen and nitrous oxide are capable of vigorously supporting combustion; flammable agents that merely burn in air may explode in a mixture of nitrous oxide and oxygen. The accumulation of these agents under surgical drapes during head and neck surgery is particularly hazardous. With the routine use of pulse oximetry, there is no reason to indiscriminately insufflate oxygen under surgical drapes.

Operating room supplies that may be combustible and serve as fuel include tracheal tubes, oxygen cannulas and masks, surgical drapes, sponges, sutures, benzoin aerosol, alcohol cleansing solutions, and even petroleum-based ointments (Lacri-Lube). If these substances ignite, they should be *immedi-*

Figure 2–9. A line isolation monitor.

Figure 2–10. Electrosurgical burn. If the intended path is compromised, the circuit may be completed through other routes. Because the current is of high frequency, recognized conductors are not essential; capacitances can complete gaps in the circuit. Current passing through the patient to a contact of small area may produce a burn. (A leg drape would not offer protection in the situation depicted.) The isolated output electrosurgical unit (ESU) is much less likely than the ground-referenced ESU to provoke burns at ectopic sites. *Ground-referenced* in this context applies to the ESU output and has nothing to do with isolated versus grounded power systems. (Modified and reproduced, with permission, from Bruner J, Leonard PF: *Electricity, Safety, and the Patient.* Mosby Year Book, 1989.)

Table 2–2. Potential contributors to operating room fires and explosions.

Flammable agents (fuels)
Solutions, aerosols, and ointments
Alcohol
Chlorhexidine
Benzoin
Mastisol
Acetone
Petrolatum products
Surgical drapes (paper and cloth)
Surgical gowns
Surgical sponges and packs
Surgical sutures and mesh
Plastic/poly(vinyl chloride)/latex products
Endotracheal tubes
Masks
Cannulas
Tubing
Intestinal gases
Hair
Gases supporting combustion (oxidizers)
Oxygen
Nitrous oxide
Air
Ignition sources (heat)
Lasers
Electrosurgical units
Fiberoptic light sources (distal tip)
Drills
External defibrillation

ately removed from the patient and extinguished. Burning surgical drapes are particularly difficult to extinguish, as they are designed to be water resistant. Hair, including eyebrows, moustaches, beards, and lanugo (the fine hair found mostly on the face), can ignite and serve as fuel. Hair near the operative site should either be shaved or rendered nonflammable by a heavy coating of water-soluble lubricant jelly. Conversely, patients should be instructed not to use facial creams and hair products that are petroleum based. Bowel gas contains methane (up to 30%) and hydrogen gas (up to 44%), which are highly flammable. Liberation of these gases from accidental perforation of the bowel during surgery could potentially result in intraabdominal ignition. Only 100% carbon dioxide should be used for gas insufflation during laparoscopy. Although the oxygen concentration in the intestines is normally low (5%) and cannot support a fire, diffusion of nitrous oxide into the bowel and the peritoneal cavity poses a potential

danger. The risk of an intestinal gas fire or explosion may therefore be reduced if nitrous oxide is not used.

Historically, static electricity was the most feared source of ignition. Hospital regulations attempted to minimize this risk in operating rooms by prohibiting the use of materials apt to cause static discharge (eg, nylon, wool), installing conductive breathing circuits and flooring, and maintaining relative humidity above 50%. Most of these antiquated guidelines are now disregarded. In fact, conductive flooring increases the risk of electrical hazards.

More contemporary sources of ignition include electrical equipment, such as the ESU or laser. The tip of a high-intensity fiberoptic light source could also potentially ignite a fire. The use of diathermy near a distended bowel or the laser in the upper airway near combustible tracheal tubes indicates that the danger of intraoperative explosion persists. Tracheal tubes can be *partially* protected from the laser by wrapping them with foil or filling the cuff with saline. Special-purpose laser-resistant tubes are also available (see Chapter 39). Ignition of the tracheal tube may also occur during tonsillectomy and tracheostomy. When the ESU is used in the tonsillar fossa, or to incise the pretracheal fascia and control bleeding on the trachea, sparks may ignite the tracheal tube in gas that leaks during ventilation. This risk may be reduced by avoiding electrocautery at that point, withholding ventilation, and/or reducing the inspired oxygen to as low a concentration as possible. **Should the tube ignite, it should be removed immediately and the patient should be ventilated by mask until reintubated or, in the case of a tracheostomy, until the tracheostomy tube is inserted.**

BURNS

Burns are a significant cause of morbidity and potential liability. In the American Society of Anesthesiologists (ASA) Closed Claims Project (Chapter 46), burns were responsible for 2% of all liability claims. Fires accounted for only about 21% of burn injury claims. Most fire-related burn claims involved the face, and in the majority of claims plastic surgery was being performed with monitored anesthesia care and supplemental oxygen.

The majority of burn injuries (58%) in the ASA Closed Claims Project were caused by warmed intravenous bags and bottles, and devices (eg, heating pads, warming blankets, and warming lights) used to warm patients. Burn injuries from warmed intravenous bags and bottles tended to be on the trunk (including axilla) and most occurred prior to 1994.

Burns from warming devices tended to be on the lower body. Cautery (ESU) burns not involving fire were responsible for 12% of burn injury claims and were either the result of a direct burn injury (high setting) or a faulty grounding pad (see Surgical Diathermy).

CASE DISCUSSION:
CHECKING OUT THE MEDICAL
GAS SYSTEM IN A NEW
OPERATING ROOM

A hospital has just dedicated its new obstetric wing, which includes two operating rooms. You are scheduled to deliver the first anesthetic.

Who is responsible for testing and certifying the medical gas delivery system?

No governmental or accreditation agency in the United States inspects hospital gas systems to enforce conformity with the National Fire Protection Association's 1999 standard (NFPA 99) for health care facilities (the Canadian Standards Association certifies independent inspection firms in Canada). Ideally, third-party testing should certify that all aspects of the medical gas supply, piping, and outlet system comply with NFPA standards before use. Hospitals should have well-defined written policies for management, testing, and control of their medical gas systems and appropriate training of personnel. Although anesthesiologists are not responsible for hospital construction, they are responsible for intraoperative patient safety. In particular, the anesthesiologist is accountable for the portion of the medical gas system that extends from the wall outlet to the patient.

Which elements of the medical gas system need to be tested?

A 24-h standing pressure test checks for system leaks and faulty pressure-relief valves. Cross-connection of pipelines is prevented by pressurizing each gas system separately and confirming that pressure is present only at corresponding gas outlets. The content purity of each pipeline is verified by analysis of samples collected from each outlet. Excessive contamination by volatile gases or water moisture can usually be removed by high-flow nitrogen

purging of the system. The anesthesiologist should double-check each ceiling outlet to make certain that the correct color-coded hose and quick-connect device are present. Gasline contents should be confirmed with an oxygen analyzer, gas chromatograph, or mass spectrometer. The vacuum system can be checked with a suction gauge capable of measuring negative pressure. Common problems include residual copper oxide particles inside the piping, improper joints, inadequate sizing, and component failure.

Can the new wing affect the preexisting operating room suites?

Whenever any new construction, remodeling, or expansion occurs near medical gas storage sites or pipelines, a high index of suspicion is justified regarding the use of medical gases throughout the hospital.

SUGGESTED READING

Dorsh JA, Dorsh SE: *Understanding Anesthesia Equipment,* 4th ed. Williams & Wilkins, 1999. A detailed discussion of compressed gases and medical gas delivery systems.

Henderson KA, Matthews IP: An environmental survey of compliance with Occupational Exposure Standards (OES) for anesthetic gases. Anaesthesia 1999;54:941. Higher levels of nitrous oxide were found in areas without scavenging equipment (ie, radiology and delivery suites) than in operating rooms.

Koch ME, Kain ZN, Ayoub C: The sedative and analgesic sparing effect of music. Anesthesiology 1998;89:300. Patients listening to their choice of music required less pharmacological sedation and analgesia.

Macdonald MR, Wong A, Walker P, Crysdale WS: Electrocautery-induced ignition of tonsillar packing. J Otolaryngol 1994;23:426. An examination of factors that can decrease the risk of airway fire including lower oxygen concentration (using a cuffed tracheal tube), completely soaked tonsil packs, and avoidance of contact between electrocautery and bismuth subgallate.

National Fire Protection Association (NFPA): *Standard for Health Care Facilities.* NFPA, 2002. An updated version of NFPA 99 standards.

WEB SITES

http://www.apsf.org

The Anesthesia Patient Safety Foundation web site provides resources and a newsletter that discusses important safety issues in anesthesia.

http://www.cganet.com

The Compressed Gas Association and its web site are dedicated to the development and promotion of safety standards and safe practices in the industrial gas industry.

http://www.ecri.org

The ECRI (formerly the Emergency Care Research Institute) is an independent nonprofit health services research agency that focuses on health care technology, health care risk and quality management, and health care environmental management.

http://www.nfpa.org

The National Fire Protection Association (NPFA) has a web site with a catalog of publications on fire, electrical, and building safety issues.

Breathing Systems

KEY CONCEPTS

 Because insufflation avoids any direct patient contact, there is no rebreathing of exhaled gases if the flow is high enough. Ventilation cannot be controlled with this technique, however, and the inspired gas contains unpredictable amounts of entrained atmospheric air.

 Long breathing tubes with high compliance increase the difference between the volume of gas delivered to a circuit by a reservoir bag or ventilator and the volume actually delivered to the patient.

 The adjustable pressure-limiting (APL) valve should be fully open during spontaneous ventilation so that circuit pressure remains negligible throughout inspiration and expiration.

 Because a fresh gas flow equal to minute ventilation is sufficient to prevent rebreathing, the Mapleson A design is the most efficient Mapleson circuit for spontaneous ventilation.

 The Mapleson D circuit is efficient during controlled ventilation, because fresh gas flow forces alveolar air away from the patient and toward the APL valve.

 The drier the soda lime, the more likely it will absorb and degrade volatile anesthetics. Desflurane can be broken down to carbon monoxide by dry barium hydroxide lime to such a degree that it is capable of causing clinically significant carbon monoxide poisoning.

 Malfunction of either unidirectional valve in a circle system may allow rebreathing of carbon dioxide, resulting in hypercapnia.

 With an absorber, the circle system prevents rebreathing of carbon dioxide at fresh gas flows that are considered low (fresh gas flow ≤ 1 L) or even fresh gas flows equal to the uptake of anesthetic gases and oxygen by the patient and the circuit itself (closed-system anesthesia).

 Because of the unidirectional valves, apparatus dead space in a circle system is limited to the area distal to the point of inspiratory and expiratory gas mixing at the Y-piece. Unlike some Mapleson circuits, the breathing-tube length of a circle system does not directly affect dead space.

 The fraction of inspired oxygen (F_{IO_2}) delivered by a resuscitator breathing system to the patient is directly proportional to the oxygen concentration and flow rate of the gas mixture supplied to the resuscitator (usually 100% oxygen) and inversely proportional to the minute ventilation delivered to the patient.

Breathing systems provide the final conduit for the delivery of anesthetic gases to the patient. Breathing circuits link a patient to an anesthesia machine (Figure 3–1). Many modifications in circuit design have been developed, each with varying degrees of efficiency, convenience, and complexity. This chapter reviews the most important breathing systems: insufflation, draw-over, Mapleson circuits, the circle system, and resuscitation systems.

Most traditional attempts to classify breathing systems artificially consolidate functional aspects (eg, the extent of rebreathing) with physical characteristics (eg, the presence of unidirectional valves). Because these often contradictory classifications (eg, open, closed, semiopen, semiclosed) tend to result in confusion rather than understanding, they are avoided in this discussion.

Figure 3–1. The relationship between the patient, the breathing system, and the anesthesia machine.

INSUFFLATION

The term insufflation usually denotes the blowing of anesthetic gases across a patient's face. Although insufflation is categorized as a breathing system, it is perhaps better considered a technique that avoids direct connection between a breathing circuit and a patient's airway. Because children often resist the placement of a face mask or an intravenous line, insufflation is particularly valuable during pediatric inductions with inhalation anesthetics (Figure 3–2). It is useful in other situations as well. Carbon dioxide accumulation under head and neck draping is a hazard of ophthalmic surgery performed with local anesthesia. Insufflation of oxygen and air across the patient's face at a high flow rate (> 10 L/min) avoids this problem (Figure 3–3). Because insufflation avoids any direct patient contact, there is no rebreathing of exhaled gases if the flow is high enough. Ventilation cannot be controlled with this technique, however, and the inspired gas contains unpredictable amounts of entrained atmospheric air.

Insufflation can also be used to maintain arterial oxygenation during brief periods of apnea (eg, during bronchoscopy; see Chapter 39). Instead of blowing gases across the face, oxygen is directed into the lungs through a device placed in the trachea.

OPEN-DROP ANESTHESIA

Although open-drop anesthesia is not used in modern medicine, its historic significance warrants a brief description here. A highly volatile anesthetic—most commonly ether or halothane—is dripped onto a gauze-covered mask (Schimmelbusch mask) applied to the patient's face. As the patient inhales, air passes through the gauze, vaporizes the liquid agent, and carries high concentrations of anesthetic to the patient. The vaporization lowers mask temperature, resulting in moisture condensation and a drop in anesthetic vapor pressure (vapor pressure is proportional to temperature).

A modern derivative of open-drop anesthesia utilizes draw-over vaporizers that depend on the patient's inspiratory efforts to draw ambient air through a vapor-

Figure 3–2. Insufflation of an anesthetic agent across a child's face during induction.

Figure 3–3. Insufflation of oxygen and air under a head drape.

ization chamber. This technique may be used in locations or situations in which compressed medical gases are unavailable (eg, developing countries and battlefields).

DRAW-OVER ANESTHESIA

Draw-over devices have nonrebreathing circuits that use ambient air as the carrier gas, though supplemental oxygen can be used if available. Despite the simplicity of these devices, the inspired vapor and oxygen concentrations are predictable and controllable. The devices can be fitted with connections and equipment that allow intermittent positive-pressure ventilation (IPPV) and passive scavenging, as well as continuous positive airway pressure (CPAP) and positive end-expiratory pressure (PEEP).

In its most basic application (Figure 3–4), air is drawn through a low-resistance vaporizer as the patient inspires. Patients spontaneously breathing room air and a volatile, halogenated agent (nitrous oxide is never used with draw-over devices) often manifest an oxygen saturation (SpO_2) < 90%, a situation treated with IPPV, supplemental oxygen, or both. The fraction of inspired oxygen (FIO_2) can be supplemented using an open-ended reservoir tube of about 400 mL, attached to a t-piece at the upstream side of the vaporizer. Across the clinical range of tidal volume and res-

piratory rate, an oxygen flow rate of 1 L/min gives an FIO_2 of 30–40%, or with 4 L/min an FIO_2 of 60–80%. There are several commercial draw-over systems available that share common properties (Table 3–1).

The greatest advantage of the draw-over systems is their simplicity and portability. There are several disadvantages. Because of the absence of a reservoir bag, the depth of tidal volume is not well appreciated during spontaneous ventilation. The presence of the nonrebreathing valve, PEEP valve, and circuit filter close to the patient's head makes the technique awkward to use for head and neck surgery and pediatric cases. If the head is draped, the nonrebreathing valve is often covered as well.

MAPLESON CIRCUITS

The insufflation and draw-over systems have several disadvantages: poor control of inspired gas concentration and depth of anesthesia, inability to assist or control ventilation, no conservation of exhaled heat or humidity, difficult airway management during head and neck surgery, and pollution of the operating room with large volumes of waste gas. The **Mapleson systems** solve some of these problems by incorporating additional components (breathing tubes, fresh gas inlets, adjustable pressure-

Figure 3–4. Schematic diagram of a draw-over anesthesia device/circuit.

Hose ≈ 400 mL volume

Nonrebreathing valve
(eg, Laerdal or AMBU)

Open air to

Patient

O_2 supply if available

Self-inflating bag

Low-resistance vaporizer
(eg, EMO, OMV, PAC)

Valve to prevent retrograde gas flow from self-inflating bag (valve must be between the vaporizing chamber and the self-inflating bag)

limiting [APL] valves, and reservoir bags) into the breathing circuit. The relative location of these components determines circuit performance and is the basis of the Mapleson classification (Table 3–2).

Components of Mapleson Circuits

A. BREATHING TUBES

Corrugated breathing tubes—made of rubber (reusable) or plastic (disposable)—connect the components of the Mapleson circuit to the patient (Figure 3–5). The large diameter of the tubes (22 mm) creates a low-resistance pathway and a potential reservoir for anesthetic gases. To minimize fresh gas flow requirements, the volume of the breathing tube in most Mapleson circuits should be at least as great as the patient's tidal volume.

The compliance of the breathing tubes partially determines the compliance of the circuit. (Compliance is defined as the change of volume produced by a change in pressure.) Long breathing tubes with high compliance increase the difference between the volume of gas delivered to a circuit by a reservoir bag or ventilator and the volume actually delivered to the patient. For example, if a breathing circuit with a compliance of 8 mL gas/cm H_2O is pressurized during delivery of a tidal volume to 20 cm H_2O, 160 mL of the tidal volume will be lost to the circuit. The 160 mL represents a combination of gas compression and breathing-tube expansion. This is an important consideration in any circuit delivering positive-pressure ventilation through breathing tubes (eg, circle systems).

B. FRESH GAS INLET

Gases (anesthetics with oxygen or air) from the anesthesia machine continuously enter the circuit through the fresh

gas inlet. As discussed below, the relative position of this component is a key differentiating factor in Mapleson circuit performance.

C. ADJUSTABLE PRESSURE-LIMITING VALVE (PRESSURE-RELIEF VALVE, POP-OFF VALVE)

As anesthetic gases enter the breathing circuit, pressure will rise if the gas inflow is greater than the combined uptake of the patient and the circuit. Allowing gases to exit the circuit through an APL valve controls this pressure buildup. Exiting gases enter the operating room atmosphere or, preferably, a waste-gas scavenging system. All APL valves allow a variable pressure threshold for venting. The APL valve should be fully open during spontaneous ventilation so that circuit pressure remains negligible throughout inspiration and expiration. Assisted and controlled ventilation require positive pressure during inspiration to expand the lungs. Partial closure of the APL valve limits gas exit, permitting positive circuit pressures during reservoir bag compressions.

Table 3–1. Properties of draw-over devices.

Portable
Robust
Low resistance to gas flow
Usable with any agent[1]
Controllable vapor output

[1]Halothane cannot be used with the Epstein Mackintosh Oxford device.

Table 3–2. Classification and characteristics of Mapleson circuits.

Mapleson Class	Other Names	Configuration[1]	Required Fresh Gas Flows		Comments
			Spontaneous	Controlled	
A	Magill attachment	FGI → Breathing tube — APL valve — Breathing bag — Mask	Equal to minute ventilation (≈ 80 mL/kg/min)	Very high and difficult to predict	Poor choice during controlled ventilation. Enclosed Magill system is a modification that improves efficiency. Coaxial Mapleson A (Lack breathing system) provides waste-gas scavenging.
B		FGI APL valve	$2 \times$ minute ventilation	$2–2\frac{1}{2} \times$ minute ventilation	
C	Waters' to-and-fro	FGI APL valve	$2 \times$ minute ventilation	$2–2\frac{1}{2} \times$ minute ventilation	
D	Bain circuit	APL valve FGI	$2–3 \times$ minute ventilation	$1–2 \times$ minute ventilation	Bain coaxial modification: fresh gas tube inside breathing tube (see Figure 3–7).
E	Ayre's T-piece	FGI	$2–3 \times$ minute ventilation	$3 \times$ minute ventilation (I:E =1:2)	Exhalation tubing should provide a larger volume than tidal volume to prevent rebreathing. Scavenging is difficult.
F	Jackson-Rees' modification	FGI APL valve	$2–3 \times$ minute ventilation	$2 \times$ minute ventilation	A Mapleson E with a breathing bag connected to the end of the breathing tube to allow controlled ventilation and scavenging.

[1]FGI, fresh gas inlet; APL, adjustable pressure-limiting (valve).

35

Figure 3–5. Components of a Mapleson circuit. APL, adjustable pressure-limiting (valve).

D. RESERVOIR BAG (BREATHING BAG)

Reservoir bags function as a reservoir of anesthetic gas and a method of generating positive-pressure ventilation. They are designed to increase in compliance as their volume increases. Three distinct phases of reservoir bag filling are recognizable (Figure 3–6). After the nominal 3-L capacity of an adult reservoir bag is achieved (phase I), pressure rises rapidly to a peak (phase II). Further increases in volume result in a plateau or even a slight decrease in pressure (phase III). This ceiling effect helps to protect the patient's lungs against high airway pressures if the APL valve is unintentionally left in the closed position while fresh gas continues to flow into the circuit.

Performance Characteristics of Mapleson Circuits

Mapleson circuits are lightweight, inexpensive, and simple. Breathing-circuit efficiency is measured by the fresh gas flow required to eliminate, as much as possible, CO_2 rebreathing. Because there are no unidirectional valves or CO_2 absorption in Mapleson circuits, rebreathing is prevented by venting exhaled gas through the APL valve before inspiration. There is usually some rebreathing in any Mapleson circuit. The flow through the circuit controls the amount. To attenuate rebreathing, high fresh gas flows are required.

Reexamine the drawing of a Mapleson A circuit in Figure 3–5. During spontaneous ventilation, alveolar gas containing CO_2 will be exhaled into the breathing tube or directly vented through an open APL valve. Before inhala-

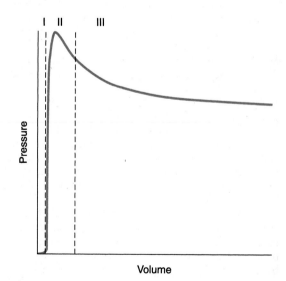

Figure 3–6. The increasing compliance and elasticity of breathing bags as demonstrated by three phases of filling. (Reproduced, with permission, from Johnstone RE, Smith TC: Rebreathing bags as pressure limiting devices. Anesthesiology 1973;38:192.)

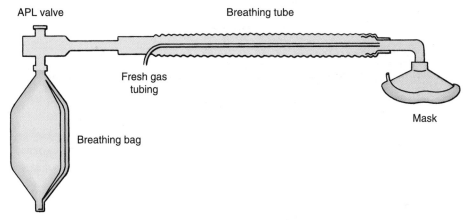

Figure 3–7. A Bain circuit is a Mapleson D circuit design with the fresh gas tubing inside the corrugated breathing tube. APL, adjustable pressure-limiting (valve). (Redrawn and reproduced, with permission, from Bain JA, Spoerel WE: Flow requirements for a modified Mapleson D system during controlled ventilation. Can Anaesth Soc J 1973;20:629.)

tion occurs, if the fresh gas flow exceeds alveolar minute ventilation, the inflow of fresh gas will force the alveolar gas remaining in the breathing tube to exit from the APL valve. If the breathing-tube volume is equal to or greater than the patient's tidal volume, the next inspiration will contain only fresh gas. Because a fresh gas flow equal to minute ventilation is sufficient to prevent rebreathing, the Mapleson A design is the most efficient Mapleson circuit for *spontaneous* ventilation.

Positive pressure during *controlled* ventilation, however, requires a partially closed APL valve. Although some alveolar and fresh gas exits through the valve during inspiration, no gas is vented during expiration. As a result, very high fresh gas flows (greater than three times minute ventilation) are required to prevent rebreathing with a Mapleson A circuit during controlled ventilation.

Interchanging the position of the APL valve and the fresh gas inlet transforms a Mapleson A into a **Mapleson D circuit** (Table 3–2). The Mapleson D circuit is efficient during controlled ventilation, since fresh gas flow forces alveolar air *away* from the patient and *toward* the APL valve. Thus, simply moving components completely alters the fresh gas requirements of the Mapleson circuits.

The **Bain circuit** is a popular modification of the Mapleson D system that incorporates the fresh gas inlet tubing inside the breathing tube (Figure 3–7). This modification decreases the circuit's bulk and retains heat and humidity better than the Mapleson D circuit as a result of partial warming of the inspiratory gas by countercurrent exchange with the warmer expired gases. A disadvantage of this coaxial circuit is the possibility of kinking or disconnection of the fresh gas inlet tubing. If unrecognized, either of these mishaps could result in significant rebreathing of exhaled gas.

THE CIRCLE SYSTEM

Although Mapleson circuits overcome some of the disadvantages of the insufflation and draw-over systems, the high fresh gas flows required to prevent rebreathing result in waste of anesthetic agent, pollution of the operating room environment, and loss of patient heat and humidity (Table 3–3). In an attempt to avoid these problems, the **circle system** adds more components to the breathing system.

Components of the Circle System

A. CARBON DIOXIDE ABSORBENT

Rebreathing alveolar gas conserves heat and humidity. However, the CO_2 in exhaled gas must be eliminated to prevent hypercapnia. CO_2 chemically combines with water to form carbonic acid. CO_2 absorbents (eg, soda lime or barium hydroxide lime) contain hydroxide salts that are capable of neutralizing carbonic acid (Table 3–4). Reaction end products include heat (the heat of neutralization), water, and calcium carbonate. **Soda lime** is the more common absorbent and is capable of absorbing up to 23 L of CO_2 per 100 g of absorbent. Its reactions are as follows:

$$CO_2 + H_2O \rightarrow H_2CO_3$$

$$H_2CO_3 + 2NaOH \rightarrow Na_2CO_3 + 2H_2O + Heat$$
$$\text{(a fast reaction)}$$

$$Na_2CO_3 + Ca(OH)_2 \rightarrow CaCO_3 + 2NaOH$$
$$\text{(a slow reaction)}$$

Table 3–3. Characteristics of breathing circuits.

	Insufflation and Open Drop	Mapleson	Circle
Complexity	Very simple	Simple	Complex
Control of anesthetic depth	Poor	Variable	Good
Ability to scavenge	Very poor	Variable	Good
Conservation of heat and humidity	No	No	Yes[1]
Rebreathing of exhaled gases	No	No[1]	Yes[1]

[1]These properties depend on the rate of fresh gas flow.

Note that the water and sodium hydroxide initially required are regenerated.

Color conversion of a pH indicator dye (eg, ethyl violet) by increasing hydrogen ion concentration signals absorbent exhaustion (Table 3–5). Absorbent should be replaced when 50–70% has changed color. Although exhausted granules may revert to their original color if rested, no significant recovery of absorptive capacity

Table 3–4. Comparison of soda lime and barium hydroxide lime.

	Soda Lime	Barium Hydroxide Lime
Mesh size[1]	4–8	4–8
Method of hardness	Silica added	Water of crystallization
Content	Calcium hydroxide Sodium hydroxide Potassium hydroxide	Barium hydroxide Calcium hydroxide
Usual indicator dye	Ethyl violet	Ethyl violet
Absorptive capacity (liters of CO_2/100 g granules)	14–23	9–18

[1]The number of openings per linear inch in a wire screen used to grade particle size.

Table 3–5. Indicator dye changes signaling absorbent exhaustion.

Indicator	Color when Fresh	Color when Exhausted
Ethyl violet	White	Purple
Phenolphthalein	White	Pink
Clayton yellow	Red	Yellow
Ethyl orange	Orange	Yellow
Mimosa 2	Red	White

occurs. Granule size is a compromise between the higher absorptive surface area of small granules and the lower resistance to gas flow of larger granules. The hydroxide salts are irritating to the skin and mucous membranes. Increasing the hardness of soda lime by adding silica minimizes the risk of inhalation of sodium hydroxide dust. Because barium hydroxide lime incorporates water into its structure (the water of crystallization), it is sufficiently hard without silica. Additional water is added to both types of absorbent during packaging to provide optimal conditions for carbonic acid formation. Commercial soda lime has a water content of 14–19%.

Absorbent granules can absorb and later release significant amounts of volatile anesthetic. This property can be responsible for delayed induction or emergence. The drier the soda lime, the more likely it will absorb and degrade volatile anesthetics. Desflurane can be broken down to carbon monoxide by dry barium hydroxide lime to such a degree that it is capable of causing clinically significant carbon monoxide poisoning.

A new carbon dioxide absorbent consisting of calcium hydroxide and calcium chloride (with calcium sulfate and polyvinylpyrrolidone added to increase hardness) has been developed. This absorbent (Amsorb) possesses greater inertness than soda lime or barium hydroxide lime, resulting in less degradation of volatile anesthetics (eg, sevoflurane into compound A or desflurane into carbon monoxide; see Chapter 7).

B. CARBON DIOXIDE ABSORBERS

The granules of absorbent are contained within one or two canisters that fit snugly between a head and base plate. Together, this unit is called an absorber (Figure 3–8). Although bulky, double canisters permit more complete CO_2 absorption, less frequent absorbent changes, and lower gas flow resistance. To ensure complete absorption, a patient's tidal volume should not exceed the air space between absorbent granules, which is roughly equal

Figure 3–8. A carbon dioxide absorber.

— Head plate

— Granules of absorbent

— Double canisters

— Base plate

— Dust trap

— Lever release

to 50% of the absorber's capacity. Indicator dye color is monitored through the absorber's transparent walls. Absorbent exhaustion typically occurs first where exhaled gas enters the absorber and along the canister's smooth inner walls. Channeling through areas of loosely packed granules is minimized by a baffle system. A trap at the base of the absorber collects dust and moisture. Newer absorbers are used until CO_2 is found in the inhaled gas on the anesthetic-gas monitor, at which time the canister(s) are replaced.

C. UNIDIRECTIONAL VALVES

Unidirectional valves, which function as check valves, contain a ceramic or mica disk resting horizontally on an annular valve seat (Figure 3–9). Forward flow displaces the disk upward, permitting the gas to proceed through the circuit. Reverse flow pushes the disk against its seat, preventing reflux. Valve incompetence is usually due to a warped disk or seat irregularities. The expiratory valve is exposed to the humidity of alveolar gas.

Inhalation opens the inspiratory valve, allowing the patient to breath a mixture of fresh and exhaled gas that has passed through the CO_2 absorber. Simultaneously, the expiratory valve closes to prevent rebreathing of exhaled gas that still contains CO_2. The subsequent flow of gas away from the patient during exhalation opens the expiratory valve. This gas is vented through the APL valve or rebreathed by the patient after passing through the absorber. Closure of the inspiratory valve during exhalation prevents expiratory gas from mixing with fresh gas in the inspiratory limb. Malfunction of either unidirectional valve may allow rebreathing of CO_2, resulting in hypercapnia.

Optimization of Circle System Design

Although the major components of the circle system (unidirectional valves, fresh gas inlet, APL valve, CO_2 absorber, and a reservoir bag) can be placed in several configurations, the following arrangement is preferred (Figure 3–10):

- Unidirectional valves are relatively close to the patient to prevent backflow into the inspiratory limb if a circuit leak develops. However, unidirectional valves are not placed in the Y-piece, as that makes it difficult to confirm proper orientation and intraoperative function.

- The fresh gas inlet is placed between the absorber and the inspiratory valve. Positioning it downstream from the inspiratory valve would allow fresh gas to bypass the patient during exhalation and be wasted. Fresh gas introduced between the expiratory valve and the absorber would be diluted by recirculating gas. Furthermore, inhalation anesthetics may be absorbed or released by soda lime granules, thus slowing induction and emergence.

- The APL valve should be placed immediately before the absorber to conserve absorption capacity and to minimize venting of fresh gas.

Disk   Transparent dome

Valve seat —

Figure 3–9. A unidirectional valve.

Inspiratory unidirectional valve

Right-angle connector

Flexible breathing tube

Fresh gas inlet

Mask

Y-connector

Expiratory unidirectional valve

APL valve

Absorber

Reservoir

Figure 3–10. A circle system. APL, adjustable pressure-limiting (valve).

• Resistance to exhalation is decreased by locating the reservoir bag in the expiratory limb. Bag compression during controlled ventilation will vent expired gas through the APL valve, conserving absorbent.

Performance Characteristics of the Circle System

A. Fresh Gas Requirement

With an absorber, the circle system prevents rebreathing of CO_2 at low fresh gas flows that are considered low (≤ 1 L) or even fresh gas flows equal to the uptake of anesthetic gases and oxygen by the patient and the circuit itself (closed-system anesthesia; see Case Discussion in Chapter 7). At fresh gas flows greater than 5 L/min, rebreathing is so minimal that a CO_2 absorber is usually unnecessary.

With low fresh gas flows, concentrations of oxygen and inhalation anesthetics can vary markedly between fresh gas (ie, gas in the fresh gas inlet) and inspired gas (ie, gas in the inspiratory limb of the breathing tubes). The latter is a mixture of fresh gas and exhaled gas that has passed through the absorber. The greater the fresh gas flow rate, the less time it will take for a change in fresh gas anesthetic concentration to be reflected in a change in inspired gas anesthetic concentration. Higher

flows speed induction and recovery, compensate for leaks in the circuit, and decrease the risks of unanticipated gas mixtures.

B. Dead Space

That part of a tidal volume that does not undergo alveolar ventilation is referred to as dead space (see Chapter 22). Thus, any increase in dead space must be accompanied by a corresponding increase in tidal volume if alveolar ventilation is to remain unchanged. Because of the unidirectional valves, apparatus dead space in a circle system is limited to the area distal to the point of inspiratory and expiratory gas mixing at the Y-piece. Unlike Mapleson circuits, the breathing-tube length does not affect dead space. Like Mapleson circuits, length does affect circuit compliance and thus the amount of tidal volume lost to the circuit during positive-pressure ventilation. Pediatric circle systems may have both a septum dividing the inspiratory and expiratory gas in the Y-piece and low-compliance breathing tubes to further reduce dead space, though they are rarely used in current practice.

C. Resistance

The unidirectional valves and absorber increase circle system resistance, especially at high respiratory rates and large tidal volumes. Nonetheless, even premature

Figure 3–11. The Laerdal resuscitator. (Courtesy of Laerdal Medical Corp.)

neonates can be successfully ventilated using a circle system.

D. HUMIDITY AND HEAT CONSERVATION

Medical gas delivery systems supply dehumidified gases to the anesthesia circuit at room temperature. Exhaled gas, on the other hand, is saturated with water at body temperature. Therefore, the heat and humidity of inspired gas depend on the relative proportion of rebreathed gas to fresh gas. High flows are accompanied by low relative humidity, whereas low flows allow greater water saturation. Absorbent granules provide a significant source of heat and moisture in the circle system.

E. BACTERIAL CONTAMINATION

The slight risk of microorganism retention in circle system components could theoretically lead to respiratory infections in subsequent patients. For this reason, bacterial filters are sometimes incorporated into the inspiratory or expiratory breathing tubes or at the Y-piece.

Disadvantages of the Circle System

Although most of the problems of Mapleson circuits are solved by the circle system, the improvements have led to other disadvantages: greater size and less portability; increased complexity, resulting in a higher risk of disconnection or malfunction; increased resistance; and the difficulty of predicting inspired gas concentrations during low fresh gas flows.

RESUSCITATION BREATHING SYSTEMS

Resuscitation bags (AMBU bags or bag-mask units) are commonly used for emergency ventilation because of their simplicity, portability, and ability to deliver almost 100% oxygen (Figure 3–11). A resuscitator is unlike a Mapleson circuit or a circle system because it contains a **nonrebreathing valve.** (Remember that a Mapleson sys-

tem is considered valveless although it contains an APL valve, whereas a circle system contains unidirectional valves that direct flow through an absorber but allow rebreathing of exhaled gases.)

High concentrations of oxygen can be delivered to a mask or tracheal tube during spontaneous or controlled ventilation if a source of high fresh gas flow is connected to the inlet nipple. The patient valve opens during controlled or spontaneous inspiration to allow gas flow from the ventilation bag to the patient. Rebreathing is prevented by venting exhaled gas to the atmosphere through exhalation ports in this valve. The compressible, self-refilling ventilation bag also contains an intake valve. This valve closes during bag compression, permitting positive-pressure ventilation. The bag is refilled by flow through the fresh gas inlet and across the intake valve. Connecting a reservoir to the intake valve helps prevent the entrainment of room air. The reservoir valve assembly is really two unidirectional valves: the inlet valve and the outlet valve. The inlet valve allows ambient air to enter the ventilation bag if fresh gas flow is inadequate to maintain reservoir filling. Positive pressure in the reservoir bag opens the outlet valve, which vents oxygen if fresh gas flow is excessive.

There are several disadvantages to resuscitator breathing systems. First, they require high fresh gas flows to achieve a high FIO_2. FIO_2 is directly proportional to the oxygen concentration and flow rate of the gas mixture supplied to the resuscitator (usually 100% oxygen) and inversely proportional to the minute ventilation delivered to the patient. For example, a Laerdal resuscitator equipped with a reservoir requires a flow of 10 L/min to achieve an inspired oxygen concentration approaching 100% if a patient with a tidal volume of 750 mL is ventilated at a rate of 12 breaths/min. The maximum achievable tidal volumes are less than those that can be achieved with a system that uses a 3-L breathing bag. In fact, most adult resuscitators have a maximum tidal volume of 1000 mL. Finally, although a normally functioning patient valve has low resistance to inspiration and expiration, exhaled moisture can cause valve sticking.

CASE DISCUSSION:
UNEXPLAINED LIGHT ANESTHESIA

An extremely obese but otherwise healthy 5-year-old girl presents for inguinal hernia repair. After uneventful induction of general anesthesia and tracheal intubation, the patient is placed on a ventilator set to deliver a tidal volume of 7 mL/kg at a rate of 16 breaths/min. Despite delivery of 2% halothane in 50% nitrous oxide, tachycardia (145 beats/min) and mild hypertension (144/94 mm Hg) are noted. To increase anesthetic depth, fentanyl (3 µg/kg) is administered. Heart rate and blood pressure continue to rise and are accompanied by frequent premature ventricular contractions.

What should be considered in the differential diagnosis of this patient's cardiovascular changes?

The combination of tachycardia and hypertension during general anesthesia should always alert the anesthesiologist to the possibility of hypercapnia or hypoxia, both of which produce signs of increased sympathetic activity. These life-threatening conditions should be quickly and immediately ruled out by end-tidal CO_2 monitoring, pulse oximetry, or arterial blood gas analysis.

A common cause of intraoperative tachycardia and hypertension is an inadequate level of anesthesia. Normally, this is confirmed by movement. If the patient is paralyzed, however, there are few reliable indicators of light anesthesia. The lack of a response to a dose of an opioid should alert the anesthesiologist to the possibility of other, perhaps more serious, causes.

Malignant hyperthermia is rare but must be considered in cases of unexplained tachycardia, especially if accompanied by premature contractions (see Case Discussion in Chapter 44). Certain drugs used in anesthesia (eg, pancuronium, ketamine, ephedrine) stimulate the sympathetic nervous system and can produce or exacerbate tachycardia and hypertension. Diabetic patients who become hypoglycemic from administration of insulin or long-acting oral hypoglycemic agents can have similar cardiovascular changes. Other endocrine abnormalities (eg, pheochromocytoma, thyroid storm, carcinoid) should also be considered.

Could any of these problems be related to an equipment malfunction?

Briefly sniffing the anesthetic gas being delivered to the patient is an easy—if not aesthetic—method of confirming the presence of a volatile agent. Nitrous oxide is more difficult to detect without sophisticated equipment, but an oxygen analyzer should provide a clue.

A misconnection of the ventilator could result in hypoxia or hypercapnia. In addition, a malfunctioning unidirectional valve will increase circuit dead space and allow rebreathing of expired CO_2. Soda lime exhaustion could also lead to rebreathing in the presence of a low fresh gas flow. Rebreathing of CO_2 can be detected during the inspiratory phase on a capnograph (see Chapter 6). If rebreathing appears to be due to an equipment malfunction, the patient should be disconnected from the anesthesia machine and ventilated with a resuscitation bag until repairs are possible.

How are unidirectional valves checked before the anesthesia machine is used?

The incidence of incompetent unidirectional valves has been found to approach 15%. There is a quick procedure for testing the function of these valves:

(1) First, disconnect the breathing tubes from the anesthesia machine, close the APL valve, and turn off all gas flow.

(2) To check inspiratory valve function, connect one end of a section of breathing tube to the inhalation outlet and occlude the exhalation outlet. If a breathing bag that is connected to its usual site fills when air is blown into the breathing tube, the inspiratory valve is incompetent (Figure 3–12A).

(3) To check expiratory valve function, connect one end of a section of breathing tube to the usual breathing bag site and cover the inhalation outlet. If a breathing bag connected to the exhalation outlet fills when air is blown into the breathing tube, the expiratory valve is incompetent (Figure 3–12B).

What are some other consequences of hypercapnia?

Hypercapnia has a multitude of effects, most of them masked by general anesthesia. Cerebral blood flow increases proportionately

Figure 3–12. How to connect the reservoir bag and corrugated tube for the competence test of inhalation (**A**) and exhalation (**B**) unidirectional valves. Heavy arrows indicate the normal direction of flow through the valves. (From Kim J, Kovac AL, Mathewson HS: A method for detection of incompetent unidirectional dome valves: a prevalent malfunction. Anesth Analg 1985;64:745. Reprinted with permission of the International Anesthesia Research Society.)

with arterial CO_2. This effect is dangerous in patients with increased intracranial pressure (eg, from brain tumor). Extremely high levels of CO_2 (> 80 mm Hg) can cause unconsciousness related to a fall in cerebrospinal fluid pH. CO_2 depresses the myocardium, but this direct effect is usually overshadowed by activation of the sympathetic nervous system. During general anesthesia, hypercarbia usually results in an increased cardiac output, an elevation in arterial blood pressure, and a propensity toward arrhythmias.

Elevated serum CO_2 concentrations can overwhelm the blood's buffering capacity, leading to respiratory acidosis. This causes other anions such as Ca^{2+} and K^+ to shift extracellularly. Acidosis also shifts the oxyhemoglobin dissociation curve to the right.

Carbon dioxide is a powerful respiratory stimulant. In fact, for each mm Hg rise of Pa_{CO_2} above baseline, normal awake subjects increase their minute ventilation by about 2–3 L/min. General anesthesia markedly decreases this response, and paralysis would eliminate it. Finally, *severe hypercapnia can produce hypoxia by displacement of oxygen from alveoli.*

SUGGESTED READING

Dobson MB: Anaesthesia for difficult locations—developing countries and military conflicts. In: *International Practice of Anaesthesia.* Prys-Roberts C, Brown BR (editors). Butterworth Heinemann, 1996.

Dorsch JA, Dorsch SE: *Understanding Anesthesia Equipment,* 4th ed. Lippincott, Williams & Wilkins, 1999. Detailed discussion of breathing systems.

Ehrenwerth J, Eisenkraft JB (editors): *Anesthesia Equipment—Principles and Applications.* Mosby Year Book, 1993. A review of anesthesia machines and monitoring equipment.

Healthcare Product Comparison System (HPCS), published by ECRI (a nonprofit agency), August 1999. This report compares several models of anesthesia machines and includes an excellent overview of breathing circuit components and potential problems.

Murray JM, Renfrew CW, Bedi A, et al: Amsorb: a new carbon dioxide absorbent for use in anesthetic breathing systems. Anesthesiology 1999;91:1342. Calcium hydroxide proves to be nonreactive with volatile anesthetic agents.

The Anesthesia Machine

4

KEY CONCEPTS

 Misuse of anesthesia gas delivery equipment is three times more common than equipment failure in causing equipment-related adverse outcomes. Lack of familiarity with the equipment and a failure to check machine function are the most frequent causes. These mishaps account for only about 2% of cases in the ASA Closed Claims Project database. The breathing circuit was the most common single source of injury (39%); nearly all incidents were related to misconnects or disconnects.

 The anesthesia machine receives medical gases from a gas supply; controls the flow of desired gases reducing their pressure, when necessary, to a safe level; vaporizes volatile anesthetics into the final gas mixture; and delivers the gases to a breathing circuit that is connected to the patient's airway. A mechanical ventilator attaches to the breathing circuit but can be excluded with a switch during spontaneous or manual (bag) ventilation.

 Whereas the oxygen supply can pass directly to its flow control valve, nitrous oxide, air, and other gases must first pass through safety devices before reaching their respective flow control valves. These devices permit the flow of other gases only if there is sufficient oxygen pressure in the safety device and help prevent accidental delivery of a hypoxic mixture in the event of oxygen supply failure.

 Another safety feature of anesthesia machines is linkage of the nitrous oxide gas flow to the oxygen gas flow; this arrangement helps ensure a minimum oxygen concentration of 21–25%.

 All modern vaporizers are agent specific, capable of delivering a constant concentration of agent regardless of temperature changes or flow through the vaporizer.

 A rise in airway pressure may signal worsening pulmonary compliance, an increase in tidal volume, or an obstruction in the breathing circuit, tracheal tube, or the patient's airway. A drop in pressure may indicate an improvement in compliance, a decrease in tidal volume, or a leak in the circuit.

 Traditionally ventilators on anesthesia machines have a double circuit system design and are pneumatically powered and electronically controlled. Newer machines also incorporate microprocessor control, which relies on sophisticated pressure and flow sensors. Some models offer anesthesia machines with ventilators that use a single circuit piston design.

 The major advantage of a piston ventilator is its ability to deliver accurate tidal volumes to patients with very poor lung compliance and to very small patients.

 Whenever a ventilator is used, "disconnect alarms" must be passively activated. Anesthesia workstations should have at least three disconnect alarms: low pressure, low exhaled tidal volume, and low exhaled carbon dioxide.

 Because the ventilator's spill valve is closed during inspiration, fresh gas flow from the machine's common gas outlet normally contributes to the tidal volume delivered to the patient.

(continued on next page)

(continued from previous page)

 Use of the oxygen flush valve during the inspiratory cycle of a ventilator must be avoided because the ventilator spill valve will be closed and the adjustable pressure-limiting (APL) valve is excluded; the surge of oxygen (600–1200 mL/s) and circuit pressure will be transferred to the patient's lungs.

 Large discrepancies between the set and actual tidal volume are often observed in the operating room during volume-controlled ventilation. Causes include breathing circuit compliance, gas compression, ventilator-fresh gas flow coupling,

and leaks in the anesthesia machine, the breathing circuit, or the patient's airway.

 Waste-gas scavengers dispose of gases that have been vented from the breathing circuit by the APL valve and ventilator spill valve. Pollution of the operating room environment with anesthetic gases may pose a health hazard to surgical personnel.

 A routine inspection of anesthesia equipment before each use increases operator familiarity and confirms proper functioning. The United States Food and Drug Administration has made available a generic checkout procedure for anesthesia gas machines and breathing systems.

No piece of equipment is more intimately associated with the practice of anesthesiology than the anesthesia machine (Figure 4–1). On the most basic level, the anesthesiologist uses the anesthesia machine to control the patient's gas exchange and administer inhalation anesthetics. Modern anesthesia machines, however, have become extremely sophisticated, incorporating many built-in safety features and devices, a breathing circuit, monitors, a mechanical ventilator, and one or more microprocessors that can enhance, integrate, and monitor all components. Monitors that are not built-in can be added externally and often still be fully integrated. Moreover, their modular designs allow a wide variety of optional configurations and features even within the same product line. The term anesthesia workstation is therefore often used for modern anesthesia machines. Use of microprocessors provides options such as sophisticated ventilator modes, automated recordkeeping, and networking with local or remote monitors as well as hospital information systems. There are two major manufacturers of anesthesia machines in the United States, Datex-Ohmeda (GE Healthcare) and Draeger Medical. Proper functioning of the machine is crucial for patient safety.

Much progress has been made in reducing the number of adverse outcomes arising from anesthetic gas delivery equipment, through redesign of equipment and education. Misuse of anesthesia gas delivery equipment is three times more common than equipment failure in causing equipment-related adverse outcomes. Equipment misuse is characterized as errors in preparation, maintenance, or deployment of a device. Preventable anesthetic mishaps are frequently traced to a lack of familiarity with the equipment and a failure to check machine function. These mishaps account for only about 2% of cases in the American Society of Anesthesiologists' (ASA) Closed Claims Project database (Chapter 46). The breathing cir-

cuit (Chapter 3) was the most common single source of injury (39%); nearly all incidents were related to misconnects or disconnects. A misconnect was defined as a nonfunctional and unconventional configuration of breathing circuit components or attachments. In decreasing frequency, other causes involved vaporizers (21%), ventilators (17%), and oxygen supply (11%). Other more basic components of the anesthesia machine were responsible in only 7% of cases. It should be noted that all malpractice claims involving the anesthesia machine, oxygen supply tanks or lines, and ventilators took place before 1990; claims involving breathing circuits and vaporizers continued to occur after 1990.

The American National Standards Institute and subsequently the ASTM (formerly the American Society for Testing and Materials, F1850–00) published standard specifications for anesthesia machines and their components. Table 4–1 lists essential features of a modern anesthesia workstation. Changes in equipment design have been directed at minimizing the probability of breathing circuit misconnects and disconnects and automating machine checks. Because of the durability and functional longevity of anesthesia machines, the ASA is developing guidelines for determining anesthesia machine obsolescence (Table 4–2). This chapter is an introduction to anesthesia machine design, function, and use.

OVERVIEW

In its most basic form, the anesthesia machine receives medical gases from a gas supply; controls the flow of desired gases reducing their pressure, when necessary, to a safe level; vaporizes volatile anesthetics into the final gas mixture; and delivers the gases to a breathing circuit (Chapter 3) that is connected to the

A

Auxiliary O$_2$ flowmeter

Flowmeters

Display

Suction regulator

Bellows assembly

Flow controls

Rebreathing bag

Breathing system

Carbon dioxide (CO$_2$) absorber

Oxygen (O$_2$) flush button

Vaporizers

System switch

Secondary gas supply pressure gauges (cylinder gauges)

Primary gas supply gauges (usually pipeline)

Brake

B

Electrical outlets with circuit breakers

Pipeline inlets

Cylinder yokes

Cylinders

Main circuit breaker

Oxygen power outlet

Waste gas receiver

Back cover

Scavenging connector

Figure 4–1. Modern anesthesia machine (Datex-Ohmeda Aestiva). ***A:*** Front. ***B:*** Back.

Table 4–1. Essential safety features on a modern anesthesia workstation.

Essential Features	Purpose
Noninterchangeable gas-specific connections to pipeline inlets (DISS)[1] with pressure gauges, filter, and check valve	Prevent incorrect pipeline attachments; detect failure, depletion, or fluctuation
Pin index safety system for cylinders with pressure gauges, and at least one oxygen cylinder	Prevent incorrect cylinder attachments; provide backup gas supply; detect depletion
Low oxygen pressure alarm	Detect oxygen supply failure at the common gas inlet
Minimum oxygen/nitrous oxide ratio controller device (hypoxic guard)	Prevent delivery of less than 21% oxygen
Oxygen failure safety device (shut-off or proportioning device)	Prevent administration of nitrous oxide or other gases when the oxygen supply fails
Oxygen must enter the common manifold downstream to other gases	Prevent hypoxia in event of proximal gas leak
Oxygen concentration monitor and alarm	Prevent administration of hypoxic gas mixtures in event of a low-pressure system leak; precisely regulate oxygen concentration
Automatically enabled essential alarms and monitors (eg, oxygen concentration)	Prevent use of the machine without essential monitors
Vaporizer interlock device	Prevent simultaneous administration of more than one volatile agent
Capnography and anesthetic gas measurement	Guide ventilation; prevent anesthetic overdose; help reduce awareness
Oxygen flush mechanism that does not pass through vaporizers	Rapidly refill or flush the breathing circuit
Breathing circuit pressure monitor and alarm	Prevent pulmonary barotrauma and detect sustained positive, high peak, and negative airway pressures
Exhaled volume monitor	Assess ventilation and prevent hypo- or hyperventilation
Pulse oximetry, blood pressure, and ECG monitoring	Provide minimal standard monitoring
Mechanical ventilator	Control alveolar ventilation more accurately and during muscle paralysis for prolonged periods
Backup battery	Provide temporary electrical power (> 30 min) to monitors and alarms in event of power failure
Scavenger system	Prevent contamination of the operating room with waste anesthetic gases

[1]DISS, diameter-index safety system.

patient's airway (Figures 4–2 and 4–3). A mechanical ventilator attaches to the breathing circuit but can be excluded with a switch during spontaneous or manual (bag) ventilation. An auxiliary oxygen supply and suction regulator are also usually built into the workstation. In addition to standard safety features (Table 4–1) top of the line anesthesia machines have additional safety features, enhancements, and built-in computer processors that integrate and monitor all components, perform automated machine checkouts, and provide options such as automated recordkeeping and networking external monitors and hospital information systems (Figure 4–4). Some machines are designed specifically for mobility (eg, Draeger Narkomed Mobile), magnetic resonance imaging (MRI) compatibility (eg, Datex-Ohmeda Aestiva/5 MRI, Draeger Narkomed MRI-2), or compactness (eg, Datex-Ohmeda/5 Avance and Aestiva S5 Compact, Draeger Fabius Tiro).

GAS SUPPLY

Most machines have gas inlets for oxygen, nitrous oxide, and air. Compact models often lack air inlets, whereas other machines may have a fourth inlet for helium, Heliox, or carbon dioxide. Separate inlets are provided for the primary pipeline gas supply that passes through the walls of healthcare facilities and the secondary cylinder gas supply. Machines therefore have two gas inlet pressure gauges for each gas: one for pipeline pressure and another for cylinder pressure.

Pipeline Inlets

Oxygen, nitrous oxide, and often air are delivered from their central supply source to the operating room through a piping network (Chapter 2). The tubing is color coded and connects to the anesthesia machine through a noninterchangeable **diameter-index safety system (DISS)** fitting that prevents incorrect hose attachment. A filter helps trap debris from the wall supply and a one-way check valve prevents retrograde flow of gases into the pipeline supplies. It should be noted that some machines have an oxygen (pneumatic) power outlet that may be used to drive the ventilator or provide an auxiliary oxygen flowmeter. The DISS fittings for the oxygen inlet and the oxygen power outlet are identical and should not be mistakenly interchanged.

Cylinder Inlets

Similarly cylinders attach to the machine via hanger-yoke assemblies that utilize a **pin index safety system** to prevent errors. The yoke assembly includes index

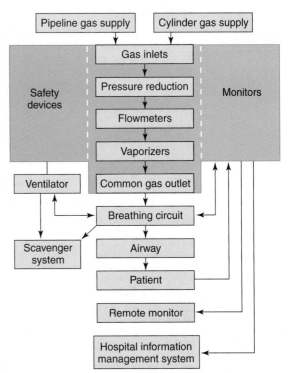

Figure 4–2. Functional schematic of an anesthesia machine/workstation.

pins, a washer, a gas filter, and a check valve that prevents retrograde gas flow. The E cylinders attached to the anesthesia machine are a high-pressure source of medical gases and are generally used only as a back-up supply in case of pipeline failure. Some machines have two oxygen cylinders so that one cylinder can be used while the other is changed. Cylinder pressure is usually measured by a Bourdon pressure gauge (Figure 4–5). A flexible tube within this gauge straightens when exposed to gas pressure, causing a gear mechanism to move a needle pointer.

FLOW CONTROL CIRCUITS

Pressure Regulators

Unlike the relatively constant pressure of the pipeline gas supply, the high and variable gas pressure in cylinders makes flow control difficult and potentially dangerous. To enhance safety and ensure optimal use of cylinder gases, machines utilize a pressure regulator to reduce the cylinder gas pressure to 45–47 psig[1] before it enters the flow valve

---

Table 4–2. Unacceptable/undesirable features of older anesthesia machines.[1]

Unacceptable features
1. Flowmeter-controlled vaporizer (eg, copper, kettle, Vernitrol)
2. More than one flow control valve for a single gas
3. Vaporizer with a rotary dial that increases concentration with clockwise rotation
4. Connections in the scavenging system that are the same size as breathing circuit connections

Undesirable features
1. Adjustable pressure-limiting (APL) valve that is not isolated during mechanical ventilation
2. Oxygen flow control knob that is not fluted or larger than other flow control knobs
3. Oxygen flush control that is unprotected from accidental activation
4. Lack of main On/Off switch for electrical power to integral monitors and alarms
5. Lack of antidisconnect device on the fresh gas hose (common gas outlet)
6. Lack of airway pressure alarms

[1]Adapted from ASA Guidelines for determining Anesthesia Machine Obsolescence.

---

[1]Pressure unit conversions: 1 kiloPascal (kP) = kg/m • s² = 1000 N/m² = 0.01 bar = 0.1013 atmospheres = 0.145 psig = 10.2 cm H_2O = 7.5 mm Hg.

Figure 4–3. Simplified internal schematic of an anesthesia machine. *A:* Datex-Ohmeda Aestiva. *B:* Draeger Narkomed.

(continued)

Figure 4–3. Continued

(Figure 4–6). This pressure, which is slightly lower than the pipeline supply, allows preferential use of the pipeline supply if a cylinder is left open (unless pipeline pressure drops below 45 psig). After passing through Bourdon pressure gauges and check valves, the pipeline gases share a common pathway with the cylinder gases. A high-pressure relief valve provided for each gas is set to open when the supply pressure exceeds the machine's maximum safety limit (95–110 psig), eg, regulator failure on a cylinder. Some machines (Datex-Ohmeda) also use a second regulator to drop both pipeline and cylinder pressure further (two-stage pressure regulation). Oxygen is reduced to 20 psig and nitrous oxide is reduced to 38 psig. This differential reduction between the two gases is important for proper functioning of the oxygen/nitrous oxide flow link-

age (Datex-Ohmeda Link-25, see below). Other machines (Draeger) do not reduce pipeline pressure so their flow valves receive gases at 45–55 psig. A second-stage pressure reduction may also be needed for an auxiliary oxygen flowmeter, the oxygen flush mechanism, or the drive gas to power a pneumatic ventilator.

Oxygen Supply Failure Protection Devices

Whereas the oxygen supply can pass directly to its flow control valve, nitrous oxide, air (in some machines), and other gases must first pass through safety devices before reaching their respective flow control valves. In some machines, such as the Aestiva (and later Datex-Ohmeda models), the

A

Ventilator "quick" function keys

Setup keys

Integrated machine monitor

ComWheel

Fresh gas flow controls

Integrated patient monitor

Ventilator bellows block

Aladin vaporizer cassette (electronic vaporizer)

Agent wheel

Compact patient circuit

Switch: ON/Standby

Anesthesia monitor central unit and modules (option)

Fresh gas outlet (optional flow indicator)

Vaporizer cassette storage slots (optional)

Drawers (optional)

Figure 4–4. Highly sophisticated anesthesia machines with full integration options. *A:* Datex-Ohmeda S/5 ADU. *B:* Draeger 6400.

(continued)

Figure 4–4. Continued

air passes directly to its flow control valve; this allows administration of air even in the absence of oxygen. These devices permit the flow of other gases only if there is sufficient oxygen pressure in the safety device and help prevent accidental delivery of a hypoxic mixture in the event of oxygen supply failure. Thus in addition to supplying the oxygen flow control valve, oxygen from the common inlet pathway is used to pressurize safety devices, oxygen flush valves, and ventilator power outlets (in some models). Safety devices sense oxygen pressure via a small "piloting pressure" line that may be derived from the gas inlet or secondary regulator. In some anesthesia machine designs (eg, Datex-Ohmeda Excel), if the piloting pressure line falls below a threshold (eg, 20 psig), shut-off valves close preventing the administration of any other gases. The terms fail-safe and nitrous cut-off valve were previously used for the nitrous oxide shut-off valve.

Most modern (particularly Datex-Ohmeda) machines use a proportioning safety device instead of a thresh-

Figure 4–5. Bourdon pressure gauge.

Adjustment screw

Regulator shell

Spring applies counter pressure

Diaphragm

Low pressure gas going out

High pressure gas going in

Full cylinder pressure

Partially full cylinder pressure

Diaphragm

Valve stem

Valve seat

Figure 4–6. Cylinder inlet regulator.

Jerry A. Dorsch, MD

ARE ANESTHESIA PROVIDERS RECEIVING ADEQUATE TRAINING IN EQUIPMENT?

Every year there are reports of accidents related to anesthesia equipment. When a problem occurs the first impulse is often to blame the equipment, but in fact only about 25% of these problems are due to equipment failure (C-392-BS, E-114-BS). In most cases, the problem is with the user and involves either failure to understand and use the equipment correctly or failure to do a proper preuse check on the equipment.

Anesthesia equipment has been undergoing a gradual evolution. Thirty years ago, anesthesia machines offered many opportunities for the inexperienced operator to make serious errors. Safety devices were almost nonexistent and monitoring equipment was rare except for cases such as cardiovascular surgery.

At that time, equipment was not considered an academic subject, partly because its function was not well known to most practitioners. Teaching about equipment function and use in most anesthesia training programs was sketchy and lacking in depth. The lack of knowledge was an important contribution to equipment-related accidents.

Fortunately things began to change in the 1970s. Dorsch and Dorsch's book, Understanding Anesthesia Equipment, first published in 1975, demystified many of the intricacies of pipeline systems, anesthesia machines, vaporizers, breathing systems, tracheal tubes, and other gadgets. The Society for Technology in Anesthesia was formed, and a more scientific approach to equipment construction and use began to be followed. The Anesthesia Patient Safety Foundation was formed and has published many articles on problems that relate to anesthesia equipment.

An important development was the introduction of safety devices for anesthesia machines. These included a system to interrupt the flow of anesthetic gases if the oxygen pressure in the machine was lost. Measured-flow vaporizers were phased out, and flowmeters in series replaced parallel flowmeters. Minimum oxygen-to-nitrous oxide ratio devices to prevent the oxygen flow from being turned off when nitrous oxide was being administered were introduced. Anesthesia machine standards were written so that new machines would include features to help overcome known problems.

old shut-off valve. These devices, either called an oxygen failure protection device (Draeger) or a balance regulator (Datex-Ohmeda), proportionately reduce the pressure of nitrous oxide and other gases except for air (Figures 4–7 and 4–8). They completely shut off nitrous oxide and other gas flow only below a set minimum oxygen pressure (eg, 0.5 psig for nitrous oxide and 10 psig for other gases).

All machines also have an oxygen supply low-pressure sensor that activates a gas whistle or electric alarm sounds when inlet gas pressure drops below a threshold value (usually 20–35 psig). It must be stressed that these safety devices do *not* protect against other possible causes of hypoxic accidents.

Flow Valves & Meters

Once the pressure has been reduced to a safe level, each gas must pass through flow-control valves and is measured by flowmeters before mixing with other

Use of electronic components further increased the safety of anesthesia machines. Devices such as the oxygen monitor and airway pressure monitor were automatically activated when the machine was turned on. These machines usually had an electronically controlled ventilator, which meant increased versatility and enabled use with difficult-to-ventilate patients.

A number of new monitoring devices became available in the 1980s. The introduction of oxygen analyzers was a significant advance. At first there was resistance to their use because they required calibration and early models required a great deal of work to get them to function properly. Fortunately, problems with reliability and calibration were largely overcome. Carbon dioxide monitoring and pulse oximetry came into use and within a short time became standards of care. An important step forward was the adoption of practice standards by the American Society of Anesthesiologists and the American Association of Nurse Anesthetists. These stipulated the types of monitors essential for the practice of anesthesia.

In 1995, the Food and Drug Administration (FDA) published an anesthesia apparatus checkout procedure, the goal of which was to uncover the most common faults in an anesthesia machine and breathing system. A feature of this procedure was that it could be used on different makes of anesthesia machines. The latest major change in equipment was the introduction of computer-driven anesthesia machines and ventilators. These machines have automated checkout procedures that cover most of the items in the FDA checkout.

Airway management has also undergone extensive changes. Disposable tracheal tubes with low-pressure cuffs became the norm. The introduction of the laryngeal mask airway in the 1990s resulted in major changes in anesthesia practice. Many devices have been developed to deal with the difficult airway. Fiberoptic endoscopy has come into widespread use.

With all the advances in anesthesia equipment, it would seem that mortality and morbidity associated with anesthesia equipment would have disappeared. Unfortunately, accidents continue to occur. Improvements in anesthesia-provider education are needed. The increased complexity of the new generation of anesthesia machines and ventilators makes improved education even more critical.

More emphasis needs to be put on teaching future anesthesia providers about equipment. One problem is that most departments standardize their equipment to minimize errors. Unfortunately, this means that graduates are not able to use the wide variety of equipment to which they will be exposed in practice. It is important for anesthesia providers who trained on one type of equipment to become familiar with other types. A common belief—that if you can use one piece of equipment you can use similar pieces of equipment—often results in human error.

Equipment education should be ongoing. When new equipment is introduced into the workplace, a formal educational process should ensure that all anesthesia providers can properly operate that equipment before it is put into use. This is particularly important with the computer-based machines that are now available and will ultimately replace the older machines. Operator error may be increased if the complexity of these new machines is not fully appreciated.

Dorsch JA, Dorsch SE: *Understanding Anesthesia Equipment*, 4th ed. Williams & Wilkins, 1999.

gases, entering the active vaporizer, and exiting the machine's common gas outlet. **Gas lines proximal to flow valves are considered to be in the high-pressure circuit whereas those between the flow valves and the common gas outlet are considered part of the low-pressure circuit of the machine.** When the knob of the flow-control valve is turned counterclockwise, a needle valve is disengaged from its seat, allowing gas to flow through the valve (Figure 4–9). Stops in the full-off and full-on positions prevent valve damage. Touch- and color-coded control knobs make it more difficult to turn the wrong gas off or on. As a safety feature the oxygen knob is usually fluted, is larger and protrudes further than the other knobs, and is positioned furthest to the right.

Flowmeters on anesthesia machines are classified as either constant-pressure variable-orifice or electronic flowmeters. In constant-pressure variable-orifice flowmeters, an indicator ball, bobbin, or float is supported by

A

Oxygen
(pressurized)

Valve open

Inlet
from
cylinder

Outlet to
flowmeter
bank

Inlet from
pipeline

B

Oxygen
(depressurized)

Valve closed

Inlet
from
cylinder

Outlet to
flowmeter
bank

Inlet from
pipeline

Figure 4–7. Draeger oxygen failure protection device (OFPD). *A:* Open. *B:* Closed.

Balance regulator

Diaphragm

Nitrous oxide
from main
output
manifold

Nitrous oxide of
balance regulator

Figure 4–8. Datex-Ohmeda balance regulator.

Figure 4–9. Gas flow control needle valve (Datex-Ohmeda). *A:* Oxygen. *B:* Nitrous oxide. Note the secondary pressure regulator in the oxygen circuit and the balance regulator in the nitrous oxide circuit.

Figure 4–10. Constant-pressure variable orifice flowmeters (Thorpe type). ***A:*** Two tube design. ***B:*** Dual taper design.

the flow of gas through a tube (Thorpe tube) whose bore (orifice) is tapered. Near the bottom of the tube, where the diameter is small, a low flow of gas will create sufficient pressure under the float to raise it in the tube. As the float rises, the orifice of the tube widens, allowing more gas to pass around the float. The float will stop rising when its weight is just supported by the difference in pressure above and below it. If flow is increased, the pressure under the float increases, raising it higher in the tube until the pressure drop again just supports the float's weight. This pressure drop is constant regardless of the flow rate or the position in the tube and depends on the float weight and tube cross-sectional area.

Flowmeters are calibrated for specific gases, as the flow rate across a constriction depends on the gas's viscosity at low laminar flows and its density at high turbulent flows. To minimize the effect of friction between them and the tube's wall, floats are designed to rotate constantly, which keeps them centered in the tube. Coating the tube's interior with a conductive substance grounds the system and reduces the effect of static electricity. Some flowmeters have two glass

tubes, one for low flows and another for high flows (Figure 4–10A); the two tubes are in series and are still controlled by one valve. A dual taper design can allow a single flowmeter to read both high and low flows (Figure 4–10B). **Causes of flowmeter malfunction include dirt in the flow tube, vertical tube misalignment, and sticking or concealment of a float at the top of a tube.**

Should a leak develop within or downstream from an oxygen flowmeter, a hypoxic gas mixture can be delivered to the patient (Figure 4–11). To reduce this risk, oxygen flowmeters are *always* positioned downstream to all other flowmeters (nearest to the vaporizer).

Some anesthesia machines have electronic flow control and measurement (eg, Datex-Ohmeda S/5 Avance, Figure 4–12). In such instances, a back-up conventional (Thorpe) auxiliary oxygen flowmeter is provided. Other models have conventional flowmeters but electronic measurement of gas flow along with Thorpe tubes (Draeger 6400) and digital (Draeger Fabius GS) or digital/graphic displays (Datex-Ohmeda S/5 ADU, see Figure 4–13). The amount of

Incorrect sequence

Datex-Ohmeda sequence

Draeger sequence

Figure 4–11. Sequence of flowmeters in a three-gas machine. ***A:*** An unsafe sequence. ***B:*** Typical Datex-Ohmeda sequence. ***C:*** Typical Draeger sequence. Note that regardless of sequence a leak in the oxygen tube or further downstream can result in delivery of a hypoxic mixture.

pressure drop caused by a flow restrictor is the basis for measurement of gas flow rate in these systems. In these machines oxygen, nitrous oxide, and air each has a separate electronic flow measurement device in the flow control section before they are mixed together.

A. MINIMUM OXYGEN FLOW

The oxygen flow valves are usually designed to deliver a minimum flow of 150 mL/min when the anesthesia machine is turned on. One method involves the use of a minimum flow resistor (Figure 4–14). This safety feature helps ensure that some oxygen enters the breathing circuit even if the operator forgets to turn on the oxygen flow. Some machines are designed to deliver minimum flow or low-flow anesthesia (< 1 L/min) and have minimum oxygen flows as low as of 50 mL/min (eg, Datex-Ohmeda Aestiva/5).

B. OXYGEN/NITROUS OXIDE RATIO CONTROLLER

 Another safety feature of anesthesia machines is linkage of the nitrous oxide gas flow to the oxygen gas flow; this arrangement helps ensure a minimum oxygen concentration of 21–25%. The oxygen/nitrous oxide ratio controller links the two flow valves either mechanically (Datex-Ohmeda, Figure 4–15), pneumatically (Draeger, Figure 4–16), or electronically (Datex-Ohmeda S/5). It should be noted that this safety device does not affect the flow of a third gas (eg, air, helium, or carbon dioxide).

Vaporizers

Volatile anesthetics (eg, halothane, isoflurane, desflurane, sevoflurane) must be vaporized before being delivered to the patient. Vaporizers have concentration-calibrated dials that precisely add volatile anesthetic agents to the combined gas flow from all flowmeters. They must be located between the flowmeters and the common gas outlet. Moreover, unless the machine accepts only one vaporizer at a time (eg, Datex-Ohmeda S/5) all anesthesia machines should have an interlocking or exclusion device that prevents the concurrent use of more than one vaporizer.

A. PHYSICS OF VAPORIZATION

At a given temperature, the molecules of a volatile agent in a closed container are distributed between the liquid and gaseous phases. The gas molecules bombard the walls of the container, creating the vapor pressure of that agent. The higher the temperature, the greater the tendency for the liquid molecules to escape into the gaseous phase and the higher the vapor pressure (Figure 4–17). Vaporization requires energy (the heat of vaporization), which is supplied as a loss of heat from the liquid. As vaporization proceeds, liquid temperature drops and vapor pressure decreases unless heat is readily available to enter the system. Vaporizers contain a chamber in which a carrier gas becomes saturated with the volatile agent.

B. COPPER KETTLE

The copper kettle vaporizer is no longer used in clinical anesthesia, however, understanding how it works provides invaluable insight into the delivery of volatile

Figure 4–12. Datex-Ohmeda S/5 Avance with electronic flow control and measurement. Note the presence of only a single alternate flowmeter for oxygen to be used in a power failure.

Figure 4–13. Graphic and digital flowmeter display of Datex-Ohmeda S/5 ADU.

Figure 4–14. A bypass tube with minimum flow resistor upstream before the oxygen flow control valve ensures minimum oxygen flow even when the needle valve is turned off. A, B, resistors.

anesthetics (Figure 4–18). It is classified as a measured-flow vaporizer (or flowmeter-controlled vaporizer). In a copper kettle, the amount of carrier gas bubbled through the volatile anesthetic is controlled by a dedicated flowmeter. This valve is turned off when the vaporizer circuit is not in use. Copper is used as the construction metal because its relatively high specific heat (the quantity of heat required to raise the temperature of 1 g of substance by 1°C) and high thermal conductivity (the speed of heat conductance through a substance) enhance the vaporizer's ability to maintain a constant temperature. All the gas entering the vaporizer passes through the anesthetic liquid and becomes saturated with vapor. One milliliter of liquid anesthetic is the equivalent of approximately 200 mL of anesthetic vapor. Because the vapor pressure of volatile anesthetics is greater than the partial pressure required for anesthesia, the saturated gas leaving a copper kettle has to be diluted before it reaches the patient.

For example, the vapor pressure of halothane is 243 mm Hg at 20°C, so the concentration of halothane exiting a copper kettle at 1 atmosphere would be 243/760, or 32%. If 100 mL of oxygen enters the kettle, roughly 150 mL of gas exits, one-

third of which would be halothane vapor. In contrast, a partial pressure of only 7 mm Hg—or less than 1% concentration (7/760) at 1 atmosphere—may be required for anesthesia. To deliver a 1% concentration of halothane, the 50 mL of halothane vapor and 100 mL of carrier gas that left the copper kettle have to be diluted with another 4850 mL of gas (5000 - 150 = 4850). Every 100 mL of oxygen passing through a halothane vaporizer translates into a 1% increase in concentration if total gas flow into the breathing circuit is 5 L/min. Therefore when total flow is fixed, flow through the vaporizer determines the ultimate concentration of anesthetic. Isoflurane has an almost identical vapor pressure, so the same relationship between copper kettle flow, total gas flow, and anesthetic concentration exists. However, if total gas flow falls unexpectedly (eg, exhaustion of a nitrous oxide cylinder), volatile anesthetic concentration rises rapidly to potentially dangerous levels.

C. Modern Conventional Vaporizers

 All modern vaporizers are agent specific, capable of delivering a constant concentration of agent regardless of temperature changes or

Figure 4–15. Draeger pneumatic linkage of oxygen and nitrous oxide gas flows (oxygen ratio controller or ORC). **A:** Noncontrolling. **B:** Controlling. **C:** Shut-off.

(continued)

Figure 4–15. Continued

Link-25 proportioning system

Link-25 chain

Nitrous oxide sprocket

Oxygen sprocket

Figure 4–16. Datex-Ohmeda mechanical linkage of oxygen and nitrous oxide gas flows (Link-25).

flow through the vaporizer (Table 4–3). Turning a single calibrated control knob counterclockwise to the desired percentage divides the total gas flow into the carrier gas, which flows over the liquid anesthetic in a vaporizing chamber, and the balance, which exits the vaporizer unchanged (Figure 4–19). Because some of

the entering gas is never exposed to anesthetic liquid, this type of agent-specific vaporizer is also known as a variable-bypass vaporizer.

Temperature compensation is achieved by a strip composed of two different metals welded together. The metal strips expand and contract differently in response

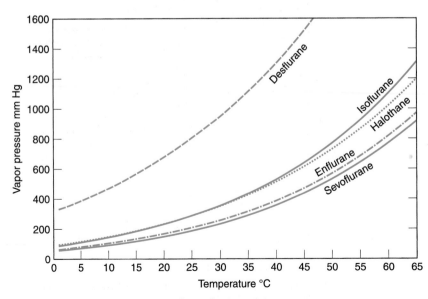

Figure 4–17. The vapor pressure of anesthetic gases.

Figure 4–18. Schematic of a copper kettle vaporizer. Note that 50 mL/min of halothane vapor is added for each 100 mL/min oxygen flow that passes through the vaporizer.

to temperature changes. When the temperature decreases differential contraction causes the strip to bend allowing more gas to pass through the vaporizer. As the temperature rises differential expansion causes the strip to bend the other way restricting gas flow into the vaporizer. Except in extreme ranges (< 250 mL/min or > 15 L/min), altering flow rates within a wide range does not significantly affect anesthetic concentration because the same proportion of gas is exposed to the liquid. Changing the gas composition, however, from

Table 4–3. Selected characteristics of modern vaporizers.

	Agent-Specific Models Available[1]	Capacity[2] (mL)	Tipping Hazard
Vapor 19.1 (Draeger)	H, E, I, S	200	Yes
Vapor 2000 (Draeger)	H, E, I, S	300	No (transport setting)
Tec 4	H, E, I, S	125	Yes
Tec 5	H, E, I, S	225	Yes
Tec 6 Plus	D	375	No (shuts off)
Tec 7	H, E, I, S	225	Yes
Aladin	H, E, I, S, D	250	No

[1]H, halothane; E, enflurane; I, isoflurane; D, desflurane; S, sevoflurane.
[2]Additional amount may be required to saturate the wick system when the vaporizer is dry.

100% oxygen to 70% nitrous oxide may transiently decrease volatile anesthetic concentration due to the greater solubility of nitrous oxide in volatile agents.

Figure 4–19. Schematic of agent-specific variable-bypass vaporizers. ***A:*** Draeger Vapor 19.n. ***B:*** Datex-Ohmeda Tec 7.

(continued)

B

Concentration dial

Bypass path

Vaporizer manifold

Carrier gas

Bi-metallic strip

Wick

Vaporizer chamber

Sump

Mixed gas to common gas manifold

Cooler temperatures

Warmer temperatures

Figure 4–19. Continued

These vaporizers are agent specific, and filling them with the wrong anesthetic must be avoided. For example, unintentionally filling an enflurane-specific vaporizer with halothane could lead to an anesthetic overdose. First, halothane's higher vapor pressure (243 mm Hg versus 175 mm Hg) will cause a 40% greater amount of anesthetic vapor to be released. Second, halothane is more than twice as potent as enflurane (see Chapter 7). Conversely, filling a halothane vaporizer with enflurane will cause an anesthetic underdose. Modern vaporizers offer agent-specific keyed filling ports to prevent filling with an incorrect agent.

Excessive tilting of older vaporizers (Tec 4, Tec 5, and Vapor 19.n) during transport may flood the bypass area and lead to dangerously high anesthetic concentrations. Fluctuations in pressure from positive-pressure ventilation in older anesthesia machines may cause a transient reversal of flow through the vaporizer, unpredictably changing agent delivery. This "pumping effect" is more pronounced with low gas flows. A one-way check valve between the vaporizers and the oxygen flush valve (Datex-Ohmeda) together with some design modifica-

tions in newer units limit the occurrence of some of these problems. **Vaporizers automatically compensate for changes in ambient pressures (ie, altitude changes).**

D. ELECTRONIC VAPORIZERS

Electronically controlled vaporizers must be utilized for desflurane and are used for all volatile anesthetics in some sophisticated anesthesia machines (eg, Datex-Ohmeda S/5 ADU).

1. Desflurane vaporizers—Desflurane's vapor pressure is so high that at sea level it almost boils at room temperature (Figure 4–17). **This high volatility, coupled with a potency only one-fifth that of other volatile agents, presents unique delivery problems.** First, the vaporization required for general anesthesia produces a cooling effect that would overwhelm the ability of conventional vaporizers to maintain a constant temperature. Second, because it vaporizes so extensively, a tremendously high fresh gas flow would be necessary to dilute the carrier gas to clinically relevant concentrations. These problems have been addressed by the

Figure 4–20. Schematic of the Datex-Ohmeda Tec 6 electronic desflurane vaporizer.

development of special desflurane vaporizers, the Tec 6, Tec 6 Plus, and D-tec (heated blender vaporizers). A reservoir containing desflurane (desflurane sump) is electrically heated to 39°C creating a vapor pressure of 2 atmospheres. Unlike a variable-bypass vaporizer, no fresh gas flows through the desflurane sump. Rather, pure desflurane vapor joins the fresh gas mixture before exiting the vaporizer (Figure 4–20). The amount of desflurane vapor released from the sump depends on the concentration selected by turning the control dial and the fresh gas flow rate. Although the Tec 6 Plus maintains a constant desflurane concentration over a wide range of fresh gas flow rates, it cannot automatically compensate for changes in elevation. Decreased ambient pressure (eg, high elevations) does not affect the concentration of agent delivered, but decreases the

partial pressure of the agent. Thus, at high elevations, the anesthesiologist must manually increase the concentration control.

2. Aladin cassette vaporizers—This vaporizer is designed for use with the Datex-Ohmeda S/5 ADU and similar machines. Gas flow from the flow control is divided into bypass flow and liquid chamber flow (Figure 4–21). The latter is conducted into an agent-specific, color-coded, cassette (Aladin cassette) in which the volatile anesthetic is vaporized. The machine accepts only one cassette at a time and recognizes the cassette through magnetic labeling. The cassette does not contain any bypass flow channels; therefore, unlike traditional vaporizers, liquid anesthetic cannot escape during handling and the cassette can be carried in any

Measurement part
(1) Bypass flow
(2) Flow through the cassette
(3) Cassette pressure
(4) Cassette temperature

Agent control
(5) Agent setting
(6) Control valve

Figure 4–21. Schematic of the electronic Datex-Ohmeda Aladin vaporizer.

position. After leaving the cassette, the now anesthetic-saturated liquid chamber flow reunites with the bypass flow before exiting the fresh gas outlet. Adjusting the ratio between the bypass flow and liquid chamber flow changes the concentration of volatile anesthetic agent delivered to the patient. In practice, the clinician changes the concentration by turning the agent wheel, which operates a digital potentiometer. Software sets the desired fresh gas agent concentration according to the number of output pulses from the agent wheel. Sensors in the cassette measure pressure and temperature, thus determining agent concentration in the gas leaving the cassette. Correct liquid chamber flow is calculated based on desired fresh gas concentration and determined cassette gas concentration.

Common (Fresh) Gas Outlet

In contrast to the multiple gas inlets, the anesthesia machine has only one common gas outlet that supplies gas to the breathing circuit. The term fresh gas outlet is also often used because of its critical role in adding new gas of fixed and known composition to the circle system. Unlike older models, some newer anesthesia machines measure and report common outlet gas flows (Ohmeda-Datex S/5 ADU and Narkomed 6400). An antidisconnect device is used to prevent accidental detachment of the gas outlet hose that connects the machine to the breathing circuit.

The oxygen flush valve provides a high flow (35–55 L/min) of oxygen directly to the common gas outlet, bypassing the flowmeters and vaporizers. It is used to rapidly refill or flush the breathing circuit, but because the oxygen may be supplied at a line pressure of 45–55 psig, there is a real potential of lung barotrauma. For this reason, the flush valve must be used cautiously whenever a patient is connected to the breathing circuit. Some machines use a second-stage regulator to drop the oxygen flush pressure to a lower level. A protective rim around the flush button limits the possibility of unintentional activation. Anesthesia machines (eg, Datex-Ohmeda Aestiva/5) may have an optional auxiliary common gas outlet that is activated with a dedicated switch. It is primarily used for performing the low-pressure circuit leak test (see Machine Checkout).

THE BREATHING CIRCUIT

The most commonly used breathing system used with anesthesia machines is the circle system (Figure 4–22); a Bain circuit is occasionally used (Chapter 3). The components and use of the circle system were discussed in Chapter 3. It is important to note that gas composition at the common gas outlet can be controlled precisely and rapidly by adjustments in flowmeters and vaporizers. In contrast, gas composition, especially volatile anesthetic concentration, in the breathing circuit is significantly affected by other factors, including anesthetic uptake in the patient's lungs, minute ventilation, total fresh gas flow, volume of the breathing circuit, and the presence of gas leaks. Use of high gas flow rates during induction and emergence decreases the effects of such variables and can diminish the magnitude of discrepancies between fresh gas outlet and circle system anesthetic concentrations (Chapter 3). Measurement of inspired and expired anesthetic gas concentration also greatly facilitates anesthetic management (Chapter 6).

In most machines the common gas outlet is attached to the breathing circuit just past the exhalation valve to prevent artificially high exhaled tidal volume measurements. When spirometry measurements

Figure 4–22. Diagram of a typical breathing circuit (Draeger Narkomed). Note gas flow during (**A**) spontaneous inspiration, (**B**) manual inspiration ("bagging"), and (**C**) exhalation (spontaneous or bag ventilation).

are made at the Y connector, fresh gas flow can enter the circuit on the patient side of the inspiratory valve (Datex-Ohmeda S/5ADU). The latter enhances CO_2 elimination and may help reduce desiccation of the CO_2 absorbent.

Newer anesthesia machines have integrated internalized breathing circuit components (Figure 4–23). The advantages of these designs include reduced probability of breathing circuit misconnects, disconnects, kinks, and leaks. The smaller volume of compact machines can also help conserve gas flow and volatile anesthetics and allow faster changes in breathing circuit gas con-

centration. Internal heating of manifolds can reduce precipitation of moisture.

Oxygen Analyzers

General anesthesia should never be administered without an oxygen analyzer in the breathing circuit. **Three types of oxygen analyzers are available: polarographic (Clark electrode), galvanic (fuel cell), and paramagnetic.** The first two techniques utilize electrochemical sensors that contain cathode and anode electrodes embedded in an electrolyte gel separated from the sam-

A

Figure 4–23. Breathing circuit design. **A:** Conventional external components. **B:** Compact design that reduces external connections and circuit volume (Draeger Fabius GS).

(continued)

B

Expiratory valve

PEEP/MAX valve connection port

Selection knob for MAN and SPONT on pressure-limiting valve

Expiration port

Connector for breathing bag

Inspiratory port

APL bypass valve connection port

Inspiratory valve

Carbon dioxide absorber

Figure 4–23. Continued

ple gas by an oxygen-permeable membrane (usually Teflon). As oxygen reacts with the electrodes, a current is generated that is proportional to the oxygen partial pressure in the sample gas. The galvanic and polarographic sensors differ in the composition of their electrodes and electrolyte gels. The components of the galvanic cell are capable of providing enough chemical energy so that the reaction does not require an external power source.

Although the initial cost of paramagnetic sensors is higher than that of electrochemical sensors, paramagnetic devices are self-calibrating and have no consumable parts. In addition, their response time is fast enough to differentiate between inspired and expired oxygen concentrations.

All oxygen analyzers should have a low-level alarm that is automatically activated by turning on the anesthesia machine. The sensor should be placed into the inspiratory or expiratory limb of the circle system's breathing circuit—but *not* into the fresh gas line. As a result of the patient's oxygen consumption, the expiratory limb has a slightly lower oxygen partial pressure than the inspiratory limb, particularly at low fresh gas flows. The increased humidity of expired gas does not significantly affect most modern sensors.

Spirometers

Spirometers, also called respirometers, are used to measure exhaled tidal volume in the breathing circuit on all anesthesia machines, typically near the

exhalation valve. Some anesthesia machines also measure the inspiratory tidal volume just past the inspiratory valve (Datex-Ohmeda Aestiva/5) or the actual delivered and exhaled tidal volumes at the Y connector that attaches to the patient's airway (eg, Datex-Ohmeda S/5 ADU).

A common method employs a rotating vane of low mass in the expiratory limb in front of the expiratory valve of the circle system (vane anemometer or Wright respirometer, Figure 4–24A).
The flow of gas across vanes within the respirometer causes their rotation, which is measured electronically, photoelectrically, or mechanically. In another variation using this turbine principle, the volumeter or displacement meter is designed to measure the movement of discrete quantities of gas over time (Figure 4–24B).

Changes in exhaled tidal volumes usually represent changes in ventilator settings, but can also be due to circuit leaks, disconnections, or ventilator malfunction. These spirometers are prone to errors caused by inertia, friction, and water condensation. Furthermore, the measurement of exhaled tidal volumes at this location in the expiratory limb includes gas that had been lost to the circuit (and not delivered to the patient; discussed below). The difference between the volume of gas delivered to the circuit and the volume of gas actually reaching the patient becomes very significant with long compliant breathing tubes, rapid respiratory rates, and high airway pressures. These problems are at least partially overcome by measuring the tidal volume at the Y connector to the patient's airway.

A

To absorber exhalation port

From breathing circuit

Forward flow

Sensor clip

Light emitting diode A

Light detector B

Light emitting diode B

Light detector A

Cartridge with vanes

B

MIN VOL 5.6
TID VOL 0.58
RR 10

Display

Processor

Armature

Hall effect transistor (A)

Magnet (4×)

Rotor

Interface panel

Volume sensor

Hall effect transistor (B)

Exhaled patient gas

Expiratory valve

Spiromed sensor

Absorber

Figure 4–24. Spirometer designs. *A:* Vane anemometer (Datex-Ohmeda). *B:* Volumeter (Draeger). *C:* Variable-orifice flowmeter (Datex-Ohmeda). *D:* Fixed orifice flowmeter (Pitot tube).

(continued)

Figure 4–24. Continued

A hot-wire anemometer (Drager Fabius GS) utilizes an electrically heated, fine platinum wire inside the gas flow. The cooling effect of increasing gas flow on the wire electrode causes a change in electrical resistance. In a constant-resistance anemometer, gas flow is determined from the current needed to maintain a constant wire temperature (and resistance). Disadvantages include an inability to detect reverse flow and the possibility that the heated wire

may be a potential ignition source for fire in the breathing manifold.

Ultrasonic flow sensors rely of discontinuities in gas flow generated by turbulent eddies in the flow stream. Upstream and downstream ultrasonic beams, generated from piezoelectric crystals, are transmitted at an angle to the gas stream. The Doppler frequency shift in the beams is proportional to the flow velocities in the breathing circuit. Major advantages include no moving parts and independence from gas density.

Machines with variable-orifice flowmeters usually employ two sensors (Figure 4–24C). One measures flow at the inspiratory port of the breathing system and the other measures flow at the expiratory port. These sensors use a change in internal diameter to generate a pressure drop that is proportional to the flow through the sensor. Clear tubes connect the sensors to differential pressure transducers inside the anesthesia machine (Datex-Ohmeda 7900 SmartVent). However, due to excessive condensation sensors can fail when used with heated humidified circuits.

A pneumotachograph is a fixed-orifice flowmeter that can function as a spirometer. A parallel bundle of small-diameter tubes in chamber (Fleisch pneumotachograph) or mesh screen provides a slight resistance to airflow. The pressure drop across this resistance is sensed by a differential pressure transducer and is proportional to the flow rate. Integration of flow rate over time yields tidal volume. Moreover, analysis of pressure, volume, and time relationships can yield potentially valuable information about airway and lung mechanics. Inaccuracies due to water condensation and temperature changes limited the clinical usefulness of these monitors until modifications in designs at least partially overcame these problems. One modification employs two Pitot tubes at the Y connection (eg, Datex-Ohmeda D-lite and Pedi-lite sensors, Figure 4–24D). Gas flowing through the sensor creates a pressure difference between the Pitot tubes. This pressure differential is used to measure flow rate, flow direction, and airway pressure. Respiratory gases are continuously sampled to correct the flow reading for changes in density and viscosity.

Circuit Pressure

A pressure gauge or electronic sensor is always used to measure breathing-circuit pressure somewhere between the expiratory and inspiratory unidirectional valves; the exact location depends on the model of anesthesia machine. Breathing-circuit pressure usually reflects airway pressure if it is measured as close to the patient's airway as possible. The most accurate measurements are from the Y connection (eg, D-lite and Pedi-lite sensors). A rise in airway pressure may signal worsening pulmonary compliance, an increase in tidal volume, or an obstruction in the breathing circuit, tracheal tube, or the patient's airway. A drop in pressure may indicate an improvement in compliance, a decrease in tidal volume, or a leak in the circuit. If circuit pressure is being measured at the CO_2 absorber, however, it will not always mirror the pressure in the patient's airway. For example, clamping the expi-

ratory limb of the breathing tubes during exhalation will prevent the patient's breath from exiting the lungs. Despite this buildup in airway pressure, a pressure gauge at the absorber will read zero because of the intervening one-way valve.

Some machines have incorporated auditory feedback for pressure changes during ventilator use (Drager "Respitone" and Datex-Ohmeda "AudiTorr").

Adjustable Pressure-Limiting Valve

The adjustable pressure-limiting (APL) valve, sometimes referred to as pressure relief or pop-off valve, is usually fully open during spontaneous ventilation but must be partially closed during manual or assisted bag ventilation (Chapter 3). The APL valve often requires fine adjustments. If it is not closed sufficiently excessive loss of circuit volume due to leaks prevents manual ventilation. At the same time if it closed too much or is fully closed a progressive rise in pressure could result in pulmonary barotrauma (eg, pneumothorax) and/or hemodynamic compromise. As an added safety feature, the APL valves on modern machines act as true pressure-limiting devices that can never be completely closed; the upper limit is usually 70–80 cm H_2O.

Humidifiers

Absolute humidity is defined as the weight of water vapor in 1 L of gas (ie, mg/L). Relative humidity is the ratio of the actual mass of water present in a volume of gas to the maximum amount of water possible at a particular temperature. At 37°C and 100% relative humidity, absolute humidity is 44 mg/L, whereas at room temperature (21°C and 100% humidity) it is 18 mg/L. Inhaled gases in the operating room are normally administered at room temperature with little or no humidification. Gases must therefore be warmed to body temperature and saturated with water by the upper respiratory tract. Tracheal intubation and high fresh gas flows bypass this normal humidification system and expose the lower airways to dry (< 10 mg H_2O/L), room temperature gases.

Prolonged humidification of gases by the lower respiratory tract leads to dehydration of mucosa, altered ciliary function, and, if excessively prolonged, could potentially lead to inspissation of secretions, atelectasis, and even ventilation/perfusion mismatching, particularly in patients with underlying lung disease. Body heat is also lost as gases are warmed and even more importantly as water is vaporized to humidify the dry gases. The heat of vaporization for water is 560 cal/g of water vaporized. Fortunately, this heat loss accounts for about only 5–10% of total intraoperative heat loss, is not significant for a short procedure (< 1 h), and usu-

HME unit

Patient
circuit

Gas
sample line

Patient circuit

Cool, dry, fresh gases
to and from the machine

HME unit
(heat and moisture exchange)

Warm, moist gases
to and from the patient

Figure 4–25. Heat and moisture exchanger (HME) functions as an "artificial nose" that attaches between the tracheal tube and the right-angle connector of the breathing circuit.

ally can easily be compensated for with a forced-air warming blanket (Chapter 6). Humidification and heating of inspiratory gases may be most important for small pediatric patients and older patients with severe underlying lung pathology, eg, cystic fibrosis.

A. Passive Humidifiers

Humidifiers added to the breathing circuit minimize water and heat loss. The simplest designs are condenser humidifiers or heat and moisture exchanger (HME) (Figure 4–25). These passive devices do not add heat or vapor but rather contain a hygroscopic material that traps exhaled humidification, which is released upon subsequent inhalation. Depending on the design, they may substantially increase apparatus dead space (more than 60 mL^3), which can cause significant rebreathing in pediatric patients. They can also increase breathing-circuit resistance and the work of breathing during spontaneous respirations. Excessive saturation of an HME with water or secretions can obstruct the breathing circuit. Some condenser humidifiers also act as effective filters that may protect the breathing circuit

and anesthesia machine from bacterial or viral cross-contamination. This may be particularly important when ventilating patients with respiratory infections or compromised immune systems.

B. Active Humidifiers

Active humidifiers add water to gas by passing the gas over a water chamber (passover humidifier) or through a saturated wick (wick humidifier), bubbling it through water (bubble-through humidifier), or mixing it with vaporized water (vapor-phase humidifier). Because increasing temperature increases the capacity of a gas to hold water vapor, heated humidifiers with thermostatically controlled elements are most effective. The hazards of heated humidifiers include thermal lung injury (inhaled gas temperature should be monitored), nosocomial infection, increased airway resistance from excess water condensation in the breathing circuit, interference with flowmeter function, and an increased likelihood of circuit disconnection. These humidifiers are particularly valuable with children as they help prevent both hypothermia and the plugging of small tracheal tubes by dried

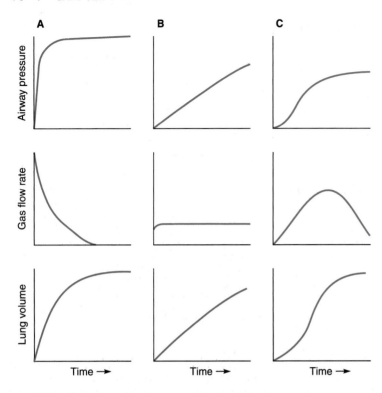

Figure 4–26. Pressure, volume, and flow profiles of different types of ventilators. **A:** Constant pressure. **B:** Constant flow. **C:** Nonconstant generator.

secretions. Of course, any design that increases airway dead space should be avoided in pediatric patients. Unlike passive humidifiers, active humidifiers do not filter respiratory gases.

VENTILATORS

Ventilators are used extensively in the operating room (OR) and the intensive care unit (ICU). All modern anesthesia machines are equipped with a ventilator. Historically OR ventilators were simpler and more compact than their ICU counterparts. This distinction has become blurred due to advances in technology together with an increasing need for "ICU-type" ventilators as more critically ill patients come to the OR. The ventilators on some modern machines are just as sophisticated as those in the ICU and have almost the same capabilities. After a general discussion of basic ventilator principles, this section reviews the use ventilators in conjunction with anesthesia machines. Chapter 49 discusses the use of ventilators in the ICU.

Overview

Ventilators generate gas flow by creating a pressure gradient between the proximal airway and the alveoli. Older units relied on the generation of negative pressure around

(and inside) the chest (eg, iron lungs), whereas modern ventilators generate positive pressure and gas flow in the upper airway. Ventilator function is best described in relation to the four phases of the ventilatory cycle: inspiration, the transition from inspiration to expiration, expiration, and the transition from expiration to inspiration. Although several classification schemes exist, the most common is based on inspiratory phase characteristics and the method of cycling from inspiration to expiration. Other classification categories may include power source (eg, pneumatic-high pressure, pneumatic-Venturi, or electric), design (single-circuit system, double-circuit system, rotary piston, linear piston), and control mechanisms (eg, electronic timer or microprocessor).

A. INSPIRATORY PHASE

During inspiration, ventilators generate tidal volumes by producing gas flow along a pressure gradient. The machine generates either a constant pressure (constant-pressure generators) or constant gas flow rate (constant-flow generators) during inspiration, regardless of changes in lung mechanics (Figure 4–26). Nonconstant generators produce pressures or gas flow rates that vary during the cycle but remain consistent from breath to breath. For instance, a ventilator that generates a flow pattern resembling a half cycle of a sine wave (eg, rotary piston ventilator) would be classified as a nonconstant-flow generator.

Figure 4–27. Rotary piston ventilator.

An increase in airway resistance or a decrease in lung compliance would increase peak inspiratory pressure but would not alter the flow rate generated by this type of ventilator (Figure 4–27).

B. TRANSITION PHASE FROM INSPIRATION TO EXPIRATION

Termination of the inspiratory phase can be triggered by a preset limit of time (fixed duration), a set inspiratory pressure that must be reached, or a predetermined tidal volume that must be delivered. Time-cycled ventilators allow tidal volume and peak inspiratory pressure to vary depending on lung compliance. Tidal volume is adjusted by setting inspiratory duration and inspiratory flow rate. Pressure-cycled ventilators will not cycle from the inspiratory phase to the expiratory phase until a preset pressure is reached. If a large circuit leak decreases peak pressures significantly, a pressure-cycled ventilator may remain in the inspiratory phase indefinitely. On the other hand, a small leak may not markedly decrease tidal volume, because cycling will be delayed until the pressure limit is met. Volume-cycled ventilators vary inspiratory duration and pressure to deliver a preset volume. In reality, modern ventilators overcome the many shortcomings of classic ventilator designs by incorporating secondary cycling parameters or other limiting mechanisms. For example, time-cycled and volume-cycled ventilators usually incorporate a pressure-limiting feature that terminates inspiration when a preset, adjustable safety

pressure limit is reached. Similarly a volume-preset control that limits the excursion of the bellows allows a time-cycled ventilator to function somewhat like a volume-cycled ventilator, depending on the selected ventilator rate and inspiratory flow rate (eg, Draeger AV2+).

C. EXPIRATORY PHASE

The expiratory phase of ventilators normally reduces airway pressure to atmospheric levels or some preset value of positive end-expiratory pressure (PEEP). Exhalation is therefore passive. Flow out of the lungs is determined primarily by airway resistance and lung compliance. PEEP is usually created with an adjustable spring valve mechanism or pneumatic pressurization of the exhalation (spill) valve (Chapter 49).

D. TRANSITION PHASE FROM EXPIRATION TO INSPIRATION

Transition into the next inspiratory phase may be based on a preset time interval or a change in pressure. The behavior of the ventilator during this phase together with the type of cycling from inspiration to expiration determines ventilator mode.

During controlled ventilation, the most basic mode of all ventilators, the next breath always occurs after a preset time interval. Thus tidal volume and rate are fixed in volume-controlled ventilation, whereas peak inspiratory pressure is fixed in pressure-controlled ventilation. Controlled ventilation modes are not designed for spontaneous breathing. In the volume-control

A

B

Figure 4–28. Ventilator controls (Datex-Ohmeda). **A:** Volume control mode. **B:** Pressure control mode.

mode, the ventilator adjusts gas flow rate and inspiratory time based on the set ventilatory rate and I:E ratio (Figure 4–28B). In the pressure-control mode, inspiratory time is also based on the set ventilator rate and inspiratory-to-expiratory (I:E) ratio, but gas flow is adjusted to maintain a constant inspiratory pressure (Figure 4–28A).

In contrast, intermittent mandatory ventilation (IMV) allows patients to breathe spontaneously between controlled breaths. Synchronized intermittent mandatory ventilation (SIMV) is a further refinement that helps prevent "fighting the ventilator" and "breath stacking"; whenever possible, the ventilator tries to time the mandatory mechanical breaths with the drops in airway pressure that occur

as the patient initiates a spontaneous breath. Chapter 49 discusses these and other ventilatory modes in more detail.

Ventilator Circuit Design

Traditionally ventilators on anesthesia machines have a double-circuit system design and are pneumatically powered and electronically controlled (Figure 4–29). Newer machines also incorporate microprocessor control that relies on sophisticated pressure and flow sensors. This feature allows multiple ventilatory modes, electronic PEEP, tidal volume modulation, and enhanced safety features. Some anesthesia machines (Draeger Fabius GS and

Figure 4–29. Double circuit pneumatic ventilator design. *A:* Datex-Ohmeda. *B:* Draeger.

6400) have ventilators that use a single-circuit piston design (Figure 4–26). Table 4–4 summarizes the important features of some anesthesia ventilators.

A. DOUBLE-CIRCUIT SYSTEM VENTILATORS

In a double-circuit system design, tidal volume is delivered from a bellows assembly that consists of a rubber or latex-free material bellows in a clear rigid plastic enclosure (Figure 4–28). A standing (ascending) bellows is preferred as it readily draws attention to a circuit disconnection by collapsing. Hanging (descending) bellows are rarely used and must not be weighted; older ventilators with weighted hanging bellows continue to fill by gravity even in the presence of a disconnect in the breathing circuit.

The bellows in a double-circuit design ventilator takes the place of the breathing bag in the anesthesia circuit. Pressurized oxygen or air from the ventilator power outlet (45–50 psig) is routed to the space between the inside wall of the plastic enclosure and the outside wall of the bellows. Pressurization of the plastic enclosure compresses the pleated bellows inside, forcing the gas inside into the breathing circuit and patient. A ventilator flow-control valve regulates drive gas flow into the pressurizing chamber. This valve is controlled by ventilator settings in the control box (Figure 4–29). Ventilators with microprocessors also utilize feedback from flow and pressure sensors. If oxygen is used for pneumatic power it will be consumed at a rate at least equal to minute

Table 4–4. Comparison of selected anesthesia machine ventilators.

	Datex-Ohmeda 7800	Datex-Ohmeda SmartVent 7900	Datex-Ohmeda 7100	Datex-Ohmeda S/5 ADU	Draeger AV2+	Draeger E-vent	Draeger Divan
Power	Pneumatic	Pneumatic	Pneumatic	Pneumatic	Pneumatic	Electric motor	Electric motor
Design type	Double-circuit ascending bellows	Double-circuit ascending bellows	Double-circuit ascending bellows	Double-circuit ascending bellows	Double-circuit ascending bellows	Piston	Piston
Control	Electronic (time-cycled, pressure-limited)	Microprocessor	Electronic (time-cycled, pressure-limited)	Microprocessor	Electronic (time-cycled, pressure-limited, volume-preset)	Microprocessor	Microprocessor
Modes[1]	VCV	VCV, PCV (SIMV, PSV options)	VCV, PCV	VCV, PCV, SIMV	VCV, PLV	VCV, PCV	VCV, PCV, SIMV
Inspiratory flow (L/min)	10–100	1–120 (80 max sustained)	2–70	≤ 80	10–100	10–75	5–75
Tidal volume (mL in VCV)	50–1500	20–1500	45–1500	20–1400	20–1500	20–1400	10–1400
Pressure limit (cm H_2O in VCV)	20–100	12–100	12–99	6–80	15–120	18–70	10–80
Inspiratory pressure (cm H_2O in PCV)	NA	5–60	5–50	5–40 (above PEEP)	NA	5–60	7–70
Pressure support range	NA	2–40	NA	5–40	NA	NA	NA
Ventilator rate	2–100	4–100	4–65	2–60	1–99	4–60	3–80
I:E ratio	2:1 to 1:99	2:1 to 1:8	2:1 to 1:6	2:1 to 1:4.5	4:1 to 1:4.5	4:1 to 1:4	5:1 to 1:5
Inspiratory pause	25%	NA	5–60%	0–60%	NA	0–50%	0–60%
PEEP (cm H_2O)	0–20 (optional)	4–30	4–30	5–20	2–15	0–20	0–20

[1]VCV, volume control ventilation; PCV, pressure control ventilation; PLV, pressure-limited ventilation; PSV, pressure support ventilation; SIMV, synchronized intermittent mandatory ventilation; I:E, inspiratory-to-expiratory; PEEP, positive end-expiratory pressure; NA, not applicable.

ventilation. Thus, if oxygen fresh gas flow is 2 L/min and a ventilator is delivering 6 L/min to the circuit, a total of at least 8 L/min of oxygen is being consumed. This should be kept in mind if the hospital's medical gas system fails and cylinder oxygen is required. Some anesthesias reduce oxygen consumption by incorporating a Venturi device that draws in room air to provide air/oxygen pneumatic power. Newer machines may offer the option of using compressed air for pneumatic power. A leak in the ventilator bellows can transmit high gas pressure to the patient's airway, potentially resulting in pulmonary barotrauma. This may be indicated by a higher than expected rise in inspired oxygen concentration (if

Figure 4–30. Modified circle system for a piston ventilator (Draeger Fabius GS).

oxygen is the sole pressurizing gas). Some machine ventilators have a built-in drive gas regulator that reduces the drive pressure (eg, to 25 psig) for added safety.

Double-circuit design ventilators also incorporate a free breathing valve that allows outside air to enter the rigid drive chamber and the bellows to collapse if the patient generates negative pressure by taking spontaneous breaths during mechanical ventilation.

B. PISTON VENTILATORS

In a piston design, the ventilator substitutes an electrically driven piston for the bellows (Figure 4–26); the ventilator requires either minimal or no pneumatic (oxygen) power. The major advantage of a piston ventilator is its ability to deliver accurate tidal volumes to patients with very poor lung compliance and to very small patients. During volume-controlled ventilation the piston moves at a constant velocity whereas during pres-

sure-controlled ventilation the piston moves with decreasing velocity. As with the bellows, the piston fills with gas from the breathing circuit. To prevent generation of significant negative pressure during the downstroke of the piston the circle system configuration has to be modified (Figure 4–30). The ventilator must also incorporate a negative-pressure relief valve (Draeger Fabius GS) or be capable of terminating the piston's downstroke if negative pressure is detected (Draeger Narkomed 6400). Introduction of a negative-pressure relief valve to the breathing circuit may introduce the risk of air entrainment and the potential for dilution of oxygen and volatile anesthetic concentrations if the patient breathes during mechanical ventilation and low fresh gas flows.

C. SPILL VALVE

Whenever a ventilator is used on an anesthesia machine, the circle system's APL valve must be functionally removed or isolated from the circuit. A bag/ventilator switch typically accomplishes this. When the switch is turned to "bag" the ventilator is excluded and spontaneous/manual (bag) ventilation is possible. When it is turned to "ventilator," the breathing bag and the APL are excluded from the breathing circuit. The APL valve may be automatically excluded in some newer anesthesia machines when the ventilator is turned on. The ventilator contains its own pressure-relief (pop-off) valve, called the spill valve, which is pneumatically closed during inspiration so that positive pressure can be generated (Figure 4–28). During exhalation, the pressurizing gas is vented out and the ventilator spill valve is no longer pressurized closed; the ventilator bellows or piston refill during expiration and the spill valve opens as circle system pressure rises. Sticking of this valve results in abnormally elevated airway pressure during exhalation.

Pressure & Volume Monitoring

Peak inspiratory pressure is the highest circuit pressure generated during an inspiratory cycle, and provides an indication of dynamic compliance. Plateau pressure is the pressure measured during an inspiratory pause (a time of no gas flow), and mirrors static compliance. During normal ventilation of a patient without lung disease, peak inspiratory pressure is equal to or only slightly greater than plateau pressure. An increase in both peak inspiratory pressure and plateau pressure implies an increase in tidal volume or a decrease in pulmonary compliance. An increase in peak inspiratory pressure without any change in plateau pressure signals an increase in airway resistance or inspiratory gas flow rate (Table 4–5). Thus, the shape of the breathing-circuit pressure waveform can provide important airway information. Many anesthesia machines graphically display breathing-circuit pressure (Figure 4–31). Airway secretions or kinking of the tracheal tube can be easily ruled out with the use of a suction catheter. Flexible fiberoptic bronchoscopy will usually provide a definitive diagnosis.

Ventilator Alarms

Alarms are an integral part of all modern anesthesia ventilators. Whenever a ventilator is used "disconnect alarms" must be passively activated. Anesthesia workstations should have at least three disconnect alarms: low peak inspiratory pressure, low exhaled tidal volume, and low exhaled carbon dioxide. The first is always built into the ventilator whereas the latter two may be in separate modules. A small leak or partial breathing-circuit disconnection

Table 4–5. Causes of increased peak inspiratory pressure (PIP), with or without an increased plateau pressure (PP).

Increased PIP and PP
Increased tidal volume
Decreased pulmonary compliance
Pulmonary edema
Trendelenburg position
Pleural effusion
Ascites
Abdominal packing
Peritoneal gas insufflation
Tension pneumothorax
Endobronchial intubation
Increased PIP and Unchanged PP
Increased inspiratory gas flow rate
Increased airway resistance
Kinked endotracheal tube
Bronchospasm
Secretions
Foreign body aspiration
Airway compression
Endotracheal tube cuff herniation

may be detected by subtle decreases in peak inspiratory pressure, exhaled volume, or end-tidal carbon dioxide before alarm thresholds are reached. Other built-in ventilator alarms include high peak inspiratory pressure, high PEEP, sustained high airway pressure, negative pressure, and low oxygen-supply pressure. Most modern anesthesia ventilators also have integrated spirometers and oxygen analyzers that provide additional alarms.

Problems Associated with Anesthesia Ventilators

A. VENTILATOR-FRESH GAS FLOW COUPLING

From the previous discussion, it is important to appreciate that because the ventilator's spill valve is closed during inspiration, fresh gas flow from the machine's common gas outlet normally contributes to the tidal volume delivered to the patient. For example, if the fresh gas flow is 6 L/min, the I:E ratio is 1:2, and the respiratory rate is 10 breaths/min, each tidal volume will include an extra 200 mL in addition to the ventilator's output:

$$\frac{(6000 \text{ mL} / \text{min}) (33\%)}{10 \text{ breaths/min}} \approx 200 \text{ mL/breath}$$

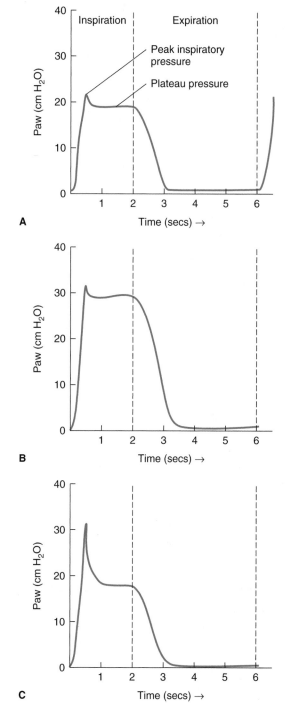

Figure 4–31. Airway pressures (Paw) can be diagrammatically presented as a function of time. **A:** In normal persons, the peak inspiratory pressure is equal to or slightly greater than the plateau pressure. **B:** An increase in peak inspiratory pressure and plateau pressure (the difference between the two remains almost constant) can be due to an increase in tidal volume or a decrease in pulmonary compliance. **C:** An increase in peak inspiratory pressure with little change in plateau pressure signals an increase in inspiratory flow rate or an increase in airway resistance.

Thus, increasing fresh gas flow increases tidal volume, minute ventilation, and peak inspiratory pressure. To avoid problems with ventilator-fresh gas flow coupling, airway pressure and exhaled tidal volume must be monitored closely and excessive fresh gas flows must be avoided.

B. EXCESSIVE POSITIVE PRESSURE

Intermittent or sustained high inspiratory pressures (> 30 mm Hg) during positive-pressure ventilation increase the risk of pulmonary barotrauma (eg, pneumothorax) and/or hemodynamic compromise during anesthesia. Excessively high pressures may arise from incorrect settings on the ventilator, ventilator malfunction, fresh gas flow coupling (above), or activation of the oxygen flush during the inspiratory phase of the ventilator. Use of the oxygen flush valve during the inspiratory cycle of a ventilator *must be avoided* because the ventilator spill valve will be closed and the APL valve is excluded; the surge of oxygen (600–1200 mL/s) and circuit pressure will be transferred to the patient's lungs.

In addition to a high-pressure alarm, all ventilators have a built-in automatic or APL valve. The mechanism of pressure limiting may be as simple as a threshold valve that opens at a certain pressure or electronic sensing that abruptly terminates the ventilator inspiratory phase.

C. TIDAL VOLUME DISCREPANCIES

Large discrepancies between the set and actual tidal volume that the patient receives are often observed in the operating room during volume control ventilation. Causes include breathing circuit compliance, gas compression, ventilator-fresh gas flow coupling (above), and leaks in the anesthesia machine, the breathing circuit, or the patient's airway.

The compliance for standard adult breathing circuits is about 5 mL/cm H_2O. Thus, if peak inspiratory pressure is 20 cm H_2O, about 100 mL of set tidal volume is lost to expanding the circuit. For this reason breathing circuits for pediatric patients are designed to be much stiffer, with compliances as small as 1.5–2.5 mL/cm H_2O.

Compression losses, normally about 3%, are due to gas compression within the ventilator bellows and may be dependent on breathing circuit volume. Thus if tidal volume is 500 mL another 15 mL of the set tidal gas may be lost. Gas sampling for capnography and anesthetic gas measurements represents additional losses in the form of gas leaks unless the sampled gas is returned to the breathing circuit, as occurs in some machines.

Accurate detection of tidal volume discrepancies is dependent on where the spirometer is placed. Sophisticated ventilators measure both inspiratory and expiratory tidal volumes. It is important to note that unless the spirometer is placed at the Y connector in the breathing circuit, compliance and compression losses will not be apparent.

Several mechanisms have been built into newer anesthesia machines to reduce tidal volume discrepancies. During the initial electronic self-checkout, some machines measure total system compliance and subsequently use this measurement to adjust the excursion of the ventilator bellows or piston; leaks may also be measured but are usually not compensated. The actual method of tidal volume compensation or modulation varies according to manufacturer and model. In one design (Datex-Ohmeda Aestiva/5), a flow sensor measures the tidal volume delivered at the inspiratory valve for the first few breaths and adjusts subsequent metered drive gas flow volumes to compensate for tidal volume losses (feedback adjustment). Another design (Datex-Ohmeda/5 ADU) continually measures fresh gas and vaporizer flow and subtracts this amount from the metered drive gas flow (preemptive adjustment). Alternately, machines that use electronic control of gas flow can decouple fresh gas flow from the tidal volume by delivery of fresh gas flow only during exhalation (Draeger Julian). Lastly, the inspiratory phase of the ventilator-fresh gas flow may be diverted through a decoupling valve into the breathing bag, which is excluded from the circle system during ventilation (Draeger Fabius GS and Narkomed 6400). During exhalation the decoupling valve opens, allowing the fresh gas that was temporarily stored in the bag to enter the breathing circuit.

WASTE-GAS SCAVENGERS

Waste-gas scavengers dispose of gases that have been vented from the breathing circuit by the APL valve and ventilator spill valve. Pollution of the operating room environment with anesthetic gases may pose a health hazard to surgical personnel (see Chapter 46). Although it is difficult to define safe levels of exposure, the National Institute for Occupational Safety and Health (NIOSH) recommends limiting the room concentration of nitrous oxide to 25 ppm and halogenated agents to 2 ppm (0.5 ppm if nitrous oxide is also being used). Reduction to these trace levels is possible only with properly functioning waste-gas scavenging systems.

To avoid the buildup of pressure, excess gas volume is vented through the APL valve in the breathing circuit and the ventilator spill valve. Both valves should be connected to hoses (transfer tubing) leading to the scavenging interface, which may be inside the machine or an external attachment (Figure 4–32).

A

Waste gas input port, 19-mm hose terminal

Safety relief valve, shown closed

Input port cap

Waste gas input port, 19-mm hose terminal

Waste gas exhaust port, 19-mm hose terminal

B

Vacuum DISS hose terminal

Lock nut

Needle valve knob

Threaded input port cap

19-mm scavenger hose terminal

Flowmeter

19-mm scavenger hose terminal

Relief port

Reservoir canister

C

Positive-pressure relief valve

Adjustment knob

Cap

Needle valve

To hospital vacuum system

Negative-pressure relief valve

Intake port for waste gases and the aestiva ventilator

Reservoir bag (3 L size)

Figure 4–32. Waste-gas scavenging systems. *A:* Closed interface with passive scavenging (Draeger). *B:* Open interface with active scavenging (Draeger). *C:* Closed interface with active scavenging (Datex-Ohmeda). *D:* Built in scavenging system that can be either active or passive; the active scavenging option has an open interface whereas the passive scavenging option has a closed interface with positive- and negative-pressure relief valves (Datex-Ohmeda).

(continued)

D

Vent engine

Scavenging reservoir

Scavenging connector

Back cover

Knob to remove back cover

Figure 4–32. Continued

The scavenging interface may be described as either open or closed.

An open interface is open to the outside atmosphere and usually requires no pressure relief valves. In contrast, a closed interface is closed to the outside atmosphere and requires negative- and positive-pressure relief valves that protect the patient from the negative pressure of the vacuum system and positive pressure from an obstruction in the disposal tubing, respectively. The outlet of the scavenging system may be a direct line to the outside via a ventilation duct beyond any point of recirculation (passive scavenging) or a connection to the hospital's vacuum system (active scavenging). A chamber or reservoir bag accepts waste-gas overflow when the capacity of the vacuum is exceeded. The vacuum control valve on an active system should be adjusted to allow the evacua-

tion of 10–15 L of waste gas per minute. This rate is adequate for periods of high fresh gas flow (ie, induction and emergence) yet minimizes the risk of transmitting negative pressure to the breathing circuit during lower flow conditions (maintenance). Unless used correctly the risk of occupational exposure for health care providers is higher with an open interface. Some machines may come with both active and passive scavenger systems.

ANESTHESIA MACHINE CHECKOUT LIST

Misuse or malfunction of anesthesia gas delivery equipment can cause major morbidity and mortality. A routine inspection of anesthesia equipment before each use increases operator familiarity and confirms proper functioning. The United States Food and Drug Administration (FDA) has made available a generic checkout procedure for anesthesia gas machines and breathing systems (Table 4–6). This procedure should be modified as necessary, depending on the specific equipment being used and the manufacturer's recommendations. Note that although the entire checkout does not need to be repeated between cases on the same day, the conscientious use of a checkout list is mandatory before each anesthetic procedure. A mandatory check-off procedure increases the likelihood of detecting anesthesia machine faults. Some anesthesia machines provide an automated system check that requires a variable amount of human intervention. These system checks may include nitrous oxide delivery (hypoxic mixture prevention), agent delivery, mechanical and manual ventilation, pipeline pressures, scavenging, breathing circuit compliance, and gas leakage.

CASE DISCUSSION: DETECTION OF A LEAK

After induction of general anesthesia and intubation of a 70-kg man for elective surgery, a standing bellows ventilator is set to deliver a tidal volume of 700 mL at a rate of 10 breaths/ min. Within a few minutes, the anesthesiologist notices that the bellows fails to rise to the top of its clear plastic enclosure during expiration. Shortly thereafter, the disconnect alarm is triggered.

Why has the ventilator bellows fallen and the disconnect alarm sounded?

Fresh gas flow into the breathing circuit is inadequate to maintain the circuit volume required for positive- pressure ventilation. In a situation in which there is no fresh gas flow, the volume in the breathing circuit will slowly fall because of the constant uptake of oxygen by the patient (metabolic oxygen consumption) and absorption of expired CO_2. An absence of fresh gas flow could be due to exhaustion of the hospital's oxygen supply (remember the function of the fail-safe valve) or failure to turn on the anesthesia machine's flow-control valves. These possibilities can be ruled out by examining the oxygen Bourdon

pressure gauge and the flowmeters. A more likely explanation is a gas leak that exceeds the rate of fresh gas flow. Leaks are particularly important in closed-circuit anesthesia (see Case Discussion, Chapter 7).

How can the size of the leak be estimated?

When the rate of fresh gas inflow equals the rate of gas outflow, the circuit's volume will be maintained. Therefore, the size of the leak can be estimated by increasing fresh gas flows until there is no change in the height of the bellows from one expiration to the next. If the bellows collapse despite a high rate of fresh gas inflow, a complete circuit disconnection should be considered. The site of the disconnection must be determined immediately and repaired to prevent hypoxia and hypercapnia. A resuscitation bag can be used to ventilate the patient if there is a delay in correcting the situation.

Where are the most likely locations of a breathing-circuit disconnection or leak?

Frank disconnections occur most frequently between the right-angle connector and the tracheal tube, whereas leaks are most commonly traced to the base plate of the CO_2 absorber. In the intubated patient, leaks often occur in the trachea around an uncuffed tracheal tube or an inadequately filled cuff. There are numerous potential sites of disconnection or leak within the anesthesia machine and the breathing circuit, however. Every addition to the breathing circuit, such as a humidifier, increases the likelihood of a leak.

How can these leaks be detected?

Leaks usually occur before the fresh gas outlet (ie, within the anesthesia machine) or after the fresh gas inlet (ie, within the breathing circuit). Large leaks within the anesthesia machine are less common and can be ruled out by a simple test. Pinching the tubing that connects the machine's fresh gas outlet to the circuit's fresh gas inlet creates a back pressure that obstructs the forward flow of fresh gas

Table 4–6. Anesthesia apparatus checkout recommendations.[1,2]

This checkout, or a reasonable equivalent, should be conducted before administration of anesthesia. These recommendations are valid only for an anesthesia system that conforms to current and relevant standards and includes an ascending bellows ventilator and at least the following monitors: capnograph, pulse oximeter, oxygen analyzer, respiratory volume monitor (spirometer), and breathing-system pressure monitor with high- and low-pressure alarms. Users are encouraged to modify this guideline to accommodate differences in equipment design and variations in local clinical practice. Such local modifications should have appropriate peer review. Users should refer to the appropriate operator manuals for specific procedures and precautions.

Emergency Ventilation Equipment
*1. Verify backup ventilation equipment is available and functioning

High-Pressure System
*2. Check O_2 cylinder supply
   a. Open O_2 cylinder and verify at least half full (about 1000 psig).
   b. Close cylinder
*3. Check central pipeline supplies; check that hoses are connected and pipeline gauges read about 50 psig.

Low-Pressure System
*4. Check initial status of low-pressure system
   a. Close flow control valves and turn vaporizers off.
   b. Check fill level and tighten vaporizers' filler caps.
*5. Perform leak check of machine low-pressure system
   a. Verify that the machine master switch and flow control valves are off.
   b. Attach suction bulb to common (fresh) gas outlet.
   c. Squeeze bulb repeatedly until fully collapsed.
   d. Verify bulb stays *fully* collapsed for at least 10 seconds.
   e. Open one vaporizer at a time and repeat steps c and d.
   f. Remove suction bulb, and reconnect fresh gas hose.
*6. Turn on machine master switch and all other necessary electrical equipment.
*7. Test flowmeters
   a. Adjust flow of all gases through their full range, checking for smooth operation of floats and undamaged flowtubes.
   b. Attempt to create a hypoxic O_2/N_2O mixture and verify correct changes in flow and/or alarm.

Scavenging System
*8. Adjust and check scavenging system
   a. Ensure proper connections between the scavenging system and both APL (pop-off) valve and ventilator relief valve.
   b. Adjust waste-gas vacuum (if possible).
   c. Fully open APL valve and occlude Y-piece.
   d. With minimum O_2 flow, allow scavenger reservoir bag to collapse completely and verify that absorber pressure gauge reads about zero.
   e. With the O_2 flush activated, allow scavenger reservoir bag to distend fully, and then verify that absorber pressure gauge reads < 10 cm H_2O.

Breathing System
*9. Calibrate O_2 monitor
   a. Ensure monitor reads 21% in room air.

   b. Verify low-O_2 alarm is enabled and functioning.
   c. Reinstall sensor in circuit and flush breathing system with O_2.
   d. Verify that monitor now reads greater than 90%.
10. Check initial status breathing system
   a. Set selector switch to Bag mode.
   b. Check that breathing circuit is complete, undamaged, and unobstructed.
   c. Verify that CO_2 absorbent is adequate.
   d. Install breathing-circuit accessory equipment (eg, humidifier, PEEP valve) to be used during the case.
11. Perform leak check of the breathing system
   a. Set all gas flows to zero (or minimum).
   b. Close APL (pop-off) valve and occlude Y-piece.
   c. Pressurize breathing system to about 30 cm H_2O with O_2 flush.
   d. Ensure that pressure remains fixed for at least 10 seconds.
   e. Open APL (pop-off) valve and ensure that pressure decreases.

Manual and Automatic Ventilation Systems
12. Test ventilation systems and unidirectional valves
   a. Place a second breathing bag on Y-piece.
   b. Set appropriate ventilator parameters for next patient.
   c. Switch to automatic-ventilation (ventilator) mode.
   d. Turn ventilator on and fill bellows and breathing bag with O_2 flush.
   e. Set O_2 flow to minimum, other gas flows to zero.
   f. Verify that during inspiration bellows deliver appropriate tidal volume and that during expiration bellows fill completely.
   g. Set fresh gas flow to about 5 L min^{-1}.
   h. Verify that the ventilator bellows and simulated lungs fill and empty appropriately without sustained pressure at end expiration.
   i. *Check for proper action of unidirectional valves.*
   j. Exercise breathing circuit accessories to ensure proper function.
   k. Turn ventilator off and switch to manual ventilation (bag/APL) mode.
   l. Ventilate manually and ensure inflation and deflation of artificial lungs and appropriate feel of system resistance and compliance.
   m. Remove second breathing bag from Y-piece.

(continued)

Table 4–6. Anesthesia apparatus checkout recommendations.[1,2] (continued)

Monitors	Final Position
13. Check, calibrate, and/or set alarm limits of all monitors: capnograph, pulse oximeter, O2 analyzer, respiratory-volume monitor (spirometer), pressure monitor with high and low airway-pressure alarms.	14. Check final status of machine a. Vaporizers off b. APL valve open c. Selector switch to Bag mode d. All flowmeters to zero (or minimum) e. Patient suction level adequate f. Breathing system ready to use

[1]Adapted from http://www.fda.gov/cdrh/humfac/anesckot.html.
[2]APL, adjust pressure-limiting; PEEP, positive end-expiratory pressure.
*If an anesthesia provider uses the same machine in successive cases, these steps need not be repeated, or they can be abbreviated after the initial checkout.

from the anesthesia machine. This is indicated by a drop in the height of the flowmeter floats. When the fresh gas tubing is released, the floats should briskly rebound and settle at their original height. If there is a substantial leak within the machine, obstructing the fresh gas tubing will not result in any back pressure, and the floats will not drop. A more sensitive test for detecting small leaks that occur before the fresh gas outlet involves attaching a suction bulb at the outlet as described in step 5 of Table 4–6. Correcting a leak within the machine usually requires removing it from service.

Leaks within a breathing circuit not connected to a patient are readily detected by closing the APL valve, occluding the Y-piece, and activating the oxygen flush until the circuit reaches a pressure of 20–30 cm H_2O. A gradual decline in circuit pressure indicates a leak within the breathing circuit (Table 4–6, step 11).

How are leaks in the breathing circuit located?

Any connection within the breathing circuit is a potential site of a gas leak. A quick survey of the circuit may reveal a loosely attached breathing tube or a cracked oxygen analyzer adaptor. Less obvious causes include detachment of the tubing used by the disconnect alarm to monitor circuit pressures, an open APL valve, or an improperly adjusted scavenging unit. Leaks can usually be identified audibly or by applying a soap solution to suspect connections and looking for bubble formation.

Leaks within the anesthesia machine and breathing circuit are usually detectable if the machine and circuit have undergone an established checkout procedure. For example, steps 5 and 11 of the FDA recommendations (Table 4–6) will reveal most significant leaks.

SUGGESTED READING

Baum JA, Nunn G: *Low Flow Anaesthesia: The Theory and Practice of Low Flow, Minimal Flow and Closed System Anaesthesia*, 2nd ed. Butterworth-Heinemann, 2001.

Block FE, Schaff C: Auditory alarms during anesthesia monitoring with an integrated monitoring system. Int J Clin Monit Comput 1996;13:81.

Caplan RA, Vistica MF, Posner KL, Cheney FW: Adverse anesthetic outcomes arising from gas delivery equipment: a closed claims analysis. *Anesthesiology* 1997;87:741.

Dorsch JA, Dorsch SE: *Understanding Anesthesia Equipment*, 4th ed. Lippincott, Williams & Wilkins, 1999. The anesthesia machine is covered in many chapters of this classic reference.

Ehrenwerth J, Eisenkraft JB (editors): *Anesthesia Equipment—Principles and Applications.* Mosby Year Book, 1993. A review of anesthesia machines and monitoring equipment.

Eisenkraft JB, Leibowitz AB: Ventilators in the operating room. Int Anesthesiol Clin 1997;35:87.

Healthcare Product Comparison System (HPCS), published by ECRI (a nonprofit agency), February 2002, pp 1–80. This report compares several models of anesthesia machines and includes an excellent overview of machine components and reported problems (including recalls).

Klopfenstein CE, Van Gessel E, Forster A: Checking the anaesthetic machine: self-reported assessment in a university hospital. Eur J Anaesthesiol 1998;15:314. Compliance with recommended safety checklists is low.

Somprakit P, Soontranan P: Low pressure leakage in anaesthetic machines: evaluation by positive and negative pressure tests. Anaesthesia 1996;51:461.

WEB SITES

http://www.apsf.org/

The Anesthesia Patient Safety Foundation web site provides resources and a newsletter that discusses important safety issues in anesthesia.

http://www.simanest.org/

An extremely useful web site of simulations in anesthesia that includes virtual anesthesia machine simulators.

Airway Management

5

KEY CONCEPTS

 1 Improper face mask technique can result in continued deflation of the anesthesia reservoir bag when the adjustable pressure-limiting valve is closed, usually indicating a substantial leak around the mask. In contrast, the generation of high breathing-circuit pressures with minimal chest movement and breath sounds implies an obstructed airway.

 2 The laryngeal mask airway partially protects the larynx from pharyngeal secretions (but not gastric regurgitation), and it should remain in place until the patient has regained airway reflexes.

 3 After insertion of a tracheal tube (TT), the cuff is inflated with the least amount of air necessary to create a seal during positive-pressure ventilation to minimize the pressure transmitted to the tracheal mucosa.

 4 Although the persistent detection of CO_2 by a capnograph is the best confirmation of tracheal placement of a TT, it cannot exclude bronchial intubation. The earliest manifestation of bronchial intubation is an increase in peak inspiratory pressure.

5 After intubation the cuff of a TT should not be felt above the level of the cricoid cartilage, because a prolonged intralaryngeal location may result in postoperative hoarseness and increases the risk of accidental extubation.

 6 Preventing unintentional esophageal intubation depends on direct visualization of the tip of the TT passing through the vocal cords, careful auscultation for the presence of bilateral breath sounds and the absence of gastric gurgling, analysis of exhaled gas for the presence of CO_2 (the most reliable method), chest radiography, or use of fiberoptic bronchoscopy.

7 Clues to the diagnosis of bronchial intubation include unilateral breath sounds, unexpected hypoxia with pulse oximetry (unreliable with high inspired oxygen concentrations), inability to palpate the TT cuff in the sternal notch during cuff inflation, and decreased breathing-bag compliance (high peak inspiratory pressures).

 8 The large negative intrathoracic pressures generated by a struggling patient in laryngospasm can result in the development of negative-pressure pulmonary edema even in healthy young adults.

Expert airway management is an essential skill for an anesthesiologist. This chapter reviews the anatomy of the upper respiratory tract, describes the necessary equipment, presents techniques, and discusses complications of laryngoscopy, intubation, and extubation. Patient safety depends on a thorough understanding of each of these topics.

ANATOMY

Other than rendering a patient insensible to pain, no characteristic better defines an anesthesiologist than the ability to "manage" an airway and a patient's breathing. Successful intubation, ventilation, cricothyrotomy, and regional anesthesia of the larynx require

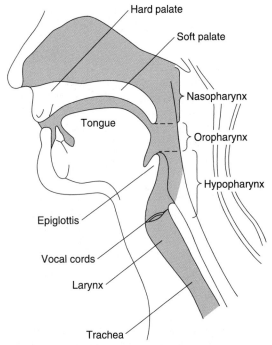

Hard palate

Soft palate

Nasopharynx

Tongue

Oropharynx

Hypopharynx

Epiglottis

Vocal cords

Larynx

Trachea

Figure 5–1. Anatomy of the airway.

detailed knowledge of airway anatomy. There are two openings to the human airway: the nose, which leads to the nasopharynx (*pars nasalis*), and the mouth, which leads to the oropharynx (*pars oralis*). These passages are separated anteriorly by the palate, but they join posteriorly in the pharynx (Figure 5–1). The pharynx is a U-shaped fibromuscular structure that extends from the base of the skull to the cricoid cartilage at the entrance to the esophagus. It opens anteriorly into the nasal cavity, the mouth, the larynx, and the nasopharynx, oropharynx, and laryngopharynx (pars laryngea), respectively. The nasopharynx is separated from the oropharynx by an imaginary plane that extends posteriorly. At the base of the tongue, the epiglottis functionally separates the oropharynx from the laryngopharynx (or hypopharynx). The epiglottis prevents aspiration by covering the glottis—the opening of the larynx—during swallowing. The larynx is a cartilaginous skeleton held together by ligaments and muscle. The larynx is composed of nine cartilages (Figure 5–2): thyroid, cricoid, epiglottic, and (in pairs) arytenoid, corniculate, and cuneiform.

The sensory supply to the upper airway is derived from the cranial nerves (Figure 5–3). The mucous membranes of the nose are innervated by the ophthalmic division (V_1) of the trigeminal nerve anteriorly (anterior ethmoidal nerve) and by the maxillary divi-

sion (V_2) posteriorly (sphenopalatine nerves). The palatine nerves provide sensory fibers from the trigeminal nerve (V) to the superior and inferior surfaces of the hard and soft palate. The lingual nerve (a branch of the mandibular division [V_3] of the trigeminal nerve) and the glossopharyngeal nerve (the ninth cranial nerve) provide general sensation to the anterior two-thirds and posterior third of the tongue, respectively. Branches of the facial nerve (VII) and glossopharyngeal nerve provide the sensation of taste to those areas, respectively. The **glossopharyngeal nerve** also innervates the roof of the pharynx, the tonsils, and the undersurface of the soft palate. The **vagus nerve** (the tenth cranial nerve) provides sensation to the airway below the epiglottis. The superior laryngeal branch of the vagus divides into an external (motor) nerve and an internal (sensory) laryngeal nerve that provide sensory supply to the larynx between the epiglottis and the vocal cords. Another branch of the vagus, the **recurrent laryngeal nerve,** innervates the larynx below the vocal cords and the trachea.

The muscles of the larynx are innervated by the recurrent laryngeal nerve with the exception of the cricothyroid muscle, which is innervated by the external (motor) laryngeal nerve, a branch of the superior laryngeal nerve. The posterior cricoarytenoid muscles abduct the vocal cords, whereas the lateral cricoarytenoid muscles are the principal adductors.

Phonation involves complex simultaneous actions by several laryngeal muscles. Damage to the motor nerves innervating the larynx leads to a spectrum of speech disorders (Table 5–1). Unilateral denervation of a cricothyroid muscle causes very subtle clinical findings. Bilateral palsy of the superior laryngeal nerve may result in hoarseness or easy tiring of the voice, but airway control is not jeopardized.

Unilateral paralysis of a recurrent laryngeal nerve results in paralysis of the ipsilateral vocal cord, causing a deterioration in voice quality. Assuming intact superior laryngeal nerves, *acute* bilateral recurrent laryngeal nerve palsy can result in stridor and respiratory distress because of the remaining unopposed tension of the cricothyroid muscles. Airway problems are less frequent in *chronic* bilateral recurrent laryngeal nerve loss because of the development of various compensatory mechanisms (eg, atrophy of the laryngeal musculature).

Bilateral injury to the vagus nerve affects both the superior and the recurrent laryngeal nerves. Thus, bilateral vagal denervation produces flaccid, midpositioned vocal cords similar to those seen after administration of succinylcholine. Although phonation is severely impaired in these patients, airway control is rarely a problem.

The blood supply of the larynx is derived from branches of the thyroid arteries. The cricothyroid artery

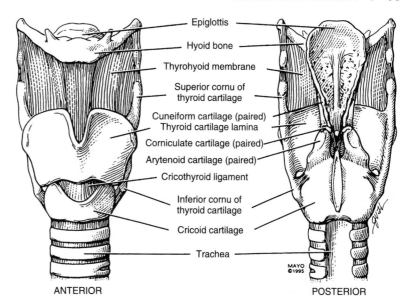

Figure 5–2. Cartilaginous structures comprising the larynx. (Modified and reproduced, with permission, from Mayo Clinic and Foundation from O'Connell F: Management of the airway and endotracheal intubation. In: *Critical Care Medicine: Perioperative Management.* Murray MJ, Coursin DB, Pearl RG, Prough DS [editors]. Lippincott-Raven Publishers, 1997.)

Epiglottis
Hyoid bone
Thyrohyoid membrane
Superior cornu of thyroid cartilage
Cuneiform cartilage (paired)
Thyroid cartilage lamina
Corniculate cartilage (paired)
Arytenoid cartilage (paired)
Cricothyroid ligament
Inferior cornu of thyroid cartilage
Cricoid cartilage
Trachea

ANTERIOR   POSTERIOR

arises from the superior thyroid artery itself, the first branch given off from the external carotid artery, and crosses the upper cricothyroid membrane, which extends from the cricoid cartilage to the thyroid cartilage. The superior thyroid artery is found along the lateral edge of the cricothyroid membrane. When planning a cricothyrotomy, the anatomy of the cricothyroid artery and the thyroid artery should be considered but rarely

V₁ Ophthalmic division of trigeminal nerve (anterior ethmoidal nerve)

V₂ Maxillary division of trigeminal nerve (sphenopalatine nerves)

V₃ Mandibular division of trigeminal nerve (lingual nerve)

IX Glossopharyngeal nerve

X Vagus nerve
    SL Superior laryngeal nerve
    IL Internal laryngeal nerve
    RL Recurrent laryngeal nerve

Figure 5–3. Sensory nerve supply of the airway.

Table 5–1. The effects of laryngeal nerve injury on the voice.

Nerve	Effect of Nerve Injury
Superior laryngeal nerve	
Unilateral	Minimal effects
Bilateral	Hoarseness, tiring of voice
Recurrent laryngeal nerve	
Unilateral	Hoarseness
Bilateral	
Acute	Stridor, respiratory distress
Chronic	Aphonia
Vagus nerve	
Unilateral	Hoarseness
Bilateral	Aphonia

should affect the practice. It is best to stay in the midline, midway between the cricoid and thyroid cartilages.

EQUIPMENT

Oral & Nasal Airways

Loss of upper airway muscle tone (eg, weakness of the genioglossus muscle) in anesthetized patients allows the tongue and epiglottis to fall back against the posterior wall of the pharynx. Repositioning the head or a jaw thrust is the preferred technique for opening the airway. To maintain the opening, though, an artificial airway can be inserted through the mouth or nose to create an air passage between the tongue and the posterior pharyngeal wall (Figure 5–4). Awake or lightly anesthetized patients may cough or even develop laryngospasm during airway insertion if laryngeal reflexes are intact. Placement of an oral airway is sometimes facilitated by suppressing airway reflexes and, in addition, sometimes by depressing the tongue with a tongue blade. Adult oral airways typically come in small (80 mm [Guedel No. 3]), medium (90 mm [Guedel No. 4]), and large (100 mm [Guedel No. 5]) sizes.

The length of a nasal airway can be estimated as the distance from the nares to the meatus of the ear, and should be approximately 2–4 cm longer than oral airways. Because of the risk of epistaxis, nasal airways should not be used in anticoagulated patients or in children with prominent adenoids. Also, nasal airways should not be used in any patient who has a basilar skull fracture. Any tube inserted through the nose (eg, nasal airways, nasogastric catheters, nasotracheal tubes) should be lubricated and advanced along the floor of the nasal passage, not as novices attempt to do—toward the apex of the nasal passage to avoid traumatizing the turbinates or the roof of the nose. Nasal airways are usually better tolerated than oral airways in lightly anesthetized patients.

Face Mask Design & Technique

The use of a face mask can facilitate delivery of oxygen or of an anesthetic gas from a breathing system to a patient by creating an airtight seal with the patient's face (Figure 5–5). The rim of the mask is contoured and conforms to a variety of facial features. The mask's 22-mm orifice attaches to the breathing circuit of the anesthesia machine through a right-angle connector. Several mask designs are available. Transparent masks allow observation of exhaled humidified gas and immediate recognition of vomiting. Black rubber masks are pliable enough to adapt to uncommon facial structures. Retaining hooks surrounding the orifice can be attached to a head strap so

Figure 5–4. A: The oropharyngeal airway in place. The airway follows the curvature of the tongue, pulling it and the epiglottis away from the posterior pharyngeal wall and providing a channel for air passage. **B:** The nasopharyngeal airway in place. The airway passes through the nose and extends to just above the epiglottis. (Modified and reproduced, with permission, from Face masks and airways. In: *Understanding Anesthesia Equipment*, 4th ed. Dorsch JA, Dorsch SE (editors). Williams & Wilkins, 1999.)

Figure 5–5. Clear adult face mask.

Figure 5–7. One-handed face mask technique.

that the mask does not have to be continually held in place. Some pediatric masks are specially designed to minimize apparatus dead space (Figure 5–6).

Effective ventilation requires both a gas-tight mask fit and a patent airway. Improper face mask technique can result in continued deflation of the anesthesia reservoir bag when the adjustable pressure-limiting valve is closed, usually indicating a substantial leak around the mask. In contrast, the generation of high breathing-circuit pressures with minimal chest movement and breath sounds implies an obstructed airway. Both these problems are usually resolved by proper technique.

If the mask is held with the left hand, the right hand can be used to generate positive-pressure ventilation by squeezing the breathing bag. The mask is held against the face by downward pressure on the mask body exerted by the left thumb and index finger (Figure 5–7). The middle and ring finger grasp the mandible to facilitate extension of the atlantooccipital joint. Finger pressure should be placed on the bony mandible and not on the soft tissues supporting the base of the tongue, which may obstruct the

airway. The little finger is placed under the angle of the jaw and used to thrust the jaw anteriorly, the most important maneuver to allow ventilation to the patient.

In difficult situations, two hands may be needed to provide adequate jaw thrust and create a mask seal. Therefore, an assistant may be needed to squeeze the anesthesia bag. In such cases, the thumbs hold the mask down and the fingertips or knuckles displace the jaw forward (Figure 5–8). Obstruction during expiration may be due to excessive downward pressure from the mask or from a ball-valve

Figure 5–6. The Rendell–Baker–Soucek pediatric face mask has a shallow body and minimal dead space.

Figure 5–8. A difficult airway can often be managed with a two-handed technique.

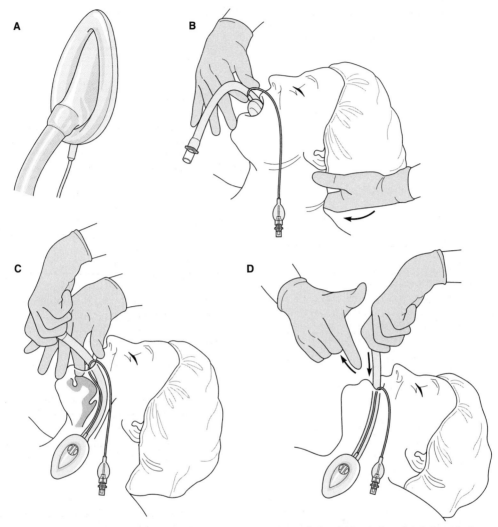

Figure 5–9. ***A:*** The laryngeal mask ready for insertion. The cuff should be deflated tightly with the rim facing away from the mask aperture. There should be no folds near the tip. ***B:*** Initial insertion of the laryngeal mask. Under direct vision, the mask tip is pressed upward against the hard palate. The middle finger may be used to push the lower jaw downward. The mask is pressed forward as it is advanced into the pharynx to ensure that the tip remains flattened and avoids the tongue. The jaw should not be held open once the mask is inside the mouth. The nonintubating hand can be used to stabilize the occiput. ***C:*** By withdrawing the other fingers and with a slight pronation of the forearm, it is usually possible to push the mask fully into position in one fluid movement. Note that the neck is kept flexed and the head extended. ***D:*** The laryngeal mask is grasped with the other hand and the index finger withdrawn. The hand holding the tube presses gently downward until resistance is encountered. (Reproduced, with permission, from LMA North America.)

effect of the jaw thrust. The former can be relieved by decreasing the pressure on the mask and the latter by releasing the jaw thrust during this phase of the respiratory cycle. It is often difficult to form an adequate mask fit with the cheeks of edentulous patients. Leaving dentures in place (not recommended) or packing the buccal cavities with gauze may help. Positive-pressure ventilation should normally be limited to 20 cm H_2O to avoid stomach inflation.

Most patients' airways can be maintained with a face mask, and an oral or nasal airway. Mask ventilation for long periods may result in pressure injury to branches of the trigeminal or facial nerves. Because of the absence of positive airway pressures during spontaneous ventilation, only minimal downward force on the face mask is required to create an adequate seal. If the face mask and mask straps are used for extended periods, the position should be regularly changed to prevent injury. Care should be used to avoid pressure on the eye, and the eyes should be taped shut to minimize the risk of **corneal abrasions.**

Laryngeal Mask Design & Technique

The laryngeal mask airway (LMA) is being increasingly used in place of a face mask or TT during administration of an anesthetic, to facilitate ventilation and passage of a TT in a patient with a difficult airway, and to aid in ventilation during fiberoptic bronchoscopy as well as placement of the bronchoscope. The LMA has surpassed the Combitube as a preferred device to manage a difficult airway. Four types of LMAs are commonly used: the reusable LMA, an improved disposable LMA, the ProSeal LMA that has an orifice through which a nasogastric tube can be inserted and that facilitates positive-pressure ventilation, and a Fastrach LMA that facilitates intubating patients with difficult airways.

An LMA consists of a wide-bore tube whose proximal end connects to a breathing circuit with a standard 15-mm connector, and whose distal end is attached to an elliptical cuff that can be inflated through a pilot tube. The deflated cuff is lubricated and inserted blindly into the hypopharynx so that, once inflated, the cuff forms a low-pressure seal around the entrance to the larynx. This requires an anesthetic depth slightly greater than required for the insertion of an oral airway. Although insertion is relatively simple (Figure 5–9), proper attention to detail will improve the success rate (Table 5–2). An ideally positioned cuff is bordered by the base of the tongue superiorly, the pyriform sinuses laterally, and the upper esophageal sphincter inferiorly. If the esophagus lies within the rim of the cuff, gastric distention and regurgitation become a distinct possibility. Anatomic variations prevent adequate functioning in some patients. However, if an LMA is not functioning properly after attempts to improve the "fit" of the LMA have failed, most practitioners will try another LMA one size larger or smaller. Because down-folding of the epiglottis or distal cuff accounts for many failures, LMA insertion under direct visualization with a laryngoscope or fiberoptic bronchoscope (FOB) may prove beneficial in difficult cases. Likewise, partial cuff inflation prior to insertion may be helpful. The shaft can be secured with tape, as a TT would be. The LMA partially protects the

Table 5–2. Successful insertion of a laryngeal mask airway depends upon attention to several details.

1. Choose the appropriate size (Table 5–3) and check for leaks before insertion.
2. The leading edge of the deflated cuff should be wrinkle-free and facing away from the aperture (Figure 5–9A).
3. Lubricate only the back side of the cuff.
4. Ensure adequate anesthesia (regional nerve block or general) before attempting insertion. Propofol with opioids provide superior conditions compared with thiopental.
5. Place patient's head in sniffing position (Figure 5–9B and Figure 5–16).
6. Use your index finger to guide the cuff along the hard palate and down into the hypopharynx until an increased resistance is felt (Figure 5–9C). The longitudinal black line should *always* be pointing directly cephalad (ie, facing the patient's upper lip).
7. Inflate with the correct amount of air (Table 5–3).
8. Ensure adequate anesthetic depth during patient positioning.
9. Obstruction after insertion is usually due to a down-folded epiglottis or transient laryngospasm.
10. Avoid pharyngeal suction, cuff deflation, or laryngeal mask removal until the patient is awake (eg, opening mouth on command).

larynx from pharyngeal secretions (but *not* gastric regurgitation), and it should remain in place until the patient has regained airway reflexes. This is usually signaled by coughing and mouth opening on command. The reusable LMA, which is autoclavable, is made of silicone rubber (ie, it is latex free) and is available in many sizes (Table 5–3).

The LMA provides an alternative to ventilation through a face mask or TT (Table 5–4). Contraindications for the LMA include patients with pharyngeal pathology (eg, abscess), pharyngeal obstruction, full stomachs (eg, pregnancy, hiatal hernia), or low pulmonary compliance (eg, restrictive airways disease) requiring peak inspiratory pressures greater than 30 cm H_2O. Traditionally, the LMA has been avoided in patients with bronchospasm or high airway resistance, but new evidence suggests that because it is not placed in the trachea, use of an LMA is associated with less bronchospasm than a TT. Although it is clearly not a substitute for tracheal intubation, the LMA has proven particularly helpful as a temporizing measure in patients with difficult airways (those who cannot be ventilated or intubated) because of its ease of insertion and relatively high success rate (95–99%). It has been used as a conduit for an intubating stylet (eg, gum-elastic bougie), ventilating jet stylet, flexible FOB, or small-diameter (6.0-mm) TT. Several LMAs are available

Table 5–3. A variety of laryngeal masks with different cuff volumes are available for different sized patients.

Mask Size	Patient Size	Weight (kg)	Cuff Volume (mL)
1	Infant	<6.5	2–4
2	Child	6.5–20	Up to 10
2½	Child	20–30	Up to 15
3	Small adult	>30	Up to 20
4	Normal adult	<70	Up to 30
5	Larger adult	>70	Up to 30

that have been modified to facilitate placement of a larger TT with or without the use of an FOB. Insertion can be performed under topical anesthesia and bilateral superior laryngeal nerve blocks if the airway must be secured while the patient is awake.

Esophageal–Tracheal Combitube Design & Technique

The esophageal–tracheal Combitube consists of two fused tubes, each with a 15-mm connector on its proximal end. The longer blue tube has an occluded distal tip that forces gas to exit through a series of side perforations. The shorter clear tube has an open tip and no side perforations. The Combitube is usually inserted blindly through the mouth and advanced until the two black rings on the shaft lie between the upper and lower teeth. The Combitube has two inflatable cuffs, a 100-mL proximal cuff and a 15-mL distal cuff, both of which should be fully inflated after placement. The distal lumen of the Combitube usually comes to lie in the esophagus approximately 95% of the time so that ventilation through the longer blue tube will force gas out of the side perforations and into the larynx. The shorter, clear tube can be used for gastric decompression. Alternatively, if the Combitube enters the trachea, ventilation through the clear tube will direct gas into the trachea. Although the Combitube is still listed as an option for managing a difficult airway in the Advanced Cardiac Life Support algorithm, it is rarely used by anesthesiologists who prefer an LMA or other devices for managing patients with difficult airways.

Tracheal Tubes

TTs can be used to deliver anesthetic gases directly into the trachea and allow the most control of ventilation and oxygenation. Standards govern TT manufacturing (American National Standard for Anesthetic Equipment; ANSI Z–79). TTs are most commonly made from polyvinyl chloride. In the past, TTs were marked "I.T." or "Z–79" to indicate that they had been implant tested to ensure nontoxicity. The shape and rigidity of TTs can be altered by inserting a stylet. The patient end

Table 5–4. Advantages and disadvantages of the laryngeal mask airway compared with face mask ventilation or tracheal intubation.[1]

	Advantages	Disadvantages
Compared with face mask	Hands-free operation	More invasive
	Better seal in bearded patients	More risk of airway trauma
	Less cumbersome in ENT surgery	Requires new skill
	Often easier to maintain airway	Deeper anesthesia required
	Protects against airway secretions	Requires some TMJ mobility
	Less facial nerve and eye trauma	N₂O diffusion into cuff
	Less operating room pollution	Multiple contraindications
Compared with tracheal intubation	Less invasive	Increased risk of gastrointestinal aspiration
	Very useful in difficult intubations	Less safe in prone or jackknife positions
	Less tooth and laryngeal trauma	Limits maximum PPV
	Less laryngospasm and bronchospasm	Less secure airway
	Does not require muscle relaxation	Greater risk of gas leak and pollution
	Does not require neck mobility	Can cause gastric distention
	No risk of esophageal or endobronchial intubation	

[1]ENT, ear, nose, and throat; TMJ, temporomandibular joint; PPV, positive pressure ventilation.

Figure 5–10. Murphy tracheal tube.

of the tube is beveled to aid visualization and insertion through the vocal cords. Murphy tubes have a hole (the Murphy eye) to decrease the risk of occlusion should the distal tube opening abut the carina or trachea (Figure 5–10).

Resistance to airflow depends primarily on tube diameter, but is also affected by tube length and curvature. TT size is usually designated in millimeters of internal diameter or, less commonly, in the French scale (external diameter in millimeters multiplied by 3). The choice of tube diameter is always a compromise between maximizing flow with a large size and minimizing airway trauma with a small size (Table 5–5).

Most adult TTs have a cuff inflation system consisting of a valve, pilot balloon, inflating tube, and cuff (Figure 5–10). The valve prevents air loss after cuff inflation. The pilot balloon provides a gross indication of cuff inflation. The inflating tube connects the valve to the cuff and is incorporated into the tube's wall. By creating a tracheal seal, TT cuffs permit positive-pressure ventilation and reduce the likelihood of aspiration. Uncuffed tubes are usually used in children to minimize the risk of pressure injury and **postintubation croup** (see Chapter 44).

There are two major types of cuffs: high pressure (low volume) and low pressure (high volume). High-pressure cuffs are associated with more ischemic damage to the tracheal mucosa and are less suitable for intubations of long duration. Low-pressure cuffs may increase the likelihood of sore throat (larger mucosal contact area), aspiration, spontaneous extubation, and difficult insertion (because of the floppy cuff). Nonetheless, because of their lower incidence of mucosal damage, low-pressure cuffs are more commonly recommended.

Cuff pressure depends on several factors: inflation volume, the diameter of the cuff in relation to the trachea, tracheal and cuff compliance, and intrathoracic pressure (cuff pressures increase with coughing). Cuff pressure may rise during general anesthesia as a result of the diffusion of nitrous oxide from the tracheal mucosa into the TT cuff.

TTs have been modified for a variety of specialized applications. Flexible, spiral-wound, wire-reinforced TTs (armored tubes) resist kinking and may prove valuable in some head and neck surgical procedures or in the prone patient. If an armored tube becomes kinked from extreme pressure (eg, an awake patient biting it), however, the lumen will tend to remain occluded and the tube will need replacement. Other specialized tubes include microlaryngeal tubes (see Chapter 39), RAE pre-

Table 5–5. Oral tracheal tube size guidelines.

Age	Internal Diameter (mm)	Cut Length (cm)
Full-term infant	3.5	12
Child	$4 + \dfrac{Age}{4}$	$14 + \dfrac{Age}{2}$
Adult		
Female	7.0–7.5	24
Male	7.5–9.0	24

Figure 5–11. A rigid laryngoscope.

Rigid Laryngoscopes

A laryngoscope is an instrument used to examine the larynx and to facilitate intubation of the trachea. The handle usually contains batteries to light a bulb on the blade tip (Figure 5–11), or alternately to power a fiberoptic bundle that terminates at the tip of the blade. Light from a fiberoptic bundle tends to be more direct and less diffuse. Also, laryngoscopes with fiberoptic light bundles in their blades can be made magnetic resonance imaging (MRI) compatible. The Macintosh and Miller blades are the most popular curved and straight designs, respectively, in the United States. The choice of blade depends on personal preference and patient anatomy. Because no blade is perfect for all situations, the clinician should become familiar and proficient with a variety of blade designs (Figure 5–12).

Specialized Laryngoscopes

In the past 15 years, two new laryngoscopes have been developed that help the anesthesiologist secure the airway in a difficult-airway patient—the Bullard laryngoscope and the Wu laryngoscope (Figure 5–13). Both have fiberoptic light sources and curved blades with elongated tips and were designed to help see the glottic opening in patients with large tongues or whose glottic opening is very anterior. Many anesthesiologists believe that these

formed tubes (see Figures 39–1 and 39–3), and double-lumen TTs (see Figure 24–8). There is now a Parker FlexTip TT that has a tapered distal opening that is more elastic. All TTs have an embedded line that is opaque on radiographs to allow visualization *in situ*.

Figure 5–12. An assortment of laryngoscope blades.

Figure 5–13. Specialized laryngoscopic blades for managing a difficult airway. *A:* Fully assembled Wu laryngoscope with a tracheal tube in the tracheal tube passage, a suction catheter in the tracheal tube lumen, and oxygen tubing connected to the oxygen port. *B:* Newer version (Elite) of the Bullard laryngoscope. The handle has been reshaped. There is a built-in focus adjustment in the eyepiece. On the viewing arm adjacent to the handle is a spring-loaded mechanism to hold the multifunctional stylet. (Courtesy of Circon Acmi, a division of Circon Corp.)

devices are preferred in patients in whom a difficult airway is anticipated. However, as with other devices used to manage patients' airways, expertise in their use should be gained in normal patients before using it urgently or emergently in a patient with a difficult airway.

Flexible Fiberoptic Bronchoscopes

In some situations—eg, patients with unstable cervical spines or with poor range of motion of the temporomandibular joint or those with certain congenital or acquired upper airway anomalies—direct laryngoscopy with a rigid laryngoscope may be undesirable or impossible. A flexible FOB allows indirect visualization of the larynx in such cases or for any situation in which awake intubation is planned (Figure 5–14). Bronchoscopes are constructed of coated glass fibers that transmit light and images by internal reflection—ie, a light beam becomes trapped within a fiber and exits unchanged at the opposite end. The insertion tube contains two bundles of fibers, each

consisting of 10,000 to 15,000 fibers. One bundle transmits light from the light source (light source bundle), which is either external to the device or contained within the handle (Figure 5–14B), whereas the other provides a high-resolution image (image bundle). Directional manipulation of the insertion tube is accomplished with an angulation wire. Aspiration channels allow suctioning of secretions, insufflation of oxygen, or instillation of local anesthetic. Aspiration channels can be difficult to clean, however; they provide a nidus for infection and, therefore, require careful cleaning and sterilization after use.

TECHNIQUES OF DIRECT LARYNGOSCOPY & INTUBATION

Indications for Intubation

Inserting a tube into the trachea has become a routine part of delivering a general anesthetic. Intubation is not a risk-free procedure, however, and not all patients

A Aspiration channel

B Light source

Light source bundle

Objective lens covering
image bundle

Insertion tube

Eyepiece

Figure 5–14. ***A:*** Cross section of a fiberoptic bronchoscope. ***B:*** A flexible fiberoptic bronchoscope with a fixed light source.

receiving general anesthesia require it, but a TT is often placed to protect the airway and for airway access. In general, intubation is indicated for patients who are at risk for aspiration and for those undergoing surgical procedures involving body cavities or the head and neck. Mask ventilation or ventilation with an LMA is usually satisfactory for short minor procedures such as cystoscopy, examination under anesthesia, inguinal hernia repairs, etc.

Preparation for Rigid Laryngoscopy

Preparation for intubation includes checking equipment and properly positioning the patient. The TT should be examined. The tube's cuff inflation system can be tested by inflating the cuff using a 10-mL syringe. Maintenance of cuff pressure *after detaching the syringe* ensures proper cuff and valve function. Some anesthesiologists cut the TT to a preset length to decrease the risk of bronchial intubation or occlusion from tube kinking (Table 5–5). The connector should be pushed into the tube as far as possible to decrease the likelihood of disconnection. If a stylet is used, it should be inserted into the TT, which is then bent to resemble a hockey stick (Figure 5–15). This shape facilitates intubation of an anteriorly positioned larynx. The desired blade is locked onto the laryngoscope handle, and bulb

function is tested. The light intensity should remain constant even if the bulb is jiggled. A blinking light signals a poor electrical contact, whereas fading indicates depleted batteries. An extra handle, blade, TT (one size smaller), and stylet should be immediately available. A functioning suction unit is needed to clear the airway in case of unexpected secretions, blood, or emesis.

Successful intubation often depends on correct patient positioning. The patient's head should be level with the anesthesiologist's waist or higher to prevent unnecessary back strain during laryngoscopy.

Stylet

Figure 5–15. A tracheal tube with a stylet bent to resemble a hockey stick.

Figure 5–16. The sniffing position and intubation with a Macintosh blade. (Modified and reproduced, with permission, from Dorsch JA, Dorsch SE: *Understanding Anesthesia Equipment: Construction, Care, and Complications.* Williams & Wilkins, 1991.)

Rigid laryngoscopy displaces pharyngeal soft tissues to create a direct line of vision from the mouth to the glottic opening. Moderate head elevation (5–10 cm above the surgical table) and extension of the atlantooccipital joint place the patient in the desired sniffing position (Figure 5–16). The lower portion of the cervical spine is flexed by resting the head on a pillow.

Preparation for induction and intubation also involves routine preoxygenation. Preoxygenation with several (four at total lung capacity) deep breaths of 100% oxygen provides an extra margin of safety in case the patient is not easily ventilated after induction. Preoxygenation can be omitted in patients who object to the face mask, who are free of pulmonary disease, and who do not have a difficult airway.

After inducing general anesthesia, the anesthesiologist becomes the patient's guardian. Because general anesthesia abolishes the protective corneal reflex, care must be taken during this period not to injure the patient's eyes by unintentionally abrading the cornea.

Thus, the eyes are routinely taped shut, often after applying a petroleum-based ophthalmic ointment.

Orotracheal Intubation

The laryngoscope is held in the left hand. With the patient's mouth opened widely, the blade is introduced into the right side of the oropharynx—with care to avoid the teeth. The tongue is swept to the left and up into the floor of the pharynx by the blade's flange. The tip of a curved blade is usually inserted into the vallecula, and the straight blade tip covers the epiglottis. With either blade, the handle is raised up and away from the patient in a plane perpendicular to the patient's mandible to expose the vocal cords (Figure 5–17). Trapping a lip between the teeth and the blade and leverage on the teeth are avoided. The TT is taken with the right hand, and its tip is passed through the abducted vocal cords. The TT cuff should lie in the upper trachea but beyond the larynx. The laryngoscope is withdrawn, again with care to

C. Philip Larson, Jr.,
MD, CM

AIRWAY MANAGEMENT

The American Society of Anesthesiologists (ASA) developed practice guidelines and an algorithm to assist anesthesiologists when faced with managing a difficult airway.[1,2] Although initially useful, the algorithm in my opinion no longer provides an effective roadmap for dealing with difficult airways for several reasons. (1) It is too complex to remember when facing an unexpectedly difficult intubation. (2) It lacks a critical distinction between a difficult intubation and a difficult ventilation (which are quite disparate). (3) It lacks specificity as to what to do next. (4) It lacks any consideration of timing, and timing is very important when facing what might be an emergency. (5) Lastly and most importantly, the algorithm cannot be practiced in its entirety on a regular basis to maintain knowledge and skill in its application.

As an alternative to the ASA algorithm, I have developed a technique that is safer, more effective, and more reliable than the algorithm. The method involves the use of four plans: Plans A, B, C, and D, which go in sequence.

Plan A: Standard laryngoscopy using the blade of choice. Experienced anesthesiologists should recognize during the first intubation attempt situations in which conventional laryngoscopy and intubation

of the trachea are not possible. A second attempt with a different blade is reasonable, but no more than two attempts should be made. Every subsequent attempt increases the risk of oral bleeding, excess secretions, inadequate anesthesia, and conversion of a can ventilate–cannot intubate to a cannot ventilate–cannot intubate situation.

Plan B: Direct laryngoscopy and insertion of a Cook (Frova) intubating catheter into the glottic opening. The Cook intubating catheter is 70 cm long; it has external distance markings every 5 cm from its tip to 40 cm, a removable stylet to maintain its curvature, a rounded distal portion with two holes, and two snap-on adaptors for attaching it to an anesthetic circuit, a gas sampling line, or a syringe. The stylet is 61 cm leaving 9 cm of the catheter flexible, which makes it safe to insert blindly without worry about tissue perforation. The Cook catheter is superior to the gum elastic bougie (ie, Eschmann) because of its length, ability to maintain its curvature, ability to insufflate oxygen, and ability to adapt it to a gas-sampling monitor.

During direct laryngoscopy, it is necessary to be able to see the epiglottis but not necessarily the glottic opening to insert the Cook catheter safely. The catheter is inserted just below the epiglottis in its midline, and the hand is dropped somewhat so that the catheter will follow the contour of the epiglottis into the glottic opening. Because the catheter tip is small (5 mm o.d.), round, and flexible, it would be extremely difficult to perforate soft tissue during blind advancement. Once the catheter is inserted, there are three ways to confirm its location in the trachea. First, an assistant who places a hand over the anterior neck can usually feel the catheter advancing through the glottis and into the trachea. Second, once the catheter reaches the carina, which is usually about 40 cm in an adult, it will not advance further; if it is in the esophagus, it will advance easily until the proximal end of the catheter is at the mouth. Third, attaching the gas monitoring sampling line to the syringe connector results in measurable carbon dioxide when the upper chest is gently

avoid tooth damage. The cuff is inflated with the least amount of air necessary to create a seal during positive-pressure ventilation to minimize the pressure transmitted to the tracheal

mucosa. Feeling the pilot balloon is *not* a reliable method of determining adequacy of cuff pressure.

After intubation, the chest and epigastrium are immediately auscultated and a capnographic tracing is compressed. Once it is established that the Cook catheter is in the larynx, a tracheal tube ranging from 5 to 8 mm can be advanced over the Cook catheter into the larynx. It is best to rotate the tracheal tube counterclockwise as it is being advanced; a distinct bump can usually be felt as the tube passes by the vocal cords. The Cook catheter will resolve most difficult intubations, and should be a readily available item of equipment.

Plan C: Insertion of a laryngeal mask airway (LMA) and attachment to the anesthetic machine. Mechanical ventilation is instituted to optimize oxygenation and carbon dioxide removal. The anesthesiologist should also call for help, and when it arrives ask for a fiberoptic bronchoscope, a 5.5- or 6.0-mm uncuffed tracheal tube, and a medium sized airway exchange catheter (one that will accept a 5.0- to 8.0-mm tracheal tube). When the equipment arrives, the 5.5- or 6.0-mm tube is inserted onto the fiberoptic bronchoscope after making certain that the tracheal tube connector is firmly on. The fiberoptic scope is then inserted into the trachea using the LMA as a guide. The tracheal tube is lubricated and gently advanced along the fiberoptic scope into the trachea. It may be necessary to rotate the tube > 90° to advance it into the trachea. The scope is then removed and the anesthetic circuit attached to the 5.5- to 6.0-mm tube. Ventilation is easy, but a high gas flow must be used to overcome the leak between the LMA and the tube. This leak can be minimized either by placing the fingers of one hand on the soft tissue between the mandible and the thyroid cartilage and pressing firmly inward or by closing the nose and mouth with one hand.

Once ventilation, oxygenation, and depth of anesthesia are adequate, the medium sized airway exchange catheter is lubricated and inserted through the 5.5- to 6.0-mm tube into the trachea. The airway exchange catheter usually meets some resistance at the tip of the tube, which is usually at the 30 cm mark on the catheter. It may be necessary to rotate the tube > 90° while pushing on the airway exchange catheter to advance the catheter beyond the 30 cm mark. This is because the catheter abuts against the anterior wall of the trachea unless the tube is rotated to change the angle of insertion of

the catheter. Once the airway exchange catheter is in position, the tube and LMA are removed en bloc, leaving only the catheter in the trachea. The final tracheal tube is then inserted over the airway exchange catheter and advanced in a counterclockwise fashion into the trachea.

Plan C should not be used only when Plan B has failed; it is also a suitable solution for establishing tracheal intubation when awake fiberoptic intubation is unsuccessful because of the inability to achieve adequate topical anesthesia. Should Plan C fail, and it has not in many hundreds of attempts, both in emergency and elective circumstances, proceed to Plan D.

Plan D: This plan has two options. The first is to cancel the operation, terminate the anesthetic, and awaken the patient. The operation would be scheduled for another day, and awake fiberoptic intubation performed. The second would be to have the surgeon perform a surgical airway (ie, tracheostomy). I have not had to resort to Plan D because of failure of Plans A–C, but it is prudent to have this alternative.

The advantage of this algorithm is that it provides a clear and decisive sequence of plans when the anesthesiologist encounters an unexpected difficult intubation in an anesthetized patient. The plans are simple to remember, effective in that they accomplish the goal of tracheal intubation, and safe because nothing of consequence is performed blindly and the patient's lungs can be ventilated and oxygenated at two intervals when resorting to Plan C. Finally, and most importantly, Plans A–C can be practiced in the anesthetized patient who is not a difficult intubation, so that when a difficult intubation is encountered, the anesthesiologist is experienced and able to perform the tasks quickly and easily.

1. Practice guidelines for management of the difficult airway: a report by the American Society of Anesthesiologists Task Force on Management of the Difficult Airway. Anesthesiology 1993;78:597.

2. Practice guidelines for management of the difficult airway: an updated report by the American Society of Anesthesiologists Task Force on Management of the Difficult Airway. Anesthesiology 2003;98:1269.

monitored to ensure intratracheal location (Figure 5–18). If there is doubt about whether the tube is in the esophagus or trachea, it is prudent to remove the tube and ventilate the patient with a mask. Otherwise, the

tube is taped or tied to secure its position. Although the persistent detection of CO_2 by a capnograph is the best confirmation of tracheal placement of a TT, it cannot exclude bronchial intubation.

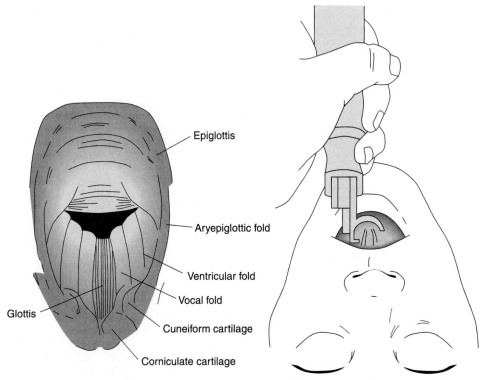

Epiglottis

Aryepiglottic fold

Ventricular fold

Vocal fold

Glottis

Cuneiform cartilage

Corniculate cartilage

Figure 5–17. Typical view of the glottis during laryngoscopy with a curved blade. (Modified and reproduced, with permission, from Barash PG: *Clinical Anesthesia,* 4th ed. Lippincott, 2001.)

The earliest manifestation of bronchial intubation is an increase in peak inspiratory pressure. Proper tube location can be reconfirmed by palpating the cuff in the sternal notch while compressing the pilot balloon with the other hand. The cuff should not be felt above the level of the cricoid cartilage, because a prolonged intralaryngeal location may result in postoperative hoarseness and increases the risk of accidental extubation. Tube position can be documented by chest radiography, but this is rarely required, except in an intensive care unit.

The description presented here assumes an unconscious patient. Oral intubation is usually poorly tolerated by patients who are awake. If necessary, in the latter case, intravenous sedation, application of a local anesthetic spray in the oropharynx, regional nerve block, and constant reassurance will improve patient acceptance.

A failed intubation should not be followed by repeated attempts that are merely more of the same. Changes must be made to increase the likelihood of success, such as repositioning the patient, decreasing the tube size, adding a stylet, selecting a different blade, attempting a nasal route, or requesting the assistance of another anesthesiologist. If the patient is also difficult to

ventilate with a mask, alternative forms of airway management (eg, LMA, Combitube, cricothyrotomy with jet ventilation, tracheostomy) must be immediately pursued. The guidelines developed by the American Society of Anesthesiologists for the management of a difficult airway include a treatment-plan algorithm (Figure 5–19).

Nasotracheal Intubation

Nasal intubation is similar to oral intubation except that the TT is advanced through the nose and nasopharynx into the oropharynx before laryngoscopy. The nostril through which the patient breathes most easily is selected in advance and prepared. Phenylephrine nose drops (0.5% or 0.25%) vasoconstrict vessels and shrink mucous membranes. However, excessive administration of nasal phenylephrine reliably leads to hypertension, tachycardia, etc. If the patient is awake, local anesthetic drops and nerve blocks can also be utilized (see the Case Discussion in this chapter).

A TT lubricated with water-soluble jelly is introduced along the floor of the nose, below the inferior turbinate, *at an angle perpendicular to the face.* The tube's bevel should be directed laterally away from the turbinates. To

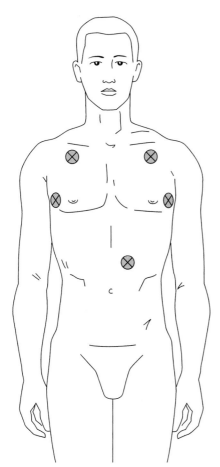

Figure 5–18. Sites for auscultation of breath sounds at the apices and over the stomach.

ensure that the tube passes along the floor of the nasal cavity, the proximal end of the TT should be pulled cephalad. The tube is gradually advanced until its tip can be visualized in the oropharynx. Laryngoscopy, as discussed, reveals the abducted vocal cords. Often the distal end of the TT can be advanced into the trachea without difficulty. If difficulty is encountered, passage of the tip of the tube through the vocal cords may be facilitated by manipulation with Magill forceps, being careful not to damage the cuff. Nasal passage of TTs, airways, or nasogastric catheters is dangerous in patients with severe midfacial trauma because of the risk of intracranial placement (Figure 5–20).

Flexible Fiberoptic Nasal Intubation

Both nostrils are prepared with vasoconstrictive drops. The nostril through which the patient breathes more easily is identified. Oxygen can be insufflated through the suction port and down the aspiration channel of the FOB to improve oxygenation and blow secretions away from the tip.

Alternatively, a large nasal airway (eg, 36F) can be inserted in the contralateral nostril. The breathing circuit can be directly connected to the end of this nasal airway to administer 100% oxygen during laryngoscopy. If the patient is unconscious and not breathing spontaneously, the mouth can be taped and ventilation attempted through the single nasal airway. When this technique is used, adequacy of ventilation and oxygenation should be confirmed by capnography and pulse oximetry. A TT is lubricated and inserted into the other nostril the length of a nasal airway. The lubricated shaft of the FOB is introduced into the TT lumen. During endoscopy, it is important to advance the scope into a *lumen*—do not advance it if only the wall of the TT or mucous membrane is seen. It is also important to keep the shaft of the bronchoscope relatively straight (Figure 5–21) so that if the head of the bronchoscope is rotated in one direction, the distal end will move to a similar degree and in the same direction. As the tip of the FOB passes through the distal end of the TT, the epiglottis or glottis should be visible. The tip of the bronchoscope is manipulated as needed to pass the abducted cords.

There is no need to hurry because an awake patient should be able to ventilate adequately and in an anesthetized patient, if either ventilation or oxygenation becomes inadequate, the FOB is withdrawn to ventilate the patient with a mask. Having an assistant thrust the jaw forward or apply cricoid pressure may improve visualization in difficult cases. If the patient is breathing spontaneously, pulling the tongue forward with a clamp may also facilitate intubation.

Once in the trachea, the FOB is advanced to within sight of the carina. The presence of tracheal rings and the carina is proof of proper positioning. The TT is pushed off the FOB. The acute angle around the arytenoid cartilage and epiglottis may prevent easy advancement of the tube. Use of an armored tube usually decreases this problem due to its greater lateral flexibility and more obtusely angled distal end. Proper TT position is confirmed by viewing the tip of the tube above the carina before the FOB is withdrawn.

TECHNIQUES OF EXTUBATION

Judging when to remove a TT is part of the art of anesthesiology that develops with experience. It is an extremely important part of the practice as more complications arise during extubation and immediately afterward than with intubation. In general, extubation is best performed when a patient is either deeply anesthetized or awake. In either case, adequate recovery

Difficult Airway Algorithm

1. Assess the likelihood and clinical impact of basic management problems.
    A. Difficult ventilation
    B. Difficult intubation
    C. Difficulty with patient cooperation or consent
    D. Difficult tracheostomy
2. Actively pursue opportunities to deliver supplemental oxygen throughout the process of difficult airway management.
3. Consider the relative merits and feasibility of basic management choices:

4. Develop primary and alternative strategies.

Figure 5–19. Difficult Airway Algorithm developed by the American Society of Anesthesiologists. *Confirm tracheal intubation or LMA placement with exhaled CO_2. (Reproduced, with permission, from the American Society of Anesthesiologists Task Force on Management of the Difficult Airway. Practice guidelines for management of the difficult airway: an updated report by the American Society of Anesthesiologists Task Force on Management of the Difficult Airway. Anesthesiology 2003;98:1269.)

Figure 5–20. Radiograph demonstrating a 7.0-mm tracheal tube placed through the cribriform plate into the cranial vault in a patient with a basilar skull fracture.

from neuromuscular blocking agents should be established prior to extubation. If blocking agents were used, the patient had controlled mechanical ventilation and therefore must be weaned from the ventilator before extubation can occur.

Extubation during a light plane of anesthesia (ie, a state between deep and awake) is avoided because of the increased risk of laryngospasm. The distinction between deep and light anesthesia is usually apparent during pharyngeal suctioning: any reaction to suctioning (eg, breath holding, coughing) signals a light plane of anesthesia, whereas no reaction is characteristic of a deep plane. Similarly, eye opening or purposeful movements imply that the patient is awake.

Extubating an awake patient is usually associated with coughing (bucking) on the TT. This reaction increases the heart rate, central venous pressure, arterial blood pressure, intracranial pressure, and intraocular pressure. It may also cause wound dehiscence and bleeding. The presence of a TT in an awake asthmatic patient often triggers bronchospasm. Although these consequences may be decreased by pretreatment with 1.5 mg/kg of intravenous lidocaine 1–2 min before suctioning and extubation, extubation during deep anesthesia may be preferable in patients who cannot tolerate

these effects. On the other hand, such extubation would be contraindicated in a patient at risk for aspiration or whose airway may be difficult to control after removal of the TT.

Regardless of whether the tube is removed when the patient is deeply anesthetized or awake, the patient's pharynx should be thoroughly suctioned before extubation to decrease the risk of aspiration or laryngospasm. In addition, patients should be ventilated with 100% oxygen in case it becomes difficult to establish an airway after the TT is removed. Just prior to extubation, the TT is untaped or untied and its cuff is deflated. Applying a small degree of positive airway pressure on an anesthesia bag connected to the TT may help blow secretions that have collected cephalad to the cuff up out of the airway into the pharynx, where they can then be suctioned. Whether the tube is removed when the patient is at end expiration or end inspiration is probably not very important. The tube is withdrawn in a single, smooth motion, and a face mask is usu-

Figure 5–21. Correct technique for manipulating a fiberoptic bronchoscope through a tracheal tube is shown in the top panel; avoid curvature in the bronchoscope, which makes manipulation difficult.

ally applied to deliver 100% oxygen until the patient is stable enough for transportation to the recovery room. In some institutions, oxygen delivery by face mask is maintained during the period of transportation.

COMPLICATIONS OF LARYNGOSCOPY & INTUBATION

The complications of laryngoscopy and intubation include hypoxia, hypercarbia, dental and airway trauma, tube malpositioning, physiological responses to airway instrumentation, or tube malfunction. These complications can occur during laryngoscopy and intubation, while the tube is in place, or following extubation (Table 5–6).

Airway Trauma

Instrumentation with a metal laryngoscope blade and insertion of a stiff TT often traumatize delicate airway tissues. Although tooth damage is the most common cause of malpractice claims against anesthesiologists, laryngoscopy and intubation can lead to a range of complications from sore throat to tracheal stenosis. Most of these are due to prolonged external pressure on sensitive airway structures. When these pressures exceed the capillary–arteriolar blood pressure (approximately 30 mm Hg), tissue ischemia can lead to a sequence of inflammation, ulceration, granulation, and stenosis. Inflation of a TT cuff to the minimum pressure that creates a seal during routine positive-pressure ventilation (usually at least 20 mm Hg) reduces tracheal blood flow by 75% at the cuff site. Further cuff inflation or induced hypotension can totally eliminate mucosal blood flow.

Postintubation croup caused by glottic, laryngeal, or tracheal edema is particularly serious in children. The efficacy of corticosteroids (eg, dexamethasone—0.2 mg/kg, up to a maximum of 12 mg) in preventing postextubation airway edema remains controversial; however, they have been demonstrated to be efficacious in children with croup from other causes. Vocal cord paralysis from cuff compression or other trauma to the recurrent laryngeal nerve results in hoarseness and increases the risk of aspiration. Some of these complications may be decreased by using a TT shaped to conform to the anatomy of the airway (eg, Lindholm Anatomical Tracheal Tube). The incidence of postoperative hoarseness appears to increase with obesity, difficult intubations, and anesthetics of long duration. Applying a water-soluble lubricant or an anesthetic-containing gel to the tip or cuff of the TT does not decrease the incidence of postoperative sore throat or hoarseness.

Table 5–6. Complications of intubation.

During laryngoscopy and intubation
  Malpositioning
    Esophageal intubation
    Bronchial intubation
    Laryngeal cuff position
  Airway trauma
    Dental damage
    Lip, tongue, or mucosal laceration
    Sore throat
    Dislocated mandible
    Retropharyngeal dissection
  Physiological reflexes
    Hypoxia, hypercarbia
    Hypertension, tachycardia
    Intracranial hypertension
    Intraocular hypertension
    Laryngospasm
  Tube malfunction
    Cuff perforation
While the tube is in place
  Malpositioning
    Unintentional extubation
    Bronchial intubation
    Laryngeal cuff position
  Airway trauma
    Mucosal inflammation and ulceration
    Excoriation of nose
  Tube malfunction
    Fire/explosion
    Obstruction
Following extubation
  Airway trauma
    Edema and stenosis (glottic, subglottic, or tracheal)
    Hoarseness (vocal cord granuloma or paralysis)
    Laryngeal malfunction and aspiration
  Laryngospasm
  Negative-pressure pulmonary edema

Smaller tubes (size 6.5 in women and size 7.0 in men) are associated with fewer complaints of postoperative sore throat. Repeated attempts at laryngoscopy during a difficult intubation may lead to periglottic edema and the inability to ventilate with a face mask, thus turning a bad situation into a life-threatening one (Figure 5–21).

Errors of Tracheal Tube Positioning

Unintentional esophageal intubation can produce catastrophic results. Prevention of this complication depends on direct visualization of the tip of the TT passing through the vocal cords, careful auscultation for the presence of bilateral breath sounds and the absence of gastric gurgling while ventilating through the TT, analysis of exhaled gas for the presence of CO_2 (the most reliable method), chest radiography, or use of an FOB.

Even though it is confirmed that the tube is in the trachea, it may not be correctly positioned. Overinsertion usually results in intubation of the right main stem bronchus because of its less acute angle with the trachea. Clues to the diagnosis of bronchial intubation include unilateral breath sounds, unexpected hypoxia with pulse oximetry (unreliable with high inspired oxygen concentrations), inability to palpate the TT cuff in the sternal notch during cuff inflation, and decreased breathing-bag compliance (high peak inspiratory pressures).

In contrast, inadequate insertion depth will position the cuff in the larynx, predisposing the patient to laryngeal trauma. Inadequate depth can be detected by palpating the cuff over the thyroid cartilage.

Because no one technique protects against all possibilities for misplacing a TT, minimal testing should include chest auscultation, routine capnography, and occasionally cuff palpation.

If the patient is repositioned, tube placement must be reconfirmed. Neck extension or lateral rotation moves a TT away from the carina, whereas neck flexion moves the tube toward the carina.

Physiological Responses to Airway Instrumentation

Laryngoscopy and tracheal intubation violate the patient's protective airway reflexes and predictably lead to hypertension and tachycardia. The insertion of an LMA is associated with less hemodynamic change. These hemodynamic changes can be attenuated by intravenous administration of drugs—lidocaine (1.5 mg/kg) 1–2 min, remifentanil (1.0 μg/kg) 1 min, alfentanil (10–20 μg/kg) 2–3 min, or fentanyl (0.5–1.0 μg/kg) 4–5 min before laryngoscopy. Hypotensive agents, including sodium nitroprusside, nitroglycerin, hydralazine, β-blockers, and calcium channel blockers, have also been shown to effectively attenuate the transient hypertensive response associated with laryngoscopy and intubation. Cardiac dysrhythmias—particularly ventricular bigeminy—are not uncommon during intubation and usually indicate light anesthesia.

Laryngospasm is a forceful involuntary spasm of the laryngeal musculature caused by sensory stimulation of the superior laryngeal nerve. Triggering stimuli include pharyngeal secretions or passing a TT through the larynx during extubation. Laryngospasm is usually prevented by extubating patients either deeply asleep or fully awake, but it can occur—albeit rarely—in an awake patient. Treatment of laryngospasm includes providing gentle positive-pressure ventilation with an anesthesia bag and mask using 100% oxygen or administering intravenous lidocaine (1–1.5 mg/kg). If laryngospasm persists and hypoxia develops, succinylcholine (0.25–1 mg/kg [usually the lower dose range]) should be given to relax the laryngeal muscles and allow controlled ventilation. The large negative intrathoracic pressures generated by a struggling patient during laryngospasm can result in the development of negative-pressure pulmonary edema even in healthy young adults.

Whereas laryngospasm represents an abnormally sensitive reflex, aspiration can result from depression of laryngeal reflexes following prolonged intubation and general anesthesia.

Bronchospasm is another reflex response to intubation and is most common in asthmatic patients. Bronchospasm can sometimes be a clue to bronchial intubation. Other pathophysiological effects of intubation include increased intracranial and intraocular pressures.

Tracheal Tube Malfunction

TTs do not always function as intended. The risk of polyvinyl chloride tube ignition in an O_2/N_2O-enriched environment was mentioned in Chapter 2. Valve or cuff damage is not unusual and should be excluded prior to insertion. TT obstruction can result from kinking, from foreign body aspiration, or from thick or inspissated secretions in the lumen.

CASE DISCUSSION:
EVALUATION & MANAGEMENT
OF A DIFFICULT AIRWAY

A 17-year-old girl presents for emergency drainage of a submandibular abscess.

What are some important anesthetic considerations during the preoperative evaluation of a patient with an abnormal airway?

Induction of general anesthesia followed by direct laryngoscopy and oral intubation is dangerous, if not impossible, in several situations (Table 5–7). To determine the optimal intubation technique, the anesthesiologist must elicit an airway history and carefully examine the patient's head and neck. Any available prior anesthesia records should be reviewed for previous problems

Table 5–7. Conditions associated with difficult intubations.

Tumors
    Cystic hygroma
    Hemangioma
    Hematoma[1]
Infections
    Submandibular abscess
    Peritonsillar abscess
    Epiglottitis
Congenital anomalies
    Pierre Robin syndrome
    Treacher Collins syndrome
    Laryngeal atresia
    Goldenhar syndrome
    Craniofacial dysostosis
Foreign body
Trauma
    Laryngeal fracture
    Mandibular or maxillary fracture
    Inhalation burn
    Cervical spine injury
Obesity
Inadequate neck extension
    Rheumatoid arthritis[2]
    Ankylosing spondylitis
    Halo traction
Anatomic variations
    Micrognathia
    Prognathism
    Large tongue
    Arched palate
    Short neck
    Prominent upper incisors

[1]Can occur postoperatively in patients who have had any neck surgery.
[2]Also affects arytenoids making them immobile.

in airway management. If a facial deformity is severe enough to preclude a good mask seal, positive-pressure ventilation may be impossible. Furthermore, patients with hypopharyngeal disease are more dependent on awake muscle tone to maintain airway patency. These two groups of patients should not be allowed to become apneic for any reason—including induction of anesthesia, sedation, or muscle paralysis—until their airway is secured.

If there is an abnormal limitation of the temporomandibular joint that may not improve with muscle paralysis, a nasal approach with an FOB should be considered. Infection confined to the floor of the mouth usually does not preclude nasal intubation. If the hypopharynx is involved to the level of the hyoid bone, however, any translaryngeal attempt will be difficult. Other clues to a potentially difficult laryngoscopy include limited neck extension (< 35°), a distance between the tip of the patient's mandible and hyoid bone of less than 7 cm, a sternomental distance of less than 12.5 cm with the head fully extended and the mouth closed, and a poorly visualized uvula during voluntary tongue protrusion (Figure 5–22). It must be stressed that because no examination technique is foolproof and the signs of a difficult airway may be subtle, the anesthesiologist must always be prepared for unanticipated difficulties.

The anesthesiologist should also evaluate the patient for signs of airway obstruction (eg, chest retraction, stridor) and hypoxia (agitation, restlessness, anxiety, lethargy). Aspiration pneumonia is more likely if the patient has recently eaten or if pus is draining from an abscess into the mouth. In either case, techniques that ablate laryngeal reflexes (eg, topical anesthesia) should be avoided.

Cervical trauma or disease is a factor that should be evaluated prior to direct laryngoscopy. Cervical arthritis or previous cervical fusion may make it difficult for the head to be put in the sniffing position; these patients are candidates for bronchoscopy to secure the airway as discussed previously. Trauma patients with unstable necks or whose neck has not yet been "cleared" are also candidates for bronchoscopy for tracheal intubation. Alternatively, if direct laryngoscopy is preferred and these individuals are skilled in airway management, one can hold the head and neck in a fixed position and the other two can ventilate and intubate the patient (Figure 5–23).

In the case under discussion, physical examination reveals extensive facial edema that limits the mandible's range of motion. Mask fit does not appear to be impaired, however. Lateral radiographs of the head and neck suggest that the infection has spread over the larynx. Frank pus is observed in the mouth.

Which intubation technique is indicated?

Routine oral and nasal intubations have been described for anesthetized patients. Both of these can also be performed in awake patients. Whether the patient is awake or asleep or

Figure 5–22. A: Mallampati classification of oral opening. *B:* Grading of the laryngeal view. A difficult orotracheal intubation (grade III or IV) may be predicted by the inability to visualize certain pharyngeal structures (class III or IV) during the preoperative examination of a seated patient. (Reproduced, with permission, from Mallampati SR: Clinical signs to predict difficult tracheal intubation [hypothesis]. Can Anaesth Soc J 1983;30:316.)

whether intubation is to be oral or nasal, it can be performed with rigid laryngoscopy, fiberoptic visualization, or a "blind" technique. Thus, there are at least 12 methods of translaryngeal intu-

bation (eg, awake/nasal/fiberoptic) possible with a TT. Alternative techniques using an LMA, a trachlite or retrograde approach, or Combitube are available, and tracheostomy or crico-

Figure 5–23. Technique for airway management of a patient with suspected spinal cord injury. One individual holds the head firmly with the patient on a backboard, the cervical collar left alone if in place, ensuring that neither the head nor neck moves with direct laryngoscopy. A second person applies cricoid pressure and the third performs direct laryngoscopy and intubation.

Figure 5–24. A tracheal tube is bent to exaggerate its curvature so that it will pass anteriorly into the larynx during a blind nasal intubation.

thyrotomy can be a lifesaving method of airway preservation.

Intubation may be difficult in this patient; however, there is pus draining into the mouth, and positive-pressure ventilation may be impossible. Induction of anesthesia should, therefore, be delayed until after the airway has been secured. The submandibular location of the abscess supports the choice of a nasal approach and probably excludes rigid laryngoscopy. Therefore, the alternatives are awake/nasal/fiberoptic intubation and awake/nasal/blind intubation. The final decision depends on the availability of an FOB and personnel experienced in its use.

Regardless of which alternative is chosen, an emergency tracheotomy may be necessary. Therefore, an experienced team including a surgeon should be in the operating room, all necessary equipment should be available and unwrapped, and the neck should be prepped and draped.

What premedication would be appropriate for this patient?

Any loss of consciousness or interference with airway reflexes could result in airway obstruction or aspiration. Glycopyrrolate would be a good choice of premedication because it minimizes upper airway secretions without crossing the blood–brain barrier (see Chapter 11). Parenteral sedatives should be very carefully titrated or omitted entirely. Psychological preparation of the patient, including explaining each step planned in securing the airway, may improve patient cooperation. Management of patients at risk for aspiration is the subject of the case discussion presented in Chapter 15.

Describe a "blind" nasotracheal intubation.

A TT is lubricated with lidocaine jelly and deformed for a few minutes to exaggerate its curvature (Figure 5–24). The patient's head should be placed in the sniffing position. After preparation of the nares, the tip of the TT is gently introduced into the naris at a plane perpendicular to the face. Air movement through the tube should be continually felt, heard, or monitored by capnography. The tube is incrementally advanced during inspiration. If the patient's respirations continue but no airflow is detected through the tube, the tip has passed the glottis and is in the esophagus. In that case, the tube must be withdrawn and advanced again. Breathholding and coughing signal close proximity to the larynx; tube advancement should continue with each inspiration.

If the tube does not easily enter the trachea, several maneuvers may enhance success. Extension of the head will also tend to guide the tube more anteriorly, whereas head rotation will move the tip laterally. Laryngeal or cricoid pressure may beneficially change the relationship between the tip and the glottis. Inflation of the TT cuff in the hypopharynx may also force the tip anteriorly. If the tube persistently slips into the esophagus, voluntary tongue protrusion will inhibit swallowing and may move the tongue and the tube anteriorly.

After intubation is confirmed, intravenous induction may proceed. At the end of the procedure, the patient should be totally awake, with protective airway reflexes intact, before extubation is attempted. Necessary equipment and personnel should be available for unexpected reintubation.

What nerve blocks could be helpful during an awake intubation?

The lingual and some pharyngeal branches of the glossopharyngeal nerve that provide sensation to the posterior third of the tongue and oropharynx are easily blocked by bilateral injection of 2 mL of local anesthetic into the base of the palatoglos-

Figure 5–25. Nerve block. While the tongue is laterally retracted with a tongue blade, the base of the palatoglossal arch is infiltrated with local anesthetic to block the lingual and pharyngeal branches of the glossopharyngeal nerve. Note that the lingual branches of the glossopharyngeal nerve are not the same as the lingual nerve, which is a branch of the trigeminal nerve.

sal arch (also known as the anterior tonsillar pillar) with a 25-gauge spinal needle (Figure 5–25).

Bilateral **superior laryngeal nerve blocks** and a transtracheal block would anesthetize the airway below the epiglottis (Figure 5–26). The hyoid bone is located, and 3 mL of 2% lidocaine is infiltrated 1 cm below each greater cornu where the internal branch of the superior laryngeal nerves penetrates the thyrohyoid membrane.

A transtracheal block is performed by identifying and penetrating the cricothyroid membrane while the neck is extended. After confirmation of an intratracheal position by aspiration of air, 4 mL of 4% lidocaine is injected into the trachea at end expiration. A deep inhalation and cough immediately following injection distribute the anesthetic throughout the trachea. Although these blocks may allow the awake patient to tolerate intubation better, they also obtund protective cough reflexes, depress the swallowing reflex, and may lead to aspiration. Topical anesthesia of the pharynx may induce a transient obstruction from the loss of reflex regulation of airway caliber at the level of the glottis.

Because of this patient's increased risk for aspiration, local anesthesia might best be limited to the nasal passages. Four percent cocaine has no advantages compared with a mixture of 4% lidocaine and 0.25% phenylephrine and can cause cardiovascular side effects. The maximum safe dose of local anesthetic should be calculated—and not exceeded (see Chapter 14). Local anesthetic is applied to the nasal mucosa with cotton-tipped applicators until a nasal airway that has been lubricated with lidocaine jelly can be placed into the naris with minimal discomfort.

Why is it necessary to be prepared for emergency tracheotomy?

Laryngospasm is always a possible complication of intubation in the nonparalyzed patient even if the patient remains awake. Laryngospasm may make positive-pressure ventilation with a mask impossible. If succinylcholine is administered to break the spasm, the consequent relaxation of pharyngeal muscles may lead to upper airway obstruction and continued inability to ventilate. In this situation, an emergency tracheotomy may be lifesaving.

What are some alternative techniques that might be successful?

Other possible strategies include the retrograde passage of a long guidewire or epidural catheter through a needle inserted across the cricothyroid membrane. The catheter is guided cephalad into the pharynx and out through the nose or mouth. A TT is passed over the catheter, which is withdrawn after the tube has entered the larynx. Variations of this technique include passing the retrograde wire through the suction

Figure 5–26. Superior laryngeal nerve block and transtracheal block.

Table 5–8. Suggested contents of the portable storage unit for difficult airway management.[1,2]

- Rigid laryngoscope blades of alternate design and size from those routinely used.
- Tracheal tubes of assorted size.
- Tracheal tube guides. Examples include (but are not limited to) semirigid stylets with or without a hollow core for jet ventilation, light wands, and forceps designed to manipulate the distal portion of the tracheal tube.
- Fiberoptic intubation equipment.
- Retrograde intubation equipment.
- At least one device suitable for emergency nonsurgical airway ventilation. Examples include (but are not limited to) a transtracheal jet ventilator, a hollow jet ventilation stylet, the laryngeal mask, and a Combitube.
- Equipment suitable for emergency surgical airway access (eg, cricothyrotomy).
- An exhaled CO_2 detector.

---

[1]Modified and used, with permission, from the American Society of Anesthesiologists: Practice guidelines for management of the difficult airway: A report by the American Society of Anesthesiologists Task Force on Management of the Difficult Airway. Anesthesiology 1993; 78:597.

[2]The items listed in this table are suggestions. The contents of the portable storage unit should be customized to meet the specific needs, preferences, and skills of the practitioner and healthcare facility.

port of a flexible FOB or the lumen of a reintubation stylet that has been preloaded with a TT. These thicker shafts help the TT negotiate the bend into the larynx more easily. Obviously, a vast array of specialized airway equipment exists and must be readily available for management of difficult airways (Table 5–8). Another possibility is cricothyrotomy, which is described in Chapter 47. Either of these techniques would have been difficult in the patient described in this case because of the swelling and anatomic distortion of the neck that can accompany a submandibular abscess.

SUGGESTED READING

Adams AP, Hewitt PB, Grande CM (editors): *Emergency Anaesthesia,* 2nd ed. Oxford University Press, 1998.

Dorsch JA, Dorsch SE: *Understanding Anesthesia Equipment,* 4th ed. Williams & Wilkins, 1999. Endotracheal tubes, laryngoscopes, face masks, and airways are described.

Hurford WE: Orotracheal intubation outside the operating room: anatomic considerations and techniques. Respir Care 1999;44:615.

Jaeger JM, Durbin CG Jr: Special purpose endotracheal tubes. Respir Care 1999;44:661.

Kim ES, Bishop MJ: Endotracheal intubation, but not laryngeal mask airway insertion, produces reversible bronchoconstriction. Anesthesiology 1999;90:391.

Langeron O, Masso E, Huraux C, et al: Prediction of difficult mask ventilation. Anesthesiology 2000;92:1217. Prospective study of more than 1500 patients. Five factors that predict difficult mask ventilation are identified: > 55 years of age, BMI > 26 kg/m², a beard, lack of teeth, and a history of snoring.

Ovassapian A (editor): *Fiberoptic Airway Endoscopy and the Difficult Airway.* Lippincott-Raven Press, 1996. Extensively illustrated.

Rosenblatt WH: Airway management. In: *Clinical Anesthesia,* 4th ed. Barash PG, Cullen BF, Stoelting RK (editors). Lippincott, Williams & Wilkins, 2001. An excellent, more in depth review of airway management issues.

Shelly MP, Nightingale P: ABC of intensive care. Respiratory support. BMJ 1999;318:1674.

Stauffer JL: Complications of endotracheal intubation and tracheostomy. Respir Care 1999;44:828.

Stix MS, O'Connor CJ Jr: Depth of insertion of the ProSeal laryngeal mask airway. Br J Anaesth 2003;90:235. As LMA variants appear, it is important to understand the differences in their characteristics. This article summarizes a study of 274 patients; all women received a #4 and the men received a #5.

Thompson AE: Issues in airway management in infants and children. Respir Care 1999;44:650.

Watson CB: Prediction of a difficult intubation: methods for successful intubation. Respir Care 1999;44:777.

Patient Monitors

6

One of the primary responsibilities of an anesthesiologist is to act as a guardian of the anesthetized patient during surgery. In fact, "vigilance" is the motto of the American Society of Anesthesiologists (ASA). Because monitoring is helpful in maintaining effective vigilance, standards for intraoperative monitoring have been adopted by the ASA (the box on Standards for Basic Anesthetic Monitoring delineates *minimum* standards). Optimal vigilance requires an understanding of the technology of sophisticated monitoring equipment—including cost–benefit considerations. This chapter reviews the indications, contraindications, techniques and devices and associated complications, and other clinical considerations for the most important and widely used anesthetic monitors.

STANDARDS FOR BASIC ANESTHETIC MONITORING[1]

(Approved by the ASA House of Delegates on October 21, 1986 and last affirmed on October 15, 2003)

These standards apply to all anesthesia care although, in emergency circumstances, appropriate life support measures take precedence. These standards may be exceeded at any time based on the judgment of the responsible anesthesiologist. They are intended to encourage quality patient care, but observing them cannot guarantee any specific patient outcome. They are subject to revision from time to time, as warranted by the evolution of technology and practice. They apply to all general anesthetics, regional anesthetics, and monitored care. This set of standards addresses only the issue of basic anesthetic monitoring, which is one component of anesthesia care. In certain rare or unusual circumstances, (1) some of these methods of monitoring may be clinically impractical, and (2) appropriate use of the described monitoring methods may fail to detect untoward clinical developments. Brief interruptions of continual[2] monitoring may be unavoidable. *Under extenuating circumstances, the responsible anesthesiologist may waive the requirements marked with an asterisk (*); it is recommended that when this is done, it should be so stated (including the reasons) in a note in the patient's medical record.* These standards are not intended for application to the care of the obstetric patient in labor or in the conduct of pain management.

STANDARD I

Qualified anesthesia personnel shall be present in the room throughout the conduct of all general anesthetics, regional anesthetics, and monitored anesthesia care.

Objective: Because of the rapid changes in patient status during anesthesia, qualified anesthesia personnel shall be continuously present to monitor the patient and provide anesthesia care. In the event there is a direct known hazard, eg, radiation, to the anesthesia personnel that might require intermittent remote observation of the patient, some provision for monitoring the patient must be made. In the event that an emergency requires the temporary absence of the person primarily responsible for the anesthetic, the best judgment of the anesthesiologist will be exercised in comparing the emergency with the anesthetized patient's condition and in the selection of the person left responsible for the anesthetic during the temporary absence.

STANDARD II

During all anesthetics, the patient's oxygenation, ventilation, circulation, and temperature shall be continually evaluated.

OXYGENATION

Objective: To ensure adequate oxygen concentration in the inspired gas and the blood during all anesthetics.

Methods:

(1) Inspired gas: During every administration of general anesthesia using an anesthesia machine, the concentration of oxygen in the patient breathing system shall be measured by an oxygen analyzer with a low oxygen concentration limit alarm in use.*

(2) Blood oxygenation: During all anesthetics, a quantitative method of assessing oxygenation such as pulse oximetry shall be employed.* Adequate illumination and exposure of the patient are necessary to assess color.

VENTILATION

Objective: To ensure adequate ventilation of the patient during all anesthetics.

■ CARDIAC MONITORS

ARTERIAL BLOOD PRESSURE

The rhythmic contraction of the left ventricle, ejecting blood into the vascular system, results in pulsatile arterial pressures. The peak pressure generated during systolic contraction is the systolic arterial blood pressure (SBP); the trough pressure during diastolic relaxation is the diastolic arterial blood pressure (DBP). Pulse pressure is the difference between the systolic and diastolic pressures. The time-weighted average of arterial pressures during a pulse cycle is the **mean arterial pressure (MAP).** MAP can be estimated by application of the following formula:

$$MAP = \frac{(SBP) + 2\,(DBP)}{3}$$

Methods:

(1) Every patient receiving general anesthesia shall have the adequacy of ventilation continually evaluated. Qualitative clinical signs such as chest excursion, observation of the reservoir breathing bag, and auscultation of breath sounds are useful. Continual monitoring for the presence of carbon dioxide shall be performed unless invalidated by the nature of the patient, procedure, or equipment. Quantitative monitoring of the volume of expired gas is strongly encouraged.*

(2) When a tracheal tube or laryngeal mask is inserted, its correct positioning must be verified by clinical assessment and by identification of carbon dioxide in the expired gas. Continual end-tidal carbon dioxide analysis, in use from the time of tracheal tube/laryngeal mask placement, until extubation/removal or initiating transfer to a postoperative care location, shall be performed using a quantitative method such as capnography, capnometry, or mass spectroscopy.*

(3) When ventilation is controlled by a mechanical ventilator, there shall be in continuous use a device that is capable of detecting disconnection of components of the breathing system. The device must give an audible signal when its alarm threshold is exceeded.

(4) During regional anesthesia and monitored anesthesia care, the adequacy of ventilation shall be evaluated, at least, by continual observation of qualitative clinical signs.

CIRCULATION

Objective: To ensure the adequacy of the patient's circulatory function during all anesthetics.

Methods:

(1) Every patient receiving anesthesia shall have the electrocardiogram continuously displayed from the beginning of anesthesia until preparing to leave the anesthetizing location.*

(2) Every patient receiving anesthesia shall have arterial blood pressure and heart rate determined and evaluated at least every 5 min.*

(3) Every patient receiving general anesthesia shall have, in addition to the above, circulatory function continually evaluated by at least one of the following: palpation of a pulse, auscultation of heart sounds, monitoring of a tracing of intraarterial pressure, ultrasound peripheral pulse monitoring, or pulse plethysmography or oximetry.

BODY TEMPERATURE

Objective: To aid in the maintenance of appropriate body temperature during all anesthetics.

Methods: Every patient receiving anesthesia shall have temperature monitored when clinically significant changes in body temperature are intended, anticipated, or suspected.

---

[1]Reproduced with permission from the American Society of Anesthesiologists. www.asahq.org/publicationsAndServices/standards/02.pdf#2, 2004.

[2]Note that "continual" is defined as "repeated regularly and frequently in steady rapid succession," whereas "continuous" means "prolonged without any interruption at any time."

Arterial blood pressure is greatly affected by where the pressure is measured. **As a pulse moves peripherally through the arterial tree, wave reflection distorts the pressure waveform, leading to an exaggeration of systolic and pulse pressures (Figure 6–1).** For example, radial artery pressures are usually higher than aortic systolic pressure because of the former's more distal location. In contrast, radial artery systolic pressures are often lower than aortic pressures following hypothermic cardiopulmonary bypass because of a decrease in the hand's vascular resistance (Figure 6–2). Vasodilating drugs (eg, isoflurane, nitroglycerin) tend to accentuate this discrepancy. The level of the sampling site relative to the heart will affect measurement of blood pressure because of the effect of gravity (Figure 6–3). In patients with severe peripheral vascular disease there may be a significant difference in blood pressure measurements between the right and left arms. The higher value should be used in these patients.

Because noninvasive (palpation, Doppler, auscultation, oscillometry, plethysmography) and invasive (arte-

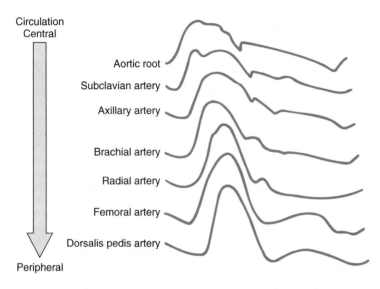

Circulation
Central

Aortic root

Subclavian artery

Axillary artery

Brachial artery

Radial artery

Femoral artery

Dorsalis pedis artery

Peripheral

Figure 6–1. Changes in configuration as a waveform moves peripherally. (Reproduced with permission from Shah N, Bedford RF: Invasive and noninvasive blood pressuring monitoring. In: *Clinical Monitoring: Practical Applications in Anesthesia and Critical Care Medicine.* Lake CL, Hines RL, Blitt CD [editors]. WB Saunders, Philadelphia, 2001, p 182.)

rial cannulation) methods of blood pressure determination differ greatly, they are discussed separately.

1. Noninvasive Arterial Blood Pressure Monitoring

Indications

The use of any anesthetic, no matter how "trivial," is an absolute indication for arterial blood pressure measurement. The techniques and frequency of pressure determination depend on the patient's condition and the type of surgical procedure. An oscillometric blood pressure measurement every 3–5 min is adequate in most cases.

Contraindications

Although some method of blood pressure measurement is mandatory, techniques that rely on a blood pressure cuff are best avoided in extremities with vascular abnormalities (eg, dialysis shunts) or with intravenous lines.

Techniques & Complications

A. PALPATION

Systolic blood pressure can be determined by (1) locating a palpable peripheral pulse, (2) inflating a blood pressure cuff proximal to the pulse until flow is occluded, (3) releasing cuff pressure by 2 or 3 mm Hg per heartbeat, and (4) measuring the cuff pressure at which pulsations are again palpable. This method tends to underestimate systolic pressure, however, because of the insensitivity of touch and the delay between flow under the cuff and distal pulsations. Palpation does not

provide a diastolic or MAP. The equipment required is simple and inexpensive.

B. DOPPLER PROBE

When a Doppler probe is substituted for the anesthesiologist's finger, arterial blood pressure measurement becomes sensitive enough to be useful in obese patients, pediatric patients, and patients in shock (Figure 6–4).

Figure 6–2. Systolic arterial pressures are higher in the radial artery than femoral artery at 15, 60, and 120 min following hypothermic cardiopulmonary bypass (CPB). This gradient increases in patients receiving nitrates and calcium channel blockers. Mean arterial pressures do not differ during the same time course. (Reproduced with permission from Maruyama K et al: Effect of combined infusion of nitroglycerin and nicardipine on femoral-to-radial arterial pressure gradient after cardiopulmonary bypass. Anesth Analg 1990;70:431.)

$$(20 \text{ cm H}_2\text{O}) \left(\frac{0.74 \text{ mm Hg}}{\text{cm H}_2\text{O}} \right) = 14.7 \text{ mm Hg}$$

Figure 6–3. The difference in blood pressure (mm Hg) at two different sites of measurement equals the height of an interposed column of water (cm H$_2$O) multiplied by a conversion factor (1 cm H$_2$O = 0.74 mm Hg).

The **Doppler effect** is the shift in the frequency of sound waves when their source moves relative to the observer. For example, the pitch of a train's whistle increases as a train approaches and decreases as it departs. Similarly, the reflection of sound waves off a moving object causes a frequency shift. A Doppler probe transmits an ultrasonic signal that is reflected by underlying tissue. As red blood cells move through an artery, a Doppler frequency shift will be detected by the probe. The difference between transmitted and received frequency causes the characteristic swishing sound, which indicates blood flow. Because air reflects ultrasound, a coupling gel (but not corrosive electrode jelly) is applied between the probe and the skin. Positioning the probe directly above an artery is crucial, since the beam must pass through the vessel wall. Interference from probe movement or electrocautery is an annoying distraction. Note that only systolic pressures can be reliably determined with the Doppler technique.

A variation of Doppler technology uses a piezoelectric crystal to detect lateral arterial wall movement to the intermittent opening and closing of vessels between systolic and diastolic pressure. This instrument thus detects both systolic and diastolic pressures.

C. AUSCULTATION

Inflation of a blood pressure cuff to a pressure between systolic and diastolic pressures will partially collapse an underlying artery, producing turbulent flow and the characteristic Korotkoff sounds. These sounds are audible through a stethoscope placed under—or just distal to—the distal third of the blood pressure cuff. The clinician measures pressure with an aneroid or mercury manometer. Because mercury is toxic in the environment, mercury sphygmomanometers are slowly being phased out of practice.

Occasionally, Korotkoff sounds cannot be heard through part of the range from systolic to diastolic pressure. This auscultatory gap is most common in hypertensive patients and can lead to an inaccurate DBP measurement. Korotkoff sounds are often difficult to auscultate

Aneroid gauge

Brachial artery

Radial artery

Doppler probe

Doppler

Figure 6–4. A Doppler probe secured over the radial artery will sense red blood cell movement as long as the blood pressure cuff is below systolic pressure. (Courtesy of Parks Medical Electronics.)

sures. Motion artifact and electrocautery interference limit the usefulness of this method.

D. OSCILLOMETRY

Arterial pulsations cause oscillations in cuff pressure. These oscillations are small if the cuff is inflated above systolic pressure. When the cuff pressure decreases to systolic pressure, the pulsations are transmitted to the entire cuff and the oscillations markedly increase. Maximal oscillation occurs at the MAP, after which oscillations decrease. Because some oscillations are present above and below arterial blood pressure, a mercury or aneroid manometer provides a gross and unreliable measurement. Automated blood pressure monitors electronically measure the pressures at which the oscillation amplitudes change (Figure 6–5). A microprocessor derives systolic, mean, and diastolic pressures using an algorithm. Machines that require identical consecutive pulse waves for measurement confirmation may be unreliable during arrhythmias (eg, atrial fibrillation). Oscillometric monitors should not be used on patients on cardiopulmonary bypass. Nonetheless, the speed, accuracy, and versatility of oscillometric devices have greatly improved, and they have become the preferred noninvasive blood pressure monitors in the United States and worldwide.

E. ARTERIAL TONOMETRY

Arterial tonometry measures beat-to-beat arterial blood pressure by sensing the pressure required to partially

during episodes of hypotension or marked peripheral vasoconstriction. In these situations, the subsonic frequencies associated with the sounds can be detected by a microphone and amplified to indicate systolic and diastolic pres-

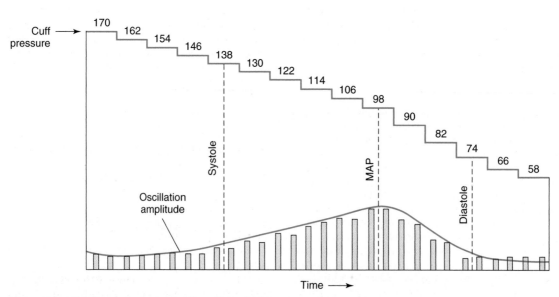

Figure 6–5. Oscillometric determination of blood pressure.

Figure 6–6. Tonometry is a method of continuous (beat-to-beat) arterial blood pressure determination. The sensors must be positioned directly over the artery.

flatten a superficial artery that is supported by a bony structure (eg, radial artery). A tonometer consisting of several independent pressure transducers is applied to the skin overlying the artery (Figure 6–6). The contact stress between the transducer directly over the artery and the skin reflects intraluminal pressure. Continuous pulse recordings produce a tracing very similar to an invasive arterial blood pressure waveform. Limitations to this technology include sensitivity to movement artifact and the need for frequent calibration.

Clinical Considerations

Adequate oxygen delivery to vital organs must be maintained during anesthesia. Unfortunately, instruments to monitor specific organ perfusion and oxygenation are complex, expensive, and often unreliable, and for that reason arterial blood pressure is assumed to reflect organ blood flow. Flow also depends on vascular resistance, however:

$$Flow = \frac{Pressure}{Resistance}$$

Even if the pressure is high, if the resistance is also high, flow can be low. Thus, arterial blood pressure should be viewed as an indicator—but not a measure—of organ perfusion.

The accuracy of any method of blood pressure measurement that involves a blood pressure cuff depends on proper cuff size (Figure 6–7). The cuff's bladder should extend at least halfway around the extremity, and the width of the cuff should be 20–50% greater than the diameter of the extremity (Figure 6–8).

Automated blood pressure monitors, using one or a combination of the methods described above, are frequently used in anesthesiology. A self-contained air pump inflates the cuff at set intervals. Incorrect or too frequent use of these automated devices has resulted in nerve palsies and extensive extravasation of intravenously administered fluids, however. In case of equipment failure, an alternative method of blood pressure determination must be immediately available.

2. Invasive Arterial Blood Pressure Monitoring

See the box on Statement on Invasive Monitoring Procedures for ASA guidelines on the use of invasive monitoring techniques.

Indications

Indications for invasive arterial blood pressure monitoring by catheterization of an artery include induced hypotension, anticipation of wide blood pressure swings, end-organ disease necessitating precise beat-to-beat blood pressure regulation, and the need for multiple arterial blood gas analyses.

Contraindications

If possible, catheterization should be avoided in arteries without documented collateral blood flow or in extremities where there is a suspicion of preexisting vascular insufficiency (eg, Raynaud's phenomenon).

Techniques & Complications

A. SELECTION OF ARTERY FOR CANNULATION

Several arteries are available for percutaneous catheterization.

1. The **radial artery** is commonly cannulated because of its superficial location and collateral flow.

STATEMENT ON INVASIVE MONITORING PROCEDURES[1]

(Approved by the House of Delegates on October 15, 2000)

A number of patients undergoing anesthesia for various surgical procedures require a more precise and sophisticated level of cardiovascular monitoring than can be obtained from standard, noninvasive techniques. Placement of an arterial catheter, central venous catheter, and/or flow-directed pulmonary artery catheter may be required to obtain additional and more precise information necessary for safe and effective anesthesia and life support in the perioperative period.

Although it is the position of the American Society of Anesthesiologists (ASA) that the interpretation of the data obtained from these "invasive" monitoring devices is accounted for in the usual anesthesia fee, their placement is not. As ASA has developed and refined its Relative Value Guide, placement of invasive monitoring devices has not been factored into basic unit values. In fact, the basic unit values for many anesthesia codes in which invasive monitoring is now common were established prior to the use of invasive devices and have not been changed. Furthermore, inclusion of additional basic units to account for invasive monitoring in some an-

esthesia codes and not in others would make the relative value system inconsistent.

The need to consider placement of invasive hemodynamic monitors as a separate service is also indicated because not all patients undergoing the same surgical procedure require the same degree of monitoring. The necessity for invasive monitoring is driven more by patient condition than by surgical procedure. For example, although most patients undergoing intestinal surgery do not require invasive monitoring, some do because of underlying cardiovascular disease or anticipated large fluid and blood loss during surgery. Similarly, most patients having carotid endarterectomy require an arterial catheter, but some who are more healthy than average do not.

USE OF INVASIVE MONITORING TECHNIQUES

(1) **Arterial Catheter (CPT code 36620).** Placement of a small catheter, usually in the radial artery, and connection of the catheter to electronic equipment allows for continuous monitoring of a patient's blood pressure. Unstable patients undergoing surgery as a result of trauma or for

Five percent of patients, however, have incomplete palmar arches and lack adequate collateral blood flow. Allen's test is a simple, but not very reliable, method for determining the adequacy of ulnar collateral circulation. In this test, the patient exsanguinates his or her hand by making a fist. While the operator occludes the radial and ulnar arteries with fingertip pressure, the patient relaxes the blanched hand. Collateral flow through the palmar arterial arch is confirmed by flushing of the thumb within 5 s after pressure on the ulnar artery is released. Delayed return of normal color (5–10 s) indicates an equivocal test or insufficient collateral circulation (>10 s). Alternatively, blood flow distal to the radial artery occlusion can be detected by palpation, Doppler probe, plethysmography, or pulse oximetry. Unlike Allen's test, these methods of determining the adequacy of collateral circulation do not require patient cooperation.

2. **Ulnar artery** catheterization is more difficult because of the artery's deeper and more tortuous course. Because of the risk of compromising blood flow to the

hand, this would not normally be considered if the ipsilateral radial artery has been punctured but unsuccessfully cannulated.

3. The **brachial artery** is large and easily identifiable in the antecubital fossa. Its proximity to the aorta provides less waveform distortion. However, being near the elbow predisposes brachial artery catheters to kinking.

4. The **femoral artery** is prone to pseudoaneurysm and formation of atheroma but often provides an excellent access. The femoral site has been associated with an increased incidence of infectious complications and arterial thrombosis. Aseptic necrosis of the head of the femur is a rare but tragic complication of femoral artery cannulation in children.

5. The **dorsalis pedis and posterior tibial arteries** are at some distance from the aorta and therefore have the most distorted waveforms. Modified Allen's tests can be performed to document adequate collateral flow around these arteries.

6. The **axillary artery** is surrounded by the axillary plexus, and nerve damage can result from a hematoma

intraabdominal pathology frequently need this form of monitoring. Patients having cardiac, vascular, chest, spine, and brain surgery are subject to rapid changes in blood pressure. Continuous monitoring greatly helps the anesthesiologist manage these patients safely. Arterial catheters also provide a reliable method for obtaining arterial blood samples frequently, thus facilitating proper management of blood gas, blood chemistry, and coagulation abnormalities.

(2) Central Venous Catheter (36489 [also 36488, 36490, 36491]) for Pressure Monitoring, Volume Replacement, or Central Drug Infusion. Placing a catheter and monitoring the pressure in a major vein returning blood to the heart allow the anesthesiologist to properly maintain and/or adjust a patient's circulating blood volume. The technique is appropriately used for patients who experience significant blood or fluid loss during surgery and have normal underlying cardiac function. Additional indications for placement of a central venous catheter are to secure a reliable means for rapid administration of large volumes of fluid or blood or to allow for administration of certain medications that are most safely and effectively administered directly into the central venous circulation.

(3) Pulmonary Artery (Swan–Ganz) Catheter (93503). This multilumen catheter is placed through a major vein and directed by blood flow through the right side of the heart and into a pulmonary artery. It has the capability to monitor the function of both sides of the heart and the vasculature. It can also be used to measure the cardiac output (amount of blood being pumped by the heart per minute) as well as other important indicators of cardiovascular function. It is used for patients whose cardiac function is, or may be, compromised either prior to or during a surgical procedure. Also, certain pulmonary artery catheters allow the heart to be temporarily paced, which may be necessary in some patients with underlying cardiac rhythm disturbances.

---

[1]Reproduced with permission from the American Society of Anesthesiologists. www.asahq.org/publicationsAndServices/standards/invasivemonitoring.htm, 2000.

or traumatic cannulation. Air or thrombi can quickly gain access to the cerebral circulation during retrograde flushing of the left axillary artery.

B. TECHNIQUE OF RADIAL ARTERY CANNULATION

One technique of radial artery cannulation is illustrated in Figure 6–9. Supination and extension of the wrist provide optimal exposure of the radial artery. The pressure-tubing-transducer system should be nearby and already flushed with heparinized saline (0.5–2.0 U of heparin/mL of saline) to ensure easy and quick connection after cannulation. The radial pulse is palpated and the artery's course is determined by lightly pressing the *tips* of the index and middle fingers of the anesthesiologist's nondominant hand over the area of maximal impulse. After preparing the skin with a bactericidal agent, 0.5 mL of lidocaine is infiltrated directly above the artery with a 25- or 27-gauge needle. An 18-gauge needle can then be used as a skin punch, facilitating entry of an 18-, 20-, or 22-gauge catheter over a needle through the skin at a 45° angle, directing it toward the point of palpation. Upon blood flashback, the needle is lowered to a 30° angle and advanced another 1–2 mm

to make certain that the tip of the catheter is well into the vessel lumen. "Spinning" the catheter often aids advancement of the catheter off the needle, which is then withdrawn. Applying firm pressure over the artery, proximal to the catheter tip, with the middle and ring fingertips prevents blood from spurting from the catheter while the tubing is being firmly connected. Waterproof tape or suture can be used to hold the catheter in place.

C. COMPLICATIONS

Complications of intraarterial monitoring include hematoma, bleeding (if the transducer tubing is not tightly affixed and separates from the catheter hub), vasospasm, arterial thrombosis, embolization of air bubbles or thrombi, necrosis of skin overlying the catheter, nerve damage, infection, loss of digits, and unintentional intraarterial drug injection. Factors associated with an increased rate of complications include prolonged cannulation, hyperlipidemia, repeated insertion attempts, female gender, extracorporeal circulation, and the use of vasopressors. The risks are minimized when the ratio of catheter to artery size is small, heparinized

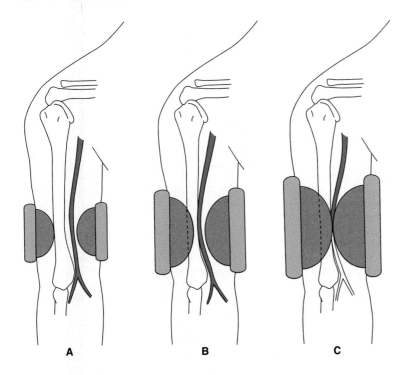

A   **B**   **C**

Figure 6–7. Blood pressure cuff width influences the pressure readings. Three cuffs, all inflated to the same pressure, are shown. The narrowest cuff (**A**) will require more pressure and the widest cuff (**C**) less pressure to occlude the brachial artery for determination of systolic pressure. Too narrow a cuff may produce a large overestimation of systolic pressure. Whereas the wider cuff may underestimate the systolic pressure, the error with a cuff 20% too wide is not as significant as the error with a cuff 20% too narrow. (Reproduced with permission from Gravenstein JS, Paulus DA: *Monitoring Practice in Clinical Anesthesia,* 2nd ed. Lippincott, Philadelphia, 1987, p 58.)

saline is continuously infused through the catheter at a rate of 2–3 mL/h, flushing of the catheter is limited, and meticulous attention is paid to aseptic technique. Adequacy of perfusion can be continually monitored during radial artery cannulation by placing a pulse oximeter on an ipsilateral finger.

Clinical Considerations

Because intraarterial cannulation allows continuous, beat-to-beat blood pressure measurement, it is considered the gold standard of blood pressure monitoring techniques. The quality of the transduced waveform, however, depends on the dynamic characteristics of the catheter-tubing-transducer system (Figure 6–10). False readings can lead to inappropriate therapeutic interventions.

A complex waveform, such as an arterial pulse wave, can be expressed as a summation of simple sine and cosine waves (Fourier analysis). For accurate measurement of pressure, the catheter-tubing-transducer system must be capable of responding adequately to the highest frequency of the arterial waveform (Figure 6–11). Stated another way, the natural frequency of the measuring system must exceed the natural frequency of the arterial pulse (approximately 16–24 Hz).

Most transducers have frequencies of several hundred Hz (> 200 Hz for disposable transducers).

The addition of tubing, stopcocks, and air in the line all decrease the frequency of the system. If the frequency response is too low, the system will be overdamped and will not faithfully reproduce the arterial waveform, underestimating the systolic pres-

100%   120–150%

Figure 6–8. The width of the blood pressure cuff should be 20–50% greater than the diameter of the patient's extremity.

Figure 6–9. Cannulation of the radial artery. **A:** Proper positioning and palpation of the artery are crucial. After skin preparation, local anesthetic is infiltrated with a 25-gauge needle. **B:** A 20- or 22-gauge catheter is advanced through the skin at a 45° angle. **C:** Flashback of blood signals entry into the artery, and the catheter-needle assembly is lowered to a 30° angle and advanced 1–2 mm to ensure an intraluminal catheter position. **D:** The catheter is advanced over the needle, which is withdrawn. **E:** Proximal pressure with middle and ring fingers prevents blood loss, while the arterial tubing Luer-lock connector is secured to the intraarterial catheter.

sure. Underdamping is also a serious problem, leading to overshoot and a falsely high SBP.

Catheter-tubing-transducer systems must also prevent **hyperresonance,** an artifact caused by reverberation of pressure waves within the system. A **damping coefficient** (β) of 0.6–0.7 is optimal. The natural fre-

quency and damping coefficient can be determined by examining tracing oscillations after a high-pressure flush (Figure 6–12).

System dynamics are improved by minimizing tubing length, eliminating unnecessary stopcocks, removing air bubbles, and using low-compliance tubing.

Figure 6–10. The catheter-tubing-transducer system.

Although smaller diameter catheters lower natural frequency, they improve underdampened systems and are less apt to result in vascular complications. If a large catheter totally occludes an artery, reflected waves can distort pressure measurements.

Pressure transducers have evolved from bulky, reusable instruments to miniaturized, disposable chips. Transducers contain a diaphragm that is distorted by an arterial pressure wave. The mechanical energy of a pressure wave is converted into an electric signal. Most transducers are resistance types that are based on the **strain gauge** principle: stretching a wire or silicone crystal changes its electrical resistance. The sensing elements are arranged as a Wheatstone bridge circuit so that the voltage output is proportionate to the pressure applied to the diaphragm (Figure 6–13).

Transducer accuracy depends on correct calibration and zeroing procedures. A stopcock at the level of the desired point of measurement—usually the midaxillary line—is opened, and the zero trigger on the monitor is activated. If the patient's position is altered by raising or lowering the operating table, the transducer must either be moved in tandem or zeroed to the new level of the midaxillary line. In a seated patient, the arterial pressure in the brain differs significantly from left ventricular pressure. In this circumstance, cerebral pressure is determined by setting the transducer to zero at the level of the ear, which approximates the circle of Willis. The transducer's zero should be checked regularly to eliminate drift.

External calibration of a transducer compares the transducer's reading with a manometer, but modern transducers rarely require external calibration.

Digital readouts of systolic and diastolic pressures are a running average of the highest and lowest mea-

Figure 6–11. An original waveform overlays a four-harmonic reconstruction (**left**) and an eight-harmonic reconstruction (**right**). Note that the higher harmonic plot more closely resembles the original waveform. (Reproduced with permission from Saidman LS, Smith WT: *Monitoring in Anesthesia.* Butterworth, 1985, p 89.)

DAMPING

Amplitude ratio $= \dfrac{D_2 \,(mm)}{D_2 \,(mm)} = \dfrac{13}{22.5} = 0.58$

Damping coefficient $\beta = \sqrt{\dfrac{\left(\ln\dfrac{D_2}{D_1}\right)^2}{\pi^2 + \left(\ln\dfrac{D_2}{D_1}\right)^2}} = 0.17$

Amplitude ratio (D_2/D_1)	Damping coefficient
.9	.034
.8	.071
.7	.113
.6	.160
.5	.215
.4	.280
.3	.358
.2	.456
.1	.591

NATURAL FREQUENCY:

Natural frequency $= fn = \dfrac{1}{2\pi}\sqrt{\dfrac{\pi D^2\, \Delta P}{4\rho\, L \Delta V}} = \dfrac{\text{Paper speed (mm/sec)}}{\text{Length of 1 cycle (mm)}}$

$= \dfrac{25 \text{ mm/sec}}{2 \text{ mm}} = 12.5 \text{ Hz}$

D = Internal diameter of tubing

ρ = Density of blood

L = Length of tubing

$\dfrac{\Delta P}{\Delta V}$ = Compliance (stiffness) of system

Figure 6–12. Damping and natural frequency of a transducer system can be determined by a high-pressure flush test.

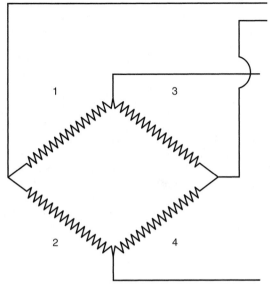

Figure 6–13. In the original strain gauge pressure transducers, a deformable diaphragm was connected to a Wheatstone bridge. When pressure was applied to the diaphragm, strain on two of the resistors (No. 2 and No. 3) increased, whereas strain on the other two (No. 1 and No. 4) decreased. The change in total resistance across the bridge was proportional to the change in blood pressure allowing direct, accurate measurement of intravascular blood pressure for the first time.

surements within a certain time interval. Because motion or cautery artifacts can result in some very misleading numbers, the arterial waveform should always be monitored. The shape of the arterial wave provides clues to several hemodynamic variables. The rate of upstroke indicates contractility, the rate of downstroke indicates peripheral vascular resistance, and exaggerated variations in size during the respiratory cycle suggest hypovolemia. MAP is calculated by integrating the area under the pressure curve.

Intraarterial catheters also provide access for intermittent arterial blood gas sampling and analysis. The development of fiberoptic sensors that can be inserted through a 20-gauge arterial catheter enables continuous blood gas monitoring. Unfortunately, these sensors are quite expensive and are often inaccurate, so they are rarely used.

ELECTROCARDIOGRAPHY

Indications & Contraindications

All patients should have intraoperative monitoring of their electrocardiogram (ECG). There are no contraindications.

Techniques & Complications

Lead selection determines the diagnostic sensitivity of the ECG. The electrical axis of lead II is approximately 60° from the right arm to the left leg, which is parallel to the electrical axis of the atria, resulting in the largest P wave voltages of any surface lead. This orientation enhances the diagnosis of arrhythmias and the detection of inferior wall ischemia. Lead V_5 lies over the fifth intercostal space at the anterior axillary line; this position is a good compromise for detecting anterior and lateral wall ischemia. A true V_5 lead is possible only on operating room ECGs with at least five lead wires, but a modified V_5 can be monitored by rearranging the standard three-limb lead placement (Figure 6–14). Ideally, because each lead provides unique information, leads II and V_5 should be monitored simultaneously. If only a single-channel machine is available, the preferred lead for monitoring depends

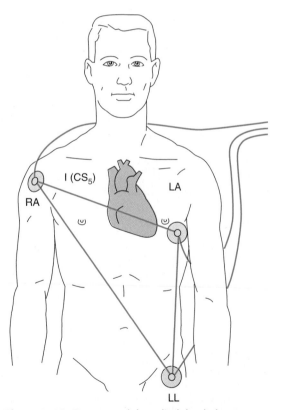

Figure 6–14. Rearranged three-limb lead placement. Anterior and lateral ischemia can be detected by placing the left arm lead (LA) at the V_5 position. When lead I is selected on the monitor, a modified V_5 lead (CS_5) is displayed. Lead II allows detection of arrhythmias and inferior wall ischemia. RA, right arm; LL, left leg.

Figure 6–15. A cross-sectional view of a silver chloride electrode.

on the location of any prior infarction or ischemia. Esophageal leads are even better than lead II for arrhythmia diagnosis but have not yet gained general acceptance in the operating room.

Electrodes are placed on the patient's body to monitor the ECG (Figure 6–15). Conductive gel lowers the skin's electrical resistance, which can be further decreased by cleansing the site with alcohol, a degreasing agent, or by mechanically exfoliating the superficial skin layer. Needle electrodes are rarely used and only if the disks are unsuitable (eg, with an extensively burned patient).

Clinical Considerations

The ECG is a recording of the electrical potentials generated by myocardial cells. Its routine use allows arrhythmias, myocardial ischemia, conduction abnormalities, pacemaker malfunction, and electrolyte disturbances to be detected. Because of the small voltage potentials being measured, artifacts remain a major problem. Patient or lead-wire movement, use of electrocautery, 60-cycle interference, and faulty electrodes can simulate arrhythmias. Monitoring filters incorporated into the amplifier may lessen artifacts, but can lead to distortion of the ST segment and impede the diagnosis of ischemia. Digital readout of heart rate may be misleading because of monitor misinterpretation of artifacts or large T waves—often seen in pediatric patients—as QRS complexes.

Depending on equipment availability, a preinduction rhythm strip can be printed or frozen on the monitor's screen to compare with intraoperative tracings. To interpret ST-segment changes properly, the ECG must be standardized so that a 1-mV signal results in a deflection of 10 mm on a standard strip monitor. Newer units continuously analyze ST segments for early detection of myocardial ischemia. Automated ST-segment analysis increases the sensitivity of ischemia detection, does not require additional physician skill or vigilance, and may help diagnose intraoperative myocardial ischemia. Unfortunately, the efficacy of automated ST-segment analysis has not been documented.

Commonly accepted criteria for diagnosing myocardial ischemia include a flat or downsloping ST-segment depression exceeding 1 mm, 60 or 80 ms after the J point (the end of the QRS complex), particularly in conjunction with T wave inversion. ST-segment elevation with peaked T waves can also represent ischemia. Wolff–Parkinson–White syndrome, bundle branch blocks, extrinsic pacemaker capture, and digoxin therapy may preclude the use of ST-segment information. The audible beep associated with each QRS complex should be loud enough to detect rate and rhythm changes when the anesthesiologist's visual attention is directed elsewhere. Some ECGs are capable of storing aberrant QRS complexes for further analysis and some can even interpret and diagnose arrhythmias. The interference caused by electrocautery units, however, has limited the usefulness of automated arrhythmia analysis in the operating room.

CENTRAL VENOUS CATHETERIZATION

Indications

Central venous catheterization is indicated for monitoring central venous pressure (CVP), for administration of fluid to treat hypovolemia and shock, for infusion of caustic drugs and total parenteral nutrition, for aspiration of air emboli, for insertion of transcutaneous pacing leads, and for gaining venous access in patients with poor peripheral veins.

Contraindications

Contraindications include renal cell tumor extension into the right atrium or fungating tricuspid valve vegetations. Other contraindications relate to the cannulation site. For example, internal jugular vein cannulation is relatively contraindicated in patients who are receiving anticoagulants or who have had an ipsilateral carotid endarterectomy, because of the possibility of unintentional carotid artery puncture.

Techniques & Complications

Central venous cannulation involves introducing a catheter into a vein so that the catheter's tip lies just above or at the junction of the superior vena cava and the right atrium. Because this location exposes the catheter tip to intrathoracic pressure, inspiration will increase or decrease CVP, depending on whether ventilation is controlled or spontaneous. Measurement of CVP is made with a water column (cm H_2O) or, preferably, an electronic transducer (mm Hg). The pressure should be measured during end expiration.

Various sites can be used for cannulation. Catheterization of the subclavian vein is associated with a significant risk of pneumothorax during insertion and with

Table 6–1. Relative rating of central venous access.[1]

	Basilic	External Jugular	Internal Jugular	Subclavian	Femoral
Ease of cannulation	1	3	2	5	3
Long-term use	4	3	2	1	5
Success rate (pulmonary artery catheter placement)	4	5	1	2	3
Complications (technique-related)	1	2	4	5	3

[1]In each category, 1 = best, 5 = worst.

line-related infection the longer the catheter stays in place. The right internal jugular vein provides a combination of accessibility and safety (Table 6–1). Left-sided catheterization increases the risk of vascular erosion, pleural effusion, and chylothorax. There are at least three cannulation techniques: a catheter over a needle (similar to peripheral catheterization), a catheter through a needle (requiring a large-bore needle stick), and a catheter over a guidewire (Seldinger's technique, Figure 6–16).

The patient is placed in the Trendelenburg position to decrease the risk of air embolism and to distend the internal jugular vein. Venous catheterization requires full aseptic technique, including sterile gloves, mask, bactericidal skin preparation, and sterile drapes. The two heads of the sternocleidomastoid muscle and the clavicle form the three sides of a triangle (Figure 6–16A). A 25-gauge needle is used to infiltrate the apex of the triangle with local anesthetic. The internal jugular vein is found by advancing the 25-gauge needle—or a 23-gauge needle in heavier patients—along the medial border of the lateral head of the sternocleidomastoid, toward the ipsilateral breast nipple at an angle of 30° to the skin. Alternatively, the vein can be located with the help of an ultrasound probe. Aspiration of venous blood confirms the vein's location. The possibility of placement of the vein dilator or catheter into the carotid artery can be decreased by transducing the vessel's pressure waveform or comparing the blood's color or PaO_2 with an arterial sample. An 18-gauge thin-wall needle is advanced along the same path as the locator needle (Figure 6–16B). When free blood flow is achieved, a J-wire with a 3-mm-radius curvature is introduced (Figure 6–16C). The needle is removed, and a pliable Silastic catheter is advanced over the wire (Figure 6–16D). The guidewire is removed, with a thumb placed over the catheter hub to prevent aspiration of air until the intravenous catheter tubing is connected to it. The catheter is then secured and a sterile dressing is applied. Correct location is confirmed with a chest radiograph. The catheter's tip should not be allowed to migrate into the heart chambers. Fluid-administration sets should be changed every 72 h.

The risks of central venous cannulation include infection, air or thrombus embolism, arrhythmias (indicating that the catheter tip is in the right atrium or ventricle), hematoma, pneumothorax, hemothorax, hydrothorax, chylothorax, cardiac perforation, cardiac tamponade, trauma to nearby nerves and arteries, and thrombosis. Some of these complications can be attributed to poor technique.

Clinical Considerations

Normal cardiac function requires adequate ventricular filling by venous blood. CVP approximates right atrial pressure, which is a major determinant of right ventricular end-diastolic volume. In healthy hearts, right and left ventricular performance is parallel, so that left ventricular filling can also be judged by CVP.

The shape of the central venous waveform corresponds to the events of cardiac contraction (Figure 6–17): *a* waves from *a*trial contraction are absent in atrial fibrillation and are exaggerated in junctional rhythms (cannon waves); *c* waves are due to tricuspid valve elevation during early ventricular contraction; *v* waves reflect *v*enous return against a closed tricuspid valve; and the *x* and *y* descents are probably caused by the downward displacement of the tricuspid valve during systole and tricuspid valve opening during diastole.

PULMONARY ARTERY CATHETERIZATION

Indications

The ASA has recently updated its guidelines for pulmonary artery catheterization. Although the effectiveness of pulmonary artery catheter (PAC) moni-

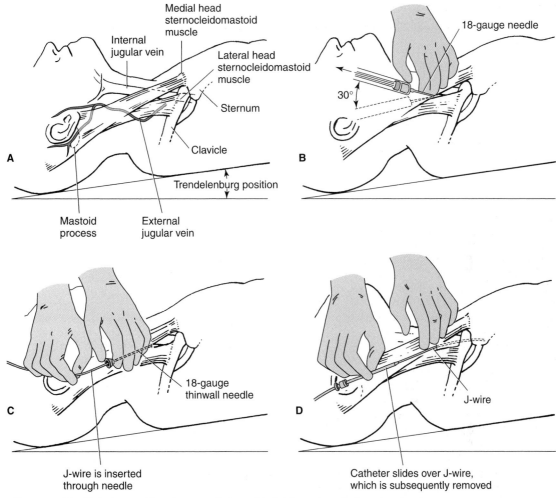

Figure 6–16. Right internal jugular cannulation with Seldinger's technique (see text).

toring remains largely unproven in many groups of surgical patients, the ASA concludes that the appropriateness of PAC use depends on the combination of risks associated with the patient, the operation, and the setting (Table 6–2).

The ASA is also a participant in the Pulmonary Artery Catheter Educational Program (PACEP: wide world http://www.pacep.org). Monitoring pulmonary artery pressure and cardiac output in critically ill patients has been shown to provide cardiovascular information that is more accurate than that obtained by clinical assessment. Basically, pulmonary artery catheterization should be considered whenever cardiac index, preload, volume status, or the degree of mixed venous blood oxygenation need to be known. These measurements might prove particularly impor-

tant in patients at high risk for hemodynamic instability (eg, recent myocardial infarction) or during surgical procedures associated with a high incidence of hemodynamic complications (eg, thoracic aortic aneurysm repair).

Contraindications

Relative contraindications to pulmonary artery catheterization include complete left bundle branch block (because of the risk of complete heart block), Wolff–Parkinson–White syndrome, and Ebstein's malformation (because of possible tachyarrhythmias). A catheter with pacing capability is better suited to these situations. A PAC may serve as a nidus of infection in bacteremic

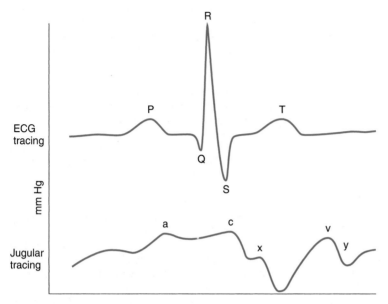

ECG tracing

mm Hg

Jugular tracing

Figure 6–17. The upward waves (*a, c, v*) and the downward descents (*x, y*) of a central venous tracing in relation to the electrocardiogram (ECG).

patients or thrombus formation in patients prone to hypercoagulation.

Techniques & Complications

Although various PACs are available, the most popular design integrates five lumens into a 7.5 FR catheter, 110 cm long, with a polyvinylchloride body (Figure 6–18). The lumens house the following: wiring to connect the thermistor near the catheter tip to a thermodilution cardiac output computer; an air channel for inflation of the balloon; a proximal port 30 cm from the tip for infusions, cardiac output injections, and measurements of right atrial pressures; a ventricular port at 20 cm for infusion of drugs; and a distal port for aspiration of mixed venous blood samples and measurements of pulmonary artery pressure.

Insertion of a PAC requires central venous access, which can be accomplished using Seldinger's technique, described above. Instead of a central venous catheter, a dilator and sheath are threaded over the guidewire. The sheath's lumen accommodates the PAC after removal of the dilator and guidewire (Figure 6–19).

Prior to insertion, the PAC is checked by inflating and deflating its balloon and irrigating all three intravascular lumens with heparinized saline. The distal port is connected to a transducer that is zeroed to the patient's midaxillary line.

The PAC is advanced through the introducer and into the internal jugular vein. At approximately 15 cm, the distal tip should enter the right atrium, and a central venous tracing that varies with respiration

confirms an intrathoracic position. The balloon is then inflated with air according to the manufacturer's recommendations (usually 1.5 mL) to protect the endocardium from the catheter tip and to

Table 6–2. Indications for pulmonary artery catheterization.

Cardiac disease
  Coronary artery disease with left ventricular dysfunction or recent infarction
  Valvular heart disease
  Heart failure (eg, cardiomyopathy, pericardial tamponade, cor pulmonale)
Pulmonary disease
  Acute respiratory failure (eg, acute respiratory distress syndrome)
  Severe chronic obstructive pulmonary disease
Complex fluid management
  Shock
  Acute renal failure
  Acute burns
  Hemorrhagic pancreatitis
Specific surgical procedures
  Pericardiectomy
  Aortic cross-clamping (eg, thoracic, aortic aneurysm repair)
  Sitting craniotomies
  Portal systemic shunts
  Liver transplants
High-risk obstetrics
  Severe toxemia
  Placental abruption

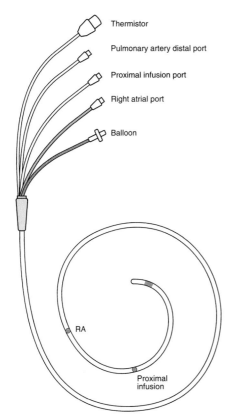

Thermistor

Pulmonary artery distal port

Proximal infusion port

Right atrial port

Balloon

RA

Proximal
infusion

Figure 6–18. Balloon-tipped pulmonary artery flotation catheter (Swan–Ganz catheter). RA, right atrium. (Reproduced with permission from Catheter Reference Manual. Baxter Healthcare Corporation, Edwards Lifesciences LLC, 1993.)

allow the right ventricle's cardiac output to direct the catheter forward. Conversely, the balloon is always deflated during withdrawal. During the catheter's advancement, the ECG should be monitored for arrhythmias. Transient ectopy from irritation of the right ventricular endocardium by the balloon and catheter tip is common but rarely requires treatment. A sudden increase in the *systolic* pressure on the distal tracing indicates a right ventricular location of the catheter tip (Figure 6–20). Entry into the pulmonary artery normally occurs by 35–45 cm and is heralded by a sudden increase in *diastolic* pressure.

To prevent catheter knotting, the balloon should be deflated and the catheter withdrawn if pressure changes do not occur at the expected distances. In particularly difficult cases (low cardiac output, pulmonary hypertension, or congenital heart anomalies), flotation of the catheter may be enhanced by having the

patient inhale deeply; by positioning the patient in a head-up, right lateral tilt position; by injecting iced saline through the proximal lumen to stiffen the catheter (which also increases the risk of perforation); or by administering a small dose of an inotropic agent to increase cardiac output.

After attaining a pulmonary artery position, minimal PAC advancement results in a pulmonary artery occlusion pressure (PAOP) waveform. The pulmonary artery tracing should reappear when the balloon is deflated. Wedging before maximal balloon inflation signals an overwedged position, and the catheter should be slightly withdrawn (with the balloon down, of course). Because **pulmonary artery rupture** carries a 50–70% mortality rate and can occur because of balloon overinflation, the frequency of wedge readings should be minimized. Pulmonary artery pressure should be continuously monitored to detect an overwedged position indicative of catheter migration. Furthermore, if the catheter has a right ventricular port 20 cm from the tip, distal migration can often be detected by a change in the pressure tracing that indicates a pulmonary artery location.

Correct catheter position can be confirmed by a lateral chest radiograph. Although most catheters migrate caudally and to the right side, occasionally a catheter will wedge anterior to the vena cava. In this position, true pulmonary capillary pressures may be less than alveolar pressures, resulting in spuriously elevated measurements during positive pressure ventilation.

The numerous complications of pulmonary artery catheterization include complications associated with central venous cannulation plus bacteremia, endocarditis, thrombogenesis, pulmonary infarction, pulmonary artery rupture, and hemorrhage (particularly in patients taking anticoagulants, elderly or female patients, or patients with pulmonary hypertension), catheter knotting, arrhythmias, conduction abnormalities, and pulmonary valvular damage (Table 6–3). Even trace hemoptysis should not be ignored, as it may herald pulmonary artery rupture. If the latter is suspected, prompt placement of a double-lumen tracheal tube may maintain adequate oxygenation by the unaffected lung. The risk of complications increases with the duration of catheterization, which usually should not exceed 72 h.

Clinical Considerations

The introduction of PACs into the operating room revolutionized the intraoperative management of critically ill patients. PACs allow more precise estimation of left ventricular preload than either CVP or physical examination. It also allows sampling of

Figure 6–19. A percutaneous introducer consisting of a vessel dilator and sheath is passed over the guidewire.

Sheath

Vessel dilator

Guidewire

mixed venous blood and detection of air embolism and myocardial ischemia. Catheters with self-contained thermistors (discussed later in this chapter) can be used to measure cardiac output, from which a multi-

tude of hemodynamic values can be derived (Table 6–4). Some catheter designs incorporate electrodes that allow intracavitary ECG recording and pacing. Optional fiberoptic bundles allow continuous mea-

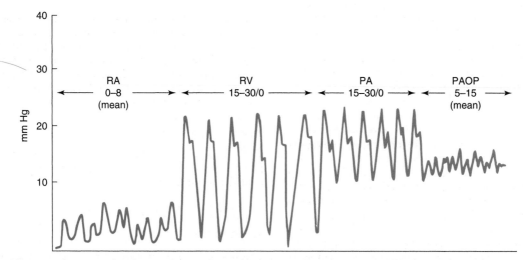

| RA | RV | PA | PAOP |
| 0–8 (mean) | 15–30/0 | 15–30/0 | 5–15 (mean) |

Figure 6–20. Normal pressure values and waveforms as a pulmonary artery catheter is advanced from the right atrium to a "wedged" position in a pulmonary artery. RA, right atrium; RV, right ventricle; PA, pulmonary artery; PAOP, pulmonary artery occlusion pressure.

Table 6–3. Reported incidence of adverse effects of pulmonary artery catheterization.[1]

Complication	Reported Incidence (%)
Central venous access	
Arterial puncture	0.1–13
Bleeding at cut-down site	5.3
Postoperative neuropathy	0.3–1.1
Pneumothorax	0.3–4.5
Air embolism	0.5
Catheterization	
Minor dysrhythmias[2]	4.7–68.9
Severe dysrhythmias (ventricular tachycardia or fibrillation)[2]	0.3–62.7
Minor increase in tricuspid regurgitation	17
Right bundle-branch block[2]	0.1–4.3
Complete heart block (in patients with prior LBBB)[2]	0–8.5
Catheter residence	
Pulmonary artery rupture[2]	0.03–1.5
Positive catheter tip cultures	1.4–34.8
Catheter-related sepsis	0.7–11.4
Thrombophlebitis	6.5
Venous thrombosis	0.5–66.7
Pulmonary infarction[2]	0.1–5.6
Mural thrombus	28–61
Valvular/endocardial vegetations or endocarditis[2]	2.2–100
Deaths[2]	0.02–1.5

[1]Reproduced with permission from Practice guidelines for pulmonary artery catheterization: An updated report by the American Society of Anesthesiologists Task Force on pulmonary artery catheterization. Anesthesiology 2003;99:999.
[2]Complications thought to be more common (or exclusively associated) with pulmonary artery catheterization than with central venous catheterization. LBBB, left bundle branch block.

surement of the oxygen saturation of mixed venous blood.

Starling demonstrated the relationship between left ventricular function and left ventricular end-diastolic muscle fiber length, which is usually proportionate to end-diastolic volume. If compliance is not abnormally decreased (eg, by myocardial ischemia, overload, ventricular hypertrophy, or pericardial tamponade), left ventricular end-diastolic pressure should reflect fiber length. In the presence of a normal mitral valve, left atrial pressure approaches left ventricular pressure during diastolic filling. The left

atrium connects with the right side of the heart through the pulmonary vasculature. The distal lumen of a correctly wedged PAC is isolated from right-sided pressures by balloon inflation. Its distal opening is exposed only to capillary pressure, which—in the absence of high airway pressures or pulmonary vascular disease—equals left atrial pressure. In fact, aspiration through the distal port during balloon inflation samples arterialized blood. These assumptions and relationships form the rationale for monitoring PAOP—ie, it is an indirect method of measuring left ventricular fiber length and, therefore, ventricular function.

Whereas central venous catheterization accurately reflects right ventricular function, a PAC is indicated if either ventricle is markedly depressed, causing disassociation of right- and left-sided hemodynamics. CVPs are not predictive of pulmonary capillary pressures in patients with ejection fractions less than 0.50. Even the PAOP does not always predict left ventricular end-diastolic pressure (Table 6–5). The relationship between left ventricular end-diastolic volume (actual preload) and PAOP (estimated preload) can become unreliable during conditions associated with changing left atrial or ventricular compliance, mitral valve function, or pulmonary vein resistance. These conditions are common immediately following major cardiac or vascular surgery and in critically ill patients who are on inotropic agents or in septic shock.

CARDIAC OUTPUT

Indications

Patients who benefit from measurements of pulmonary artery pressure also benefit from determination of cardiac output. In fact, to use the information available from PACs most effectively, cardiac output must be obtained (see Table 6–4). Perfection of noninvasive techniques may eventually lead to routine intraoperative cardiac output monitoring.

Contraindications

There are no contraindications for cardiac output measurement by thermodilution other than those for pulmonary artery catheterization.

Techniques & Complications

A. THERMODILUTION

The injection of a quantity (2.5, 5, or 10 mL) of fluid that is below body temperature (usually room temperature or iced) into the right atrium changes the temperature of blood in contact with the ther-

Table 6–4. Hemodynamic variables derived from pulmonary artery catheterization data.[1]

Variable	Formula	Normal	Units
Cardiac index	$\dfrac{\text{Cardiac output (L/min)}}{\text{Body surface area } (m^2)}$	2.2–4.2	L/min/m^2
Total peripheral resistance	$\dfrac{(\text{MAP} - \text{CVP}) \times 80}{\text{Cardiac output (L/min)}}$	1200–1500	dynes • s cm^{-5}
Pulmonary vascular resistance	$\dfrac{(\overline{\text{PA}} - \text{PAOP}) \times 80}{\text{Cardiac output (L/min)}}$	100–300	dynes • s cm^{-5}
Stroke volume	$\dfrac{\text{Cardiac output (L/min)} \times 1000}{\text{Heart rate (beats/min)}}$	60–90	mL/beat
Stroke index (SI)	$\dfrac{\text{Stroke volume (mL/beat)}}{\text{Body surface area } (m^2)}$	20–65	mL/beat/m^2
Right ventricular stroke-work index	$0.0136 (\overline{\text{PA}} - \text{CVP}) \times \text{SI}$	30–65	g-m/beat/m^2
Left ventricular stroke-work index	$0.0136 (\text{MAP} - \text{PAOP}) \times \text{SI}$	46–60	g-m/beat/m^2

[1]g-m, gram meter; MAP, mean arterial pressure; CVP, central venous pressure; $\overline{\text{PA}}$, mean pulmonary artery pressure; PAOP, pulmonary artery occlusion pressure.

mistor at the tip of the PAC. The degree of change is inversely proportionate to cardiac output: Temperature change is minimal if there is a high blood flow but pronounced if flow is low. Plotting the temperature change as a function of time produces a **thermodilution curve.** Cardiac output is determined by a computer program that integrates the area under the curve. Accurate measurements of cardiac output depend on rapid and smooth injection, precisely known injectant temperature and volume, correct entry of the calibration factors for the specific type of PAC into the cardiac output

Table 6–5. Pulmonary artery occlusion pressure (PAOP) can wrongly estimate left ventricular end-diastolic pressure (LVEDP) in certain conditions.

PAOP > LVEDP
   Mitral stenosis
   Left atrial myxoma
   Pulmonary venous obstruction
   Elevated alveolar pressure
PAOP < LVEDP
   Decreased left ventricular compliance (stiff ventricle or LVEDP > 25 mm Hg)
   Aortic insufficiency

computer, and avoidance of measurements during electrocautery. Tricuspid regurgitation and cardiac shunts invalidate results because only right ventricular output is actually being measured. Rapid infusion of the iced injectant has rarely resulted in cardiac arrhythmias.

A modification of the thermodilution technique allows continuous cardiac output measurement with a special catheter and monitor system. The catheter contains a thermal filament that introduces small pulses of heat into the blood proximal to the pulmonic valve and a thermistor that measures changes in pulmonary artery blood temperature. A computer in the monitor determines cardiac output by cross-correlating the amount of heat input with the changes in blood temperature.

B. Dye Dilution

If indocyanine green dye (or another indicator such as lithium) is injected through a central venous catheter, its appearance in the systemic arterial circulation can be measured by analyzing arterial samples with an appropriate detector, for example, a densitometer for indocyanine green. The area under the resulting **dye indicator curve** is related to cardiac output. By analyzing arterial blood pressure and integrating it with cardiac output, systems that use lithium also calculate beat-to-beat stroke volume. The dye-dilution technique, however, introduces the problems of indicator recirculation, arterial blood sampling, and background tracer buildup.

C. ULTRASONOGRAPHY

A two-dimensional image of the heart can be obtained with an ultrasound probe in the esophagus. Transesophageal echocardiography (TEE) assesses left ventricular filling (end-diastolic volume and end-systolic volume), ejection fraction, wall motion abnormalities, and contractility. Because ischemic myocardium does not exhibit normal inward movement or thickening during systole, TEE has proved to be a very sensitive indicator of intraoperative myocardial ischemia. In addition, air bubbles are easily recognized during air embolism (including paradoxic air embolism). Limitations include the need for the patient to be anesthetized before insertion (thus it is not useful during induction and intubation), difficulty distinguishing increased afterload from myocardial ischemia, and variability of interpretation. Oversized esophageal probes can cause aortic compression in infants and small children.

Pulsed Doppler is a related technology that can be used to measure the velocity of aortic blood flow. Combined with TEE, which determines the aortic cross-sectional area, this technique can measure stroke volume and cardiac output. Further applications of ultrasonography include transesophageal Doppler color-flow mapping, which evaluates valvular function and intracardiac shunting. Information on blood flow is represented by color (indicating flow direction) and intensity (indicating flow velocity). The major limitations of these systems are their relative complexity and expense.

Continuous-wave suprasternal Doppler also measures aortic blood velocity. Instead of requiring TEE, it uses a nomogram based on the patient's age, sex, and weight to estimate the aortic cross-sectional area for cardiac output calculations. Although considerably less expensive, the use of a nomogram introduces the possibility of error, particularly in patients with aortic disease.

Transtracheal Doppler consists of a Doppler transducer attached to the distal end of a tracheal tube. Cardiac output is derived from the ascending aorta diameter and blood velocity. Accurate results depend on a properly positioned probe.

D. THORACIC BIOIMPEDANCE

Changes in thoracic volume cause changes in thoracic resistance (bioimpedance). If thoracic changes in bioimpedance are measured following ventricular depolarization, stroke volume can be continuously determined.

This noninvasive technique requires four pairs of ECG electrodes to inject microcurrents and to sense bioimpedance on both sides of the chest. Disadvantages of thoracic bioimpedance include susceptibility to electrical interference and reliance upon correct electrode positioning. As with both suprasternal and transtracheal Doppler, the accuracy of this technique is questionable in several groups of patients, including those with aortic valve disease or previous heart surgery.

E. FICK PRINCIPLE

The amount of oxygen consumed by an individual ($\dot{V}O_2$) equals the difference between arterial and venous (a–v) oxygen content (C) (CaO_2 and CvO_2) multiplied by cardiac output (CO). Therefore

$$CO = \frac{\text{Oxygen consumption}}{\text{a–v } O_2 \text{ content difference}} = \frac{\dot{V}O_2}{CaO_2\text{-}CvO_2}$$

Mixed venous and arterial oxygen content are easily determined if a PAC and an arterial line are in place. Oxygen consumption can also be calculated from the difference between the oxygen content in inspired and expired gas. Variations of the Fick principle are the basis of all indicator-dilution methods of determining cardiac output.

Clinical Considerations

Cardiac output measurements allow calculation of many indices that reflect the function of the entire circulatory system. Pulmonary artery pressures are difficult to interpret without knowing cardiac output. For instance, a patient with normal blood pressure and PAOP may have poor vital organ perfusion because of a low cardiac output and a high systemic vascular resistance. Effective pharmacological manipulation of preload, afterload, and contractility depends on accurate determination of cardiac output.

■ PULMONARY MONITORS

PRECORDIAL & ESOPHAGEAL STETHOSCOPES

Indications

Many anesthesiologists believe that all anesthetized patients should be monitored with a precordial or esophageal stethoscope, though this practice is gradually changing as anesthesiologists rely on capnography and pulse oximetry to monitor pulmonary function.

Contraindications

Instrumentation of the esophagus should be avoided in patients with esophageal varices or strictures.

Techniques & Complications

A precordial stethoscope (Wenger chestpiece) is a heavy, bell-shaped piece of metal placed over the chest or suprasternal notch. Although its weight tends to maintain its position, double-sided adhesive disks provide an acoustic seal to the patient's skin. Various chestpieces are available, but the child size works well for most patients. The bell is connected to the anesthesiologist by extension tubing.

The esophageal stethoscope is a soft plastic catheter (8–24F) with balloon-covered distal openings (Figure 6–21). Although the quality of breath and heart sounds is much better than with a precordial stethoscope, its use is limited to intubated patients. Temperature probes, ECG leads, ultrasound probes, and even atrial pacemaker electrodes have been incorporated into esophageal stethoscopes. Placement through the mouth or nose can occasionally cause mucosal irritation and bleeding. Rarely, the stethoscope slides into the trachea instead of the esophagus, resulting in a gas leak around the tracheal tube cuff.

Clinical Considerations

The information provided by a precordial or esophageal stethoscope includes confirmation of ventilation, quality of breath sounds (eg, stridor, wheezing), regularity of heart rate, and quality of heart tones (muffled tones are associated with decreased cardiac output).

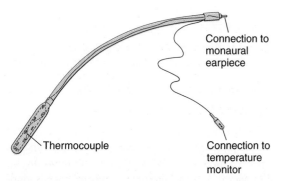

Figure 6–21. Esophageal stethoscope.

Connection to monaural earpiece

Thermocouple

Connection to temperature monitor

The confirmation of bilateral breath sounds after tracheal intubation, however, is made with a binaural stethoscope.

PULSE OXIMETRY

Indications & Contraindications

Pulse oximeters are mandatory monitors for any anesthetic including cases of moderate sedation. They are particularly useful when patient oxygenation must be measured frequently because of preexisting lung disease (eg, bleomycin toxicity), the nature of the surgical procedure (eg, hiatal hernia repair), or the requirements of a special anesthetic technique (eg, one-lung anesthesia). Pulse oximeters are also helpful in monitoring neonates at risk for the retinopathy of prematurity. There are no contraindications.

Techniques & Complications

Pulse oximeters combine the principles of oximetry and plethysmography to noninvasively measure oxygen saturation in arterial blood. A sensor containing light sources (two or three light-emitting diodes) and a light detector (a photodiode) is placed across a finger, toe, earlobe, or any other perfused tissue that can be transilluminated.

Oximetry depends on the observation that oxygenated and reduced hemoglobin differ in their absorption of red and infrared light (Lambert–Beer law). Specifically, oxyhemoglobin (HbO_2) absorbs more infrared light (960 nm), whereas deoxyhemoglobin absorbs more red light (660 nm) and thus appears blue, or cyanotic, to the naked eye. The change in light absorption during arterial pulsations is the basis of oximetric determinations (Figure 6–22). The ratio of the absorptions at the red and infrared wavelengths is analyzed by a microprocessor to provide the oxygen saturation (SpO_2) of arterial blood. Arterial pulsations are identified by plethysmography, allowing corrections for light absorption by nonpulsating venous blood and tissue. Heat from the light source or sensor pressure may, rarely, result in tissue damage if the monitor is not periodically moved. No user calibration is required.

Clinical Considerations

In addition to SpO_2, pulse oximeters provide an indication of tissue perfusion (pulse amplitude) and measure heart rate. Because SpO_2 is normally close to 100%, only gross abnormalities are detectable in most anesthetized patients. Depending on a particular patient's oxygen–hemoglobin dissociation curve, a 90% saturation may indicate a PaO_2 of less than 65 mm Hg. This compares with clinically detectable

Figure 6–22. Oxyhemoglobin and deoxyhemoglobin differ in their absorption of red and infrared light.

cyanosis, which requires 5 g of desaturated hemoglobin and usually corresponds to an SpO_2 of less than 80%. Bronchial intubation will usually go undetected by pulse oximetry in the absence of lung disease or low fraction of inspired oxygen concentrations (FIO_2).

Because carboxyhemoglobin (COHb) and HbO_2 absorb light at 660 nm identically, pulse oximeters that compare only two wavelengths of light will register a falsely high reading in patients with carbon monoxide poisoning. Methemoglobin has the same absorption coefficient at both red and infrared wavelengths. The resulting 1:1 absorption ratio corresponds to a saturation reading of 85%. **Thus, methemoglobinemia causes a falsely low saturation reading when SaO_2 is actually greater than 85% and a falsely high reading if SaO_2 is actually less than 85%.**

Most pulse oximeters are inaccurate at low SpO_2, and all demonstrate a delay between changes in SaO_2 and SpO_2. **Other causes of pulse oximetry artifact include excessive ambient light, motion, methylene blue dye, venous pulsations in a dependent limb, low perfusion (eg, low cardiac output, profound anemia, hypothermia, increased systemic vascular resistance), malpositioned sensor, and leakage of light from the light-emitting diode to the photodiode, bypassing the arterial bed (optical shunting).** Nevertheless, pulse oximetry can be an invaluable aid to the rapid diagnosis

of hypoxia, which may occur in unrecognized esophageal intubation, and it furthers the goal of monitoring oxygen delivery to vital organs. In the recovery room, pulse oximetry helps identify postoperative pulmonary problems such as severe hypoventilation, bronchospasm, and atelectasis.

Two extensions of pulse oximetry technology are mixed venous blood oxygen saturation (SvO_2) and noninvasive brain oximetry. The former requires the placement of a PAC containing fiberoptic sensors that continuously determine SvO_2 in a manner analogous to pulse oximetry. Because SvO_2 varies with changes in hemoglobin concentration, cardiac output, arterial oxygen saturation, and whole-body oxygen consumption, its interpretation is somewhat complex. A variation of this technique involves placing the fiberoptic sensor in the internal jugular vein, which provides measurements of jugular bulb oxygen saturation in an attempt to assess the adequacy of cerebral oxygen delivery.

Noninvasive brain oximetry monitors regional oxygen saturation (rSO_2) of hemoglobin in the brain. A sensor placed on the forehead emits light of specific wavelengths and measures the light reflected back to the sensor (near-infrared optical spectroscopy). Unlike pulse oximetry, brain oximetry measures venous and capillary blood oxygen saturation in addition to arterial blood saturation. Thus, its oxygen saturation readings represent the average oxygen saturation of all regional microvascular hemoglobin (approximately 70%). Cardiac arrest, cerebral embolization, deep hypothermia, or severe hypoxia causes a dramatic decrease in rSO_2.

CAPNOGRAPHY

Indications & Contraindications

Determination of end-tidal CO_2 ($ETCO_2$) concentration to confirm adequate ventilation is useful during all anesthetic procedures, but particularly so for general anesthesia. A rapid fall of $ETCO_2$ is a sensitive indicator of air embolism, a major complication of sitting craniotomies. There are no contraindications.

Techniques & Complications

Capnography is a valuable monitor of the pulmonary, cardiovascular, and anesthetic breathing systems. Both types of capnographs in common use rely on the absorption of infrared light by CO_2 (Figure 6–23).

A. NONDIVERTING (FLOWTHROUGH)

Nondiverting (mainstream) capnographs measure CO_2 passing through an adaptor placed in the breathing circuit (Figure 6–24). Infrared light transmission through the gas is measured and CO_2 concentration is determined by the monitor. Because of problems with drift,

Figure 6–23. Absorption spectrum for CO_2. (Reproduced with permission from Hill DW: Methods of analysis in the gaseous and vapour phase. In: *Scientific Foundations of Anesthesia.* Scurr C, Feldman S [editors]. Year Book, 1982, p 85.)

older flowthrough models self-zeroed during inspiration. Thus, they were incapable of detecting inspired CO_2, such as would occur with a breathing circuit malfunction (eg, absorbent exhaustion, sticking unidirectional valves). The weight of the sensor causes traction on the tracheal tube, and its generation of radiant heat can cause skin burns. Newer designs address these problems.

B. DIVERTING (ASPIRATION)

Diverting (sidestream) capnographs continuously suction gas from the breathing circuit into a sample cell within the monitor. CO_2 concentration is determined by comparing infrared light absorption in the sample cell with a chamber free of CO_2. Continuous aspiration of anesthetic gas essentially represents a leak in the breathing circuit that will contaminate the operating room unless it is scavenged or returned to the breathing system. High aspiration rates (up to 250 mL/min) and low-dead-space sampling tubing usually increase sensitivity and decrease lag time. If tidal volumes (VT) are small (eg, pediatric patients), however, a high rate of aspiration may entrain fresh gas from the circuit and dilute $ETCO_2$ measurement. Low aspiration rates (less than 50 mL/min) can retard $ETCO_2$ measurement and underestimate it during rapid ventilation. New units autocalibrate, but older units must be zeroed to room air and against a known CO_2 concentration (usually 5%). Diverting units are prone to water precipitation in the aspiration tube and sampling cell that can cause obstruction of the sampling line and erroneous readings. Expiratory valve malfunction is detected by the presence of CO_2 in inspired gas. Although inspiratory valve failure also results in rebreathing CO_2, this is not as readily apparent because part of the inspiratory volume will still be free of CO_2, causing the monitor to read zero during part of the inspiratory phase.

Clinical Considerations

Other gases (eg, nitrous oxide) also absorb infrared light, leading to a pressure-broadening effect. To minimize the error introduced by nitrous oxide, various modifications and filters have been incorporated into monitor design. Capnographs rapidly and reliably indicate esophageal intubation—a common cause of anesthetic catastrophe—but do not reliably detect bronchial intubation. Although there may be some CO_2 in the stomach from swallowing expired air, this should be washed out within a few breaths. Sudden cessation of CO_2 during the expiratory

Figure 6–24. A nondiverting sensor placed in-line analyzes CO_2 concentration at the sampling site.

End-tidal CO_2 monitor

Infrared transducer

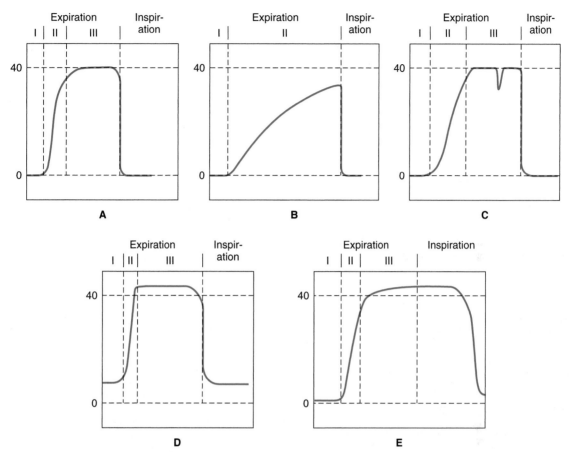

Figure 6–25. *A:* A normal capnograph demonstrating the three phases of expiration: phase I—dead space; phase II—mixture of dead space and alveolar gas; phase III—alveolar gas plateau. *B:* Capnograph of a patient with severe chronic obstructive pulmonary disease. No plateau is reached before the next inspiration. The gradient between end-tidal CO_2 and arterial CO_2 is increased. *C:* Depression during phase III indicates spontaneous respiratory effort. *D:* Failure of the inspired CO_2 to return to zero may represent an incompetent expiratory valve or exhausted CO_2 absorbent. *E:* The persistence of exhaled gas during part of the inspiratory cycle signals the presence of an incompetent inspiratory valve.

phase may indicate a circuit disconnection. The increased metabolic rate caused by malignant hyperthermia causes a marked rise in $ETCO_2$.

The gradient between $PaCO_2$ and $ETCO_2$ (normally 2–5 mm Hg) reflects alveolar dead space (alveoli that are ventilated but not perfused). Any significant reduction in lung perfusion (eg, air embolism, decreased cardiac output, or decreased blood pressure) increases alveolar dead space, dilutes expired CO_2, and lessens $ETCO_2$. True capnographs (as opposed to capnometers) display a waveform of CO_2 concentration that allows recognition of a variety of conditions (Figure 6–25).

ANESTHETIC GAS ANALYSIS

Indications

Analysis of anesthetic gases is useful during any procedure requiring inhalation anesthesia. There are no contraindications to analyzing these gases.

Techniques

Techniques for analyzing multiple anesthetic gases involve mass spectrometry, Raman spectroscopy, infrared spectrophotometry, or piezoelectric crystal (quartz) oscillation. Mass spectrometry and Raman spectroscopy are primarily of historical interest as most anesthetic gases are now measured by infrared absorption analysis.

Infrared units use a variety of techniques similar to that described for capnography. Variations of infrared absorption include acoustic sensing, near-infrared optical sensing, and far-infrared optical sensing. These devices are all based on the Beer–Lambert law, which provides a formula for measuring an unknown gas within inspired gas because the absorption of infrared light passing through a solvent (inspired or expired gas) is proportional to the amount of the unknown gas. Nonpolar gases such as oxygen and nitrogen do not absorb infrared light. There are a number of commercially available devices that use a single- or dual-beam infrared light source and positive or negative filtering. Because oxygen molecules do not absorb infrared light, their concentration cannot be measured with monitors that rely on infrared technology and, hence, it must be measured by other means (see below).

Clinical Considerations

A. Piezoelectric Analysis

The piezoelectric method uses oscillating quartz crystals, one of which is covered with lipid. Volatile anesthetics dissolve in the lipid layer and change the frequency of oscillation, which, when compared to the frequency of oscillation of an uncovered crystal, allows the concentration of the volatile anesthetic to be calculated. Neither these devices nor infrared photoacoustic analysis allow different anesthetic agents to be distinguished. New dual-beam infrared optical analyzers do allow gases to be separated and an improperly filled vaporizer to be detected.

B. Oxygen Analysis

To measure the FIO_2 of inhaled gas, manufacturers of anesthesia machines have relied on two technologies.

C. Galvanic Cell

Galvanic cell (fuel cell) contains a lead anode and gold cathode bathed in potassium chloride. At the gold terminal, hydroxyl ions are formed that react with the lead electrode (thereby gradually consuming it) to produce lead oxide, causing current, which is proportional to the amount of oxygen being measured, to flow. Because the lead electrode is consumed, monitor life can be prolonged by exposing it to room air when not in use. These are the oxygen monitors used on many anesthesia machines in the inspiratory limb.

D. Paramagnetic Analysis

Oxygen is a nonpolar gas, but it is paramagnetic and when placed in a magnetic field, the gas will expand, contracting when the magnet is turned off. By switching the field on and off and comparing the resulting change in volume (or pressure or flow) to a known standard, the amount of oxygen can be measured.

E. Polarographic Electrode

A polarographic electrode has a gold (or platinum) cathode and a silver anode, both based in an electrolyte, separated from the gas to be measured by a semipermeable membrane. Unlike the galvanic cell, a polarographic electrode works only if a small voltage is applied to two electrodes. The amount of current that flows is proportional to the amount of oxygen present.

F. Spirometry

Newer anesthesia machines can measure (and therefore manage) airway pressures, volume, and flow, to calculate resistance and compliance, and to display the relationship of these variables as flow–volume or pressure–volume loops. Measurements of flow and volume are made by mechanical devices that are usually fairly lightweight and are often placed in the inspiratory limb of the anesthesia circuit.

The most fundamental measurements include low peak inspiratory pressure and high peak inspiratory pressure, which indicate either a ventilator or circuit disconnect, or an airway obstruction, respectively. By measuring V_T and breathing frequency (f), exhaled minute ventilation (V_E) can be calculated, providing some sense of security that ventilation requirements are being met.

Spirometric loops and waveforms are characteristically altered by certain disease processes and events. If a normal loop is observed shortly after induction of anesthesia and a subsequent loop is different, the observant anesthesiologist is alerted to the fact that something has occurred. Spirometric loops are usually displayed as flow versus volume and volume versus pressure. (Figure 6–26). There are characteristic changes with obstruction, bronchial intubation, reactive airways disease, etc.

■ NEUROLOGICAL SYSTEM MONITORS

ELECTROENCEPHALOGRAPHY

Indications & Contraindications

The electroencephalogram (EEG) is occasionally used during cerebrovascular surgery to confirm the adequacy of cerebral oxygenation. Monitoring the depth of anesthesia with a full 16-lead, 8-channel EEG is not warranted, considering the availability of simpler techniques. There are no contraindications.

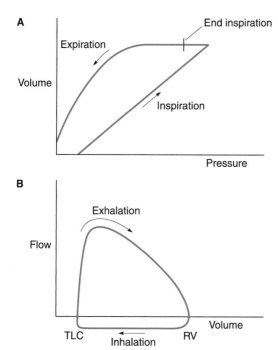

A: Normal volume–pressure loop. **B:** Normal flow–volume loop.

Figure 6–26. **A:** Normal volume–pressure loop. **B:** Normal flow–volume loop.

Techniques & Complications

The EEG is a recording of electrical potentials generated by cells in the cerebral cortex. Although standard ECG electrodes can be used, silver disks containing a conductive gel are preferred. Platinum or stainless steel needle electrodes traumatize the scalp and have high impedance (resistance); however, they can be sterilized and placed in a surgical field. Electrode position (montage) is governed by the international 10–20 system (Figure 6–27). Electric potential differences between combinations of electrodes are filtered, amplified, and displayed by an oscilloscope or pen recorder.

New two-channeled processed EEG devices pass the EEG signal through a fast Fourier transform (bispectral analysis) leading to a traditional power spectrum. The Bispectral Index (BIS) represents a numerical value that has been correlated with the patient's current hypnotic state (see below).

Clinical Considerations

Acceptance of intraoperative EEG monitoring has been limited by requirements of space, difficulty of interpretation, equivocal efficacy, and the need to avoid high concentrations of anesthetic agents. Its accuracy has proved questionable in patients who have sustained prior brain damage

(eg, stroke). The EEG changes that accompany ischemia, such as high-frequency activity, can be mimicked by hypothermia, anesthetic agents, electrolyte disturbances, and marked hypocapnia. Detection of changes in the EEG in an anesthetized patient should lead to an immediate review of possible causes of cerebral ischemia before irreversible brain damage occurs.

To perform a bispectral analysis, data measured by EEG are taken through a number of steps (Figure 6–28) to calculate a single number that correlates with depth of anesthesia/hypnosis.

BIS values of 65–85 have been advocated as a measure of sedation, whereas values of 40–65 have been recommended for general anesthesia (Figure 6–29). Bispectral analysis may reduce patient awareness during anesthesia, an issue that is important to the public. It may also reduce resource utilization because less drug is required to ensure amnesia, facilitating a faster wake-up time and perhaps a shorter stay in the recovery room.

Many of the initial studies of its use were not prospective, randomized, controlled trials, but were primarily observational in nature. Artifacts can be a problem. The monitor, in and of itself, costs several thousand dollars and the electrodes are approximately $10 to $15 per anesthetic and cannot be reused.

Some cases with awareness have been identified as having a BIS less than 65. However, in other cases of awareness, either there were problems with the recordings or

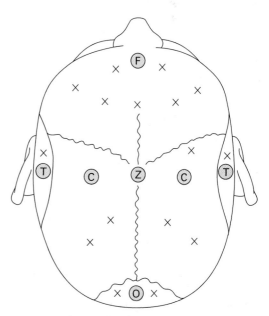

Figure 6–27. International 10–20 system. Montage letters refer to cranial location. F, frontal; C, coronal; T, temporal; O, occipital; Z, middle.

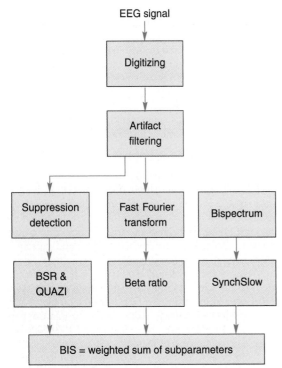

EEG signal

Digitizing

Artifact filtering

Suppression detection | Fast Fourier transform | Bispectrum

BSR & QUAZI | Beta ratio | SynchSlow

BIS = weighted sum of subparameters

Figure 6–28. Calculation of the Bispectral Index. EEG, electroencephalogram; BSR, burst suppression ratio; BIS, Bispectral Index Scale. (Reproduced with permission from Rampil IJ: A primer for EEG signal processing in anesthesia. Anesthesiology 1998;89:980.)

awareness could not be related to any specific time or BIS value. Whether this monitoring technique becomes a standard of care in the future remains to be seen.

EVOKED POTENTIALS

Indications

Indications for intraoperative monitoring of **evoked potentials** (EPs) include surgical procedures associated with possible neurological injury: spinal fusion with instrumentation, spine and spinal cord tumor resection, brachial plexus repair, thoracoabdominal aortic aneurysm repair, epilepsy surgery, and cerebral tumor resection. Ischemia in the spinal cord or cerebral cortex can be detected by EPs. EP monitoring facilitates probe localization during stereotactic neurosurgery.

Contraindications

Although there are no specific contraindications for somatosensory-evoked potentials (SEPs), this modality

is severely limited by the availability of monitoring sites, equipment, and trained personnel. Sensitivity to anesthetic agents can also be a limiting factor, particularly in children. Motor-evoked potentials (MEPs) are contraindicated in patients with retained intracranial metal, with a skull defect, after seizures, and after any major cerebral insult.

Techniques & Complications

EP monitoring noninvasively assesses neural function by measuring electrophysiological responses to sensory or motor pathway stimulation. Commonly monitored EPs are brain stem auditory evoked responses (BAERs), SEPs, and increasingly MEPs (Table 6–6).

For SEPs, a brief electrical current is delivered to a sensory or mixed peripheral nerve by a pair of elec-

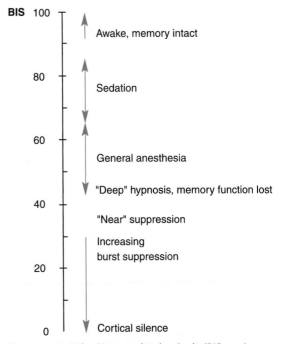

Figure 6–29. The Bispectral Index Scale (BIS versions 3.0 and higher) is a dimensionless scale from 0 (complete cortical electroencephalographic suppression) to 100 (awake). BIS values of 65–85 have been recommended for sedation, whereas values of 40–65 have been recommended for general anesthesia. At BIS values lower than 40, cortical suppression becomes discernible in a raw electroencephalogram as a burst suppression pattern. (Reproduced with permission from Johansen JW et al: Development and clinical application of electroencephalographic bispectrum monitoring. Anesthesiology 2000;93:1337.)

Table 6–6. Characteristics and uses of evoked potentials.

Type	Stimulus	Method of Delivering Stimulus	Surgical Procedure
Auditory	Clicks, tones	Ear transducer	Cerebellopontine angle tumor resection
Somatosensory	Electric current	Electrodes	Spinal or thoracoabdominal aortic aneurysm surgery
Motor	Electric current/magnetic field	Electrodes	Spinal or thoracoabdominal aortic aneurysm surgery

trodes. If the intervening pathway is intact, a nerve action potential will be transmitted to the contralateral sensory cortex to produce an EP. This potential can be measured by cortical surface electrodes, but is usually measured by scalp electrodes. To distinguish the cortical response to a specific stimulus, multiple responses are averaged and background noise is eliminated. EPs are represented by a plot of voltage versus time. The resulting waveforms are analyzed for their poststimulus latency (the time between stimulation and potential detection) and peak amplitude. These are compared with baseline tracings. Technical and physiological causes of a change in an EP must be distinguished from changes due to neural damage. Complications of EP monitoring are rare but include skin irritation and pressure ischemia at the sites of electrode application.

Clinical Considerations

EPs are altered by many variables other than neural damage. The effect of anesthetics is complex and not easily summarized. In general, balanced anesthetic techniques (nitrous oxide, neuromuscular blocking agents, and opioids) cause minimal changes, whereas volatile agents (halothane, sevoflurane, desflurane, and isoflurane) are best avoided or used at a constant low dose. Early-occurring (specific) EPs are less affected by anesthetics than are late-occurring (nonspecific) responses. Changes in BAERs may provide a measure of the depth of anesthesia. Physiological (eg, blood pressure, temperature, and oxygen saturation) and pharmacological factors should be kept as constant as possible.

Persistent obliteration of EPs is predictive of postoperative neurological deficit. Although SEPs usually identify spinal cord damage, because of their different anatomic pathways, *sensory* (dorsal spinal cord) EP preservation does not guarantee normal *motor* (ventral spinal cord) function (false negative). Furthermore, SEPs elicited from posterior tibial nerve stimulation cannot distinguish between peripheral and central ischemia (false positive). Techniques that elicit MEPs by using transcranial magnetic stimulation or percutaneous cer-

vical spinal cord stimulation by inserting needle electrodes in the cervical region are being used clinically in a number of institutions. The advantage of using MEPs as opposed to SEPs for spinal cord monitoring is that the MEPs monitor the ventral spinal cord, and if sensitive and specific enough, can be used to indicate which patients might develop a postoperative motor deficit. The same considerations for SEPs are applicable to MEPs in that they are affected by volatile inhalational agents, high-dose benzodiazepines, and moderate hypothermia (temperatures less than 32°C). Monitoring of MEPs may require monitoring of the level of neuromuscular blockade.

■ MISCELLANEOUS MONITORS

TEMPERATURE

Indications

The temperature of patients undergoing general anesthesia should be monitored. Very brief procedures (eg, less than 15 min) may be an exception to this guideline.

Contraindications

There are no contraindications, though a particular monitoring site may be unsuitable in certain patients.

Techniques & Complications

Intraoperatively, temperature is usually measured using a thermistor or thermocouple. Thermistors are semiconductors whose resistance decreases predictably with warming. A thermocouple is a circuit of two dissimilar metals joined so that a potential difference is generated when the metals are at different temperatures. Disposable thermocouple and thermistor probes are available for monitoring the temperature of the tympanic membrane, nasopharynx, esophagus, bladder, rectum, and

John R. Moyers, MD

APPLICATION OF THE BASIC PHYSICAL EXAMINATION TO INTRAOPERATIVE MONITORING

An observer in today's operating rooms would be struck by the devotion of the anesthesiologist to the complex array of sophisticated electronics that comprise the present operating room monitoring system. Anesthesiologists sit enthralled by the display screens, often with their backs to a patient whose head is completely covered, arms carefully tucked at the side, and eyelids meticulously taped closed.[1] The observer then witnesses at exact 5-min intervals the careful, but unanalytical and uncritical recording on the anesthesia record, of every value displayed on each of the monitors. I suggest that applying the basics of the physical examination learned in medical school to intraoperative monitoring enhances patient care and safety.

Several examples may lead to a better understanding of this premise. Basic monitoring variables include assessment of depth of anesthesia, ventilation, oxygenation, circulation, and temperature. Monitoring of capillary refill and palpation of a peripheral pulse can enable the anesthesiologist to assess the circulatory system and confirm the more objective and sophisticated data gleaned from electronic monitoring devices. A finding of a warm and pink nose, brisk capillary refill, warm extremities, and bounding peripheral pulses provides a great deal of information about circulatory status. Conversely, a patient who has skin that appears gray and mottled, cold extremities, poor capillary refill, and a weak pulse needs some attention to circulatory status regardless of the data displayed by the electronic monitoring devices.

Similarly, after placement of a double-lumen tracheal tube, the anesthesiologist often immediately inserts a fiberoptic bronchoscope through the lumen of the tube to assess proper placement. Alternatively, or prior to fiberoptic bronchoscopy, ventilation and tube placement (albeit with less precision) can be assessed by inspection, palpation, and auscultation of the chest. With some experience ventilation of one hemithorax can be detected by each of these methods of physical examination. After this assessment of ventilation, there is time to proceed safely with bronchoscopy and to correct any difficulties with tube placement that may have occurred. Also, using physical examination trains the anesthesiologist to obtain a quick assessment of single-lung ventilation, or to recognize rapidly when a single-lumen tube has been placed improperly. It is currently popular among some to rely upon the index derived from bispectral

---

skin. Complications of temperature monitoring are usually related to trauma caused by the probe (eg, rectal or tympanic membrane perforation).

Clinical Considerations

Hypothermia, usually defined as a body temperature less than 36°C, occurs frequently during anesthesia and surgery. Because hypothermia reduces metabolic oxygen requirements, it has proved to be protective during times of cerebral or cardiac

ischemia. **Unintentional hypothermia has several deleterious physiological effects, however (Table 6–7).** In fact, perioperative hypothermia has been associated with an increased mortality rate.

Postoperative shivering increases oxygen consumption as much as 5-fold, decreases arterial oxygen saturation, and has been shown to correlate with an increased risk of myocardial ischemia and angina. Although postoperative shivering can be effectively treated with intravenous meperidine (25 mg), the best solution remains prevention by maintaining normothermia. The inci-

analysis of the electroencephalogram to assess depth of anesthesia and to prevent awareness.[2] Nonetheless, the bispectral index does have its disadvantages. It is not as reliable as one would like with all anesthetic agents, and in many situations it may be neither sensitive nor specific enough to evaluate depth reliably.[3] I once applied bispectral index electrodes to a serving of cherry gelatin with fruit cocktail from our cafeteria and recorded an index of 22. More appropriately and convincingly, a recent review by Drummond suggests that the peer-reviewed literature does not support the belief that such a device can serve to either monitor depth of anesthesia or prevent awareness.[4] With application of the physical examination, using papillary response, ventilatory pattern, muscle tone, response to command, or movement, it is also possible to assess depth of anesthesia. Again, clinical observation and judgment in concert with sophisticated monitoring provide a fuller and more accurate assessment of patient responsiveness to anesthesia than does monitoring alone.

Indeed, sophisticated and complex monitoring techniques are necessary for good anesthesia practice. Simpler assessments are not always available or useful. Many patients are paralyzed with neuromuscular blocking agents necessitating controlled ventilation, which precludes the use of muscle tone or respiratory pattern to assess depth of anesthesia. It is difficult without sophisticated tools to monitor depth of anesthesia in a hypothermic patient in whom a cardiopulmonary bypass technique has been instituted. Adequacy of oxygenation does not lend itself very well to observation. A patient with a normal hemoglobin level will usually not appear cyanotic until the reading on the pulse oximeter is below about 75%. For many procedures the anesthesiologist is remote from some or all of the patient's body, making direct contact difficult or impossible. Also, complex

monitors free up time for other activities and allow objective measurement. Finally, other extremely important monitors measure parameters beyond our senses or quantitate otherwise inaccessible variables. For example, it is impossible to assess blood pH by physical examination.

Applying the physical examination to monitoring in the operating room adds no cost and leads to more patient contact and focus. There is no substitute for vigilance and common sense. Astute observation of the patient in the operating room can minimize recording of either incorrect or unnecessarily complex information and tends to eliminate a false sense of security that may result with blithe devotion to electronic monitors. Judgment based upon both electronic monitors and aspects of the physical examination is usually a better assessment of patient status than judgment based on either alone. There is comfort in assessing the same variable by more than one method and obtaining a similar answer. That is why our local television weatherman once told me that he always looks out the window before he gives the weather report. Because human error plays a major role in most anesthesia disasters, applying the tenets of physical examination and common sense to monitoring may help to provide safer anesthetic care.

1. Hamilton WK: Do we monitor enough? We monitor too much. J Clin Monitoring 1986;2:246.
2. Kissin I: Ambulatory anesthesia: depth of anesthesia and bispectral index monitoring. Anesth Analg 2000;90:1114.
3. Vuyk J, Lichtenbelt BJ, Vieveen J, et al: Low bispectral index values in awake volunteers receiving a combination of propofol and midazolam. Anesthesiology 2004;100:179.
4. Drummond JC: Monitoring depth of anesthesia with emphasis on the application of the bispectral index and the middle latency auditory evoked response to the prevention of recall. Anesthesiology 2000;93:876.

dence of unintentional perioperative hypothermia increases with extremes of age, abdominal surgery, procedures of long duration, and cold ambient operating room temperature.

Core temperature (central blood temperature) usually decreases 1 or 2°C during the first hour of general anesthesia (phase I), followed by a more gradual decline during the ensuing 3–4 h (phase II), eventually reaching a point of steady state or equilibrium (phase III). Redistribution of heat from warm central compartments (eg, abdomen, thorax)

to cooler peripheral tissues (eg, arms, legs) from anesthetic-induced vasodilation explains most of the initial decrease in temperature, with actual heat loss being a minor contributor. Continuous heat loss to the environment appears to be primarily responsible for the slower subsequent decline. During steady-state equilibrium, heat loss equals metabolic heat production (Figure 6–30).

Normally the hypothalamus maintains core body temperature within a very narrow range (the interthreshold range). Raising body temperature a fraction of a

Table 6–7. Deleterious effects of hypothermia.

Cardiac arrhythmias and ischemia
Increased peripheral vascular resistance
Left shift of the hemoglobin–oxygen saturation curve
Reversible coagulopathy (platelet dysfunction)
Postoperative protein catabolism and stress response
Altered mental status
Impaired renal function
Decreased drug metabolism
Poor wound healing
Increased incidence of infection

degree induces sweating and vasodilation, whereas lowering temperature triggers vasoconstriction and shivering. During general anesthesia, however, the body cannot compensate for hypothermia because anesthetics inhibit central thermoregulation by interfering with hypothalamic function. For example, isoflurane produces a dose-dependent decrease in the vasoconstrictive threshold (3°C for each percent of inhaled isoflurane).

Spinal and epidural anesthesia also lead to hypothermia by causing vasodilation and subsequent internal redistribution of heat (phase I). The accompanying thermoregulatory impairment from regional anesthesia that allows continued heat loss (phase II) appears to be due to an altered perception of temperature in the blocked dermatomes by the hypothalamus—as opposed to a central drug effect as seen with general anesthetics. Thus, both general and regional anesthesia increase the interthreshold range, albeit by different mechanisms.

Prewarming for half an hour with convective forced-air warming blankets effectively prevents phase I hypothermia by eliminating the central-peripheral temperature gradient. Methods to minimize phase II hypothermia from heat loss include use of forced-air warming blankets and warm-water blankets, heated humidification of inspired gases, warming of intravenous fluids, and raising ambient operating room temperature. Passive insulators such as heated cotton blankets or so-called space blankets have little utility unless most of the body is covered.

Each monitoring site has advantages and disadvantages. The tympanic membrane theoretically reflects brain temperature because the auditory canal's blood supply is the external carotid artery. Trauma during insertion and cerumen insulation detract from the routine use of tympanic probes. Rectal temperatures have a slow response to changes in core temperature. Nasopharyngeal probes are prone to cause epistaxis but accurately measure core temperature if placed adjacent to the nasopharyngeal mucosa. The thermistor on a pulmonary artery catheter also measures core temperature. There is a variable correlation between axillary temperature and core temperature, depending on skin perfusion. Liquid crystal adhesive strips placed on the skin are inadequate indicators of core body temperature during surgery. Esophageal temperature sensors, often incorporated into esophageal stethoscopes, provide the best combination of economy, performance, and safety. To avoid measuring the temperature of tracheal gases, the temperature sensor should be positioned behind the heart in the lower third of the esophagus. Conveniently, heart sounds are most prominent at this location.

URINARY OUTPUT

Indications

Urinary bladder catheterization is the only reliable method of monitoring urinary output. Insertion of a urinary catheter is indicated in patients with congestive heart failure, renal failure, advanced hepatic disease, or shock. Catheterization is routine in some surgical procedures such as cardiac surgery, aortic or renal vascular surgery, craniotomy, major abdominal surgery, or procedures in which large fluid shifts are expected. Lengthy surgeries and intraoperative diuretic administration are other possible indications. Occasionally, postoperative bladder catheterization is indicated in patients having difficulty voiding in the recovery room after general or regional anesthesia.

Contraindications

Bladder catheterization should be done with utmost care in patients at high risk for infection.

Figure 6–30. Unintentional hypothermia during general anesthesia follows a typical pattern: a steep drop in core temperature during the first hour (phase I redistribution), followed by a gradual decline during the next 3–4 h (phase II heat loss), eventually reaching a steady state (phase III equilibrium).

Techniques & Complications

Bladder catheterization is usually performed by surgical or nursing personnel. To avoid unnecessary trauma, a urologist should catheterize patients suspected of having abnormal urethral anatomy. A soft rubber Foley catheter is inserted into the bladder transurethrally and connected to a disposable calibrated collection chamber. To avoid urine reflux and minimize the risk of infection, the chamber should remain at a level below the bladder. Complications of catheterization include urethral trauma and urinary tract infections. Rapid decompression of a distended bladder can cause hypotension. Suprapubic catheterization of the bladder with plastic tubing inserted through a large-bore needle is an uncommon alternative.

Clinical Considerations

An additional advantage of placing a Foley catheter is the ability to include a thermistor in the catheter tip so that bladder temperature can be monitored. As long as urinary output is high, bladder temperature accurately reflects core temperature. An added value with more widespread use of urometers is the ability to electronically monitor and record urinary output and temperature.

Urinary output is a reflection of kidney perfusion and function and an indicator of renal, cardiovascular, and fluid volume status. Inadequate urinary output (oliguria) is often arbitrarily defined as urinary output of less than 0.5 mL/kg/h, but actually is a function of the patient's concentrating ability and osmotic load. Urine electrolyte composition, osmolality, and specific gravity aid in the differential diagnosis of oliguria (see Chapter 31).

PERIPHERAL NERVE STIMULATION

Indications

Because of the variation in patient sensitivity to neuromuscular blocking agents, the neuromuscular function of all patients receiving intermediate- or long-acting neuromuscular blocking agents should be monitored. In addition, peripheral nerve stimulation is helpful in assessing paralysis during rapid-sequence inductions or during continuous infusions of short-acting agents. Furthermore, peripheral nerve stimulators can help locate nerves to be blocked by regional anesthesia.

Contraindications

There are no contraindications to neuromuscular monitoring, although certain sites may be precluded by the surgical procedure.

Techniques & Complications

A peripheral nerve stimulator delivers a current of variable frequency and amplitude to a pair of either ECG silver chloride pads or subcutaneous needles placed over a peripheral motor nerve. The evoked mechanical or electrical response of the innervated muscle is observed. Although electromyography provides a fast, accurate, and quantitative measure of neuromuscular transmission, visual or tactile observation of muscle contraction is usually relied upon in clinical practice. Ulnar nerve stimulation of the adductor pollicis muscle and facial nerve stimulation of the orbicularis oculi are most commonly monitored (Figure 6–31). Because it is the inhibition of the neuromuscular receptor that needs to be monitored, direct stimulation of muscle should be avoided by placing electrodes over the course of the nerve and not over the muscle itself. To deliver a supramaximal stimulation to the underlying nerve, peripheral nerve stimulators must be capable of generating at least a 50-mA current across a 1000-Ω load. This cur-

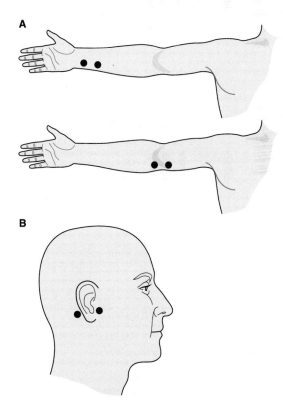

Figure 6–31. **A:** Stimulation of the ulnar nerve causes contraction of the adductor pollicis muscle. **B:** Stimulation of the facial nerve leads to orbicularis oculi contraction. The orbicularis oculi recovers from neuromuscular blockade before the adductor pollicis. (Reproduced with permission from Dorsch JA, Dorsch SE: *Understanding Anesthesia Equipment,* 4th ed. Williams & Wilkins, 1999.)

rent is uncomfortable for a conscious patient. Complications of nerve stimulation are limited to skin irritation and abrasion at the site of electrode attachment.

Clinical Considerations

The degree of neuromuscular blockade is monitored by applying various patterns of electrical stimulation (Figure 6–32). All stimuli are 200 μs in duration, of square-wave pattern, and of equal current intensity. A twitch is a single pulse that is delivered from every 1 to every 10 s (1–0.1 Hz). Increasing block results in decreased evoked response to stimulation.

Train-of-four stimulation denotes four successive 200-μs stimuli in 2 s (2 Hz). The twitches in a train-of-four pattern progressively fade as relaxation increases. The ratio of the responses to the first and fourth twitches is a sensitive indicator of nondepolarizing muscle paralysis. Because it is difficult to estimate the train-of-four ratio, it is more convenient to visually observe the sequential disappearance of the twitches, as this also correlates with the extent of blockade. Disappearance of the fourth twitch represents a 75% block, the third twitch an 80% block, and the second twitch a 90% block. Clinical relaxation usually requires 75–95% neuromuscular blockade.

Tetany at 50 or 100 Hz is a sensitive test of neuromuscular function. Sustained contraction for 5 s indicates adequate—but not necessarily complete—reversal from neuromuscular blockade. Double-burst stimulation (DBS) represents two variations of tetany that are less painful to the patient. The DBS$_{3,3}$ pattern of nerve stimulation consists of three short (200-μs) high-frequency bursts separated by 20-ms intervals (50 Hz) followed 750 ms later by another three bursts. DBS$_{3,2}$ consists of three 200-μs impulses at 50 Hz followed 750 ms later by two such impulses. DBS is more sensitive than train-of-four stimulation for the clinical (ie, visual) evaluation of fade.

Because muscle groups differ in their sensitivity to neuromuscular blocking agents, use of the peripheral nerve stimulator cannot replace direct observation of the muscles (eg, the diaphragm) that need to be relaxed for a specific surgical procedure. Furthermore, recovery of adductor pollicis function does not exactly parallel recovery of muscles required to maintain an airway. **The diaphragm, rectus abdominis, laryngeal adductors, and orbicularis oculi muscles recover from neuromuscular blockade sooner than the adductor pollicis.** Other indicators of adequate recovery include sustained (≥ 5 s) head lift, the ability to generate an inspiratory pressure of at least –25 cm H_2O, and a forceful hand grip. Twitch tension is reduced by hypothermia of the monitored muscle group (6%/°C). Peripheral nerve stimulation is considered further in Chapter 9.

CASE DISCUSSION: MONITORING DURING MAGNETIC RESONANCE IMAGING

A 50-year-old man with recent onset of seizures is scheduled for magnetic resonance imaging (MRI). A prior MRI attempt was unsuccessful because of the patient's severe claustrophobic reaction. The radiologist requests your help in providing either sedation or general anesthesia.

Why does the MRI suite pose special problems for the patient and the anesthesiologist?

MRI studies tend to be long (often more than 1 h) and most scanners totally surround the body, causing a high incidence of claustrophobia in patients already anxious about their health. Good imaging requires immobility, something that is difficult to achieve in many patients without sedation or general anesthesia.

Because the MRI uses a powerful magnet, no ferromagnetic objects can be placed near the scanner. This includes implanted prosthetic joints, artificial pacemakers, surgical clips, batteries, ordinary anesthesia machines, watches, pens, or credit cards. Ordinary metal lead wires for pulse oximeters or electrocardiography act as antennas and may attract enough radiofrequency energy to distort the MRI image or even cause patient burns. In addition, the scanner's magnetic field causes severe monitor artifact. The more powerful the scanner's magnet as measured in Tesla units (1 T = 10,000 gauss), the greater the potential problem. Other obstacles include poor access to the patient during the imaging (particularly the patient's airway), hypothermia in pediatric patients, dim lighting within the patient tunnel, and very loud noise (up to 100 dB).

How have these monitoring and anesthesia machine problems been addressed?

Equipment manufacturers have modified monitors so that they are compatible with the MRI environment. These modifications include nonferromagnetic electrocardiographic electrodes, graphite and copper cables, extensive filtering and gating of signals, extra-long blood pressure cuff tubing, and use of fiberoptic technologies. Anesthesia machines with no ferromagnetic components (eg, aluminum gas cylinders) have been fitted with MRI-compatible ventilators and

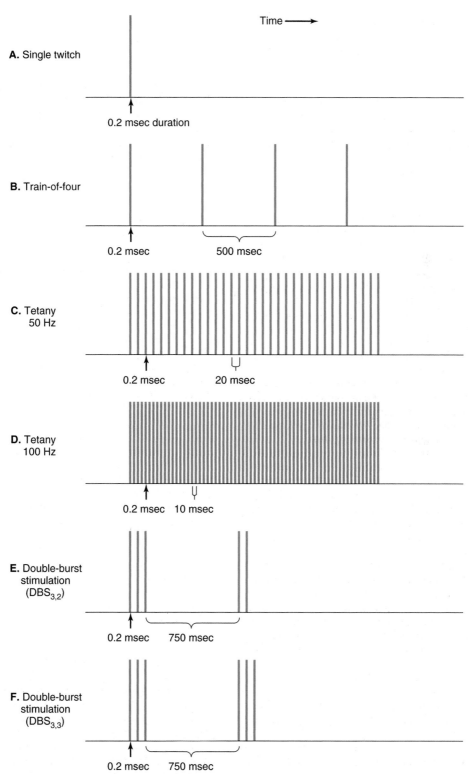

Figure 6–32. Peripheral nerve stimulators can generate various patterns of electrical impulses.

long circle systems or Mapleson D breathing circuits.

What factors influence the choice between general anesthesia and intravenous sedation?

Although most patients will tolerate an MRI study with sedation, head injured and pediatric patients present special challenges and will often require general anesthesia. Because of machine and monitoring limitations, an argument could be made that sedation, when possible, would be a safer choice. On the other hand, loss of airway control from deep sedation could prove catastrophic because of poor patient access and delayed detection. Other important considerations include the monitoring modalities available at a particular facility and the general medical condition of the patient.

Which monitors should be considered mandatory in this case?

The patient should receive at least the same level of monitoring and care in the MRI suite as in the operating room for a similarly noninvasive procedure. Thus, the American Society of Anesthesiologists Standards for Basic Anesthetic Monitoring apply as they would to a patient undergoing general anesthesia.

The MRI suite itself precludes some monitoring methods commonly used during intravenous sedation and requires modification of others. Pulse oximetry is recommended. Continuous auscultation of breath sounds with a plastic (not metal) precordial stethoscope can help identify airway obstruction caused by excessive sedation. Palpation of a peripheral pulse or listening for Korotkoff sounds is impractical in this setting. Ensuring adequacy of circulation depends on electrocardiographic and oscillometric blood pressure monitoring. Although not mandatory, aspiration end-tidal carbon dioxide analyzers can be adapted to sedation cases by connecting the sampling line to a site near the patient's mouth or nose. Because room air entrainment precludes exact measurements, this technique provides a qualitative indicator of ventilation. Whenever sedation is planned, equipment for emergency conversion to gener-

al anesthesia (eg, tracheal tubes, resuscitation bag) must be immediately available.

Is the continuous presence of anesthesia personnel required during these cases?

Absolutely yes. Sedated patients need to have continuous monitored anesthesia care to prevent a multitude of unforeseen complications, such as apnea or emesis.

SUGGESTED READING

Bernard GR, Sopko G, Cerra F, et al: Pulmonary artery catheterization and clinical outcomes. National Heart, Lung, and Blood Institute and Food and Drug Administration Workshop Report. JAMA 2000;19:2568.

Cope DK: Monitoring in the 19th century: from blood-letting to blood-flow measurements. Am Soc Anesthesiol Newslett 2002;66:6. Excellent review of the history of monitoring in this specialty.

Dorsch JA, Dorsch SE: *Understanding Anesthesia Equipment*, 4th ed. Williams & Wilkins, 1999. Includes an excellent discussion on capnography and anesthetic gas monitors.

Fenelly M: Spinal cord monitoring. Anaesthesia 1998;53:41.

Hamilton TT, Huber LM, Jessen ME: PulseCO: a less-invasive method to monitor cardiac output from arterial pressure after cardiac surgery. Ann Thorac Surg 2002;74:S1408. Discusses a new method for measuring cardiac output using pulse contour compared to lithium dilution (used in over 100 centers in the United States) versus thermodilution with a pulmonary artery catheter.

Jubran A: Advances in respiratory monitoring during mechanical ventilation. Chest 1999;116:1416.

Keenan SP, Guyatt GH, Sibbald WJ, et al: How to use articles about diagnostic technology: gastric tonometry. Crit Care Med 1999;27:1726.

Lake CL, Hines RL, Blitt CD: *Clinical Monitoring: Practical Applications for Anesthesia and Critical Care*. WB Saunders, 2001.

McGee DC, Gould MK: Preventing complications of central venous catheterization. N Engl J Med 2003;348:1123. A recent review of the complications of central venous cannulation.

O'Grady NP, Alexander M, Dellinger EP, et al: Guidelines for the prevention of intravascular catheter-related infections. Infect Control Hosp Epidemiol 2002;23:759.

Practice guidelines for pulmonary artery catheterization: An updated report by the American Society of Anesthesiologists Task Force on pulmonary artery catheterization. Anesthesiology 2003;99:999.

Schell RM, Cole DJ: Cerebral monitoring: jugular venous oximetry. Anesth Analg 2000;90:559.

SECTION II
Clinical Pharmacology

Inhalation Anesthetics

7

KEY CONCEPTS

 The study of the relationship between a drug's dose, tissue concentration, and elapsed time is called pharmacokinetics (how a body affects a drug). The study of drug action, including toxic responses, is called pharmacodynamics (how a drug affects a body).

 The greater the uptake of anesthetic agent, the greater the difference between inspired and alveolar concentrations, and the slower the rate of induction.

 Three factors affect anesthetic uptake: solubility in the blood, alveolar blood flow, and the difference in partial pressure between alveolar gas and venous blood.

 Low-output states predispose patients to overdosage with soluble agents, as the rate of rise in alveolar concentrations will be markedly increased.

Many of the factors that speed induction also speed recovery: elimination of rebreathing, high fresh gas flows, low anesthetic-circuit volume, low absorption by the anesthetic circuit, decreased solubility, high cerebral blood flow, and increased ventilation.

 General anesthesia is an altered physiological state characterized by reversible loss of consciousness, analgesia of the entire body, amnesia, and some degree of muscle relaxation.

 The unitary hypothesis proposes that all inhalation agents share a common mechanism of action at the molecular level. This is supported by the observation that the anesthetic potency of inhalation agents correlates directly with their lipid solubility (Meyer–Overton rule).

 The minimum alveolar concentration (MAC) is the alveolar concentration of an inhaled anesthetic that prevents movement in 50% of patients in response to a standardized stimulus (eg, surgical incision).

 Prolonged exposure to anesthetic concentrations of nitrous oxide can result in bone marrow depression (megaloblastic anemia) and even neurological deficiencies (peripheral neuropathies and pernicious anemia).

(continued on next page)

(continued from previous page)

 Halothane hepatitis is extremely rare (1 per 35,000 cases). Patients exposed to multiple halothane anesthetics at short intervals, middle-aged obese women, and persons with a familial predisposition to halothane toxicity or a personal history of toxicity are considered to be at increased risk.

 Isoflurane dilates coronary arteries, but is not nearly as potent a dilator as nitroglycerin or adenosine. Dilation of normal coronary arteries could theoretically divert blood away from fixed stenotic lesions. There have been conflicting reports about whether the coronary steal syndrome causes regional myocardial ischemia during episodes of tachycardia or drops in perfusion pressure.

 The low solubility of desflurane in blood and body tissues causes a very rapid washin and washout of anesthetic.

 Rapid increases in desflurane concentration lead to transient but sometimes worrisome elevations in heart rate, blood pressure, and catecholamine levels that are more pronounced than occur with isoflurane, particularly in patients with cardiovascular disease.

 Nonpungency and rapid increases in alveolar anesthetic concentration make sevoflurane an excellent choice for smooth and rapid inhalation inductions in pediatric and adult patients.

Nitrous oxide, chloroform, and ether were the first universally accepted general anesthetics. Ethyl chloride, ethylene, and cyclopropane were also used; the latter was particularly popular because of the fast induction associated with its use. Recovery from cyclopropane was notable; because of its rapidity of effect and the fact that it did not result in delirium, patients were more clear headed. Toxicity and flammability of these drugs led to their withdrawal from the market.

Methoxyflurane and enflurane, two halogenated agents in use for many years, are no longer used because of their toxicity and efficacy. Methoxyflurane was the most potent inhalation agent, but its high solubility and low vapor pressure limited its rate of induction and emergence. Up to 50% of it was metabolized by cytochrome P-450 enzymes to free fluoride (F⁻), oxalic acid, and other nephrotoxic compounds. Methoxyflurane was associated with a vasopressin-resistant, high-output, renal failure that was most commonly seen when F^- levels increased to greater than 50 μmol/L. Enflurane has a nonpungent odor and is nonflammable at clinical concentrations. It depresses myocardial contractility and sensitizes the myocardium to epinephrine. It also increases the secretion of cerebrospinal fluid (CSF) and the resistance to CSF outflow. During deep anesthesia, high-voltage, high-frequency electroencephalographic changes can progress to a spike-and-wave pattern that culminates in tonic–clonic seizures.

Although chloroform, ether, methoxyflurane, and enflurane are no longer used in the United States (chiefly because of problems with toxicity and flammability), five inhalation agents continue to be used in clinical anesthesiology: nitrous oxide, halothane, isoflurane, desflurane, and sevoflurane.

The course of general anesthesia can be divided into three phases: (1) induction, (2) maintenance, and (3) emergence. Inhalation anesthetics are particularly useful in the induction of pediatric patients in whom it may be difficult to start an intravenous line. In contrast, adults usually prefer rapid induction with intravenous agents, although the nonpungency and rapid onset of sevoflurane have made inhalation induction practical for adults. Regardless of the patient's age, anesthesia is often maintained with inhalation agents. Emergence depends primarily upon the pulmonary elimination of these agents.

Because of their unique route of administration, inhalation anesthetics have useful pharmacological properties not shared by other anesthetic agents. For instance, exposure to the pulmonary circulation allows a more rapid appearance of the drug in arterial blood than does intravenous administration. The study of the relationship between a drug's dose, tissue concentration, and elapsed time is called pharmacokinetics (how a body affects a drug). The study of drug action, including toxic responses, is called pharmacodynamics (how a drug affects a body).

After a general description of the pharmacokinetics and pharmacodynamics of inhalation anesthetics, this chapter presents the clinical pharmacology of individual agents.

■ PHARMACOKINETICS OF INHALATION ANESTHETICS

Although the mechanism of action of inhalation anesthetics remains unknown, it is assumed that their ultimate effect depends on attainment of a therapeutic tissue concentration in the central nervous system. There are many steps, however, between the administration of an anesthetic from a vaporizer and its deposition in the brain (Figure 7–1).

FACTORS AFFECTING INSPIRATORY CONCENTRATION (FI)

The fresh gas leaving the anesthesia machine mixes with gases in the breathing circuit before being inspired by the patient. Therefore, the patient is not necessarily receiving the concentration set on the vaporizer. The actual composition of the inspired gas mixture depends mainly on the fresh gas flow rate, the volume of the breathing system, and any absorption by the machine or breathing circuit. The higher the fresh gas flow rate, the smaller the breathing system volume, and the lower the circuit absorption, the closer the inspired gas concentration will be to the fresh gas concentration. Clinically, these attributes translate into faster induction and recovery times.

FACTORS AFFECTING ALVEOLAR CONCENTRATION (FA)

Uptake

If there were no uptake of anesthetic agent by the body, the alveolar gas concentration (FA) would rapidly approach the inspired gas concentration (FI). Because anesthetic agents are taken up by the pulmonary circulation during induction, alveolar concentrations lag behind inspired concentrations (FA/FI < 1.0). The greater the uptake, the slower the rate of rise of the alveolar concentration and the lower the FA:FI ratio.

Because the concentration of a gas is directly proportional to its partial pressure, the alveolar partial pres-

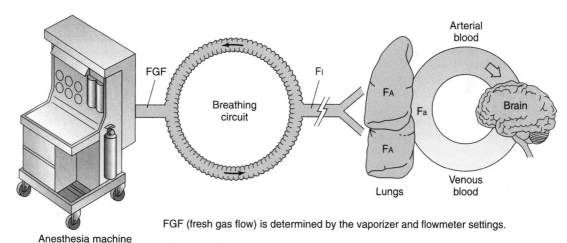

FGF (fresh gas flow) is determined by the vaporizer and flowmeter settings.

FI   (inspired gas concentration) is determined by (1) FGF rate; (2) breathing-circuit volume; and (3) circuit absorption.

FA   (alveolar gas concentration) is determined by (1) uptake (uptake = $\lambda_{b/g} \times C(A-V) \times Q$); (2) ventilation; and (3) the concentration effect and second gas effect:
    a) concentrating effect
    b) augmented inflow effect

Fa   (arterial gas concentration) is affected by ventilation/perfusion mismatching.

Figure 7–1. Inhalation anesthetic agents must pass through many barriers between the anesthesia machine and the brain.

Table 7-1. Partition coefficients of volatile anesthetics at 37°C.[1]

Agent	Blood/Gas	Brain/Blood	Muscle/Blood	Fat/Blood
Nitrous oxide	0.47	1.1	1.2	2.3
Halothane	2.4	2.9	3.5	60
Isoflurane	1.4	2.6	4.0	45
Desflurane	0.42	1.3	2.0	27
Sevoflurane	0.65	1.7	3.1	48

[1]These values are averages derived from multiple studies and should be used for comparison purposes, not as exact numbers.

sure will also be slow to rise. The alveolar partial pressure is important because it determines the partial pressure of anesthetic in the blood and, ultimately, in the brain. Similarly, the partial pressure of the anesthetic in the brain is directly proportional to its brain tissue concentration, which determines clinical effect.

Therefore, the greater the uptake of anesthetic agent, the greater the difference between inspired and alveolar concentrations, and the slower the rate of induction.

Three factors affect anesthetic uptake: solubility in the blood, alveolar blood flow, and the difference in partial pressure between alveolar gas and venous blood.

Insoluble agents, such as nitrous oxide, are taken up by the blood less avidly than soluble agents, such as halothane. As a consequence, the alveolar concentration of nitrous oxide rises faster than that of halothane, and induction is faster. The relative solubilities of an anesthetic in air, blood, and tissues are expressed as partition coefficients (Table 7–1). Each coefficient is the ratio of the concentrations of the anesthetic gas in each of two phases at equilibrium. Equilibrium is defined as equal partial pressures in the two phases. For instance, the blood/gas partition coefficient ($\lambda_{b/g}$) of nitrous oxide at 37°C is 0.47. In other words, at equilibrium, 1 mL of blood contains 0.47 as much nitrous oxide as does 1 mL of alveolar gas, even though the partial pressures are the same. Stated another way, blood has 47% of the capacity for nitrous oxide as alveolar gas. Nitrous oxide is much less soluble in blood than is halothane, which has a blood/gas partition coefficient at 37°C of 2.4. Thus, almost five times more halothane than nitrous oxide must be dissolved to raise the partial pressure of blood. The higher the blood/gas coefficient, the greater the anesthetic's solubility and the greater its uptake by the pulmonary circulation. As a consequence of this high solubility, alveolar partial pressure rises more slowly, and induction is prolonged. Because fat/blood partition coefficients are greater than 1, it is not surprising

that blood/gas solubility is increased by postprandial lipidemia and is decreased by anemia.

The second factor that affects uptake is alveolar blood flow, which—in the absence of pulmonary shunting—is essentially equal to cardiac output. If the cardiac output drops to zero, so will anesthetic uptake. As cardiac output increases, anesthetic uptake increases, the rise in alveolar partial pressure slows, and induction is delayed. The effect of changing cardiac output is less pronounced for insoluble anesthetics, as so little is taken up regardless of alveolar blood flow. Low-output states predispose patients to overdosage with soluble agents, as the rate of rise in alveolar concentrations will be markedly increased. Higher than anticipated levels of a volatile anesthetic, which is also a myocardial depressant (eg, halothane), may create a positive feedback loop by lowering cardiac output even further.

The final factor affecting uptake of anesthetic by the pulmonary circulation is the partial pressure difference between alveolar gas and venous blood. This gradient depends on tissue uptake. If anesthetics did not pass into organs such as the brain, venous and alveolar partial pressures would become identical and there would be no pulmonary uptake. The transfer of anesthetic from blood to tissues is determined by three factors analogous to systemic uptake: tissue solubility of the agent (tissue/blood partition coefficient), tissue blood flow, and the difference in partial pressure between arterial blood and the tissue.

Tissues can be divided into four groups based on their solubility and blood flow (Table 7–2). The highly perfused vessel-rich group (brain, heart, liver, kidney, and endocrine organs) is the first to take up appreciable amounts of anesthetic. Moderate solubility and small volume limit the capacity of this group, so it is also the first to fill (ie, arterial and tissue partial pressures are equal). The muscle group (skin and muscle) is not as well perfused, so uptake is slower. In addition, it has a greater capacity due to a larger volume, and uptake will be sustained for hours.

Table 7–2. Tissue groups based on perfusion and solubilities.

Characteristic	Vessel Rich	Muscle	Fat	Vessel Poor
Percentage of body weight	10	50	20	20
Percentage of cardiac output	75	19	6	0
Perfusion (mL/min/100 g)	75	3	3	0
Relative solubility	1	1	20	0

Perfusion of the fat group nearly equals that of the muscle group, but the tremendous solubility of anesthetic in fat leads to a total capacity (tissue/blood solubility × tissue volume) that would take days to fill. The minimal perfusion of the vessel-poor group (bones, ligaments, teeth, hair, and cartilage) results in insignificant uptake.

Anesthetic uptake produces a characteristic curve that relates the rise in alveolar concentration to time (Figure 7–2). The shape of this graph is determined by the uptakes of individual tissue groups (Figure 7–3). The initial steep rate of uptake is due to unopposed filling of the alveoli by ventilation. The rate of rise slows as the vessel-rich group—and eventually the muscle group—reach their capacity.

Ventilation

The lowering of alveolar partial pressure by uptake can be countered by increasing alveolar ventilation. In other words, constantly replacing anesthetic taken up by the pulmonary bloodstream results in better maintenance of alveolar concentration. The effect of increasing ventilation will be most obvious in raising the FA/FI for soluble anesthetics, as they are more subject to uptake. Because the FA/FI is already high for insoluble agents, increasing ventilation has minimal effect. In contrast to the effect of anesthetics on cardiac output, anesthetics that depress ventilation (eg, halothane) will decrease the rate of rise in alveolar concentration and create a negative feedback loop.

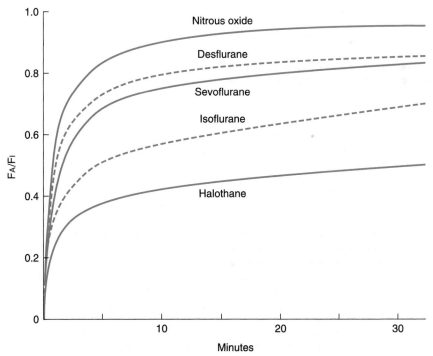

Figure 7–2. FA rises toward FI faster with nitrous oxide (an insoluble agent) than with halothane (a soluble agent). See Figure 7–1 for an explanation of FA and FI. (Modified and reproduced, with permission, from Eger EL II: *Isoflurane [Forane]: A Reference and Compendium.* Ohio Medical Products, 1981.)

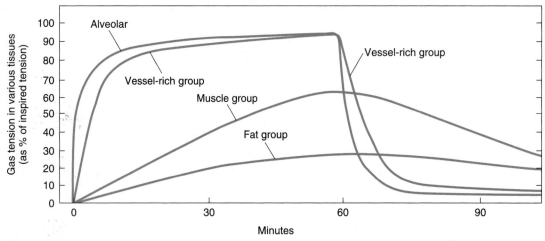

Figure 7–3. The rise and fall in alveolar partial pressure precedes that of other tissues. (Modified and reproduced, with permission, from Cowles AL et al: Uptake and distribution of inhalation anesthetic agents in clinical practice. Anesth Analg 1968;4:404.)

Concentration

The effects of uptake can also be reduced by increasing the inspired concentration. Interestingly, increasing the inspired concentration not only increases the alveolar concentration but also increases its rate of rise (ie, increases FA/FI). This has been termed the concentration effect (see Figure 7–1), which is really the result of two phenomena. The first is confusingly called the concentrating effect. If 50% of an anesthetic is taken up by the pulmonary circulation, an inspired concentration of 20% (20 parts of anesthetic per 100 parts of gas) will result in an alveolar concentration of 11% (10 parts of anesthetic remaining in a total volume of 90 parts of gas). On the other hand, if the inspired concentration is raised to 80% (80 parts of anesthetic per 100 parts of gas), the alveolar concentration will be 67% (40 parts of anesthetic remaining in a total volume of 60 parts of gas.). Thus, even though 50% of the anesthetic is taken up in both examples, a higher inspired concentration results in a disproportionately higher alveolar concentration. In this example, increasing the inspired concentration 4-fold results in a 6-fold increase in alveolar concentration. The extreme case is an inspired concentration of 100% (100 parts of 100), which, despite a 50% uptake, will result in an alveolar concentration of 100% (50 parts of anesthetic remaining in a total volume of 50 parts of gas).

The second phenomenon responsible for the concentration effect is the augmented inflow effect. Using the example above, the 10 parts of absorbed gas must be replaced by an equal volume of the 20% mixture to prevent alveolar collapse. Thus, the alveolar concentration becomes 12% (10 plus 2 parts of anesthetic in a total of 100 parts of gas). In contrast, after absorption of 50% of the anesthetic in the 80% gas mixture, 40 parts of 80% gas must be inspired. This further increases the alveolar concentration from 67% to 72% (40 plus 32 parts of anesthetic in a volume of 100 parts of gas).

The concentration effect is more significant with nitrous oxide than with the volatile anesthetics, as the former can be used in much higher concentrations. Nonetheless, a high concentration of nitrous oxide will augment (by the same mechanism) not only its own uptake but theoretically that of a concurrently administered volatile anesthetic. The concentration effect of one gas upon another is called the second gas effect, which is probably insignificant in the clinical practice of anesthesiology.

FACTORS AFFECTING ARTERIAL CONCENTRATION (Fa)

Ventilation/Perfusion Mismatch

Normally, alveolar and arterial anesthetic partial pressures are assumed to be equal, but in fact the arterial partial pressure is consistently less than end-expiratory gas would predict. Reasons for this may include venous admixture, alveolar dead space, and nonuniform alveolar gas distribution. Furthermore, the existence of ventilation/perfusion mismatching will increase the alveolar–arterial difference. Mismatch acts as a restriction to flow: It raises the pressure in front of the restriction, lowers the pressure beyond the restriction, and reduces the flow through the restriction. The overall effect is an increase in the alveolar partial pressure (particularly for highly soluble agents) and a decrease in the arterial partial pressure (particularly for poorly soluble agents). Thus, a bronchial intubation or a right-to-left intracardiac shunt will slow the rate of induction with nitrous oxide more than with halothane.

FACTORS AFFECTING ELIMINATION

Recovery from anesthesia depends on lowering the concentration of anesthetic in brain tissue. Anesthetics can be eliminated by biotransformation, transcutaneous loss, or exhalation. Biotransformation usually accounts for a minimal increase in the rate of decline of alveolar partial pressure. Its greatest impact is on the elimination of soluble anesthetics that undergo extensive metabolism (eg, methoxyflurane). The greater biotransformation of halothane compared with isoflurane accounts for halothane's faster elimination, even though it is more soluble. The cytochrome P-450 (CYP) group of isozymes (specifically CYP 2EI) appears to be important in the metabolism of some volatile anesthetics. Diffusion of anesthetic through the skin is insignificant.

The most important route for elimination of inhalation anesthetics is the alveolus. Many of the factors that speed induction also speed recovery: elimination of rebreathing, high fresh gas flows, low anesthetic-circuit volume, low absorption by the anesthetic circuit, decreased solubility, high cerebral blood flow (CBF), and increased ventilation. Elimination of nitrous oxide is so rapid that alveolar oxygen and CO_2 are diluted. The resulting **diffusion hypoxia** is prevented by administering 100% oxygen for 5–10 min after discontinuing nitrous oxide. The rate of recovery is usually faster than induction because tissues that have not reached equilibrium will continue to take up anesthetic until the alveolar partial pressure falls below the tissue partial pressure. For instance, fat will continue to take up anesthetic and hasten recovery until the partial pressure exceeds the alveolar partial pressure. This redistribution is not as available after prolonged anesthesia—thus, the speed of recovery also depends on the length of time the anesthetic has been administered.

■ PHARMACODYNAMICS OF INHALATION ANESTHETICS

THEORIES OF ANESTHETIC ACTION

General anesthesia is an altered physiological state characterized by reversible loss of consciousness, analgesia of the entire body, amnesia, and some degree of muscle relaxation. The multitude of substances capable of producing general anesthesia is remarkable: inert elements (xenon), simple inorganic compounds (nitrous oxide), halogenated hydrocarbons (halothane), and complex organic structures (barbiturates). A unifying theory explaining anesthetic action would have to accommodate this diversity of structure. In fact, the various agents probably produce anesthesia by different methods (agent-specific theory). For example, opioids are known to interact with stereospecific receptors, whereas inhalation agents do not have a predominant structure–activity relationship (opiate receptors may mediate some minor inhalation anesthetic effects).

There does not appear to be a single macroscopic site of action that is shared by all inhalation agents. Specific brain areas affected by various anesthetics include the reticular activating system, the cerebral cortex, the cuneate nucleus, the olfactory cortex, and the hippocampus. Anesthetics have also been shown to depress excitatory transmission in the spinal cord, particularly at the level of the dorsal horn interneurons that are involved in pain transmission. Differing aspects of anesthesia may be related to different sites of anesthetic action. For example, unconsciousness and amnesia are probably mediated by cortical anesthetic action, whereas the suppression of purposeful withdrawal from pain may be related to subcortical structures such as the spinal cord or brain stem. One study in rats revealed that removal of the cerebral cortex did not alter the potency of the anesthetic!

At a microscopic level, synaptic transmission is much more sensitive to general anesthetic agents than axonal conduction, though small-diameter nerve axons may be vulnerable. Both presynaptic and postsynaptic mechanisms are plausible.

The unitary hypothesis proposes that all inhalation agents share a common mechanism of action at the molecular level. This is supported by the observation that the anesthetic potency of inhalation agents correlates directly with their lipid solubility (Meyer–Overton rule). The implication is that anesthesia results from molecules dissolving at specific lipophilic sites. Of course, not all lipid-soluble molecules are anesthetics (some are actually convulsants), and the correlation between anesthetic potency and lipid solubility is only approximate (Figure 7–4).

Neuronal membranes contain a multitude of hydrophobic sites in their phospholipid bilayer. Anesthetic binding to these sites could expand the bilayer beyond a critical amount, altering membrane function (critical volume hypothesis). Although this theory is probably an oversimplification, it explains an interesting phenomenon: the reversal of anesthesia by increased pressure. Laboratory animals exposed to elevated hydro-

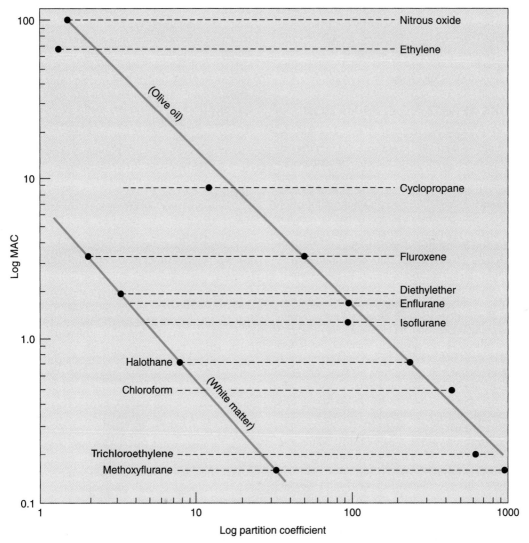

Figure 7–4. There is a good but not perfect correlation between anesthetic potency and lipid solubility. MAC, minimum alveolar concentration. (Modified and reproduced, with permission, from Lowe HJ, Hagler K: *Gas Chromatography in Biology and Medicine.* Churchill, 1969.)

static pressure develop a resistance to anesthetic effects. Perhaps the pressure is displacing a number of molecules from the membrane, increasing anesthetic requirements.

Anesthetic binding might significantly modify membrane structure. Two theories suggest disturbances in membrane form (the fluidization theory of anesthesia and the lateral phase separation theory); another theory proposes decreases in membrane conductance. Altering membrane structure could produce anesthesia in a number of ways. For instance, electrolyte perme-

ability could be changed by disrupting ion channels. Alternatively, hydrophobic membrane proteins might undergo conformational changes. In either event, synaptic function could be inhibited.

General anesthetic action could be due to alterations in any one of several cellular systems including ligand-gated ion channels, second messenger functions, or neurotransmitter receptors. For example, many anesthetics enhance γ-aminobutyric acid (GABA) inhibition of the central nervous system. Furthermore, GABA receptor agonists appear to enhance anesthesia, whereas

GABA antagonists reverse some anesthetic effects. There appears to be a strong correlation between anesthetic potency and potentiation of GABA receptor activity. Thus, anesthetic action may relate to hydrophobic binding to channel proteins (GABA receptors).

Modulation of GABA function may prove to be a principal mechanism of action for many anesthetic drugs.

The glycine receptor α_1-subunit, whose function is enhanced by inhalation anesthetics, is another receptor that is being extensively investigated.

Amino acids within an anesthetic-binding pocket could be modified by inhalation agents to conformationally change the receptor itself, or transduce an effect at a distant site.

Other ligand-gated ion channels whose modulation may play a role in anesthetic action include nicotinic acetylcholine receptors (see Chapter 10) and N-methyl-D-aspartate receptors.

MINIMUM ALVEOLAR CONCENTRATION

The minimum alveolar concentration (MAC) of an inhaled anesthetic is the alveolar concentration that prevents movement in 50% of patients in response to a standardized stimulus (eg, surgical incision). MAC is a useful measure because it mirrors brain partial pressure, allows comparisons of potency between agents, and provides a standard for experimental evaluations (Table 7–3). Nonetheless, it should be considered a statistical average with limited value in managing individual patients, particularly during times of rapidly changing alveolar concentrations (eg, induction).

The MAC values for different anesthetics are roughly additive. For example, a mixture of 0.5 MAC of nitrous oxide (53%) and 0.5 MAC of halothane (0.37%) approximates the degree of central nervous depression of 1.0 MAC of isoflurane (1.7%). In con-

Table 7–3. Properties of modern inhalation anesthetics.

Agent	Structure	MAC%[1]	Vapor Pressure (mm Hg at 20°C)
Nitrous oxide	$N=N$ — O	105[2]	—
Halothane (Fluothane)	F—C—C—H (with F, Cl, F, Br)	0.75	243
Isoflurane (Forane)	H—C—O—C—C—F (with F, H, F, Cl, F)	1.2	240
Desflurane (Suprane)	H—C—O—C—C—F (with F, H, F, F, F)	6.0	681
Sevoflurane (Ultane)	H—C—O—C with F—C—F groups	2.0	160

[1]These minimum alveolar concentration (MAC) values are for 30- to 55-year-old human subjects and are expressed as a percentage of 1 atmosphere. High altitude requires a higher inspired concentration of anesthetic to achieve the same partial pressure.

[2]A concentration greater than 100% means that hyperbaric conditions are required to achieve 1.0 MAC.

trast to central nervous system depression, the degree of myocardial depression may not be equivalent at the same MAC: 0.5 MAC of halothane causes more myocardial depression than 0.5 MAC of nitrous oxide. MAC represents only one point on the dose–response curve—it is the equivalent of a median effective dose (ED_{50}). MAC multiples are clinically useful if the dose–response curves of the anesthetics being compared are parallel, straight, and continuous for the effect being predicted. Roughly 1.3 MAC of any of the volatile anesthetics (eg, for halothane: $1.3 \times 0.74\%$ = 0.96%) has been found to prevent movement in about 95% of patients (an approximation of the ED_{95}); 0.3–0.4 MAC is associated with awakening from anesthesia (MAC awake).

MAC can be altered by several physiological and pharmacological variables (Table 7–4). **One of the most striking is the 6% decrease in MAC per decade of age, regardless of volatile anesthetic.** MAC is relatively unaffected by species, sex, or duration of anesthesia. Surprisingly, MAC is not altered after hypothermic spinal cord transection in rats, leading to the hypothesis that the site of anesthetic inhibition of motor responses lies in the spinal cord.

■ CLINICAL PHARMACOLOGY OF INHALATION ANESTHETICS

NITROUS OXIDE

Physical Properties

Nitrous oxide (N_2O; laughing gas) is the only inorganic anesthetic gas in clinical use (see Table 7–3). It is colorless and essentially odorless. Although nonexplosive and nonflammable, nitrous oxide is as capable as oxygen of supporting combustion. Unlike the potent volatile agents, nitrous oxide is a gas at room temperature and ambient pressure. It can be kept as a liquid under pressure because its critical temperature lies above room temperature (see Chapter 2). Nitrous oxide is a relatively inexpensive anesthetic, however, concerns regarding its safety have led to continued interest in alternatives such as **xenon** (Table 7–5).

Effects on Organ Systems

A. CARDIOVASCULAR

The circulatory effects of nitrous oxide are explained by its tendency to stimulate the sympathetic nervous system. Even though nitrous oxide directly depresses myocardial contractility in vitro, arterial blood pressure, cardiac output, and heart rate are essentially unchanged or slightly elevated in vivo because of its stimulation of catecholamines (Table 7–6). Myocardial depression may be unmasked in patients with coronary artery disease or severe hypovolemia. The resulting drop in arterial blood pressure may occasionally lead to myocardial ischemia. Constriction of pulmonary vascular smooth muscle increases pulmonary vascular resistance, which results in an elevation of right ventricular end-diastolic pressure. Despite vasoconstriction of cutaneous vessels, peripheral vascular resistance is not significantly altered. Because nitrous oxide increases endogenous catecholamine levels, it may be associated with a higher incidence of epinephrine-induced arrhythmias.

B. RESPIRATORY

Nitrous oxide increases respiratory rate (tachypnea) and decreases tidal volume as a result of central nervous system stimulation and, perhaps, activation of pulmonary stretch receptors. The net effect is a minimal change in minute ventilation and resting arterial CO_2 levels. Hypoxic drive, the ventilatory response to arterial hypoxia that is mediated by peripheral chemoreceptors in the carotid bodies, is markedly depressed by even small amounts of nitrous oxide. This has serious implications in the recovery room, where low arterial oxygen tensions in patients may go unrecognized.

C. CEREBRAL

By increasing CBF and cerebral blood volume, nitrous oxide produces a mild elevation of intracranial pressure. Nitrous oxide also increases cerebral oxygen consumption ($CMRO_2$). Levels of nitrous oxide below MAC provide analgesia in dental surgery and other minor procedures.

D. NEUROMUSCULAR

In contrast to other inhalation agents, nitrous oxide does not provide significant muscle relaxation. In fact, at high concentrations in hyperbaric chambers, nitrous oxide causes skeletal muscle rigidity. Nitrous oxide is probably not a triggering agent of malignant hyperthermia.

E. RENAL

Nitrous oxide appears to decrease renal blood flow by increasing renal vascular resistance. This leads to a drop in glomerular filtration rate and urinary output.

F. HEPATIC

Hepatic blood flow probably falls during nitrous oxide anesthesia, but to a lesser extent than with the other volatile agents.

Table 7–4. Factors affecting MAC.[1]

Variable	Effect on MAC	Comments
Temperature		
Hypothermia	↓	
Hyperthermia	↓	↑ if > 42°C
Age		
Young	↑	
Elderly	↓	
Alcohol		
Acute intoxication	↓	
Chronic abuse	↑	
Anemia		
Hematocrit < 10%	↓	
Pao$_2$		
< 40 mm Hg	↓	
Paco$_2$		
> 95 mm Hg	↓	Caused by < pH in CSF
Thyroid		
Hyperthyroid	No change	
Hypothyroid	No change	
Blood pressure		
MAP < 40 mm Hg	↓	
Electrolytes		
Hypercalcemia	↓	
Hypernatremia	↑	Caused by altered CSF[2]
Hyponatremia	↓	Caused by altered CSF
Pregnancy	↓	MAC decreased by one-third at 8 weeks' gestation; normal by 72 h postpartum
Drugs		
Local anesthetics	↓	Except cocaine
Opioids	↓	
Ketamine	↓	
Barbiturates	↓	
Benzodiazepines	↓	
Verapamil	↓	
Lithium	↓	
Sympatholytics		
Methyldopa	↓	
Clonidine	↓	
Dexmedetomidine	↓	
Sympathomimetics		
Amphetamine		
Chronic	↓	
Acute	↑	
Cocaine	↑	
Ephedrine	↑	

[1]These conclusions are based on human and animal studies.
[2]CSF, cerebrospinal fluid.

Table 7–5. Advantages and disadvantages of xenon (Xe) anesthesia.

Advantages
Inert (probably nontoxic with no metabolism)
Minimal cardiovascular effects
Low blood solubility
Rapid induction and recovery
Does not trigger malignant hyperthermia
Environmentally friendly
Nonexplosive
Disadvantages
High cost
Low potency (MAC = 70%)[1]
No commercially available anesthesia equipment

[1]MAC, minimum alveolar concentration.

G. Gastrointestinal

Some studies have suggested that nitrous oxide is a cause of postoperative nausea and vomiting, presumably as a result of activation of the chemoreceptor trigger zone and the vomiting center in the medulla. Other studies, particularly in children, have failed to demonstrate any association between nitrous oxide and emesis.

Biotransformation & Toxicity

During emergence, almost all nitrous oxide is eliminated by exhalation. A small amount diffuses out through the skin. Biotransformation is limited to the less than 0.01% that undergoes reductive metabolism in the gastrointestinal tract by anaerobic bacteria.

By irreversibly oxidizing the cobalt atom in vitamin B_{12}, nitrous oxide inhibits enzymes that are vitamin B_{12} dependent. These enzymes include methionine synthetase, which is necessary for myelin formation, and thymidylate synthetase, which is necessary for DNA synthesis. Prolonged exposure to anesthetic concentrations of nitrous oxide can result in bone marrow depression (megaloblastic anemia) and even neurological deficiencies (peripheral neuropathies and pernicious anemia). However, administration of nitrous oxide for bone marrow harvest does not appear to affect the viability of bone marrow mononuclear cells. Because of possible teratogenic effects, nitrous oxide is often avoided in patients who are pregnant. Nitrous oxide may also alter the immunological response to infection by affecting chemotaxis and motility of polymorphonuclear leukocytes.

Contraindications

Although nitrous oxide is insoluble in comparison with other inhalation agents, it is 35 times more soluble than nitrogen in blood. Thus, it tends to diffuse into air-containing cavities more rapidly than nitrogen is absorbed by the bloodstream. For instance, if a patient with a 100-mL pneumothorax inhales 50% nitrous oxide, the gas content of the pneumothorax will tend to approach that of the bloodstream. Because nitrous oxide will diffuse into the cavity more rapidly than the air (principally nitrogen) diffuses out, the pneumothorax expands until it contains 100 mL of air and 100 mL of nitrous oxide. If the walls surrounding the cavity are rigid, pressure rises instead of volume. **Examples of conditions in which nitrous oxide might be hazardous include air embolism, pneumothorax, acute intestinal obstruction, intracranial air (tension pneumocephalus following dural closure or pneumoencephalography), pulmonary air cysts, intraocular air bubbles, and tympanic membrane grafting.** Nitrous oxide will even diffuse into tracheal tube cuffs, increasing the pressure against the tracheal mucosa.

Because of the effect of nitrous oxide on the pulmonary vasculature, it should be avoided in patients with pulmonary hypertension. Obviously, nitrous oxide is of limited value in patients requiring high inspired oxygen concentrations.

Drug Interactions

Because the relatively high MAC of nitrous oxide prevents its use as a complete general anesthetic, it is frequently used in combination with the more potent volatile agents. The addition of nitrous oxide decreases the requirements of these other agents (65% nitrous oxide decreases the MAC of the volatile anesthetics by approximately 50%). Although nitrous oxide should not be considered a benign carrier gas, it does attenuate the circulatory and respiratory effects of volatile anesthetics in adults. Nitrous oxide potentiates neuromuscular blockade, but less so than the volatile agents (see Chapter 9). The concentration of nitrous oxide flowing through a vaporizer can influence the concentration of volatile anesthetic delivered. For example, decreasing nitrous oxide concentration (ie, increasing oxygen concentration) increases the concentration of volatile agent despite a constant vaporizer setting. This disparity is due to the relative solubilities of nitrous oxide and oxygen in liquid volatile anesthetics. The second gas effect was discussed earlier.

HALOTHANE

Physical Properties

Halothane is a halogenated alkane (see Table 7–3). The carbon–fluoride bonds are responsible for its nonflammable and nonexplosive nature. Thymol preservative and amber-colored bottles retard spon-

Table 7–6. Clinical pharmacology of inhalational anesthetics.

	Nitrous Oxide	Halothane	Isoflurane	Desflurane	Sevoflurane
Cardiovascular					
Blood pressure	N/C[1]	↓↓	↓↓	↓↓	↓
Heart rate	N/C	↓	↑	N/C or ↑	N/C
Systemic vascular resistance	N/C	N/C	↓↓	↓↓	↓
Cardiac output[2]	N/C	↓	N/C	N/C or ↓	↓
Respiratory					
Tidal volume	↓	↓↓	↓↓	↓	↓
Respiratory rate	↑	↑↑	↑	↑	↑
Paco₂					
Resting	N/C	↑	↑	↑↑	↑
Challenge	↑	↑	↑	↑↑	↑
Cerebral					
Blood flow	↑	↑↑	↑	↑	↑
Intracranial pressure	↑	↑↑	↑	↑	↑
Cerebral metabolic rate	↑	↓	↓↓	↓↓	↓↓
Seizures	↓	↓	↓	↓	↓
Neuromuscular					
Nondepolarizing blockade[3]	↑	↑↑	↑↑↑	↑↑↑	↑↑
Renal					
Renal blood flow	↓↓	↓↓	↓↓	↓	↓
Glomerular filtration rate	↓↓	↓↓	↓↓	↓	↓
Urinary output	↓↓	↓↓	↓↓	↓	↓
Hepatic					
Blood flow	↓	↓↓	↓	↓	↓
Metabolism[4]	0.004%	15–20%	0.2%	< 0.1%	5%

[1]N/C, no change.
[2]Controlled ventilation.
[3]Depolarizing blockage is probably also prolonged by these agents, but this is usually not clinically significant.
[4]Percentage of absorbed anesthetic undergoing metabolism.

taneous oxidative decomposition. Halothane is the least expensive volatile anesthetic, and because of its safety profile (see below), continues to be used worldwide.

Effects on Organ Systems

A. CARDIOVASCULAR

A dose-dependent reduction of arterial blood pressure is due to direct myocardial depression; 2.0 MAC of halothane results in a 50% decrease in blood pressure and cardiac output. Cardiac depression—from interference with sodium–calcium exchange and intracellular calcium utilization—causes an increase in right atrial pressure. Although halothane is a coronary artery vasodilator, coronary blood flow decreases, due to the drop in systemic arterial pressure. Adequate myocardial perfusion is usually maintained, as oxygen demand also drops. Normally, hypotension inhibits baroreceptors in the aortic arch and carotid bifurcation, causing a decrease in vagal stimulation and a compensatory rise in heart rate. Halothane blunts this reflex. Slowing of sinoatrial node conduction may result in a junctional rhythm or bradycardia. In infants, halothane decreases cardiac output by a combination of decreased heart rate and depressed myocardial contractility. Halothane sensitizes the heart to the arrhythmogenic effects of epinephrine, so that doses of epinephrine above 1.5 μg/kg should be avoided. This phenomenon may be a result of halothane interfering with slow calcium channel conductance. Although organ blood flow is redistributed, systemic vascular resistance is unchanged.

B. Respiratory

Halothane typically causes rapid, shallow breathing. The increased respiratory rate is not enough to counter the decreased tidal volume, so alveolar ventilation drops and resting $PaCO_2$ is elevated. **Apneic threshold,** the highest $PaCO_2$ at which a patient remains apneic, also rises because the difference between it and resting $PaCO_2$ is not altered by general anesthesia. Similarly, halothane limits the increase in minute ventilation that normally accompanies a rise in $PaCO_2$. Halothane's ventilatory effects are probably due to central (medullary depression) and peripheral (intercostal muscle dysfunction) mechanisms. These changes are exaggerated by preexisting lung disease and attenuated by surgical stimulation. The increase in $PaCO_2$ and the decrease in intrathoracic pressure that accompany spontaneous ventilation with halothane partially reverse the depression in cardiac output, arterial blood pressure, and heart rate described above. Hypoxic drive is severely depressed by even low concentrations of halothane (0.1 MAC).

Halothane is considered a potent bronchodilator, as it often reverses asthma-induced bronchospasm. In fact, halothane may be the best bronchodilator among the currently available volatile anesthetics. This action is not inhibited by propranolol, a β-adrenergic blocking agent. Halothane attenuates airway reflexes and relaxes bronchial smooth muscle by inhibiting intracellular calcium mobilization. Halothane also depresses clearance of mucus from the respiratory tract (mucociliary function), promoting postoperative hypoxia and atelectasis.

C. Cerebral

By dilating cerebral vessels, halothane lowers cerebral vascular resistance and increases CBF. **Autoregulation,** the maintenance of constant CBF during changes in arterial blood pressure, is blunted. Concomitant rises in intracranial pressure can be prevented by establishing hyperventilation *prior to* administration of halothane. Cerebral activity is decreased, leading to electroencephalographic slowing and modest reductions in metabolic oxygen requirements.

D. Neuromuscular

Halothane relaxes skeletal muscle and potentiates nondepolarizing neuromuscular-blocking agents (NMBA). Like the other potent volatile anesthetics, it is a triggering agent of malignant hyperthermia.

E. Renal

Halothane reduces renal blood flow, glomerular filtration rate, and urinary output. Part of this decrease can be explained by a fall in arterial blood pressure and cardiac output. Because the reduction in renal blood flow is greater than the reduction in glomerular filtration

rate, the filtration fraction is increased. Preoperative hydration limits these changes.

F. Hepatic

Halothane causes hepatic blood flow to decrease in proportion to the depression of cardiac output. Hepatic artery vasospasm has been reported during halothane anesthesia. The metabolism and clearance of some drugs (eg, fentanyl, phenytoin, verapamil) appear to be impaired by halothane. Other evidence of hepatic cellular dysfunction includes sulfobromophthalein (BSP) dye retention and minor liver transaminase elevations.

Biotransformation & Toxicity

Halothane is oxidized in the liver by a particular isozyme of cytochrome P-450 (2EI) to its principal metabolite, trifluoroacetic acid. This metabolism can be inhibited by pretreatment with disulfiram. Bromide, another oxidative metabolite, has been incriminated in but is an improbable cause of postanesthetic changes in mental status. In the absence of oxygen, reductive metabolism may result in a small amount of hepatotoxic end products that covalently bind to tissue macromolecules. This is more apt to occur following enzyme induction by phenobarbital. Elevated fluoride levels signal significant anaerobic metabolism.

Postoperative hepatic dysfunction has several causes: viral hepatitis, impaired hepatic perfusion, preexisting liver disease, hepatocyte hypoxia, sepsis, hemolysis, benign postoperative intrahepatic cholestasis, and drug-induced hepatitis. **Halothane hepatitis** is extremely rare (1 per 35,000 cases). Patients exposed to multiple halothane anesthetics at short intervals, middle-aged obese women, and persons with a familial predisposition to halothane toxicity or a personal history of toxicity are considered to be at increased risk. Signs include increased serum alanine and aspartate transferase, elevated bilirubin (leading to jaundice), and encephalopathy.

The hepatic lesion seen in humans—centrilobular necrosis—also occurs in rats pretreated with an enzyme inducer (phenobarbital) and exposed to halothane under hypoxic conditions ($FIO_2 < 14\%$). This *halothane hypoxic model* implies hepatic damage from reductive metabolites or hypoxia.

More recent evidence points to an immune mechanism. For instance, some signs of the disease indicate an allergic reaction (eg, eosinophilia, rash, fever) and do not appear until a few days after exposure. Furthermore, an antibody that binds to hepatocytes previously exposed to halothane has been isolated from patients with halothane-induced hepatic dysfunction. This antibody response may involve liver microsomal proteins that have been modified by trifluoroacetic acid as the triggering antigens (trifluoroacetylated liver proteins such as microsomal carboxylesterase).

Contraindications

It is prudent to withhold halothane from patients with unexplained liver dysfunction following previous exposure. Because halothane hepatitis appears to affect primarily adults and children past puberty, some anesthesiologists choose other volatile anesthetics in these patients. There is no compelling evidence associating halothane with worsening of preexisting liver disease.

Halothane should be used with great caution in patients with intracranial mass lesions because of the possibility of intracranial hypertension.

Hypovolemic patients and some patients with severe cardiac disease (aortic stenosis) may not tolerate halothane's negative inotropic effects. Sensitization of the heart to catecholamines limits the usefulness of halothane when exogenous epinephrine is administered or in patients with pheochromocytoma.

Drug Interactions

The myocardial depression seen with halothane is exacerbated by β-adrenergic-blocking agents (eg, propranolol) and calcium channel-blocking agents (eg, verapamil). Tricyclic antidepressants and monoamine oxidase inhibitors have been associated with fluctuations in blood pressure and arrhythmias, although neither represents an absolute contraindication. The combination of halothane and aminophylline has resulted in serious ventricular arrhythmias.

ISOFLURANE

Physical Properties

Isoflurane is a nonflammable volatile anesthetic with a pungent ethereal odor. Although it is a chemical isomer of enflurane, it has different physicochemical properties (see Table 7–3).

Effects on Organ Systems

A. CARDIOVASCULAR

Isoflurane causes minimal cardiac depression in vivo. Cardiac output is maintained by a rise in heart rate due to partial preservation of carotid baroreflexes. Mild β-adrenergic stimulation increases skeletal muscle blood flow, decreases systemic vascular resistance, and lowers arterial blood pressure. Rapid increases in isoflurane concentration lead to transient increases in heart rate, arterial blood pressure, and plasma levels of norepinephrine. Isoflurane dilates coronary arteries, but is not nearly as potent a dilator as nitroglycerin or

adenosine. Dilation of normal coronary arteries could theoretically divert blood away from fixed stenotic lesions. There have been conflicting reports regarding whether this coronary steal syndrome causes regional myocardial ischemia during episodes of tachycardia or drops in perfusion pressure. Despite the negative results of several large outcome studies, some anesthesiologists still avoid isoflurane in patients with coronary artery disease.

B. RESPIRATORY

Respiratory depression during isoflurane anesthesia resembles that of other volatile anesthetics, except that tachypnea is less pronounced. The net effect is a more pronounced fall in minute ventilation. Even low levels of isoflurane (0.1 MAC) blunt the normal ventilatory response to hypoxia and hypercapnia. Despite a tendency to irritate upper airway reflexes, isoflurane is considered a good bronchodilator, but may not be as potent a bronchodilator as halothane.

C. CEREBRAL

At concentrations greater than 1 MAC, isoflurane increases CBF and intracranial pressure. These effects are thought to be less pronounced than with halothane and are reversed by hyperventilation. In contrast to halothane, the hyperventilation does not have to be instituted prior to the use of isoflurane to prevent intracranial hypertension. Isoflurane reduces cerebral metabolic oxygen requirements, and at 2 MAC it produces an electrically silent electroencephalogram (EEG). EEG suppression probably provides some degree of brain protection during episodes of cerebral ischemia.

D. NEUROMUSCULAR

Isoflurane relaxes skeletal muscle.

E. RENAL

Isoflurane decreases renal blood flow, glomerular filtration rate, and urinary output.

F. HEPATIC

Total hepatic blood flow (hepatic artery and portal vein flow) is reduced during isoflurane anesthesia. Hepatic oxygen supply may be better maintained with isoflurane than with halothane, however, because hepatic artery perfusion and hepatic venous oxygen saturation are preserved. Liver function tests are minimally affected.

Biotransformation & Toxicity

Isoflurane is metabolized to trifluoroacetic acid. Although serum fluoride fluid levels may rise, nephrotoxicity is extremely unlikely even in the presence of enzyme inducers. Prolonged sedation (> 24 h at 0.1–0.6% isoflurane) of critically ill patients has resulted in elevated

Gerald A. Gronert, MD

MALIGNANT HYPERTHERMIA

Genetics

The most fascinating genetic aspect of malignant hyperthermia (MH) is the single-point ryanodine receptor mutation in all susceptible swine (eg, Poland China, Pietrain, Landrace), featuring extreme muscularity, hybrid vigor, and susceptibility to stress. This single-point mutation is shared by muscular breeds in all countries (South and North America, Europe, Asia, Australia, South Africa, and Japan). This implies that a boar (or sow), perhaps 150 years ago, developed this mutation, with its desirable heavy musculature, and bred true. Because swine breeders shared stock, the mutation became widespread, despite difficult transportation. It seems inconceivable that this mutation arose de novo in multiple areas. This shared mutation permits DNA testing of blood to guide breeding and to prevent what used to be a several hundred million dollar annual loss in abattoir pork. Stresses of slaughter triggered unrealized excessive metabolism and the meat rotted during the 45-min delay to refrigeration. David MacLennan's laboratory at the University of Toronto isolated the mutation,[1] and testing of litters has provided substantial university income.

Humans, with uncontrolled breeding, have multiple mutations in the ryanodine receptor, per-

haps 40–50; selection of subjects can provide about a 50% detection rate for susceptibility using DNA analysis of blood or a cheek swab.[2] The gold standard for testing remains the vastus muscle contracture test, but there are problems related to testing. The patient must travel to a test center, for the specimen must be viable, ie, twitch to electrical stimuli. In Europe, there are many test centers, well situated for convenient patient travel. The cost to the patient, shared by governments and universities, is minimal. In North America, there are only about six centers, widely dispersed; testing is costly (eg, $4000–$6000 per patient), with poor coverage by medical insurance and/or government. In addition, few patients can afford the costs of travel. Contractures are the initial basic test in Europe; however, the expense is prohibitive in North America. DNA testing in North America is presently focused on patients who have undergone contracture testing in the past and identifies mutations on this continent.

Heat Stroke—Awake MH?

Some MH-susceptible patients do not tolerate exposure to heat, but cases of heat stroke are rare: a 12-year-old boy with a fractured humerus developed MH during sevoflurane anesthesia.[3] He recovered with appropriate therapy, but had a fatal heat stroke 8 months later. While playing football in humid warm (26°C) weather, he became hot and sweaty, hyperventilated, seized, arrested, and died (rectal temperature >108°F [42.2°C]; arterial blood gas: pH 6.76, P_{CO_2} 115, P_{O_2} 22, K^+ 8.8, increasing to 14.5 mEq/L). DNA analysis on him and his father demonstrated a typical MH ryanodine mutation, C487T, in both, substituting arginine for 163 cysteine. Swine are excitable and easily triggered in the awake state, but this is rare in humans.

Statins

Skeletal muscle is abnormal in MH-susceptible persons even though the myopathy is subclinical. Statins alter skeletal muscle permeability and metabolism via inhibition of the formation of mevalonate—a cholesterol precursor; in addition, they can inhibit mitochondrial production of ATPase, thus impairing energy metabolism. These can result in increased creatine kinase (CK), and, in time, muscle breakdown, *or rhabdomyolysis. This response occurs in some normal patients, but there is no direct evidence that it is more likely in MH patients. However, professional athletes with familial hypercholesterolemia rarely tolerate statin treatment because of muscular problems.[4] Sixteen of 22 athletes who had been followed for 8 years could not tolerate statins. Do professional athletes as a group (admittedly small) respond like this because of extreme conditioning or an acquired muscle sensitivity? Or are they athletes because they have a myopathy that lends itself to great performance? MH patients may react adversely to conditions that alter muscle permeability or metabolism, but I know of no examples other than anesthesia.*

MH Episodes

Episodes of MH now occur less frequently for three reasons: (1) the decreased use of triggers, eg, the potent volatile agents and succinylcholine (SCh), (2) delay in triggering of MH by volatile agents, due to the use of nondepolarizers, tranquilizers, sedatives, opioids, or barbiturates,[5] and (3) the protective effect of minor hypothermia.[6] MH is now detected earlier because of better awareness and more sophisticated monitoring, eg, end-expired CO_2. Early signs include tachycardia or rigidity. Treatment involves notifying the surgeon, discontinuing volatile agents or SCh, giving 100% O_2, stopping anesthesia or continuing with nontriggers, dantrolene 2.5 mg/kg, hyperventilation for respiratory acidosis, bicarbonate for metabolic acidosis, cooling for high temperatures, diuresis for pigmenturia, and calcium if there is dangerous hyperkalemia. Dantrolene should be continued for 24 h, 1 mg/kg every 6 h, as there is a 50% recurrence rate.[7] It is important to remember to fill out an American Medical Record Association (AMRA) form for Malignant Hyperthermia of the US (MHAUS) and the North American MH Registry. This is easy to forget once the excitement and confusion are gone.

Temperature Monitoring

There are cogent reasons to monitor temperature, particularly for procedures longer than an hour. For patients who are well covered by almost impervious plastic drapes, eg, head, neck, or limb procedures, and who are being warmed, the temperature may increase. Without ongoing data, the terminal acid–base and vital signs of iatrogenic hyperthermia resemble those of MH. Monitoring of temperature is best done via esophageal stethoscope/thermistor, bladder, rectum, tympanic membrane, or other areas of access to core values. Of four such cases that I know of—a 7-year-old for tympanoplasty, a teenager for sinus surgery, a husky athletic young adult for rhinoplasty, and a mother for breast augmentation—three died. We do not know which were actually MH.

Rhabdomyolysis & Sudden Cardiac Arrest

Patients with unsuspected myopathies may react to potent volatile agents or SCh with sudden muscle breakdown, with release of myoglobin, potassium, and CK. With rapid breakdown, potassium cannot be quickly redistributed, and difficult-to-treat hyperkalemia may result.[8] Myoglobin is a renal toxin, but has a slower less critical onset. Statins can be a factor in this response.

Anesthetic Routine

Necessities for detecting problems in anesthesia include analysis of expired gas, monitoring temperature, vital signs (including stethoscope), dantrolene, bicarbonate, and calcium, and access to laboratory facilities (for blood gases and electrolytes).

1. Fujii J, Otsu K, Zorzato F, et al: Identification of a mutation in porcine ryanodine receptor associated with malignant hyperthermia. Science 1991;253:448.

2. Girard T, Treves S, Voronkov E, et al: Molecular genetic testing for malignant hyperthermia susceptibility. Anesthesiology 2004;100:1076.

3. Tobin JR, Jason DR, Nelson TE, Sambuughin N: Malignant hyperthermia and apparent heat stroke. JAMA 2001;286:168.

4. Sinzinger H, O'Grady J: Professional athletes suffering from familial hypercholesterolaemia rarely tolerate statin treatment because of muscular problems. Br J Clin Pharmacol 2004;57:525.

5. Gronert GA, Milde JH: Variations in onset of porcine malignant hyperthermia. Anesth Analg 1981;60:499.

6. Nelson TE: Porcine malignant hyperthermia: critical temperatures for in vivo and in vitro responses. Anesthesiology 1990;73:449.

7. Brandom BW, Larach MG, North American MH Registry: Reassessment of the safety and efficacy of dantrolene. Anesthesiology 2002;97:A1199.

8. Gronert GA: Cardiac arrest after succinylcholine. Mortality greater with rhabdomyolysis than receptor upregulation. Anesthesiology 2001;94:523.

plasma fluoride levels (15–50 µmol/L) without evidence of renal impairment. Similarly, up to 20 MAC-hours of isoflurane may lead to fluoride levels exceeding 50 µmol/L without detectable postoperative renal dysfunction. Its limited metabolism also minimizes any possible risk of significant hepatic dysfunction.

Contraindications

Isoflurane presents no unique contraindications. Patients with severe hypovolemia may not tolerate its vasodilating effects.

Drug Interactions

Epinephrine can be safely administered in doses up to 4.5 µg/kg. Nondepolarizing NMBAs are potentiated by isoflurane.

DESFLURANE

Physical Properties

The structure of desflurane is very similar to that of isoflurane. In fact, the only difference is the substitution of a fluorine atom for isoflurane's chlorine atom. That "minor" change has profound effects on the physical properties of the drug, however. For instance, because the vapor pressure of desflurane at 20°C is 681 mm Hg, at high altitudes it boils at room temperature (eg, Denver, Colorado). This problem necessitated the development of a special desflurane vaporizer (see Chapter 4). Furthermore, the low solubility of desflurane in blood and body tissues causes a very rapid washin and washout of anesthetic. Therefore, the alveolar concentration of desflurane approaches the inspired concentration much more rapidly than the other volatile agents, giving the anesthesiologist tighter control over anesthetic levels. **Wakeup times are approximately 50% less than those observed following isoflurane.** This is principally attributable to a blood/gas partition coefficient (0.42) that is even lower than that of nitrous oxide (0.47). Although desflurane is roughly one-fourth as potent as the other volatile agents, it is 17 times more potent than nitrous oxide. A high vapor pressure, an ultrashort duration of action, and moderate potency are the most characteristic features of desflurane.

Effects on Organ Systems

A. CARDIOVASCULAR

The cardiovascular effects of desflurane appear to be similar to those of isoflurane. Increasing the dose is associated with a decline in systemic vascular resistance that leads to a fall in arterial blood pressure. Cardiac output remains relatively unchanged or slightly depressed at 1–2

MAC. There is a moderate rise in heart rate, central venous pressure, and pulmonary artery pressure that often does not become apparent at low doses. Rapid increases in desflurane concentration lead to transient but sometimes worrisome elevations in heart rate, blood pressure, and catecholamine levels that are more pronounced than occur with isoflurane, particularly in patients with cardiovascular disease. These cardiovascular responses to rapidly increasing desflurane concentration can be attenuated by fentanyl, esmolol, or clonidine. Unlike isoflurane, desflurane does not increase coronary artery blood flow.

B. RESPIRATORY

Desflurane causes a decrease in tidal volume and an increase in respiratory rate. There is an overall decrease in alveolar ventilation that causes a rise in resting $PaCO_2$. Like other modern volatile anesthetic agents, desflurane depresses the ventilatory response to increasing $PaCO_2$. Pungency and airway irritation during desflurane induction can be manifested by salivation, breath-holding, coughing, and laryngospasm. These problems make desflurane less than ideally suited for inhalation inductions.

C. CEREBRAL

Like the other volatile anesthetics, desflurane directly vasodilates the cerebral vasculature, increasing CBF and intracranial pressure at normotension and normocapnia. Countering the decrease in cerebral vascular resistance is a marked decline in the cerebral metabolic rate of oxygen ($CMRO_2$) that tends to cause cerebral vasoconstriction and moderate any increase in CBF. The cerebral vasculature remains responsive to changes in $PaCO_2$, however, so that intracranial pressure can be lowered by hyperventilation. Cerebral oxygen consumption is decreased during desflurane anesthesia. Thus, during periods of desflurane-induced hypotension (mean arterial pressure = 60 mm Hg), CBF is adequate to maintain aerobic metabolism despite a low cerebral perfusion pressure. The effect on the EEG is similar to that of isoflurane.

D. NEUROMUSCULAR

Desflurane is associated with a dose-dependent decrease in the response to train-of-four and tetanic peripheral nerve stimulation.

E. RENAL

There is no evidence of any nephrotoxic effects caused by exposure to desflurane.

F. HEPATIC

Hepatic function tests are unaffected, and there is no evidence of hepatic injury following desflurane anesthesia.

Biotransformation & Toxicity

Desflurane undergoes minimal metabolism in humans. Serum and urine inorganic fluoride levels following desflurane anesthesia are essentially unchanged from preanesthetic levels. There is insignificant percutaneous loss. Desflurane, more than other volatile anesthetics, is degraded by desiccated carbon dioxide absorbent (particularly barium hydroxide lime, but also sodium and potassium hydroxide) into potentially clinically significant levels of carbon monoxide. Carbon monoxide poisoning is difficult to diagnose under general anesthesia, but the presence of carboxyhemoglobin may be detectable by arterial blood gas analysis or lower than expected pulse oximetry readings (although still falsely high). Disposing of dried out absorbent or use of calcium hydroxide (see Chapter 3) can minimize the risk of carbon monoxide poisoning.

Contraindications

Desflurane shares many of the contraindications of other modern volatile anesthetics: severe hypovolemia, malignant hyperthermia, and intracranial hypertension.

Drug Interactions

Desflurane potentiates nondepolarizing neuromuscular blocking agents to the same extent as isoflurane. Epinephrine can be safely administered in doses up to 4.5 μg/kg as desflurane does not sensitize the myocardium to the arrhythmogenic effects of epinephrine. Although emergence is more rapid following desflurane anesthesia than after isoflurane anesthesia, switching from isoflurane to desflurane toward the end of anesthesia does not significantly accelerate recovery nor does faster emergence translate into faster discharge times from the postanesthesia care unit. Desflurane emergence has been associated with delirium in some pediatric patients.

SEVOFLURANE

Physical Properties

Like desflurane, sevoflurane is halogenated with fluorine. Sevoflurane combines a solubility in blood slightly greater than desflurane ($\lambda_{b/g}$ 0.65 versus 0.42) (see Table 7–3). Nonpungency and rapid increases in alveolar anesthetic concentration make sevoflurane an excellent choice for smooth and rapid inhalation inductions in pediatric and adult patients. In fact, inhalation induction with 4–8% sevoflurane in a 50% mixture of nitrous oxide and oxygen can be achieved in approximately 1–3 min. Likewise, its low blood solubility results in a rapid fall in alveolar anesthetic concentration upon discontinuation and a more rapid emergence compared with isoflurane (although not an earlier discharge from the postanesthesia care unit). As with desflurane, this faster emergence has been associated with a greater incidence of delirium in some pediatric populations, which can be successfully treated with 1.0–2.0 μg/kg of fentanyl. Sevoflurane's modest vapor pressure permits the use of a conventional variable bypass vaporizer.

Effects on Organ Systems

A. CARDIOVASCULAR

Sevoflurane mildly depresses myocardial contractility. Systemic vascular resistance and arterial blood pressure decline slightly less than with isoflurane or desflurane. Because sevoflurane causes little, if any, rise in heart rate, cardiac output is not maintained as well as with isoflurane or desflurane. There is no evidence associating sevoflurane with coronary steal syndrome. Sevoflurane may prolong the QT interval, the clinical significance of which is unknown.

B. RESPIRATORY

Sevoflurane depresses respiration and reverses bronchospasm to an extent similar to that of isoflurane.

C. CEREBRAL

Similar to isoflurane and desflurane, sevoflurane causes slight increases in CBF and intracranial pressure at normocarbia, although some studies show a decrease in cerebral blood flow. High concentrations of sevoflurane (> 1.5 MAC) may impair autoregulation of CBF, thus allowing a drop in CBF during hemorrhagic hypotension. This effect on CBF autoregulation appears to be less pronounced than with isoflurane. Cerebral metabolic oxygen requirements decrease, and seizure activity has not been reported.

D. NEUROMUSCULAR

Sevoflurane produces adequate muscle relaxation for intubation of children following an inhalation induction.

E. RENAL

Sevoflurane slightly decreases renal blood flow. Its metabolism to substances associated with impaired renal tubule function (eg, decreased concentrating ability) is discussed below.

F. HEPATIC

Sevoflurane decreases portal vein blood flow, but increases hepatic artery blood flow, thereby maintaining total hepatic blood flow and oxygen delivery.

Biotransformation & Toxicity

The liver microsomal enzyme P-450 (specifically the 2E1 isoform) metabolizes sevoflurane at a rate one-fourth that of halothane (5% versus 20%), but 10 to 25 times that of isoflurane or desflurane and may be induced with ethanol or phenobarbital pretreatment. The potential nephrotoxicity of the resulting rise in inorganic fluoride (F^-) was discussed earlier. Serum fluoride concentrations exceed 50 μmol/L in approximately 7% of patients who receive sevoflurane, yet clinically significant renal dysfunction has not been associated with sevoflurane anesthesia. The overall rate of sevoflurane metabolism is 5%, or 10 times that of isoflurane. Nonetheless, there has been no association with peak fluoride levels following sevoflurane and any renal concentrating abnormality.

Alkali such as barium hydroxide lime or soda lime (but not calcium hydroxide—see Chapter 3) can degrade sevoflurane, producing another proven (at least in rats) nephrotoxic end product (*compound A*, fluoromethyl-2,2-difluoro-1-[trifluoromethyl]vinyl ether). Accumulation of compound A increases with increased respiratory gas temperature, low-flow anesthesia (see Case Discussion, following), dry barium hydroxide absorbent (Baralyme), high sevoflurane concentrations, and anesthetics of long duration.

Most studies have not associated sevoflurane with any detectable postoperative impairment of renal function that would indicate toxicity or injury. Nonetheless, some clinicians recommend that fresh gas flows be at least 2 L/min for anesthetics lasting more than a few hours and that sevoflurane not be used in patients with preexisting renal dysfunction.

Sevoflurane can also be degraded into hydrogen fluoride by metal and environmental impurities present in manufacturing equipment, glass bottle packaging, and anesthesia equipment. Hydrogen fluoride can produce an acid burn on contact with respiratory mucosa. The risk of patient injury has been substantially reduced by inhibition of the degradation process by adding water to sevoflurane during the manufacturing process and packaging it in a special plastic container. The manufacturer has also distributed a "Dear Provider" letter warning of isolated incidents of fire in the respiratory circuits of anesthesia machines with desiccated CO_2 absorbent when sevoflurane was used.

Contraindications

Contraindications include severe hypovolemia, susceptibility to malignant hyperthermia, and intracranial hypertension.

Drug Interactions

Like other volatile anesthetics, sevoflurane potentiates NMBAs. It does not sensitize the heart to catecholamine-induced arrhythmias.

CASE DISCUSSION: CLOSED-CIRCUIT ANESTHESIA[1]

A 22-year-old man weighing 70 kg is scheduled for shoulder reconstruction under general anesthesia. You are considering a closed-circuit anesthetic technique.

Describe closed-circuit anesthesia and indicate how it differs from other techniques.

Anesthesia systems can be classified as nonrebreathing, partial rebreathing, or total rebreathing systems. In nonrebreathing systems (open systems), the fresh gas flow into the breathing circuit exceeds the patient's minute ventilation. All gases not absorbed by the patient are exhausted through the adjustable pressure-relief valve, there is no flow through the CO_2 absorber, and no gas is rebreathed by the patient.

In partial rebreathing systems (semiopen or semiclosed), the fresh gas flow into the breathing circuit is less than the minute ventilation provided to the patient but greater than the rate of uptake of all gases by the patient. The difference between the fresh gas flow and patient uptake is equal to the exhaust volume from the pressure-relief valve. Therefore, exhaled gas can take one of three courses: It can be evacuated by the pressure-relief valve, absorbed by the CO_2 absorber, or rebreathed by the patient.

A total rebreathing system (closed system) does not evacuate any gas through the adjustable pressure-relief valve. This implies that all exhaled gases except CO_2 are rebreathed, expired CO_2 must be eliminated by the CO_2 absorber to prevent hypercapnia, and the total amount of fresh gas delivered to the system must nearly equal the amount of gas taken up by the patient's lungs. The fresh gas flow required to maintain the desired alveolar partial pressure of anesthetic agent and oxygen depends upon anesthetic uptake and metabolic rate. This flow rate is achieved by maintaining both a constant circuit volume, as reflected in an unchanging end-expiratory breathing-bag volume or ventilator-bellows height, and a constant expired oxygen concentration.

[1]The authors would like to thank Harry J. Lowe, MD, for his contribution to this Case Discussion.

What are the advantages and disadvantages of closed-circuit anesthesia?

Rebreathing anesthetic gases conserves heat and humidity, decreases anesthetic pollution, demonstrates the principles of anesthetic uptake, and allows early detection of circuit leaks and metabolic changes. Flow rates are a major determinant of volatile anesthetic cost. Some anesthesiologists, however, consider that closed-circuit techniques impose a greater risk of hypoxia, hypercapnia, and anesthetic overdose. Without question, closed-circuit anesthesia requires a high level of vigilance and a comprehensive understanding of pharmacokinetics. Some anesthetic machines cannot deliver low flows because they have mandatory oxygen flow rates greater than metabolic oxygen consumption or do not allow the administration of potentially hypoxic gas mixtures.

What factors determine the cost of delivering an inhalation anesthetic?

Fresh gas flow rates are only one factor that determines consumption of anesthetic agent. Other considerations include potency, blood and tissue solubility, and the amount of vapor produced per milliliter of liquid anesthetic. Obviously, the price charged to the pharmacy by the manufacturer plays an important role, as would any special equipment required for delivery or monitoring. Less obvious are the indirect factors that influence discharge from the recovery room or hospital: time to awakening, incidence of vomiting, and so on.

Is any special equipment necessary for closed-circuit anesthesia?

General anesthesia should never be performed without an oxygen analyzer in the breathing circuit. During low-flow anesthesia, the oxygen concentrations in the expiratory limb may be significantly lower than in the inspiratory limb because of the patient's oxygen consumption. Therefore, it has been suggested that expiratory oxygen concentration be measured whenever the anesthesia system is closed. Gas leaks in the anesthetic system will interfere with estimates of nitrous oxide and oxygen consumption. These leaks are proportional to mean airway pressure and inspiratory time. Modern

circle systems have more than 20 potential sites of leaks, including the absorber, tubing connections, unidirectional valves, rubber hoses, and breathing bag (see Case Discussion, Chapter 4). Vaporizers and flow meters must be accurate at low flows and varying circuit pressures. An alternative to a vaporizer is the direct injection of volatile agent into the expiratory limb of the breathing circuit.*

How are oxygen requirements predicted during closed-circuit anesthesia?

Anesthesia establishes a basal metabolic rate that is dependent upon the patient's weight and body temperature. Basal metabolic oxygen consumption ($\dot{V}O_2$) equals 10 times a patient's weight in kilograms to the three-quarters power:

$$\dot{V}O_2 = 10 \text{ kg}^{3/4}$$

For a 70-kg patient, oxygen consumption is

$$\dot{V}O_2 = 10 \times (24.2) = 242 \text{ mL O}_2/\text{min}$$

Oxygen requirements decrease by 10% for each degree below 37.6°C:

$$\dot{V}O_2 \text{ at } 36.6°C = 242 - 24 = 218 \text{ mL O}_2/\text{min}$$

$$\dot{V}O_2 \text{ at } 35.6°C = 218 - 22 = 196 \text{ mL O}_2/\text{min}$$

This is only a model for prediction. Actual oxygen requirements vary, and must be determined for each patient. For example, hypovolemic shock, hypothyroidism, and aortic cross-clamping are associated with decreased metabolic oxygen consumption. In contrast, malignant hyperthermia, hyperthyroidism, and thermal burns lead to greater than predicted oxygen requirements. Increasing depth of anesthesia does not significantly alter basal metabolic rate unless tissue perfusion is compromised.

What is the relationship between oxygen consumption and CO_2 production?

Carbon dioxide production is approximately 80% of oxygen consumption (ie, respiratory ratio = 0.8):

$$\dot{V}CO_2 = 8 \text{ kg}^{3/4} = 194 \text{ mL CO}_2/\text{min}$$

How much ventilation is required to maintain normocapnia?

Minute ventilation is the sum of alveolar ventilation and ventilation of anatomic dead space and equipment dead space. Normocapnia is approximately a 5.6% alveolar concentration of CO_2:

$$\frac{40 \text{ mm Hg}}{760 \text{ mm Hg} - 47 \text{ mm Hg}} = 5.6\%$$

Therefore, alveolar ventilation must be sufficient to dilute the 194 mL of expired CO_2 to a concentration of 5.6%:

$$\dot{V}_A = \frac{\dot{V}_{CO_2}}{5.6\%} = \frac{194 \text{ mL/min}}{5.6\%} = 3393 \text{ mL/min}$$

Anatomic dead space is estimated as 1 mL/kg/breath:

Anatomic dead space = Weight × 1 mL/kg
= 70 mL/breath

Equipment dead space consists primarily of the ventilation lost to expansion of the breathing circuit during positive-pressure ventilation. This can be estimated if the circuit compliance and peak airway pressure are known:

Equipment dead space
= Compliance × Pressure
= (10 mL/cm H_2O) × (20 cm H_2O)
= 200 mL/breath

Therefore, at a respiratory rate of 10 breaths/min, total ventilation as measured by a spirometer should be $\dot{V}_T = 3393 + 700 + 2000 = 6093$ mL/min, and tidal volume would equal 609 mL.

How is the uptake of a volatile anesthetic predicted?

Anesthetic uptake by the pulmonary circulation depends upon the agent's blood/gas partition coefficient ($\lambda_{b/g}$), the alveolar/venous difference (C_{A-V}), and the cardiac output ($\dot{Q}$):

$$\text{Uptake} = \lambda_{b/g} \times C_{(A-V)} \times (\dot{Q})$$

The blood/gas partition coefficients of anesthetic agents have been experimentally deter-

mined (see Table 7–1). At the beginning of an anesthetic procedure, the venous concentration of anesthetic is zero, so the alveolar–venous difference is equal to the alveolar concentration. The alveolar concentration required for surgical anesthesia is typically 1.3 MAC (see Table 7–3). Cardiac output (dL/min) is related to metabolic rate and oxygen consumption:

$$\dot{Q} = 2 \text{ kg}^{3/4}$$

Thus, the rate of halothane uptake ($\dot{Q}_{an}$) by the pulmonary circulation at the end of the first minute of anesthesia can be predicted:

$$\dot{Q}_{an} \text{ at 1 min} = (2.4) \times (1.3)(.75) \times (2)(24.2)$$
$$= 113 \text{ mL of vapor}$$

As organs fill with anesthetic, the rate of uptake declines. An empiric mathematical model that closely fits observed uptake demonstrates that the fall in uptake is inversely proportionate to the square root of time (the square-root-of-time model). In other words, the uptake at 4 min is one-half that at 1 min and twice that at 16 min. Thus, the rate of uptake in our example would be 112 mL/min (112 ÷ 1) at the end of the first minute, 56 mL/min (112 ÷ 2) at the end of the fourth minute, and 28 mL/min (112 ÷ 4) at the end of minute 16. In general, the rate of uptake at any time (t) is

$$\dot{Q}_{an} \text{ at } t \text{ min} = (\dot{Q}_{an} \text{ at 1 min}) \times t^{-1/2}$$

How can the amount of anesthetic taken up be predicted from the rate of uptake?

The cumulative anesthetic dose at any time t can be determined by integrating the rate function (finding the area under the F_A/F_I curve):

$$\text{Cumulative uptake} = 2 \times (\dot{Q}_{an} \text{ at 1 min}) \times t^{+1/2}$$

Therefore, at 1 min the total amount of anesthetic that has been taken up is 224 mL; a total of 448 mL is taken up by 4 min; and 672 mL is taken up by 9 min. Stated another way, 224 mL is required to maintain a constant alveolar concentration during each square-root-of-time interval. This quantity is called the unit dose.

What is a priming dose?

The breathing circuit, the patient's functional residual capacity, and the arterial circulation must be primed with anesthetic before tissue uptake can begin. The amount of anesthetic required to prime the breathing circuit and the functional residual capacity is equal to their combined volume (approximately 100 dL) multiplied by the desired alveolar concentration (1.3 MAC). Similarly, the amount of anesthetic required to prime the arterial circulation is equal to the blood volume—roughly equal to cardiac output—multiplied by the desired concentration and the blood/gas partition coefficient. For simplicity, these two priming doses are considered to be equal to one unit dose. Thus, during the first minute of anesthesia, two unit doses are administered: one as a priming dose and the other for tissue uptake.

By what methods can a unit dose of anesthetic be administered during a square-root-of-time interval?

The 224 mL of halothane vapor can be administered by a copper kettle vaporizer or an agent-specific variable bypass vaporizer, or it can be directly injected as a liquid into the expiratory limb of the anesthesia circuit. Because the vapor pressure of halothane is 243 mm Hg at 20°C, the concentration of halothane exiting a copper kettle is 243 ÷ 760, or 32%. Therefore, 477 mL of oxygen must enter a copper kettle during one interval for 224 mL of halothane vapor to exit (see the vapor output equation in Chapter 4):

$$224 \text{ mL} \times \frac{760 - 243}{243} = 477 \text{ mL}$$

Modern agent-specific vaporizers deliver a constant concentration of agent regardless of flow. Therefore, if the total flow (nitrous oxide, oxygen, and anesthetic vapor) is 5 L during one time interval, a 4.5% concentration is required:

$$\frac{224 \text{ mL}}{5000 \text{ mL}} = 4.5\%$$

Direct injection into the circuit from a glass syringe with a metal stopcock is an easy way to administer volatile agents. Each milliliter of liquid halothane, isoflurane, desflurane, or sevoflurane represents approximately 200 mL (±10%) of vapor. Therefore, a little more than 1 mL needs to be injected during one time interval:

$$\frac{224 \text{ mL vapor}}{200 \text{ mL vapor/mL liquid}} = 1.12 \text{ mL liquid}$$

Can nitrous oxide uptake be predicted in a similar manner?

Similar predictions can be made for nitrous oxide—with two qualifications. First, 1.3 MAC (approximately 137% N_2O) cannot be delivered at atmospheric pressure because of the certainty of hypoxia. Second, because 30% of the blood supply to highly perfused organs is shunted, only 70% of the predicted nitrous oxide is actually taken up by blood recirculating through the lungs. This introduces a shunt factor of 0.7 into the uptake equation:

$$\text{Uptake } N_2O = 0.7 \times 0.47 \times \%N_2O \times \dot{Q}$$

For a 70-kg patient at 65% nitrous oxide:

$$\dot{Q}_{an} \text{ at 1 min} = 0.7 \times 0.47 \times 65 \times (2)(24.2)$$
$$= 1035 \text{ mL/min}$$

The unit dose for nitrous oxide would be

$$\text{Unit dose} = 2 \times \dot{Q}_{an} \text{ at 1 min} = 2070 \text{ mL}$$

A large priming dose is required:

Circuit prime = (FRC + Circuit volume) × 65%
= (100 dL)(0.65) = 65 dL
Arterial prime = Blood volume × $\lambda_{b/g}$ × 65%
= (50 dL)(0.45)(0.65) = 15 dL
Total prime = 80 dL = 8L

Therefore, several liters of nitrous oxide would be administered in the first minute of a nitrous oxide anesthetic procedure. In clinical practice, nitrous oxide is empirically administered in amounts sufficient to maintain circuit volume as judged by constant breathing bag size or the height of a ventilator's standing bellows. If the expired oxygen concentration falls below acceptable levels, the metabolic oxygen flow (242 mL/min) is increased. Sixty-five percent nitrous oxide anesthesia would be supplemented with intravenous or volatile agents. Because MAC is additive, 0.65 MAC of volatile anesthetic is required to attain a total of 1.3 MAC.

Briefly describe the first few minutes of a closed-circuit anesthetic procedure with nitrous oxide and halothane.

After preoxygenation, intravenous induction, and intubation, oxygen flow is set to the predicted metabolic oxygen requirement (242 mL/min). At the same time, nitrous oxide is administered at 6–8 L/min to prime the circuit and the patient's functional residual capacity. When expired oxygen drops to 40%, the nitrous oxide is reduced to match the calculated rate of uptake (2070 mL per square-root-of-time interval), and the adjustable pressure-relief valve is closed. If the ventilator bellows or breathing bag indicates an increasing or decreasing circuit volume, the nitrous oxide flowmeter is adjusted accordingly. If the expired oxygen concentration falls too low, the oxygen flow rate is increased. The priming and unit doses of volatile anesthetic can be administered by either of the methods described. Dosing intervals and amounts are only predictions. The correct dose for each patient is determined by the clinical signs of anesthetic depth: blood pressure, heart rate, respiratory rate, tearing, pupillary changes, diaphoresis, movement, and the like.

SUGGESTED READING

Cittanova M-L, Lelongt B, Verpont M-C: Fluoride ion toxicity in human kidney collecting duct cells. Anesthesiology 1996;84:428. A reexamination of the mechanism of methoxyflurane metabolism and nephrotoxicity.

Ebert TJ: Myocardial ischemia and adverse cardiac outcomes in cardiac patients undergoing noncardiac surgery with sevoflurane and isoflurane. Anesth Analg 1997;85:993. This article by the Sevoflurane Ischemia Study Group concludes that there is no difference in the incidence of myocardial ischemia between sevoflurane and isoflurane.

Eger EI, Bowland T, Ionescu P: Recovery and kinetic characteristics of desflurane and sevoflurane in volunteers after 8-h exposure, including kinetics of degradation products. Anesthesiology 1997;87:527. An excellent overview of the pharmacokinetics of these agents.

Evers AS, Maze M: *Anesthetic Pharmacology. Physiologic Principles and Clinical Practice.* Churchill Livingstone, 2004. An excellent pharmacological review of all anesthetic drugs including the inhalation agents.

Ghatge S, Lee J, Smith I: Sevoflurane: an ideal agent for adult daycase anesthesia? Acta Anaesthesiol Scand 2003;47:917. Excellent review of sevoflurane, concluding that some of its characteristics make it desirable for outpatient surgical procedures. Costs and institutional practices must be taken into account. There is no evidence of earlier postanesthesia care unit discharge with sevoflurane.

Njoku D, Laster MJ, Gong DH: Biotransformation of halothane, enflurane, isoflurane, and desflurane to trifluoroacetylated liver proteins: association between protein acylation and hepatic injury. Anesth Analg 1997;84:173. A review of the hepatotoxicity of several volatile anesthetic agents and its relationship to their metabolism.

Stoelting RK: *Pharmacology and Physiology in Anesthetic Practice,* 3rd ed. Lippincott, 1999. One of the best discussions of the clinical pharmacology of volatile anesthetic agents.

Summors AC, Gupta AK, Matta BF: Dynamic cerebral autoregulation during sevoflurane anesthesia: a comparison with isoflurane. Anesth Analg 1999;88:341. This study confirms the decreased effects of sevoflurane on cerebral autoregulation.

Sun X, Su F, Shi Y, Lee C: The "second gas effect" is not a valid concept. Anesth Analg 1999;88:188. This study failed to show any increase in volatile anesthetic concentration due to nitrous oxide administration.

Nonvolatile Anesthetic Agents

8

KEY CONCEPTS

 As plasma concentration falls, some drug leaves the highly perfused organs to maintain equilibrium. This redistribution from the vessel-rich group is responsible for termination of effect of many anesthetic drugs. For example, awakening from the effects of thiopental is not due to metabolism or excretion but rather to redistribution of the drug from brain to muscle.

 Non–protein-bound drugs freely cross from plasma into the glomerular filtrate. The nonionized fraction of drug is reabsorbed in the renal tubules, whereas the ionized portion is excreted in urine.

 Elimination half-life of a drug is proportional to the volume of distribution and inversely proportional to the rate of clearance.

 The plasma concentration of a drug with long half-lives may still fall rapidly if distribution accounts for the vast majority of the decline and elimination is a relatively insignificant contributor. Therefore, the rate of clinical recovery from a drug cannot be predicted by its half-lives alone.

 Repetitive administration of barbiturates saturates the peripheral compartments, so that redistribution cannot occur and the duration of action becomes more dependent on elimination.

 Barbiturates constrict the cerebral vasculature. This effect may protect the brain from transient episodes of focal ischemia (eg, cerebral embolism) but probably not from global ischemia (eg, cardiac arrest).

 Although apnea may be less common after benzodiazepine induction than after barbiturate induction, even small intravenous doses of diazepam and midazolam have resulted in respiratory arrest. Ventilation must be monitored in all patients receiving intravenous benzodiazepines, and resuscitation equipment must be immediately available.

 The accumulation of morphine metabolites (morphine 3-glucuronide and morphine 6-glucuronide) in patients with renal failure has been associated with narcosis and ventilatory depression lasting several days.

 Opioids (particularly fentanyl, sufentanil, and alfentanil) can induce chest wall rigidity severe enough to prevent adequate ventilation.

 The stress response to surgical stimulation is measured in terms of the secretion of specific hormones, including catecholamines, antidiuretic hormone, and cortisol. Opioids block the release of these hormones more completely than volatile anesthetics.

 In sharp contrast to other anesthetic agents, ketamine increases arterial blood pressure, heart rate, and cardiac output. These indirect cardiovascular effects are due to central stimulation of the sympathetic nervous system and inhibition of the reuptake of norepinephrine.

 Induction doses of etomidate transiently inhibit enzymes involved in cortisol and aldosterone synthesis. Long-term infusions lead to adrenocortical suppression that may be associated with an increased mortality rate in critically ill patients.

(continued on next page)

(continued from previous page)

 Propofol formulations can support the growth of bacteria, so good sterile technique must be observed in preparation and handling. Sepsis and death have been linked to contaminated propofol preparations.

 Droperidol is a potent antiemetic; however, delayed awakening limits its intraoperative use to low doses (0.05 mg/kg, to a maximum of 2.5 mg). The antidopaminergic activity of droperidol rarely precipitates extrapyramidal reactions (eg, oculogyric crises, torticollis, agitation), which can be treated with diphenhydramine. Nonetheless, droperidol should be avoided in patients with Parkinson disease.

General anesthesia is not limited to the use of inhalation agents. Numerous drugs that are administered orally, intramuscularly, and intravenously augment or produce an anesthetic state within their therapeutic dosage range. Preoperative sedation, the topic of this chapter's case study, is traditionally accomplished by way of oral or intravenous routes. Induction of anesthesia in adult patients usually involves intravenous administration, and the development of EMLA (eutectic [easily melted] mixture of local anesthetic) cream, LMX (plain lidocaine cream 4% and 5%), and 2% lidocaine jelly (see Chapter 14) has significantly increased the popularity of intravenous inductions in children. Even maintenance of general anesthesia can be achieved with a total intravenous anesthesia technique (see Case Discussion, Chapter 46). This chapter begins with a review of the pharmacological principles of pharmacokinetics and pharmacodynamics and how they apply to this class of drugs. The clinical pharmacology of several anesthetic agents is presented: barbiturates, benzodiazepines, opioids, ketamine, etomidate, propofol, and droperidol.

■ PHARMACOLOGICAL PRINCIPLES

PHARMACOKINETICS

As explained in Chapter 7, pharmacokinetics is the study of the relationship of a drug's dose, concentration in tissue, and time since administration. Simply stated, it describes how the body affects a drug. Pharmacokinetics is defined by four parameters: absorption, distribution, biotransformation, and excretion. Elimination implies drug removal by both biotransformation and excretion. Clearance is a measurement of the rate of elimination.

Absorption

There are many possible routes of systemic drug absorption: oral, sublingual, rectal, inhalation, transdermal, subcutaneous, intramuscular, and intravenous. Absorption, the process by which a drug leaves its site of administration to enter the bloodstream, is affected by the physical characteristics of the drug (solubility, pK_a, and concentration) and the site of absorption (circulation, pH, and surface area). Absorption differs from bioavailability, which is the fraction of unchanged drug that reaches the systemic circulation. For instance, nitroglycerin is well absorbed by the gastrointestinal tract. It has low bioavailability when administered orally, as it is extensively metabolized by the liver before it can reach the systemic circulation and the myocardium (first-pass hepatic metabolism).

Oral administration is convenient, economical, and relatively tolerant of dosage error. However, it is unreliable as it depends on patient cooperation, exposes the drug to first-pass hepatic metabolism, and allows interference by gastric pH, enzymes, motility, food, and other drugs.

The nonionized forms of drugs are preferentially absorbed. Therefore, an acidic environment favors the absorption of acidic drugs ($A^- + H^+ \rightarrow AH$), whereas an alkaline environment favors basic drugs ($BH^+ \rightarrow H^+ + B$). Regardless of considerations of ionization, the large surface area of the small intestine provides a preferential site of absorption for most drugs compared with the stomach.

Because the veins of the mouth drain into the superior vena cava, sublingual or buccal drug absorption bypasses the liver and first-pass metabolism. Rectal administration is an alternative to oral medication in patients who are uncooperative (eg, pediatric patients) or unable to tolerate oral ingestion. Because the venous drainage of the rectum bypasses the liver, first-pass metabolism is less significant than with small intestinal absorption. Rectal absorption can be erratic, however, and many drugs cause irritation of the rectal mucosa. Absorption of inhalation agents is discussed in Chapter 7.

Transdermal drug administration has the advantage of prolonged and continuous absorption with a minimal total drug dose. The stratum corneum serves as an effective barrier to all but small, lipid-soluble drugs (eg, clonidine, nitroglycerin, scopolamine).

Parenteral injection includes subcutaneous, intramusclular, and intravenous routes of administration. Subcutaneous and intramuscular absorption depends on diffusion from the site of injection to the circulation. The rate of diffusion depends on the blood flow to the area and the carrier vehicle (solutions are absorbed faster than suspensions). Irritating preparations can cause pain and tissue necrosis. Intravenous injection completely bypasses the process of absorption, because the drug is placed directly into the bloodstream.

Distribution

Distribution plays a key role in clinical pharmacology because it is a major determinant of end-organ drug concentration. A drug's distribution depends primarily on organ perfusion, protein binding, and lipid solubility.

After absorption, a drug is distributed by the bloodstream throughout the body. Highly perfused organs (the vessel-rich group) take up a disproportionately large amount of drug compared with less perfused organs (the muscle, fat, and vessel-poor groups). Thus, even though the total mass of the vessel-rich group is small, it can account for substantial initial drug uptake (Table 8–1).

Table 8–1. Tissue group composition, relative body mass, and percentage of cardiac output.

Tissue Group	Composition	Body Mass (%)	Cardiac Output (%)
Vessel-rich	Brain, heart, liver, kidney, endocrine glands	10	75
Muscle	Muscle, skin	50	19
Fat	Fat	20	6
Vessel-poor	Bone, ligament, cartilage	20	0

As long as a drug is bound to a plasma protein, it is unavailable for uptake by an organ regardless of the extent of perfusion to that organ. Albumin often binds acidic drugs (eg, barbiturates), whereas α_1-acid glycoprotein (AAG) binds basic drugs (local anesthetics). If these proteins are diminished or if the protein-binding sites are occupied (eg, other drugs), the amount of free drug available for tissue uptake is increased. Renal disease, liver disease, chronic congestive heart failure, and malignancies decrease albumin production. Trauma (including surgery), infection, myocardial infarction, and chronic pain increase AAG levels.

Availability of a drug to a specific organ does not ensure uptake by that organ. For instance, the permeation of the central nervous system by ionized drugs is limited by pericapillary glial cells and endothelial cell tight junctions, which constitute the blood–brain barrier. Lipid-soluble, nonionized molecules pass freely through lipid membranes. Other factors, such as molecular size and tissue binding—particularly by the lung—can also influence drug distribution.

After the highly perfused organs are saturated during initial distribution, the greater mass of the less perfused organs continue to take up drug from the bloodstream. As plasma concentration falls, some drug leaves the highly perfused organs to maintain equilibrium. This redistribution from the vessel-rich group is responsible for termination of effect of many anesthetic drugs. For example, awakening from the effects of thiopental is not due to metabolism or excretion but rather to redistribution of the drug from brain to muscle. As a corollary, if the less perfused organs are saturated from repeated doses of drug, redistribution cannot occur and awakening depends to a greater extent on drug elimination. Thus, rapid-acting drugs such as thiopental and fentanyl will become longer acting after repeated administration or when a large single dose is given. The *apparent* volume into which a drug has been distributed is called its volume of distribution (V_d) and is determined by dividing the dose of drug administered by the resulting plasma concentration:

$$V_d = \frac{Dose}{Concentration}$$

This calculation is complicated by the need to adjust for the effects of drug elimination and continual redistribution. A small V_d implies relative confinement of the drug to the intravascular space, which leads to a high plasma concentration (eg, the V_d of pancuronium = 10 L in a 70-kg person). Causes for a small V_d include high protein binding or ionization. On the other hand, the apparent V_d may exceed total body water (approximately 40 L). Explanations for this include high solubility or binding of the drug in tissues other than plasma (eg, the V_d of fentanyl = 350 L). Therefore, the V_d does not represent a real volume but rather reflects the volume of plasma that would be necessary to account for the observed plasma concentration.

Biotransformation

Biotransformation is the alteration of a substance by metabolic processes. The liver is the primary organ of biotransformation. The end products of biotransformation are usually—but not necessarily—inactive and water soluble. The latter property allows excretion by the kidney.

Metabolic biotransformation can be divided into phase I and phase II reactions. Phase I reactions convert a parent drug into more polar metabolites through oxidation, reduction, or hydrolysis. Phase II reactions couple (conjugate) a parent drug or a phase I metabolite with an endogenous substrate (eg, glucuronic acid) to form a highly polar end product that can be eliminated in the urine. Although this is usually a sequential process, phase I metabolites may be excreted without undergoing phase II biotransformation, and a phase II reaction can precede a phase I reaction.

Hepatic clearence is the rate of elimination of a drug as a result of liver biotransformation. More specifically, clearance is the volume of plasma cleared of drug per unit of time and is expressed as milliliters per minute. The hepatic clearance depends on the hepatic blood flow and the fraction of drug removed from the blood by the liver (hepatic extraction ratio). Drugs that are efficiently cleared by the liver have a high hepatic extraction ratio, and their clearance is proportionate to hepatic blood flow. On the other hand, drugs with a low hepatic extraction ratio are poorly cleared by the liver, and their clearance is limited by the capacity of the hepatic enzyme systems. Therefore, the effect of liver disease on drug pharmacokinetics depends on the drug's hepatic extraction ratio and the disease's propensity to alter hepatic blood flow or hepatocellular function.

Excretion

The kidney is the principal organ of excretion. Non–protein-bound drugs freely cross from plasma into the glomerular filtrate. The nonionized fraction of drug is reabsorbed in the renal tubules, whereas the ionized portion is excreted in urine. Thus, alterations in urine pH can alter renal excretion. The kidney also actively secretes some drugs. Renal clearance is the rate of elimination of a drug from kidney excretion. Renal failure changes the pharmacokinetics of many drugs by altering protein binding, volumes of distribution, and clearance rates.

Relatively few drugs depend on biliary excretion, as they are usually reabsorbed in the intestine and are consequently excreted in the urine. Delayed toxic effects from some drugs (eg, fentanyl) may be due to this enterohepatic recirculation.

The lungs are responsible for excretion of volatile agents, such as inhalation anesthetics (see Chapter 7).

Compartment Models

Compartment models offer a simple way to characterize the distribution and elimination of drugs in the body. A compartment can be conceptualized as a group of tissues that possesses similar pharmacokinetics. For example, plasma and the vessel-rich group could represent the central compartment, whereas muscle, fat, and skin could represent the peripheral compartment. However, it must be stressed that compartments are *conceptual* and do not represent actual tissues.

A two-compartment model correlates well with the distribution and elimination phases of many drugs (Figure 8–1). After an intravenous bolus, the plasma concentration of a drug will instantaneously rise. The initial rapid decline in plasma concentration, called the distribution phase or alpha (α) phase, corresponds to the redistribution of drug from the plasma and the vessel-rich group of the central compartment to the less perfused tissues of the peripheral compartment. As distribution slows, elimination of drug from the central compartment is responsible for a continued—but less steep—decline in plasma concentration, called the elimination phase or beta (β) phase. Elimination half-life of a drug is proportional to the volume of distribution (V_d) and inversely proportional to the rate of clearance. The plasma concentration curves of many drugs are better characterized by a three-compartment model consist-

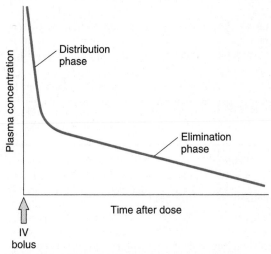

Figure 8–1. Two-compartment model demonstrates the distribution phase (α phase) and the elimination phase (β phase). During the distribution phase, the drug moves from the central compartment to the peripheral compartment. The elimination phase consists of metabolism and excretion.

ing of a central compartment and two peripheral compartments.

Plasma concentration (C_p) following a bolus administration of a drug can be expressed by a triexponential equation:

$$C_p(t) = Ae^{-\alpha t} + Be^{-\beta t} + Ce^{-\gamma t}$$

where $C_p(t)$ equals plasma concentration at time t, and A, B, and C are fractional coefficients that denote the relative contributions of each of three hybrid rate constants (α corresponding to the rapid distribution half-life, β to the slow distribution half-life, and γ to the terminal elimination half-life). Because the fractional coefficients quantify the amount that each half-life contributes to the overall decline in drug concentration, they are as important as half-lives in predicting termination of drug action. For example, drug x may have longer distribution and elimination half-lives than does drug y, but its plasma concentration may fall more rapidly if its fractional coefficient of distribution (A) is greater. Stated another way, the plasma concentration of a drug with long half-lives may still fall rapidly if distribution accounts for the vast majority of the decline and elimination is a relatively insignificant contributor. Therefore, the rate of clinical recovery from a drug cannot be predicted by its half-lives alone.

Rates of distribution and biotransformation can usually be described in terms of first-order kinetics. In other words, a constant fraction or percentage of drug is distributed or metabolized per unit of time, regardless of plasma concentration. For instance, 10% of a drug may be biotransformed hourly whether the plasma concentration is 10 or 100 μg/mL. If the concentration of drug exceeds the biotransformation capacity, however, then a constant amount of drug may be metabolized per unit of time (zero-order kinetics). Using a similar example, 500 μg of drug might be metabolized each hour regardless of whether the plasma concentration was 10 or 100 μg/mL. Metabolism of alcohol can be predicted by zero-order kinetics.

PHARMACODYNAMICS

Pharmacodynamics is the study of the therapeutic and toxic organ system effects of drugs (how a drug affects a body). The extent of these effects determines a drug's efficacy, potency, and therapeutic ratio. Pharmacodynamics also inquires into mechanisms of action, drug interactions, and structure–activity relationships. Understanding dose–response curves and drug receptors provides a framework to help explain these diverse parameters of pharmacodynamics.

Dose–Response Curves

Dose–response curves express the relationship between drug dose and pharmacological effect. Drug dose or

steady-state plasma concentration is plotted on the abscissa (x axis) and is represented in linear (Figure 8–2A) or logarithmic scale (Figure 8–2B). Pharmacological effect is plotted on the ordinate (y axis) in terms of absolute units (Figure 8–2A) or as a fraction of maximal effect (Figure 8–2B). The position of the dose–response curve along the abscissa is an indication of drug potency. The maximal effect of the drug relates to its efficacy. The slope of the dose–response curve reflects receptor-binding characteristics. The influence of pharmacokinetics on dose–response curves can be minimized by studying the relationship of blood concentration to pharmacological response.

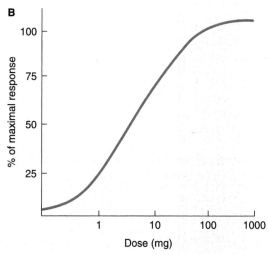

Figure 8–2. The shape of the dose–response curve depends on whether the dose or steady-state plasma concentration (C_{cpss}) is plotted on a linear **(A)** or logarithmic **(B)** scale. MAP, mean arterial pressure.

The median effective dose (ED_{50}) is the dose of drug required to produce a given effect in 50% of the population. Note that the ED_{50} is *not* the dose required to produce one-half the maximal effect. The ED_{50} of inhalation anesthetics is the same as the minimum alveolar concentration (see Chapter 7). The median lethal dose (LD_{50}) is the dose that results in death in 50% of the population exposed to that dose. The therapeutic index is the ratio of the median lethal dose to the median effective dose (LD_{50}:ED_{50}).

Drug Receptors

Drug receptors are macromolecules—usually proteins embedded into cell membranes—that interact with a drug to mediate characteristic intracellular changes. The mechanism of action of several (not all) drugs depends on interaction with a receptor. Endogenous substances (eg, hormones) or exogenous substances (eg, drugs) that directly change cell function by binding to receptors are called agonists. Antagonists also bind to the receptors but do not cause a direct effect on the cell. The pharmacological effect of antagonist drugs depends on the subsequent inability of agonist substances to activate the receptors. Competitive antagonists bind reversibly to receptors and can be displaced by higher concentrations of agonists. Noncompetitive (irreversible) antagonists bind to the receptor with such affinity that even high concentrations of agonists cannot reverse the receptor blockade. Competition of two drugs for the same receptor is one source of drug interactions.

Receptors affect cell function either directly (eg, by changing transmembrane ion flux) or by controlling the production of another regulatory molecule (eg, the second-messenger cyclic adenosine monophosphate). Individual variability in response to receptor binding is a significant cause of inconsistency in drug responsiveness. Continued activation of a receptor often leads to hyporeactivity, whereas lack of stimulation results in hyperreactivity. Chemical structure determines the degree of affinity between a drug and a receptor (structure–activity relationship). Minor changes in molecular configuration can have dramatic effects on clinical pharmacology.

■ SPECIFIC NONVOLATILE ANESTHETIC AGENTS

BARBITURATES

Mechanisms of Action

Barbiturates depress the reticular activating system—a complex polysynaptic network of neurons and regulatory centers—located in the brain stem that controls several vital functions, including consciousness. In clinical concentrations, barbiturates preferentially affect the function of nerve synapses rather than axons. They suppress transmission of excitatory neurotransmitters (eg, acetylcholine) and enhance transmission of inhibitory neurotransmitters (eg, γ-aminobutyric acid [GABA]). Specific mechanisms include interfering with transmitter release (presynaptic) and stereoselectively interacting with receptors (postsynaptic).

Structure–Activity Relationships

Barbiturates are barbituric acid derivatives (Figure 8–3). Substitution at the number 5 carbon (C_5) determines hypnotic potency and anticonvulsant activity. For example, a long-branched chain conveys more potency than does a short straight chain. Likewise, the phenyl group in *pheno*barbital is anticonvulsive, whereas the methyl group in *metho*hexital is not. Replacing the oxygen at C_2 (*oxy*barbiturates) with a sulfur atom (*thio*barbiturates) increases lipid solubility. As a result, thiopental and thiamylal have a greater potency, more rapid onset of action, and shorter durations of action than pentobarbital and secobarbital. The short duration of action of methohexital is related to the methyl substitution at N_1. The sodium salts of the barbiturates are water soluble but markedly alkaline (pH of 2.5% thiopental > 10) and relatively unstable (2-week shelf-life for 2.5% thiopental solution). Concentrations higher than recommended cause an unacceptable incidence of both pain on injection and venous thrombosis.

Pharmacokinetics

A. ABSORPTION

In clinical anesthesiology, barbiturates are most frequently administered intravenously for induction of general anesthesia in adults and children with an intravenous line. Exceptions include rectal thiopental or methohexital for induction in children and intramuscular pentobarbital or secobarbital for premedication of all age groups.

B. DISTRIBUTION

The duration of action of highly lipid-soluble barbiturates (thiopental, thiamylal, and methohexital) is determined by redistribution, not metabolism or elimination. For example, although thiopental is highly protein bound (80%), its great lipid solubility and high nonionized fraction (60%) account for maximal brain uptake within 30 s. If the central compartment is contracted (eg, hypovolemic shock), if the serum albumin is low (eg, severe liver disease), or if the nonionized fraction is increased (eg, acidosis), higher brain and heart concentrations will be

BARBITURIC ACID

Figure 8–3. Barbiturates share the structure of barbituric acid and differ in the C_2, C_3, and N_1 substitutions.

achieved for a given dose. Subsequent redistribution to the peripheral compartment—specifically, the muscle group—lowers plasma and brain concentration to 10% of peak levels within 20–30 min (Figure 8–4). This pharmacokinetic profile correlates with clinical experience—patients typically lose consciousness within 30 s and awaken within 20 min. Induction doses of thiopental depend on body weight and age. Lower induction doses in elderly patients is a reflection of higher peak plasma levels because of slower redistribution. In contrast to the rapid initial distribution half-life of a few minutes, the elimination half-life of thiopental ranges from 3–12 h. Thiamylal and methohexital have similar distribution patterns, whereas less lipid-soluble barbiturates have

much longer distribution half-lives and durations of action. Repetitive administration of barbiturates saturates the peripheral compartments, so that redistribution cannot occur and the duration of action becomes more dependent on elimination.

C. Biotransformation

Biotransformation of barbiturates principally involves hepatic oxidation to inactive water-soluble metabolites. Because of greater hepatic extraction, methohexital is cleared by the liver three to four times more rapidly than thiopental or thiamylal. Although redistribution is responsible for the awakening from a single dose of any of these lipid-soluble barbiturates, full recovery of psy-

Figure 8–4. Distribution of thiopental from plasma to the vessel-rich group (VRG), to the muscle group (MG), and finally to the fat group (FG). (Modified and reproduced, with permission, from Price HL et al: The uptake of thiopental by body tissues and its relation to the duration of narcosis. Clin Pharmacol Ther 1960;1:16.)

chomotor function is more rapid following use of methohexital due to its enhanced metabolism.

D. EXCRETION

High protein binding decreases barbiturate glomerular filtration, whereas high lipid solubility tends to increase renal tubular reabsorption. Except for the less protein-bound and less lipid-soluble agents such as phenobarbital, renal excretion is limited to water-soluble end products of hepatic biotransformation. Methohexital is excreted in the feces.

Effects on Organ Systems

A. CARDIOVASCULAR

Induction doses of intravenously administered barbiturates cause a fall in blood pressure and an elevation in heart rate. Depression of the medullary vasomotor center vasodilates peripheral capacitance vessels, which increases peripheral pooling of blood and decreases venous return to the right atrium. The tachycardia is probably due to a central vagolytic effect. Cardiac output is often maintained by a rise in heart rate and increased myocardial contractility from compensatory baroreceptor reflexes. Sympathetically induced vasoconstriction of resistance vessels may actually increase peripheral vascular resistance. However, in the absence of an adequate baroreceptor response (eg, hypovolemia, congestive heart failure, β-adrenergic blockade), **cardiac output and arterial blood pressure may fall dramatically due to uncompensated peripheral pooling and unmasked direct myocardial depression.** Patients with poorly controlled hypertension are particularly prone to wide

swings in blood pressure during induction. The cardiovascular effects of barbiturates therefore vary markedly, depending on volume status, baseline autonomic tone, and preexisting cardiovascular disease. A slow rate of injection and adequate preoperative hydration attenuate these changes in most patients.

B. RESPIRATORY

Barbiturate depression of the medullary ventilatory center decreases the ventilatory response to hypercapnia and hypoxia. Barbiturate sedation typically leads to upper airway obstruction; apnea usually follows an induction dose. During awakening, tidal volume and respiratory rate are decreased. Barbiturates do not completely depress noxious airway reflexes, and bronchospasm in asthmatic patients or laryngospasm in lightly anesthetized patients is not uncommon following airway instrumentation. Laryngospasm and hiccuping are more common after use of methohexital than after thiopental. Bronchospasm following induction with thiopental may be due to cholinergic nerve stimulation (which would be preventable by pretreatment with atropine), histamine release, or direct bronchial smooth muscle stimulation.

C. CEREBRAL

 Barbiturates constrict the cerebral vasculature, causing a decrease in cerebral blood flow and intracranial pressure. The drop in intracranial pressure exceeds the decline in arterial blood pressure, so that cerebral perfusion pressure (CPP) is usually increased. (CPP equals cerebral artery pressure minus the greater of cerebral venous pressure or intracranial pressure.) The decrease in cerebral blood flow is not detrimental, as barbiturates induce an even greater decline in cerebral oxygen consumption (up to 50% of normal). Alterations in cerebral activity and oxygen requirements are reflected by changes in the electroencephalogram (EEG), which progresses from low-voltage fast activity with small doses to high-voltage slow activity and electrical silence (suppression) with very large doses of barbiturate (a bolus of 15–40 mg/kg of thiopental followed by an infusion of 0.5 mg/kg/min). This effect of barbiturates may protect the brain from transient episodes of focal ischemia (eg, cerebral embolism) but probably not from global ischemia (eg, cardiac arrest). Furthermore, doses required for EEG suppression have been associated with prolonged awakening, delayed extubation, and the need for inotropic support.

The degree of central nervous system depression induced by barbiturates ranges from mild sedation to unconsciousness, depending on the dose administered (Table 8–2). Some patients relate a taste sensation of garlic or onions during induction with thiopental. Unlike opioids, barbiturates do not selectively impair the perception

Table 8–2. Uses and dosages of commonly used barbiturates.

Agent	Use	Route[1]	Concentration (%)	Dose (mg/kg)
Thiopental, thiamylal	Induction	IV	2.5	3–6
	Sedation	IV	2.5	0.5–1.5
Methohexital	Induction	IV	1	1–2
	Sedation	IV	1	0.2–0.4
	Induction	Rectal (children)	10	25
Secobarbital, pentobarbital	Premedication	Oral	5	2–4[2]
		IM		2–4[2]
		Rectal suppository		3

[1]IV, intravenous; IM, intramuscular.
[2]Maximum dose is 150 mg.

of pain. In fact, they sometimes appear to have an antianalgesic effect by lowering the pain threshold. Small doses occasionally cause a state of excitement and disorientation that can be disconcerting when sedation is the objective. Barbiturates do not produce muscle relaxation, and some induce involuntary skeletal muscle contractions (eg, methohexital). Relatively small doses of thiopental (50–100 mg intravenously) rapidly control most grand mal seizures. Unfortunately, acute tolerance and physiological dependence on the sedative effect of barbiturates develop quickly.

D. Renal

Barbiturates reduce renal blood flow and glomerular filtration rate in proportion to the fall in blood pressure.

E. Hepatic

Hepatic blood flow is decreased. Chronic exposure to barbiturates has opposing effects on drug biotransformation. Induction of hepatic enzymes increases the rate of metabolism of some drugs (eg, digitoxin), whereas combination with the cytochrome P-450 enzyme system interferes with the biotransformation of others (eg, tricyclic antidepressants). The induction of aminolevulinic acid synthetase stimulates the formation of **porphyrin** (an intermediary in heme synthesis), which may precipitate acute intermittent porphyria or variegate porphyria in susceptible individuals.

F. Immunological

Anaphylactic and anaphylactoid allergic reactions are rare. Sulfur-containing thiobarbiturates evoke mast cell histamine release *in vitro*, whereas oxybarbiturates do not. For this reason, some anesthesiologists prefer methohexital over thiopental or thiamylal in asthmatic or atopic patients.

Drug Interactions

Contrast media, sulfonamides, and other drugs that occupy the same protein-binding sites as thiopental will increase the amount of free drug available and potentiate the organ system effects of a given dose.

Ethanol, opioids, antihistamines, and other central nervous system depressants potentiate the sedative effects of barbiturates. The common clinical impression that chronic alcohol abuse is associated with increased thiopental requirements lacks scientific proof.

BENZODIAZEPINES

Mechanisms of Action

Benzodiazepines interact with specific receptors in the central nervous system, particularly in the cerebral cortex. Benzodiazepine–receptor binding enhances the inhibitory effects of various neurotransmitters. For example, benzodiazepine-receptor binding facilitates GABA–receptor binding, which increases the membrane conductance of chloride ions. This causes a change in membrane polarization that inhibits normal neuronal function. **Flumazenil** (an imidazobenzodiazepine) is a specific benzodiazepine–receptor antagonist that effectively reverses most of the central nervous system effect of benzodiazepines (see Chapter 15).

Structure–Activity Relationships

The chemical structure of benzodiazepines includes a benzene ring and a seven-member diazepine ring (Figure 8–5). Substitutions at various positions on these rings affect potency and biotransformation. The imidazole ring of midazolam contributes to its water solubility at low pH. The insolubility of diazepam and lorazepam in water

Figure 8–5. The structures of commonly used benzodiazepines and their antagonist, flumazenil, share a seven-member diazepine ring. (Modified and reproduced, with permission, from White PF: Pharmacologic and clinical aspects of preoperative medication. Anesth Analg 1986;65:963. With permission from the International Anesthesia Research Society.)

requires that parenteral preparations contain propylene glycol, which has been associated with venous irritation.

Pharmacokinetics

A. ABSORPTION

Benzodiazepines are commonly administered orally, intramuscularly, and intravenously to provide sedation or induction of general anesthesia (Table 8–3). Diazepam and lorazepam are well absorbed from the gastrointestinal tract, with peak plasma levels usually achieved in 1 and 2 h, respectively. Although oral midazolam has not been approved by the U.S. Food and Drug Administration, this route of administration has been popular for pediatric premedication. Likewise, intranasal (0.2–0.3 mg/kg), buccal

(0.07 mg/kg), and sublingual (0.1 mg/kg) midazolam provide effective preoperative sedation.

Intramuscular injection of diazepam is painful and unreliable. In contrast, midazolam and lorazepam are well absorbed after intramuscular injection, with peak levels achieved in 30 and 90 min, respectively. Induction of general anesthesia with midazolam requires intravenous administration of the drug.

B. DISTRIBUTION

Diazepam is quite lipid soluble and rapidly penetrates the blood–brain barrier. Although midazolam is water soluble at low pH, its imidazole ring closes at physiological pH, causing an increase in its lipid solubility (Figure 8–5). The moderate lipid solubility of

Table 8–3. Uses and doses of commonly used benzodiazepines.

Agent	Use	Route[1]	Dose (mg/kg)
Diazepam	Premedication	Oral	0.2–0.5[2]
	Sedation	IV	0.04–0.2
	Induction	IV	0.3–0.6
Midazolam	Premedication	IM	0.07–0.15
	Sedation	IV	0.01–0.1
	Induction	IV	0.1–0.4
Lorazepam	Premedication	Oral	0.053
		IM	0.03–0.05[3]
	Sedation	IV	0.03–0.04[3]

[1]IV, intravenous; IM, intramuscular.
[2]Maximum dose 15 mg.
[3]Not recommended for children.

lorazepam accounts for its slower brain uptake and onset of action. Redistribution is fairly rapid for the benzodiazepines (the initial distribution half-life is 3–10 min) and, like the barbiturates, is responsible for awakening. Although midazolam is frequently used as an induction agent, none of the benzodiazepines can match the rapid onset and short duration of action of thiopental. All three benzodiazepines are highly protein bound (90–98%).

C. BIOTRANSFORMATION

The benzodiazepines rely on the liver for biotransformation into water-soluble glucuronide end products. The phase I metabolites of diazepam are pharmacologically active.

Slow hepatic extraction and a large V_d result in a long elimination half-life for diazepam (30 h). Although lorazepam also has a low hepatic extraction ratio, its lower lipid solubility limits its V_d, resulting in a shorter elimination half-life (15 h). Nonetheless, the clinical duration of lorazepam is often quite prolonged due to a very high receptor affinity. In contrast, midazolam shares diazepam's V_d, but its elimination half-life (2 h) is the shortest of the group because of its high hepatic extraction ratio.

D. EXCRETION

The metabolites of benzodiazepine biotransformation are excreted chiefly in the urine. Enterohepatic circulation produces a secondary peak in diazepam plasma concentration 6–12 h following administration. Renal failure may lead to prolonged sedation in patients

receiving midazolam due to the accumulation of a conjugated metabolite (α-hydroxymidazolam).

Effects on Organ Systems

A. CARDIOVASCULAR

The benzodiazepines display minimal cardiovascular depressant effects even at induction doses. Arterial blood pressure, cardiac output, and peripheral vascular resistance usually decline slightly, whereas heart rate sometimes rises. Midazolam tends to reduce blood pressure and peripheral vascular resistance more than diazepam. Changes in heart rate variability during midazolam sedation suggest decreased vagal tone (ie, drug-induced vagolysis).

B. RESPIRATORY

Benzodiazepines depress the ventilatory response to CO_2. This depression is usually insignificant unless the drugs are administered intravenously or in association with other respiratory depressants. Although apnea may be less common after benzodiazepine induction than after barbiturate induction, even small intravenous doses of diazepam and midazolam have resulted in respiratory arrest. The steep dose–response curve, slightly prolonged onset (compared with thiopental or diazepam), and high potency of midazolam necessitate careful titration to avoid overdosage and apnea. Ventilation must be monitored in all patients receiving intravenous benzodiazepines, and resuscitation equipment must be immediately available.

C. CEREBRAL

Benzodiazepines reduce cerebral oxygen consumption, cerebral blood flow, and intracranial pressure but not to the extent the barbiturates do. They are very effective in preventing and controlling grand mal seizures. Oral sedative doses often produce antegrade amnesia, a useful premedication property. The mild muscle-relaxant property of these drugs is mediated at the spinal cord level, not at the neuromuscular junction. The antianxiety, amnesic, and sedative effects seen at low doses progress to stupor and unconsciousness at induction doses. Compared with thiopental, induction with benzodiazepines is associated with a slower loss of consciousness and a longer recovery. Benzodiazepines have no direct analgesic properties.

Drug Interactions

Cimetidine binds to cytochrome P-450 and reduces the metabolism of diazepam. Erythromycin inhibits metabolism of midazolam and causes a 2- to 3-fold prolongation and intensification of its effects. Heparin displaces diazepam from protein-binding sites and increases the free

J. G. Reves, MD

RATIONAL ADMINISTRATION OF INTRAVENOUS ANESTHESIA

General anesthesia requires that adequate levels of anesthetic drugs be rapidly attained in the brain and that they be maintained during the time required for surgery. This is a concept that applies equally well to anesthesia achieved by inhalation anesthetics, intravenous drugs, or both. However, the routine clinical practice of anesthesia by many clinicians seems to approach the goal of maintaining therapeutic levels of anesthesia differently depending on whether inhalation or intravenous anesthetics are used. This mystifies me. Why do clinicians continuously administer inhalation drugs with the aid of a vaporizer, but intermittently administer intravenous drugs by bolus injections?

With inhalation drugs the minimum alveolar concentration (MAC) is known and is achieved relatively quickly (usually by giving more than the desired brain concentration— "overpressurized") and then equilibration of inspired to expired gaseous anesthetic occurs. Maintenance of inhalation anesthesia is achieved by continuously administering the drug with this equilibrium. With intravenous drugs a bolus (usually a large "overdose") is given to induce anesthesia rapidly. However, maintenance of intravenous anesthesia is conventionally done by an inconstant infusion (intermittent bolus) or by a constant fixed/dose infusion that seldom achieves equilibrium betwe0en blood and brain. There usually is an ever changing blood and consequent brain level in contrast to the equilibrium achieved with an inhalation anesthetic.

It has never seemed rational to administer intravenous drugs intermittently and not by continuous infu-

sion. Ideally the infusion rate would be determined by the known pharmacokinetics of the drug to achieve constant blood–brain levels. Figure 1 shows the contrast between continuous infusion and intermittent bolus administration. Problems with a bolus technique are obvious: there are great variations in the blood levels, which cause anesthesia to be too deep right after the bolus and then too light before the next bolus. Repeated bolus administrations also tend to promote drug accumulation in patients, making it more difficult to arouse patients at the conclusion of surgery.

It has not previously been routine to administer intravenous drugs continuously for two principal reasons: (1) most anesthetic drugs were not suited for continuous infusions, and (2) infusion pumps were not simple and easy to operate. These reasons are no longer valid. Drugs such as midazolam, propofol, alfentanil, and remifentanil are ideally suited to continuous infusion. Likewise, infusion technology has advanced to the point that sophisticated pumps with preset programs make it easy to set a precise, individualized infusion rate for continuous infusion.

Another important advance in infusion anesthesia has been the use of a computer to administer anesthetics continuously using pharmacokinetic principles.[1,2] This technology is called "target-controlled infusion" (TCI). The pharmacokinetics of the anesthetic drug to be used are in a "chip" within the computer-controlled syringe pump. The clinician sets a desired therapeutic

Figure 1. The goal of anesthesiologists is to maintain a safe, constant therapeutic level of drug throughout the surgical period. Using intravenous drugs, this can be done in one of three ways: by bolus injection (solid line), by bolus injection followed by constant infusion (BET, dotted line), or by computer-assisted continuous infusion (CACI, hatched line). CACI provides the most constant plasma and brain concentrations.

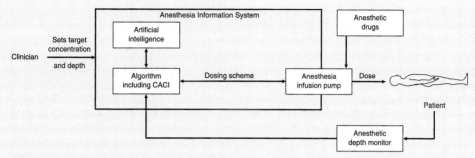

Figure 2. Future intravenous anesthesia drug delivery systems will involve automation and closed-loop drug administration. The clinician will use the appropriate drug concentration, and the desired level of unconsciousness (anesthesia) using an automated EEG monitor. The anesthetic dose and depth for that patient will then be maintained at the prescribed level by closed-loop technology. CACI, computer-assisted continuous infusion. (Reproduced, with permission, from Reves JG, Greene MN: Anesthesiology and the academic medical center: Place and promise at the start of the new millennium. Int Anesthesiol Clin 2000;38:iii. With permission from Lippincott, Williams & Wilkins.)

blood or brain (effect site) level of anesthetic and the computer infuses the drug, first by rapid infusion to attain a therapeutic level, and then by continuous infusion at an exponentially declining rate to maintain a constant drug level in the patient. This technology has been described for propofol,[3,4] and has been used worldwide with the Diprifusor in over 13 million patients.[5]

What is the advantage of TCI over other continuous infusion methods? The differences between TCI and continuous manual infusion are not great, but TCI is superior to an intermittent bolus.[6] The major advantage of TCI is that it produces a stable intravenous anesthetic that permits the clinician to titrate to the required level with less chance of overdosing or underdosing the patient. This is the same advantage that the vaporizer provides the clinician using an inhalation anesthetic: relatively constant blood (brain) levels are easily titrated to the desired effect.

At some point in the future, intravenous anesthetic drugs will be delivered by intelligent infusion pumps that are able to individualize the administration based on the pharmacokinetics of the drug in that patient, and maintain a desired brain concentration based on a feedback signal. Sophisticated systems of the future will include a "closed-loop" intravenous and inhalation anesthesia system (Figure 2). The clinician would activate the system by choosing a desired drug level utilizing the processed electroencephalographic (EEG) reading. Processed EEG signaling similar to the existing bispectral (BIS) system now available will undoubtedly be used to close the loop.[7] Such an automated system will be able to administer anesthetic drugs to rapidly attain and maintain the patient at the desired level of anesthesia. The depth of anesthesia or sedation (in

nongeneral anesthesia settings) will be maintained automatically, akin to cruise control of an automobile. This technology will also have applications in intensive care units, in emergency departments, and in a host of other nonoperating room settings.

Anesthesiologists will teach others the science behind the seemingly simple patient care applications of these new drug delivery technologies. This "robotic-like" approach to anesthesia and sedation cannot be viewed as a threat to the practice of anesthesia, but must be embraced as another step in the progress of the field of anesthesiology.[7] It will allow anesthesiologists to improve patient care in multiple settings even when not personally present!

1. Schuttler J, Schwilden H, Stockel H: Pharmacokinetics as applied to total intravenous anesthesia: Practical implications. Anaesthesia 1983;38:53.

2. Alvis JM, Reves JG, Govier AV, et al: Computer-assisted continuous infusions of fentanyl during cardiac anesthesia: Comparison with a manual method. Anesthesiology 1985;63:41.

3. White M, Kenny DNC: Intravenous propofol using a computerized infusion system. Anaesthesia 1990;45:204.

4. Glass PSA, Shafer SL, Jacobs JR, Reves JG: Intravenous drug delivery systems. In: *Anesthesia,* 4th ed. Miller RD (editor). Churchill Livingstone, 2000, pp 377–411.

5. Egan TD, Shafer SL: Target-controlled infusions for intravenous anesthetics. Anesthesiology 2003;99:1039.

6. Theil DR, Stanley TE, White WD, et al: Midazolam and fentanyl continuous intravenous anesthesia for cardiac surgery: A comparison of two infusion systems. J Cardiothorac Vasc Anesth 1993;7:300.

7. Reves JG, Green MN: Anesthesiology and the academic medical center: Place and promise at the start of the new millennium. Int Anesthesiol Clin 2000;38:iii.

drug concentration (200% increase after 1000 units of heparin).

The combination of opioids and diazepam markedly reduces arterial blood pressure and peripheral vascular resistance. This synergistic interaction is particularly pronounced in patients with ischemic or valvular heart disease.

Benzodiazepines reduce the minimum alveolar concentration of volatile anesthetics as much as 30%.

Ethanol, barbiturates, and other central nervous system depressants potentiate the sedative effects of the benzodiazepines.

OPIOIDS

Mechanisms of Action

Opioids bind to specific receptors located throughout the central nervous system and other tissues. Four major types of opioid receptor have been identified (Table 8–4): mu (μ, with subtypes μ-1 and μ-2), kappa (κ), delta (δ), and sigma (σ). Although opioids provide some degree of sedation, they are most effective at producing analgesia. The pharmacodynamic properties of specific opioids depend on which receptor is bound, the binding affinity, and whether the receptor is activated. Although both opioid agonists and antagonists bind to opioid receptors, only agonists are capable of receptor activation. Agonists–antag-

onists (eg, nalbuphine, nalorphine, butorphanol, and pentazocine) are drugs that have opposite actions at different receptor types. The pure opioid antagonist naloxone is discussed in Chapter 15.

Endorphins, enkephalins, and dynorphins are endogenous peptides that bind to opioid receptors. These three families of opioid peptides differ in their protein precursors, anatomic distributions, and receptor affinities.

Opiate–receptor activation inhibits the presynaptic release and postsynaptic response to excitatory neurotransmitters (eg, acetylcholine, substance P) from nociceptive neurons. The cellular mechanism for this neuromodulation may involve alterations in potassium and calcium ion conductance. Transmission of pain impulses can be interrupted at the level of the dorsal horn of the spinal cord with intrathecal or epidural administration of opioids. Modulation of a descending inhibitory pathway from the periaqueductal gray through the nucleus raphe magnus to the dorsal horn of the spinal cord may also play a role in opioid analgesia. Although opioids exert their greatest effect within the central nervous system, opiate receptors have also been isolated from somatic and sympathetic peripheral nerves.

Structure–Activity Relationships

Opiate–receptor interaction is shared by a chemically diverse group of compounds. Nonetheless, there are common structural characteristics, which are shown in Figure 8–6. Small molecular changes can convert an agonist into an antagonist. Note that the levorotatory isomers are generally more potent than the dextrorotatory isomers.

Pharmacokinetics

A. ABSORPTION

Rapid and complete absorption follows the intramuscular injection of morphine and meperidine, with peak plasma levels usually reached after 20–60 min. Oral transmucosal fentanyl citrate absorption (fentanyl "lollipop") is an effective method of producing analgesia and sedation and provides rapid onset (10 min) of analgesia and sedation in children (15–20 μg/kg) and adults (200–800 μg).

The low molecular weight and high lipid solubility of fentanyl also allow transdermal absorption (the fentanyl patch). The amount of fentanyl released depends primarily on the surface area of the patch but can vary with local skin conditions (eg, blood flow). Establishing a reservoir of drug in the upper dermis delays systemic absorption for the first few hours. Serum concentrations of fentanyl reach a plateau within 14–24 h of application (peak levels occur later

Table 8–4. Classification of opioid receptors.[1]

Receptor	Clinical Effect	Agonists
μ	Supraspinal analgesia (μ-1) Respiratory depression (μ-2) Physical dependence Muscle rigidity	Morphine Met-enkephalin[2] β-endorphin[2] Fentanyl
κ	Sedation Spinal analgesia	Morphine Nalbuphine Butorphanol Dynorphin[2] Oxycodone
δ	Analgesia Behavioral Epileptogenic	Leu-enkephalin[2] β-endorphin[2]
σ	Dysphoria Hallucinations Respiratory stimulation	Pentazocine Nalorphine Ketamine?

[1]Note: The relationships among receptor, clinical effect, and agonist are more complex than indicated in this table. For example, pentazocine is an antagonist at μ receptors, a partial agonist at κ receptors, and an agonist at σ receptors.
[2]Endogenous opioid.

Figure 8-6. Opioid agonists and antagonists share part of their chemical structure, which is outlined in bold.

in elderly patients than in young adult patients) and remain constant for up to 72 h. Continued absorption from the dermal reservoir accounts for a prolonged fall in serum levels after patch removal. A high incidence of nausea and variable blood levels have limited the acceptance of fentanyl patches for postoperative relief of pain.

Experimental studies have explored the possibility of an inhalation delivery of liposome-encapsulated fentanyl.

B. DISTRIBUTION

Table 8–5 summarizes the physical characteristics that determine distribution and uptake of opioid analgesics. The distribution half-lives of all of the opioids are fairly rapid (5–20 min). The low fat solubility of morphine slows passage across the blood–brain barrier, however, so that its onset of action is slow and its duration of action is prolonged. This contrasts with the high lipid solubility of fentanyl and sufentanil, which allows a rapid onset and short duration of action. Interestingly, alfentanil has a more rapid onset of action and shorter duration of action than fentanyl following a bolus injection, even though it is less lipid soluble than fentanyl. The high nonionized fraction of alfentanil at physiological pH and its small V_d increase the amount of drug available for binding in the brain. Significant amounts of lipid-soluble opioids can be retained by the lungs (first-pass uptake) and later diffuse back into the systemic circulation. The amount of pulmonary uptake depends on prior accumulation of another drug (decreases), a history of tobacco use (increases), and coincident inhalation anesthetic administration (decreases). Redistribution terminates the action of small doses of all of these drugs, whereas larger doses must depend on biotransformation to adequately lower plasma levels.

Table 8–5. Physical characteristics of opioids that determine distribution.[1]

Agent	Nonionized Fraction	Protein Binding	Lipid Solubility
Morphine	++	++	+
Meperidine	+	+++	++
Fentanyl	+	+++	++++
Sufentanil	++	++++	++++
Alfentanil	++++	++++	+++
Remifentanil	+++	+++	++

[1]+, very low; ++, low; +++, high; ++++, very high.

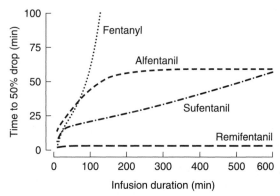

Figure 8–7. In contrast to other opioids, the time necessary to achieve a 50% decrease in the plasma concentration of remifentanil (its **context-sensitive half-time**) is very short and is not influenced by the duration of the infusion. (Reproduced, with permission, from Egan TD: The pharmacokinetics of the new short-acting opioid remifentanil [GI87084B] in healthy adult male volunteers. Anesthesiology 1993;79:881.)

C. BIOTRANSFORMATION

Most opioids depend primarily on the liver for biotransformation. Because of their high hepatic extraction ratio, their clearance depends on liver blood flow. The small V_d of alfentanil is responsible for a short elimination half-life (1.5 h). Morphine undergoes conjugation with glucuronic acid to form morphine 3-glucuronide and morphine 6-glucuronide. Meperidine is N-demethylated to normeperidine, an active metabolite associated with seizure activity. The end products of fentanyl, sufentanil, and alfentanil are inactive.

The unique ester structure of remifentanil, an ultrashort-acting opioid with a terminal elimination half-life of less than 10 min, makes it susceptible to rapid ester hydrolysis by nonspecific esterases in blood (red cells) and tissue (see Figure 8–6) in a manner similar to esmolol (see Chapter 12). Biotransformation is so rapid and so complete that the duration of a remifentanil infusion has little effect on wake-up time (Figure 8–7). Its **context/sensitive half-time** (the time required for the plasma drug concentration to decline by 50% after termination of an infusion) is approximately 3 min regardless of the duration of infusion. This lack of drug accumulation following repeated boluses or prolonged infusions differs from other currently available opioids. Extrahepatic hydrolysis also implies the absence of metabolite toxicity in patients with hepatic dysfunction. Patients with pseudocholinesterase deficiency have a normal response to remifentanil.

D. EXCRETION

The end products of morphine and meperidine biotransformation are eliminated by the kidneys, with less than 10% undergoing biliary excretion. Because 5–10% of morphine is excreted unchanged in the urine, renal failure prolongs its duration of action. The accumulation of morphine metabolites (morphine 3-glucuronide and morphine 6-glucuronide) in patients with renal failure has been associated with narcosis and ventilatory depression lasting several days. In fact, morphine 6-glucuronide is a more potent and longer-lasting opioid agonist than morphine. **Similarly, renal dysfunction increases the chance of toxic effects from normeperidine accumulation.** Normeperidine has an excitatory effect on the central nervous system, leading to myoclonic activity and seizures that are not reversed by naloxone. A late secondary peak in fentanyl plasma levels occurs up to 4 h after the last intravenous dose and may be explained by enterohepatic recirculation or mobilization of sequestered drug. Metabolites of sufentanil are excreted in urine and bile. The main metabolite of remifentanil is eliminated renally but is several thousand times less potent than its parent compound, and thus is unlikely to produce any noticeable opioid effects. Even severe liver disease does not affect the pharmacokinetics or pharmacodynamics of remifentanil.

Effects on Organ Systems

A. CARDIOVASCULAR

In general, opioids do not seriously impair cardiovascular function. Meperidine tends to increase heart rate (it is structurally similar to atropine), whereas high doses of morphine, fentanyl, sufentanil, remifentanil, and alfentanil are associated with a vagus-mediated bradycardia. With the exception of meperidine, the opioids do not depress cardiac contractility. Nonetheless, arterial blood pressure often falls as a result of bradycardia, venodilation, and decreased sympathetic reflexes, sometimes requiring vasopressor (eg, ephedrine) support. Furthermore, meperidine and morphine evoke histamine release in some individuals that can lead to profound drops in systemic vascular resistance and arterial blood pressure. The effects of histamine release can be minimized in susceptible patients by slow opioid infusion, adequate intravascular volume, or pretreatment with H_1 and H_2 histamine antagonists.

Intraoperative hypertension during opioid anesthesia, particularly morphine and meperidine, is not uncommon. It is often attributable to inadequate anesthetic depth and can be controlled with the addition of vasodilators or volatile anesthetic agents. The combination of opioids with other anesthetic drugs (eg, nitrous oxide, benzodiazepines, barbiturates, volatile agents) can result in significant myocardial depression.

Figure 8–8. Opioids depress ventilation. This is graphically displayed by a shift of the CO_2 curve downward and to the right.

B. RESPIRATORY

Opioids depress ventilation, particularly respiratory rate. Resting $PaCO_2$ increases and the response to a CO_2 challenge is blunted, resulting in a shift of the CO_2 response curve downward and to the right (Figure 8–8). These effects are mediated through the respiratory centers in the brain stem. **The apneic threshold—the highest $PaCO_2$ at which a patient remains apneic—is elevated, and hypoxic drive is decreased.** Gender differences may exist in these effects, with women demonstrating more respiratory depression. Morphine and meperidine can cause histamine-induced bronchospasm in susceptible patients. **Opioids (particularly fentanyl, sufentanil, and alfentanil) can induce chest wall rigidity severe enough to prevent adequate ventilation.** This centrally mediated muscle contraction is most frequent after large drug boluses and is effectively treated with neuromuscular blocking agents. Opioids can effectively blunt the bronchoconstrictive response to airway stimulation such as occurs during intubation.

C. CEREBRAL

The effects of opioids on cerebral perfusion and intracranial pressure appear to be variable. In general, opioids reduce cerebral oxygen consumption, cerebral blood flow, and intracranial pressure, but to a much lesser extent than barbiturates or benzodiazepines. These effects presume a maintenance of normocarbia by artificial ventilation; however, there are some reports of mild—and usually transient—increases in cerebral artery blood flow velocity and intracranial pressure following opioid boluses in patients with brain tumors or head trauma. Because opioids also tend to produce a mild decrease in mean arterial pressure, the resulting fall in CPP may be significant in some patients with abnormal intracranial elastance. Any small rise in intracranial pressure that opioids may cause must be compared with the potentially large increases in intracranial pressure during intubation in an inadequately anesthetized patient. The effect of most opioids on the EEG is minimal, although high doses are associated with slow δ-wave activity. High doses of fentanyl may rarely cause seizure activity; however, some cases may actually be severe opioid-induced muscle rigidity. EEG activation has been attributed to meperidine.

Stimulation of the medullary chemoreceptor trigger zone is responsible for a high incidence of nausea and vomiting. Physical dependence is a significant problem associated with repeated opioid administration. Unlike the barbiturates or benzodiazepines, relatively large doses of opioids are required to render patients unconscious (Table 8–6). Regardless of the dose, however, opioids do not reliably produce amnesia. Intravenous opioids have been the mainstay of pain control for more than a century. The relatively recent use of opioids in epidural and subdural spaces has revolutionized pain management (see Chapter 18).

Unique among opioids, meperidine and structurally similar sameridine have local anesthetic qualities when administered into the subarachnoid space. Meperidine's clinical use has been limited by classic opioid side effects (nausea, sedation, and pruritus), which may not be as pronounced with sameridine. **Intravenous meperidine (25 mg) has been found to be the most effective opioid for decreasing shivering.**

D. GASTROINTESTINAL

Opioids slow gastric emptying time by reducing peristalsis. Biliary colic may result from opioid-induced contraction of the sphincter of Oddi. Biliary spasm, which can mimic a common bile duct stone on cholangiography, is effectively reversed with the pure opioid antagonist naloxone. Patients receiving long-term opioid therapy (for cancer pain, for example) usually become tolerant to most of the side effects, except constipation because of the decreased gastrointestinal motility.

E. ENDOCRINE

The stress response to surgical stimulation is measured in terms of the secretion of specific hormones, including catecholamines, antidiuretic hormone, and cortisol. Opioids block the release of these hormones more completely than volatile anesthetics. This is particularly true of the more potent opioids such as fentanyl, sufentanil, alfentanil, and remifen-

Table 8–6. Uses and doses of common opioids.

Agent	Use	Route[1]	Dose[2]
Morphine	Premedication	IM	0.05–0.2 mg/kg
	Intraoperative anesthesia	IV	0.1–1 mg/kg
	Postoperative analgesia	IM	0.05–0.2 mg/kg
		IV	0.03–0.15 mg/kg
Meperidine	Premedication	IM	0.5–1 mg/kg
	Intraoperative anesthesia	IV	2.5–5 mg/kg
	Postoperative analgesia	IM	0.5–1 mg/kg
		IV	0.2–0.5 mg/kg
Fentanyl	Intraoperative anesthesia	IV	2–150 µg/kg
	Postoperative analgesia	IV	0.5–1.5 µg/kg
Sufentanil	Intraoperative anesthesia	IV	0.25–30 µg/kg
Alfentanil	Intraoperative anesthesia		
	Loading dose	IV	8–100 µg/kg
	Maintenance infusion	IV	0.5–3 µg/kg/min
Remifentanil	Intraoperative anesthesia		
	Loading dose	IV	1.0 µg/kg
	Maintenance infusion	IV	0.5–20 µg/kg/min
	Postoperative analgesia/ sedation	IV	0.05–0.3 µg/kg/min

[1]IM, intramuscular; IV, intravenous.
[2]**Note:** The wide range of opioid doses reflects a large therapeutic index and depends upon which other anesthetics are simultaneously administered. For obese patients, dose should be based on ideal body weight or lean body mass, not total body weight. Tolerance can develop rapidly (ie, within 2 h) during IV infusion of opioids, necessitating higher infusion rates. Dose correlates with other variables besides body weight that need to be considered (eg, age). The relative potencies of fentanyl, sufentanil, and alfentanil are estimated to be 1:9:1/7.

tanil. In particular, patients with ischemic heart disease may benefit from attenuation of the stress response.

Drug Interactions

The combination of opioids—particularly meperidine—and monoamine oxidase inhibitors may result in respiratory arrest, hypertension or hypotension, coma, and hyperpyrexia. The cause of this dramatic interaction is not understood.

Barbiturates, benzodiazepines, and other central nervous system depressants can have synergistic cardiovascular, respiratory, and sedative effects with opioids.

The biotransformation of alfentanil, but not sufentanil, may be impaired following a 7-day course of erythromycin, leading to prolonged sedation and respiratory depression.

KETAMINE

Mechanisms of Action

Ketamine has multiple effects throughout the central nervous system, including blocking polysynaptic reflexes in the spinal cord and inhibiting excitatory neurotransmitter effects in selected areas of the brain. In contrast to the depression of the reticular activating system induced by the barbiturates, ketamine functionally "dissociates" the thalamus (which relays sensory impulses from the reticular activating system to the cerebral cortex) from the limbic cortex (which is involved with the awareness of sensation). Although some brain neurons are inhibited, others are tonically excited. Clinically, this state of dissociative anesthesia causes the patient to appear conscious (eg, eye opening, swallowing, muscle contracture) but unable to process or respond to sensory input. Ketamine has been demonstrated to be an *N*-methyl-D-aspartate receptor (a subtype of the glutamate receptor) antagonist. The existence of specific ketamine receptors and interactions with opioid receptors has been postulated.

Structure–Activity Relationships

Ketamine (Figure 8–9) is a structural analogue of phencyclidine. It is one-tenth as potent, yet retains many of phencyclidine's psychotomimetic effects. Even subtherapeutic doses of ketamine can cause hallucinogenic effects. The increased anesthetic potency and decreased psychotomimetic side effects of one isomer (S[+] versus R[–]) imply the existence of stereospecific receptors.

Pharmacokinetics

A. ABSORPTION

Ketamine is administered intravenously or intramuscularly (Table 8–7). Peak plasma levels are usually achieved within 10–15 min after intramuscular injection.

B. DISTRIBUTION

Ketamine is more lipid soluble and less protein bound than thiopental; it is equally ionized at physiological pH. These characteristics, along with a ketamine-induced

increase in cerebral blood flow and cardiac output, lead to rapid brain uptake and subsequent redistribution (the distribution half-life is 10–15 min). Once again, awakening is due to redistribution to peripheral compartments.

C. BIOTRANSFORMATION

Ketamine is biotransformed in the liver to several metabolites, some of which (eg, norketamine) retain anesthetic activity. Induction of hepatic enzymes may partially explain the development of tolerance in patients who receive multiple doses of ketamine. Extensive hepatic uptake (hepatic extraction ratio of 0.9) explains ketamine's relatively short elimination half-life (2 h).

D. EXCRETION

End products of biotransformation are excreted renally.

Effects on Organ Systems

A. CARDIOVASCULAR

In sharp contrast to other anesthetic agents, ketamine increases arterial blood pressure, heart rate, and cardiac output (Table 8–8). These indirect cardiovascular effects are due to central stimulation of the sympathetic nervous system and inhibition of the reuptake of norepinephrine. Accompanying these changes are increases in pulmonary artery pressure and myocardial work. For these reasons, ketamine should be avoided in patients with coronary artery disease, uncontrolled hypertension, congestive heart failure, and arterial aneurysms. The **direct myocardial depressant** effects of large doses of ketamine, probably due to inhibition of calcium transients, are unmasked by sympathetic blockade (eg, spinal cord transection) or exhaustion of catecholamine stores (eg, severe end-stage shock). On the other hand, ketamine's **indirect stimulatory effects** are often beneficial to patients with acute hypovolemic shock.

B. RESPIRATORY

Ventilatory drive is minimally affected by the customary induction doses of ketamine, although rapid intravenous bolus administration or pretreatment with opioids occasionally produces apnea. Ketamine is a potent bronchodilator, making it a good induction agent for asthmatic patients. Although upper airway reflexes remain largely intact, patients at increased risk for aspiration pneumonia should be intubated (see Case Discussion, Chapter 15). The increased salivation associated with ketamine can be attenuated by premedication with an anticholinergic agent.

C. CEREBRAL

Consistent with its cardiovascular effects, ketamine increases cerebral oxygen consumption, cerebral blood

Figure 8–9. The structures of ketamine, etomidate, propofol, and droperidol. Note the similarities between ketamine and phencyclidine and between droperidol and haloperidol.

flow, and intracranial pressure. These effects preclude its use in patients with space-occupying intracranial lesions. Myoclonic activity is associated with increased subcortical electrical activity, which is not apparent on surface EEG. Undesirable psychotomimetic side effects (eg, illusions, dis-turbing dreams, and delirium) during emergence and recovery are less common in children and in patients pre-medicated with benzodiazepines. Of the nonvolatile agents, ketamine may be the closest to being a "complete" anes-thetic as it induces analgesia, amnesia, and unconsciousness.

Table 8–7. Uses and doses of ketamine, etomidate, propofol, and droperidol.

Agent	Use	Route[1]	Dose
Ketamine	Induction	IV	1–2 mg/kg
		IM	3–5 mg/kg
Etomidate	Induction	IV	0.2–0.5 mg/kg
Propofol	Induction	IV	1–2.5 mg/kg
	Maintenance infusion	IV	50–200 μg/kg/min
	Sedation infusion	IV	25–100 μg/kg/min
Droperidol	Premedication	IM	0.04–0.07 mg/kg
	Sedation	IV	0.02–0.07 mg/kg
	Antiemetic	IV	0.05 mg/kg[2]

[1]IV, intravenous; IM, intramuscular.
[2]Maximum adult dose without prolonging emergence is 1.25–2.5 mg.

Drug Interactions

Nondepolarizing neuromuscular blocking agents are potentiated by ketamine (see Chapter 9). The combination of theophylline and ketamine may predispose patients to seizures. Diazepam attenuates ketamine's cardiostimulatory effects and prolongs its elimination half-life. Propranolol, phenoxybenzamine, and other sympathetic antagonists unmask the direct myocardial depressant effects of ketamine. Ketamine produces myocardial depression when given to patients anesthetized with halothane or, to a lesser extent, other volatile anesthetics. Lithium may prolong the duration of action of ketamine.

ETOMIDATE

Mechanisms of Action

Etomidate depresses the reticular activating system and mimics the inhibitory effects of GABA. Specifically, etomidate (particularly the R[+] isomer) appears to bind to a subunit of the GABA type A receptor, increasing its affinity for GABA. Unlike barbiturates, it may have disinhibitory effects on the parts of the nervous system that control extrapyramidal motor activity. This disinhibition is responsible for a 30–60% incidence of myoclonus.

Structure–Activity Relationships

Etomidate, which contains a carboxylated imidazole, is structurally unrelated to other anesthetic agents (see Figure 8–9). The imidazole ring provides water solubility in acidic solutions and lipid solubility at physiologi-

cal pH. Etomidate is dissolved in propylene glycol. This solution often causes pain on injection that can be lessened by a prior injection of lidocaine.

Pharmacokinetics

A. Absorption

Etomidate is available only for intravenous administration and is used primarily for induction of general anesthesia (see Table 8–7).

B. Distribution

Although it is highly protein bound, etomidate is characterized by a very rapid onset of action due to its high lipid solubility and large nonionized fraction at physiological pH. Redistribution is responsible for decreasing the plasma concentration to awakening levels.

C. Biotransformation

Hepatic microsomal enzymes and plasma esterases rapidly hydrolyze etomidate to an inactive metabolite. The rate of biotransformation is five times greater for etomidate than for thiopental.

D. Excretion

The end product of hydrolysis is primarily excreted in the urine.

Effects on Organ Systems

A. Cardiovascular

Etomidate has minimal effects on the cardiovascular system. A mild reduction in peripheral vascular resistance is responsible for a slight decline in arterial blood pressure. Myocardial contractility and cardiac output are usually unchanged. Etomidate does not release histamine.

B. Respiratory

Ventilation is affected less with etomidate than with barbiturates or benzodiazepines. Even induction doses usually do not result in apnea unless opioids have also been administered.

C. Cerebral

Etomidate decreases the cerebral metabolic rate, cerebral blood flow, and intracranial pressure to the same extent as thiopental. Because of minimal cardiovascular effects, CPP is well maintained. Although changes on EEG resemble those associated with barbiturates, etomidate enhances somatosensory evoked potentials. Postoperative nausea and vomiting are more common

Table 8–8. Summary of nonvolatile anesthetic effects on organ systems.[1]

Agent	Cardiovascular		Respiratory		Cerebral		
	HR	MAP	Vent	B'dil	CBF	CMRO$_2$	ICP
Barbiturates							
Thiopental	↑↑	↓↓	↓↓↓	↓	↓↓↓	↓↓↓	↓↓↓
Thiamylal	↑↑	↓↓	↓↓↓	↓	↓↓↓	↓↓↓	↓↓↓
Methohexital	↑↑	↓↓	↓↓↓	0	↓↓↓	↓↓↓	↓↓↓
Benzodiazepines							
Diazepam	0/↑	↓	↓↓	0	↓↓	↓↓	↓↓
Lorazepam	0/↑	↓	↓↓	0	↓↓	↓↓	↓↓
Midazolam	↑	↓↓	↓↓	0	↓↓	↓↓	↓↓
Opioids							
Meperidine[2]	↑	—[2]	↓↓↓	—[2]	↓	↓	↓
Morphine[2]	↓	—[2]	↓↓↓	—[2]	↓	↓	↓
Fentanyl	↓↓	↓	↓↓↓	0	↓	↓	↓
Sufentanil	↓↓	↓	↓↓↓	0	↓	↓	↓
Alfentanil	↓↓	↓↓	↓↓↓	0	↓	↓	↓
Remifentanil	↓↓	↓↓	↓↓↓	0	↓	↓	↓
Ketamine	↑↑	↑↑	↓	↑↑↑	↑↑↑	↑	↑↑↑
Etomidate	0	↓	↓	0	↓↓↓	↓↓↓	↓↓↓
Propofol	0	↓↓↓	↓↓↓	0	↓↓↓	↓↓↓	↓↓↓
Droperidol	↑	↓↓	0	0	↓	0	↓

[1]HR, heart rate; MAP, mean arterial pressure; Vent, ventilatory drive; B'dil, bronchodilation; CBF, cerebral blood flow; CMRO$_2$, cerebral oxygen consumption; ICP, intracranial pressure; 0, no effect; 0/↑, no change or mild increase; ↓, decrease (mild, moderate, marked); ↑, increase (mild, moderate, marked).
[2]The effects of meperidine and morphine on MAP and bronchodilation depend upon the extent of histamine release.

than following barbiturate induction, but can be minimized by antiemetic medications. Etomidate is a sedative-hypnotic but lacks analgesic properties.

D. ENDOCRINE

Induction doses of etomidate transiently inhibit enzymes involved in cortisol and aldosterone synthesis. Long-term infusions lead to **adrenocortical suppression** that may be associated with an increased mortality rate in critically ill patients.

Drug Interactions

Fentanyl increases the plasma level and prolongs the elimination half-life of etomidate.

Opioids decrease the myoclonus characteristic of an etomidate induction.

PROPOFOL

Mechanisms of Action

The mechanism by which propofol induces a state of general anesthesia may involve facilitation of inhibitory neurotransmission mediated by GABA.

Structure–Activity Relationships

Propofol (2,6-diisopropylphenol) consists of a phenol ring with two isopropyl groups attached (Figure 8–9). Altering the side-chain length of this alkylphenol influences potency, induction, and recovery characteristics. Propofol is not water soluble, but a 1% aqueous solution (10 mg/mL) is available for intravenous administration as an oil-in-water emulsion containing soybean oil, glycerol, and egg lecithin. A history of egg allergy does not necessarily contraindicate the use of propofol because most egg allergies involve a reaction to egg white (egg albumin), whereas egg lecithin is extracted from egg yolk. This formulation can cause pain during injection (less common in elderly patients) that can be decreased by prior injection of lidocaine or by mixing lidocaine with propofol prior to injection (2 mL of 1% lidocaine in 18 mL propofol). Other formulations of propofol (eg, 1% propofol in 16% polyoxyethylated castor oil) may decrease injection discomfort. Propofol formulations can support the growth of bacteria, so good sterile technique must be observed in preparation and handling, including cleaning the rubber stopper or ampule neck surface with an alcohol swab prior to opening it. Administration should be completed within 6 h of opening the ampule. Sepsis and death have been linked to contaminated propofol preparations. Current formulations of propofol contain 0.005% disodium edetate or 0.025% sodium metabisulfite to help retard the rate of growth of microorganisms; however, these are still not antimicrobially preserved products under United States Pharmacopeia standards.

Pharmacokinetics

A. ABSORPTION

Propofol is available only for intravenous administration for the induction of general anesthesia and for moderate to deep sedation (see Table 8–7).

B. DISTRIBUTION

The high lipid solubility of propofol results in an onset of action that is almost as rapid as that of thiopental (one-arm-to-brain circulation time). Awakening from a single bolus dose is also rapid due to a very short initial distribution half-life (2–8 min). Most investigators believe that recovery from propofol is more rapid and is accompanied by less hangover than recovery from methohexital, thiopental, or etomidate. This makes it a good agent for outpatient anesthesia. A lower induction dose is recommended in elderly patients because of their smaller V_d. Women may require a higher dose of propofol than men and appear to awaken faster.

C. BIOTRANSFORMATION

The clearance of propofol exceeds hepatic blood flow, implying the existence of extrahepatic metabolism. This exceptionally high clearance rate (10 times that of thiopental) probably contributes to relatively rapid recovery after a continuous infusion. Conjugation in the liver results in inactive metabolites that are eliminated by renal clearance. The pharmacokinetics of propofol do not appear to be affected by moderate cirrhosis. Use of propofol infusion for long-term sedation of children who are critically ill or young adult neurosurgical patients has been associated with cases of lipemia, metabolic acidosis, and death.

D. EXCRETION

Although metabolites of propofol are primarily excreted in the urine, chronic renal failure does not affect clearance of the parent drug.

Effects on Organ Systems

A. CARDIOVASCULAR

The major cardiovascular effect of propofol is a decrease in arterial blood pressure due to a drop in systemic vascular resistance (inhibition of sympathetic vasoconstrictor activity), cardiac contractility, and preload. Hypotension is more pronounced than with thiopental but is usually reversed by the stimulation accompanying laryngoscopy and intubation. Factors exacerbating the hypotension include large doses, rapid injection, and old age. Propofol markedly impairs the normal arterial baroreflex response to hypotension, particularly in conditions of normocarbia or hypocarbia. Rarely, a marked drop in preload may lead to a vagally mediated reflex bradycardia. Changes in heart rate and cardiac output are usually transient and insignificant in healthy patients but may be severe enough to lead to asystole, particularly in patients at the extremes of age, on negative chronotropic medications, or undergoing surgical procedures associated with the oculocardiac reflex (see Chapter 38). Patients with impaired ventricular function may experience a significant drop in cardiac output as a result of decreases in ventricular filling pressures and contractility. Although myocardial oxygen consumption and coronary blood flow decrease to a similar extent, coronary sinus lactate production increases in some patients. This indicates a regional mismatch between myocardial oxygen supply and demand.

B. RESPIRATORY

Like the barbiturates, propofol is a profound respiratory depressant that usually causes apnea following an induction dose. Even when used for conscious sedation in subanesthetic doses, propofol infusion inhibits hypoxic ventilatory drive and depresses the normal response to hypercarbia. As a result, only properly trained personnel should use this technique. Propofol-induced depression of upper airway reflexes exceeds that of thiopental and can prove helpful during intubation or laryngeal mask placement in the absence of paralysis. Although propofol can cause histamine release, induction with propofol is accompanied by a lower incidence of wheezing in asthmatic and nonasthmatic patients compared with barbiturates or etomidate and is not contraindicated in asthmatic patients.

C. CEREBRAL

Propofol decreases cerebral blood flow and intracranial pressure. In patients with elevated intracranial pressure, propofol can cause a critical reduction in CPP (< 50 mm Hg) unless steps are taken to support mean arterial blood pressure. Propofol and thiopental probably provide a similar degree of cerebral protection during focal ischemia. Unique to propofol are its antipruritic properties. Its antiemetic effects (requiring a blood propofol concentration of 200 ng/mL) make it a preferred drug for outpatient anesthesia. Induction is occasionally accompanied by excitatory phenomena such as muscle twitching, spontaneous movement, opisthotonus, or hiccupping possibly due to subcortical glycine antagonism. Although these reactions may occasionally mimic tonic–clonic seizures, propofol appears to have predominantly anticonvulsant properties (ie, burst suppression), has been successfully used to terminate status epilepticus, and may be safely administered to epileptic patients. Propofol decreases intraocular pressure. Tolerance does not develop after long-term propofol infusions.

Drug Interactions

Nondepolarizing neuromuscular blocking agents may be potentiated by previous formulations of propofol, which contained Cremophor. Newer formulations do not share this interaction.

Fentanyl and alfentanil concentrations may be increased by concomitant administration of propofol. Some clinicians administer a small amount of midazolam (eg, 30 μg/kg) prior to induction with propofol; they believe the combination produces synergistic effects (eg, faster onset and lower total dose requirements). However, this technique of "coinduction" has questionable efficacy.

DROPERIDOL

Mechanisms of Action

Droperidol antagonizes the activation of dopamine receptors. For example, in the central nervous system, the caudate nucleus and the medullary chemoreceptor trigger zone are affected. Droperidol also interferes with transmission mediated by serotonin, norepinephrine, and GABA. These central actions account for the tranquilizer and antiemetic properties of droperidol. Peripheral actions include α-adrenergic blockade.

Structure–Activity Relationships

Droperidol, a butyrophenone, is structurally related to haloperidol (see Figure 8–9). Structural differences between the two drugs explain the neuroleptic characteristics of the former and the antipsychotic activity of the latter.

Pharmacokinetics

A. Absorption

Although droperidol is occasionally administered intramuscularly as part of a premedication regimen, it is usually given intravenously (see Table 8–7).

B. Distribution

Despite a rapid distribution phase ($t_{1/2}$ = 10 min), the sedative effects of droperidol are delayed by a relatively high molecular weight and extensive protein binding, which hinder penetration of the blood–brain barrier. A prolonged duration of action (3–24 h) may be explained by tenacious receptor binding.

C. Biotransformation

Droperidol is extensively metabolized in the liver, as evidenced by a hepatic clearance as rapid as that of ketamine and etomidate.

D. Excretion

The end products of biotransformation are excreted primarily in the urine.

Effects on Organ Systems

A. Cardiovascular

Droperidol's mild α-adrenergic blocking effects decrease arterial blood pressure by peripheral vasodilation. Hypovolemic patients can experience exaggerated declines in blood pressure. The α-adrenergic blocking actions may be responsible for an antiarrhythmic effect. In fact, droperidol has been associated with QT interval prolongation and torsades de pointes. Because there have been several deaths associated with droperidol use, the U.S. Food and Drug Administration has published a black box warning. Prior to administering droperidol, a 12-lead electrocardiogram should be recorded. If the QT measures greater than 440 ms for men or greater than 450 ms for women, droperidol should not be given. If the QT interval is normal and droperidol is given, the electrocardiogram should be monitored for 2–3 h.

Patients with pheochromocytoma should not receive droperidol because it can induce catecholamine release from the adrenal medulla, resulting in severe hypertension.

B. Respiratory

Droperidol, administered alone and in usual doses, does not significantly depress respiration and may actually stimulate hypoxic ventilatory drive.

C. Cerebral

Droperidol decreases cerebral blood flow and intracranial pressure by inducing cerebral vasoconstriction. However, droperidol does not reduce cerebral oxygen consumption—unlike the barbiturates, benzodiazepines, and etomidate. The EEG is not markedly changed. Droperidol is a potent antiemetic; however, delayed awakening limits its intraoperative use to low doses (0.05 mg/kg, to a maximum of 2.5 mg). The **antidopaminergic activity of droperidol rarely precipitates extrapyramidal** reactions (eg, oculogyric crises, torticollis, agitation), **which can be treated with diphenhydramine.** Nonetheless, droperidol should be avoided in patients with Parkinson disease, restless leg syndrome, or perhaps any patient with a neurologically mediated movement disorder.

Although patients premedicated with droperidol appear placid and sedated, they are often extremely apprehensive and fearful. For this reason, droperidol has fallen into disfavor as a sole premedication. The addition of an opioid decreases the incidence of dysphoria. Droperidol is a tranquilizer, and it does not produce analgesia, amnesia, or unconsciousness at usual doses. The combination of fentanyl and droperidol (Innovar) produces a state characterized by analgesia, immobility, and variable amnesia (classically referred to as neuroleptanalgesia). The addition of nitrous oxide or a hypnotic agent leads to unconsciousness and general anesthesia (neuroleptanalgesia) similar to the dissociative state induced by ketamine.

Drug Interactions

Droperidol antagonizes the effects of levodopa and may precipitate parkinsonian symptoms. The renal effects of dopamine are countered by droperidol.

Theoretically, droperidol could antagonize the central α-adrenergic action of clonidine and precipitate rebound hypertension.

Droperidol attenuates the cardiovascular effects of ketamine.

CASE DISCUSSION: PREMEDICATION OF THE SURGICAL PATIENT

An extremely anxious 17-year-old woman presents for uterine dilatation and curettage. She demands to be asleep before going to the operating room and does not want to remember anything.

What are the goals of administering preoperative medication?

Anxiety is a normal emotional response to impending surgery. Minimizing anxiety is usually the major goal of preoperative medication. For many patients, the preoperative interview with the anesthesiologist allays fears more effectively than sedative drugs. Other psychological objectives of preoperative medication include relief of preoperative pain and perioperative amnesia.

There may also be specific medical indications for preoperative medication: prophylaxis against postoperative nausea and vomiting (5-HT₃s) and against aspiration pneumonia (eg, antacids), prevention of allergic reactions (eg, antihistamines), or decreasing

upper airway secretions (eg, anticholinergics). The goals of preoperative medication depend on many factors, including the health and emotional status of the patient, the proposed surgical procedure, and the anesthetic plan. For this reason, the choice of anesthetic premedication is not routine and must follow a thorough preoperative evaluation.

What is the difference between sedation and anxiety relief?

This distinction is well illustrated by the paradoxic effects of droperidol. Patients may appear to an observer to be adequately sedated but on questioning may be quite anxious. Anxiety relief can be measured only by the patient.

Do all patients require preoperative medication?

No—customary levels of preoperative anxiety do not harm most patients. Some patients dread intramuscular injections, and others find altered states of consciousness more unpleasant than nervousness. If the surgical procedure is brief, the effects of some sedatives may extend into the postoperative period and prolong recovery time. This is particularly troublesome for patients undergoing ambulatory surgery. Specific contraindications for sedative premedication include severe lung disease, hypovolemia, impending airway obstruction, increased intracranial pressure, and depressed baseline mental status. Premedication with sedative drugs should never be given before informed consent has been obtained.

Which patients are most likely to benefit from preoperative medication?

Some patients are quite anxious despite the preoperative interview. Separation of young children from their parents is often a traumatic ordeal, particularly if they have endured multiple prior surgeries. Chronic drug abusers may benefit from premedication to decrease the risk of withdrawal reactions. Medical conditions such as coronary artery disease or hypertension may be aggravated by psychological stress.

How does preoperative medication influence the induction of general anesthesia?

Some preoperative medications (eg, opioids) decrease anesthetic requirements and can smooth induction. Intravenous administration of these medications just prior to induction is a more reliable method of achieving the same benefits, however.

What governs the choice between the preoperative medications commonly administered?

After the goals of premedication have been determined, the clinical effects of the agents dictate choice. For instance, in a patient experiencing preoperative pain from a femoral fracture, the analgesic effects of an opioid (eg, fentanyl, morphine, meperidine) will decrease the discomfort associated with transportation to the operating room and positioning on the operating room table. Respiratory depression (drops in oxygen saturation), orthostatic hypotension, and nausea and vomiting make opioid premedication less desirable.

Barbiturates are effective sedatives but lack analgesic properties and can produce respiratory depression. Benzodiazepines relieve anxiety, often provide amnesia, and are relatively free of side effects. Like barbiturates, however, they are not analgesics. Diazepam and lorazepam are available orally. Intramuscular midazolam has a rapid onset (30 min) and short duration (90 min), but intravenous midazolam has an even better pharmacokinetic profile. Dysphoria, prolonged sedation, and α-adrenergic blockade limit the clinical usefulness of droperidol. Other preoperative medications are discussed in subsequent chapters: anticholinergics in Chapter 11 and antihistamines, antiemetics, and antacids in Chapter 15.

Which factors must be considered in selecting the anesthetic premedication for this patient?

First, it must be made clear to the patient that for safety reasons, anesthesia is not induced outside the operating room. Long-acting agents such as morphine or droperidol would not be a good choice for an outpatient procedure. Lorazepam and diazepam can also affect mental function for several hours. One alternative is to establish an intravenous line in the preoperative holding area and titrate small doses of midazolam, with or without fentanyl, using slurred speech as an end point. At that time, the patient can be taken to the operating room. Vital signs—particularly respiratory rate—must be continuously monitored.

SUGGESTED READING

Bissonnette B, Swan H, Ravussin P, Un V: Neuroleptanesthesia: Current status. Can J Anesth 1999;46:154. This article discusses several intravenous drugs used for moderate sedation.

Cammarano WB, Pittet J, Weitz S: Acute withdrawal syndrome related to the administration of analgesic and sedative medications in adult intensive care unit patients. Crit Care Med 1998;26:676. Symptoms of acute withdrawal are not uncommon in ICU patients receiving prolonged continuous infusions of opioids and benzodiazepines.

Evers AS, Maze M: Anesthetic pharmacology. *Physiologic Principles and Clinical Practice. A Companion to Miller's Anesthesia.* Churchill Livingstone, 2004. Several chapters address noninhalation drug pharmacology, providing outstanding basic science and clinical information.

Fragen RJ (editor): *Drug Infusions in Anesthesiology,* 2nd ed. Lippincott, Williams & Wilkins, 1996. The pharmacokinetic and hardware information necessary to fully utilize intravenous drug delivery systems.

Gan TJ, Glass PS, Sigl J: Women emerge from general anesthesia with propofol/alfentanil/nitrous oxide faster than men. Anesthesiology 1999;90:1283. Faster recovery may result in a higher incidence of intraoperative recall in women.

Jensen LS, Merry AF, Webster CS, et al: Evidence-based strategies for preventing drug administration errors during anaesthesia. Anaesthesia 2004;59:493. Provides evidence-based recommendations for the minimization of errors in intravenous drug administration in anesthesia from a systematic review of the literature that identified 98 relevant references (14 with experimental designs or reports and 19 with reports of cases or case series).

O'Hare R, McAtamney D, Mirakhur RK, et al: Bolus dose remifentanil for control of haemodynamic response to tracheal intubation during rapid sequence induction of anaesthesia. Br J Anaesth 1999;82:283. This article indicates that a dose of 1 μg/kg effectively blunted the cardiovascular response to intubation 1 min later.

Quinlan JJ, Homanics GE, Firestone LL: Anesthesia sensitivity in mice that lack the beta-3 subunit of the gamma aminobutyric acid type A receptor. Anesthesiology 1998;88:775. Mice that lack this subunit appear resistant to the obtunding effects of midazolam and etomidate but not pentobarbital, enflurane, or halothane.

Raeder J: Ketamine, revival of a versatile intravenous anaesthetic. Adv Exp Med Biol 2003;523:269. Excellent, up-to-date review of ketamine.

Short TG, Young R: Toxicity of intravenous anaesthetics. Best Pract Res Clin Anaesthesiol 2003;17:77. Wonderful review of the toxicity of several intravenous anesthetics.

Stoelting RK: *Pharmacology and Physiology in Anesthetic Practice,* 3rd ed. Lippincott, 1999.

Tesniere A, Servin F: Intravenous techniques in ambulatory anesthesia. Anesthesiol Clin North Am 2003;21:273. The growing importance of ambulatory surgery during the past decade has led to the development of efficient anesthetic techniques in terms of quality and safety of anesthesia and recovery. In these challenging objectives, intravenous techniques, which are well reviewed in this article, have played an important role, as they provide safe, efficient, and cost-effective anesthesia in the ambulatory setting.

Neuromuscular Blocking Agents

9

KEY CONCEPTS

 1 It is important to realize that muscle relaxation does not ensure unconsciousness, amnesia, or analgesia.

2 Depolarizing muscle relaxants act as acetylcholine (ACh) receptor agonists, whereas nondepolarizing muscle relaxants function as competitive antagonists.

3 Because depolarizing muscle relaxants are not metabolized by acetylcholinesterase, they diffuse away from the neuromuscular junction and are hydrolyzed in the plasma and liver by another enzyme, pseudocholinesterase (nonspecific cholinesterase, plasma cholinesterase, or butyrylcholinesterase).

4 With the exception of mivacurium, nondepolarizing agents are not significantly metabolized by either acetylcholinesterase or pseudocholinesterase. Reversal of their blockade depends on redistribution, gradual metabolism, and excretion of the relaxant by the body, or administration of specific reversal agents (eg, cholinesterase inhibitors) that inhibit acetylcholinesterase enzyme activity.

 5 Muscle relaxants owe their paralytic properties to mimicry of ACh. For example, succinylcholine consists of two joined ACh molecules.

 6 Compared with patients with low enzyme levels or heterozygous atypical enzyme in whom blockade duration is doubled or tripled, patients with homozygous atypical enzyme will have a very long blockade (eg, 4–6 h) following succinylcholine administration.

 7 Succinylcholine is considered contraindicated in the routine management of children and adolescents because of the risk of hyperkalemia, rhabdomyolysis, and cardiac arrest in children with undiagnosed myopathies.

 8 Normal muscle releases enough potassium during succinylcholine-induced depolarization to raise serum potassium by 0.5 mEq/L. Although this is usually insignificant in patients with normal baseline potassium levels, a life-threatening potassium elevation is possible in patients with burn injury, massive trauma, neurological disorders, and several other conditions.

 9 As a general rule, the more potent the nondepolarizing muscle relaxant the longer its speed of onset.

 10 Doxacurium, pancuronium, vecuronium, and pipecuronium are partially excreted by the kidneys, and their action is prolonged in patients with renal failure.

 11 Cirrhotic liver disease and chronic renal failure often result in an increased volume of distribution and a lower plasma concentration for a given dose of water-soluble drugs, such as muscle relaxants. On the other hand, drugs dependent on hepatic or renal excretion may demonstrate prolonged clearance. Thus, depending on the drug, a greater initial dose—but smaller maintenance doses—might be required in these diseases.

 12 Atracurium and cisatracurium undergo degradation in plasma at physiological pH and temperature by organ-independent Hofmann elimination. The resulting metabolites (a monoquaternary acrylate and laudanosine) have no intrinsic neuromuscular blocking effects.

 13 Mivacurium, like succinylcholine, is metabolized by pseudocholinesterase. It is only minimally metabolized by true cholinesterase.

(continued on next page)

(continued from previous page)

Hypertension and tachycardia may occur in patients given pancuronium. These cardiovascular effects are caused by the combination of vagal blockade and catecholamine release from adrenergic nerve endings.

Long-term administration of vecuronium to patients in intensive care units has resulted in prolonged neuromuscular blockade (up to several days), possibly

from accumulation of its active 3-hydroxy metabolite, changing drug clearance, or the development of a polyneuropathy.

Rocuronium (0.9–1.2 mg/kg) has an onset of action that approaches succinylcholine (60–90 s), making it a suitable alternative for rapid-sequence inductions, but at the cost of a much longer duration of action.

Skeletal muscle relaxation can be produced by deep inhalational anesthesia, regional nerve block, or neuromuscular blocking agents (commonly called *muscle relaxants*). In 1942, Harold Griffith published the results of a study using a refined extract of curare (a South American arrow poison) during anesthesia. Muscle relaxants rapidly became a routine part of the anesthesiologist's drug arsenal. As Griffith noted, it is important to realize that neuromuscular junction blocking agents produce paralysis, not anesthesia. In other words, muscle relaxation does not ensure unconsciousness, amnesia, or analgesia. This chapter reviews the principles of neuromuscular transmission and presents the mechanisms of action, physical structures, routes of elimination, recommended dosages, and side effects of several muscle relaxants.

receptors, but activation of only about 500,000 receptors is required for normal muscle contraction.

The structure of ACh receptors varies in different tissues and at different times in development. Each ACh receptor in the neuromuscular junction normally consists of five protein subunits, two α subunits and single β, δ, and ϵ subunits. Only the two identical α subunits are capable of binding ACh molecules. If both binding sites are occupied by ACh, a conformational change in the subunits briefly (1 ms) opens an ion channel in the core of the receptor (Figure 9–2). The channel will not open if ACh is only on one site. In contrast to the normal (or mature) junctional ACh receptor, another isoform con-

■ NEUROMUSCULAR TRANSMISSION

The region of approximation between a motor neuron and a muscle cell is the neuromuscular junction (Figure 9–1). The cell membranes of the neuron and muscle fiber are separated by a narrow (20-nm) gap, the synaptic cleft. As a nerve's action potential depolarizes its terminal, an influx of calcium ions through voltage-gated calcium channels into the nerve cytoplasm allows storage vesicles to fuse with the terminal membrane and release their contents of acetylcholine (ACh). The ACh molecules diffuse across the synaptic cleft to bind with nicotinic cholinergic receptors on a specialized portion of the muscle membrane, the motor end-plate. Each neuromuscular junction contains approximately 5 million of these

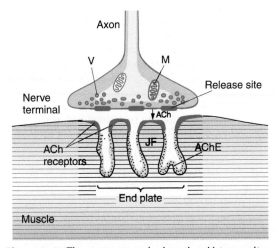

Figure 9–1. The neuromuscular junction. V, transmitter vesicle; M, mitochondrion; ACh, acetylcholine; AChE, acetylcholinesterase; JF, junctional folds. (Reproduced, with permission, from Drachman DB: Myasthenia gravis. N Engl J Med 1978;298:135.)

A

Center channel

B

ACh

Nicotinic cholinergic receptor

Na+

Ca2+

Ion channel

K+

Figure 9–2. ***A:*** Structure of the ACh receptor. Note the two α subunits that actually bind ACh and the center channel. ***B:*** Binding of ACh to receptors on muscle end-plate causes channel opening and ion flux.

tains a γ subunit instead of the ε subunit. This isoform is referred to as the fetal or immature receptor because it is in the form initially expressed in fetal muscle. It is also often referred to as extrajunctional because, unlike the mature isoform, expressed in adults, it may be located anywhere in the muscle membrane, inside or outside the neuromuscular junction.

Cations flow through the open ACh receptor channel (sodium and calcium in; potassium out), generating an **end-plate potential.** The contents of a single vesicle, a quantum of ACh (10^4 molecules per quantum), produce a miniature end-plate potential. The number of quanta released by each nerve impulse, normally at least 200, is very sensitive to extracellular ionized calcium concentration; increasing calcium concentration increases the number of quanta released. When enough receptors are occupied by ACh, the end-plate potential will be sufficiently strong to depolarize the perijunctional membrane. Sodium channels within this portion of the muscle membrane open when a threshold voltage is developed across them, as opposed to end-plate receptors that open when ACh is applied (Figure 9–3).

Perijunctional areas of muscle membrane have a higher density of sodium channels than other parts of the membrane. The resulting action potential propagates along the muscle membrane and T-tubule system, opening sodium channels and releasing calcium from the sarcoplasmic reticulum. This intracellular calcium allows the contractile proteins actin and myosin to interact, bringing about muscle contraction. The amount of ACh usually released and the number of receptors subsequently activated normally far exceed the minimum required for the initiation of an action potential. The nearly 10-fold margin of safety is overwhelmed in Eaton–Lambert myasthenic syndrome (decreased release of ACh) and myasthenia gravis (decreased number of receptors).

ACh is rapidly hydrolyzed into acetate and choline by the substrate-specific enzyme acetylcholinesterase. This enzyme (also called specific cholinesterase or true cholinesterase) is embedded into the motor end-plate membrane immediately adjacent to the ACh receptors. Eventually, the receptors' ion channels close, causing the end-plate to repolarize. When generation of action potential ceases,

A

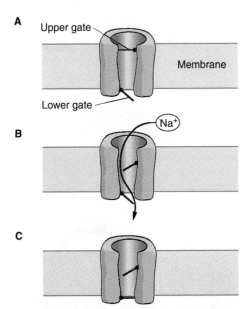

Figure 9–3. Schematic of the sodium channel. The sodium channel is a transmembrane protein that has two functional gates. Sodium ions pass only when both gates are open. Opening of the lower (inactivation) gate is time dependent, whereas the upper gate is voltage dependent. The channel therefore possesses three functional states. At rest the lower gate is open but the upper gate is closed (**A**). When the muscle membrane reaches threshold voltage depolarization, the upper gate opens and sodium can pass (**B**). Shortly after the upper gate opens the time-dependent lower gate closes (**C**). When the membrane repolarizes to its resting voltage the upper gate closes and the lower gate opens (**A**).

the sodium channels in the muscle membrane also close. Calcium is resequestered in the sarcoplasmic reticulum, and the muscle cell relaxes.

■ DISTINCTIONS BETWEEN DEPOLARIZING & NONDEPOLARIZING BLOCKADE

Neuromuscular blocking agents are divided into two classes: depolarizing and nondepolarizing (Table 9–1). This division reflects distinct differences in the mechanism of action, response to peripheral nerve stimulation, and reversal of block.

Table 9–1. Depolarizing and nondepolarizing muscle relaxants.

Depolarizing	Nondepolarizing
Short-acting	Short-acting
Succinylcholine	Mivacurium
	Intermediate-acting
	Atracurium
	Cisatracurium
	Vecuronium
	Rocuronium
	Long-acting
	Doxacurium
	Pancuronium
	Pipecuronium

MECHANISM OF ACTION

Similar to ACh, all neuromuscular blocking agents are quaternary ammonium compounds whose positively charged nitrogen imparts an affinity to nicotinic ACh receptors. Whereas most agents have two quaternary ammonium atoms, a few have one quaternary ammonium cation and one tertiary nitrogen that is protonated at physiological pH.

Depolarizing muscle relaxants very closely resemble ACh and therefore readily bind to ACh receptors, generating a muscle action potential. Unlike ACh, however, these drugs are *not* metabolized by acetylcholinesterase, and their concentration in the synaptic cleft does not fall as rapidly, resulting in a prolonged depolarization of the muscle end-plate.

Continuous end-plate depolarization causes muscle relaxation because opening of the lower gate in the perijunctional sodium channels is time limited (Figure 9–3). After the initial excitation and opening (Figure 9–3B), these sodium channels close (Figure 9–3C) and cannot reopen until the end-plate repolarizes. The end-plate cannot repolarize as long as the depolarizing muscle relaxant continues to bind to ACh receptors; this is called a phase I block. After a period of time, prolonged end-plate depolarization can cause ionic and conformational changes in the ACh receptor that result in a phase II block, which clinically resembles that of nondepolarizing muscle relaxants.

Nondepolarizing muscle relaxants bind ACh receptors but are incapable of inducing the conformational change necessary for ion channel opening. Because ACh is prevented from binding to its receptors, no end-plate potential develops. Neuromuscular blockade occurs even if only one α subunit is blocked.

 Thus, depolarizing muscle relaxants act as ACh receptor agonists, whereas nondepolarizing muscle relaxants function as competitive antagonists. This basic difference in mechanism of action explains their varying effects in certain disease states. For example, conditions associated with a chronic decrease in ACh release (eg, muscle denervation injuries) stimulate a compensatory increase in the number of ACh receptors within muscle membranes. These states also promote the expression of the immature (extrajunctional) isoform of the ACh receptor, which displays low channel conductance properties and prolonged open-channel time. This up-regulation causes an exaggerated response to depolarizing muscle relaxants (with more receptors being depolarized), but a resistance to nondepolarizing relaxants (more receptors that must be blocked). In contrast, conditions associated with fewer ACh receptors (eg, down-regulation in myasthenia gravis) demonstrate a resistance to depolarizing relaxants and an increased sensitivity to nondepolarizing relaxants.

NONCLASSICAL MECHANISMS OF NEUROMUSCULAR BLOCKADE

Some drugs may interfere with the function of the ACh receptor without acting as an agonist or antagonist. They interfere with normal functioning of the ACh receptor-binding site or with the opening and closing of the receptor channel. These may include inhaled anesthetic agents, local anesthetics, and ketamine. The ACh receptor–lipid membrane interface may be an important site of action.

Drugs may also cause either closed or open channel blockade. During closed channel blockade, the drug physically plugs up the channel, preventing passage of cations whether or not ACh has activated the receptor. Open channel blockade is use dependent, because the drug enters and obstructs the ACh receptor channel only after it is opened by ACh binding. The clinical relevance of channel blockade is that increasing the concentration of ACh with a cholinesterase inhibitor does not overcome neuromuscular blockade. Drugs that may cause channel block include neostigmine, some antibiotics, cocaine, and quinidine.

Prejunctional nicotinic ACh receptors have been identified on nerve endings at the neuromuscular junction. Although their physiological role is not entirely clear, the prejunctional actions for some muscle relaxants may be significant.

REVERSAL OF NEUROMUSCULAR BLOCKADE

Because depolarizing muscle relaxants are not metabolized by acetylcholinesterase, they diffuse away from the neuromuscular junction and are hydrolyzed in the plasma and liver by another enzyme, pseudocholinesterase (nonspecific cholinesterase, plasma cholinesterase, or butyrylcholinesterase). Fortunately, this is a fairly rapid process, because no specific agent to reverse a depolarizing blockade is available.

With the exception of mivacurium, nondepolarizing agents are not significantly metabolized by either acetylcholinesterase or pseudocholinesterase. Reversal of their blockade depends on redistribution, gradual metabolism, and excretion of the relaxant by the body, or administration of specific reversal agents (eg, cholinesterase inhibitors) that inhibit acetylcholinesterase enzyme activity (see Chapter 10). Because this inhibition increases the amount of ACh that is available at the neuromuscular junction and can compete with the nondepolarizing agent, clearly, the reversal agents are of no benefit in reversing a depolarizing block. In fact, by increasing neuromuscular junction ACh concentration and inhibiting pseudocholinesterase, *cholinesterase inhibitors can prolong depolarization blockade.*

RESPONSE TO PERIPHERAL NERVE STIMULATION

The use of peripheral nerve stimulators to monitor neuromuscular function is discussed in Chapter 6. Four patterns of electrical stimulation with supramaximal square-wave pulses are considered:

Tetany: A sustained stimulus of 50–100 Hz, usually lasting 5 s.

Twitch: A single pulse 0.2 ms in duration.

Train-of-four: A series of four twitches in 2 s (2-Hz frequency), each 0.2 ms long.

Double-burst stimulation (DBS): Three short (0.2 ms) high-frequency stimulations separated by a 20-ms interval (50 Hz) and followed 750 ms later by two ($DBS_{3,2}$) or three ($DBS_{3,3}$) additional impulses (see Figure 6–32).

The occurrence of fade, a gradual diminution of evoked response during prolonged or repeated nerve stimulation, is indicative of a nondepolarizing block (Table 9–2). Fade may be due to a prejunctional effect of nondepolarizing relaxants that reduces the amount of ACh in the nerve terminal available for release during stimulation (blockade of ACh mobilization). Adequate clinical recovery correlates well with the absence of fade. Because fade is more obvious during sustained tetanic stimulation or double-burst stimulation than following a train-of-four pattern or repeated twitches, the first two patterns are the preferred methods for determining adequacy of recovery from a nondepolarizing block.

The ability of tetanic stimulation during a partial nondepolarizing block to increase the evoked response to a subsequent twitch is termed posttetanic potentiation. This phenomenon may relate to a transient increase in ACh mobilization following tetanic stimulation.

In contrast, a phase I depolarization block does not exhibit fade during tetanus or train-of-four; neither does it demonstrate posttetanic potentiation. If enough depolarizer

Table 9–2. Evoked responses during depolarizing (phase I and phase II) and nondepolarizing block.

Normal Evoked Stimulus	Depolarizing Block		Nondepolarizing Block
	Phase I	Phase II	
Train-of-four	Constant but diminished	Fade	Fade
Tetany	Constant but diminished	Fade	Fade
Double-burst stimulation (DBS$_{3,2}$)	Constant but diminished	Fade	Fade
Posttetanic potentiation	Absent	Present	Present

is administered, however, the quality of the block changes to resemble a nondepolarizing block (phase II block).

◼ DEPOLARIZING MUSCLE RELAXANTS

SUCCINYLCHOLINE

The only depolarizing muscle relaxant in clinical use today is succinylcholine.

Physical Structure

 Succinylcholine—also called diacetylcholine or suxamethonium—consists of two joined ACh molecules (Figure 9–4). This copycat structure of ACh is responsible for succinylcholine's mechanism of action, side effects, and metabolism.

Metabolism & Excretion

The popularity of succinylcholine is due to its rapid onset of action (30–60 s) and short duration of action (typically less than 10 min). Its rapid onset of action is largely due to its low lipid solubility (all muscle relax-

Figure 9–4. Chemical structures of neuromuscular blocking agents.

Table 9–3. Drugs known to decrease pseudocholinesterase activity.

Drug	Description
Echothiophate	Organophosphate use for glaucoma
Neostigmine Pyridostigmine	Cholinesterase inhibitors
Phenelzine	Monoamine oxidase inhibitor
Cyclophosphamide	Antineoplastic agent
Metoclopramide	Antiemetic/prokinetic agent
Esmolol	β-Blocker
Pancuronium	Nondepolarizing muscle relaxant
Oral contraceptives	Various agents

ants are highly charged and water soluble) and the relative overdose that is usually administered. As succinylcholine enters the circulation, most of it is rapidly metabolized by pseudocholinesterase into succinylmonocholine. This process is so efficient that only a small fraction of the injected dose ever reaches the neuromuscular junction. As drug serum levels fall, succinylcholine molecules diffuse away from the neuromuscular junction, limiting the duration of action. The duration of action is prolonged by high doses or by abnormal metabolism. The latter may result from hypothermia, low pseudocholinesterase levels, or a genetically aberrant enzyme. Hypothermia decreases the rate of hydrolysis. Low levels of pseudocholinesterase (measured as units per liter) accompany pregnancy, liver disease, renal failure, and certain drug therapies (Table 9–3). Low pseudocholinesterase levels generally produce only modest prolongation of succinylcholine's actions (2–20 min).

One in 50 patients has one normal and one abnormal (atypical) pseudocholinesterase gene, resulting in a slightly prolonged block (20–30 min). Even fewer (1 in 3000) patients have two abnormal genes (homozygous atypical) that produce an enzyme with little or no affinity for succinylcholine. In contrast to the doubling or tripling of blockade duration seen in patients with low enzyme levels or heterozygous atypical enzyme, patients with homozygous atypical enzyme will have a *very* long blockade (eg, 4–8 h) following administration of succinylcholine. Of the recognized abnormal pseudocholinesterase genes, the dibucaine-resistant (variant) gene, which displays 1/100 of normal affinity for succinylcholine, is the most common. Other variants include fluoride-resistant and silent (no activity).

Dibucaine, a local anesthetic, inhibits normal pseudocholinesterase activity by 80% but inhibits atypical enzyme activity by only 20%. Serum from an individual who is heterozygous for the atypical enzyme is characterized by an intermediate 40–60% inhibition. The percentage of inhibition of pseudocholinesterase activity is termed the **dibucaine number.** The dibucaine number is proportional to pseudocholinesterase function and independent of the amount of enzyme. Therefore, adequacy of pseudocholinesterase can be determined in the laboratory quantitatively in units per liter (a minor factor) and qualitatively by dibucaine number (the major factor). **Prolonged paralysis from succinylcholine caused by abnormal pseudocholinesterase (atypical cholinesterase) should be treated with continued mechanical ventilation until muscle function returns to normal.**

Drug Interactions

The effects of muscle relaxants can be modified by concurrent drug therapy (Table 9–4). Succinylcholine is involved in two interactions deserving special comment.

A. Cholinesterase Inhibitors

Although cholinesterase inhibitors reverse nondepolarizing paralysis, they markedly prolong a depolarizing phase I block by two mechanisms: By inhibiting acetylcholinesterase, they lead to a higher ACh concentration at the nerve terminal, which intensifies depolarization. They also reduce the hydrolysis of succinylcholine by inhibiting pseudocholinesterase. Organophosphate pesticides, for example, cause an irreversible inhibition of acetylcholinesterase and can prolong the action of succinylcholine by 20–30 min.

B. Nondepolarizing Relaxants

In general, small doses of nondepolarizing relaxants antagonize a depolarizing phase I block. Because the drugs occupy some ACh receptors, depolarization by succinylcholine is partially prevented. An exception to this interaction is pancuronium, which augments succinylcholine blockade by inhibiting pseudocholinesterase.

Intubating doses of succinylcholine consistently reduce some nondepolarizer (atracurium and rocuronium) requirements for about 30 min; no effect is reported with mivacurium, pancuronium, or pipecuronium. Similarly, if enough depolarizing agent is administered to develop a phase II block, a nondepolarizer will potentiate paralysis.

Dosage

Because of the rapid onset, short duration, and low cost of succinylcholine, many clinicians believe that it is still a good choice for routine intubation in

Table 9-4. Potentiation (+) and resistance (-) of neuromuscular blocking agents by other drugs.

Drug	Effect on Depolarizing Blockade	Effect on Nondepolarizing Blockade	Comments
Antibiotics	+	+	Streptomycin, aminoglycosides, kanamycin, neomycin, colistin, polymyxin, tetracycline, lincomycin, clindamycin
Anticonvulsants	?	-	Phenytoin, carbamazepine, primidone, sodium valproate
Antiarrhythmics	+	+	Quinidine, calcium channel blockers
Cholinesterase inhibitors	+	-	Neostigmine, pyridostigmine
Dantrolene	?	+	Used in treatment of malignant hyperthermia (has quaternary ammonium group)
Inhalational anesthetics	+	+	Volatile anesthetics
Ketamine	?	+	
Local anesthetics	+	+	High doses only
Lithium carbonate	+	?	Prolongs onset and duration of succinylcholine
Magnesium sulfate	+	+	Doses used to treat preeclampsia and eclampsia of pregnancy

adults. The usual adult dose of succinylcholine needed for intubation is 1–1.5 mg/kg intravenously. Doses as small as 0.5 mg/kg may provide acceptable intubating conditions if a defasciculating dose of a nondepolarizer is not used. Repeated small boluses (10 mg) or a succinylcholine drip (1 g in 500 or 1000 mL, titrated to effect) can be used during surgical procedures that require brief but intense paralysis (eg, otolaryngological endoscopies). Methylene blue indicator dye is often added to succinylcholine drips to prevent confusion with other intravenous fluids. In addition, neuromuscular function should be constantly monitored with a nerve stimulator to prevent overdosing and the development of phase II block. The availability of short-acting nondepolarizing muscle relaxants (eg, mivacurium) has reduced the popularity of this technique.

Because succinylcholine is not lipid soluble, its distribution is limited to the extracellular space. Per kilogram, infants and neonates have a larger extracellular space than adults. Therefore, dosage requirements for pediatric patients are often greater than for adults. If succinylcholine is administered *intramuscularly* to children, a dose as high as 4–5 mg/kg does not always produce complete paralysis.

Succinylcholine should be stored under refrigeration (2–8°C), and should generally be used within 14 days after removal from refrigeration and exposure to room temperature.

Side Effects & Clinical Considerations

Succinylcholine is a relatively safe drug— assuming that its many potential complications are understood and avoided. Because of the risk of hyperkalemia, rhabdomyolysis, and cardiac arrest in children with undiagnosed myopathies, however, succinylcholine is considered contraindicated in the routine management of children and adolescent patients. In the absence of a difficult airway or full stomach, many clinicians have also abandoned the routine use of succinylcholine for adults. None of the presently available nondepolarizing muscle relaxants has the very rapid onset and short duration of succinylcholine. Clinicians continue to wait for such a drug.

A. CARDIOVASCULAR

Because of the resemblance of muscle relaxants to ACh, it is not surprising that they affect cholinergic receptors in addition to those at the neuromuscular junction. The entire parasympathetic nervous system and parts of the sympathetic nervous system (sympathetic ganglions, adrenal medulla, and sweat glands) depend on ACh as a neurotransmitter.

Succinylcholine not only stimulates nicotinic cholinergic receptors at the neuromuscular junction, it stimulates all ACh receptors. Succinylcholine's cardiovascular actions are therefore very complex. Stimulation of nicotinic receptors in parasympathetic and sympathetic ganglia and muscarinic receptors in the sinoatrial node of the heart can increase or decrease blood pressure and heart rate. Low doses of succinylcholine can produce negative chronotropic and inotropic effects, but higher doses usually increase heart rate and contractility and elevate circulating catecholamine levels.

Children are particularly susceptible to profound bradycardia following administration of succinylcholine. Bradycardia typically occurs in adults only if a second bolus of succinylcholine is administered approximately 3–8 min after the first dose. A succinylcholine metabolite, succinylmonocholine, appears to sensitize muscarinic cholinergic receptors in the sinoatrial node to the second dose of succinylcholine, resulting in bradycardia. Intravenous atropine (0.02 mg/kg in children, 0.4 mg in adults) is normally given prophylactically to children prior to the first dose and *always* before a second dose of succinylcholine. Other arrhythmias such as nodal bradycardia and ventricular ectopy have been reported.

B. Fasciculations

The onset of paralysis by succinylcholine is usually signaled by visible motor unit contractions called fasciculations. These can be prevented by pretreatment with a small dose of nondepolarizing relaxant. Because this pretreatment usually antagonizes a depolarizing block, a higher dose of succinylcholine is subsequently required (1.5 mg/kg). Fasciculations are typically not observed in young children and elderly patients.

C. Hyperkalemia

 Normal muscle releases enough potassium during succinylcholine-induced depolarization to raise serum potassium by 0.5 mEq/L. Although this is usually insignificant in patients with normal baseline potassium levels, it can be life-threatening in patients with preexisting hyperkalemia or those with burn injury, massive trauma, neurological disorders, and several other conditions (Table 9–5). Subsequent cardiac arrest can prove to be quite refractory to routine cardiopulmonary resuscitation, requiring calcium, insulin, glucose, bicarbonate, epinephrine, cation-exchange resin, dantrolene, and even cardiopulmonary bypass to reduce metabolic acidosis and serum potassium levels.

Following denervation injuries, the immature isoform of the ACh receptor may be expressed inside and outside the neuromuscular junction (up-regulation). These extrajunctional receptors allow succinylcholine to effect widespread depolarization and extensive potassium release. Life-threatening potassium release is *not* reliably prevented by pretreatment with a nondepolarizer. The risk of hyperkalemia usually appears to peak in 7–10 days following the injury, but the exact time of onset and the duration of the risk period vary.

Table 9–5. Conditions causing susceptibility to succinylcholine-induced hyperkalemia.

Burn injury
Massive trauma
Severe intraabdominal infection
Spinal cord injury
Encephalitis
Stroke
Guillain-Barré syndrome
Severe Parkinson's disease
Tetanus
Prolonged total body immobilization
Ruptured cerebral aneurysm
Polyneuropathy
Closed head injury
Hemorrhagic shock with metabolic acidosis
Myopathies (eg, Duchenne's dystrophy)

D. Muscle Pains

Patients who have received succinylcholine have an increased incidence of postoperative myalgia. This complaint is most common in females and outpatients. Pregnancy and extremes of age seem to be protective. The efficacy of nondepolarizing pretreatment is controversial but most clinicians feel it is effective. Administration of rocuronium 0.06–0.1 mg/kg prior to succinylcholine has been reported to be effective in preventing fasciculations and reducing postoperative myalgias. The relationship between fasciculations and postoperative myalgias is also inconsistent. The myalgias are theorized to be due to the initial unsynchronized contraction of muscle groups; myoglobinemia and increases in serum creatine kinase can be detected following administration of succinylcholine. Perioperative use of nonsteroidal antiinflammatory drugs may reduce the incidence and severity of myalgias.

E. Intragastric Pressure Elevation

Abdominal wall muscle fasciculations increase intragastric pressure, which is offset by an increase in lower esophageal sphincter tone. Therefore, the risk of gastric reflux or pulmonary aspiration is probably not increased by succinylcholine. Although pretreatment with nondepolarizers abolishes the rise in gastric pressure, it also prevents the increase in lower esophageal sphincter tone.

F. Intraocular Pressure Elevation

Extraocular muscle differs from other striated muscle in that it has multiple motor end-plates on each cell. Prolonged membrane depolarization and contraction of extraocular muscles following administration of succinylcholine transiently raise intraocular pressure and could compromise an injured eye (see Case Discussion, Chapter 38). The elevation in intraocular pressure is not always prevented by pretreatment with a nondepolarizer.

G. MASSETER MUSCLE RIGIDITY

Succinylcholine transiently increases muscle tone in the masseter muscles. Some difficulty may initially be encountered in opening the mouth because of incomplete relaxation of the jaw. A marked increase in tone preventing laryngoscopy is abnormal and may be a premonitory sign of malignant hyperthermia.

H. MALIGNANT HYPERTHERMIA

Succinylcholine is a potent triggering agent in patients susceptible to malignant hyperthermia, a hypermetabolic disorder of skeletal muscle (see Case Discussion, Chapter 44). Although the signs and symptoms of neuroleptic malignant syndrome (NMS) resemble those of malignant hyperthermia, the pathogenesis is completely different and there is no need to avoid use of succinylcholine in patients with NMS.

I. GENERALIZED CONTRACTIONS

Patients afflicted with myotonia may develop myoclonus after administration of succinylcholine.

J. PROLONGED PARALYSIS

As discussed above, patients with low levels of normal pseudocholinesterase may have a longer than normal duration of action, whereas patients with atypical pseudocholinesterase will experience markedly prolonged paralysis.

K. INTRACRANIAL PRESSURE

Succinylcholine may lead to an activation of the electroencephalogram and slight increases in cerebral blood flow and intracranial pressure in some patients. Muscle fasciculations stimulate muscle stretch receptors, which subsequently increase cerebral activity. The increase in intracranial pressure can be attenuated by maintaining good airway control and instituting hyperventilation. It can be prevented by pretreating with a nondepolarizing muscle relaxant and administering intravenous lidocaine (1.5–2.0 mg/kg) 2–3 min prior to intubation. The effects of intubation on intracranial pressure far outweigh any increase caused by succinylcholine.

L. HISTAMINE RELEASE

Slight histamine release may be observed following succinylcholine in some patients.

■ NONDEPOLARIZING MUSCLE RELAXANTS

Unique Pharmacological Characteristics

In contrast to depolarizing muscle relaxants, there is a wide selection of nondepolarizers (Tables 9–6 and 9–7). Chemically they are either benzylisoquinolines or steroidal compounds. Choice of a particular drug depends on its unique characteristics, which are often related to its structure. For example, steroidal compounds tend to be vagolytic, whereas benzylisoquinolines tend to release histamine. Because of structural similarities,

Table 9–6. A summary of the pharmacology of nondepolarizing muscle relaxants.

Relaxant	Chemical Structure[1]	Metabolism	Primary Excretion	Onset[2]	Duration[3]	Histamine Release[4]	Vagal Blockade[5]
Atracurium	B	+++	Insignificant	++	++	+	0
Cisatracurium	B	+++	Insignificant	++	++	0	0
Mivacurium	B	+++	Insignificant	++	+	+	0
Doxacurium	B	Insignificant	Renal	+	+++	0	0
Pancuronium	S	+	Renal	++	+++	0	++
Pipecuronium	S	+	Renal	++	+++	0	0
Vecuronium	S	+	Biliary	++	++	0	0
Rocuronium	S	Insignificant	Biliary	+++	++	0	+

[1]B, benzylisoquinolone; S, steroidal.
[2]Onset: +, slow; ++, moderately rapid; +++, rapid.
[3]Duration: +, short; ++, intermediate; +++, long.
[4]Histamine release: 0, no effect; +, slight effect; ++, moderate effect; +++, marked effect.
[5]Vagal blockade: 0, no effect; +, slight effect; ++, moderate effect.

UPCOMING IMPROVEMENTS IN RELAXATION & REVERSAL

John J. Savarese, MD

Throughout the history of the basic and clinical sciences in which surgical relaxation has been studied (neuromuscular blockade is now our most commonly employed option), ideal circumstances have been envisioned and foreseen. The ideal situation might simply be conceptualized as the ability to induce or remove neuromuscular blockade rapidly and safely at any time, without concern for negative outcome.

The clinician's view of the utility of a neuromuscular blocking drug most likely involves four considerations: what are the onset of effect, the duration of effect, the side effects, and the "reversibility" of the drug in question? These factors underlie the clinician's feelings of convenience, confidence, suitability, and versatility in the application of a specific neuromuscular blocking drug in a particular procedure. It still all resolves to one fundamental issue, which, after all, is the underlying guideline in anesthetic practice: safety, as related to outcome.

Drug developers may improve the safety of neuromuscular blocking drugs with respect to clinical practice by improving the above clinical features, so that the practitioner can make more appropriate choices for neuromuscular blockade and so feel more confident and versatile in terms of safe practice and reduced negative outcomes.

Three or possibly four new drugs will most likely become available in the next 3 years or so, to bring clinical practice closer to ideal circumstances as far as relaxation is concerned. These features could only be imagined 10 years ago.

First, as well known for over 50 years, a replacement for succinylcholine is needed. Look for GW 280430A (AV 430A) to supply that need in about 2 years. Its onset, duration, and offset are almost identi-

---

an allergic history to one muscle relaxant strongly suggests the possibility of allergic reactions to other muscle relaxants.

A. SUITABILITY FOR INTUBATION

None of the currently available nondepolarizing muscle relaxants equals succinylcholine's rapid onset of action or short duration; however, the onset of nondepolarizing relaxants can be quickened by using either a larger dose or a priming dose. The ED_{95} is the effective dose of a drug in 95% of individuals. One to two times the ED_{95} is usually used for intubation. Although a larger intubating dose speeds onset, it exacerbates side effects and prolongs the duration of blockade. For example, a dose of 0.15 mg/kg of pancuronium may produce intubating conditions in 90 s, but at the cost of more pronounced hypertension and tachycardia—and a block that may be irreversible for more than 60 min. The

consequence of a long duration of action is the ensuing difficulty in completely reversing the blockade and a subsequent increased incidence of postoperative pulmonary complications, particularly in elderly patients and those undergoing abdominal surgery. As a general rule, the more potent the nondepolarizing muscle relaxant the longer its speed of onset; presumably greater potency necessitates a lower dose, which in turn decreases drug delivery to the neuromuscular junction.

The introduction of short- and intermediate-acting agents has resulted in the greater use of priming doses. Theoretically, giving 10–15% of the usual intubating dose 5 min before induction will occupy enough receptors so that paralysis will quickly follow when the balance of relaxant is administered. Use of a priming dose can produce conditions suitable for intubation as soon as 60 s following administration of rocuronium or 90 s cal to succinylcholine's pattern of blockade. 430A is the first nondepolarizer to provide all these features. As a nondepolarizer, 430A will not stimulate the autonomic nervous system, induce cardiac dysrhythmias, or be a trigger for malignant hyperthermia. But perhaps its greatest advantage is its degradation process.

Unlike succinylcholine, which is hydrolyzed and inactivated enzymatically by pseudocholinesterase, AV 430A undergoes chemical degradation at pH 7.4 by two mechanisms: pH-sensitive hydrolysis and cysteine adduction. The former mechanism is strictly chemical and occurs with a $t_{1/2}$ of about 15 min at pH 7.4. The latter mechanism results in a condensation product of AV 430A and cysteine, which is inactive. This condensation is also a chemical reaction requiring no catalyst, and has a $t_{1/2}$ of only 1–2 min. This is most likely the basis for the ultrashort duration of action of AV 430A.

Administration of excess cysteine speeds up the reaction to cause very rapid inactivation of 430A. For example, doses of 5–10 mg/kg cysteine will "reverse" 100% block within 1–2 min in monkeys. Therefore, this mechanism also "provides" an innocuous rapidly acting reversal agent that has no side effects of its own, which will enable the restoration of normal neuromuscular function within 2 min even from deep levels of paralysis such as 100% twitch inhibition.

Cysteine itself, therefore, constitutes a second drug that we can expect: a specific antagonist for AV 430A, which rapidly converts the neuromuscular blocking drug into its inactive metabolite, thereby "reversing"

paralysis. Cysteine, a normal amino acid building block for protein synthesis, has no side effects of its own. Its antagonistic effect seems to be generic for the group of compounds (the asymmetrical bis-onium chlorofumarates) of which AV 430A is a member.

The steroidal neuromuscular blocking drugs now have their own specific antagonist as well. The steroidal relaxants may be viewed as pie-shaped lipophilic molecules with two positive charges on the outer edge of the pie. ORG 25969, a doughnut-shaped cyclodextrin, has been synthesized specifically to accommodate the rocuronium steroidal structure within its lipophilic center, and to bind the quaternary groups to its negatively charged periphery. This new reversal agent will antagonize rocuronium-induced block within 2–3 min by a process of chelation. ORG 25969 is effective at higher dosage, for antagonism of the blocking effects of other steroidal relaxant molecules as well, such as vecuronium. The side effects of ORG 25969 seem to be minimal.

With the above three new drugs in hand, anesthesiologists will be able to intubate the trachea within 60 s without the problems of succinylcholine. Two specific antagonists will be available that will convert the neuromuscular blockers into inactive forms, at any point during the administration of relaxants, without side effects. Succinylcholine and the anticholinesterase drugs will become obsolete. The options available to anesthesiologists to induce and remove paralysis will increase, and the safety of clinical practice will improve.

following administration of other intermediate-acting nondepolarizers. A priming dose does not usually lead to clinically significant paralysis, which requires that 75–80% of the receptors be blocked (a neuromuscular margin of safety). In some patients, however, the priming dose occupies enough receptors to produce distressing dyspnea, diplopia, or dysphagia; in such instances, the patient should be reassured and induction of anesthesia should proceed without delay. Priming can additionally cause significant deterioration in respiratory function (eg, decreased forced vital capacity) and may lead to oxygen desaturation in patients with marginal pulmonary reserve. These negative side effects are more common in elderly patients.

It is important to keep in mind that muscle groups vary in their sensitivity to muscle relaxants (see Chapter 6 and the section on Muscle Groups below). For example, the laryngeal muscles—whose relaxation is important during intubation—recover from blockade more quickly than the adductor pollicis, which is commonly monitored by the peripheral nerve stimulator.

B. SUITABILITY FOR PREVENTING FASCICULATIONS

To prevent fasciculations, 10–15% of a nondepolarizer intubating dose can be administered 5 min before succinylcholine. Although most nondepolarizers have been successfully used for this purpose, tubocurarine and rocuronium appear to be particularly efficacious (precurarization); tubocurarine is no longer available in the United States. Because of the antagonism between most nondepolarizers and a phase I block, the subsequent dose of succinylcholine should be raised to 1.5 mg/kg.

C. MAINTENANCE RELAXATION

Following intubation, muscle paralysis may need to be continued to facilitate surgery, eg, abdominal

Table 9–7. Clinical characteristics of nondepolarizing muscle relaxants.

Drug	ED$_{95}$ for Adductor Pollicis During N$_2$/O$_2$ Anesthesia (mg/kg)	Intubation Dose (mg/kg)	Onset of Action for Intubating Dose (min)	Duration of Intubating Dose (min)	Maintenance Dosing by Boluses (mg/kg)	Maintenance Dosing by Infusion (μg/kg/min)
Succinylcholine	0.5	1.0	0.5	5–10	0.15	2–15 mg/min
Rocuronium	0.3	0.8	1.5	35–75	0.15	9–12
Mivacurium	0.08	0.2	2.5–3.0	15–20	0.05	4–15
Atracurium	0.2	0.5	2.5–3.0	30–45	0.1	5–12
Cisatracurium	0.05	0.2	2.0–3.0	40–75	0.02	1–2
Vecuronium	0.05	0.12	2.0–3.0	45–90	0.01	1–2
Pancuronium	0.07	0.12	2.0–3.0	60–120	0.01	—
Pipecuronium	0.05	0.1	2.0–3.0	80–120	0.01	—
Doxacurium	0.025	0.07	4.0–5.0	90–150	0.05	—

operations, or anesthetic management, eg, hemodynamic compromise precluding deepening anesthesia or the need to control ventilation. The variability between patients in dose responses to muscle relaxants cannot be overemphasized. Monitoring neuromuscular function with a nerve stimulator (Chapter 6) helps prevent over- and underdosing, as well as serious residual muscle paralysis in the recovery room. Maintenance doses whether by intermittent boluses or continuous infusion (Table 9–7) should be guided by the nerve stimulator *and* clinical signs (eg, spontaneous respiratory efforts or movement). In some instances clinical signs may precede twitch recovery because of differing sensitivities to muscle relaxants between muscle groups or technical problems with the nerve stimulator. Some return of neuromuscular transmission should be evident prior to administering each maintenance dose. When an infusion is used for maintenance, the rate should be adjusted at or just above the rate that allows some return of neuromuscular transmission.

D. POTENTIATION BY INHALATIONAL ANESTHETICS

Volatile agents decrease nondepolarizer dosage requirements by at least 15%. The actual degree of this postsynaptic augmentation depends on both the inhalational anesthetic (desflurane > sevoflurane > isoflurane and enflurane > halothane > N$_2$O/O$_2$/narcotic) and the muscle relaxant employed (pancuronium > vecuronium and atracurium). Volatile anesthetic-induced enhanced affinity for nondepolarizing relaxants has been proposed.

E. POTENTIATION BY OTHER NONDEPOLARIZERS

Some combinations of nondepolarizers (eg, mivacurium and pancuronium) produce a greater than additive neuromuscular blockade. The lack of augmentation by closely related compounds (eg, vecuronium and pancuronium) lends credence to the theory that potentiation results from slightly differing mechanisms of action.

F. AUTONOMIC SIDE EFFECTS

In clinical doses, the nondepolarizers can significantly differ in their effects on nicotinic and muscarinic cholinergic receptors. Some older agents (tubocurarine and, to a lesser extent, metocurine) blocked autonomic ganglia, compromising the ability of the sympathetic nervous system to increase heart contractility and rate in response to hypotension and other intraoperative stresses. In contrast, pancuronium (and gallamine) block vagal muscarinic receptors in the sinoatrial node, resulting in tachycardia. All newer nondepolarizing relaxants, including atracurium, cisatracurium, mivacurium, doxacurium, vecuronium, and pipecuronium, are devoid of significant autonomic effects in their recommended dosage ranges.

G. HISTAMINE RELEASE

Histamine release from mast cells can result in bronchospasm, skin flushing, and hypotension from peripheral vasodilation. Both atracurium and mivacurium are capable of triggering histamine release, particularly at higher doses. Slow injection rates and

H_1 and H_2 antihistamine pretreatment ameliorate these side effects.

H. HEPATIC CLEARANCE

Only pancuronium and vecuronium are metabolized to any significant degree by the liver. Active metabolites likely contribute to their clinical effect. Vecuronium and rocuronium depend heavily on biliary excretion. Clinically, liver failure prolongs pancuronium and rocuronium blockade, with less effect on vecuronium, and no effect on pipecuronium. Atracurium, cisatracurium, and mivacurium, although extensively metabolized, depend on extrahepatic mechanisms. Severe liver disease does not significantly affect clearance of atracurium or cisatracurium, but the associated decrease in pseudocholinesterase levels may slow the metabolism of mivacurium.

I. RENAL EXCRETION

Doxacurium, pancuronium, vecuronium, and pipecuronium are partially excreted by the kidneys, and their action is prolonged in patients with renal failure. The elimination of atracurium, cisatracurium, mivacurium, and rocuronium is independent of kidney function.

General Pharmacological Characteristics

Some variables affect all nondepolarizing muscle relaxants.

A. TEMPERATURE

Hypothermia prolongs blockade by decreasing metabolism (eg, mivacurium, atracurium, and cisatracurium) and delaying excretion (eg, pancuronium and vecuronium).

B. ACID–BASE BALANCE

Respiratory acidosis potentiates the blockade of most nondepolarizing relaxants and antagonizes its reversal. This could prevent complete neuromuscular recovery in a hypoventilating postoperative patient. Conflicting findings regarding the neuromuscular effects of other acid–base changes may be due to coexisting alterations in extracellular pH, intracellular pH, electrolyte concentrations, or structural differences between drugs (eg, monoquaternary versus bisquaternary; steroidal versus isoquinolinium).

C. ELECTROLYTE ABNORMALITIES

Hypokalemia and hypocalcemia augment a nondepolarizing block. The response of a patient with hypercalcemia is unpredictable. Hypermagnesemia, as may be seen in preeclamptic patients being managed with magnesium sulfate, potentiates a nondepolarizing blockade by competing with calcium at the motor end-plate.

D. AGE

Neonates have an increased sensitivity to nondepolarizing relaxants because of their immature neuromuscular junctions. This sensitivity does not necessarily decrease dosage requirements, as the neonate's greater extracellular space provides a larger volume of distribution.

E. DRUG INTERACTIONS

As noted earlier, many drugs augment nondepolarizing blockade (see Table 9–4). They have multiple sites of interaction: prejunctional structures, postjunctional cholinergic receptors, and muscle membranes.

F. CONCURRENT DISEASE

The presence of neurological or muscular disease can have profound effects on an individual's response to muscle relaxants (Table 9–8). Cirrhotic liver disease and chronic renal failure often result in an increased volume of distribution and a lower plasma concentration for a given dose of water-soluble drugs, such as muscle relaxants. On the other hand, drugs dependent on hepatic or renal excretion may demonstrate prolonged clearance. Thus, depending on the drug chosen, a greater initial (loading) dose—but smaller maintenance doses—might be required in these diseases.

G. MUSCLE GROUPS

The onset and intensity of blockade vary among muscle groups. This may be due to differences in blood flow, distance from the central circulation, or different fiber types. Furthermore, the relative sensitivity of a muscle group may depend on the choice of muscle relaxant. In general, the diaphragm, jaw, larynx, and facial muscles (orbicularis oculi) respond to and recover from muscle relaxation sooner than the thumb. Although they are a fortuitous safety feature, persistent diaphragmatic contractions can be disconcerting in the face of complete adductor pollicis paralysis. Glottic musculature is also quite resistant to blockade, as is often confirmed during laryngoscopy. The ED_{95} for laryngeal muscles is nearly two times that for the adductor pollicis muscle. Good intubating conditions are usually associated with visual loss of the orbicularis oculi twitch response.

Considering the multitude of factors influencing the duration and magnitude of muscle relaxation, it becomes clear that an individual's response to neuromuscular blocking agents should be monitored. Dosage recommendations, including those in this chapter, should be considered guidelines that require modification for individual patients. Wide variability in sensitivity to nondepolarizing muscle relaxants is often encountered in clinical practice.

Table 9–8. Diseases with altered responses to muscle relaxants.

Disease	Response to Depolarizers	Response to Nondepolarizers
Amyotrophic lateral sclerosis	Contracture	Hypersensitivity
Autoimmune disorders (systemic lupus erythematosus, polymyositis, dermatomyositis)	Hypersensitivity	Hypersensitivity
Burn injury	Hyperkalemia	Resistance
Cerebral palsy	Slight hypersensitivity	Resistance
Familial periodic paralysis (hyperkalemic)	Myotonia and hyperkalemia	Hypersensitivity?
Guillain–Barré syndrome	Hyperkalemia	Hypersensitivity
Hemiplegia	Hyperkalemia	Resistance on affected side
Muscular denervation (peripheral nerve injury)	Hyperkalemia and contracture	Normal response or resistance
Muscular dystrophy (Duchenne type)	Hyperkalemia and malignant hyperthemia	Hypersensitivity
Myasthenia gravis	Resistance and proneness to phase II block	Hypersensitivity
Myasthenic syndrome	Hypersensitivity	Hypersensitivity
Myotonia (dystrophica, congenita, paramyotonia)	Generalized muscular contractions	Normal or hypersensitivity
Severe chronic infection (tetanus, botulism)	Hyperkalemia	Resistance

ATRACURIUM

Physical Structure

Like all muscle relaxants, atracurium has a quaternary group; however, a benzylisoquinoline structure is responsible for its unique method of degradation. The drug is a mixture of 10 stereoisomers.

Metabolism & Excretion

Atracurium is so extensively metabolized that its pharmacokinetics are independent of renal and hepatic function, and less than 10% is excreted unchanged by renal and biliary routes. Two separate processes are responsible for metabolism.

A. ESTER HYDROLYSIS

This action is catalyzed by nonspecific esterases, not by acetylcholinesterase or pseudocholinesterase.

B. HOFMANN ELIMINATION

A spontaneous nonenzymatic chemical breakdown occurs at physiological pH and temperature.

Dosage

A dose of 0.5 mg/kg is administered intravenously over 30–60 s for intubation. Intraoperative relaxation is achieved with 0.25 mg/kg initially, then in incremental doses of 0.1 mg/kg every 10–20 min. An infusion of 5–10 μg/kg/min can effectively replace intermittent boluses.

Although dosage requirements do not significantly vary with age, atracurium may be shorter-acting in children and infants than in adults.

Atracurium is available as a solution of 10 mg/mL. It must be stored at 2–8°C, as it loses 5–10% of its potency for each month it is exposed to room temperature. At room temperature it should be used within 14 days to preserve potency.

Side Effects & Clinical Considerations

Atracurium triggers dose-dependent histamine release that becomes significant at doses above 0.5 mg/kg.

A. HYPOTENSION AND TACHYCARDIA

Cardiovascular side effects are unusual unless doses in excess of 0.5 mg/kg are administered. Atracurium may also cause a transient drop in systemic vascular resistance and an increase in cardiac index independent of any histamine release. A slow rate of injection minimizes these effects.

B. BRONCHOSPASM

Atracurium should be avoided in asthmatic patients. Nonetheless, severe bronchospasm is possible even in patients without a history of asthma.

C. LAUDANOSINE TOXICITY

Laudanosine, a tertiary amine, is a breakdown product of atracurium's Hofmann elimination and has been associated with central nervous system excitation, resulting in elevation of the minimum alveolar concentration and even precipitation of seizures. These are probably irrelevant considerations unless a patient has received an extremely high total dose or has hepatic failure. Laudanosine is metabolized by the liver and excreted in urine and bile.

D. TEMPERATURE AND pH SENSITIVITY

Because of its unique metabolism, atracurium's duration of action can be markedly prolonged by hypothermia and to a lesser extent by acidosis.

E. CHEMICAL INCOMPATIBILITY

Atracurium will precipitate as a free acid if it is introduced into an intravenous line containing an alkaline solution such as thiopental.

F. ALLERGIC REACTIONS

Rare anaphylactoid reactions to atracurium have been described. Proposed mechanisms include direct immunogenicity and acrylate-mediated immune activation. IgE-mediated antibody reactions directed against substituted ammonium compounds, including muscle relaxants, have been described. Reactions to acrylate, a metabolite of atracurium and a structural component of some dialysis membranes, have also been reported in patients undergoing hemodialysis.

CISATRACURIUM

Physical Structure

Cisatracurium is a stereoisomer of atracurium that is four times more potent. Atracurium contains approximately 15% cisatracurium.

Metabolism & Excretion

Like atracurium, cisatracurium undergoes degradation in plasma at physiological pH and temperature by organ-independent Hofmann elimination. The resulting metabolites (a monoquaternary acrylate and laudanosine) have no intrinsic neuromuscular blocking effects. Because of its higher potency the amount of laudanosine produced is significantly less than atracurium. Nonspecific esterases do not appear to be involved in the metabolism of cisatracurium. Metabolism and elimination appear to be independent of renal or liver failure. Minor variations in pharmacokinetic patterns due to age do not tend to result in clinically significant changes in duration of action.

Dosage

Cisatracurium produces good intubating conditions following a dose of 0.1–0.15 mg/kg within 2 min and results in muscle blockade of intermediate duration. The average infusion rate ranges from 1.0–2.0 μg/kg/min. Thus, it is equipotent with vecuronium and more potent than atracurium.

Cisatracurium should be stored under refrigeration (2–8°C), and should be used within 21 days after removal from refrigeration and exposure to room temperature.

Side Effects & Clinical Considerations

Unlike atracurium, cisatracurium does not produce a consistent, dose-dependent increase in plasma histamine levels following administration. Cisatracurium does not affect heart rate or blood pressure, nor does it produce autonomic effects, even at doses as high as eight times ED_{95}.

Cisatracurium shares with atracurium the considerations discussed above with regard to laudanosine toxicity (although levels appear to be lower due to its greater potency), pH and temperature sensitivity, and chemical incompatibility.

MIVACURIUM

Physical Structure

Mivacurium is a benzylisoquinoline derivative.

Metabolism & Excretion

Mivacurium, like succinylcholine, is metabolized by pseudocholinesterase. It is only minimally metabolized by true cholinesterase. This introduces the possibility of prolonged action in patients with low pseudocholinesterase levels (see Table 9–3) or variants of the pseudocholinesterase gene. In fact, patients who are heterozygous for the atypical gene will experience a block approximately twice the normal duration, whereas atypical homozygous patients will remain paralyzed for hours. Because atypical homozygotes cannot metabolize mivacurium, the neuromuscular blockade may last 3–4 h. In contrast to succinylcholine-induced paralysis in these patients, pharmacological antagonism with cholinesterase inhibitors will quicken reversal of mivacurium blockade once some response to nerve stimulation becomes apparent. Edrophonium more effectively reverses mivacurium blockade than neostigmine because neostigmine inhibits plasma cholinesterase activity (see Chapter 10). Although mivacurium metabolism and excretion do not directly depend on the kidneys or liver, duration of action can be prolonged in patients with renal or hepatic failure or in patients who are pregnant or postpartum as a result of decreased plasma cholinesterase levels.

Dosage

The usual intubating dose of mivacurium is 0.15–0.2 mg/kg. Steady-state infusion rates for intraoperative relaxation vary with pseudocholinesterase levels but can be initiated at 4–10 µg/kg/min. Children require higher dosages than adults if dosage is calculated in terms of body weight, but not if based on surface area. Mivacurium has a shelf-life of 18 months when stored at room temperature.

Side Effects & Clinical Considerations

Mivacurium releases histamine to about the same degree as atracurium. The consequent cardiovascular side effects can be minimized by slow injection over 1 min. Nonetheless, patients with cardiac disease may rarely experience a significant drop in arterial blood pressure after doses larger than 0.15 mg/kg, despite a slow injection rate. The onset time of mivacurium is similar to that of atracurium (2–3 min). Its principal advantage is its brief duration of action (20–30 min), which is still two to three times longer than a phase I block from succinylcholine—but half the duration of atracurium, vecuronium, or rocuronium. Children tend to exhibit a faster onset and shorter duration of action than adults. Despite relatively rapid recovery after mivacurium, neuromuscular function must be monitored in all patients to determine whether pharmacological reversal is necessary. The short duration of action of mivacurium can be markedly prolonged by prior administration of pancuronium.

DOXACURIUM

Physical Structure

Doxacurium is a benzylisoquinoline compound closely related to mivacurium and atracurium.

Metabolism & Excretion

This potent, long-acting relaxant undergoes a minor degree of slow hydrolysis by plasma cholinesterase. Like other long-acting muscle relaxants, however, its primary route of elimination is renal excretion. Predictably, the duration of action of doxacurium is prolonged and more variable in patients with renal disease. Hepatobiliary excretion appears to play a minor role in doxacurium clearance.

Dosage

Adequate conditions for tracheal intubation within 5 min require 0.05 mg/kg. Intraoperative relaxation is achieved with an initial dose of 0.02 mg/kg followed by

doses of 0.005 mg/kg. Doxacurium may be given in similar weight-adjusted dosages to young and elderly patients, although the latter demonstrate a prolonged duration of action.

Side Effects & Clinical Considerations

Doxacurium is essentially devoid of cardiovascular and histamine-releasing side effects. Because of its greater potency, doxacurium has an onset of action slightly slower than that of other long-acting nondepolarizing relaxants (4–6 min). Its duration of action is similar to that of pancuronium (60–90 min).

PANCURONIUM

Physical Structure

Pancuronium consists of a steroid ring on which two modified ACh molecules are positioned (a bisquaternary relaxant). To an ACh receptor, pancuronium resembles ACh enough to bind—but not enough to open—the lock.

Metabolism & Excretion

Pancuronium is metabolized (deacetylated) by the liver to a limited degree. Its metabolic products have some neuromuscular blocking activity. Excretion is primarily renal (40%), although some of the drug is cleared by the bile (10%). Not surprisingly, elimination of pancuronium is slowed and neuromuscular blockade is prolonged by renal failure. Patients with cirrhosis may require a higher initial dose due to an increased volume of distribution but have lower maintenance requirements because of a decreased rate of plasma clearance.

Dosage

A dose of 0.08–0.12 mg/kg of pancuronium provides adequate relaxation for intubation in 2–3 min. Intraoperative relaxation is achieved by administering 0.04 mg/kg initially followed every 20–40 min by 0.01 mg/kg.

Children may require moderately higher doses of pancuronium. Pancuronium is available as a solution of 1 or 2 mg/mL and is stored at 2–8°C but may be stable for up to 6 months at normal room temperature.

Side Effects & Clinical Considerations

A. HYPERTENSION AND TACHYCARDIA

These cardiovascular effects are caused by the combination of vagal blockade and sympathetic stimulation. The latter is due to a combination of ganglionic stimulation, catecholamine release from adrenergic nerve endings, and decreased catecholamine reuptake. Pancuronium should be given with caution to patients in whom an increased heart rate would be particularly detrimental (eg, coronary artery disease, idiopathic hypertrophic subaortic stenosis).

B. ARRHYTHMIAS

Increased atrioventricular conduction and catecholamine release increase the likelihood of ventricular dysrhythmias in predisposed individuals. The combination of pancuronium, tricyclic antidepressants, and halothane has been reported to be particularly arrhythmogenic.

C. ALLERGIC REACTIONS

Patients who are hypersensitive to bromides may exhibit allergic reactions to pancuronium (pancuronium bromide).

PIPECURONIUM

Physical Structure

Pipecuronium has a bisquaternary steroidal structure very similar to that of pancuronium.

Metabolism & Excretion

For pipecuronium, metabolism plays a very minor role. Elimination depends on excretion, which is primarily renal (70%) and secondarily biliary (20%). The duration of action is increased in patients with renal failure, but not in those with hepatic insufficiency.

Dosage

Pipecuronium is slightly more potent than pancuronium, and the usual intubating dose ranges from 0.06–0.1 mg/kg. Likewise, maintenance relaxation doses can be reduced by approximately 20% compared with pancuronium. Infants require less pipecuronium on a per kilogram basis than children or adults. Pipecuronium's pharmacological profile is relatively unchanged in elderly patients.

Side Effects & Clinical Considerations

The principal advantage of pipecuronium over pancuronium is its lack of cardiovascular side effects due to a decreased binding to cardiac muscarinic receptors. Like other steroidal relaxants, pipecuronium is not associated with histamine release. The onset of action and duration of action are similar to pancuronium.

VECURONIUM

Physical Structure

Vecuronium is pancuronium minus a quaternary methyl group (a monoquaternary relaxant). This minor structural change beneficially alters side effects without affecting potency.

Metabolism & Excretion

Vecuronium is metabolized to a small extent by the liver. It depends primarily on biliary excretion and secondarily (25%) on renal excretion. Although it is a satisfactory drug for patients with renal failure, its duration of action is somewhat prolonged. Vecuronium's brief duration of action is explained by its shorter elimination half-life and more rapid clearance compared with pancuronium. Long-term administration of vecuronium to patients in intensive care units has resulted in prolonged neuromuscular blockade (up to several days), possibly from accumulation of its active 3-hydroxy metabolite, changing drug clearance, or the development of a polyneuropathy. Risk factors appear to include female gender, renal failure, long-term or high-dose corticosteroid therapy, and sepsis. Thus, these patients must be closely monitored and the dose of vecuronium carefully titrated. Long-term relaxant administration and the subsequent prolonged lack of ACh binding at the postsynaptic nicotinic ACh receptors may mimic a chronic denervation state and cause lasting receptor dysfunction and paralysis. The neuromuscular effects of vecuronium may be prolonged in patients with AIDS. Tolerance to nondepolarizing muscle relaxants can also develop after long-term use.

Dosage

Vecuronium is equipotent with pancuronium, and the intubating dose is 0.08–0.12 mg/kg. A dose of 0.04 mg/kg initially followed by increments of 0.01 mg/kg every 15–20 min provides intraoperative relaxation. Alternatively, an infusion of 1–2 μg/kg/min produces good maintenance of relaxation.

Age does not affect initial dose requirements, although subsequent doses are required less frequently in neonates and infants. Women appear to be approximately 30% more sensitive than men to vecuronium as evidenced by a greater degree of blockade and longer duration of action (this has also been seen with pancuronium and rocuronium). The cause for this sensitivity may be related to gender-related differences in fat and muscle mass, protein binding, volume of distribution, or metabolic activity. The duration of action of vecuronium may be further prolonged in postpartum patients due to alterations in hepatic blood flow or liver uptake.

Vecuronium is packaged as 10 mg of powder, which is reconstituted with 5 or 10 mL of preservative-free water immediately before use. Unused portions are discarded after 24 h. Vecuronium and thiopental can form a precipitate that can obstruct flow through an intravenous line and lead to particulate pulmonary emboli.

Side Effects & Clinical Considerations

A. CARDIOVASCULAR

Even at doses of 0.28 mg/kg, vecuronium is devoid of significant cardiovascular effects. Potentiation of opioid-induced bradycardia may be observed in some patients.

B. LIVER FAILURE

Although it is dependent on biliary excretion, the duration of action of vecuronium is usually not significantly prolonged in patients with cirrhosis unless doses greater than 0.15 mg/kg are given. Vecuronium requirements are reduced during the anhepatic phase of liver transplantation.

ROCURONIUM

Physical Structure

This monoquaternary steroid analogue of vecuronium was designed to provide a rapid onset of action.

Metabolism & Excretion

Rocuronium undergoes no metabolism and is eliminated primarily by the liver and slightly by the kidneys. Its duration of action is not significantly affected by renal disease, but it is modestly prolonged by severe hepatic failure and pregnancy. Because rocuronium does not have active metabolites, it may be a better choice than vecuronium for prolonged infusions (eg, the intensive care unit setting). Elderly patients may experience a prolonged duration of action due to decreased liver mass.

Dosage

Rocuronium is less potent than most other steroidal muscle relaxants (potency appears to be inversely related to speed of onset). It requires 0.45–0.9 mg/kg intravenously for intubation and 0.15 mg/kg boluses for maintenance. A lower dose of 0.4 mg/kg may allow reversal as soon as 25 min after intubation. Intramuscular rocuronium (1 mg/kg for infants; 2 mg/kg for children) provides adequate vocal cord and diaphragmatic paralysis for intubation, but not until after 3–6 min (deltoid injection has a faster onset than quadriceps), and can be reversed after about 1 h. The infusion requirements for rocuronium range from 5–12 µg/kg/min. Rocuronium can produce a prolonged duration of action in elderly patients. Initial dosage requirements are modestly increased in patients with advanced liver disease, presumably due to a larger volume of distribution.

Side Effects & Clinical Considerations

 Rocuronium (at a dose of 0.9–1.2 mg/kg) has an onset of action that approaches succinylcholine (60–90 s), making it a suitable alternative for rapid-sequence inductions, but at the cost of a much longer duration of action. This intermediate duration of action is comparable to vecuronium or atracurium.

Some clinicians compensate for rocuronium's longer onset of action (compared with that of succinylcholine) by administering it 20 s before propofol or thiopental (the "timing principle"). Disadvantages to this technique include the possibility of delayed administration of induction agent (eg, due to intravenous line precipitate) resulting in a conscious but paralyzed patient.

Rocuronium (0.1 mg/kg) has been shown to be a rapid (90 s) and effective agent (decreased fasciculations and postoperative myalgias) for precurarization prior to administration of succinylcholine. It has slight vagolytic tendencies.

OTHER RELAXANTS

Muscle relaxants primarily of historical interest are either no longer manufactured or not clinically used. They include tubocurarine, metocurine, gallamine, alcuronium, rapacuronium, and decamethonium. Tubocurarine, the first muscle relaxant used clinically, often produced hypotension and tachycardia through histamine release; its ability to block autonomic ganglia was of secondary importance. Histamine release could also produce or exacerbate bronchospasm. Tubocurarine is not metabolized significantly and its elimination is primarily renal and secondarily biliary. Metocurine, a closely related agent, shares many of the side effects of tubocurarine. It is primarily dependent on renal function for elimination. Patients allergic to iodine (eg, shellfish allergies) could exhibit hypersensitivity to metocurine preparations as they too contain iodide. Gallamine has potent vagolytic properties and is entirely dependent on renal function for elimination. Alcuronium, a long-acting nondepolarizer with mild vagolytic properties, is also primarily dependent on renal function for elimination. Rapacuronium has a rapid onset of action, minimal cardiovascular side effects, and a short duration of action. It was withdrawn by the manufacturer following several reports of serious bronchospasm, including a few unexplained fatalities. Histamine release may have been a factor. Decamethonium was an older depolarizing agent.

CASE DISCUSSION: DELAYED RECOVERY FROM GENERAL ANESTHESIA

A 72-year-old man has undergone general anesthesia for transurethral resection of the prostate. Twenty minutes after conclusion of the procedure, he is still intubated and shows no evidence of spontaneous respiration or consciousness.

What is your general approach to this diagnostic dilemma?

Clues to the solution of complex clinical problems are usually found in a pertinent review of the medical and surgical history, the history of drug ingestions, the physical examination, and laboratory results. In this case, the perioperative anesthetic management should also be considered.

What medical illnesses predispose a patient to delayed awakening or prolonged paralysis?

Chronic hypertension alters cerebral blood flow autoregulation and decreases the brain's tolerance to episodes of hypotension. Liver disease reduces hepatic drug metabolism and biliary excretion, resulting in prolonged drug action. Reduced serum albumin levels increase free drug (active drug) availability. Hepatic encephalopathy can alter consciousness. Kidney disease decreases the renal excretion of many drugs. Uremia can also affect consciousness. Diabetic patients are prone to hypoglycemia and hyperosmotic, hyperglycemic, and nonketotic coma. A prior stroke or symptomatic carotid bruit increases the risk of intraoperative cerebral vascular accident. Right-to-left heart shunts, particularly in children with congenital heart disease, allow air emboli to pass directly from the venous circulation to the systemic (possibly cerebral) arterial circulation. A paradoxic air embolism can result in permanent brain damage. Severe hypothyroidism is associated with impaired drug metabolism and, rarely, myxedema coma.

Does an uneventful history of general anesthesia narrow the differential?

Hereditary atypical pseudocholinesterase is ruled out by uneventful prior general anesthesia, assuming succinylcholine was administered. Decreased levels of normal enzyme would not result in postoperative apnea unless the surgery was of very short duration. Malignant hyperthermia does not typically present as delayed awakening, although prolonged somnolence is not unusual. Uneventful prior anesthetics do not, however, rule out malignant hyperthermia. Persons unusually sensitive to anesthetic agents

(eg, geriatric patients) may have a history of delayed emergence.

How do drugs that a patient takes at home affect awakening from general anesthesia?

Drugs that decrease minimum alveolar concentration, such as methyldopa, predispose patients to anesthetic overdose. Acute ethanol intoxication decreases barbiturate metabolism and acts independently as a sedative. Drugs that decrease liver blood flow, such as cimetidine, will limit hepatic drug metabolism. Antiparkinsonian drugs and tricyclic antidepressants have anticholinergic side effects that augment the sedation produced by scopolamine. Long-acting sedatives, such as the benzodiazepines, can delay awakening.

Does anesthetic technique alter awakening?

Preoperative medications can affect awakening. In particular, anticholinergics (with the exception of glycopyrrolate, which does not cross the blood–brain barrier), opioids, and sedatives can interfere with postoperative recovery. Patients with low cardiac output may have delayed absorption of intramuscular injections.

Anesthetic maintenance techniques influence the recovery rate. Specifically, nitrous-narcotic (eg, N_2O/fentanyl) techniques tend to be associated with rapid return of early signs of awakening, such as eye opening or response to verbal commands. Nitrous-narcotic and volatile anesthetics do not significantly differ in the time required for complete recovery, however.

Intraoperative hyperventilation is a common cause of postoperative apnea. Because volatile agents raise the apneic threshold, the $Paco_2$ level at which spontaneous ventilation ceases, moderate postoperative hypoventilation may be required to stimulate the respiratory centers. Severe intraoperative hypotension or hypertension may lead to cerebral hypoxia and edema.

Hypothermia decreases minimum alveolar concentration, antagonizes muscle relaxation reversal, and limits drug metabolism. Arterial hypoxia or severe hypercapnia ($Paco_2 > 70$ mm Hg) can alter consciousness.

Certain surgical procedures, such as carotid endarterectomy, cardiopulmonary bypass, and intracranial procedures, are associated with an increased incidence of postoperative neurological deficits. Transurethral resection of the prostate is associated with hyponatremia from the dilutional effects of absorbed irrigating solution.

What clues does a physical examination provide?

Pupil size is not always a reliable indicator of central nervous system integrity. Fixed and dilated pupils in the absence of anticholinergic medication or ganglionic blockade (eg, trimethaphan), however, may be an ominous sign. Response to physical stimulation, such as a forceful jaw thrust, may differentiate somnolence from paralysis. Peripheral nerve stimulation also differentiates paralysis from coma.

What specific laboratory findings would you order?

Arterial blood gases and serum electrolytes, particularly sodium, may be helpful. Computed tomographic scanning may be recommended by a neurological consultant.

What therapeutic interventions should be considered?

Supportive mechanical ventilation should be continued in the unresponsive patient. Naloxone, flumazenil, physostigmine, doxapram, or aminophylline may be indicated, depending on the probable cause of the delayed emergence.

SUGGESTED READING

Berg H, Viby-Morgensen J, Chraemmer Jorgensen B, et al: Residual neuromuscular block is a risk factor for postoperative pulmonary complications. A prospective, randomized, and blinded study of postoperative pulmonary complications after atracurium, vecuronium, and pancuronium. Acta Anaesthesiol Scand 1997;41:1095.

Caldwell JE: The problem with long-acting muscle relaxants? They cost more! [Editorial] Anesth Analg 1997;85:473.

Donati F: The right dose of succinylcholine. Anesthesiology 2003;99:1037.

Feldman S: *Neuromuscular Blockade.* Butterworth-Heinemann, 1996. Excellent chapters on neuromuscular transmission, acetylcholine pharmacology, and mechanisms of muscle relaxant actions.

Haywood PT, Divekar N, Karalliedde LD: Concurrent medication and the neuromuscular junction. Eur J Anaesthesiol 1999;16:77.

Kopman AF, Yee PS, and Neuman GG: Relationship of train-of-four fade to clinical signs and symptoms of residual paralysis in awake volunteers. Anesthesiology 1997;86:765.

Kopman AF, Klewicka MM, Koman DJ: Molar potency is predictive of the speed of onset of neuromuscular block for agents of intermediate, short, and ultrashort duration. Anesthesiology 1999;90:425.

Lee C: Structure, conformation, and action of neuromuscular blocking drugs. Br J Anaesth 2001;87:755.

Moore EW, Hunter JM: The new neuromuscular blocking agents: Do they offer any advantages? Br J Anaesth 2001;87:912.

Naguib M, Flood P, McArdle JJ, Brenner HR: Advances in the neurobiology of the neuromuscular junction. Anesthesiology 2002;96:202.

Naguib M, Samarkandi A, Riad W, Alharby SW: Optimal dose of succinylcholine revisited. Anesthesiology 2003;99:1045.

Schow AJ, Libarsky DA, Olson RP: Can succinylcholine be used safely in hyperkalemic patients? Anesth Analg 2002;95:119.

Cholinesterase Inhibitors

10

KEY CONCEPTS

 The primary clinical use of cholinesterase inhibitors, also called anticholinesterases, is to reverse nondepolarizing muscle blockade.

 Acetylcholine is the neurotransmitter for the entire parasympathetic nervous system (parasympathetic ganglions and effector cells), parts of the sympathetic nervous system (sympathetic ganglions, adrenal medulla, and sweat glands), some neurons in the central nervous system, and somatic nerves innervating skeletal muscle.

 Neuromuscular transmission is blocked when nondepolarizing muscle relaxants compete with acetylcholine to bind to nicotinic cholinergic receptors. The cholinesterase inhibitors indirectly increase the amount of acetylcholine available to compete with the nondepolarizing agent, thereby reestablishing neuromuscular transmission.

 In excessive doses, acetylcholinesterase inhibitors can paradoxically potentiate a nondepolarizing neuromuscular blockade. In addition, these drugs prolong the depolarization blockade of succinylcholine.

 Any prolongation of action of a nondepolarizing muscle relaxant from renal or hepatic insufficiency will probably be accompanied by a corresponding increase in the duration of action of a cholinesterase inhibitor.

 The time required to fully reverse a nondepolarizing block depends on several factors, including the choice and dose of cholinesterase inhibitor administered, the muscle relaxant being antagonized, and the extent of the blockade before reversal.

 A reversal agent should be routinely given to patients who have received nondepolarizing muscle relaxants unless full reversal can be demonstrated or the postoperative plan includes continued intubation and ventilation.

 In monitoring a patient's recovery from neuromuscular blockade, the suggested end points are sustained tetanus for 5 s in response to a 100-Hz stimulus in anesthetized patients or sustained head lift in awake patients. If neither of these end points is achieved, the patient should remain intubated and ventilation should be continued.

The primary clinical use of cholinesterase inhibitors, also called anticholinesterases, is to reverse nondepolarizing muscle blockade. However, this group of drugs has effects on cholinergic receptors beyond the neuromuscular end plate. This chapter reviews cholinergic pharmacology, explores the mechanisms of acetylcholinesterase inhibition, and presents the clinical pharmacology of commonly used cholinesterase inhibitors (neostigmine, edrophonium, pyridostigmine, and physostigmine).

CHOLINERGIC PHARMACOLOGY

The term cholinergic refers to the effects of the neurotransmitter acetyl*choline,* as opposed to the adrenergic effects of nor*adrenaline* (norepinephrine). Acetylcholine is synthesized in the nerve terminal by the enzyme cho-

ACETYL-CoA

+

CHOLINE   HO—CH₂—CH₂—⁺N—CH₃

$$CHOLINE\quad HO-CH_2-CH_2-{}^+N-CH_3$$

with side groups CH_3, CH_3

↓ Choline
Acetyltransferase

$$ACETYLCHOLINE\quad CH_3-C-O-CH_2-CH_2-{}^+N-CH_3$$

↓ Acetylcholinesterase

$$ACETATE\quad CH_3-C-OH$$

+

CHOLINE

Figure 10–1. The synthesis and hydrolysis of acetylcholine.

line acetyltransferase, which catalyzes the reaction between acetylcoenzyme A and choline (Figure 10–1). After its release, acetylcholine is rapidly hydrolyzed by acetylcholinesterase (true cholinesterase) into acetate and choline.

Acetylcholine is the neurotransmitter for the entire parasympathetic nervous system (parasympathetic ganglions and effector cells), parts of the sympathetic nervous system (sympathetic ganglions, adrenal medulla, and sweat glands), some neurons in the central nervous system, and somatic nerves innervating skeletal muscle (Figure 10–2).

Cholinergic receptors have been subdivided into two major groups based on their reaction to the alkaloids muscarine and nicotine (Figure 10–3). Nicotine stimulates the autonomic ganglia and skeletal muscle receptors (nicotinic receptors), whereas muscarine activates end-organ effector cells in bronchial smooth muscle, salivary glands, and the sinoatrial node (muscarinic receptors). The central nervous system has both nicotinic and muscarinic receptors. Nicotinic receptors are blocked by muscle relaxants (also called neuromuscular blockers, Chapter 9), and muscarinic receptors are blocked by anticholinergic drugs such as atropine (see Chapter 11). Although nicotinic and muscarinic receptors differ in their response to some agonists (eg, nicotine, muscarine) and some antagonists (eg, pancuronium, atropine), they both respond to acetylcholine (Table 10–1). Clinically available cholinergic agonists resist hydrolysis by cholinesterase. Methacholine and

bethanechol are primarily muscarinic agonists, whereas carbachol has both muscarinic and nicotinic agonist activities. Methacholine by inhalation has been used as a provocative test in asthma, bethanechol is used for bladder atony, and carbachol may be used topically for wide-angle glaucoma.

When reversing neuromuscular blockade, the primary goal is to maximize nicotinic transmission and minimize muscarinic side effects.

MECHANISM OF ACTION

Normal neuromuscular transmission critically depends on acetylcholine binding to nicotinic cholinergic receptors on the motor end plate. Nondepolarizing muscle relaxants act by competing with acetylcholine for these binding sites, thereby blocking neuromuscular transmission. Reversal of blockade depends on gradual diffusion, redistribution, metabolism, and excretion from the body of the nondepolarizing relaxant (*spontaneous reversal*) or on the administration of specific reversal agents (*pharmacological reversal*). Cholinesterase inhibitors *indirectly* increase the amount of acetylcholine available to compete with the nondepolarizing agent, thereby reestablishing normal neuromuscular transmission.

Cholinesterase inhibitors inactivate acetylcholinesterase by reversibly binding to the enzyme. The stability of the bond influences the duration of action: The electrostatic attraction and hydrogen bonding of edrophonium are short-lived; the covalent bonds of neostigmine and pyridostigmine are longer lasting.

Organophosphates, a special class of cholinesterase inhibitors, form very stable, irreversible bonds to the enzyme. They are used in ophthalmology and more commonly as pesticides. The clinical duration of the cholinesterase inhibitors used in anesthesia, however, is probably most influenced by the rate of drug disappearance from the plasma. Differences in duration of action can be overcome by dosage adjustments. Thus, the normally short duration of action of edrophonium can be partially overcome by increasing dosage. Cholinesterase inhibitors are also used in the diagnosis and treatment of myasthenia gravis (Chapter 37).

Mechanisms of action other than acetylcholinesterase inactivation may contribute to the restoration of neuromuscular function. Edrophonium appears to have prejunctional effects that enhance the release of acetylcholine. Neostigmine has a direct (but weak) agonist effect on nicotinic receptors. Acetylcholine mobilization and release by the nerve may also be enhanced (a presynaptic mechanism).

In excessive doses, however, acetylcholinesterase inhibitors paradoxically potentiate a nondepolarizing neuromuscular blockade. Neostig-

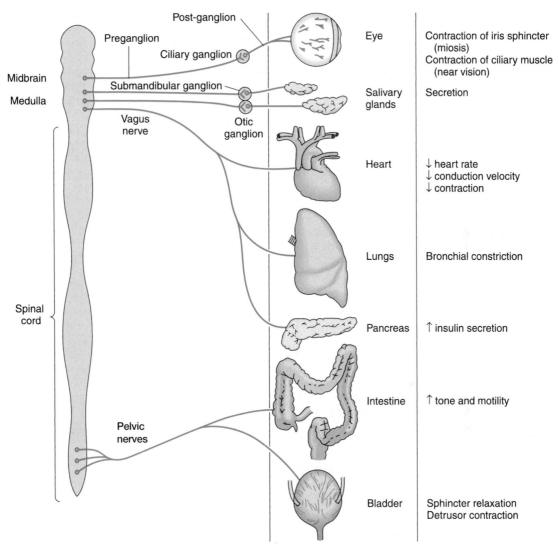

Figure 10–2. The parasympathetic nervous system uses acetylcholine as a preganglionic and postganglionic neurotransmitter.

mine in high doses may cause acetylcholine channel blockade (Chapter 9). In addition, these drugs prolong the depolarization blockade of succinylcholine. Two mechanisms may explain this latter effect: an increase in acetylcholine (which increases motor end plate depolarization) and inhibition of pseudocholinesterase activity. Neostigmine and to some extent pyridostigmine display some limited pseudocholinesterase-inhibiting activity, but their effect on acetylcholinesterase is much greater. Edrophonium has little or no effect on pseudocholinesterase. Thus, although neostigmine could slow the metabolism of mivacurium slightly, its net effect is to speed the reversal of mivacurium blockade. In large doses, neostigmine can cause a weak depolarizing neuromuscular blockade.

CLINICAL PHARMACOLOGY

General Pharmacological Characteristics

The increase in acetylcholine caused by cholinesterase inhibitors affects more than the nicotinic receptors of skeletal muscle (Table 10–2). Cholinesterase inhibitors can act at cholinergic receptors of several other organ systems, including the following.

NICOTINE

MUSCARINE

Figure 10–3. The molecular structures of nicotine and muscarine. Compare these alkaloids with acetylcholine (Figure 10–1).

Cardiovascular receptors—The predominant muscarinic effect on the heart is a vagal-like bradycardia that can progress to sinus arrest. **This effect has even been reported in the newly transplanted (denervated) heart but is more likely to occur in a heart transplanted more than 6 months earlier (reinnervated).**

Pulmonary receptors—Muscarinic stimulation can result in bronchospasm (smooth muscle contraction) and increased respiratory tract secretions.

Cerebral receptors—Physostigmine is a cholinesterase inhibitor that crosses the blood–brain barrier and can cause diffuse activation of the electroencephalogram by stimulating muscarinic and nicotinic receptors within the central nervous system (CNS). Inactivation of nicotinic acetylcholine receptors in the CNS may play a role in the action of general anesthetics (see Chapter 7).

Gastrointestinal receptors—Muscarinic stimulation increases peristaltic activity (esophageal, gastric, and intestinal) and glandular secretions (eg, salivary, parietal). Perioperative bowel anastomotic leakage, nausea and vomiting, and fecal incontinence have been attributed to the use of cholinesterase inhibitors.

Unwanted muscarinic side effects are minimized by prior or concomitant administration of anticholinergic medications such as atropine sulfate or glycopyrrolate (see Chapter 11).

The duration of action is similar among the cholinesterase inhibitors. Clearance is due to both hepatic metabolism (25–50%) and renal excretion (50–75%). Thus, any prolongation of action of a nondepolarizing muscle relaxant from renal or hepatic insufficiency will probably be accompanied by a corresponding increase in the duration of action of a cholinesterase inhibitor.

Dosage requirements of cholinesterase inhibitors depend on the degree of neuromuscular block that is being reversed. This is usually estimated by the response to peripheral nerve stimulation. As a rule, no amount of cholinesterase inhibitor can immediately reverse a block that is so intense that there is no response to tetanic peripheral nerve stimulation. Moreover, the absence of any palpable single twitches following 5 s of tetanic stimulation at 50 Hz implies very intensive blockade that cannot be reversed. Excessive doses of cholinesterase inhibitors may actually prolong recovery. Some evidence of spontaneous recovery (ie, the first twitch of the train of four [TOF], see Chapter 6) must be present before reversal is attempted. The posttetanic count (the number of palpable twitches after tetanus) generally correlates with the time of return of the first twitch of the TOF and therefore the ability to reverse intense paralysis. For intermediate-acting agents such as atracurium and vecuronium, a palpable posttetanic twitch appears about 10 min before spontaneous recovery of the first twitch of the TOF. In contrast, for longer-acting agents such as pancuronium, the first twitch of the TOF appears about 40 min after a palpable posttetanic twitch.

 The time required to fully reverse a nondepolarizing block depends on several factors, including the choice and dose of cholinesterase

Table 10–1. Characteristics of cholinergic receptors.

	Nicotinic	Muscarinic
Location	Autonomic ganglia Sympathetic ganglia Parasympathetic ganglia Skeletal muscle	Glands Lacrimal Salivary Gastric Smooth muscle Bronchial Gastrointestinal Bladder Blood vessels Heart Sinoatrial node Atrioventricular node
Agonists	Acetylcholine Nicotine	Acetylcholine Muscarine
Antagonists	Nondepolarizing relaxants	Antimuscarinics Atropine Scopolamine Glycopyrrolate

Table 10–2. Muscarinic side effects of cholinesterase inhibitors.

Organ System	Muscarinic Side Effects
Cardiovascular	Decreased heart rate, bradyarrhythmias
Pulmonary	Bronchospasm, bronchial secretions
Cerebral	Diffuse excitation[1]
Gastrointestinal	Intestinal spasm, increased salivation
Genitourinary	Increased bladder tone
Ophthalmological	Pupillary constriction

[1]Applies only to physostigmine.

inhibitor administered, the muscle relaxant being antagonized, and the extent of the blockade before reversal. For example, reversal with edrophonium is usually faster than with neostigmine; large doses of neostigmine lead to faster reversal than small doses; intermediate-acting relaxants reverse sooner than long-acting relaxants; and a shallow block is easier to reverse than a deep block (ie, twitch height > 10%). Short- and intermediate-acting muscle relaxants therefore require a lower dose of reversal agent (for the same degree of blockade) than long-acting agents, and concurrent excretion or metabolism provides a proportionally faster reversal of the short- and intermediate-acting agents. These advantages can be lost in conditions associated with severe end-organ disease (eg, the use of vecuronium in a patient with liver failure) or enzyme deficiencies (eg, mivacurium in a patient with homozygous atypical pseudocholinesterase). Depending on the dose of muscle relaxant that has been given, spontaneous recovery to a level adequate for pharmacological reversal may take more than 1 h with long-acting muscle relaxants because of their insignificant metabolism and slow excretion. Factors associated with faster reversal are also associated with a lower incidence of residual paralysis in the recovery room and a lower risk of postoperative respiratory complications.

A reversal agent should be routinely given to patients who have received nondepolarizing muscle relaxants unless full reversal can be demonstrated or the postoperative plan includes continued intubation and ventilation. In the latter situation, adequate sedation must also be provided.

A peripheral nerve stimulator (Chapters 6 and 9) should also be used to monitor the progress and confirm the adequacy of reversal. In general, the higher the frequency of stimulation, the greater the sensitivity of the test (100-Hz tetany > 50-Hz tetany or TOF > single-

twitch height). Because peripheral nerve stimulation is uncomfortable, double-burst stimulation and alternative tests of neuromuscular function must be used in awake patients. These also vary in sensitivity (sustained head lift > inspiratory force > vital capacity > tidal volume). Therefore, the suggested end points of recovery are sustained tetanus for 5 s in response to a 100-Hz stimulus in anesthetized patients or sustained head lift in awake patients. If neither of these end points is achieved, the patient should remain intubated and ventilation should be continued.

SPECIFIC CHOLINESTERASE INHIBITORS

NEOSTIGMINE

Physical Structure

Neostigmine consists of a carbamate moiety and a quaternary ammonium group (Figure 10–4). The former provides covalent bonding to acetylcholinesterase. The latter renders the molecule lipid insoluble, so that it cannot pass through the blood–brain barrier.

Dosage & Packaging

The maximum recommended dose of neostigmine is 0.08 mg/kg (up to 5 mg in adults), but smaller amounts often suffice (Table 10–3). Neostigmine is most commonly packaged as 10 mL of a 1 mg/mL solution, although 0.5 mg/mL and 0.25 mg/mL concentrations are also available.

Clinical Considerations

The effects of neostigmine (0.04 mg/kg) are usually apparent in 5–10 min, peak at 10 min, and last more than 1 h. If reversal in not complete in 10 min after 0.08 mg/kg, the time for full recovery of neuromuscular function will depend on the nondepolarizing agent used and the intensity of blockade. In practice, many clinicians use a dose of 0.04 mg/kg if the preexisting blockade is mild to moderate and a dose of 0.08 mg/kg if intense paralysis is being reversed. Pediatric and elderly patients appear to be more sensitive to its effects, experiencing a more rapid onset and requiring a smaller dose. The duration of action is prolonged in geriatric patients. Muscarinic side effects are minimized by prior or concomitant administration of an anticholinergic agent. The onset of action of glycopyrrolate (0.2 mg glycopyrrolate per 1 mg of neostigmine) is similar to that of neostigmine and is associated with less tachycardia than is experienced with atropine (0.4 mg of atropine per 1 mg of neostigmine). It has been reported that neo-

PROFILES IN ANESTHETIC PRACTICE

Jennifer M. Hunter, MD

OVERDOSING WITH NEUROMUSCULAR BLOCKING DRUGS: A UNIVERSAL FOIBLE

What is it in the psyche of anesthesiologists that makes them use much more of a drug than is necessary to produce the desired effect? Is it simply a human failing or just laziness? Why is it that although the recommended dose of, for instance, atracurium is 0.5 mg/kg, so many anesthesiologists give at least 0.6–0.9 mg/kg at the beginning of anesthesia? Is it because they want a more rapid onset of action? Undoubtedly, it will be slightly faster, albeit only by a matter of seconds, with the larger dose. Do they want a longer clinical duration of action (25% recovery of the twitch response) of about 47 min after atracurium 0.9 mg/kg instead of 32 min after atracurium 0.6 mg/kg for any particular patient? I doubt it. It is "bucket anesthesia": rapidly and carelessly pouring an excessive, and inexact, amount of the requisite drug into a patient, as if to cover every eventuality, without any consideration of how long that dose is likely to produce a clinical effect. Do they give any thought to the variability of effect of a dose of any nondepolarizing drug given on a weight-related basis? Do they acknowledge that the standard deviation of 20% recovery (when an incremental dose can be given or reversal effected) from atracurium 0.5 mg/ kg is 11 min, for a mean time of 43 min?[1] How do they know that their patient is not at the upper end of that range of effect? They are probably relying on the spontaneous breakdown of the drug in the plasma by Hofmann degradation and ester hydrolysis. Remember the variable effect Katz showed in 1967 with tubocurarine 0.1 mg/kg. In 7% of patients, complete abla-

tion of the four twitches of the train-of-four (TOF) response occurred, even with this very low dose.[2]

Only recently, it has been clearly demonstrated that all anesthesiologists use an unnecessarily large dose of succinylcholine.[3] Succinylcholine 0.6 mg/kg will still have a rapid onset (81 s) and even 0.4 mg/kg may suffice, with maximum block at a mean of 105 s. More importantly, clinical recovery will be faster at 6.6 min after succinylcholine 0.4 mg/kg and 7.6 min after 0.6 mg/kg, compared with 9.3 min after succinylcholine 1.0 mg/kg.[3] Thus, following preoxygenation, recovery of respiration could occur before hypoxic damage ensued if a smaller dose of succinylcholine had been used and intubation had failed. Even with succinylcholine, however, there is a range in the clinical recovery times of 5–6 min.[3]

The practice of using an excessive dose of muscle relaxant is made worse by the tendency to give a generous increment every 30 min ("on the half hour" in UK terminology). No thought is given to monitoring neuromuscular block to determine the degree of recovery prior to the increment. Nor is detection of the second twitch of the TOF response ascertained, as it should be, before another often excessive bolus is given, for instance, atracurium 15–20 mg.

It is not surprising that when surgery finishes somewhat earlier than expected, which occasionally happens, and an anticholinesterase such as neostigmine has been given, recovery from block is slow and incomplete, with all the potential complications that have been described.[4] For if neostigmine 2.5 mg is given when the first twitch of the TOF response has recovered to 10% after vecuronium 0.1 mg/kg, it takes 3.9 min for T_1/T_0 to reach 70% and 9.2 min for the TOF ratio to reach 0.7, when the patient can probably be extubated safely. How many anesthesiologists wait 10 min after giving neostigmine before they extubate their patient? But if neostigmine 2.5 mg is not given until $T_1/T_0 = 0.5$, it takes only 1.2 min for T_1/T_0 to reach 0.7, and only 2.1 min for the TOF ratio to do so.[5]

Anesthesiologists should realize that the art of their practice is to give a sufficient amount, but no more, of a neuromuscular blocking drug and its antagonist, and to give both drugs at an appropriate time. Only then will the desired effect of the drug be achieved and fewer side effects encountered. For instance, anesthesiologists do not want to produce unnecessary histamine release and subsequent hypotension from mivacurium by giving too large a dose (0.3 mg/kg) too rapidly, over 10–15 s.[6] A 33% fall in mean arterial pressure can be an-

ticipated in such circumstances. Nor do they wish to see the tachycardia and hypertension that result from administration of a large dose of that now archaic drug, pancuronium. Do they want an incomplete reversal when too much vecuronium has been given too frequently to a patient with either acute or chronic renal dysfunction?[8] I see about three such cases a year in my hospital, so such occurrences must be common.

The tendency to encourage the use of larger doses of a nondepolarizing muscle relaxant, such as rocuronium 1.2 mg/kg or cisatracurium 0.4 mg/kg,[8] to increase the rate of onset of block may at first seem attractive. But do not forget that prolonged neuromuscular block is then being produced. Twenty-five percent recovery of the first twitch of the TOF, when it is appropriate to give an anticholinesterase, takes 67 ± 25 (mean ± SD) min[10] following rocuronium 1.2 mg/kg and 91 ± 3.3 (mean ± SE) min after cisatracurium 0.4 mg/kg.[8] Few anesthesiologists appreciate the length of action of the neuromuscular blocking drugs they use.

Never forget the old days of recurarization. This phenomenon should no longer occur except in patients with undiagnosed neuromuscular disorders such as myasthenia gravis and amyotrophic lateral sclerosis, or in the hypothyroid patient. It could be considered a sign of negligence for a patient to experience residual curarization in the recovery room. For now there are drugs that are broken down independent of organ function, such as atracurium, cisatracurium, and mivacurium. If the correct dose of these drugs is used, neuromuscular block is monitored, and the anticholinesterase is given only when the second twitch of the TOF response is detectable; then residual block should never be seen. In the days of tubocurarine and pancuronium, it was more understandable if patients had impaired clearance of these long-acting drugs from reduced renal or hepatic function (which can occur in the hypovolemic shocked patient as well as in the patient with chronic organ dysfunction).

Remember too that organ function deteriorates with increasing age. The older the patient, the lower the rate of clearance and the longer the elimination half time of a neuromuscular blocking drug, even if it primarily undergoes organ-independent elimination. How many anesthesiologists consider the age of their patients before selecting the dose of a neuromuscular blocking drug? It is inappropriate to use the same dose in a 20-year-old patient as in an 80-year-old patient, even if they are of the same sex and weight. If succinylcholine is given to intubate a patient, the duration of action of the nondepolarizing agent will also be potentiated.

The clearance of many nondepolarizing neuromuscular blocking drugs is lower in women, so they may need a smaller dose to achieve an effect similar to that in men.[9] Ethnicity is also important; different races metabolize drugs at different rates. This difference is augmented by the different rates of alcohol consumption and cigarette smoking in different cultures, as these substances stimulate hepatic enzyme induction and faster metabolism of drugs cleared by the liver. Thus the nonsmoking, non–alcohol-consuming, nonwhite, vegetarian lady will be more sensitive to the effect of a neuromuscular blocking drug than an overweight white man who smokes and who drinks a large amount of alcohol every day. In addition, it is uncertain whether in adults it is necessary to give a dose of neuromuscular blocking drugs such as atracurium, which undergo organ-independent elimination on a weight-related basis. Atracurium 25 mg will be sufficient in most adult females, and atracurium 30 mg in adult males.

So remember, there is no rationale for using excessive doses of neuromuscular blocking drugs. By taking pride in giving a good anesthetic in which the dose of all drugs used is tailored to a particular patient, anesthesiologists can achieve an ideal effect, for both the well-being of their patients and the smooth running of their practice.

"Right conduct can never, except by some rare accident, be promoted by ignorance or hindered by knowledge" (Bertram Russell, 1929).

1. Hunter JM, Jones RS, Utting JE: Comparison of vecuronium, atracurium and tubocurarine in normal patients and in patients with no renal function. Br J Anaesth 1984;56:941.
2. Katz RL: Neuromuscular effects of d-tubocurarine, edrophonium and neostigmine in man. Anesthesiology 1967;28:327.
3. Kopman AF, Zhaku B, Laik S: The intubating dose of succinylcholine: The effect of decreasing doses on recovery time. Anesthesiology 2003;99:1050.
4. Savarese JJ: A current practice of relaxation. In: *Clinical Anesthesiology*, 3rd ed. McGraw-Hill, 2002 (Chapter 9).
5. Jones JE, Hunter JM, Utting JE: Use of neostigmine in the antagonism of residual neuromuscular blockade produced by vecuronium. Br J Anaesth 1987;59:1454.
6. Savarese JJ, Ali HH, Basta SJ, et al: The cardiovascular effects of mivacurium chloride (BW B1090U) in patients receiving nitrous oxide–opiate-barbiturate anesthesia. Anesthesiology 1989;70:386.
7. Cody MW, Dormon FM: Recurarization after vecuronium in a patient with renal failure. Anaesthesia 1987;42:993.
8. Belmont MR, Lien CA, Quessy S, et al: The clinical neuromuscular pharmacology of 51W89 in patients receiving nitrous oxide/opioid/barbiturate anesthesia. Anesthesiology 1995;82:1139.
9. Parker CJR, Hunter JM, Snowdon SL: Effect of age, sex and anaesthetic technique on the pharmacokinetics of atracurium. Br J Anaesth 1992;69:439.

NEOSTIGMINE

PYRIDOSTIGMINE

EDROPHONIUM

PHYSOSTIGMINE

Figure 10–4. Molecular structures of neostigmine, pyridostigmine, edrophonium, and physostigmine.

stigmine crosses the placenta resulting in fetal bradycardia. Thus, atropine may be a better choice of an anticholinergic agent than glycopyrrolate in pregnant patients receiving neostigmine. Neostigmine is also used to treat myasthenia gravis, urinary bladder atony, and paralytic ileus. Neostigmine (50–100 μg) has been used as an adjunct to intrathecal anesthesia causing a prolongation of sensory and motor blockade, presumably by inhibiting the breakdown of spinal cord acetylcholine. However, side effects include nausea, vomiting, fecal incontinence, delayed recovery room discharge, and atropine-resistant bradycardia at higher doses (200 μg).

PYRIDOSTIGMINE

Physical Structure

Pyridostigmine is structurally similar to neostigmine except that the quaternary ammonium is incorporated

into the phenol ring. Pyridostigmine shares neostigmine's covalent binding to acetylcholinesterase and its lipid insolubility.

Dosage & Packaging

Pyridostigmine is 20% as potent as neostigmine and may be administered in doses up to 0.4 mg/kg (a total of 20 mg in adults). It is available as a solution of 5 mg/mL.

Clinical Considerations

The onset of action of pyridostigmine is slower (10–15 min) than that of neostigmine, and its duration is slightly longer (> 2 h). Glycopyrrolate (0.05 mg per 1 mg of pyridostigmine) or atropine (0.1 mg per 1 mg of pyridostigmine) must also be administered to prevent bradycardia. Glycopyrrolate is preferred because its

Table 10–3. The choice and dose of cholinesterase inhibitor determine the choice and dose of anticholinergic.

Cholinesterase Inhibitor	Usual Dose of Cholinesterase Inhibitor	Recommended Anticholinergic	Usual Dose of Anticholinergic per mg of Cholinesterase Inhibitor
Neostigmine	0.04–0.08 mg/kg	Glycopyrrolate	0.2 mg
Pyridostigmine	0.1–0.4 mg/kg	Glycopyrrolate	0.05 mg
Edrophonium	0.5–1 mg/kg	Atropine	0.014 mg
Physostigmine[1]	0.01–0.03 mg/kg	Usually not necessary	NA

[1]Not used to reverse muscle relaxants.

slower onset of action better matches that of pyridostigmine, again resulting in less tachycardia.

EDROPHONIUM

Physical Structure

Because it lacks a carbamate group, edrophonium must rely on noncovalent bonding to the acetylcholinesterase enzyme. The quaternary ammonium group limits lipid solubility.

Dosage & Packaging

Edrophonium is less than 10% as potent as neostigmine. The recommended dosage is 0.5–1 mg/kg. Edrophonium is available as a solution containing 10 mg/mL; it is available with atropine as a combination drug (Enlon-Plus; 10 mg edrophonium and 0.14 mg atropine per milliliter).

Clinical Considerations

Edrophonium has the most rapid onset of action (1–2 min) and the shortest duration of effect of any of the cholinesterase inhibitors. Low doses should not be used, because longer-acting muscle relaxants may outlast the effects of edrophonium. Higher doses prolong the duration of action to more than 1 h. Patients at the extremes of age are not more sensitive to edrophonium reversal (unlike the case with neostigmine). Edrophonium may not be as effective as neostigmine at reversing intense neuromuscular blockade, but may be more effective in reversing a mivacurium blockade. In equipotent doses, muscarinic effects of edrophonium are less pronounced than those of neostigmine or pyridostigmine, requiring only half the amount of anticholinergic agent. Edrophonium's rapid onset is well matched to that of atropine (0.014 mg of atropine per 1 mg of edrophonium). Although glycopyrrolate (0.007 mg per 1 mg of edrophonium) can also be used, it should be given several minutes prior to edrophonium to avoid the possibility of bradycardia.

PHYSOSTIGMINE

Physical Structure

Physostigmine, a tertiary amine, has a carbamate group but no quaternary ammonium. Therefore, it is lipid soluble and is the only clinically available cholinesterase inhibitor that freely passes the blood–brain barrier.

Dosage & Packaging

The dose of physostigmine is 0.01–0.03 mg/kg. It is packaged as a solution containing 1 mg/mL.

Clinical Considerations

The lipid solubility and CNS penetration of physostigmine limit its usefulness as a reversal agent for nondepolarizing blockade, but make it effective in the treatment of central anticholinergic toxicity caused by overdoses of atropine or scopolamine (see Chapter 11). In addition, it reverses some of the CNS depression and delirium associated with use of benzodiazepines and volatile anesthetics. Physostigmine (0.04 mg/kg) has been shown to be effective in preventing postoperative shivering. It reportedly partially antagonizes morphine-induced respiratory depression, presumably because morphine reduces acetylcholine release in the brain. These effects are transient, and repeated doses may be required. Bradycardia is infrequent in the recommended dosage range, but atropine or glycopyrrolate should be immediately available. Because glycopyrrolate does not cross the blood–brain barrier, it will not reverse the CNS effects of physostigmine (see Chapter 11). Other possible muscarinic side effects include excessive salivation, vomiting, and convulsions. In contrast to other cholinesterase inhibitors, physostigmine is almost completely metabolized by plasma esterases, so renal excretion is not important.

CASE DISCUSSION:
RESPIRATORY FAILURE
IN THE RECOVERY ROOM

A 66-year-old woman weighing 85 kg is brought to the recovery room following cholecystectomy. The anesthetic technique included the use of isoflurane and vecuronium for muscle relaxation. At the conclusion of the procedure, the anesthesiologist administered 6 mg of morphine sulfate for postoperative pain control and 3 mg of neostigmine with 0.6 mg of glycopyrrolate to reverse any residual neuromuscular blockade. The dose of cholinesterase inhibitor was empirically based on clinical judgment. Although the patient was apparently breathing normally on arrival in the recovery room, her tidal volume progressively diminished. Arterial blood gas measurements revealed a Pa_{CO_2} of 62 mm Hg, a Pa_{O_2} of 110 mm Hg, and a pH of 7.26 on a fraction of inspired oxygen (F_{IO_2}) of 40%.

Which drugs administered to this patient could explain her hypoventilation?

Isoflurane, morphine sulfate, and pancuronium all interfere with a patient's ability to maintain a normal ventilatory response to an elevated Pa_{CO_2}.

Why would the patient's breathing worsen in the recovery room?

Possibilities include the delayed onset of action of morphine sulfate, a lack of sensory stimulation in the recovery area, fatigue of respiratory muscles, and splinting as a result of upper abdominal pain.

Could the patient still have residual neuromuscular blockade?

If the dose of neostigmine was not determined by the response to a peripheral nerve stimulator, or if the recovery of muscle function was inadequately tested after the reversal drugs were given, persistent neuromuscular blockade is possible. Assume, for example, that the patient had minimal or no response to initial tetanic stimulation at 100 Hz. Even the maximal dose of neostigmine (5 mg) might not yet have adequately reversed the paralysis. Because of enormous patient variability, the response to peripheral nerve stimulation must always be monitored when intermediate- or long-acting muscle relaxants are administered. Even if partial reversal is achieved, paralysis may worsen if the patient hypoventilates. **Other factors (in addition to respiratory acidosis) that impair the reversal of nondepolarizing muscle relaxants include intense neuromuscular paralysis, electrolyte disturbances (hypermagnesemia, hypokalemia, and hypocalcemia), hypothermia (temperature < 32°C), drug interactions (see Table 9–4), metabolic alkalosis (from accompanying hypokalemia and hypocalcemia), and coexisting diseases (see Table 9–7).**

How could the extent of reversal be tested?

Tetanic stimulation is a sensitive but uncomfortable test of neuromuscular transmission in an awake patient. Because of its shorter duration, double-burst stimulation is tolerated better than tetany by conscious patients. Many other tests of neuromuscular transmission, such as vital capacity and tidal volume, are insensitive as they may still appear normal when 70–80% of receptors are blocked. In fact, 70% of receptors may remain blocked despite an apparently normal response to TOF stimulation. The ability to sustain a head lift for 5 s, however, indicates that fewer than 33% of receptors are occupied by muscle relaxant.

What treatment would you suggest?

Ventilation should be assisted to reduce the respiratory acidosis. Even if diaphragmatic function appears to be adequate, residual blockade can lead to airway obstruction and poor airway protection. More neostigmine (with an anticholinergic) could be administered up to a maximum recommended dose of 5 mg. If this does not adequately reverse paralysis, mechanical ventilation and airway protection should be instituted and continued until neuromuscular function is fully restored.

SUGGESTED READING

Bevan DR, Donati F, Kopman AF: Reversal of neuromuscular blockade. Anesthesiology 1992;77:785. This article covers methods of determining adequacy of reversal, anticholinesterase pharmacology, and clinical conditions affecting reversal.

Bevan JC, Collins L, Fowler C, et al: Early and late reversal of rocuronium and vecuronium with neostigmine in adults and children. Anesth Analg 1999;89:333. One study demonstrating no advantage to delaying reversal of blockade until some degree of spontaneous reversal.

Evers AS, Maze M: *Anesthetic Pharmacology: Physiologic Principles and Clinical Practice.* Elsevier Churchill Livingstone, 2004.

Fuchs-Buder T, Ziegenfub T, Lysakowski K, Tassonyi E: Antagonism of vecuronium-induced neuromuscular block in patients pretreated with magnesium sulphate: Dose-effect relationship of neostigmine. Br J Anaesth 1999;82:61. Magnesium sulfate treatment prolongs neuromuscular blockade by slowing spontaneous reversal but does not appear to affect reversal of blockade by neostigmine.

Joshi GP, Garg SA, Hailey A, Yu SY: The effects of antagonizing residual neuromuscular blockade by neostigmine and glycopyrrolate on nausea and vomiting after ambulatory surgery. Anesth Analg 1999;89:628. Reversal with neostigmine did not increase the incidence of nausea and vomiting or the need for antiemetic therapy in outpatient surgery.

Klamt JG, Garcia LV, Prado WA: Analgesic and adverse effects of a low dose of intrathecally administered hyperbaric neostigmine alone or combined with morphine in patients submitted to spinal anesthesia: pilot studies. Anaesthesia 1999; 54:27. Multiple side effects of intrathecal neostigmine, even at relatively low doses, are described.

Stoelting RK: *Pharmacology and Physiology in Anesthetic Practice,* 3rd ed. Lippincott, William & Wilkins, 1999.

Taylor P: Anticholinesterase agents. In: *Goodman and Gilman's Pharmacological Basis of Therapeutics,* 10th ed. Hardman JG (editor). McGraw-Hill, 2002. An excellent overview of this drug class.

Anticholinergic Drugs

11

KEY CONCEPTS

1 *Ester linkage is essential for effective binding of the anticholinergics to the acetylcholine receptors. This competitively blocks binding by acetylcholine and prevents receptor activation. The cellular effects of acetylcholine, which are mediated through second messengers such as cyclic guanosine monophosphate (cGMP), are inhibited.*

2 *Anticholinergics relax the bronchial smooth musculature, which reduces airway resistance and increases anatomic dead space.*

3 *Atropine has particularly potent effects on the heart and bronchial smooth muscle and is the most efficacious anticholinergic for treating bradyarrhythmias.*

4 *Ipratropium solution (0.5 mg in 2.5 mL) appears particularly effective in the treatment of acute chronic obstructive pulmonary disease when combined with a β-agonist drug (eg, albuterol).*

5 *Scopolamine is a more potent antisialagogue than atropine and causes greater central nervous system effects.*

6 *Because of a quaternary structure, glycopyrrolate cannot cross the blood–brain barrier and is almost always devoid of central nervous system and ophthalmic activity.*

One group of cholinergic antagonists has already been discussed: the nondepolarizing neuromuscular-blocking agents (see Chapter 9). These drugs act primarily at the nicotinic receptors in skeletal muscle. This chapter presents the pharmacology of drugs that block muscarinic receptors. Although the classification *anticholinergic* usually refers to this latter group, a more precise term would be *antimuscarinic*.

In this chapter, the mechanism of action and clinical pharmacology are introduced for three common anticholinergics: atropine, scopolamine, and glycopyrrolate. The clinical uses of these drugs in anesthesia relate to their effect on the cardiovascular, respiratory, cerebral, gastrointestinal, and other organ systems (Table 11–1).

MECHANISMS OF ACTION

Anticholinergics are esters of an aromatic acid combined with an organic base (Figure 11–1). The ester linkage is essential for effective bind-

ing of the anticholinergics to the acetylcholine receptors. **This competitively blocks binding by acetylcholine and prevents receptor activation.** The cellular effects of acetylcholine, which are mediated through second messengers such as cyclic guanosine monophosphate (cGMP), are inhibited. The tissue receptors vary in their sensitivity to blockade. In fact, muscarinic receptors are not homogeneous, and receptor subgroups have been identified: neuronal (M_1), cardiac (M_2), and glandular (M_3) receptors.

CLINICAL PHARMACOLOGY

General Pharmacological Characteristics

In clinical doses, only muscarinic receptors are blocked by the anticholinergic drugs discussed in this chapter. The extent of the anticholinergic effect depends on the degree of baseline vagal tone. Several organ systems are affected.

Table 11–1. Pharmacological characteristics of anticholinergic drugs.[1]

	Atropine	Scopolamine	Glycopyrrolate
Tachycardia	+++	+	++
Bronchodilatation	++	+	++
Sedation	+	+++	0
Antisialagogue effect	++	+++	+++

[1]0, no effect; +, minimal effect; ++, moderate effect; +++, marked effect.

A. CARDIOVASCULAR

Blockade of muscarinic receptors in the sinoatrial node results in tachycardia. This effect is especially useful in reversing bradycardia due to vagal reflexes (eg, baroreceptor reflex, peritoneal stimulation, or oculocardiac reflex). A transient slowing of heart rate in response to low doses of anticholinergics has been reported. The mechanism of this paradoxic response may be a weak peripheral agonist effect, suggesting that these drugs are not pure antagonists. Facilitation of conduction through the atrioventricular node shortens the P–R interval on the electrocardiogram and often decreases heart block caused by vagal activity. Atrial arrhythmias and nodal (junctional) rhythms occasionally occur. Anticholinergics generally have little effect on ventricular function or peripheral vasculature because of the paucity of direct cholinergic innervation of these areas despite the presence of cholinergic receptors. Presynaptic muscarinic receptors on adrenergic nerve terminals are known to inhibit norepinephrine release, so muscarinic antagonists may in fact modestly enhance sympathetic activity. Large doses of anticholinergic agents can result in dilation of cutaneous blood vessels (atropine flush).

B. RESPIRATORY

The anticholinergics inhibit the secretions of the respiratory tract mucosa, from the nose to the bronchi. This drying effect was more important before the advent of less irritating inhalational agents. Relaxation of the bronchial smooth musculature reduces airway resistance and increases anatomic dead space. These effects are particularly pronounced in patients with chronic obstructive pulmonary disease or asthma.

C. CEREBRAL

Anticholinergic medications can cause a spectrum of central nervous system effects ranging from stimulation to depression, depending on drug choice and dosage. Stimulation may present as excitation, restlessness, or hallucinations. Depression can cause sedation and amnesia. Physostigmine, a cholinesterase inhibitor that crosses the blood–brain barrier, promptly reverses these actions (see Chapter 10).

D. GASTROINTESTINAL

Salivary secretions are markedly reduced by anticholinergic drugs. Gastric secretions are also decreased, but larger doses are necessary. Decreased intestinal motility and peristalsis prolong gastric emptying time. Lower esophageal sphincter pressure is reduced. Overall, the anticholinergic drugs are not very advantageous in the prevention of aspiration pneumonia (see Case Discussion, Chapter 15).

E. OPHTHALMIC

Anticholinergics cause mydriasis (pupillary dilation) and cycloplegia (an inability to accommodate to near vision); acute angle-closure glaucoma is unlikely following systemic administration of most anticholinergic drugs.

F. GENITOURINARY

Anticholinergics may decrease ureter and bladder tone as a result of smooth muscle relaxation and lead to urinary retention, particularly in elderly men with prostatic hypertrophy.

G. THERMOREGULATION

Inhibition of sweat glands may lead to a rise in body temperature (atropine fever).

H. IMMUNE-MEDIATED HYPERSENSITIVITY

Decreasing intracellular cGMP would theoretically be useful in the treatment of hypersensitivity reactions. Clinically, anticholinergics appear to have little efficacy in these situations.

Figure 11–1. Physical structures of anticholinergic drugs.

■ SPECIFIC ANTICHOLINERGIC DRUGS

ATROPINE

Physical Structure

Atropine is a tertiary amine consisting of tropic acid (an aromatic acid) and tropine (an organic base). The naturally occurring levorotatory form is active, but the commercial mixture is racemic (Figure 11–1).

Dosage & Packaging

As a premedication, atropine is administered intravenously or intramuscularly in a range of 0.01–0.02 mg/kg up to the usual adult dose of 0.4–0.6 mg. Larger intravenous doses up to 2 mg may be required to completely block the cardiac vagal nerves in treating severe bradycardia. The appropriate dose for minimizing the side effects of cholinesterase inhibitors during reversal of nondepolarizing blockade is shown in Table 10–3. Atropine sulfate is available in a multitude of concentrations.

Clinical Considerations

Atropine has particularly potent effects on the heart and bronchial smooth muscle and is the most efficacious anticholinergic for treating bradyarrhythmias. Patients with coronary artery disease may not tolerate the increased myocardial oxygen demand and decreased oxygen supply associated with the tachycardia caused by atropine. A derivative of atropine, ipratropium bromide, is available in a metered-dose inhaler for the treatment of bronchospasm. Its quaternary ammonium structure significantly limits systemic absorption. Ipratropium solution (0.5 mg in 2.5 mL) appears particularly effective in the treatment of acute chronic obstructive pulmonary disease when combined with a β-agonist drug (eg, albuterol). The central nervous system effects of atropine are minimal after the usual doses, even though this tertiary amine can rapidly cross the blood–brain barrier. Atropine has been associated with mild postoperative memory deficits, and toxic doses are usually associated with excitatory reactions. An intramuscular dose of 0.01–0.02 mg/kg reliably provides an antisialagogue effect. Atropine should be used cautiously in patients with narrow-angle glaucoma, prostatic hypertrophy, or bladder-neck obstruction.

SCOPOLAMINE

Physical Structure

Scopolamine differs from atropine by incorporating an oxygen bridge into the organic base to form scopine.

Dosage & Packaging

The premedication dose of scopolamine is the same as that of atropine, and it is usually given intramuscularly. Scopolamine hydrobromide is available as solutions containing 0.3, 0.4, and 1 mg/mL.

Clinical Considerations

 Scopolamine is a more potent antisialagogue than atropine and causes greater central nervous system effects. Clinical dosages usually result in drowsiness and amnesia, although restlessness and delirium are possible. The sedative effects may be desirable for premedication but can interfere with awakening following short procedures. Scopolamine has the added virtue of preventing motion sickness. The lipid solubility allows transdermal absorption. Because of its pronounced ocular effects, scopolamine is best avoided in patients with closed-angle glaucoma.

GLYCOPYRROLATE

Physical Structure

Glycopyrrolate is a synthetic quaternary ammonium containing mandelic acid in the place of tropic acid.

Dosage & Packaging

The usual dose of glycopyrrolate is one-half that of atropine. For instance, the premedication dose is 0.005–0.01 mg/kg up to 0.2–0.3 mg in adults. Glycopyrrolate for injection is packaged as a solution of 0.2 mg/mL.

Clinical Considerations

Because of a quaternary structure, glycopyrrolate cannot cross the blood–brain barrier and is almost always devoid of central nervous system and ophthalmic activity. Potent inhibition of salivary gland and respiratory tract secretions is the primary rationale for using glycopyrrolate as a premedication. Heart rate usually increases after intravenous—but not intramuscular—administration. Glycopyrrolate has a longer duration of action than atropine (2–4 h versus 30 min after intravenous administration).

CASE DISCUSSION: CENTRAL ANTICHOLINERGIC SYNDROME

An elderly patient is scheduled for enucleation of a blind, painful eye. Scopolamine, 0.4 mg intramuscularly, is administered as premedication. In the preoperative holding area, the patient becomes agitated and disoriented. The only other medication the patient has received is 1% atropine eye drops.

How many milligrams of atropine are in one drop of a 1% solution?

A 1% solution contains 1 g dissolved in 100 mL, or 10 mg/mL. Eyedroppers vary in the number of drops formed per milliliter of solution but average 20 drops/mL. Therefore, one drop usually contains 0.5 mg of atropine.

How are ophthalmic drops systemically absorbed?

Absorption by vessels in the conjunctival sac is similar to subcutaneous injection. More rapid absorption is possible by the nasolacrimal duct mucosa.

What are the signs and symptoms of anticholinergic poisoning?

*Reactions from an overdose of anticholinergic medication involve several organ systems. The **central anticholinergic syndrome** refers to central nervous system changes that range from unconsciousness to hallucinations. Agitation and delirium are not unusual in elderly patients. Other systemic manifestations include dry mouth, tachycardia, atropine flush, atropine fever, and impaired vision.*

What other drugs possess anticholinergic activity that could predispose patients to the central anticholinergic syndrome?

Tricyclic antidepressants, antihistamines, and antipsychotics have antimuscarinic properties that could potentiate the side effects of anticholinergic drugs.

What drug is an effective antidote to anticholinergic overdosage?

Cholinesterase inhibitors indirectly increase the amount of acetylcholine available to compete with anticholinergic drugs at the muscarinic receptor. Neostigmine, pyridostigmine, and edrophonium possess a quaternary ammonium group that prevents penetration of the blood–brain barrier. Physostigmine, a tertiary amine, is lipid soluble and effectively reverses central anticholinergic toxicity. An initial dose of 0.01–0.03 mg/kg may have to be repeated after 15–30 min.

Should this case be canceled or allowed to proceed?

Enucleation to relieve a painful eye is clearly an elective procedure. The most important question that must be addressed for elective cases is whether the patient is optimally medically managed. In other words, would canceling surgery allow further fine-tuning of any medical problems? For example, if this anticholinergic overdose were accompanied by tachycardia, it would probably be prudent to postpone surgery in this elderly patient. On the other hand, if the patient's mental status responds to physostigmine and there appear to be no other significant anticholinergic side effects, surgery could proceed.

SUGGESTED READING

Brown JH, Taylor P: Muscarinic receptor agonists and antagonists. Chapter 7 in: *Goodman and Gilman's The Pharmacological Basis of Therapeutics,* 10th ed. Hardman JG (editor). McGraw-Hill, 2002. Mechanisms of action, structure-activity relationships, and therapeutic uses are included.

Katzung BG (editor): Cholinoceptor-blocking drugs. Chapter 8 in: *Basic and Clinical Pharmacology,* 8th ed. McGraw-Hill, 2001.

Naguib M, Yaksh TL: Characterization of muscarinic receptor subtypes that mediate antinociception in the rat spinal cord. Anesth Analg 1997;85:847. A discussion of the function of muscarinic receptor subtypes.

Adrenergic Agonists & Antagonists

KEY CONCEPTS

 Adrenergic agonists can be categorized as direct or indirect. Direct agonists bind to the receptor, whereas indirect agonists increase endogenous neurotransmitter activity.

 The primary effect of phenylephrine is peripheral vasoconstriction with a concomitant rise in systemic vascular resistance and arterial blood pressure.

 Clonidine appears to decrease anesthetic and analgesic requirements and to provide sedation and anxiolysis.

 Dexmedetomidine is a novel lipophilic α-methylol derivative with a higher affinity for α_2-receptors than clonidine. It has sedative, analgesic, and sympatholytic effects that blunt many of the cardiovascular responses seen during the perioperative period.

 Long-term use of these agents, particularly clonidine and dexmedetomidine, leads to supersensitization and up-regulation of receptors; with abrupt discontinuation of either drug, an acute withdrawal syndrome manifested by a hypertensive crisis can occur.

 Ephedrine is commonly used as a vasopressor during anesthesia. As such, its administration should be viewed as a temporizing measure while the cause of hypotension is determined and remedied.

 Small doses ($\leq 2\ \mu g/kg/min$) of dopamine (DA) have minimal adrenergic effects but activate dopaminergic receptors. Stimulation of these nonadrenergic receptors (specifically, DA_1 receptors) vasodilates the renal vasculature and promotes diuresis.

 Favorable effects on myocardial oxygen balance make dobutamine a good choice for patients with the combination of congestive heart failure and coronary artery disease, particularly if peripheral vascular resistance and heart rate are already elevated.

 Labetalol lowers blood pressure without reflex tachycardia because of its combination of α- and β-effects.

 Esmolol is an ultrashort-acting selective β_1-antagonist that reduces heart rate and, to a lesser extent, blood pressure.

 Discontinuation of β-blocker therapy for 24–48 h may trigger a withdrawal syndrome characterized by hypertension, tachycardia, and angina pectoris.

The three previous chapters presented the pharmacology of drugs that affect cholinergic activity. This chapter introduces an analogous group of agents that interacts at adrenergic receptors—adrenoceptors. The clinical effects of these drugs can be deduced from an understanding of adrenoceptor physiology and a knowledge of which receptors each drug activates or blocks.

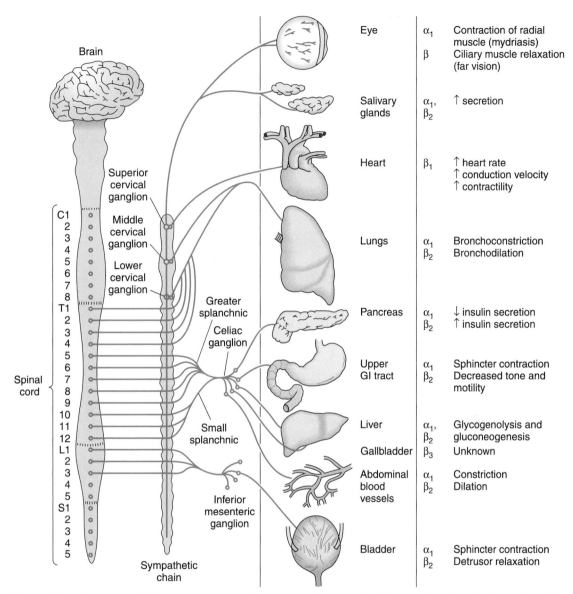

Figure 12–1. The sympathetic nervous system. Organ innervation, receptor type, and response to stimulation. The origin of the sympathetic chain is the thoracoabdominal (T1–L3) spinal cord, in contrast to the craniosacral distribution of the parasympathetic nervous system. Another anatomic difference is the greater distance from the sympathetic ganglion to the visceral structures.

ADRENOCEPTOR PHYSIOLOGY

The term adrenergic originally referred to the effects of epinephrine (*adren*aline), as opposed to the cholinergic effects of acetyl*choline.* It is now known that norepinephrine (noradrenaline) is the neurotransmit-

ter responsible for most of the adrenergic activity of the sympathetic nervous system. With the exception of eccrine sweat glands and some blood vessels, norepinephrine is released by postganglionic sympathetic fibers at end-organ tissues (Figure 12–1). In contrast, as was explained in Chapter 10, acetylcholine is

Figure 12–2. The synthesis of norepinephrine. Hydroxylation of tyrosine to dopa is the rate-limiting step. Dopamine is actively transported into storage vesicles. Norepinephrine can be converted to epinephrine in the adrenal medulla.

released by preganglionic sympathetic fibers and all parasympathetic fibers.

Norepinephrine is synthesized in the cytoplasm and packaged into vesicles of sympathetic postganglionic fibers (Figure 12–2). After release by a process of exocytosis, the action of norepinephrine is terminated by reuptake into the postganglionic nerve ending (inhibited by tricyclic antidepressants), diffusion from receptor sites, or metabolism by monoamine oxidase (inhibited by monoamine oxidase inhibitors) and catechol-O-methyltransferase (Figure 12–3). Prolonged adrenergic acti-

vation leads to desensitization and hyporesponsiveness to further stimulation.

Adrenergic receptors are divided into two general categories: α and β. Each of these has been further subdivided into at least two subtypes: α_1 and α_2, and β_1, β_2, and β_3. The α-receptors have been further divided using molecular cloning techniques into α_{1A}, α_{1B}, α_{1D}, α_{2A}, α_{2B}, and α_{2C}. These receptors are linked to G proteins (Figure 12–4; Drs. Rodbell and Gilman received the Nobel Prize in physiology medicine in 1994 for their discovery)—heterotrimeric receptors with α, β, and γ sub-

Figure 12–3. Sequential metabolism of norepinephrine and epinephrine. Monoamine oxidase (MAO) and catechol-*O*-methyltransferase (COMT) produce a common end product, vanillylmandelic acid (VMA).

units. The different adrenoreceptors are linked to specific G proteins, each with a unique effector, but each using guanosine triphosphate (GTP) as a cofactor. α_1 is linked to G_q, which activates phospholipases, α_2 is linked to G_i, which inhibits adenylate cyclase, and β is linked to G_s, which activates adenylate cyclase.

α_1-Receptors

α_1-Receptors are postsynaptic adrenoceptors located in smooth muscle throughout the body, in the eye, lung, blood vessels, uterus, gut, and genitourinary system. Activation of these receptors increases intracellular calcium ion concentration, which leads to muscle contraction. Thus, α_1-agonists are associated with mydriasis (pupillary dilation due to contraction of the radial eye muscles), bronchoconstriction, vasoconstriction, uterine contracture, and contraction of sphincters in the gastrointestinal and genitourinary tracts. α_1-Stimulation also inhibits insulin secretion and lipolysis. The myocardium possesses α_1-receptors that have slightly positive inotropic and negative chronotropic effects. During myocardial ischemia, enhanced α_1-receptor coupling with agonists is observed. Nonetheless, the most important cardiovascular effect of α_1-stimulation is vasoconstriction, which increases peripheral vascular resistance, left ventricular afterload, and arterial blood pressure.

α_2-Receptors

In contrast to α_1-receptors, α_2-receptors are located primarily on the presynaptic nerve terminals. Activation of these adrenoceptors inhibits adenylate cyclase activity. This decreases the entry of calcium ions into the neuronal terminal, which limits subsequent exocytosis of storage vesicles containing norepinephrine. Thus, α_2-receptors create a negative feedback loop that inhibits further norepinephrine release from the neuron. In addition, vascular smooth muscle contains postsynaptic α_2-receptors that produce vasoconstriction. More important, stimulation of postsynaptic α_2-receptors in the central nervous system causes sedation and reduces sympathetic outflow, which leads to peripheral vasodilation and lower blood pressure.

β_1-Receptors

The most important β_1-receptors are located on postsynaptic membranes in the heart. Stimulation of these receptors activates adenylate cyclase, which converts adenosine triphosphate to cyclic adenosine monophosphate and initiates a kinase phosphorylation cascade. Initiation of

Figure 12–4. The adrenoreceptor is a transmembrane-spanning receptor made up of seven subunits, which is linked to a G protein. G proteins are trimeric endoplasmic membrane proteins made of α, β, and γ units. With activation, GTP on the α-subunit is replaced by GDP, stimulating a conformational change, disassociating the α, β, and γ units. Either the Gα or G$\beta\gamma$ subunits can activate (or inhibit) the enzyme effector for that adrenoceptor. M1–M7, membrane-spanning units; α, β, γ, subunits of G protein; GTP, guanosine triphosphate; P_i, inorganic phosphate—quickly assimilated; GDP, guanosine diphosphate; E effector, cyclophosphatase for G_q, adenylate cyclase for G_i, and G_s.

the cascade has positive chronotropic (increased heart rate), dromotropic (increased conduction), and inotropic (increased contractilty) effects.

β_2-Receptors

β_2-Receptors are primarily postsynaptic adrenoceptors located in smooth muscle and gland cells. They share a common mechanism of action with β_1-receptors: adenylate cyclase activation. Despite this commonality, β_2-stimulation relaxes smooth muscle, resulting in bronchodilation, vasodilation, and relaxation of the uterus (tocolysis), bladder, and gut. Glycogenolysis, lipolysis, gluconeogenesis, and insulin release are stimulated by β_2-receptor activation. β_2-Agonists also activate the sodium–potassium pump, which drives potassium intracellularly and can induce hypokalemia and dysrhythmias.

β_3-Receptors

β_3-Receptors are found in the gallbladder and in brain adipose tissue. Their role in gallbladder physiology is unknown, but they are thought to play a role in lipolysis and thermogenesis in brown fat.

■ ADRENERGIC AGONISTS

Adrenergic agonists interact with varying specificity (selectivity) at α- and β-adrenoceptors (Table 12–1).

Table 12–1. Receptor selectivity of adrenergic agonists.[1]

Drug	α_1	α_2	β_1	β_2	DA$_1$	DA$_2$
Phenylephrine	+++	+	+	0	0	0
Methyldopa	+	+	0	0	0	0
Clonidine	+	++	0	0	0	0
Dexmedetomidine	+	+++	0	0	0	0
Epinephrine[2]	++	++	+++	++	0	0
Ephedrine[3]	++	?	++	+	0	0
Fenoldopam	0	0	0	0	+++	0
Norepinephrine[2]	++	++	++	0	0	0
Dopamine[2]	++	++	++	+	+++	+++
Dopexamine	0	0	+	+++	++	+++
Dobutamine	0/+	0	+++	+	0	0
Terbutaline	0	0	+	+++	0	0

[1]0, no effect; +, agonist effect (mild, moderate, marked); ?, unknown effect; DA$_1$ and DA$_2$, dopaminergic receptors.
[2]The α_1-effects of epinephrine, norepinephrine, and dopamine become more prominent at high doses.
[3]The primary mode of action of ephedrine is indirect stimulation.

Figure 12–5. Adrenergic agonists that have a 3,4-dihydroxybenzene structure are known as catecholamines. Substitutions at the R_1, R_2, and R_3 sites affect activity and selectivity.

Overlapping of activity complicates the prediction of clinical effects. For example, epinephrine stimulates α_1-, α_2-, β_1-, and β_2-adrenoceptors. Its net effect on arterial blood pressure depends on the balance between α_1-vasoconstriction, α_2- and β_2-vasodilation, and β_1-inotropic influences. Moreover, this balance changes at different doses.

Adrenergic agonists can be categorized as direct or indirect. Direct agonists bind to the receptor, whereas indirect agonists increase endogenous neurotransmitter activity. Mechanisms of indirect action include increased release or decreased reuptake of norepinephrine. The differentiation between direct and indirect mechanisms of action is particularly important in patients who have abnormal endogenous norepinephrine stores, as may occur with use of some antihypertensive medications or monoamine oxidase inhibitors. Intraoperative hypotension in these patients should be treated with direct agonists, as their response to indirect agonists will be altered.

Another feature distinguishing adrenergic agonists from each other is their chemical structure. Adrenergic agonists that have a 3,4-dihydroxybenzene structure (Figure 12–5) are known as catecholamines. These drugs are typically short acting because of their metabolism by monoamine oxidase and catechol-O-methyltransferase. Patients taking monoamine oxidase inhibitors or tricyclic antidepressants may therefore demonstrate an exaggerated response to catecholamines. The naturally occurring catecholamines are epinephrine, norepinephrine, and dopamine. Changing the side-chain structure (R_1, R_2, R_3) of naturally occurring catecholamines has led to the development of synthetic catecholamines (eg, isoproterenol and dobutamine), which tend to be more receptor specific.

Adrenergic agonists commonly used in anesthesiology are discussed individually below. Note that the recommended doses for continuous infusion are expressed as µg/kg/min for some agents and µg/min for others. In either case, these recommendations should be regarded only as guidelines, as individual responses are quite variable.

PHENYLEPHRINE

Clinical Considerations

Phenylephrine is a noncatecholamine with predominantly direct α_1-agonist activity (high doses may stimulate α_2- and β-receptors). The primary effect of phenylephrine is peripheral vasoconstriction with a concomitant rise in systemic vascular resistance and arterial blood pressure. Reflex bradycardia can reduce cardiac output. Coronary blood flow increases because any direct vasoconstrictive effect of phenylephrine on the coronary arteries is overridden by vasodilation induced by the release of metabolic factors (Table 12–2).

Dosing & Packaging

Small intravenous boluses of 50–100 µg (0.5–1 µg/kg) of phenylephrine rapidly reverse reductions in blood pressure caused by peripheral vasodilation (eg, spinal anesthesia). A continuous infusion (100 µg/mL at a rate of 0.25–1 µg/kg/min) will maintain arterial blood pressure but at the expense of renal blood flow. Tachyphylaxis occurs with phenylephrine infusions requiring upward titration of the infusion. Phenylephrine must be diluted from a 1% solution (10 mg/1-mL ampule), usually to a 100 µg/mL solution.

α_2-AGONISTS

Clinical Considerations

Methyldopa, a prototypical drug, is an analogue of levodopa. Methyldopa enters the norepinephrine-synthesis pathway and is converted to α-methylnorepinephrine and α-methylepinephrine. These false transmitters activate α-adrenoceptors, particularly central α_2-receptors. As a result, norepinephrine release and sympathetic tone are diminished. A fall in peripheral vascular resistance is responsible for a drop in arterial blood pressure (peak effect within 4 h). Renal blood flow is maintained or increased. Because methyldopa relies on metabolites to be effective, it is being replaced by drugs with direct α_2-activity, although it is still recommended for treating high blood pressure in pregnancy.

Clonidine is an α_2-agonist that is now commonly used for its antihypertensive (decreased systemic vascular resistance) and negative chronotropic effects. More recently, it and other α_2-agonists have been found to have sedative properties. Investigational studies have examined the anesthetic effects of oral (3–5 µg/kg), intramuscular (2 µg/kg), intravenous (1–3 µg/kg), transdermal (0.1–0.3 mg released per day), intrathecal (75–150 µg), and epidural (1–2 µg/kg) clonidine administration. In general, clonidine appears to decrease anesthetic and analgesic

Table 12–2. Effects of adrenergic agonists on organ systems.[1]

Drug	Heart Rate	Mean Arterial Pressure	Cardiac Output	Peripheral Vascular Resistance	Bronchodilation	Renal Blood Flow
Phenylephrine	↓	↑↑↑	↓	↑↑↑	0	↓↓↓
Epinephrine	↑↑	↑	↑↑	↑/↓	↑↑	↓↓
Ephedrine	↑↑	↑↑	↑↑	↑	↑↑	↓↓
Fenoldopam	↑↑	↓↓↓	↓/↑	↓↓	0	↑↑↑
Norepinephrine	↓	↑↑↑	↓/↑	↑↑↑	0	↓↓↓
Dopamine	↑/↑↑	↑	↑↑↑	↑	0	↑↑↑
Dopexamine	↑/↑↑	↓/↑	↑↑	↑	0	↑
Isoproterenol	↑↑↑	↓	↑↑↑	↓↓	↑↑↑	↓/↑
Dobutamine	↑	↑	↑↑↑	↓	0	↑

[1]0, no effect; ↑, increase (mild, moderate, marked); ↓, decrease (mild, moderate, marked); ↓/↑, variable effect; ↑/↑↑, mild-to-moderate increase.

requirements (decreases MAC) and to provide sedation and anxiolysis. During general anesthesia, clonidine reportedly enhances intraoperative circulatory stability by reducing catecholamine levels. During regional anesthesia, including peripheral nerve block, clonidine prolongs the duration of the block. Direct effects on the spinal cord may be mediated by α_2-postsynaptic receptors within the dorsal horn. Other possible benefits include decreased postoperative shivering, inhibition of opioid-induced muscle rigidity, attenuation of opioid withdrawal symptoms, and the treatment of some chronic pain syndromes. Side effects include bradycardia, hypotension, sedation, respiratory depression, and dry mouth.

Dexmedetomidine is a novel lipophylic α-methylol derivative with a higher affinity for α_2-receptors than clonidine. It has sedative, analgesic, and sympatholytic effects that blunt many of the cardiovascular responses seen during the perioperative period. When used intraoperatively, it reduces intravenous and volatile anesthetic requirements; when used postoperatively, it reduces concurrent analgesic and sedative requirements. Patients remain sedated when undisturbed but arouse readily with stimulation. Similar to methyldopa and clonidine, dexmedetomidine is a sympatholytic because sympathetic outflow is reduced. It may be a useful agent for decreasing intraoperative anesthetic requirements and for sedating ventilated patients postoperatively in the postanesthesia care unit and in the intensive care unit because of its anxiolytic and analgesic effects. It does so without significant ventilatory depression. Rapid administration

may elevate blood pressure, but hypotension and bradycardia may occur during ongoing therapy.

Although these agents are adrenergic agonists, they are also considered to be sympatholytic because sympathetic outflow is reduced. Long-term use of these agents, particularly clonidine and dexmedetomidine, leads to supersensitization and upregulation of receptors; with abrupt discontinuation of either drug, an acute withdrawal syndrome manifested by a hypertensive crisis can occur. Because of the increased affinity of dexmedetomidine compared to clonidine for the α_2-receptor, this syndrome may manifest after only 48 h of dexmedetomidine use when the drug is discontinued.

Dosing & Packaging

Clonidine is available as an oral, transdermal, or parenteral preparation (see Clinical Considerations in the α_2-Agonists section for dosages). The latter is approved only for epidural or intrathecal use as an adjunct to regional analgesia/anesthesia. However, it is widely used in Europe at an intravenous bolus dose of 50 µg for blood pressure or heart rate control. It has a slow onset of action.

EPINEPHRINE

Clinical Considerations

Direct stimulation of β_1-receptors by epinephrine raises cardiac output and myocardial oxygen demand by increasing contractility and heart rate (increased rate of spontaneous phase IV depolarization). α_1-Stimulation decreases splanchnic and renal blood flow but increases coronary and cerebral perfusion pressure. Systolic blood pressure rises, although β_2-mediated vasodilation in skeletal muscle may lower diastolic pressure. β_2-Stimulation also relaxes bronchial smooth muscle.

Administration of epinephrine is the principal pharmacological treatment for anaphylaxis and can be used to treat ventricular fibrillation (see Chapters 47 and 48). Complications include cerebral hemorrhage, coronary ischemia, and ventricular dysrhythmias. Volatile anesthetics, particularly halothane, potentiate the dysrhythmic effects of epinephrine.

Dosing & Packaging

In emergency situations (eg, shock and allergic reactions), epinephrine is administered as an intravenous bolus of 0.05–1 mg depending on the severity of cardiovascular compromise. To improve myocardial contractility or heart rate, a continuous infusion is prepared (1 mg in 250 mL dextrose 5% in water [D_5W; 4 μg/mL]) and run at a rate of 2–20 μg/min. Some local anesthetic solutions containing epinephrine at a concentration of 1:200,000 (5 μg/mL) or 1:400,000 (2.5 μg/mL) are characterized by less systemic absorption and a longer duration of action. Epinephrine is available in vials at a concentration of 1:1000 (1 mg/mL) and prefilled syringes at a concentration of 1:10,000 (0.1 mg/mL [100 μg/mL]). A 1:100,000 (10 μg/mL) concentration is available for pediatric use.

EPHEDRINE

Clinical Considerations

The cardiovascular effects of ephedrine are similar to those of epinephrine: increase in blood pressure, heart rate, contractility, and cardiac output. Likewise, ephedrine is also a bronchodilator. There are important differences, however: ephedrine has a longer duration of action because it is a noncatecholamine, is much less potent, has indirect and direct actions, and stimulates the central nervous system (it raises minimum alveolar concentration). The indirect agonist properties of ephedrine may be due to central stimulation, peripheral postsynaptic norepinephrine release, or inhibition of norepinephrine reuptake.

Ephedrine is commonly used as a vasopressor during anesthesia. As such, its administration should be viewed as a temporizing measure while the cause of hypotension is determined and remedied. Unlike direct-acting α_1-agonists, ephedrine does not decrease uterine blood flow. This makes it the preferred vasopressor for most obstetric uses. Ephedrine has also been reported to possess antiemetic properties, particularly in association with hypotension following spinal

anesthesia. Clonidine premedication augments the effects of ephedrine.

Dosing & Packaging

In adults, ephedrine is administered as a bolus of 2.5–10 mg; in children it is given as a bolus of 0.1 mg/kg. Subsequent doses are increased to offset the development of tachyphylaxis, which is probably due to depletion of norepinephrine stores. Ephedrine is available in 1-mL ampules containing 25 or 50 mg of the agent.

NOREPINEPHRINE

Clinical Considerations

Direct α_1-stimulation in the absence of β_2-activity induces intense vasoconstriction of arterial and venous vessels. Increased myocardial contractility from β_1-effects may contribute to a rise in arterial blood pressure, but increased afterload and reflex bradycardia prevent any elevation in cardiac output. Decreased renal blood flow and increased myocardial oxygen requirements limit the usefulness of norepinephrine to the treatment of refractory shock, which requires potent vasoconstriction to maintain tissue perfusion pressure. Norepinephrine has been used with an α-blocker (eg, phentolamine) in an attempt to take advantage of its β-activity without the profound vasoconstriction caused by its α-stimulation. Extravasation of norepinephrine at the site of intravenous administration can cause tissue necrosis.

Dosing & Packaging

Norepinephrine is administered as a bolus (0.1 μg/kg) or as a continuous infusion (4 mg of drug to 500 mL D_5W [8 μg/mL]) at a rate of 2–20 μg/min. Ampules contain 4 mg of norepinephrine in 4 mL of solution.

DOPAMINE

Clinical Considerations

The clinical effects of dopamine (DA), a nonselective direct and indirect adrenergic agonist, vary markedly with the dose. Small doses ($\leq$ 2 μg/kg/min) of DA have minimal adrenergic effects but activate dopaminergic receptors. Stimulation of these nonadrenergic receptors (specifically, DA_1 receptors) vasodilates the renal vasculature and promotes diuresis. At moderate doses (2–10 μg/kg/min), β_1-stimulation increases myocardial contractility, heart rate, and cardiac output. Myocardial oxygen demand typically increases more than supply. α_1-Effects become prominent at higher doses (10–20 μg/kg/min), causing an increase in peripheral vascular resistance and a fall in renal blood flow. The indirect effects of DA are due to release of norepinephrine, which it resembles at doses above 20 μg/kg/min.

DA is commonly used in the treatment of shock to improve cardiac output, support blood pressure, and maintain renal function. It is often used in combination with a vasodilator (eg, nitroglycerin or nitroprusside), which reduces afterload and further improves cardiac output (see Chapter 13). The chronotropic and dysrhythmogenic effects of DA limit its usefulness in some patients.

Dosing & Packaging

DA is administered as a continuous infusion (400 mg in 1000 mL D_5W; 400 µg/mL) at a rate of 1–20 µg/kg/min. It is most commonly supplied in 5-mL ampules containing 200 or 400 mg of DA.

ISOPROTERENOL

Isoproterenol is of interest because it is a pure β-agonist. $β_1$-Effects increase heart rate, contractility, and cardiac output. $β_2$-Stimulation decreases peripheral vascular resistance and diastolic blood pressure. Myocardial oxygen demand increases while oxygen supply falls, making isoproterenol or any pure β-agonist a poor inotropic choice in most situations. Isoproterenol's availability is decreasing in the United States.

DOBUTAMINE
Clinical Considerations

Dobutamine is a relatively selective $β_1$-agonist. Its primary cardiovascular effect is a rise in cardiac output as a result of increased myocardial contractility. A slight decline in peripheral vascular resistance caused by $β_2$-activation usually prevents much of a rise in arterial blood pressure. Left ventricular filling pressure decreases, whereas coronary blood flow increases. Heart rate increases are less marked than with other β-agonists. Favorable effects on myocardial oxygen balance make dobutamine a good choice for patients with the combination of congestive heart failure and coronary artery disease, particularly if peripheral vascular resistance and heart rate are already elevated.

Dosing & Packaging

Dobutamine is administered as an infusion (1 g in 250 mL [4 mg/mL]) at a rate of 2–20 µg/kg/min. It is supplied in 20-mL vials containing 250 mg.

DOPEXAMINE
Clinical Considerations

Dopexamine is a structural analogue of DA that has potential advantages over dopamine because it has less $β_1$-adrenergic (arrhythmogenic) and α-adrenergic effects. Because of the decreased β-adrenergic effects and its specific effect on renal perfusion, it may have advantages over dobutamine. The drug has been clinically available since 1990 but has not gained widespread acceptance in practice.

Dosing & Packaging

Dopexamine comes in a concentration of 50 mg/mL and should be diluted in D_5W. The infusion should be started at a rate of 0.5 µg/kg/min, increasing to 1 µg/kg/min at intervals of 10– 15 min to a maximum infusion rate of 6 µg/kg/min.

FENOLDOPAM
Clinical Considerations

Fenoldopam is a selective DA_1-receptor agonist that has many of the benefits of DA but with little or no α- or β-adrenoceptor or DA_2-receptor agonist activity. Fenoldopam has been shown to exert hypotensive effects characterized by a decrease in peripheral vascular resistance, along with an increase in renal blood flow, diuresis, and natriuresis. It is indicated for patients undergoing cardiac surgery and aortic aneurysm repair, because of its antihypertensive and renal-sparing properties. It is also indicated for patients who have severe hypertension, particularly those with renal impairment.

Dosing & Packaging

Fenoldopam is supplied in 1-, 2-, and 5-mL ampules, 10 mg/mL. It is started as a continuous infusion of 0.1 µg/kg/min, increased by increments of 0.1 µg/kg/min at 15- to 20-min intervals until target blood pressure is achieved. Lower doses have been associated with less reflex tachycardia.

■ ADRENERGIC ANTAGONISTS

Adrenergic antagonists bind but do not activate adrenoceptors. They act by preventing adrenergic agonist activity. Like the agonists, the antagonists differ in their spectrum of receptor interaction (Table 12–3).

α-BLOCKERS—PHENTOLAMINE
Clinical Considerations

Phentolamine produces a competitive (reversible) blockade of α-receptors. $α_1$-Antagonism and direct smooth

Table 12–3. Receptor selectivity of adrenergic antagonists.[1]

Drug	α_1	α_1	β_1	β_2
Prazosin	–	0	0	0
Phenoxybenzamine	–	–	0	0
Phentolamine	–	–	0	0
Labetalol[2]		–	0	–	–
Metoprolol	0	0	–	–
Esmolol	0	0	–	–
Propranolol	0	0	–	–

[1]0, no effect; –, antagonist effect (mild, moderate, marked).
[2]Labetalol may also have some β_2-agonist activity.

muscle relaxation are responsible for peripheral vasodilation and a decline in arterial blood pressure. The drop in blood pressure provokes reflex tachycardia. This tachycardia is augmented by antagonism of α_2-receptors in the heart because α_2-blockade promotes norepinephrine release by eliminating negative feedback. These cardiovascular effects are usually apparent within 2 min and last up to 15 min. As with all of the adrenergic antagonists, the extent of the response to receptor blockade depends on the degree of existing sympathetic tone. Reflex tachycardia and postural hypotension limit the usefulness of phentolamine to the treatment of hypertension caused by excessive α-stimulation (eg, pheochromocytoma, clonidine withdrawal).

Dosing & Packaging

Phentolamine is administered intravenously as intermittent boluses (1–5 mg in adults) or as a continuous infusion (10 mg in 100 mL D_5W [100 µg/mL]). To prevent tissue necrosis following extravasation of intravenous fluids containing an α-agonist (eg, norepinephrine), 5–10 mg of phentolamine in 10 mL of normal saline can be locally infiltrated. Phentolamine is packaged as a lyophilized powder (5 mg).

MIXED ANTAGONISTS—LABETALOL

Clinical Considerations

Labetalol blocks α_1-, β_1-, and β_2-receptors. The ratio of α-blockade to β-blockade has been estimated to be approximately 1:7 following intravenous administration. This mixed blockade reduces peripheral vascular resistance and arterial blood pressure. Heart rate and

cardiac output are usually slightly depressed or unchanged. Thus, labetalol lowers blood pressure without reflex tachycardia because of its combination of α- and β-effects. Peak effect usually occurs within 5 min after an intravenous dose. Left ventricular failure, paradoxical hypertension, and bronchospasm have been reported.

Dosing & Packaging

The initial recommended dose of labetalol is 0.1–0.25 mg/kg administered intravenously over 2 min. Twice this amount may be given at 10-min intervals until the desired blood pressure response is obtained. Labetalol can also be administered as a slow continuous infusion (200 mg in 250 mL D_5W) at a rate of 2 mg/min. However, due to its long elimination half-life (> 5 h), prolonged infusions are not recommended. Labetalol (5 mg/mL) is available in 20- and 40-mL multidose containers and in 4- and 8-mL single-dose prefilled syringes.

β-BLOCKERS

β-Receptor blockers have variable degrees of selectivity for the β_1-receptors. Those that are more β_1 selective have less influence on bronchopulmonary and vascular β_2-receptors (Table 12–4). Theoretically, a selective β_1-blocker would have less of an inhibitory effect on β_2-receptors and, therefore, might be preferred in patients with chronic obstructive lung disease or peripheral vascular disease. Patients with peripheral vascular disease could potentially have a decrease in blood flow if β_2-receptors, which are dilating the arterioles, are blocked.

β-Blockers are also classified by the amount of intrinsic sympathomimetic activity (ISA) they have. Many of the β-blockers have some slight agonist activity; although they would not produce effects similar to full agonists, such as epinephrine, β-blockers with ISA may not be as beneficial as β-blockers without ISA in treating patients with cardiovascular disease.

β-Blockers can be further classified as those that are eliminated by hepatic metabolism (such as atenolol or metoprolol), those that are excreted by the kidneys unchanged (such as atenolol), or those that are hydrolyzed in the blood (such as esmolol).

ESMOLOL

Clinical Considerations

Esmolol is an ultrashort-acting selective β_1-antagonist that reduces heart rate and, to a lesser extent, blood pressure. **It has been successfully used to prevent tachycardia and hypertension in response to perioperative stimuli, such as intubation, surgical stimulation, and emergence. For example, esmolol (1 mg/kg)**

Table 12–4. Pharmacology of β-blockers.[1]

	Selectivity for β₁-Receptors	ISA	α₂-Blockade	Hepatic Metabolism	t½
Atenolol	+	0	0	0	6–7
Esmolol	+	0	0	0	$-\frac{1}{4}$
Labetalol	0		+	+	4
Metoprolol	+	0	0	+	3–4
Propranolol	0		0	+	4–6

[1]ISA, intrinsic sympathomimetic activity; +, mild effect; 0, no effect.

attenuates the rise in blood pressure and heart rate that usually accompanies electroconvulsive therapy, without affecting seizure duration. Esmolol is as effective as propranolol in controlling the ventricular rate of patients with atrial fibrillation or flutter. Although esmolol is considered to be cardioselective, at higher doses it inhibits β₂-receptors in bronchial and vascular smooth muscle.

The short duration of action of esmolol is due to rapid redistribution (the distribution half-life is 2 min) and hydrolysis by red blood cell esterase (the elimination half-life is 9 min). Side effects can be reversed within minutes by discontinuing its infusion. As with all β₁-antagonists, esmolol should be avoided in patients with sinus bradycardia, heart block greater than first degree, cardiogenic shock, or overt heart failure.

Dosing & Packaging

Esmolol is administered as a bolus (0.2–0.5 mg/kg) for short-term therapy, such as attenuating the cardiovascular response to laryngoscopy and intubation. Long-term treatment is typically initiated with a loading dose of 0.5 mg/kg administered over 1 min, followed by a continuous infusion of 50 μg/kg/min to maintain the therapeutic effect. If this fails to produce a sufficient response within 5 min, the loading dose may be repeated and the infusion increased by increments of 50 μg/kg/min every 5 min to a maximum of 200 μg/kg/min.

Esmolol is supplied as multidose vials for bolus administration containing 10 mL of drug (10 mg/mL). Ampules for continuous infusion (2.5 g in 10 mL) are also available but must be diluted prior to administration to a concentration of 10 mg/mL.

PROPRANOLOL

Clinical Considerations

Propranolol nonselectively blocks β₁- and β₂-receptors. Arterial blood pressure is lowered by several mecha-

nisms, including decreased myocardial contractility, lowered heart rate, and diminished renin release. Cardiac output and myocardial oxygen demand are reduced. Propranolol is particularly useful during myocardial ischemia related to increased blood pressure and heart rate. Impedance of ventricular ejection is beneficial in patients with obstructive cardiomyopathy and aortic aneurysm. Propranolol slows atrioventricular conduction and stabilizes myocardial membranes, although the latter effect may not be significant at clinical doses. Propranolol is particularly effective in slowing the ventricular response to supraventricular tachycardia, and it occasionally controls recurrent ventricular tachycardia or fibrillation caused by myocardial ischemia. Propranolol blocks the β-adrenergic effects of thyrotoxicosis and pheochromocytoma.

Side effects of propranolol include bronchospasm (β₂-antagonism), congestive heart failure, bradycardia, and atrioventricular heart block (β₁-antagonism). Propranolol may worsen the myocardial depression of volatile anesthetics (eg, halothane) or unmask the negative inotropic characteristics of indirect cardiac stimulants (eg, isoflurane). Concomitant administration of propranolol and verapamil (a calcium channel blocker) can synergistically depress heart rate, contractility, and atrioventricular node conduction.

Discontinuation of β-blocker therapy for 24–48 h may trigger a withdrawal syndrome characterized by hypertension (rebound hypertension), tachycardia, and angina pectoris. This effect appears to be caused by an increase in the number of β-adrenergic receptors (up-regulation). Propranolol is extensively protein bound and is cleared by hepatic metabolism. Its elimination half-life of 100 min is quite long compared with that of esmolol.

Dosing & Packaging

Individual dosage requirements of propranolol depend on baseline sympathetic tone. Generally, propranolol is titrated to the desired effect, beginning with 0.5 mg and progressing by 0.5-mg increments every 3–5 min. Total doses rarely exceed 0.15 mg/kg. Propranolol is supplied in 1-mL ampules containing 1 mg.

CASE DISCUSSION: PHEOCHROMOCYTOMA

A 45-year-old man with a history of paroxysmal attacks of headache, hypertension, sweating, and palpitations is scheduled for resection of an abdominal pheochromocytoma.

What is a pheochromocytoma?

A pheochromocytoma is a vascular tumor of chromaffin tissue (most commonly the adrenal medulla) that produces and secretes norepinephrine and epinephrine. The diagnosis and management of pheochromocytoma are based on the effects of abnormally high circulating levels of these endogenous adrenergic agonists.

How is the diagnosis of pheochromocytoma made in the laboratory?

Urinary excretion of vanillylmandelic acid (an end product of catecholamine metabolism), norepinephrine, and epinephrine is often markedly increased. Elevated levels of urinary catecholamines and metanephrines (Figure 12–3) provide a highly accurate diagnosis. Fractionated plasma-free metanephrine levels may be superior to urinary studies in making the diagnosis. The location of the tumor can be determined by magnetic resonance imaging or computed tomographic scan with or without contrast.

What pathophysiology is associated with chronic elevations of norepinephrine and epinephrine?

α_1-Stimulation increases peripheral vascular resistance and arterial blood pressure. Hypertension can lead to intravascular volume depletion (increasing hematocrit), renal failure, and cerebral hemorrhage. Elevated peripheral vascular resistance also increases myocardial work, which predisposes patients to myocardial ischemia, ventricular hypertrophy, and congestive heart failure. Prolonged exposure to epinephrine and norepinephrine may lead to a catecholamine-induced cardiomyopathy. Hyperglycemia results from decreased insulin secretion in the face of increased glycogenolysis and gluconeogenesis. β_1-Stimulation increases automaticity and ventricular ectopy.

Which adrenergic antagonists might be helpful in controlling the effects of norepinephrine and epinephrine hypersecretion?

Phenoxybenzamine, an α_1-antagonist (see Table 12–3), effectively reverses the vasoconstriction, resulting in a drop in arterial blood pressure and an increase in intravascular volume (hematocrit drops). Glucose intolerance is often corrected. Phenoxybenzamine can be administered orally and is longer-acting than phentolamine, another α_1-antagonist. For these reasons, phenoxybenzamine is often administered preoperatively to control symptoms.

Intravenous phentolamine is often used intraoperatively to control hypertensive episodes. Compared with some other hypotensive agents (see Chapter 13), however, phentolamine has a slow onset and long duration of action; furthermore, tachyphylaxis often develops.

β_1-Blockade with an agent such as labetalol is recommended for patients with tachycardia or ventricular arrhythmias.

Why should α_1-receptors be blocked with phenoxybenzamine before administration of a β-antagonist?

If β-receptors are blocked first, norepinephrine and epinephrine will produce unopposed α-stimulation. β_2-Mediated vasodilation will not be able to offset α_1-vasoconstriction, and peripheral vascular resistance would increase. This may explain the paradoxical hypertension that has been reported in a few patients with pheochromocytoma treated only with labetalol. Finally, the myocardium might not be able to handle its already elevated workload without the inotropic effects of β_1-stimulation.

Which anesthetic agents should be specifically avoided?

Succinylcholine-induced fasciculations of the abdominal musculature will increase intraabdominal pressure, which might cause release of catecholamines from the tumor. Ketamine is a sympathomimetic and would exacerbate the effects of adrenergic agonists. Halothane sensitizes the myocardium to the arrhythmogenic effects of epinephrine. Vagolytic drugs (eg, anticholinergics and pancuronium) will worsen the imbalance of autonomic tone. Because histamine provokes catecholamine secretion by the tumor, drugs associated with histamine release (eg, tubocurarine, atracurium, morphine sulfate, and meperidine) are best avoided. Vecuronium, rocuronium, pipecuronium, and doxacurium are probably the neuromuscular blocking agents of choice. Although droperidol is an α-antagonist, it has been associated with hypertensive crises in some patients with pheochromocytoma.

Would an epidural or spinal technique effectively block sympathetic hyperactivity?

A major regional block—such as an epidural or spinal anesthetic—could block sensory (afferent) nerves and sympathetic (efferent) discharge in the area of the surgical field. The catecholamines released from a pheochromocytoma during surgical manipulation would still be able to bind and activate adrenergic receptors throughout the body, however. Therefore, these regional techniques cannot block the sympathetic hyperactivity associated with pheochromocytoma, which is further discussed in Chapter 36.

SUGGESTED READING

Bonet S, Agusti A, Arnau JM, et al: β-Adrenergic blocking agents in heart failure: Benefits of vasodilating and nonvasodilating agents according to patients' characteristics: A meta-analysis of clinical trials. Arch Intern Med 2000;160:621.

Ebert TJ: Is gaining control of the autonomic nervous system important to our specialty? Anesthesiology 1999;90:651.

Insel PA: Adrenergic receptors—evolving concepts and clinical implications. N Engl J Med 1996;334:580. Excellent, up-to-date review of advances in receptor physiology and pathophysiology.

Evers AS, Maze M: *Anesthetic Pharmacology. Physiologic Principles and Clinical Practice. A Companion to Miller's Anesthesia.* Churchill Livingstone, 2004. Chapters on autonomic function and sympathomimetic and lytic drugs are excellent reviews of basic science that contain much useful information on clinical pharmacology of this important class of drugs.

Moss J, Renz C: The autonomic nervous system. Chapter 14 in: *Anesthesia,* 5th ed. Miller RD (editor). Churchill Livingstone, 2000. Excellent discussion of the autonomic nervous system and drugs with adrenergic activity.

Piper SN, Boldt J, Schmidt CC, et al: Influence of dopexamine on hemodynamics, intramucosal pH, and regulators of the macrocirculation and microcirculation in patients undergoing abdominal aortic surgery. J Cardiothorac Vasc Anesth 2000;14:281.

Stoelting RK: *Pharmacology and Physiology in Anesthetic Practice,* 3rd ed. Lippincott-Raven, 1999. Chapter 12 contains an excellent review and discussion of sympathomimetic drugs. Chapter 14 contains an excellent summary of the α- and β-adrenergic receptor antagonists and blockers. Chapter 42 reviews the physiology of the autonomic nervous system.

Hypotensive Agents

KEY CONCEPTS

 Clinical trials have shown that inhaled nitric oxide is a selective pulmonary vasodilator that may be beneficial in the treatment of reversible pulmonary hypertension. By improving perfusion only in ventilated areas of the lung, inhaled nitric oxide may improve oxygenation in patients with acute respiratory distress syndrome or during one-lung ventilation.

 Acute cyanide toxicity is characterized by metabolic acidosis, cardiac arrhythmias, and increased venous oxygen content (as a result of the inability to utilize oxygen). Another early sign of cyanide toxicity is the acute resistance to the hypotensive effects of increasing doses of sodium nitroprusside (tachyphylaxis).

 By dilating pulmonary vessels, sodium nitroprusside may prevent the normal vasoconstrictive response of the pulmonary vasculature to hypoxia (hypoxic pulmonary vasoconstriction).

 Preload reduction makes nitroglycerin an excellent drug for the relief of cardiogenic pulmonary edema.

 Hydralazine relaxes arteriolar smooth muscle, causing dilatation of precapillary resistance vessels.

 The body reacts to a hydralazine-induced fall in blood pressure by increasing heart rate, myocardial contractility, and cardiac output. These compensatory responses can be detrimental to patients with coronary artery disease and are minimized by the concurrent administration of a β-adrenergic antagonist.

 Adenosine slows atrioventricular (AV) conduction (increases the P–R interval) and can interrupt reentrant dysrhythmias that involve the AV node.

 Fenoldopam mesylate (infusion rates studied in clinical trials range from 0.01–1.6 μg/kg/min) reduces systolic and diastolic blood pressure in patients with malignant hypertension to an extent comparable to nitroprusside.

A multitude of drugs are capable of lowering blood pressure, including volatile anesthetics (see Chapter 7), sympathetic antagonists and agonists (see Chapter 12), and calcium channel blockers and angiotensin-converting enzyme inhibitors (see Chapter 20). This chapter examines additional agents that may be useful to the anesthesiologist for intraoperative control of arterial blood pressure: nitrates, adenosine, and fenoldopam (Figure 13–1 and Table 13–1). Although all these drugs lower blood pressure by dilating peripheral vessels, they are not identical in their mechanisms of action, clinical uses, routes of metabolism, effects on organ systems, or drug interactions. Trimethaphan, the only ganglionic blocker, is no longer being manufactured and will not be discussed.

Figure 13–1. Structures of hypotensive agents.

SODIUM NITROPRUSSIDE

Mechanism of Action

Sodium nitroprusside relaxes both arteriolar and venous smooth muscle. Its primary mechanism of action is shared with other nitrates (eg, hydralazine and nitroglycerin). As these drugs are metabolized, they release **nitric oxide**, which activates guanylyl cyclase. This enzyme is responsible for the synthesis of cyclic guanosine 3',5'-monophosphate (cGMP), which controls the phosphorylation of several proteins, including some involved in control of free intracellular calcium and smooth muscle contraction.

Nitric oxide, a naturally occurring potent vasodilator released by endothelial cells (endothelium-derived relaxing factor), plays an important role in regulating vascular tone throughout the body. Its ultrashort half-life (< 5 s) provides sensitive endogenous control of regional blood flow. Clinical trials have shown that *inhaled* nitric oxide is a selective pulmonary vasodilator that may be beneficial in the treatment of reversible pulmonary hypertension. By improving perfusion only in ventilated areas of the lung, inhaled nitric oxide may improve oxygenation in patients with acute respiratory distress syndrome

(ARDS) or during one-lung ventilation. Nitric oxide may also have antiinflammatory effects that could promote lung healing.

Clinical Uses

Sodium nitroprusside is a potent and reliable antihypertensive. It is usually diluted to a concentration of $100~\mu g/mL$ and administered as a continuous intravenous infusion (0.5–10 μg/kg/min). Its extremely rapid onset of action (1–2 min) and fleeting duration of action allow precise titration of arterial blood pressure. A bolus of 1–2 μg/kg minimizes blood pressure elevation during laryngoscopy but can cause transient hypotension in some patients. The potency of this drug requires frequent blood pressure measurements—or, preferably, intraarterial monitoring—and the use of mechanical infusion pumps. Solutions of sodium nitroprusside must be protected from light because of photodegradation.

Metabolism

After parenteral injection, sodium nitroprusside enters red blood cells, where it receives an electron from the iron (Fe^{2+}) of oxyhemoglobin. This nonenzymatic elec-

Table 13–1. Comparative pharmacology of hypotensive agents.[1]

	Nitroprusside	Nitroglycerin	Hydralazine	Trimethaphan	Adenosine	Fenoldopam
Organ effects						
Heart rate	↑↑	↑	↑↑↑	↑	↑	↑↑
Preload	↓↓	↓↓↓	0	↓↓	0	?
Afterload	↓↓↓	↓↓	↓↓↓	↓↓	↓↓	↓↓
Cerebral blood flow, intracranial pressure	↑↑	↑↑	↑↑	0	↑↑	?
Kinetics						
Onset	1 min	1 min	5–10 min	3 min	< 1 min	< 15 min
Duration	5 min	5 min	2–4 h	10 min	1 min	1 h
Metabolism	Blood, kidney	Blood, liver	Liver	Blood?	Blood	Liver
Dose						
Bolus	50–100 µg	50–100 µg	5–20 mg	NA	6–12 mg	NA
Infusion (µg/kg/min)	0.5–10	0.5–10	0.25–1.5	10–100	60–120	0.01–1.6
Relative cost[2]	Low	Low	Low	Moderate	High	Very high

[1]0, no change; ↑, increase (slight, moderate, marked); ↓, decrease (slight, moderate, marked); ?, Incomplete data or variable results reported; NA, not applicable.
[2]Based on cost of 1-h infusion.

tron transfer results in an unstable nitroprusside radical and methemoglobin (Hgb Fe^{3+}). The former moiety spontaneously decomposes into five cyanide ions and the active nitroso (N═O) group.

The cyanide ions can be involved in one of three possible reactions: binding to methemoglobin to form **cyanmethemoglobin;** undergoing a reaction in the liver and kidney catalyzed by the enzyme rhodanase (thiosulfate + cyanide → thiocyanate); or binding to tissue cytochrome oxidase, which interferes with normal oxygen utilization (Figure 13–2).

The last of these reactions is responsible for the development of **acute cyanide toxicity,** characterized by metabolic acidosis, cardiac arrhythmias, and increased venous oxygen content (as a result of the inability to utilize oxygen). Another early sign of cyanide toxicity is the acute resistance to the hypotensive effects of increasing doses of sodium nitroprusside (tachyphylaxis). It should be noted that tachyphylaxis implies acute tolerance to the drug following multiple rapid injections, as opposed to tolerance, which is caused by more chronic exposure. Cyanide toxicity can usually be avoided if the cumulative dose of sodium nitroprusside is less than 0.5 mg/kg/h. Patients with cyanide toxicity should be mechanically ventilated with 100% oxygen to maximize oxygen availability. The pharmacological treatment of cyanide toxicity depends

on increasing the kinetics of the two reactions by administering sodium thiosulfate (150 mg/kg over 15 min) or 3% sodium nitrate (5 mg/kg over 5 min), which oxidizes hemoglobin to methemoglobin. Hydroxocobalamin, an experimental drug, combines with cyanide to form cyanocobalamin (vitamin B_{12}).

Thiocyanate is slowly cleared by the kidney. Accumulation of large amounts of thiocyanate (eg, in patients with renal failure) may result in a milder toxic reaction that includes thyroid dysfunction, muscle weakness, nausea, hypoxia, and an acute toxic psychosis. The risk of cyanide toxicity is not increased by renal

SNP + Oxyhemoglobin ⟶ (SNP)⁻ + Methemoglobin
(SNP)⁻ ⟶ 5CN⁻

CN⁻ + Methemoglobin ⟶ Cyanmethemoglobin

or

CN⁻ + Thiosulfate $\xrightarrow{\text{Rhodanase, vitamin } B_{12}}$ Thiocyanate

or

CN⁻ + Cytochrome oxidase ⟶ Cyanide toxicity

Figure 13–2. The metabolism of sodium nitroprusside.

failure, however. Methemoglobinemia from excessive doses of sodium nitroprusside or sodium nitrate can be treated with methylene blue (1–2 mg/kg of a 1% solution over 5 min), which reduces methemoglobin to hemoglobin.

Effects on Organ Systems

A. CARDIOVASCULAR

The combined dilation of venous and arteriolar vascular beds by sodium nitroprusside results in reductions of preload and afterload. Arterial blood pressure falls due to the decrease in peripheral vascular resistance. Although cardiac output is usually unchanged in normal patients, the reduction in afterload may increase cardiac output in patients with congestive heart failure, mitral regurgitation, or aortic regurgitation. In contrast to the pure afterload reduction produced by hydralazine, sodium nitroprusside primarily reduces preload, which decreases myocardial work and the likelihood of ischemia. In opposition to any favorable changes in myocardial oxygen requirements are reflex-mediated responses to the fall in arterial blood pressure. These include tachycardia (less pronounced than with hydralazine) and increased myocardial contractility. In addition, dilation of coronary arterioles by sodium nitroprusside may result in an **intracoronary** steal of blood flow away from ischemic areas that are already maximally dilated.

B. CEREBRAL

Sodium nitroprusside dilates cerebral vessels and abolishes cerebral autoregulation. Cerebral blood flow is maintained or increases unless arterial blood pressure is markedly reduced. The resulting increase in cerebral blood volume tends to increase intracranial pressure, particularly in patients with reduced intracranial compliance (eg, brain tumors). This intracranial hypertension can be minimized by slow administration of sodium nitroprusside and institution of hypocapnia.

C. RESPIRATORY

The pulmonary vasculature also dilates in response to sodium nitroprusside infusion. Reductions in pulmonary artery pressure may decrease the perfusion of some normally ventilated alveoli, increasing physiological dead space. By dilating pulmonary vessels, sodium nitroprusside may prevent the normal vasoconstrictive response of the pulmonary vasculature to hypoxia (hypoxic pulmonary vasoconstriction). Both these effects tend to mismatch pulmonary ventilation to perfusion and decrease arterial oxygenation.

D. RENAL

In response to decreased arterial blood pressure, renin and catecholamines are released during administration of nitroprusside. This hormonal response, which can lead to a pressure rebound after discontinuation of the drug, is blocked by propranolol or a high epidural block (T1 level). Renal function is fairly well maintained during sodium nitroprusside infusion despite moderate drops in arterial blood pressure and renal perfusion.

Drug Interactions

Sodium nitroprusside does not directly interact with neuromuscular blocking agents. Nonetheless, a decrease in muscle blood flow caused by arterial hypotension could indirectly delay the onset and prolong the duration of neuromuscular blockade. By inhibiting phosphodiesterase, aminophylline increases cGMP and potentiates the hypotensive effects of these agents.

NITROGLYCERIN

Mechanism of Action

Nitroglycerin relaxes vascular smooth muscle, with venous dilation predominating over arterial dilation. Its mechanism of action is presumably similar to sodium nitroprusside: metabolism to nitric oxide, which activates guanylyl cyclase, leading to increased cGMP, decreased intracellular calcium, and vascular smooth muscle relaxation.

Clinical Uses

Nitroglycerin relieves myocardial ischemia, hypertension, and ventricular failure. Like sodium nitroprusside, nitroglycerin is commonly diluted to a concentration of 100 μg/mL and administered as a continuous intravenous infusion (0.5–10 μg/kg/min). Glass containers and special intravenous tubing are recommended because of the adsorption of nitroglycerin to polyvinylchloride. Nitroglycerin can also be administered by a sublingual (peak effect in 4 min) or transdermal (sustained release for 24 h) route. Some patients appear to require higher than expected doses of nitroglycerin to achieve a given drop in blood pressure, particularly after chronic administration (tolerance). Tolerance may be due to depletion of reactants necessary for nitric oxide formation, compensatory secretion of vasoconstrictive substances, or volume expansion. Dosing regimens that provide for intermittent periods of low or no drug exposure may minimize the development of tolerance.

Metabolism

Nitroglycerin undergoes rapid reductive hydrolysis in the liver and blood by glutathione-organic nitrate reductase. One metabolic product is nitrite, which can convert hemoglobin to methemoglobin. Significant methemoglobinemia is rare and can be treated with intravenous methylene blue (1–2 mg/kg over 5 min).

Effects on Organ Systems

A. CARDIOVASCULAR

Nitroglycerin reduces myocardial oxygen demand and increases myocardial oxygen supply by several mechanisms:

- The pooling of blood in the large-capacitance vessels reduces venous return and preload. The accompanying decrease in ventricular end-diastolic pressure reduces myocardial oxygen demand and increases endocardial perfusion.
- Any afterload reduction from arteriolar dilation will decrease both end-systolic pressure and oxygen demand. Of course, a fall in diastolic pressure may lower coronary perfusion pressure and actually decrease myocardial oxygen supply.
- Nitroglycerin redistributes coronary blood flow to ischemic areas of the subendocardium.
- Coronary artery spasm may be relieved.
- Nitroglycerin decreases platelet aggregation and may improve the patency of coronary vessels.

The beneficial effect of nitroglycerin in patients with coronary artery disease contrasts with the coronary steal phenomenon seen with sodium nitroprusside. Preload reduction makes nitroglycerin an excellent drug for the relief of cardiogenic pulmonary edema. Heart rate is unchanged or minimally increased. Rebound hypertension is less likely after discontinuation of nitroglycerin than following discontinuation of sodium nitroprusside. The prophylactic administration of low-dose nitroglycerin (0.5–2.0 µg/kg/min) during anesthesia of patients at high risk for perioperative myocardial ischemia remains controversial.

B. CEREBRAL

The effects of nitroglycerin on cerebral blood flow and intracranial pressure are similar to those of sodium nitroprusside. Headache from dilation of cerebral vessels is a common side effect of nitroglycerin.

C. RESPIRATORY

In addition to the dilating effects on the pulmonary vasculature (previously described for sodium nitroprusside), nitroglycerin relaxes bronchial smooth muscle.

D. OTHER

Nitroglycerin (50–100 µg boluses) has been demonstrated to be an effective but transient uterine relaxant that can be beneficial during certain obstetrical procedures if the placenta is still present in the uterus (eg, retained placenta, uterine inversion, uterine tetany, breech extraction, and external version of the second

twin). Nitroglycerin therapy has been shown to diminish platelet aggregation, an effect enhanced by administration of *N*-acetylcysteine.

Drug Interactions

Nitroglycerin has been reported to potentiate the neuromuscular blockade produced by pancuronium.

HYDRALAZINE

Mechanism of Action

 Hydralazine relaxes arteriolar smooth muscle, causing dilation of precapillary resistance vessels. The mechanism of this effect may be interference with calcium utilization or activation of guanylyl cyclase.

Clinical Uses

Intraoperative hypertension is usually controlled with an intravenous dose of 5–20 mg of hydralazine. The onset of action is within 15 min, and the antihypertensive effect usually lasts 2–4 h. Continuous infusions (0.25–1.5 µg/kg/min) are less frequently used due to their rather slow onset and long duration of action. Hydralazine is frequently used to control pregnancy-induced hypertension (see Chapter 43).

Metabolism

Hydralazine undergoes acetylation and hydroxylation in the liver.

Effects on Organ Systems

A. CARDIOVASCULAR

 The lowering of peripheral vascular resistance causes a drop in arterial blood pressure. The body reacts to a hydralazine-induced fall in blood pressure by increasing heart rate, myocardial contractility, and cardiac output. These compensatory responses can be detrimental to patients with coronary artery disease and are minimized by the concurrent administration of a β-adrenergic antagonist. Conversely, the decline in afterload often proves beneficial to patients in congestive heart failure.

B. CEREBRAL

Hydralazine is a potent cerebral vasodilator and inhibitor of cerebral blood flow autoregulation. Unless blood pressure is markedly reduced, cerebral blood flow and intracranial pressure will rise.

C. RENAL

Because renal blood flow is usually maintained or increased by hydralazine, it is often selected for patients with renal disease. Renin secretion by juxtaglomerular cells is stimulated.

ADENOSINE

Mechanism of Action

Adenosine, a purine endogenous to all cells of the body, acts on specific adenosine receptors located in several vascular beds and on the atrioventricular (AV) node. Its mechanism of action may involve activation of adenylate cyclase and depression of action potentials. Specifically, adenosine is thought to open potassium channels, hyperpolarizing nodal tissue and making it less likely to fire. This leads to an AV block and a slowing of the sinus rate in patients with supraventricular tachycardia. Adenosine has little effect on atrial or ventricular muscle tissue.

Clinical Uses

Adenosine is a potent vasodilator that can be used to reduce arterial blood pressure during anesthesia. It selectively affects arteriolar resistance vessels (afterload), with little effect on venous capacitance (preload). Because of a very short half-life (< 10 s), a continuous infusion (60–120 µg/kg/min) is required for controlled hypotension.

Currently, the only indication approved by the Food and Drug Administration for adenosine is conversion to sinus rhythm of paroxysmal supraventricular tachycardia, including that associated with Wolff–Parkinson–White syndrome, by an intravenous bolus injection of 6 mg over 1–2 s (6 mg/2 mL). If this proves ineffective, a 12-mg bolus should be administered and may be repeated once. Its ultrashort duration of action prevents cumulative effects after repeat doses. **Intravenous bolus of adenosine for paroxysmal supraventricular tachycardia can induce the onset of atrial fibrillation and thus should be administered only in an appropriate setting (eg, cardioversion capability).** Wide complex tachycardias arising in the ventricle, as opposed to the AV node, will not be affected by adenosine. Similarly, atrial arrhythmias (eg, atrial fibrillation, atrial flutter, multifocal atrial tachycardia) will demonstrate only a transient slowing of ventricular rate. Intrathecal adenosine (0.5–1.0 mg) has undergone successful preliminary study for the treatment of chronic neuropathic pain.

Metabolism

Erythrocytes and vascular endothelial cells rapidly take up adenosine from the circulation and metabolize it to inosine and adenosine monophosphate.

Effects on Organ Systems

A. CARDIOVASCULAR

Adenosine decreases arterial blood pressure by lowering systemic vascular resistance. Cardiac index, heart rate, and stroke volume increase. Myocardial blood flow increases as a result of coronary vasodilation without an increase in oxygen consumption or work. Unfavorable changes in distribution of regional coronary blood flow (intracoronary steal) have led to myocardial ischemia in patients with coronary artery disease, however—which may greatly limit its usefulness during anesthesia.

Adenosine slows AV conduction (increases the P–R interval) and can interrupt reentrant arrhythmias that involve the AV node. **Large doses of adenosine depress sinus node and ventricular automaticity, leading to brief periods of sinus pause that resolve spontaneously.** Although it is best avoided in patients with second- or third-degree heart block or sick sinus syndrome, adverse reactions are rare and of brief duration. Hypotension has not been reported to be a significant side effect of bolus administration of the dose recommended for treatment of paroxysmal supraventricular tachycardia.

B. PULMONARY

Adenosine decreases pulmonary vascular resistance, increases intrapulmonary shunt, and can lead to a drop in arterial oxygen saturation as a result of the inhibition of pulmonary hypoxic vasoconstriction. Adenosine may rarely cause bronchospasm in predisposed individuals.

C. RENAL

Surprisingly, adenosine causes renal vasoconstriction with a resulting drop in renal blood flow, glomerular filtration rate, filtration fraction, and urinary output.

Drug Interactions

Methylxanthines (eg, aminophylline) competitively antagonize adenosine, whereas blockers of nucleoside transport (eg, dipyridamole) potentiate its actions.

FENOLDOPAM

Mechanism of Action

Fenoldopam mesylate causes rapid vasodilation by selectively activating D_1-dopamine receptors. It has also demonstrated moderate affinity for α_2-adrenoceptors. The R-isomer is responsible for the racemic mixture's biological activity due to its much greater receptor affinity, compared with the S-isomer.

Clinical Uses

 Fenoldopam mesylate (infusion rates studied in clinical trials range from 0.01–1.6 µg/kg/min) reduces systolic and diastolic blood pressure in patients with malignant hypertension to an extent comparable to nitroprusside. Side effects include headache, flushing, nausea, tachycardia, hypokalemia, and hypotension. The onset of the hypotensive effect occurs within 15 min and discontinuation of an infusion quickly reverses this effect without rebound hypertension. There may be some degree of tolerance that develops after 48 h of infusion. As with most new drugs, fenoldopam's clinical profile has yet to be fully determined. However, its eventual place in anesthetic practice may be greatly influenced by its very high cost.

Metabolism

Fenoldopam undergoes conjugation without participation of the cytochrome P-450 enzymes, and its metabolites are inactive. Clearance of fenoldopam remains unaltered despite the presence of renal or hepatic failure, and no dosage adjustments are necessary for these patients.

Effects on Organ Systems

A. Cardiovascular

Fenoldopam decreases systolic and diastolic blood pressure. Heart rate typically increases. Low initial doses (0.03–0.1 µg/kg/min) titrated slowly have been associated with less reflex tachycardia than higher doses (> 0.3 µg/kg/min). Tachycardia decreases over time but remains substantial at higher doses.

B. Ophthalmic

Fenoldopam can lead to rises in intraocular pressure and should be administered with caution or avoided in patients with a history of glaucoma or intraocular hypertension.

C. Renal

As would be expected from a D_1-dopamine receptor agonist, fenoldopam markedly increases renal blood flow. Despite a drop in arterial blood pressure, glomerular filtration rate is well maintained. Fenoldopam increases urinary flow rate, urinary sodium extraction, and creatinine clearance compared with sodium nitroprusside.

Warnings

The preservative sodium metabisulfite may cause allergic reactions and even anaphylactic reactions. Patients with asthma and those with a history of sulfite sensitivity appear to be at higher risk.

Drug Interactions

To date, there have been no formal interaction studies; however, fenoldopam has been safely administered with digitalis and sublingual nitroglycerin.

CASE DISCUSSION: CONTROLLED HYPOTENSION

A 59-year-old man is scheduled for total hip arthroplasty under general anesthesia. The surgeon requests a controlled hypotensive technique.

What is controlled hypotension, and what are its advantages?

Controlled hypotension is the elective lowering of arterial blood pressure. The primary advantages of this technique are minimization of surgical blood loss and better surgical visualization.

How is controlled hypotension achieved?

The primary methods of electively lowering blood pressure are proper positioning, positive-pressure ventilation, and the administration of hypotensive drugs. Positioning involves elevation of the surgical site so that the blood pressure at the wound is selectively reduced. The increase in intrathoracic pressure that accompanies positive-pressure ventilation lowers venous return, cardiac output, and mean arterial pressure. Numerous pharmacological agents effectively lower blood pressure: volatile anesthetics, sympathetic antagonists, calcium channel blockers, angiotensin-converting enzyme inhibitors, and the peripheral vasodilators discussed in this chapter. Due to their rapid onset and short duration of action, sodium nitroprusside and nitroglycerin have the advantage of precise control. An additional method of producing hypotension is creation of a high sympathetic block with an epidural or spinal anesthetic.

What surgical procedures might benefit most from a controlled hypotensive technique?

Controlled hypotension has been successfully used during cerebral aneurysm repair, brain tu-

mor resection, total hip arthroplasty, radical neck dissection, radical cystectomy, and other operations associated with significant blood loss. Controlled hypotension may allow safer surgery of patients whose religious beliefs prohibit blood transfusions (eg, Jehovah's Witnesses; see Case Discussion, Chapter 40). Decreasing extravasation of blood may improve the result of some plastic surgery procedures.

What are some relative contraindications to controlled hypotension?

Some patients have predisposing illnesses that decrease the margin of safety for adequate organ perfusion: severe anemia, hypovolemia, atherosclerotic cardiovascular disease, renal or hepatic insufficiency, cerebrovascular disease, or uncontrolled glaucoma.

What are the possible complications of controlled hypotension?

As the above list of contraindications suggests, the risks of low arterial blood pressure include cerebral thrombosis, hemiplegia (due to decreased spinal cord perfusion), acute tubular necrosis, massive hepatic necrosis, myocardial infarction, cardiac arrest, and blindness (from retinal artery thrombosis or ischemic optic neuropathy). These complications are more likely in patients with co-existing anemia.

What is a safe level of hypotension?

This depends on the patient. Healthy young individuals tolerate mean arterial pressures as low as 50–60 mm Hg without complications. On the other hand, chronically hypertensive patients have altered autoregulation of cerebral blood flow and may tolerate a mean arterial pressure no more than 20–30% lower than baseline. Patients with a history of transient ischemic attacks may not tolerate any decline in cerebral perfusion.

What special monitoring is indicated during controlled hypotension?

Intraarterial blood pressure monitoring and electrocardiography with ST-segment analysis are strongly recommended. Central venous monitoring and measurement of urinary output by an indwelling catheter are indicated if extensive surgery is anticipated. Monitors of neurological function (eg, electroencephalography) have not gained widespread acceptance.

SUGGESTED READING

Lauretti GR, de Oliveira R, Reis MP: Transdermal nitroglycerine enhances spinal sufentanil postoperative analgesia following orthopedic surgery. Anesthesiology 1999;90:734. Nitroglycerin possesses analgesic properties.

Marshman LAG, Morice AH, Thompson JS: Increased efficacy of sodium nitroprusside in middle cerebral arteries following acute subarachnoid hemorrhage: Indications for its use after rupture. J Neurosurg Anesthesiol 1998;10:171.

Oates JA: Antihypertensive agents and the drug therapy of hypertension. Chapter 33 in: *Goodman and Gilman's The Pharmaceutical Basis of Therapeutics*, 10th ed. Gilman AG et al (editors). McGraw-Hill, 2001.

Parker JD, Parker JO: Nitrate therapy for stable angina pectoris. N Engl J Med 1998;338:520. A comprehensive review of organic nitrates including nitroglycerin and isosorbide dinitrate.

Tobias JD: Fenoldopam: Applications in anesthesiology, perioperative medicine, and critical care medicine. Am J Anesthesiol 2000;27:395.

Van Aken H, Miller ED: Deliberate hypotension. Chapter 41, in: *Anesthesia*, 5th ed. Miller RD (editor). Churchill Livingstone, 2000.

Williams-Russo P, Sharrock NE, Mattis S: Randomized trial of hypotensive epidural anesthesia in older adults. Anesthesiology 1999;91:926. Cognitive outcome following hip arthroplasty did not differ between a low blood pressure group (mean arterial pressure [MAP] 45–55 mm Hg) and higher blood pressure group (MAP 55–70 mm Hg).

Local Anesthetics

14

KEY CONCEPTS

 Most local anesthetics block voltage-gated sodium channels from inside the cell, preventing subsequent channel activation and interfering with the large transient sodium influx associated with membrane depolarization. Impulse conduction slows, the rate of rise and the magnitude of the action potential decrease, and the threshold for excitation is raised progressively until an action potential can no longer be generated and impulse propagation is abolished.

 Not all nerve fibers are equally affected by local anesthetics. Sensitivity to blockade is determined by axonal diameter, degree of myelination, and various other anatomic and physiological factors.

 Potency correlates with lipid solubility, that is, the ability of the local anesthetic molecule to penetrate membranes, a hydrophobic environment.

Onset of action depends on many factors, including lipid solubility and the relative concentration of the nonionized lipid-soluble form (B) and the ionized water-soluble form (BH⁺), expressed by the pK_a. Local anesthetics with a pK_a closest to physiological pH will have a higher concentration of nonionized base that can pass through the nerve cell membrane, and generally a more rapid onset.

Duration of action is generally correlated with lipid solubility. Highly lipid-soluble local anesthetics have a longer duration of action, presumably because they are less likely to be cleared by blood flow.

 Because local anesthetics are typically injected or applied very close to their intended site of action their pharmacokinetic profiles are generally more important determinants of elimination and toxicity than is their desired clinical effect.

 The rate of systemic absorption is proportionate to the vascularity of the site of injection: intravenous > tracheal > intercostal > caudal > paracervical > epidural > brachial plexus > sciatic > subcutaneous.

 Ester local anesthetics are predominantly metabolized by pseudocholinesterase. Amide local anesthetics are metabolized (N-dealkylation and hydroxylation) by microsomal P-450 enzymes in the liver.

 The central nervous system is the site of premonitory signs of overdose in awake patients. Early symptoms are circumoral numbness, tongue paresthesia, and dizziness. Sensory complaints may include tinnitus and blurred vision. Excitatory signs (eg, restlessness, agitation, nervousness, paranoia) often precede central nervous system depression (eg, slurred speech, drowsiness, unconsciousness). Muscle twitching heralds the onset of tonic–clonic seizures.

 Major cardiovascular toxicity usually requires about three times the concentration of blood that produces seizures. Cardiac arrhythmia or circulatory collapse is therefore the usual presenting sign of local anesthetic overdose during general anesthesia.

(continued on next page)

(continued from previous page)

 Unintentional intravascular injection of bupivacaine during regional anesthesia produces severe cardiotoxic reactions, including hypotension, atrioventricular heart block, idioventricular rhythms, and life-threatening arrhythmias such as ventricular tachycardia and fibrillation.

True hypersensitivity reactions to local anesthetic agents—as distinct from systemic toxicity caused by excessive plasma concentration—are quite uncommon. Esters are more likely to induce an allergic reaction because they are derivatives of p-aminobenzoic acid, a known allergen.

Local and regional anesthesia techniques depend on a group of drugs—local anesthetics—that produces transient loss of sensory, motor, and autonomic function when the drugs are injected or applied in proximity to neural tissue. This chapter presents the mechanism of action, structure–activity relationships, and clinical pharmacology of local anesthetic drugs. Commonly used nerve blocks are presented in Section III (see Chapters 16 and 17).

THEORIES OF LOCAL ANESTHETIC ACTION

Like other cells, neurons maintain a resting membrane potential by active transport and passive diffusion of ions. An electrogenic sodium–potassium pump (Na$^+$-K$^+$-ATPase) couples the transport of three sodium ions out of the cell for every two potassium ions it moves into the cell. This creates a concentration gradient that favors the extracellular diffusion of potassium and the intracellular diffusion of sodium. The cell membrane is normally much more permeable to potassium than to sodium, however, so a relative excess of negatively charged ions (anions) accumulates intracellularly. This accounts for the negative resting potential difference (–70 mV polarization).

Unlike most other types of tissue, neurons have membrane-bound, voltage-gated sodium and potassium channels that produce membrane depolarization following chemical, mechanical, or electrical stimuli. If the depolarization exceeds a threshold level (about –55 mV), voltage-gated sodium channels are activated, allowing a sudden and spontaneous influx of sodium ions and generating an **action potential** (Figure 14–1) that is normally conducted as is an impulse along the nerve axon. The increase in sodium permeability causes a relative excess of positively charged ions (cations) intracellularly, resulting in a reversal of membrane potential to +35 mV. However, a subsequent rapid drop in sodium permeability (caused by inactivation of voltage-gated sodium channels) along with a transient increase in potassium conductance through voltage-gated potassium channels (allowing more potassium to

exit the cell) return the membrane to its resting potential. Baseline concentration gradients are eventually reestablished by the sodium–potassium pump.

Sodium channels are membrane-bound proteins that are composed of one large α-subunit, through which sodium ions pass, and one or two smaller β-subunits. Voltage-gated sodium channels exist in three states—resting, activated (open), and inactivated (Figure 14–2).

 Most local anesthetics bind the α-subunit and block voltage-gated sodium channels from inside the cell, preventing subsequent channel activation and interfering with the large transient sodium influx associated with membrane depolarization. This does not alter the resting membrane potential, but with increasing concentrations of local anesthetic, impulse conduction slows, the rate of rise and the magnitude of the action potential decrease, and the threshold for excitation is raised progressively until an action potential can no longer be generated and impulse propagation is abol-

Figure 14–1. The complete action potential of a large mammalian myelinated fiber, drawn without time or voltage distortion to show the proportions of the components. (Redrawn, with permission, from Ganong WS: *Review of Medical Physiology,* 21st ed. McGraw-Hill, 2003.)

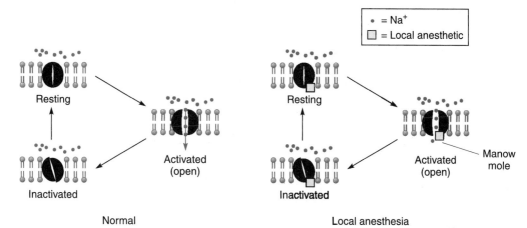

Figure 14–2. Voltage-gated sodium channels exist in three states—resting, activated (open), and inactivated. Note that the local anesthetic binds and blocks the voltage-gated sodium channel from inside the cell, interfering with the large transient sodium influx associated with membrane depolarization.

ished. Local anesthetics have a much greater affinity for the channel in the activated and inactivated state than in the resting state. As a result, local anesthetic action is both voltage and time dependent; their effect is greatest when nerve fibers are firing rapidly.

Local anesthetics may also block calcium and potassium channels and N-methyl-D-aspartate (NMDA) receptors to varying degrees. Differences in these additional actions may be responsible for clinically observed differences between agents. Conversely, other classes of drugs, most notably tricyclic antidepressants (amitriptyline), meperidine, volatile anesthetics, and ketamine also have sodium channel-blocking properties. Tetrodotoxin is a poison that specifically binds sodium channels but from outside the cell membrane (site 1). Systemic toxicity has prevented its use, but animal studies have suggested that when used in low doses with vasoconstrictors and other local anesthetics it can significantly prolong the duration of the anesthesia.

Not all nerve fibers are equally affected by local anesthetics. Sensitivity to blockade is determined by axonal diameter, degree of myelination, and various other anatomic and physiological factors. Table 14–1 lists the most commonly used classification for nerve fibers. Small diameter and lack of myelin enhance sensitivity to local anesthetics. Thus, in spinal nerves sensitivity to local anesthetics is autonomic > sensory > motor.

STRUCTURE–ACTIVITY RELATIONSHIPS

Local anesthetics consist of a lipophilic group—usually a benzene ring—separated from a hydrophilic group—usually a tertiary amine—by an intermediate chain that includes an ester or amide linkage. Local anesthetics are weak bases that usually carry a positive charge at the tertiary amine group at physiological pH. The nature of the intermediate chain is the basis of the classification of local anesthetics as either esters or amides (Table 14–2). Physicochemical properties of local anesthetics depend on the substitutions in the aromatic ring, the type of linkage in the intermediate chain, and the alkyl groups attached to the amine nitrogen.

Potency correlates with lipid solubility, that is, the ability of the local anesthetic molecule to penetrate membranes, a hydrophobic environment. In general, potency and lipid solubility increase with an increase in the total number of carbon atoms in the molecule (molecular size). More specifically, potency is increased by adding a halide to the aromatic ring (2-chloroprocaine as opposed to procaine), an ester linkage (procaine versus procainamide), and large alkyl groups on the tertiary amide nitrogen. There are multiple measurements of local anesthetic potency that are analogous to the minimum alveolar concentration (MAC) of inhalation anesthetics, but none is commonly used clinically. C_m is the minimum concentration of local anesthetic that will block nerve impulse conduction. This measure of relative potency is affected by several factors, including fiber size, type, and myelination; pH (acidic pH antagonizes block); frequency of nerve stimulation; and electrolyte concentrations (hypokalemia and hypercalcemia antagonize blockade).

Onset of action depends on many factors, including lipid solubility and the relative concentration of the nonionized lipid-soluble form (B) and the ionized water-soluble form (BH⁺), expressed by the pK_a. This measurement is the pH at

Table 14–1. Nerve fiber classification.[1]

Fiber Type	Sensory Classification	Modality Served	Diameter (mm)	Conduction (m/s)	Local Anesthetic Sensitivity	Myelination
Aα		Motor	12–20	70–120	+	Yes
Aα	Type Ia	Proprioception	12–20	70–120	++	Yes
Aα	Type Ib	Proprioception	12–30	70–120	++	Yes
Aβ	Type II	Touch pressure Proprioception	5–12	30–70	++	Yes
Aγ		Motor (muscle spindle)	3–6	15–30	++	Yes
Aδ	Type III	Pain Cold temperature Touch	2–5	12–30	+++	Yes
B		Preganglionic autonomic fibers	< 3	3–14	++++	Some
C Dorsal root	Type IV	Pain Warm and cold temperature Touch	0.4–1.2	0.5–2	++++	No
C Sympathetic		Postganglionic sympathetic fibers	0.3–1.3	0.7–2.3	++++	No

[1]Peripheral nerve fibers and their respective neurons are classified from A to C according to axonal diameter, covering (myelinated or unmyelinated), and conduction velocity. Sensory fibers also are categorized as I–IV. Type C (sensory type IV) are unmyelinated fibers, whereas type Aδ fibers are lightly myelinated.

which the amount of ionized and nonionized drug is equal. Less lipid-soluble agents generally have a faster onset.

Local anesthetics with a pK_a closest to physiological pH will have a higher concentration of nonionized base that can pass through the nerve cell membrane, and generally a more rapid onset. However, the charged cation more avidly binds the sodium channel inside the cell; it is the lipid-soluble form that more readily diffuses across the neural sheath (epineurium) and passes through the nerve membrane. Once inside the cell, the nonionized base reaches equilibrium with its ionized form. For instance, the pK_a of lidocaine is 7.8. Thus, at physiological pH (7.40) more than half the lidocaine will exist as the charged cation form (BH+). The onset of action of local anesthetics in *isolated* nerve fiber preparations directly correlates with pK_a. However, *clinical* onset of action is not necessarily identical for local anesthetics with the same pK_a. Other factors, such as ease of diffusion through connective tissue, can affect the onset of action *in vivo*. A notable exception is the relatively rapid onset of chloroprocaine, which has a high pK_a. Moreover, not all local anesthetics exist in a charged form (eg, benzocaine); these anesthetics probably act by alternate mechanisms (eg, expanding the lipid membrane).

The importance of the ionized and nonionized forms has many clinical implications. Local anesthetic solutions are prepared commercially as water-soluble hydrochloride salt (pH 6–7). Because epinephrine is unstable in alkaline environments, commercially available, epinephrine-containing, local anesthetic solutions are made even more acidic (pH 4–5). As a direct consequence, these preparations have a lower concentration of free base and a slower onset than when the epinephrine is added by the clinician at the time of use. Similarly, the extracellular base-to-cation ratio is decreased and onset is delayed when local anesthetics are injected into acidic (eg, infected) tissues. Tachyphylaxis—the decreased efficacy of repeated doses—may be at least partly explained by the eventual consumption of the local extracellular buffering capacity by repeat injections of the acidic local anesthetic solution. Conversely, if carbonated solutions of local anesthetic rather than

Table 14–2. Physicochemical properties of local anesthetics.

Generic (Proprietary)	Ring	Structure Chain	Amine	Potency and Lipid Solubility	pK_a	Duration and Protein Binding
Amides						
Bupivacaine (Marcaine) and levobupivacaine	CH_3 / CH_3 ring	NHCO	C_4H_9–N (piperidine)	++++	8.1	++++
Etidocaine (Duranest)	CH_3 / CH_3 ring	NHCOCH (C_2H_5)	N (C_2H_5, C_3H_7)	++++	7.7	++++
Lidocaine (Xylocaine)	CH_3 / CH_3 ring	$NHCOCH_2$	N (C_2H_5, C_2H_5)	++	7.8	++
Mepivacaine (Carbocaine)	CH_3 / CH_3 ring	NHCO	CH_3–N (piperidine)	++	7.6	++
Prilocaine (Citanest)	CH_3 ring	NHCOCH (CH_3)	N (H, C_3H_7)	++	7.8	++
Ropivacaine	CH_3 / CH_3 ring	NHCO	C_3H_7–N (piperidine)	++++	8.1	++++
Esters						
Chloroprocaine (Nesacaine)[1]	Cl / H_2N ring	$COOCH_2CH_2$	N (C_2H_5, C_2H_5)	+	9.0	+

(continued)

Table 14–2. Physicochemical properties of local anesthetics. (continued)

Generic (Proprietary)	Ring	Structure Chain	Amine	Potency and Lipid Solubility	pK_a	Duration and Protein Binding
Cocaine				++	8.7	++
Procaine				+	8.9	+
Tetracaine (Pontocaine)				++++	8.2	+++

[1]Chloroprocaine is metabolized too rapidly to measure lipid solubility or protein binding. It has a rapid onset of action despite a high pK_a.

the hydrochloride salts are used, the onset of action may be shortened. Although it is controversial, some researchers have reported that alkalinization of local anesthetic solutions (particularly commercially prepared, epinephrine-containing ones) by the addition of sodium bicarbonate (eg, 1 mL 8.4% sodium bicarbonate per 10 mL 1% lidocaine) speeds onset, improves the quality of the block, and prolongs blockade by increasing the amount of free base available. Interestingly, alkalinization also decreases pain during subcutaneous infiltration.

Duration of action is generally correlated with lipid solubility. Highly lipid-soluble local anesthetics have a longer duration of action, presumably because they are less likely to be cleared by blood flow. Local anesthetics that are highly lipid soluble also exhibit a high degree of plasma protein binding, mostly to α_1-acid glycoprotein and to a lesser extent to albumin; as a direct consequence, their elimination is prolonged. Sustained-release systems using liposomal encapsulation or microspheres for delivery of local anesthetics can significantly prolong their duration of action.

Differential sensory blockade may be a desirable property in selecting a local anesthetic that allows anesthesia with preservation of motor function. Unfortu-nately, only bupivacaine and ropivacaine display *some* selectively for sensory nerves; the concentrations required for surgical anesthesia almost always result in some motor blockade.

CLINICAL PHARMACOLOGY

Pharmacokinetics

Because local anesthetics are typically injected or applied very close to their intended site of action their pharmacokinetic profiles are generally more important determinants of elimination and toxicity than is their desired clinical effect.

A. ABSORPTION

Most mucous membranes (eg, ocular conjunctiva, tracheal mucosa) provide a weak barrier to local anesthetic penetration, leading to a rapid onset of action. Intact skin, on the other hand, requires a high water concentration for its penetration and a high concentration of lipid-soluble local anesthetic base to ensure analgesia. EMLA cream (a eutectic [easily melted] mixture of local anesthetic) consists of a 1:1 mixture of 5% lidocaine and 5% prilocaine in an oil-in-water emulsion. Dermal analgesia sufficient for beginning an intravenous line requires a contact time of at least 1 h under an occlusive dressing. Depth of penetration (usually 3–5 mm), duration of action (usually 1–2 h), and amount of drug absorbed depend on application time, dermal blood flow, keratin thickness, and total dose administered. Typically, 1–2 g of cream is applied per 10-cm^2 area of skin, with a maximum application area of 2000 cm^2 in an adult (100 cm^2 in children weighing less than 10 kg). Split-thickness skin-graft harvesting, laser removal of portwine stains, lithotripsy, and circumcision have been successfully performed with EMLA cream. Side effects include skin blanching, erythema, and edema. EMLA cream should not be used on mucous membranes, broken skin, infants less than 1 month old, or patients with a predisposition to methemoglobinemia (see Metabolism, below).

Systemic absorption of injected local anesthetics depends on blood flow, which is determined by the following factors.

1. Site of injection—The rate of systemic absorption is proportionate to the vascularity of the site of injection: intravenous > tracheal > intercostal > caudal > paracervical > epidural > brachial plexus > sciatic > subcutaneous.

2. Presence of vasoconstrictors—The addition of epinephrine—or less commonly phenylephrine—causes vasoconstriction at the site of administration. The consequent decreased absorption increases neuronal uptake, enhances the quality of analgesia, prolongs the duration of action, and limits toxic side effects. The effects of vasoconstrictors are more pronounced with shorter-acting agents. For example, the addition of epinephrine to lidocaine usually extends the duration of anesthesia by at least 50%, but epinephrine has little or no significant effect when added to bupivacaine, whose long duration of action is due to a high degree of protein binding. Epinephrine can also augment and prolong analgesia through activation of α_2-adrenergic receptors.

3. Local anesthetic agent—Local anesthetics that are highly tissue bound are more slowly absorbed. The agents also vary in their intrinsic vasodilator properties.

B. DISTRIBUTION

Distribution depends on organ uptake, which is determined by the following factors.

1. Tissue perfusion—The highly perfused organs (brain, lung, liver, kidney, and heart) are responsible for the initial rapid uptake (α phase), which is followed by a slower redistribution (β phase) to moderately perfused tissues (muscle and gut). In particular, the lung extracts significant amounts of local anes-

thetic; consequently, the threshold for systemic toxicity involves much lower doses following arterial injections than venous injections.

2. Tissue/blood partition coefficient—Strong plasma protein binding tends to retain anesthetic in the blood, whereas high lipid solubility facilitates tissue uptake.

3. Tissue mass—Muscle provides the greatest reservoir for local anesthetic agents because of its large mass.

C. METABOLISM AND EXCRETION

The metabolism and excretion of local anesthetics differ depending on their structure.

 1. Esters—Ester local anesthetics are predominantly metabolized by pseudocholinesterase (plasma cholinesterase or butyrylcholinesterase). Ester hydrolysis is very rapid, and the water-soluble metabolites are excreted in the urine. Procaine and benzocaine are metabolized to p-aminobenzoic acid (PABA), which has been associated with allergic reactions. Patients with genetically abnormal pseudocholinesterase are at increased risk for toxic side effects, as metabolism is slower. Cerebrospinal fluid lacks esterase enzymes, so the termination of action of intrathecally injected ester local anesthetics, eg, tetracaine, depends on their absorption into the bloodstream. In contrast to other ester anesthetics, cocaine is partially metabolized (N-methylation and ester hydrolysis) in the liver and partially excreted unchanged in the urine.

2. Amides—Amide local anesthetics are metabolized (N-dealkylation and hydroxylation) by microsomal P-450 enzymes in the liver. The rate of amide metabolism depends on the specific agent (prilocaine > lidocaine > mepivacaine > ropivacaine > bupivacaine), but overall is much slower than ester hydrolysis. Decreases in hepatic function (eg, cirrhosis of the liver) or liver blood flow (eg, congestive heart failure, vasopressors, or H_2-receptor blockers) will reduce the metabolic rate and predispose patients to systemic toxicity. Very little drug is excreted unchanged by the kidneys, although the metabolites are dependent on renal clearance.

Metabolites of prilocaine (o-toluidine derivatives), which accumulate after large doses of drug (> 10 mg/kg), convert hemoglobin to methemoglobin. Neonates of mothers who have received prilocaine epidural anesthesia during labor and patients with limited cardiopulmonary reserve are particularly susceptible to the alteration in oxygen transport. **Benzocaine, a common ingredient in local anesthetic sprays, can also cause methemoglobinemia.** Treatment of significant methemoglobinemia includes intravenous administration of methylene blue (1–2 mg/kg of a 1% solution over 5 min). Methylene blue reduces methemoglobin (Fe^{3+}) to hemoglobin (Fe^{2+}).

Table 14–3. Clinical use of local anesthetic agents.

Agent	Techniques	Concentrations Available	Maximum Dose (mg/kg)	Typical Duration of Neural Blockade[1] (h)
Esters				
Benzocaine	Topical	20%	NA[2]	0.5–1
Chloroprocaine	Epidural, infiltration, peripheral nerve block	1%, 2%, 3%	12	0.5–1
Cocaine	Topical	4%, 10%	3	0.5–1
Procaine	Spinal, infiltration, peripheral nerve block	1%, 2%, 10%	12	0.5–1
Tetracaine (amethocaine)	Spinal, topical	0.2%, 0.3%, 0.5%, 1%, 2%	3	1.5–6
Amides				
Bupivacaine	Epidural, spinal, infiltration, peripheral nerve block	0.25%, 0.5%, 0.75%	3	1.5–8
Lidocaine (lignocaine)	Epidural, spinal infiltration, peripheral nerve block, intravenous regional, topical	0.5%, 1%, 1.5%, 2%, 4%, 5%	4.5 7 (with epinephrine)	0.75–2
Mepivacaine	Epidural, infiltration, peripheral nerve block	1%, 1.5%, 2%, 3%	4.5 7 (with epinephrine)	1–2
Prilocaine	Peripheral nerve block (dental)	4%	8	0.5–1
Ropivacaine	Epidural, spinal, infiltration, peripheral nerve block	0.2%, 0.5%, 0.75%, 1%	3	1.5–8

[1]Wide variation depending on concentration, location, technique, and whether combined with a vasoconstrictor (epinephrine).
[2]NA, not available.

Effects on Organ Systems

Because blockade of voltage-gated sodium channels affects action potential propagation throughout the body, it is not surprising that local anesthetics have the ability for systemic toxicity. Although organ system effects are discussed for these drugs as a group, it must be recognized that individual drugs differ in their pharmacology.

Toxicity is often directly proportionate to potency. Maximum safe doses are listed in Table 14–3. Mixtures of local anesthetics should be considered to have roughly additive toxic effects: A solution containing 50% of the toxic dose of lidocaine and 50% of the toxic dose of bupivacaine will have roughly 100% of the toxic effects of either drug.

A. NEUROLOGICAL

The central nervous system is particularly vulnerable to local anesthetic toxicity and is the site of premonitory signs of overdose in awake patients. Early symptoms are circumoral numbness, tongue paresthesia, and dizziness. Sensory complaints may include tinnitus and blurred vision. Excitatory signs (eg, restlessness, agitation, nervousness, paranoia) often precede central nervous system depression (eg, slurred speech, drowsiness, unconsciousness). Muscle twitching heralds the onset of tonic–clonic seizures. Respiratory arrest often follows. The excitatory reactions are a result of selective blockade of inhibitory pathways. Potent, highly lipid-soluble, local anesthetics produce seizures at lower blood concentrations than less potent agents. By decreasing cerebral blood flow and drug exposure, benzodiazepines and hyperventilation raise the threshold of local anesthetic-induced seizures. Thiopental (1–2 mg/kg) quickly and reliably terminates seizure activity. Adequate ventilation and oxygenation must be maintained.

Intravenous lidocaine (1.5 mg/kg) decreases cerebral blood flow and attenuates the rise in intracranial pressure that accompanies intubation in patients with decreased intracranial compliance. Infusions of lidocaine and procaine have been used to supplement general anesthetic techniques, as they are capable of reducing the MAC of volatile anesthetics by up to 40%.

Cocaine stimulates the central nervous system and usually causes a sense of euphoria. An overdose is heralded by restlessness, emesis, tremors, convulsions, and respiratory failure.

Local anesthetics only temporarily block neuronal function. **Nonetheless, large volumes of chloroprocaine unintentionally injected into the subarachnoid instead of the epidural space have caused prolonged neurological deficit.** The cause of this neural toxicity may be direct neurotoxicity or the low pH of the combination of chloroprocaine and a preservative, sodium bisulfate, which has been replaced with an antioxidant, a derivative of disodium ethylenediaminetetraacetic acid (EDTA). Chloroprocaine has also been associated with severe back pain following epidural administration. Possible etiologies include large volumes (> 40 mL) of, or local infiltration with, chloroprocaine; low pH; and the EDTA preservative. Chloroprocaine has more recently become available in a preservative-free formulation, which should be used for epidural blockade.

Repeated doses of 5% lidocaine and 0.5% tetracaine may be responsible for neurotoxicity (cauda equina syndrome) following infusion through small-bore catheters used in continuous spinal anesthesia. This may be due to pooling of drug around the cauda equina, resulting in high concentrations and permanent neuronal damage. Animal data suggest that the extent of histological evidence of neurotoxicity following repeat intrathecal injection is lidocaine = tetracaine > bupivacaine > ropivacaine. Some animal data also suggest repeated administration of preservative-free chloroprocaine via an intrathecal catheter can produce neurotoxicity.

Transient neurological symptoms, which consist of dysesthesia, burning pain, and aching in the lower extremities and buttocks, have been reported following spinal anesthesia with a variety of local anesthetic agents. The etiology for these symptoms has been attributed to radicular irritation, and the symptoms typically resolve within 1 week. Risk factors include lidocaine (versus mepivacaine, bupivacaine, or tetracaine), lithotomy position, obesity, and outpatient status.

B. RESPIRATORY

Lidocaine depresses hypoxic drive (the ventilatory response to low PaO_2). Apnea can result from phrenic and intercostal nerve paralysis or depression of the medullary respiratory center following direct exposure to local anesthetic agents (eg, postretrobulbar apnea syndrome; see Chapter 38). Local anesthetics relax bronchial smooth muscle. Intravenous lidocaine (1.5 mg/kg) may be effective in blocking the reflex bronchoconstriction sometimes associated with intubation. Lidocaine administered as an aerosol can lead to bronchospasm in some patients with reactive airway disease.

C. CARDIOVASCULAR

In general, all local anesthetics depress myocardial automaticity (spontaneous phase IV depolarization) and reduce the duration of the refractory period. Myocardial contractility and conduction velocity are also depressed at higher concentrations. These effects result from direct cardiac muscle membrane changes (ie, cardiac sodium channel blockade) and inhibition of the autonomic nervous system. All local anesthetics except for cocaine produce smooth muscle relaxation, which causes some degree of arteriolar vasodilatation. The ensuing combination of bradycardia, heart block, and hypotension may culminate in cardiac arrest. Major cardiovascular toxicity usually requires about three times the concentration of blood that produces seizures. Cardiac arrhythmia or circulatory collapse is therefore the usual presenting sign of local anesthetic overdose during general anesthesia. Transient cardiovascular stimulation (tachycardia and hypertension) may occur earlier and reflect central nervous system excitation.

Lower concentrations of lidocaine provide effective treatment for some types of ventricular arrhythmias. Myocardial contractility and arterial blood pressure are generally unaffected by the usual intravenous doses. The hypertension associated with laryngoscopy and intubation is attenuated in some patients by intravenous administration of lidocaine (1.5 mg/kg) 1–3 min prior to instrumentation.

Unintentional intravascular injection of bupivacaine during regional anesthesia produces severe cardiotoxic reactions, including hypotension, atrioventricular heart block, idioventricular rhythms, and life-threatening arrhythmias such as ventricular tachycardia and fibrillation. Pregnancy, hypoxemia, and respiratory acidosis are predisposing risk factors. Young children may also be at increased risk of toxicity. Electrophysiologic studies have demonstrated that bupivacaine is associated with more pronounced changes in depolarization than lidocaine. The R(+) isomer of bupivacaine avidly blocks cardiac sodium channels and dissociates very slowly; its high and prolonged degree of protein binding makes resuscitation prolonged and difficult. At high doses calcium and potassium channels may also be blocked. Resuscitation from bupivacaine-induced cardiac toxicity often requires high doses of vasopressors and prolonged therapy.

Ropivacaine, a relatively new amide local anesthetic, shares many physicochemical properties with bupiv-

John Butterworth, MD

UNRESOLVED ISSUES IN LOCAL ANESTHETIC MECHANISMS & TOXICITY

The western concept of local anesthesia dates from 1884 when Koller reported the topical use of cocaine as an anesthetic for the cornea. However, the medicinal properties of cocaine were well known and widely used by the Incas long before explorers brought cocaine back to Europe. In the 1950s, local anesthetics (LAs) were found to inhibit sodium (Na) currents. Na channels are now known to initiate and propagate action potentials in axons, dendrites, and muscle tissue, and to shape and filter synaptic inputs. They also initiate and maintain membrane potential oscillations in heart and brain cells. The interactions of LAs with Na channels and other binding sites underlie many unresolved issues in local and regional anesthesia.

Speed of Onset of LAs

For most LAs, the onset of anesthesia in isolated nerves is inversely associated with increasing LA lipid solubility and increasing pK_a. At any pH, the percentage of LA molecules present in the uncharged form, largely responsible for membrane permeability, decreases with increasing pK_a. The rate of onset of LAs is associated with the aqueous diffusion rate, which is inversely related to molecular weight. However, contrary to textbook teaching, of the two LAs of fastest onset, etidocaine has one of the largest

molecular weights and is highly lipid soluble and chloroprocaine has a high pK_a.

Differential Sensory Nerve Block

Clinicians seek an LA that selectively inhibits sensory nerve fibers; nevertheless, sensory anesthesia sufficient for skin incision usually cannot be obtained without motor impairment. All LAs will block smaller diameter fibers at concentrations lower than required to block larger fibers of the same type. Bupivacaine and ropivacaine are relatively selective for sensory fibers. Bupivacaine produces more rapid onset of sensory block than motor block, whereas the closely related chemical mepivacaine demonstrates no differential onset of block.[1]

Cardiovascular Toxicity

The cardiovascular (CV) toxicity of LAs remains a vexing problem. Much is known about the actions of LAs on the heart, but the relationship between these pharmacological and biophysical findings and clinical CV toxicity remains speculative. All LAs bind and inhibit cardiac NA channels, but bupivacaine binds more avidly and longer than lidocaine. The bupivacaine R(+) isomer binds cardiac Na channels more avidly than the S(−) isomer. This finding led to the development of levobupivacaine and ropivacaine.

In addition to Na channels, LAs bind to many different sites, including K and Ca channels, enzymes, N-methyl-D-aspartate (NMDA) receptors, β-adrenergic receptors, and nicotinic acetylcholine receptors. The binding of LAs to these other sites could underlie the production of spinal or epidural analgesia by LAs and could contribute to toxic side effects.[2] LAs produce dose-dependent myocardial depression, which may relate to their interference with Ca signaling mechanisms within the cardiac muscle. Inhibition of epinephrine-stimulated cyclic AMP formation by LAs could explain the refractoriness of bupivacaine CV toxicity to standard resuscitation measures.[3]

Not all LAs produce CV toxicity by the same mechanisms. In a recent series of canine experiments, programmed electrical stimulation elicited more arrhythmias with bupivacaine and levobupivacaine than with lidocaine or ropivacaine.[4,5] In addition, dogs receiving bupivacaine were more susceptible to epinephrine-induced ventricular fibrillation. Thus, the pattern of CV toxicity differs among the LAs.

Another vexing issue relates to the neurotoxic effects of 2-chloroprocaine and lidocaine. During the 1980s, 2-chloroprocaine (at that time formulated with Na metabisulfite at an acidic pH) produced cauda equina syndrome when large doses were accidentally injected into spinal fluid during attempts at epidural anesthesia. Reports of neurotoxicity all but disappeared when the compound was reformatted, but have now returned following the introduction of generic products containing the original metabisulfite and pH. Whether the toxin is 2-chloroprocaine or metabisulfite has not been determined: 2-chloroprocaine is now being tested as a substitute for lidocaine in human spinal anesthesia.[6] At the same time, other investigators have linked neurotoxic reactions to 2-chloroprocaine rather than to metabisulfite.

Presently, there is controversy about transient neurological symptoms and persisting sacral deficits after use of lidocaine for spinal anesthesia. The deficit controversy initially arose when 5% lidocaine was used for continuous spinal anesthesia via 32-gauge spinal catheters. More recently, transient neurological symptoms have been observed after use of single-injection lidocaine as a spinal anesthetic, particularly with patients undergoing arthroscopy while in the lithotomy position. What makes lidocaine different? Unlike other spinal LA solutions, 5% lidocaine permanently interrupts conduction when applied to isolated nerves or to isolated neurons.[7] This may be the result of lidocaine-induced increases in intracellular calcium, unrelated to Na channel blockade. I believe that (reduced metabisulfite, less acidic) 2-chloroprocaine may replace lidocaine for short-duration spinal anesthesia once additional studies and publications narrow the confidence limits for the possible incidence of human neurotoxic side effects.

Treatment of LA Toxicity

Treatment of adverse LA reactions depends on their severity. Minor reactions can be allowed to resolve spontaneously. LA-induced seizures should be managed by protecting the airway and providing oxygen. Seizures may be terminated with intravenous thiopental, midazolam, or propofol. If LA intoxication produces cardiac arrest, the guidelines for advanced cardiac life support (ACLS) are reasonable[8]; however, I suggest that amiodarone and vasopressin be substituted for lidocaine and epinephrine, respectively. With unresponsive bupivacaine cardiac toxicity, intravenous lipid or cardiopulmonary bypass may be considered. Recent animal experiments demonstrate the remarkable ability of intravenous lipid infusion to effect resuscitation from bupivacaine overdosage, even after 10 min of unsuccessful "conventional" resuscitative efforts.[9]

After nearly 120 years of use in western medicine, LAs remain important tools for the twenty-first–century physician. Although we are certain that peripheral nerve blocks arise from LA inhibition of Na channels in neuronal membranes, the mechanisms of spinal and epidural anesthesia remain unclear. Why one agent has a faster onset of action than another is less clear than is often assumed. The mechanism by which LAs produce CV toxicity likely varies: the more potent agents (eg, bupivacaine) may promote arrhythmias through Na channel mechanisms, whereas the less potent agents (eg, lidocaine) may produce myocardial depression through other pathways. Clinical experience will determine whether intravenous lipids will prove as useful for humans as for rats after LA overdosage. Finally, whether 2-chloroprocaine may safely be substituted for lidocaine for spinal anesthesia of short duration remains undetermined.

1. Butterworth J, Ririe DG, Thompson RB, et al: Differential onset of median nerve block: Randomized, double-blind comparison of mepivacaine and bupivacaine in healthy volunteers. Br J Anaesth 1998;81:515.

2. McCaslin PP, Butterworth J: Bupivacaine suppresses [CA(2+)](i) oscillations in neonatal rat cardiomyocytes with increased extracellular K+ and is reversed with increased extracellular Mg(2+). Anesth Analg 2000;91:82.

3. Butterworth JF IV, Brownlow RC, Leith JP, et al: Bupivacaine inhibits cyclic-3',5'-adenosine monophosphate production. A possible contributing factor to cardiovascular toxicity. Anesthesiology 1993;79:88.

4. Groban L, Deal DD, Vernon JC, et al: Ventricular arrhythmias with or without programmed electrical stimulation after incremental overdosage with lidocaine, bupivacaine, levobupivacaine, and ropivacaine. Anesth Analg 2000;91:1103.

5. Groban L, Deal DD, Vernon JC, et al: Cardiac resuscitation after incremental overdosage with lidocaine, bupivacaine, levobupivacaine, and ropivacaine in anesthetized dogs. Anesth Analg 2001;92:37.

6. Kouri ME, Kopacz DJ: Spinal 2-chloroprocaine: A comparison with lidocaine in volunteers. Anesth Analg 2004;98:75.

7. Lambert LA, Lambert DH, Strichartz GR: Irreversible conduction block in isolated nerve by high concentrations of local anesthetics. Anesthesiology 1994;80:1082.

8. Guidelines 2000 for cardiopulmonary resuscitation and emergency cardiovascular care. Circulation 2000;102 (Suppl 1):I-1.

9. Groban L, Butterworth J: Lipid reversal of bupivacaine toxicity: has the silver bullet been identified? Reg Anesth Pain Med 2003;28:167.

acaine, except that it is half as lipid soluble. Onset time and duration of action are similar, but ropivacaine provides less motor block, which may reflect an overall lower potency as demonstrated by some studies. Most notably, ropivacaine has a larger therapeutic index because it is 70% less likely to cause severe cardiac arrhythmias than bupivacaine. Ropivacaine has been associated with greater central nervous system tolerance. This improved safety profile likely reflects its lower lipid solubility or its availability as a pure S(–) isomer, as opposed to bupivacaine's racemic mixture. Levobupivacaine, the S(–) isomer of bupivacaine, which is no longer available in the United States, was reported to have fewer cardiovascular and cerebral side effects than the racemic mixture; studies suggest its cardiovascular effects may approximate those of ropivacaine.

Cocaine's cardiovascular reactions are unlike those of any other local anesthetic. Adrenergic nerve terminals normally reabsorb norepinephrine after its release. Cocaine inhibits this reuptake, thereby potentiating the effects of adrenergic stimulation. Cardiovascular responses to cocaine include hypertension and ventricular ectopy. The latter contraindicates its use in patients anesthetized with halothane. **Cocaine-induced arrhythmias** have been successfully treated with adrenergic and calcium channel antagonists. Cocaine produces vasoconstriction when applied topically.

D. IMMUNOLOGICAL

True hypersensitivity reactions to local anesthetic agents—as distinct from systemic toxicity caused by excessive plasma concentration—are uncommon. Esters are more likely to induce an allergic reaction because they are derivatives of *p*-aminobenzoic acid, a known allergen. Commercial multidose preparations of amides often contain **methylparaben,** which has a chemical structure similar to that of PABA. This preservative may be responsible for most of the rare allergic responses to amide agents. The signs and treatment of allergic drug reactions are discussed in Chapter 47. Local anesthetics may help reduce the inflammatory response to surgery by inhibiting the effect of lysophosphatidic acid in activating neutrophils.

E. MUSCULOSKELETAL

When directly injected into skeletal muscle (eg, trigger-point injection), local anesthetics are myotoxic (bupivacaine > lidocaine > procaine). Histologically, myofibril hypercontraction progresses to lytic degeneration, edema, and necrosis. Regeneration usually occurs after 3–4 weeks. Concomitant steroid or epinephrine injection worsens the myonecrosis. Animal data suggest that ropivacaine produces less severe muscle injury than bupivacaine.

F. HEMATOLOGICAL

It has been demonstrated that lidocaine decreases coagulation (prevention of thrombosis and decreased platelet aggregation) and enhances fibrinolysis of whole blood as measured by thromboelastography. These effects may relate to the reduced efficacy of an epidural autologous blood patch shortly following local anesthetic administration and the lower incidence of embolic events in patients receiving epidural anesthetics.

Drug Interactions

Local anesthetics potentiate nondepolarizing muscle relaxant blockade.

Succinylcholine and ester local anesthetics depend on pseudocholinesterase for metabolism. Concurrent administration may potentiate the effects of both drugs.

Dibucaine, an amide local anesthetic, inhibits pseudocholinesterase and is used to detect genetically abnormal enzyme (see Chapter 9).

Pseudocholinesterase inhibitors can lead to decreased metabolism of ester local anesthetics (see Table 9–3).

Cimetidine and propranolol decrease hepatic blood flow and lidocaine clearance. Higher lidocaine blood levels increase the potential for systemic toxicity.

Opioids (eg, fentanyl, morphine) and α_2-adrenergic agonists (eg, epinephrine, clonidine) potentiate local anesthetic pain relief. Epidural chloroprocaine may interfere with the analgesic actions of intraspinal morphine.

CASE DISCUSSION: LOCAL ANESTHETIC OVERDOSE

An 18-year-old woman in the active stage of labor requests an epidural anesthetic for delivery. Immediately following the epidural injection of 12 mL of 2% lidocaine, the patient complains of lip numbness and becomes very apprehensive.

What is your presumptive diagnosis?

The temporal relationship of the numbness and apprehension to the administration of local anesthetic suggests an unintentional intravascular injection. These prodromal signs do not always precede a seizure.

What prophylactic measures should be immediately taken?

Because hypocapnia increases the seizure threshold of local anesthetics, the patient should be instructed to hyperventilate. Simultaneously, a very small dose of thiopental sodium (50 mg) could be administered intravenously. Unconsciousness should be strictly avoided, because pregnant patients are considered to have a full stomach. The patient should already be receiving supplemental oxygen.

If symptoms progress to a generalized convulsion, what treatment should be initiated?

The laboring patient is always considered to be at risk for aspiration (see Chapter 43). Therefore, protecting the airway is of utmost importance. Immediate administration of succinylcholine should be followed by a rapid-sequence intubation (see Case Discussion, Chapter 15). Although the succinylcholine will eliminate tonic–clonic activity, it will not address the underlying cerebral excitability. An anticonvulsant such as diazepam (2.5–10 mg) or thiopental sodium (50–75 mg) should be administered. It is clear from this sequence of events that whenever large doses of local anesthetic are administered, the same drugs and equipment must be available as for a general anesthetic.

What could have been expected if a large dose of bupivacaine—instead of lidocaine—had been given intravascularly?

Bupivacaine is more cardiotoxic than lidocaine, particularly in the presence of acute respiratory acidosis. Ventricular arrhythmias and conduction disturbances may lead to cardiac arrest and death. Bupivacaine is considered a more potent cardiac sodium channel blocker because the channels recover more slowly than after lidocaine blockade. Amiodarone and possibly bretylium should be considered as the preferred alternative to lidocaine in the treatment of local anesthetic-induced ventricular tachyarrhythmias. Vasopressors may include epinephrine, norepinephrine, and vasopressin. Isoproterenol may ef-

fectively reverse some of the electrophysiological abnormalities characteristic of bupivacaine toxicity. The reason for the higher incidence of cardiotoxicity during pregnancy is unclear. Although total dose rather than concentration determines toxicity, the Food and Drug Administration no longer recommends 0.75% bupivacaine for anesthesia during labor.

What could have prevented the toxic reaction described?

The risk of intravascular injection of toxic doses of local anesthetic during epidural anesthesia is minimized by using an adequate test dose (see Chapter 16), fractionation of the therapeutic dose into safe aliquots, and administering the minimum total dose of local anesthetic possible.

SUGGESTED READING

Covino BG, Wildsmith JAW: Clinical pharmacology of local anesthetic agents. In: *Neural Blockade in Clinical Anesthesia and Management of Pain,* 3rd ed. Cousins MJ (editor). Lippincott, Williams & Wilkins, 1998.

Evers AS, Maze M: *Anesthetic Pharmacology—Physiologic Principles and Clinical Practice.* Churchill Livingstone, 2004.

Freedman JM: Transient neurologic symptoms after spinal anesthesia: an epidemiologic study of 1,863 patients. Anesthesiology 1998;89:633. Conclusions of the Spinal Anesthesia Study Group that include the increased incidence of neurological symptoms following spinal anesthesia with lidocaine compared with bupivacaine or tetracaine.

Hadzic A, Vloka J: *Peripheral Nerve Blocks: Principles and Practice.* McGraw-Hill, 2004. Includes discussions of the selection of local anesthetic agents.

Hardman J, Limbird L, Gilman A: *Goodman and Gilman's The Pharmacological Basis of Therapeutics,* 10th ed. McGraw-Hill, 2002. Chapter 15 has an excellent discussion of local anesthetics.

Scholz A: Mechanisms of (local) anaesthetics on voltage-gated sodium and other ion channels. Br J Anaesth 2002;89:52.

Tetzlaff JE: *Clinical Pharmacology of Local Anesthetics.* Butterworth-Heinemann, 2000.

Adjuncts to Anesthesia

15

KEY CONCEPTS

 Diphenhydramine is an example of a diverse group of drugs that competitively blocks H_1-receptors. Many drugs with H_1-receptor antagonist properties have considerable antimuscarinic, or atropine-like, activity (eg, dry mouth), or antiserotonergic activity (antiemetic).

 H_2-blockers reduce the perioperative risk of aspiration pneumonia by decreasing gastric fluid volume and raising the pH of gastric contents.

 Metoclopramide increases lower esophageal sphincter tone, speeds gastric emptying, and lowers gastric fluid volume by enhancing the stimulatory effects of acetylcholine on intestinal smooth muscle.

 Ondansetron, granisetron, and dolasetron selectively block serotonin 5-HT_3 receptors, with little or no effect on dopamine receptors. 5-HT_3 receptors, which are located peripherally and centrally, appear to play an important role in the initiation of the vomiting reflex.

 Ketorolac is a parenterally administered nonsteroidal antiinflammatory drug that provides analgesia by inhibiting prostaglandin synthesis.

 Clonidine is a commonly used antihypertensive agent but in anesthesia it is used as an adjunct for epidural infusions in pain management. It is most useful in the management of patients with neuropathic pain who become increasingly resistant to epidural opioid infusions.

 Dexmedetomidine is a parenteral selective α_2-agonist with sedative properties. It appears to be more selective for the α_2-receptor than clonidine.

 Selective activation of carotid chemoreceptors by low doses of doxapram stimulates hypoxic drive, producing an increase in tidal volume and a slight increase in respiratory rate. However, doxapram is not a specific reversal agent and should not replace standard supportive therapy (ie, mechanical ventilation).

 Naloxone reverses the agonist activity associated with endogenous or exogenous opioid compounds.

 Flumazenil is useful in the reversal of benzodiazepine sedation and the treatment of benzodiazepine overdose.

 Aspiration does not necessarily result in aspiration pneumonia. The seriousness of the lung damage depends on the volume and composition of the aspirate. Patients are at risk if their gastric volume is greater than 25 mL (0.4 mL/kg) and their gastric pH is less than 2.5.

This final pharmacology chapter describes several drugs of particular interest to the anesthesiologist. Because some of these are histamine-receptor antagonists, the physiology of histamine is briefly reviewed. Diphenhydramine represents the classic antihistaminic drug. Cimetidine, ranitidine, and famotidine are helpful in the preoperative preparation of patients at risk for aspiration pneumonia. The chapter reviews other drugs (eg, metoclopramide, antacids, and proton pump inhibitors) that may be used to decrease the risk of aspiration as well as serotonin antagonists, which have proved to be potent antiemetics. The α_2-adrenergic agonists clonidine and dexmedetomidine are also

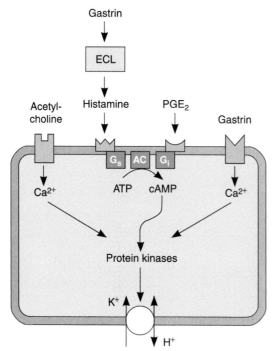

Gastrin

ECL

Acetyl-
choline   Histamine   PGE$_2$

Gastrin

G$_s$ AC G$_i$

Ca^{2+} ATP   cAMP   Ca^{2+}

Protein kinases

K$^+$

H$^+$

Figure 15–1. Secretion of hydrochloric acid is normally mediated by gastrin-induced histamine release from enterochromaffin-like cells in the stomach. Note that acid secretion by gastric parietal cells can also be increased indirectly by acetylcholine via stimulation of M$_3$ receptors and directly by gastrin through an increase in intracellular Ca^{2+} concentration. Prostaglandin E$_2$ can inhibit acid secretion by decreasing cAMP activity.

reviewed. The chapter concludes with a discussion of a respiratory stimulant (doxapram), an opioid antagonist (naloxone), and a benzodiazepine antagonist (flumazenil).

HISTAMINE-RECEPTOR ANTAGONISTS

Histamine Physiology

Histamine is found in the central nervous system, in the gastric mucosa, and in other peripheral tissues. It is synthesized by decarboxylation of the amino acid histidine. Histaminergic neurons are primarily located in the posterior hypothalamus but have wide projections in the brain. Histamine also normally plays a major role in the secretion of hydrochloric acid by parietal cells in the stomach (Figure 15–1). The highest concentrations of histamine are found in the storage granules of circulating basophils and mast cells throughout the body. Mast cells tend to be concentrated in connective tissue just beneath epithelial (mucosal) surfaces. Histamine release (degranulation) from these cells

can be triggered by chemical, mechanical, or immunological stimulation (Chapter 46).

Two receptors, H$_1$ and H$_2$, mediate the effects of histamine. The H$_1$-receptor activates phospholipase C, whereas the H$_2$-receptor increases intracellular cyclic adenosine monophosphate (cAMP). An H$_3$-receptor is primarily located on histamine-secreting cells and mediates negative feedback, inhibiting the synthesis and release of additional histamine. Histamine-*N*-methyltransferase metabolizes histamine to inactive metabolites that are excreted in the urine. This enzymatic reaction is inhibited by droperidol.

A. CARDIOVASCULAR

Histamine reduces arterial blood pressure but increases heart rate and myocardial contractility. H$_1$-Receptor stimulation increases capillary permeability and enhances ventricular irritability, whereas H$_2$-receptor stimulation increases heart rate and increases contractility. Both types of receptors mediate peripheral arteriolar dilation and some coronary vasodilation.

B. RESPIRATORY

Histamine constricts bronchiolar smooth muscle via the H$_1$-receptor. H$_2$-Receptor stimulation may produce mild bronchodilation. Histamine has variable effects on the pulmonary vasculature; the H$_1$-receptor appears to mediate some pulmonary vasodilation, whereas the H$_2$-receptor may be responsible for histamine-mediated pulmonary vasoconstriction.

C. GASTROINTESTINAL

Activation of H$_2$-receptors in parietal cells increases gastric acid secretion. Stimulation of H$_1$-receptors leads to contraction of intestinal smooth muscle.

D. DERMAL

The classic wheal-and-flare response of the skin to histamine results from increased capillary permeability and vasodilation and is primarily via H$_1$-receptor activation.

E. IMMUNOLOGICAL

Histamine is a major mediator of type 1 hypersensitivity reactions (see Chapter 46). H$_1$-Receptor stimulation attracts leukocytes and induces synthesis of prostaglandin. In contrast, the H$_2$-receptor appears to activate suppressor T lymphocytes.

1. H$_1$-Receptor Antagonists

Mechanism of Action

 Diphenhydramine (an ethanolamine) is an example of a diverse group of drugs that competitively blocks H$_1$-receptors (Table 15–1).

Table 15–1. Properties of commonly used H_1-receptor antagonists.[1]

Drug	Route	Dose (mg)	Duration (h)	Sedation	Antiemesis
Diphenhydramine (Benadryl)	PO, IM, IV	25–100	3–6	+++	++
Dimenhydrinate (Dramamine)	PO, IM, IV	50–100	3–6	+++	++
Chlorpheniramine (Chlor-Trimeton)	PO IM, IV	2–12 5–20	4–8	++	0
Hydroxyzine (Atarax, Vistaril)	PO, IM	25–100	4–12	+++	++
Promethazine (Phenergan)	PO, IM, IV	12.5–50	4–12	+++	+++
Cetirizine (Zyrtec)	PO	5–10	24	+	
Cyproheptadine (Periactin)	PO	4	6–8	++	
Dimenhydrinate (Dramamine)	PO	50	6–12	++	
Fexofenadine (Allegra)	PO	30–60	12	0	
Meclizine (Antivert)	PO	12.5–50	8–24	+	
Loratadine (Claritin)	PO	10	24	0	

[1]0, no effect; ++, moderate activity; +++, marked activity.

Many drugs with H_1-receptor antagonist properties have considerable antimuscarinic, or atropine-like, activity (eg, dry mouth), or antiserotonergic activity (antiemetic). Promethazine is a phenothiazine derivative with H_1-receptor antagonist activity as well as antidopaminergic and α-adrenergic–blocking properties.

Clinical Uses

Like other H_1-receptor antagonists, diphenhydramine has a multitude of therapeutic uses: suppression of allergic symptoms (eg, urticaria, rhinitis, conjunctivitis); vertigo, nausea, and vomiting (eg, motion sickness, Ménière's disease); sedation; suppression of cough; and dyskinesia (eg, parkinsonism, drug-induced extrapyramidal side effects). Some of these actions are predictable from an understanding of histamine physiology, whereas others are the result of the drugs' antimuscarinic and antiserotoninergic effects (Table 15–1). Although H_1-blockers prevent the bronchoconstrictive response to histamine, they are ineffective in treating bronchial asthma, which is primarily due to other mediators (see Chapters 23 and 46). Likewise, H_1-blockers will not completely prevent the hypotensive effect of histamine unless an H_2-blocker is administered concomitantly. Thus, the usefulness of H_1-blockers during an acute anaphylactic reaction is quite limited; epinephrine is the treatment of choice.

The antiemetic and mild hypnotic effects of antihistaminic drugs (particularly diphenhydramine, promethazine, and hydroxyzine) have led to their use for premedication.

Although many H_1-blockers cause significant sedation, ventilatory drive is usually unaffected in the absence of other sedative medications. Promethazine and hydroxyzine are often combined with opioids to potentiate analgesia. Newer (second-generation) antihistamines tend to produce little or no sedation because of limited penetration across the blood–brain barrier. This group of drugs is available only in oral preparations that are used primarily for allergic rhinitis and urticaria. They include loratadine, fexofenadine, and cetirizine. Many preparations for allergic rhinitis often also contain vasoconstrictors such as pseudoephedrine. Meclizine and dimenhydrinate are used primarily as an antiemetic, particularly for motion sickness, and in the management of vertigo. Cyproheptadine, which also has significant serotonin antagonist activity, has been used in the management of Cushing's syndrome, carcinoid syndrome, and vascular (cluster) headaches.

Dosage

The usual adult dose of diphenhydramine is 25–50 mg (0.5–1.5 mg/kg) orally, intramuscularly, or intravenously every 4–6 h. The doses of other H_1-receptor antagonists are listed in Table 15–1.

Drug Interactions

The sedative effects of H_1-receptor antagonists can potentiate other central nervous system depressants such as barbiturates, benzodiazepines, and opioids.

Table 15–2. Pharmacology of aspiration pneumonia prophylaxis.[1]

Drug	Route	Dose	Onset	Duration	Acidity	Volume	LES Tone
Cimetidine (Tagamet)	PO IV	300–800 mg 300 mg	1–2 h	4–8 h	↓↓↓	↓↓	0
Ranitidine (Zantac)	PO IV	150–300 mg 50 mg	1–2 h	10–12 h	↓↓↓	↓↓	0
Famotidine (Pepcid)	PO IV	20–40 mg 20 mg	1–2 h	10–12 h	↓↓↓	↓↓	0
Nizatidine (Axid)	PO	150–300 mg	0.5–1 h	10–12 h	↓↓↓	↓↓	0
Nonparticulate antacids (Bicitra, Polycitra)	PO	15–30 mL	5–10 min	30–60 min	↓↓↓	↑	0
Metoclopramide (Reglan)	IV PO	10 mg 10–15 mg	1–3 min	1–2 h 30–60 min[2]	0	↓↓	↑↑

[1]0, no effect; ↓↓, moderate decrease; ↓↓↓, marked decrease; ↑, slight increase; ↑↑, moderate increase; LES, lower esophageal sphincter.
[2]Oral metoclopramide has a quite variable onset of action and duration of action.

2. H_2-Receptor Antagonists

Mechanism of Action

H_2-Receptor antagonists include cimetidine, famotidine, nizatidine, and ranitidine (Table 15–2). These agents competitively inhibit histamine binding to H_2-receptors, thereby reducing gastric acid output and raising gastric pH. Nizatidine is available only in an oral formulation.

Clinical Uses

All H_2-receptor antagonists are equally effective in the treatment of peptic duodenal and gastric ulcers, hypersecretory states (Zollinger–Ellison syndrome), and gastroesophageal reflux disease (GERD). Intravenous preparations are also used to prevent stress ulceration in critically ill patients (see Chapter 49). Duodenal and gastric ulcers are usually associated with *Helicobacter pylori* infection, which is also treated with combinations of bismuth, tetracycline, and metronidazole. Ranitidine bismuth citrate with clarithromycin may also be used for peptic ulcers associated with *H pylori* infection. By decreasing gastric fluid volume and hydrogen ion content, H_2-blockers reduce the perioperative risk of aspiration pneumonia. These drugs affect the pH of only those gastric secretions that occur after their administration.

The combination of H_1- and H_2-receptor antagonists provides some protection against drug-induced allergic reactions (eg, intravenous radiocontrast, chymopapain injection for lumbar disk disease, protamine).

Although pretreatment with these agents does not reduce histamine release, it does decrease subsequent hypotension.

Side Effects

Rapid intravenous injection of cimetidine and ranitidine has been rarely associated with hypotension, bradycardia, arrhythmias, and cardiac arrest. These adverse cardiovascular effects are more frequent following the administration of cimetidine to critically ill patients. In contrast, famotidine can be safely injected intravenously over a 2-min period. H_2-Receptor antagonists change the gastric flora by virtue of their pH effects. The clinical significance of this alteration has yet to be determined. Complications of long-term cimetidine therapy include hepatotoxicity (elevated serum transaminases), interstitial nephritis (elevated serum creatinine), granulocytopenia, and thrombocytopenia. Cimetidine also binds to androgen receptors, occasionally causing gynecomastia and impotence. Finally, cimetidine has been associated with changes in mental status ranging from lethargy and hallucinations to seizures, particularly in elderly patients. In contrast, ranitidine, nizatidine, and famotidine do not affect androgen receptors and penetrate the blood–brain barrier poorly.

Dosage

As a premedication to reduce the risk of aspiration pneumonia, H_2-receptor antagonists should be administered at bedtime and again at least 2 h before surgery

(Table 15–2). Because all four drugs are eliminated primarily by the kidneys, the dose should be reduced in patients with significant renal dysfunction.

Drug Interactions

Cimetidine may reduce hepatic blood flow and binds to the cytochrome P-450 mixed-function oxidases. These effects slow the metabolism of a multitude of drugs, including lidocaine, propranolol, diazepam, theophylline, phenobarbital, warfarin, and phenytoin. Ranitidine is a weak inhibitor of the cytochrome P-450 system, and no significant drug interactions have been demonstrated. Famotidine and nizatidine do not appear to affect the cytochrome P-450 system.

ANTACIDS

Mechanism of Action

Antacids neutralize the acidity of gastric fluid by providing a base (usually hydroxide, carbonate, bicarbonate, citrate, or trisilicate) that reacts with hydrogen ions to form water.

Clinical Uses

Common uses of antacids include the treatment of gastric and duodenal ulcers, GERD, and Zollinger–Ellison syndrome. In anesthesiology, antacids provide protection against the harmful effects of aspiration pneumonia by raising the pH of gastric contents. Unlike H_2-receptor antagonists, antacids have an immediate effect. Unfortunately, they increase intragastric volume. Aspiration of particulate antacids (aluminum or magnesium hydroxide) produces abnormalities in lung function comparable to those that occur following acid aspiration. Nonparticulate antacids (sodium citrate or sodium bicarbonate) are much less damaging to lung alveoli if aspirated. Furthermore, nonparticulate antacids mix with gastric contents better than particulate solutions. Timing is critical, as nonparticulate antacids lose their effectiveness 30–60 min after ingestion.

Dosage

The usual adult dose of a 0.3 M solution of sodium citrate—Bicitra (sodium citrate and citric acid) or Polycitra (sodium citrate, potassium citrate, and citric acid)—is 15–30 mL orally, 15–30 min prior to induction.

Drug Interactions

Because antacids alter gastric and urinary pH, they change the absorption and elimination of many drugs. The rate of absorption of digoxin, cimetidine, and ranitidine is slowed, whereas the rate of phenobarbital elimination is quickened.

METOCLOPRAMIDE

Mechanism of Action

Metoclopramide acts peripherally as a cholinomimetic (ie, facilitates acetylcholine transmission at selective muscarinic receptors) and centrally as a dopamine antagonist. Its action as a prokinetic agent in the upper gastrointestinal (GI) tract is not dependent on vagal innervation but is abolished by anticholinergic agents. It does not stimulate secretions.

Clinical Uses

 By enhancing the stimulatory effects of acetylcholine on intestinal smooth muscle, metoclopramide increases lower esophageal sphincter tone, speeds gastric emptying, and lowers gastric fluid volume. These properties account for its efficacy in the treatment of patients with diabetic gastroparesis and GERD, as well as prophylaxis for those at risk for aspiration pneumonia. Metoclopramide does not affect the secretion of gastric acid or the pH of gastric fluid.

Metoclopramide produces an antiemetic effect by blocking dopamine receptors in the chemoreceptor trigger zone of the central nervous system. Its usefulness as an antiemetic agent during cancer chemotherapy is better documented than when it is used as the sole agent for prevention of postoperative nausea and vomiting (PONV).

Metoclopramide may provide some degree of analgesia in conditions associated with smooth muscle spasm (eg, renal or biliary colic, uterine cramping), presumably because of its cholinergic and dopaminergic effects. It may also reduce the analgesic requirements in patients undergoing prostaglandin-induced termination of pregnancy.

Side Effects

Rapid intravenous injection may cause abdominal cramping, and metoclopramide is contraindicated in patients with complete intestinal obstruction. It can induce a hypertensive crisis in patients with pheochromocytoma by releasing catecholamines from the tumor. Sedation, nervousness, and extrapyramidal signs from dopamine antagonism (eg, akathisia) are uncommon and reversible. Nonetheless, metoclopramide is best avoided in patients with Parkinson's disease. Metoclopramide-induced increases in aldosterone and prolactin secretion are probably inconsequential during short-term therapy. Metoclopramide may rarely result in hypotension and arrhythmias.

Dosage

An adult dose of 10–20 mg of metoclopramide (0.25 mg/kg) is effective orally, intramuscularly, or intravenously (injected over 5 min). Higher doses (1–2 mg/kg) have been used to prevent emesis during chemotherapy. The onset of action is much more rapid following parenteral (3–5 min) than oral (30–60 min) administration. Because metoclopramide is excreted in the urine, its dose should be decreased in patients with renal dysfunction.

Drug Interactions

Antimuscarinic drugs (eg, atropine, glycopyrrolate) block the GI effects of metoclopramide. Metoclopramide decreases the absorption of orally administered cimetidine. Concurrent use of phenothiazines or butyrophenones (droperidol) increases the likelihood of extrapyramidal side effects. Metoclopramide decreases dosage requirements for thiopental induction of anesthesia. It does not reverse the effects of low-dose dopamine infusion on the renal vasculature.

PROTON PUMP INHIBITORS

Mechanism of Action

These agents, including omeprazole (Prilosec), lansoprazole (Prevacid), rabeprazole (Aciphex), and pantoprazole (Protonix), bind to the proton pump of parietal cells in the gastric mucosa and inhibit secretion of hydrogen ions.

Clinical Uses

Proton pump inhibitors are indicated for the treatment of duodenal ulcer, GERD, and Zollinger–Ellison syndrome. They may heal peptic ulcers and erosive GERD faster than H_2-receptor blockers. The use of proton pump inhibitors in aspiration prophylaxis prior to general anesthesia is limited. Some studies have shown that compared with omeprazole, H_2-receptor blockers are more reliable in consistently raising gastric pH and reducing gastric volume; lansoprazole may be as effective as H_2-receptor blockers. Two doses of lansoprazole (the evening before surgery and the morning of surgery) appear to be more effective than a single-dose prophylaxis. Data on the use of newer intravenous agents (pantoprazole) for aspiration prophylaxis are limited.

Side Effects

Proton pump inhibitors are generally well tolerated causing few side effects. Adverse side effects are primarily GI (nausea, abdominal pain, constipation, and diarrhea). On rare occasions, they have been associated with myalgias, anaphylaxis, angioedema, and severe dermatological reactions. Long-term treatment has also been associated with gastric enterochromaffin-like cell hyperplasia.

Dosage

Recommended oral doses for adults are omeprazole 20 mg, lansoprazole 15 mg, rabeprazole 20 mg, and pan-

toprazole 40 mg. Only pantoprazole is available for intravenous use in the United States. Because these drugs are primarily eliminated by the liver, repeat doses should be decreased in patients with severe liver impairment.

Drug Interactions

Omeprazole interferes with hepatic P-450 enzymes and decreases the clearance of diazepam, warfarin, and phenytoin. Other agents do not appear to have significant drug interactions.

5-HT$_3$ RECEPTOR ANTAGONISTS

Serotonin Physiology

Serotonin, 5-hydroxytryptamine (5-HT), is present in large quantities in platelets and the GI tract (enterchromaffin cells and the myenteric plexus). It is also an important neurotransmitter in many areas of the central nervous system, including the retina, limbic system, hypothalamus, cerebellum, and spinal cord. Serotonin is formed by hydroxylation and decarboxylation of tryptophan. Monoamine oxidase inactivates serotonin into 5-hydroxyindoleacetic acid (5-HIAA). The physiology of serotonin is very complex because there are at least seven receptor types, most with multiple subtypes. The 5-HT$_3$ receptor mediates vomiting and is found in the GI tract and the brain (area postrema). The 5-HT$_{2A}$ receptors are responsible for smooth muscle contraction and platelet aggregation, the 5-HT$_4$ receptors in the GI tract mediate secretion and peristalsis, and the 5-HT$_6$ and 5-HT$_7$ receptors are located primarily in the limbic system where they appear to play a role in depression. Many antidepressant drugs (Chapters 18 and 27) bind 5-HT$_6$ receptors. All except the 5-HT$_3$ receptor are coupled to G proteins and affect either adenylyl cyclase or phospholipase C; the 5-HT$_3$ receptor is an ion channel.

A. CARDIOVASCULAR

Except in the heart and skeletal muscle, serotonin is a powerful vasoconstrictor of arterioles and veins. Its vasodilator effect in the heart is critically dependent on the endothelium. When the myocardial endothelium is damaged following injury, serotonin produces vasoconstriction. The pulmonary and renal vasculatures are very sensitive to the arterial vasoconstrictive effects of serotonin. Modest and transient increases in cardiac contractility and heart rate may occur following serotonin release; reflex bradycardia often follows. Vasodilatation in skeletal muscle can subsequently cause hypotension.

B. RESPIRATORY

Contraction of smooth muscle increases airway resistance. Bronchoconstriction is often a prominent feature of carcinoid syndrome (Chapter 36).

ONDANSETRON

5-HYDROXYTRYPTAMINE (serotonin)

Figure 15–2. Ondansetron is structurally related to serotonin.

C. GASTROINTESTINAL

Direct smooth muscle contraction (via 5-HT$_2$ receptors) and serotonin-induced release of acetylcholine in the myenteric plexus (via 5-HT$_3$ receptors) greatly augment peristalsis. Secretions are unaffected.

D. HEMATOLOGICAL

Activation of 5-HT$_2$ receptors causes platelet aggregation.

Mechanism of Action

Ondansetron (Zofran), granisetron (Kytril), and dolasetron (Anzemet) selectively block serotonin 5-HT$_3$ receptors, with little or no effect on dopamine receptors (Figure 15–2). 5-HT$_3$ receptors, which are located peripherally (abdominal vagal afferents) and centrally (chemoreceptor trigger zone of the area postrema and the nucleus tractus solitarius), appear to play an important role in the initiation of the vomiting reflex. Unlike metoclopramide, these agents do not affect GI motility or lower esophageal sphincter tone.

Clinical Uses

All these agents have proved to be effective antiemetics in the postoperative period. In some studies, 5-HT$_3$ receptor antagonists, as single agents, provided superior antiemetic prophylaxis compared with metoclopramide or droperidol alone. Other studies suggest that metoclopramide and droperidol together can provide equivalent prophylaxis to ondansetron alone. Some clinicians believe that because of

their expense, 5-HT$_3$ receptor antagonists should not be used for routine prophylaxis but rather should be reserved for symptomatic treatment of nausea or vomiting. Indeed, studies indicate no differences in outcome when antiemetics are administered either for symptomatic treatment or prophylactically. Prophylaxis should, however, be seriously considered in patients who have a prior history of postoperative nausea, who are undergoing procedures at high risk for nausea (eg, laparoscopy), in whom nausea and vomiting must be avoided (eg, neurosurgery), and who are experiencing nausea and vomiting, to prevent further episodes.

Side Effects

5-HT$_3$ receptor antagonists are essentially devoid of serious side effects, even in amounts several times the recommended dose. They do not appear to cause sedation, extrapyramidal signs, or respiratory depression. The most commonly reported side effect is headache. All three drugs can slightly prolong the QT interval on the electrocardiogram. This effect may be more frequent with dolasetron, although it has not been associated with any adverse arrhythmias. Nonetheless, these drugs, particularly dolasetron, should be used cautiously in patients who are taking antiarrhythmic drugs or who have a prolonged QT interval.

Dosage

The recommended adult intravenous dose of ondansetron for prevention of perioperative nausea and vomiting is 4 mg either prior to the induction of anesthesia or at the end of surgery. Postoperative nausea and vomiting can also be treated with a 4 mg dose, repeated as needed every 4–8 h. Ondansetron undergoes extensive metabolism in the liver via hydroxylation and conjugation by cytochrome P-450 enzymes. Liver failure impairs clearance several-fold, and the dose should be reduced accordingly. The recommended intravenous dose is 12.5 mg for dolasetron and 1 mg for granisetron. All three drugs are available in oral formulations for PONV prophylaxis. The oral dose is the same as the parenteral preparation for ondansetron and granisetron, whereas it is 100 mg for dolasetron.

Drug Interactions

No significant drug interactions with 5-HT$_3$ receptor antagonists have been reported.

KETOROLAC

Mechanism of Action

Ketorolac is a parenterally administered nonsteroidal antiinflammatory drug (NSAID) that provides analgesia by inhibiting prostaglandin synthesis.

Clinical Uses

Ketorolac is indicated for the short-term (less than 5 days) management of pain, and appears to be particularly useful in the immediate postoperative period. A standard dose of ketorolac provides analgesia equivalent to 6–12 mg of morphine administered by the same route. Its time to onset is also similar to morphine, but ketorolac has a longer duration of action (6–8 h).

Ketorolac, a peripherally acting drug, has become a popular alternative to opioids for postoperative analgesia because of its minimal central nervous system side effects. Specifically, ketorolac does not cause respiratory depression, sedation, or nausea and vomiting. In fact, ketorolac does not cross the blood–brain barrier to any significant degree. Numerous studies have shown that oral and parenteral NSAIDs have an opioid-sparing effect. They may be most beneficial in patients at increased risk for postoperative respiratory depression or emesis. The analgesic effects of ketorolac may be more pronounced following orthopedic and gynecological procedures than following intraabdominal surgery.

Side Effects

As with other NSAIDs, ketorolac inhibits platelet aggregation and prolongs bleeding time. It and other NSAIDs should therefore be used with caution in patients at risk for postoperative hemorrhage. Long-term administration may lead to renal toxicity (eg, papillary necrosis) or GI tract ulceration with bleeding and perforation. Because ketorolac depends on elimination by the kidneys, it should not be given to patients in renal failure. Ketorolac is contraindicated in patients allergic to aspirin or NSAIDs. Patients with asthma have an increased incidence of aspirin sensitivity (approximately 10%), particularly if they also have a history of nasal polyps (approximately 20%).

Dosage

Ketorolac has been approved for administration as either a 60 mg intramuscular or 30 mg intravenous loading dose; a maintenance dose of 15–30 mg every 6 h is recommended. Elderly patients clear ketorolac more slowly and should receive reduced doses.

Drug Interactions

Aspirin decreases the protein binding of ketorolac, increasing the amount of active unbound drug. Ketorolac does not affect minimum alveolar concentration of inhalation anesthetic agents, and its administration does not alter the hemodynamics of anesthetized patients. It decreases the postoperative requirement for opioid analgesics.

Other Parenteral NSAIDs

NSAIDs that have been used parenterally include diclofenac, ketoprofen, and parecoxib. Whereas ketorolac and diclofenac are nonspecific cyclooxygenase (COX) inhibitors, parecoxib is a selective COX-2 inhibitor (Chapter 18). COX-2 inhibitors appear to have lower toxicity, in particular fewer GI side effects, and have little effect on platelet aggregation. Diclofenac has been administered at a dose of 1 mg/kg intravenously, whereas for parecoxib the dose has been 20–40 mg intravenously to adults.

CLONIDINE

Mechanism of Action

Clonidine (Catapres and Duraclon) is an imidazoline derivative with predominantly α_2-adrenergic agonist activity (Chapter 12). It is highly lipid soluble and readily penetrates the blood–brain barrier and the placenta. Studies indicate that binding of clonidine to receptors is highest in the rostral venterolateral medulla in the brain stem (the final common pathway for sympathetic outflow) where it activates inhibitory neurons. The overall effect is to decrease sympathetic activity, enhance parasympathetic tone, and reduce circulating catecholamines. There is also evidence that much of clonidine's antihypertensive action occurs via binding to a nonadrenergic (imidazoline) receptor. In contrast, its analgesic effects, particularly in the spinal cord, are mediated entirely via pre- and possibly postsynaptic α_2-adrenergic receptors that block nociceptive transmission.

Clinical Uses

 Clonidine is a commonly used antihypertensive agent (Chapters 12 and 20), but in anesthesia it is used as an adjunct for epidural infusions in pain management (Chapter 18). It is most useful in the management of patients with neuropathic pain who become increasingly resistant to epidural opioid infusions. When given epidurally, the analgesic effect of clonidine is segmental, being localized to the level at which it is injected or infused. When used for the acute or chronic management of hypertension, the reduction in sympathetic tone decreases systemic vascular resistance, heart rate, and blood pressure.

Unlabeled/investigational uses include serving as an adjunct in premedication, control of withdrawal syndromes (nicotine, opioids, alcohol, and vasomotor symptoms of menopause), and treatment of glaucoma as well as various psychiatric disorders.

Side Effects

Sedation, dizziness, bradycardia, and dry mouth are common side effects. Less commonly, bradycardia, orthostatic hypotension, nausea, and diarrhea may be observed. Abrupt discontinuation of clonidine following long-term administration (> 1 month) can produce a withdrawal phenomenon characterized by rebound hypertension, agitation, and sympathetic overactivity.

Dosage

Epidural clonidine is usually started at 30 μg/h in a mixture with an opioid and/or local anesthetic (Chapter 18). Oral clonidine is readily absorbed, has a 30–60 min onset, and lasts 6–12 h. In the treatment of acute hypertension, 0.1 mg can be given orally every hour until the blood pressure is controlled, or up to a maximum of 0.6 mg; the maintenance dose is 0.1–0.3 mg twice a day. Transdermal preparations of clonidine can also be used for maintenance therapy. They are available as 0.1, 0.2, and 0.3 mg/day patches that are replaced every 7 days. Clonidine is metabolized by the liver and excreted renally. Dosages should be reduced for patients with renal insufficiency.

Drug Interactions

Clonidine enhances and prolongs sensory and motor blockade from epidural local anesthetics. Additive effects with hypnotic agents, general anesthetics, and sedatives can potentiate sedation, hypotension, and bradycardia. The drug should be used cautiously, if at all, in patients on β-adrenergic blockers and in those with significant cardiac conduction system abnormalities. Lastly, clonidine can mask the symptoms of hypoglycemia in diabetic patients (Chapter 36).

DEXMEDETOMIDINE

Mechanism of Action

Dexmedetomidine (Precedex) is a parenteral selective α_2-agonist with sedative properties (Chapter 12). It appears to be more selective for the α_2-receptor than clonidine. At higher doses it loses its selectivity and also stimulates α_1-adrenergic receptors.

Clinical Uses

Dexmedetomidine causes dose-dependent sedation anxiolysis and some analgesia and blunts the sympathetic response to surgery and other stress. Most importantly, it has an opioid-sparing effect and does not significantly depress respiratory drive; excessive sedation, however, can cause airway obstruction. The drug is used for short-term (< 24 h), intravenous sedation of mechanically ventilated patients. Discontinuation after more prolonged use can potentially cause a withdrawal phenomenon similar to that of clonidine. It has also been used for intraoperative sedation and as an adjunct to general anesthetics.

Side Effects

The principal side effects are bradycardia, heart block, and hypotension. It may also cause nausea.

Dosage

The recommended initial loading dose is 1 μg/kg intravenously over 10 min with a maintenance infusion rate of 0.2–0.7 μg/kg/h. Dexmedetomidine has a rapid onset and terminal half-life of 2 h. The drug is metabolized in the liver and its metabolites are eliminated in the urine. Dosage should be reduced in patients with renal insufficiency or hepatic impairment.

Drug Interactions

Caution should be used when dexmedetomidine is administered with vasodilators, cardiac depressants, and drugs that decrease heart rate. Reduced requirements of hypnotics/anesthetic agents should prevent excessive hypotension.

DOXAPRAM

Mechanism of Action

Doxapram is a peripheral and central nervous system stimulant. Selective activation of carotid chemoreceptors by low doses of doxapram stimulates hypoxic drive, producing an increase in tidal volume and a slight increase in respiratory rate. At higher doses, the central respiratory centers in the medulla are stimulated.

Clinical Uses

Because doxapram mimics a low PaO_2, it may be useful in patients with chronic obstructive pulmonary disease who are dependent on hypoxic drive yet require supplemental oxygen. Drug-induced respiratory and central nervous system depression, including that seen immediately postoperatively, can be *temporarily* overcome. Doxapram is not a specific reversal agent, however, and should not replace standard supportive therapy (mechanical ventilation). For example, doxapram will not reverse paralysis caused by muscle relaxants, although it may transiently mask respiratory failure. The most common cause of postoperative hypoventilation—airway obstruction—will not be alleviated by doxapram. For these reasons, many anesthesiologists believe that the usefulness of doxapram is very limited.

Side Effects

Stimulation of the central nervous system leads to a variety of possible side effects: changes in mental status (confusion, dizziness, seizures), cardiac abnormalities (tachycardia, dysrhythmias, hypertension), and pulmonary dysfunction (wheezing, tachypnea). Vomiting and laryngospasm are of particular concern to the anesthesiologist in the postoperative period. Doxapram should not be used in patients with a history of epilepsy, cerebrovascular disease, acute head injury, coronary artery disease, hypertension, or bronchial asthma.

Dosage

Bolus intravenous administration (0.5–1 mg/kg) results in transient increases in minute ventilation (the onset of action is 1 min; the duration of action is 5–12 min). Continuous intravenous infusions (1–3 mg/min) provide longer-lasting effects (the maximum dose is 4 mg/kg).

Drug Interactions

The sympathetic stimulation produced by doxapram may exaggerate the cardiovascular effects of monoamine oxidase inhibitors or adrenergic agents. Doxapram should not be used in patients awakening from halothane anesthesia, as halothane sensitizes the myocardium to catecholamines.

NALOXONE

Mechanism of Action

Naloxone is a competitive antagonist at opioid receptors. Its affinity for μ receptors appears to be much greater than for κ or δ receptors (see Chapter 8). Naloxone has no significant agonist activity.

Clinical Uses

Naloxone reverses the agonist activity associated with endogenous (enkephalins, endorphins) or exogenous opioid compounds. A dramatic example is the reversal of unconsciousness that occurs in a patient with opioid overdose who has received naloxone. Perioperative respiratory depression caused by overzealous opioid administration is rapidly antagonized (1–2 min). Some degree of opioid analgesia can often be spared if the dose of naloxone is limited to the minimum required to maintain adequate ventilation. Low doses of intravenous naloxone reverse the side effects of epidurally administered opioids (see Chapter 18) without necessarily reversing the analgesia.

Side Effects

Abrupt reversal of opioid analgesia can result in sympathetic stimulation (tachycardia, ventricular irritability, hypertension, pulmonary edema) caused by pain perception, an acute withdrawal syndrome in patients who are opioid dependent or vomiting. The extent of these side effects is proportional to the amount of opioid being reversed and the speed of the reversal.

Dosage

In postoperative patients experiencing respiratory depression from excessive opioid administration, intravenous naloxone (0.4 mg/mL vial diluted to 0.04 mg/mL) can be titrated in increments of 0.5–1 μg/kg every 3–5 min until adequate ventilation and alertness are achieved. Intravenous doses in excess of 0.2 mg are rarely indicated. The brief duration of action of intravenous naloxone (30–45 min) is due to rapid redistribution from the central nervous system. A more prolonged effect is almost always necessary to prevent the recurrence of respiratory depression from longer-acting opioids. Therefore, intramuscular naloxone (twice the required intravenous dose) or a continuous infusion (4–5 μg/kg/h) is recommended. Neonatal respiratory depression resulting from maternal opioid administration is treated with 10 μg/kg, repeated in 2 min if necessary. Neonates of opioid-dependent mothers will exhibit withdrawal symptoms if given naloxone. The primary treatment of respiratory depression is always airway establishment and artificial ventilation.

Drug Interactions

The effect of naloxone on nonopioid anesthetic agents such as nitrous oxide is controversial and probably insignificant. Naloxone may antagonize the antihypertensive effect of clonidine.

Other Opioid Antagonists

Nalmefene (Revex) and naltrexone (ReVia) are also pure opioid antagonists with a high affinity for the μ receptor. Both have significantly longer half-lives than naloxone. Nalmefene is used for suspected opioid overdose and complete or partial reversal of perioperative, opioid-induced respiratory depression. It may be given intravenously, intramuscularly, or subcutaneously. To reverse opioid-induced postoperative respiratory depression, nalmefene is administered intravenously in 0.25 μg/kg increments every 2–5 min up to a total of 1 μg/kg. For a suspected opioid overdose the recommended dose of nalmefene is 0.5 mg/70 kg, up to a maximum of 1.5 mg/70 kg. Naltrexone is used orally for maintenance treatment of opioid addicts and for ethanol abuse. In the latter instance, it appears to block some of the pleasant effects of alcohol in some individuals.

FLUMAZENIL

Mechanism of Action

Flumazenil, an imidazobenzodiazepine, is a specific and competitive antagonist of benzodiazepines at benzodiazepine receptors (see Figure 8–5).

Clinical Uses

 Flumazenil is useful in the reversal of benzodiazepine sedation and the treatment of benzodiazepine overdose. Although it promptly (onset < 1 min) reverses the hypnotic effects of benzodiazepines, amnesia has proved to be less reliably prevented. Some evidence of respiratory depression may linger despite an alert and awake appearance. Specifically, tidal volume and minute ventilation return to normal, but the slope of the carbon dioxide response curve remains depressed (see Figure 8–8). Elderly patients appear to be particularly difficult to reverse fully and are more prone to resedation.

Side Effects & Drug Interactions

Rapid administration of flumazenil may cause anxiety reactions in previously sedated patients and symptoms of withdrawal in those on long-term benzodiazepine therapy. Flumazenil reversal has been associated with increases in intracranial pressure in patients with head injuries and abnormal intracranial compliance. Flumazenil may induce seizure activity if benzodiazepines have been given as anticonvulsants or in conjunction with an overdose of tricyclic antidepressants. Flumazenil reversal following a midazolam–ketamine anesthetic technique may increase the incidence of emergence dysphoria and hallucinations. Nausea and vomiting are not uncommon following administration of flumazenil. The reversal effect of flumazenil is based on its strong affinity for benzodiazepine receptors, a *pharmacodynamic* (not pharmacokinetic) effect. Flumazenil does not affect the minimum alveolar concentration of inhalation anesthetics.

Dosage

Gradual titration of flumazenil is usually accomplished by intravenous administration of 0.2 mg/min until reaching the desired degree of reversal. The usual total dose is 0.6–1.0 mg. Because of flumazenil's rapid hepatic clearance, repeat doses may be required after 1–2 h to avoid resedation and premature recovery room or outpatient discharge. A continuous infusion (0.5 mg/h) may be helpful in the case of an overdose of a longer-acting benzodiazepine. Liver failure prolongs the clearance of flumazenil and benzodiazepines.

CASE DISCUSSION: MANAGEMENT OF PATIENTS AT RISK FOR ASPIRATION PNEUMONIA

A 58-year-old man is scheduled for elective inguinal hernia repair. His past history reveals a persistent problem with heartburn and passive regurgitation of gastric contents into the pharynx. He has been told by his internist that these symptoms are due to a hiatal hernia.

Why would a history of hiatal hernia concern the anesthesiologist?

Perioperative aspiration of gastric contents (Mendelson's syndrome) is a potentially fatal complication of anesthesia. Hiatal hernia is commonly associated with symptomatic GERD, which is considered a predisposing factor for aspiration. Mild or occasional heartburn may not significantly increase the risk of aspiration. In contrast, symptoms related to passive reflux of gastric fluid, such as acid taste or sensation of refluxing liquid into the mouth, should alert the clinician to a high risk of pulmonary aspiration. Paroxysms of coughing and/or wheezing, particularly at night or when the patient is flat, may be indicative of chronic aspiration. Aspiration can occur on induction, during maintenance, or upon emergence from anesthesia.

Which patients are predisposed to aspiration?

Patients with altered airway reflexes (eg, drug intoxication, general anesthesia, encephalopathy, neuromuscular disease) or abnormal pharyngeal or esophageal anatomy (eg, large hiatal hernia, Zenker's diverticulum, scleroderma, pregnancy, obesity) are prone to pulmonary aspiration.

Does aspiration consistently result in aspiration pneumonia?

Not necessarily. The seriousness of the lung damage depends on the volume and composition of the aspirate. Traditionally, patients are considered to be at risk if their gastric volume is greater than 25 mL (0.4 mL/kg) and their gastric pH is less than 2.5. Some investigators believe that controlling acidity is more important than volume and that the criteria should be revised to a pH less than 3.5 with a volume greater than 50 mL.

Patients who have eaten immediately prior to emergency surgery are obviously at risk. Traditionally, "NPO after midnight" implied a preoperative fast of at least 6 h. Current opinion allows clear liquids until 2–4 h before induction of anesthesia, although solids are still taboo for 6 h in adult patients. Some patients who have fasted for 8 h or more before elective surgery also meet the at-risk criteria, however. Certain patient populations are particularly likely to have large volumes of acidic gastric fluid: patients with an acute abdomen or peptic ulcer disease, children, the elderly, diabetic patients, pregnant women, and obese patients. Furthermore, pain, anxiety, or opioid-agonists may delay gastric emptying. Note that pregnancy and obesity place patients in double jeopardy by increasing the chance of aspiration (increased intra-abdominal pressure and distortion of the lower esophageal sphincter) and the risk of aspiration pneumonia (increased acidity and volume of gastric contents). Aspiration is more common in patients undergoing esophageal, upper abdominal, or emergency laparoscopic surgery.

Which drugs lower the risk of aspiration pneumonia?

H_2-Receptor antagonists decrease gastric acid secretion. Although they will not affect gastric contents already in the stomach, they will inhibit further acid production. Both gastric pH and volume are affected. In addition, the long duration of action of ranitidine and famotidine may provide protection in the recovery room.

Metoclopramide shortens gastric emptying time, increases lower esophageal sphincter tone, and is an antiemetic. It does not affect gastric pH, and it cannot clear large volumes of food in a few hours. Nonetheless, metoclopramide with ranitidine is a good combination for most at-risk patients. Antacids usually raise gastric fluid pH, but, at the same time, they increase gastric volume. Although antacid administration technically removes a patient from the at-risk category, aspiration of a substantial volume of particulate matter will lead to serious physiological damage. For this reason, clear antacids (eg, sodium citrate) are strongly preferred. In contrast to H_2 antagonists, antacids are immediately effective and alter the acidity of existing gastric contents. Thus, they are useful in emergency situations and in patients who have recently eaten.

Anticholinergic drugs (see Chapter 11), particularly glycopyrrolate, decrease gastric secretions if large doses are administered; however, lower esophageal sphincter tone is reduced. Overall, anticholinergic drugs do not reliably reduce the risk of aspiration pneumonia and can reverse the protective effects of metoclopramide. The role of proton pump inhibitors is not clear; they are generally as effective as H_2 antagonists.

What anesthetic techniques are used in full-stomach patients?

If the full stomach is due to recent food intake and the surgical procedure is elective, the operation should be postponed. If the risk factor is not reversible (eg, large hiatal hernia) or the case is emergent, proper anesthetic technique can minimize the risk of aspiration pneumonia. Regional anesthesia with minimal sedation should be considered in patients at increased risk for aspiration pneumonia. If local anesthetic techniques are impractical, the patient's airway must be protected. Delivering anesthesia by mask or laryngeal mask airway is contraindicated. As in every anesthetic case, the availability of suction must be confirmed before induction. If there are signs suggesting a difficult airway, intubation should precede induction (see Case Discussion, Chapter 5). Otherwise, a rapid-sequence induction is indicated.

How does a rapid-sequence induction differ from a routine induction?

- The patient is always preoxygenated prior to induction. Four maximal breaths of oxygen are sufficient to denitrogenate normal lungs. Patients with lung disease require 3–5 min of preoxygenation.
- Prior curarization with a nondepolarizing muscle relaxant may prevent the increase in intra-abdominal pressure that accompanies the fasciculations caused by succinylcholine. This step is often omitted, however, as it can decrease lower esophageal sphincter tone. If rocuronium has been selected for relaxation, a small priming dose (0.1 mg/kg) given 2–3 min prior to induction may speed its onset of action.
- A wide assortment of blades and endotracheal tubes are prepared in advance. It is prudent to begin with a stylet and an endotracheal tube one-half size smaller than usual to maximize the chances of an easy intubation.
- An assistant applies firm pressure over the cricoid cartilage prior to induction (Sellick's maneuver). Because the cricoid cartilage forms an uninterrupted and incompressible ring, pressure over it is transmitted to underlying tissue. The esophagus is collapsed, and passively regurgitated gastric fluid cannot reach the hypopharynx. Excessive cricoid pressure

(beyond what can be tolerated by a conscious person) applied during active regurgitation has been associated with rupture of the posterior wall of the esophagus.

- Usually propofol or thiopental is used. In the latter instance, no test dose of thiopental is given. The induction dose is given as a bolus. Obviously, this dose must be modified if there is any indication that the patient's cardiovascular system is unstable. Other rapid-acting induction agents can be substituted (eg, etomidate, ketamine).

- Succinylcholine (1.5 mg/kg) or rocuronium (0.9–1.2 mg/kg) is administered immediately following the thiopental, even if the patient has not yet lost consciousness.

- The patient is not artificially ventilated, to avoid filling the stomach with gas and thereby increasing the risk of emesis. Once spontaneous efforts have ceased or muscle response to nerve stimulation has disappeared, the patient is rapidly intubated. Cricoid pressure is maintained until the endotracheal tube cuff is inflated and tube position is confirmed. A modification of the classic rapid-sequence induction allows gentle ventilation as long as cricoid pressure is maintained.

- If the intubation proves difficult, cricoid pressure is maintained and the patient is gently ventilated with oxygen until another intubation attempt can be performed. If intubation is still unsuccessful, spontaneous ventilation should be allowed to return and an awake intubation performed (see Figure 5–21).

- After surgery, the patient should remain intubated until airway reflexes have returned and consciousness has been regained.

What are the relative contraindications to rapid-sequence inductions?

Rapid-sequence inductions are usually associated with increases in intracranial pressure, arterial blood pressure, and heart rate. Contraindications to succinylcholine also apply (eg, thermal burns).

Describe the pathophysiology and clinical findings associated with aspiration pneumonia.

The pathophysiological changes depend on the composition of the aspirate. Acid solutions cause atelectasis, alveolar edema, and loss of surfactant. Particulate aspirate will also result in small-airway obstruction and alveolar necrosis. Granulomas may form around food or antacid particles. The earliest physiological change following aspiration is intrapulmonary shunting, resulting in hypoxia. Other changes may include pulmonary edema, pulmonary hypertension, and hypercapnia.

Wheezing, rhonchi, tachycardia, and tachypnea are common physical findings. Decreased lung compliance can make ventilation difficult. Hypotension signals significant fluid shifts into the alveoli and is associated with massive lung injury. Chest roentgenography may not demonstrate diffuse bilateral infiltrates for several hours after the event. Arterial blood gases reveal hypoxemia, hypercapnia, and respiratory acidosis.

What is the treatment for aspiration pneumonia?

As soon as regurgitation is suspected, the patient should be placed in a head-down position so that gastric contents drain out of the mouth instead of into the trachea. The pharynx and, if possible, the trachea should be thoroughly suctioned. The mainstay of therapy in patients who subsequently become hypoxic is positive-pressure ventilation. Intubation and the institution of positive end-expiratory pressure or continuous positive airway pressure are often required. Bronchoscopy, pulmonary lavage, and broad-spectrum antibiotics are usually not indicated except possibly when particulate aspiration has occurred. Use of corticosteroids is generally not recommended.

SUGGESTED READING

Birmacombe JR, Berry AM: Cricoid pressure. Can J Anaesth 1997;44:414.

Bovill JG, Howie MB: *Clinical Pharmacology for Anaesthetists.* W.B. Saunders, 1999.

Evers AS, Maze M: *Anesthetic Pharmacology—Physiologic Principles and Clinical Practice.* Churchill Livingstone, 2004.

Ferrari LR, Rooney FM, Rockoff MA: Preoperative fasting practices in pediatrics. Anesthesiology 1999;90:978.

Kovac AL: Prevention and treatment of postoperative nausea and vomiting. Drugs 2000;59:213.

Practice guidelines for preoperative fasting and the use of pharmacologic agents to reduce the risk of pulmonary aspiration: Application to healthy patients undergoing elective procedures. A report by the American Society of Anesthesiologists Task Force on Preoperative Fasting. Anesthesiology 1999;90:896.

Schreiner MS: Gastric fluid volume: Is it really a risk factor for pulmonary aspiration? Anesth Analg 1998;86:754.

Warner MA, Warner ME, Warner DO, et al: Clinical significance of pulmonary aspiration during the perioperative period. Anesthesiology 1993;78:56.

Whitwam JG, Amrein R: Pharmacology of flumazenil. Acta Anaesthesiol Scand Suppl 1995;108:3.

SECTION III
Regional Anesthesia & Pain Management

Spinal, Epidural, & Caudal Blocks

16

Wayne Kleinman, MD, & Maged Mikhail, MD*

KEY CONCEPTS

 1 Spinal, epidural, and caudal blocks are also known as neuraxial anesthesia. Each of these blocks can be performed as a single injection or with a catheter to allow intermittent boluses or continuous infusions.

 2 Performing a lumbar (subarachnoid) puncture below L1 in an adult (L3 in a child) avoids potential needle trauma to the cord.

 3 The principal site of action for neuraxial blockade is the nerve root.

 4 Differential blockade typically results in sympathetic blockade (judged by temperature sensitivity) that may be two segments higher than the sensory block (pain, light touch), which in turn is usually two segments higher than the motor blockade.

 5 Interruption of efferent autonomic transmission at the spinal nerve roots can produce sympathetic and some parasympathetic blockade.

 6 Neuraxial blocks typically produce variable decreases in blood pressure that may be accompanied by a decrease in heart rate and cardiac contractility.

 7 Deleterious cardiovascular effects should be anticipated and steps undertaken to minimize the degree of hypotension. Volume loading with 10–20 mL/kg of intravenous fluid for a healthy patient will partially compensate for the venous pooling.

 8 Excessive or symptomatic bradycardia should be treated with atropine, and hypotension should be treated with vasopressors.

 9 Major contraindications to neuraxial anesthesia are patient refusal, bleeding diathesis, severe hypovolemia, elevated intracranial pressure, infection at the site of injection, and severe stenotic valvular heart disease or ventricular outflow obstruction.

(continued on next page)

---

*Director of Obstetric Anesthesia, Encino-Tarzana Regional Medical Center, Los Angeles, California.

(continued from previous page)

 For epidural anesthesia, a sudden loss of resistance is encountered as the needle penetrates the ligamentum flavum and enters the epidural space. For spinal anesthesia, the needle is advanced further through the epidural space and penetrates the dura–subarachnoid membranes as signaled by free flowing cerebrospinal fluid.

 Epidural anesthesia is a neuraxial technique offering a range of applications wider than the typical all-or-nothing spinal anesthetic. An epidural block can be performed at the lumbar, thoracic, or cervical level.

 Epidural techniques are widely used for operative anesthesia, obstetric analgesia, postoperative pain control, and chronic pain management.

 Epidural anesthesia is slower in onset (10–20 min) and may not be as dense as spinal anesthesia.

 The quantity (volume and concentration) of local anesthetic needed for epidural anesthesia is very large compared with spinal anesthesia. Significant toxicity can occur if this amount is injected intrathecally or intravascularly. Safeguards against this include the epidural test dose and incremental dosing.

 Caudal epidural anesthesia is one of the most commonly used regional techniques in pediatric patients.

Spinal, caudal, and epidural blocks were first used for surgical procedures at the turn of the twentieth century (see Chapter 1). These central blocks were widely used prior to the 1940s until increasing reports of permanent neurological injury appeared. However, a large-scale epidemiological study conducted in the 1950s indicated that complications were rare when these blocks were performed skillfully with attention to asepsis and when newer, safer local anesthetics were used. A resurgence in the use of central blocks ensued, and today they are once again widely used in clinical practice.

Spinal, epidural, and caudal blocks are also known as neuraxial anesthesia. Each of these blocks can be performed as a single injection or with a catheter to allow intermittent boluses or continuous infusions. Neuraxial anesthesia greatly expands the anesthesiologists' armamentarium, providing alternatives to general anesthesia when appropriate. They may also be used simultaneously with general anesthesia or afterward for postoperative analgesia and for the management of acute and chronic pain disorders (see Chapter 18).

Neuraxial techniques have proved to be extremely safe when managed well; however, there is still a risk for complications. Adverse reactions and complications range from self-limited back soreness to debilitating permanent neurological deficits and even death. The practitioner must therefore have a good understanding of the anatomy involved, be thoroughly familiar with the pharmacology and toxic dosages of the agents employed, dili-

gently employ sterile techniques, and anticipate and quickly treat physiological derangements.

THE ROLE OF NEURAXIAL ANESTHESIA IN ANESTHETIC PRACTICE

Almost all operations below the neck can be performed under neuraxial anesthesia. However, because intrathoracic, upper abdominal, and laparoscopic operations can significantly impair ventilation, general anesthesia with endotracheal intubation is also necessary. So why do a regional anesthetic for these cases, or for any other cases?

Some clinical studies suggest that postoperative morbidity—and possibly mortality—may be reduced when neuraxial blockade is used either alone or in combination with general anesthesia in some settings. Neuraxial blocks may reduce the incidence of venous thrombosis and pulmonary embolism, cardiac complications in high-risk patients, bleeding and transfusion requirements, vascular graft occlusion, and pneumonia and respiratory depression following upper abdominal or thoracic surgery in patients with chronic lung disease. Neuraxial blocks may also allow earlier return of gastrointestinal function following surgery. Proposed mechanisms include amelioration of the hypercoagulable state associated with surgery, sympathectomy-mediated increases in tissue blood flow, improved oxygenation from decreased splinting, enhanced peristalsis, and suppression of the neuroendocrine stress response to surgery. For patients with coronary artery disease, a decreased stress response may result in less perioperative ischemia and reduced morbidity and mortality. The increasing use of perioperative β-blockade to reduce perioperative cardiac complications, however, may minimize or eliminate the potential advantage of neuraxial anesthesia in this setting. Reduction of parenteral opioid requirements may decrease the incidence of atelectasis, hypoventilation, and aspiration pneumonia. Postoperative epidural analgesia may also significantly reduce the time until extubation and reduce the need for mechanical ventilation after major abdominal or thoracic surgery.

The Sick Elderly Patient

Anesthesiologists are all too familiar with situations in which a consultant "clears" a sick elderly patient with significant cardiac disease for surgery "under spinal anesthesia." But is a spinal anesthetic really safer than general anesthesia for such a patient? A spinal anesthetic with no intravenous sedation may reduce the likelihood of postoperative delirium or cognitive dysfunction, which is sometimes seen in the elderly. Unfortunately, some, if not most, patients require some sedation during the course of the procedure, either for comfort or to facilitate cooperation. And is spinal anesthesia always safer for a patient with severe coronary artery disease or a decreased ejection fraction? Ideally an anesthetic technique in such a patient should not involve either hypotension (which decreases myocardial perfusion pressure) or hypertension or tachycardia (which increase myocardial oxygen consumption), and should not require large fluid infusion (which can precipitate congestive heart failure). Unfortunately, a spinal anesthetic is often associated with hypotension and bradycardia, which may be rapid in onset and is sometimes profound. Moreover, treatment may require rapid administration of intravenous fluid, vasopressors, and/or an anticholinergic, which can cause fluid overload (when the vasodilatation wears off), rebound hypertension, and tachycardia. The slower onset of hypotension and bradycardia following epidural anesthesia may give the anesthesiologist more time to correct hemodynamic changes, although they still occur. Some clinicians avoid epidural anesthesia in elderly patients who may have spinal stenosis, fearing the mass effect of the bolus of anesthetic might compromise spinal cord perfusion. General anesthesia, on the other hand, also poses potential problems for patients with cardiac compromise. Most general anesthetics are cardiac depressants and many cause vasodilatation. Deep anesthesia can readily cause hypotension, whereas light anesthesia relative to the level of stimulation causes hypertension and tachycardia. Insertion of a laryngeal mask airway causes less of a stress response than endotracheal intubation, but deeper levels of general anesthesia are still required to blunt the response to surgical stimulation.

Thus arguments can be made for and against neuraxial and regional anesthesia in this setting. Perhaps then it is not the technique that is critical as much as the careful execution of whatever anesthetic technique is planned.

The Obstetric Patient

Neuraxial anesthesia has had a great impact in obstetrics (see Chapter 43). Currently, epidural anesthesia is widely used for analgesia in women in labor and during vaginal delivery. Cesarean section is most commonly performed under epidural or spinal anesthesia. Both blocks allow a mother to remain awake and experience the birth of her child. Large population studies in Great Britain and in the United States have shown that regional anesthesia for cesarean section is associated with less maternal morbidity and mortality than is general anesthesia. This may be largely due to a reduction in the incidence of pulmonary aspiration and failed intubation.

◼ ANATOMY

THE VERTEBRAL COLUMN

The spine is composed of the vertebral bones and fibrocartilaginous intervertebral disks (Figure 16–1). There are 7 cervical, 12 thoracic, and 5 lumbar vertebra (Figure 16–2). The sacrum is a fusion of 5 sacral vertebra, and there are small rudimentary coccygeal vertebra. The spine as a whole provides structural support for the body and protection for the spinal cord and nerves, and allows a degree of mobility in several spatial planes. At each vertebral level, paired spinal nerves exit the central nervous system (Figure 16–2).

Vertebra differ in shape and size at the various levels. The first cervical vertebra, the atlas, lacks a body and has unique articulations with the base of the skull and the second vertebra. The second vertebra, also called the axis, consequently has atypical articulating surfaces. All 12 thoracic vertebrae articulate with their corresponding rib. Lumbar vertebrae have a large anterior cylindrical vertebral body. A hollow ring is defined anteriorly by the vertebral body, laterally by the pedicles and transverse processes, and posteriorly by the lamina and spinous processes (Figure 16–1B and C). The laminae extend between the transverse processes and the spinous processes and the pedicle extends between the vertebral body and the transverse processes. When stacked vertically, the hollow rings become the spinal canal in

Figure 16–1. Sagittal section through lumbar vertebrae (**A**). Common features of vertebrae (**B, C**).

which the spinal cord and its coverings sit. The individual vertebral bodies are connected by the intervertebral disks. There are four small synovial joints at each vertebra, two articulating with the vertebra above it and two with the vertebra below. These are the facet joints, which are adjacent to the transverse processes (Figure 16–1C). The pedicles are notched superiorly and inferiorly, these notches forming the intervertebral foramina, from which the spinal nerves exit. Sacral vertebrae normally fuse into one large bone, the sacrum, but each one retains discrete anterior and posterior intervertebral foramina. The laminae of S5 and all or part of S4 normally do not fuse, leaving a caudal opening to the spinal canal, the sacral hiatus (Figure 16–3).

The spinal column normally forms a double C, being convex anteriorly in the cervical and lumbar regions (Figure 16–2). Ligamentous elements provide structural support and together with supporting muscles help maintain the unique shape. Ventrally, the vertebral bodies and intervertebral disks are connected and supported by the

Figure 16–2. The vertebral column. (Adapted, with permission, from Waxman SG: *Correlative Neuroanatomy*, 24th ed. McGraw-Hill, 2000.)

anterior and posterior longitudinal ligaments (Figure 16–1A). Dorsally, the ligamentum flavum, interspinous ligament, and supraspinous ligament provide additional stability. Using the midline approach, a needle passes through these three dorsal ligaments and through an oval space between the bony lamina and spinous processes of adjacent vertebra (Figure 16–4).

THE SPINAL CORD

The spinal canal contains the spinal cord with its coverings (the meninges), fatty tissue, and a venous plexus (Figure 16–5). The meninges are composed of three layers: the pia mater, the arachnoid mater, and the dura mater; all are contiguous with their cranial counterparts (Figure 16–6). The pia mater is closely adherent to the spinal cord, whereas the arachnoid mater is usually closely adherent to the thicker and denser dura mater. Cerebrospinal fluid (CSF) is contained between the pia and arachnoid maters in the subarachnoid space (see Chapter 25). The spinal subdural space is generally a poorly demarcated, potential space that exists between the dura and arachnoid membranes. The epidural space is a better defined potential space within the spinal canal that is bounded by the dura and the ligamentum flavum (Figures 16–1 and 16–5). The anatomy of the spinal cord is further discussed in Chapter 18.

The spinal cord normally extends from the foramen magnum to the level of L1 in adults (Figure 16–7). In children, the spinal cord ends at L3 and moves up as they grow older. The anterior and posterior nerve roots at each spinal level join one another and exit the intervertebral foramina forming spinal nerves from C1 to S5 (Figure 16–2). At the cervical level, the nerves arise above their respective vertebrae, but starting at T1 they exit below their vertebrae. As a result, there are eight cervical nerve roots but only seven cervical vertebrae. The cervical and upper thoracic nerve roots emerge from the spinal cord and exit the vertebral foramina nearly at the same level (Figure 16–2). But because the spinal cord normally ends at L1, lower nerve roots course some distance before exiting the intervertebral foramina. These lower spinal nerves form the cauda equina ("horse's tail"; Figure 16–2). Therefore, performing a lumbar (subarachnoid) puncture below L1 in an adult (L3 in a child) avoids potential needle trauma to the cord; damage to the cauda equina is unlikely as these nerve roots float in the dural sac below L1 and tend to be pushed away (rather than pierced) by an advancing needle.

A dural sheath invests most nerve roots for a small distance even after they exit the spinal canal (Figure 16–5). Nerve blocks close to the intervertebral foramen therefore carry a risk of subdural or subarachnoid injection (see Chapter 17). The dural sac and the subarachnoid and subdural spaces usually extend to S2 in adults and often to S3 in children. Because of this fact and the smaller body size,

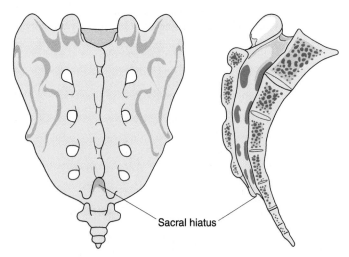

Figure 16–3. Posterior and sagittal views of the sacrum and coccyx.

caudal anesthesia carries a greater risk of subarachnoid injection in children than in adults. An extension of the pia mater, the filum terminale, penetrates the dura and attaches the terminal end of the spinal cord (conus medullaris) to the periostium of the coccyx (Figure 16–7).

The blood supply to the spinal cord and nerve roots is derived from a single anterior spinal artery and paired posterior spinal arteries (Figure 16–8). The anterior spinal artery is formed from the vertebral artery at the base of the skull and courses down along the anterior surface of the cord. The anterior spinal artery supplies the anterior two-thirds of the cord, whereas the two posterior spinal arteries supply the posterior one-third. The posterior spinal arteries arise from the posterior inferior cerebellar arteries and

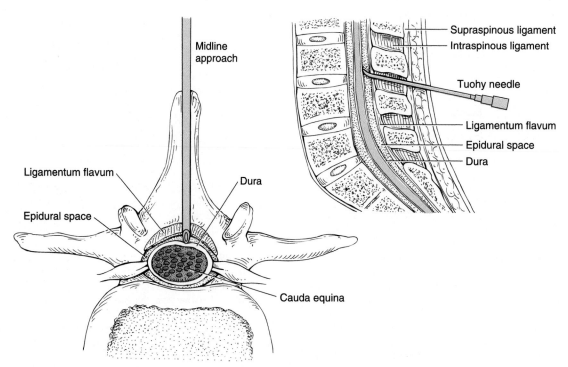

Figure 16–4. Lumbar epidural anesthesia; midline approach.

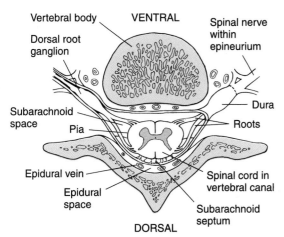

Vertebral body
VENTRAL
Dorsal root ganglion
Spinal nerve within epineurium
Subarachnoid space
Pia
Dura
Roots
Epidural vein
Epidural space
Spinal cord in vertebral canal
Subarachnoid septum
DORSAL

Figure 16–5. **Exit of the spinal nerves.** (Adapted, with permission, from Waxman SG: *Correlative Neuroanatomy,* 24th ed. McGraw-Hill, 2000.)

course down along the dorsal surface of the cord medial to the dorsal nerve roots (see Chapter 25). The anterior and posterior spinal arteries receive additional blood flow from the intercostal arteries in the thorax and the lumbar arteries in the abdomen. One of these radicular arteries is typically large, the artery of Adamkiewicz, or arteria radicularis magna, arising from the aorta (Figures 16–8A). It is typically unilateral and nearly always arises on the left side, providing the major blood supply to the anterior, lower two-thirds of the spinal cord. Injury to this artery can result in the anterior spinal artery syndrome (see Chapters 21 and 33).

■ MECHANISM OF ACTION

The principal site of action for neuraxial blockade is the nerve root. Local anesthetic is injected into CSF (spinal anesthesia) or the epidural space (epidural and caudal anesthesia) and bathes the nerve root in the subarachnoid space or epidural space, respectively. Direct injection of local anesthetic into CSF for spinal anesthesia allows a relatively small dose and volume of local anesthetic to achieve dense sensory and motor blockade. In contrast, the same local anesthetic concentration is achieved at nerve roots only with much higher volumes and quantities of local anesthetic with epidural and caudal anesthesia. Moreover, the injection site (level) for epidural anesthesia must generally be close to the nerve roots that must be anesthetized. Blockade of neural transmission (conduction) in the posterior nerve

root fibers interrupts somatic and visceral sensation, whereas blockade of anterior nerve root fibers prevents efferent motor and autonomic outflow (see Chapter 18).

SOMATIC BLOCKADE

By interrupting the transmission of painful stimuli and abolishing skeletal muscle tone, neuraxial blocks can provide excellent operating conditions. Sensory blockade interrupts both somatic and visceral painful stimuli, whereas motor blockade produces skeletal muscle relaxation. The mechanism of action for local anesthetic agents is discussed in Chapter 14. The effect of local anesthetics on nerve fibers varies according to the size of the nerve fiber, whether it is myelinated, and the con-

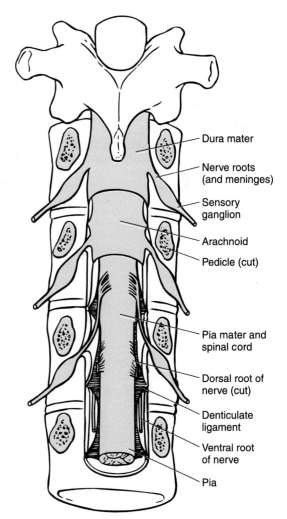

Dura mater
Nerve roots (and meninges)
Sensory ganglion
Arachnoid
Pedicle (cut)
Pia mater and spinal cord
Dorsal root of nerve (cut)
Denticulate ligament
Ventral root of nerve
Pia

Figure 16–6. **The spinal cord.**

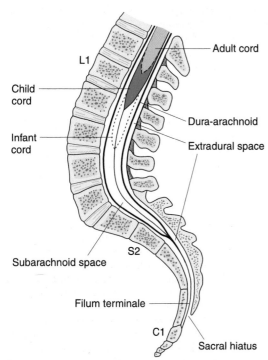

Figure 16–7. Sagittal view through the lumbar vertebrae and sacrum. Note the end of the spinal cord rises with development from approximately L3 to L1. The dural sac normally ends at S2.

centration achieved and the duration of contact (Chapter 14). Spinal nerve roots contain varying mixtures of these fiber types. Smaller and myelinated fibers are generally more easily blocked than larger and unmyelinated ones. This, and the fact that the concentration of local anesthetic decreases with increasing distance from the level of injection, explains the phenomenon of differential blockade. Differential blockade typically results in sympathetic blockade (judged by temperature sensitivity) that may be two segments higher than the sensory block (pain, light touch), which in turn is usually two segments higher than the motor blockade.

AUTONOMIC BLOCKADE

Interruption of efferent autonomic transmission at the spinal nerve roots can produce sympathetic and some parasympathetic blockade (see Chapters 11 and 12). Sympathetic outflow from the spinal cord may be described as thoracolumbar, whereas parasympathetic outflow is craniosacral. Sympathetic preganglionic nerve fibers (small, myelinated B

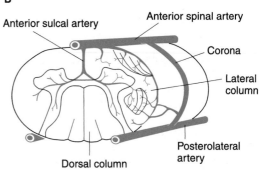

Figure 16–8. Arterial supply to the spinal cord. Anterior view showing principal sources of blood supply (**A**). Cross-sectional view through the spinal cord showing paired posterior spinal arteries and a single anterior spinal artery (**B**). (Adapted, with permission, from Waxman SG: *Correlative Neuroanatomy*, 24th ed. McGraw-Hill, 2000.)

fibers) exit the spinal cord with the spinal nerves from T1 to the L2 level and may course many levels up or down the sympathetic chain before synapsing with a postganglionic cell in a sympathetic ganglia. In contrast, parasympathetic preganglionic fibers exit the spinal cord with the cranial and sacral nerves. Neuraxial anesthesia does not block the vagus nerve (tenth cranial nerve). The physiological responses of neuraxial blockade therefore result from decreased sympathetic tone and/or unopposed parasympathetic tone.

Cardiovascular Manifestations

Neuraxial blocks typically produce variable decreases in blood pressure that may be accompanied by a decrease in heart rate and cardiac contractility. These effects are generally proportional to the degree (level) of the sympathectomy. Vasomotor tone is primarily determined by sympathetic fibers arising from T5 to L1, innervating arterial and venous smooth muscle. Blocking these nerves causes vasodilation of the venous capacitance vessels, pooling of blood, and decreased venous return to the heart; in some instances, arterial vasodilation may also decrease systemic vascular resistance. The effects of arterial vasodilation may be minimized by compensatory vasoconstriction above the level of the block. A high sympathetic block not only prevents compensatory vasoconstriction but also blocks the sympathetic cardiac accelerator fibers that arise at T1–T4 (see Chapter 12). Profound hypotension may result from vasodilation combined with bradycardia and decreased contractility. These effects are exaggerated if venous return is further compromised by a head-up position or by the weight of a gravid uterus. Unopposed vagal tone may explain the sudden cardiac arrest sometimes seen with spinal anesthesia (see Chapter 46).

Deleterious cardiovascular effects should be anticipated and steps undertaken to minimize the degree of hypotension. Volume loading with 10–20 mL/kg of intravenous fluid for a healthy patient will partially compensate for the venous pooling. Left uterine displacement in the third trimester of pregnancy helps minimize physical obstruction to venous return (see Chapter 42). Despite these efforts, hypotension may still occur and should be treated promptly. Fluid administration can be increased, and autotransfusion may be accomplished by placing the patient in a head-down position. Excessive or symptomatic bradycardia should be treated with atropine, and hypotension should be treated with vasopressors. Direct α-adrenergic agonists (such as phenylephrine) increase venous tone and produce arteriolar constriction, increasing both venous return and systemic vascular resistance. Ephedrine has direct β-adrenergic effects that increase heart rate and contractility and indirect effects that also produce some vasoconstriction. If profound hypotension and/or bradycardia persist despite these interventions, epinephrine (5–10 μg intravenously) should be administered promptly.

Pulmonary Manifestations

Clinically significant alterations in pulmonary physiology are usually minimal with neuraxial blocks because the diaphragm is innervated by the phrenic nerve with fibers originating from C3–C5. Even with high thoracic levels, tidal volume is unchanged; there is only a small decrease in vital capacity, which results from a loss of the abdominal muscles' contribution to forced expiration. Phrenic nerve block may not occur even with total spinal anesthesia as apnea often resolves with hemodynamic resuscitation, suggesting that brain stem hypoperfusion is responsible rather than phrenic nerve block. The concentration of local anesthetic, even with a cervical sensory level, is reported to be below that required to block the large Aα fibers of the phrenic nerve.

Patients with severe chronic lung disease may rely upon accessory muscles of respiration (intercostal and abdominal muscles) to actively inspire or exhale. High levels of neural blockade will impair these muscles. Similarly, effective coughing and clearing of secretions require these muscles for expiration. For these reasons, neuraxial blocks should be used with caution in patients with limited respiratory reserve. These deleterious effects need to be weighed against the advantages of avoiding airway instrumentation and positive-pressure ventilation. For surgical procedures above the umbilicus, a pure regional technique may not be the best choice for patients with severe lung disease. On the other hand, these patients may benefit from the effects of thoracic epidural analgesia (with dilute local anesthetics and opioids) in the postoperative period, particularly following upper abdominal or thoracic surgery. Thoracic or upper abdominal surgery is associated with decreased diaphragmatic function postoperatively (from decreased phrenic nerve activity) and decreased functional residual capacity (FRC), which can lead to atelectasis and hypoxia via ventilation/perfusion (V̇/Q̇) mismatch. Some evidence suggests that postoperative thoracic epidural analgesia in high-risk patients can improve pulmonary outcome by decreasing the incidence of pneumonia and respiratory failure, improving oxygenation, and decreasing the duration of mechanical ventilatory support.

Gastrointestinal Manifestations

Sympathetic outflow originates at the T5–L1 level. Neuraxial block–induced sympathectomy allows vagal tone dominance and results in a small, contracted gut with active peristalsis. This can provide excellent operative conditions for some laparoscopic procedures when used as an adjunct to general anesthesia. Postoperative epidural analgesia has been shown to hasten return of gastrointestinal function.

Hepatic blood flow will decrease with reductions in mean arterial pressure from any anesthetic technique. For intraabdominal surgery, the decrease in hepatic perfusion is related more to surgical manipulation than to anesthetic technique (see Chapter 34).

Urinary Tract Manifestations

Renal blood flow is maintained through autoregulation, and there is little clinical effect upon renal function from neuraxial blockade. Neuraxial anesthesia at the lumbar and sacral levels blocks both sympathetic and parasympathetic control of bladder function. Loss of autonomic bladder control results in urinary retention until the block wears off. If no urinary catheter is anticipated perioperatively, it is prudent to use the shortest acting and smallest amount of drug necessary for the surgical procedure and limit the amount of intravenous fluid administration (if possible). The patient should be monitored for urinary retention to avoid bladder distention following neuraxial anesthesia.

Metabolic & Endocrine Manifestations

Surgical trauma produces a neuroendocrine response via a localized inflammatory response and activation of somatic and visceral afferent nerve fibers. This response includes increases in adrenocorticotropic hormone, cortisol, epinephrine, norepinephrine, and vasopressin levels as well as activation of the renin–angiotensin–aldosterone system. Clinical manifestations include intraoperative and postoperative hypertension, tachycardia, hyperglycemia, protein catabolism, suppressed immune responses, and altered renal function. Neuraxial blockade can partially suppress (during major invasive surgery) or totally block (during lower extremity surgery) this stress response. By reducing catecholamine release, neuraxial blocks may decrease perioperative arrhythmias and possibly reduce the incidence of ischemia. To maximize this blunting of the neuroendocrine stress response, neuraxial block should precede incision and extend into the postoperative period.

■ CLINICAL CONSIDERATIONS COMMON TO SPINAL & EPIDURAL BLOCKS

Indications

Neuraxial blocks may be used alone or in conjunction with general anesthesia for most procedures below the neck. Indeed in some European centers, cardiac surgery has been routinely performed under thoracic epidural anesthesia (typically with light general anesthesia). As a primary anesthetic, neuraxial blocks have proved most useful for lower abdominal, inguinal, urogenital, rectal, and lower extremity surgery. Lumbar spinal surgery may also be performed under spinal anesthesia. Upper abdominal procedures (eg, cholecystectomy) can be performed with spinal or epidural anesthesia, but it can be difficult to achieve a sensory level adequate for patient comfort yet avoid the complications of a high block. Spinal anesthesia has been used for neonatal surgery.

If a neuraxial anesthetic is being considered, the risks and benefits need to be discussed with the patient, and an informed consent should be obtained. It is important to ascertain that the patient is mentally prepared for neuraxial anesthesia, that the choice of anesthesia is appropriate for the type of surgery, and that there are no contraindications. Patients should understand that they will have little or no motor function until the block resolves. Procedures that involve major blood loss, maneuvers that might compromise respiratory function, or unusually prolonged surgery should generally be performed under general endotracheal anesthesia with or without neuraxial blockade.

Contraindications

Major contraindications to neuraxial anesthesia are patient refusal, bleeding diathesis, severe hypovolemia, elevated intracranial pressure, infection at the site of injection, and severe stenotic valvular heart disease or ventricular outflow obstruction.

Relative and controversial contraindications are also listed in (Table 16–1). Physical examination of the back can reveal important information, such as the presence of surgical scars, scoliosis, skin lesions, and whether the spinous processes are palpable. Although no preoperative screening tests are required for healthy patients undergoing neuraxial blockade, coagulation studies and platelet count should be checked when the clinical history suggests the possibility of a bleeding diathesis. Neuraxial anesthesia in the presence of sepsis or bacteremia could theoretically predispose patients to hematogenous spread of the infectious agents into the epidural or subarachnoid space.

Patients with preexisting neurological deficits or demyelinating diseases may report that their symptoms are worse following a block. It may be impossible to discern effects or complications of the block from preexisting deficits or unrelated exacerbation of preexisting disease. For these reasons, many practitioners argue against neuraxial anesthesia in such patients.

Regional anesthesia requires at least some degree of patient cooperation. This may be difficult or impossible for patients with dementia, psychosis, or emotional instability. The decision needs to be individualized. Young

Table 16–1. Contraindications to neuraxial blockade.

Absolute
  Infection at the site of injection
  Patient refusal
  Coagulopathy or other bleeding diathesis
  Severe hypovolemia
  Increased intracranial pressure
  Severe aortic stenosis
  Severe mitral stenosis
Relative
  Sepsis
  Uncooperative patient[1]
  Preexisting neurological deficits
    Demyelinating lesions
  Stenotic valvular heart lesions
  Severe spinal deformity
Controversial
  Prior back surgery at the site of injection
  Inability to communicate with patient[1]
  Complicated surgery[1]
    Prolonged operation
    Major blood loss
    Maneuvers that compromise respiration

---

[1]May be performed in conjunction with general anesthesia.

children may similarly not be suitable for pure regional techniques.

Neuraxial Blockade in the Setting of Anticoagulants & Antiplatelet Agents

Whether a block should be performed in the setting of anticoagulants and antiplatelet agents can be problematic.

A. ORAL ANTICOAGULANTS

If neuraxial anesthesia is to be used in patients on long-term warfarin therapy, it must be stopped and a normal prothrombin time (PT) and international normalized ratio (INR) should be documented prior to the block. For perioperative thromboembolic prophylaxis, if the initial dose was given more than 24 h prior to the block or if more than one dose was given, the PT and INR need to be checked. If only one dose was given within 24 h, it should be safe to proceed. Removing an epidural catheter from patients receiving low-dose warfarin (5 mg/d) is reported to be safe.

B. ANTIPLATELET DRUGS

By themselves, most antiplatelet (aspirin and nonsteroidal antiinflammatory drugs [NSAIDs]) drugs do not appear to increase the risk of spinal hematoma from neuraxial anesthesia or epidural catheter removal. This

assumes a normal patient with a normal coagulation profile who is not receiving other medications that might affect clotting mechanisms. In contrast, more potent agents should be stopped and neuraxial blockade should generally be administered only after their effects have worn off. The waiting period depends on the specific agent: for ticlopidine (Ticlid) it is 14 days, clopidogrel (Plavix) 7 days, abciximab (Rheopro) 48 h, and eptifibatide (Integrilin) 8 h.

C. STANDARD (UNFRACTIONATED) HEPARIN

Minidose subcutaneous prophylaxis is not a contraindication to neuraxial anesthesia. For patients who are to receive heparin intraoperatively, blocks may be performed 1 h or more before heparin administration. A bloody epidural or spinal does not necessarily require cancellation of surgery but discussion of the risks with the surgeon and careful postoperative monitoring is needed. Removal of an epidural catheter should occur 1 h prior to, or 4 h following, subsequent heparin dosing.

Neuraxial anesthesia should be avoided in patients on therapeutic doses of heparin and with increased partial thromboplastin time (PTT). If the patient is started on heparin after the placement of an epidural catheter, the catheter should be removed only after discontinuation or interruption of heparin infusion and evaluation of the coagulation status. The risk of spinal hematoma is undetermined in the setting of full anticoagulation for cardiac surgery.

D. LOW-MOLECULAR-WEIGHT HEPARIN (LMWH)

Many cases of spinal hematoma associated with neuraxial anesthesia followed the introduction of enoxaparin (Lovenox) in the United States in 1993. **Many of these cases involved intraoperative or early postoperative LMWH use, and several patients were receiving concomitant antiplatelet medication.** If bloody needle or catheter placement occurs, LMWH should be delayed until 24 h postoperatively, because this trauma may significantly increase the risk of spinal hematoma. If postoperative LMWH thromboprophylaxis will be utilized, epidural catheters should be removed 2 h prior to the first LMWH dose. If already present, the catheter should be removed at least 10 h after a dose of LMWH and subsequent dosing should not occur for another 2 h.

E. FIBRINOLYTIC OR THROMBOLYTIC THERAPY

Neuraxial anesthesia is best avoided if a patient has received fibrinolytic or thrombolytic therapy.

Awake or Asleep?

Should regional anesthesia, to be used in conjunction with general anesthesia, be performed before or after induction of general anesthesia? This is very controversial. The major arguments for having the patient asleep are that (1) most patients, if given a choice, would prefer to be asleep, and (2) the possibility of sudden patient movement causing injury is markedly diminished. It may, however, be difficult to achieve ideal spinal flexion in some patients under general anesthesia. The major argument for neuraxial blockade while the patient is still awake is that the patient can alert the clinician to paresthesias and pain on injection, both of which have been associated with postoperative neurological deficits. A few anecdotal reports of needle injections into the spinal cord during neuraxial (epidural) blocks and interscalene nerve blocks in anesthetized patients have strengthened the latter argument, but studies documenting an increased incidence of neurological complications in anesthetized patients are lacking. Pediatric neuraxial blocks, particularly caudal blocks, are usually performed under general anesthesia.

Technical Considerations

Neuraxial blocks should be performed only in a facility in which all the equipment and drugs needed for intubation and resuscitation are immediately available. Regional anesthesia is greatly facilitated by adequate patient premedication. Nonpharmacological patient preparation is also very helpful. The patient should be told what to expect so as to minimize anxiety. This is particularly important in situations in which premedication is not used, as is typically the case in obstetric anesthesia. Supplemental oxygen via a face mask or nasal cannula helps avoid hypoxemia, particularly if sedation is used. Minimum monitoring requirements include blood pressure and pulse oximetry for labor analgesia. Monitoring for blocks rendered for surgical anesthesia is the same as for general anesthesia. Epidural steroid injections for management of pain (no local anesthetic) frequently do not require continuous monitoring.

Surface Anatomy

Spinous processes are generally palpable over the spine and help define the midline. The spinous processes of the cervical and lumbar spine are nearly horizontal, whereas those in the thoracic spine slant in a caudal direction and can overlap significantly (Figure 16–2). Therefore, when performing a lumbar or cervical epidural block (with maximum spinal flexion), the needle is directed with only a slight cephalad angle, whereas for a thoracic block the needle must be angled significantly more cephalad to enter the thoracic epidural space. In the cervical area, the first palpable spinous process is that of C2, but the most prominent one is that of C7 (vertebra prominens). With the arms at the side, the spinous process of T7 is usually at the same level as the inferior angle of the scapulae (Figure 16–9). A line drawn between the highest points of both iliac crests (Tuffier's line) usually crosses either the body of L4 or the L4–L5 interspace. Counting spinous processes up or down from these reference points identifies other spinal levels. A parallel line drawn connecting the posterior superior iliac spine crosses the S2 posterior

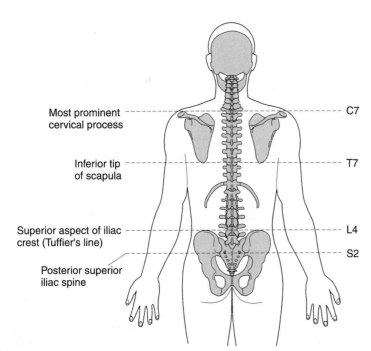

Most prominent cervical process — C7

Inferior tip of scapula — T7

Superior aspect of iliac crest (Tuffier's line) — L4

— S2

Posterior superior iliac spine

Figure 16–9. Surface landmarks for identifying spinal levels.

Figure 16–10. Sitting position for neuraxial blockade. Note an assistant helps in obtaining maximal spinal flexion.

foramina. In slender persons, the sacrum is easily palpable, and the sacral hiatus is felt as a depression just above or between the gluteal clefts and above the coccyx.

Patient Positioning

A. SITTING POSITION

The anatomic midline is often easier to appreciate when the patient is sitting than when the patient is in the lateral decubitus position (Figure 16–10). This is particularly true with very obese patients. Patients sit with their elbows resting on their thighs or a bedside table or they can hug a pillow. Flexion of the spine (arching the back "like a mad cat" maximizes the "target" area between adjacent spinous processes and brings the spine closer to the skin surface (Figure 16–11).

B. LATERAL DECUBITUS

Many clinicians prefer the lateral position for central blocks (Figure 16–12). Patients lie on their side with

their knees flexed and pulled high against the abdomen or chest, assuming a "fetal position." An assistant can help the patient assume and hold this position.

C. PRONE POSITION

This position may be used for anorectal procedures utilizing a hypobaric anesthetic solution (see below). The advantage is that the block is done in the same position as the operative procedure (jackknife) so that the patient does not have to be moved following the block. The disadvantage is that CSF will not freely flow through the needle, so that correct subarachnoid needle tip placement will need to be confirmed by CSF aspiration. The prone position is also used whenever fluoroscopic guidance is required.

Anatomic Approach

Anatomic landmarks for the desired level of the block are first identified (see Surface Anatomy). A sterile field is established with a povidone–iodine or similar solution that is applied with three abrasive sponges. The solution is applied starting at the anticipated injection site and proceeding outward in a widening circle. A fenestrated sterile drape is applied. After the preparation solution has dried, it should be wiped away with sterile gauze to avoid introduction of this solution into the subarachnoid space, which may cause a chemical meningitis. A skin wheal is raised at the level of the chosen interspace with local anesthetic using a small (25-gauge) needle. A longer (22-gauge) needle can then be used for deeper local anesthetic infiltration.

A. MIDLINE APPROACH

The spine is palpated and the patient's body position is examined to ensure that the plane of the back is perpendicular to that of the floor. This ensures that a needle passed parallel to the floor will stay midline as it courses deeper (Figure 16–4). The depression between the spinous processes of the vertebra above and below the level to be used is palpated; this will be the needle entry site. After prepping and anesthetizing the skin as above, the procedure needle is introduced in the midline. Remembering that the spinous processes course downward from the spine toward the skin, the needle will be directed slightly cephalad. The subcutaneous tissues offer little feeling of resistance to the needle. As the needle courses deeper, it will enter the supraspinous and interspinous ligaments, felt as an increase in tissue density. The needle also feels more firmly implanted in the back. If bone is contacted superficially, a midline needle is likely hitting the lower spinous process. Contact with bone at a deeper depth usually indicates the needle is in the midline and hitting the upper spinous process or it is lateral to the midline and hitting a lamina. In either case the needle must be redirected. As the needle

A

Extension   Flexion

B

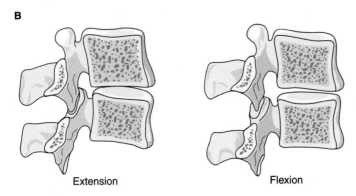

Extension   Flexion

Figure 16–11. The effect of flexion on adjacent vertebrae. Posterior view (**A**). Lateral view (**B**). Note the target area (interlaminar foramen) for neuraxial blocks increases in size with flexion.

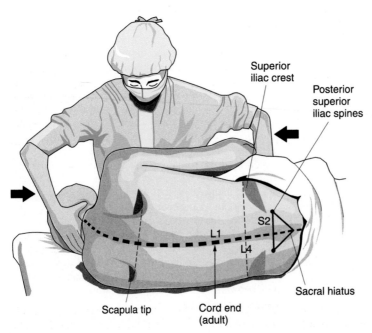

Figure 16–12. Lateral decubitus position for neuraxial blockade. Note again the assistant helping to provide maximal spine flexion.

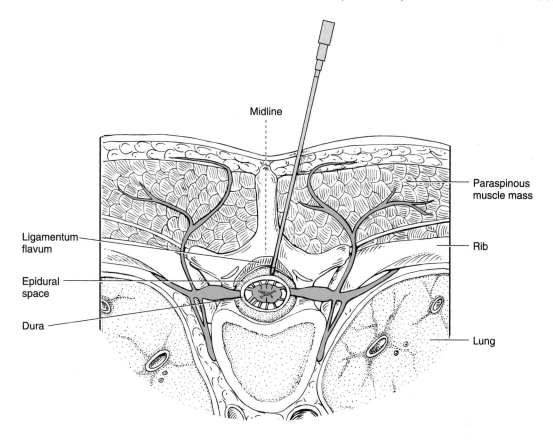

Figure 16–13. Lumbar spinal anesthesia; paramedian approach.

penetrates the ligamentum flavum an obvious increase in resistance is usually encountered. At this point, the procedures for spinal and epidural anesthesia differ (see Spinal Anesthesia and Epidural Anesthesia). For epidural anesthesia, a sudden loss of resistance is encountered as the needle penetrates the ligamentum flavum and enters the epidural space. For spinal anesthesia, the needle is advanced further through the epidural space and penetrates the dura–subarachnoid membranes as signaled by free flowing CSF.

B. PARAMEDIAN APPROACH

The paramedian technique may be selected if epidural or subarachnoid block is difficult, particularly in patients who cannot be positioned easily (eg, severe arthritis, kyphoscoliosis, or prior lumbar spine surgery) (Figure 16–13). The skin wheal for a paramedian approach is raised 2 cm lateral to the inferior aspect of the superior spinous process of the desired level. Because this approach is lateral to most of the

interspinous ligaments and penetrates the paraspinous muscles, the needle may encounter little resistance initially and may not seem to be in firm tissue. The needle is directed and advanced at a 10–25° angle toward the midline. Identification of the ligamentum flavum and entry into the epidural space with loss of resistance are often more subtle than with the midline approach. If bone is encountered at a shallow depth with the paramedian approach, the needle is likely in contact with the medial part of the lower lamina and should be redirected mostly upward and perhaps slightly more laterally. On the other hand, if bone is encountered deeply, the needle is usually in contact with the lateral part of the lower lamina and should be redirected only slightly upward, more toward the midline (Figure 16–14).

C. ASSESSING LEVEL OF BLOCKADE

With knowledge of the sensory dermatomes (see inside rear cover), the sensory level achieved by a block can be

A

Flexion

a   b

B

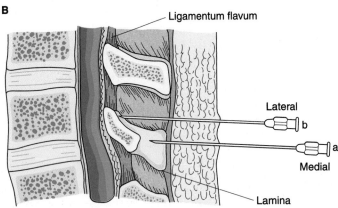

Ligamentum flavum

Lateral
b

Medial
a

Lamina

Figure 16–14. Paramedian approach. A needle that encounters bone at a shallow depth (*a*) is usually hitting the medial lamina, whereas one that encounters bone deeply (*b*) is further lateral from the midline. Posterior view (***A***). Parasagittal view (***B***).

assessed by a blunted needle (pinprick), whereas the level of sympathectomy is assessed by measuring skin temperature sensation.

SPINAL ANESTHESIA

Spinal anesthesia blocks nerve roots as they course through the subarachnoid space. The spinal subarachnoid space extends from the foramen magnum to the S2 in adults and S3 in children. Injection of local anesthetic below L1 in adults and L3 in children helps avoid direct trauma to the spinal cord. Spinal anesthesia is also referred to a subarachnoid block or intrathecal injection.

Spinal Needles

Spinal needles are commercially available in an array of sizes (16–30 gauge), lengths, and bevel and tip designs (Figure 16–15). All should have a tightly fitting removable

stylet that completely occludes the lumen to avoid tracking epithelial cells into the subarachnoid space. Broadly, they can be divided into either sharp (cutting)-tipped or blunt-tipped needles. The Quincke needle is a cutting needle with end injection. The introduction of blunt tip (pencil-point) needles has markedly decreased the incidence of postdural puncture headache; in general the smaller the gauge needle the lower the incidence of headache. The Whitacre and other pencil-point needles have rounded points and side injection. The Sprotte is a side-injection needle with a long opening. It has the advantage of more vigorous CSF flow compared with similar gauge needles. However, this can lead to a failed block if the distal part of the opening is subarachnoid (with free flow CSF), the proximal part is not past the dura, and the full dose of medication is not delivered.

Spinal Catheters

Very small subarachnoid catheters are currently no longer approved by the U.S. Food and Drug Administration (FDA). The withdrawal of these catheters was

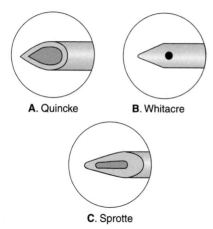

A. Quincke   **B.** Whitacre

C. Sprotte

Figure 16–15. Spinal needles.

Table 16–2. Factors affecting the level of spinal anesthesia.

Most important factors
Baricity of anesthetic solution
Position of the patient
During injection
Immediately after injection
Drug dosage
Site of injection
Other factors
Age
Cerebrospinal fluid
Curvature of the spine
Drug volume
Intraabdominal pressure
Needle direction
Patient height
Pregnancy

prompted by their association with cauda equina syndrome. Larger catheters designed for epidural use are associated with relatively high complication rates when placed subarachnoid.

Specific Technique for Spinal Anesthesia

The midline, paramedian, or prone approach can be used for spinal anesthesia. As previously discussed, the needle is advanced from skin through the deeper structures until two "pops" are felt. The first is penetration of the ligamentum flavum and the second is penetration of the dura–arachnoid membrane. Successful dural puncture is confirmed by withdrawing the stylet to verify free flow of CSF. With small-gauge needles (< 25 g), particularly in the presence of low CSF pressure (eg, a dehydrated patient), aspiration may be necessary to detect CSF. If initially free flow occurs but then CSF cannot be aspirated after attaching the syringe, the needle may have moved. Persistent paresthesia or pain upon injection should alert the clinician to withdraw and redirect the needle.

Factors Influencing Level of Block

Table 16–2 lists factors that have been shown to affect level of neural blockade following spinal anesthesia. The most important determinants are baricity, position of the patient during and immediately after injection, and drug dosage. In general, the higher the dosage or site of injection, the higher the level of anesthesia obtained. Moreover, migration of the local anesthetic cephalad in CSF depends on its specific gravity relative to CSF (baricity). CSF has a specific gravity of 1.003–1.008 at 37°C. Table 16–3 lists the specific gravity of commonly used local anesthetic solutions. A hyperbaric solution of local anesthetic is denser (heavier) than CSF, whereas a hypobaric

solution is less dense (lighter) than CSF. The local anesthetic solutions can be made hyperbaric by the addition of glucose or hypobaric by the addition of sterile water. Thus, with a head-down position, a hyperbaric solution spreads cephalad and a hypobaric anesthetic solution moves caudad. A head-up position causes a hyperbaric solution to settle caudad and a hypobaric solution to ascend cephalad. Similarly, in a lateral position, a hyperbaric spinal solution will have a greater effect on the dependent (down) side, whereas a hypobaric solution will achieve a higher level on the nondependent (up) side. An isobaric solution tends to remain at the level of injection. Anesthetic agents are mixed with CSF (at least 1:1) to

Table 16–3. Specific gravities of some spinal anesthetic agents.

Agent	Specific Gravity
Bupivacaine	
0.5% in 8.25% dextrose	1.0227–1.0278
0.5% plain	0.9990–1.0058
Lidocaine	
2% plain	1.0004–1.0066
5% in 7.5% dextrose	1.0262–1.0333
Procaine	
10% plain	1.0104
2.5% in water	0.9983
Tetracaine	
0.5% in water	0.9977–0.9997
0.5% in D_5W	1.0133–1.0203

Takefumi Sakabe, MD

NEUROTOXICITY OF LOCAL ANESTHETICS: WHAT DRUG DO YOU CHOOSE FOR SPINAL ANESTHESIA?

Spinal anesthesia has been used since anesthesia was first performed using cocaine in 1898. Many local anesthetics have since been developed and successfully used with reasonable safety. However, persistent neurological complications such as cauda equina syndrome are well known. Nevertheless, the real cause of this complication remains undetermined and for a long time little attention was given to the neurotoxicity of drugs administered intrathecally. In 1985, Ready et al[1] reported that local anesthetics at concentrations higher than clinically used provoked histopathological changes in the spinal cord and neurological deficits in rabbits. Since then many experimental studies have indicated that local anesthetics may be neurotoxic.

Clinically, in 1991 four cases of cauda equina syndrome were reported after continuous spinal anesthesia with 5% lidocaine or 1% tetracaine,[2] which generated concern about the neurotoxicity of local anesthetics given intrathecally. Two years later, transient neurological symptoms (TNS), characterized by pain and/or dysesthesia in the buttocks, thighs, or lower limbs, were reported after spinal anesthesia, but not necessarily after continuous spinal anesthesia or repeated injections.[3] Although it is still not known if the persistent neurological injury and TNS are caused by the same mechanism, it is possible that TNS repre-

sent the lower end of a spectrum of toxicity. Accumulated data suggest that the incidence of TNS appears to be higher with lidocaine than with other local anesthetics.[4]

Many questions have been raised. What is the mechanism for neurotoxicity? What drugs should be used? Should we stop using lidocaine? We have no satisfactory answers to these questions at present. This is probably due to the fact that the precise mechanism for neurological injury is still obscure.

Accumulated data indicate that the effects of pH, osmolarity, and the addition of glucose to local anesthetics are not causes of neurotoxicity. In addition, the toxic effect does not appear to be related to Na channel blocking, but may be related to an increase in intracellular calcium.[5] A recent study in rabbits showed increases of an excitatory amino acid, glutamate, in lumbar cerebrospinal fluid (CSF) after intrathecal administration of tetracaine (1, 2, and 4%) in association with hindlimb motor dysfunction in a dose-dependent manner.[6] Histological examination showed vacuolation in the dorsal funiculus and central chromatolysis of motor neurons in the spinal cord.[6] The results may be compatible with the established concept that excessive release of glutamate causes neuronal damage due to an increase in intracellular calcium.

The increase in glutamate can be observed with lidocaine and other local anesthetics (bupivacaine, ropivacaine) at high concentrations. In a subsequent study in rabbits using 2% tetracaine, 10% lidocaine, 2% bupivacaine, or 2% ropivacaine, sensory and motor dysfunctions in the lidocaine group were significantly worse than in the other groups, although the increase in glutamate concentration revealed no significant difference among the drugs.[7] Although the concentrations used are larger than those used clinically, the results suggest that the margin of safety may be smallest with lidocaine. Should TNS represent the lower end of a spectrum of toxicity, these results have substantial clinical relevance.

What clinical decisions should now be made?

My first experience with spinal anesthesia, more than 30 years ago, was the use of 0.3% dibucaine. Until recently dibucaine was the most popular local anesthetic used intrathecally in Japan. Although dibucaine has been considered highly toxic, I personally have no experience with neurological symptoms *that may suggest neurotoxicity. However, this does not mean that dibucaine is not neurotoxic. Because bupivacaine is now commercially available in Japan, I believe dibucaine will soon disappear from use.*

Is decreasing the concentration of local anesthetics an effective way to decrease neurological complications? The use of the lowest effective concentration is the rule in clinical practice. After the animal study mentioned above, I started using a lower concentration of tetracaine (0.4% instead of 0.5%). However, the report showed that dilution of lidocaine to even 0.5% did not decrease the risk of TNS.[8] This means that dilution does not guarantee a decrease in the incidence of risk. Repeat injection after failed spinal anesthesia is a common practice. I do repeat the injection, but I do not use lidocaine, even though, in Japan, the commercially available lidocaine concentration for spinal anesthesia is 3%.

Is the addition of epinephrine to local anesthetics to prolong the duration of anesthesia safe? I think the addition might be deleterious because it prolongs the exposure of nerve tissue to a potentially toxic drug. A recent study demonstrated that the addition of epinephrine to a high concentration of tetracaine (1%) given intrathecally sustained large concentrations of glutamate in the CSF, worsened histological injury, and exacerbated sensory and motor dysfunction.[9] I believe the addition of epinephrine to lidocaine to prolong the duration of anesthesia is unnecessary because we now have less toxic drugs, such as bupivacaine, with longer durations of action.

A major question concerns the risk factors for the occurrence of TNS. The incidence of TNS is reported to be higher when surgery is performed on patients in the lithotomy position or on outpatients. It is not known why. The nerve root may be stretched and vulnerability increased. Preferential damage to nerve roots after intrathecal administration of local anesthetics has been demonstrated. Takenami et al[10] showed that tetracaine most often induced neuronal destruction at sites at which glial sheaths were interrupted, and suggested that neurotoxicity could be derived from direct toxicity to neurites. It has been reported that oligodendrocytes are vulnerable to 2-(aminomethyl)phenylacetic acid/kainate receptor-mediated excitotoxicity. The increase in glutamate produced by local anesthetics may damage oligodendrocytes. This could be related to the neurotoxic-

ity of local anesthetics. We recently demonstrated that the Obersteiner–Redlich (OR) zone is the area that is damaged at an early stage after intrathecal injection of large concentrations of local anesthetics (unpublished data). Oligodendrocytes, which constitute the central part of the OR zone, appear to be vulnerable to local anesthetics. Although it is only speculative, when the nerve is stretched, the OR zone might have greater opportunity to be exposed to local anesthetics, which would result in injury. This could be the cause of the higher incidence of neurological deficits in patients undergoing surgery in the lithotomy position.

Further basic research is warranted to elucidate the mechanisms for neurotoxicity and to develop less toxic drugs. In the meantime, I recommend the administration of anesthetic at the lowest effective concentration. Lidocaine should be avoided, particularly when surgery is to be done in the lithotomy position.

1. Ready LB, Plumer MH, Haschke RH, et al: Neurotoxicity of intrathecal local anesthetics in rabbits. Anesthesiology 1985;63:364.

2. Rigler ML, Drasner K, Krejcie TC, et al: Cauda equina syndrome after continuous spinal anesthesia. Anesth Analg 1991;72:275.

3. Schneider M, Ettlin T, Kaufmann M, et al: Transient neurologic toxicity after hyperbaric subarachnoid anesthesia with 5% lidocaine. Anesth Analg 1993;76:1154.

4. Hampl KF, Schneider MC, Drasner K: Toxicity of spinal local anesthetics. Curr Opin Anaesthesiol 1999;12:559.

5. Gold MS, Reichling DB, Hampl KF, et al: Lidocaine toxicity in primary afferent neurons from the rat. J Pharmacol Exp Ther 1998;285:413.

6. Ohtake K, Matsumoto M, Wakamatsu H, et al: Glutamate release and neuronal injury after intrathecal injection of local anesthetics. NeuroReport 2000;11:1105.

7. Yamashita A, Matsumoto M, Matsumoto S, et al: A comparison of the neurotoxic effects on the spinal cord of tetracaine, lidocaine, bupivacaine, and ropivacaine administered intrathecally in rabbits. Anesth Analg 2003;97:512.

8. Pollock JE, Liu SS, Neal JM, Stepheson CA: Dilution of spinal lidocaine does not alter the incidence of transient neurologic symptoms. Anesthesiology 1999;90:445.

9. Oka S, Matsumoto M, Ohtake K, et al: The addition of epinephrine to tetracaine injected intrathecally sustains an increase in glutamate concentrations in the cerebrospinal fluid and worsens neuronal injury. Anesth Analg 2001;93:1050.

10. Takenami T, Yagishita S, Asato F, Hoka S: Neurotoxicity of intrathecally administered tetracaine commences at the posterior roots near entry into the spinal cord. Reg Anesth Pain Med 2000;25:372.

A

B

Figure 16–16. The position of the spinal canal in the supine position (***A***) and lateral decubitus position (***B***). Note the lowest point is usually between T5 and T7 where a hyperbaric solution tends to settle once the patient is placed supine.

make their solutions isobaric. Other factors affecting the level of neural blockade include the level of injection and the patient's height and vertebral column anatomy. The direction of the needle bevel or injection port may also play a role; higher levels of anesthesia are achieved if the injection is directed cephalad than if the point of injection is oriented laterally or caudad.

Hyperbaric solutions tend to move to the most dependent area of the spine (normally T4–T8 in the supine position). With normal spinal anatomy, the apex of the thoracolumbar curvature is T4 (Figure 16–16). In the supine position, this should limit a hyperbaric solution to produce a level of anesthesia at or below T4. Abnormal curvatures of the spine, such as scoliosis and kyphoscoliosis, have multiple effects on spinal anesthesia. Placing the block becomes more difficult because of the rotation and angulation of the vertebral bodies and spinous processes. Finding the midline and the interlaminar space may be difficult. The paramedian approach to lumbar puncture may be preferable in patients with severe scoliosis and kyphoscoliosis, particularly if there is associated degenerative joint disease. The paramedian approach is easiest for spinal anesthesia at the L5–S1 level. In the Taylor approach, a variant of the standard paramedian approach described previously, the needle enters 1 cm medial and 1 cm inferior to the posterior superior iliac spine and is directed cephalad and toward the midline. Reviewing radiographs of the spine before attempting the block may be useful. Spinal curvature affects the ultimate level by changing the contour of the subarachnoid space. Previous spinal surgery can similarly result in technical difficulties in placing a block. Correctly identifying the interspinous and interlaminar spaces may be difficult at the

levels of previous laminectomy or spinal fusion. The paramedian approach may be easier, or a level above the surgical site can be chosen. The block may be incomplete, or the level may be different than anticipated, due to postsurgical anatomic changes.

CSF volume inversely correlates with level of anesthesia. Increased intraabdominal pressure or conditions that cause engorgement of the epidural veins, thus decreasing CSF volume, are associated with higher blocks. This would include conditions such as pregnancy, ascites, and large abdominal tumors. In these clinical situations, higher levels of anesthesia are achieved with a given dose of local anesthetic than would otherwise be expected. For spinal anesthesia on a term parturient, the dosage of anesthetic can be reduced by one-third compared with a nonpregnant patient (see Chapters 42 and 43). Age-related decreases in CSF volume are likely responsible for the higher anesthetic levels achieved in the elderly for a given dosage of spinal anesthetic. Severe kyphosis or kyphoscoliosis can also be associated with a decreased volume of CSF and often results in a higher than expected level, particularly with a hypobaric technique or rapid injection. Conflicting opinion exists as to whether increased CSF pressure caused by coughing or straining, or turbulence on injection has any effect on the spread of local anesthetic in the CSF.

Spinal Anesthetic Agents

Many local anesthetics have been used for spinal anesthesia in the past, but only a few are currently in use (Table 16–4). There is renewed interest in some older medications because of reports documenting an increased inci-

Table 16–4. Dosages and actions of commonly used spinal anesthetic agents.

Drug	Preparation	Doses (mg)			Duration (min)	
		Perineum, Lower Limbs	Lower Abdomen	Upper Abdomen	Plain	Epinephrine
Procaine	10% solution	75	125	200	45	60
Bupivacaine	0.75% in 8.25% dextrose	4–10	12–14	12–18	90–120	100–150
Tetracaine	1% solution in 10% glucose	4–8	10–12	10–16	90–120	120–240
Lidocaine[1]	5% in 7.5% glucose	25–50	50–75	75–100	60–75	60–90
Ropivacaine[2]	0.2–1% solution	8–12	12–16	16–18	90–120	90–120

[1]No longer recommended. It should be diluted to 2.5% or less.
[2]Off-label use.

dence of transient neurological symptoms with 5% lidocaine (see Complications of Neuraxial Anesthesia). Only preservative-free local anesthetic solutions are used. Addition of vasoconstrictors (α-adrenergic agonists) and opioids may enhance the quality and/or prolong the duration of spinal anesthesia (see Chapter 18). Vasoconstrictors include epinephrine (0.1–0.2 mg) and phenylephrine (1–2 mg). Both agents appear to decrease the uptake and clearance of local anesthetics from CSF and may have weak spinal analgesic properties. Clonidine and neostigmine also have spinal analgesic properties, but experience with them as additives for spinal anesthesia is limited.

Hyperbaric bupivacaine and tetracaine are two of the most commonly used agents for spinal anesthesia. Both are relatively slow in onset (5–10 min) and have a prolonged duration (90–120 min). Although both agents produce similar sensory levels, spinal tetracaine generally produces more motor blockade than the equivalent dose of bupivacaine. Addition of epinephrine to spinal bupivacaine prolongs its duration only modestly. In contrast, epinephrine can prolong the duration of tetracaine anesthesia by more than 50%. Phenylephrine also prolongs tetracaine anesthesia but has no effect on bupivacaine spinal blocks. Ropivacaine has also been used for spinal anesthesia, but experience with it is more limited. A 12-mg intrathecal dose of ropivacaine is roughly equivalent to 8 mg of bupivacaine, but it appears to have no particular advantages for spinal anesthesia. Lidocaine and procaine have a rapid onset (3–5 min) and short duration of action (60–90 min). There are conflicting data as to whether their duration is prolonged by vasoconstrictors; any effect appears to be modest. Although lidocaine for spinal anesthesia has been used worldwide, some caution its use in light of the phenomenon of transient neurological symptoms (TNS) and cauda equina syndrome (see below). Some experts suggest that lidocaine can be safely used as a spinal anesthetic if the total

dose is limited to 60 mg and diluted to 2.5% or less with an opioid and/or CSF prior to injection. **Repeat doses following an initial "failed" block should be avoided as perhaps should the use of epinephrine with lidocaine.**

Hyperbaric spinal anesthesia is more commonly used than the hypobaric or isobaric techniques. The level of anesthesia is then dependent on the patient's position during and immediately following the injection. In the sitting position, "saddle block" can be achieved by keeping the patient sitting for 3–5 min following injection so that only the lower lumbar nerves and sacral nerves are blocked. If the patient is moved from a sitting position to a supine position immediately after injection, the agent will move more cephalad to the dependent region defined by the thoracolumbar curve, as full protein binding has not yet occurred. Hyperbaric anesthetics injected intrathecally with the patient in a lateral decubitus position are useful for unilateral lower extremity procedures. The patient is placed laterally with the extremity to be operated on in a dependent position. If the patient is kept in this position for about 5 min following injection, the block will tend to be denser and achieve a higher level on the operative dependent side.

If regional anesthesia is chosen for surgical procedures involving hip or lower extremity fracture, hypobaric spinal anesthesia can be useful because the patient need not lie on the fractured extremity.

EPIDURAL ANESTHESIA

 Epidural anesthesia is a neuraxial technique offering a range of applications wider than the typical all-or-nothing spinal anesthetic. An epidural block can be performed at the lumbar, thoracic, or cervical level. Sacral epidural anesthesia is referred to as a caudal block and is described at the end of this chapter. Epidural techniques are widely used for operative anesthesia, obstetric analgesia, postoperative pain control, and chronic pain management. It can be used as a single shot technique or with a catheter that allows intermittent boluses and/or continuous infusion. The motor block can range from none to complete. All these variables are controlled by the choice of drug, concentration, dosage, and level of injection.

The epidural space surrounds the dura mater posteriorly, laterally, and anteriorly. Nerve roots travel in this space as they exit laterally through the foramen and course outward to become peripheral nerves. Other contents of the epidural space include fatty connective tissue, lymphatics, and a rich venous (Batson's) plexus. Recent fluoroscopic studies have suggested the presence of septa or connective tissue bands. Epidural anesthesia is slower in onset (10–20 min) and may not be as dense as spinal anesthesia. This can be manifested as a more pronounced differential block or a segmental block, a feature that can be useful clinically. For example, by using relatively dilute concentrations of a local anesthetic combined with an opioid, an epidural can block the smaller sympathetic and sensory fibers and spare the larger motor fibers, providing analgesia without motor block. This is commonly employed for labor and postoperative analgesia. Moreover, a segmental block is possible because the anesthetic is not spread readily by CSF and can be confined close to the level at which it was injected. A segmental block is characterized by a well-defined band of anesthesia at certain nerve roots; nerve roots above *and* below are not blocked. This can be seen with a thoracic epidural that provides upper abdominal anesthesia while sparing cervical and lumbar nerve roots.

Epidural anesthesia and analgesia is most often performed in the lumbar region. The midline (Figure 16–4) or paramedian approach (Figure 16–13) can be used. Lumbar epidural anesthesia can be used for any procedure below the diaphragm. Because the spinal cord typically terminates at the L1 level, there is an extra measure of safety in performing the block in the lower lumbar interspaces, particularly if an inadvertent dural puncture occurs (see Complications).

Thoracic epidural blocks are technically more difficult to accomplish than lumbar blocks because of greater angulation and marked overlapping of the spinous processes at the vertebral level (Figure 16–17). Moreover, the potential risk of spinal cord injury with inadvertent dural puncture, although small with good technique, may be greater than that at the lumbar level. Thoracic epidural blocks can be accomplished with either a midline or paramedian approach. Rarely used for primary anesthesia, the thoracic epidural technique is most commonly used for intra- and postoperative analgesia. Single shot or catheter techniques are used for management of chronic pain. Infusions via an epidural catheter are very useful for providing analgesia and may obviate or shorten postoperative ventilation for patients with underlying lung disease and following chest surgery.

Cervical blocks are usually performed with the patient sitting, with the neck flexed, using the midline approach. Clinically, they are used primarily for management of pain (see Chapter 18).

Epidural Needles

The standard epidural needle is typically 17–18 gauge, 3 or 3.5 inches long, and has a blunt bevel with a gentle curve of 15–30° at the tip. The Tuohy needle is most commonly used (Figure 16–18). The blunt, curved tip helps push away the dura after passing through the ligamentum flavum instead of penetrating it. Straight needles without a curved tip (Crawford needles) may have a higher incidence of dural puncture but facilitate passage of an epidural catheter. Needle modifications include winged tips and introducer devices set into the hub designed for guiding catheter placement.

Epidural Catheters

Placing a catheter into the epidural space allows for continuous infusion or intermittent bolus techniques. In addition to extending the duration of the block, it may allow a lower total dose of anesthetic to be used, and, therefore, decrease the hemodynamic insults if incremental initial dosing is used.

Epidural catheters are useful for intraoperative epidural anesthesia and/or postoperative analgesia. Typically, a 19- or 20-gauge catheter is introduced through a 17- or 18-gauge epidural needle. When using a curved tipped needle, the bevel opening is directed either cephalad or caudad, and the catheter is advanced 2–6 cm into the epidural space. The shorter the distance the catheter is advanced, the more likely it is to become dislodged. Conversely, the further the catheter is advanced, the greater the chance of a unilateral block, due to the catheter tip either exiting the epidural space via an intervertebral foramen or coursing into the anterolateral recesses of the epidural space. After advancing the catheter the desired depth, the needle is removed, leaving the catheter in place. The catheter can be taped or otherwise secured along the back. Catheters have either a single port at the distal end or multiple side ports close to a closed tip. Some have a stylet for easier insertion. Spiral wire-reinforced cathe-

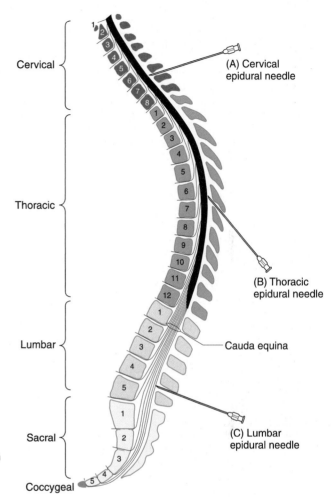

Figure 16–17. Angulation of the epidural needle at the cervical (**A**), thoracic (**B**), and lumbar (**C**) levels. Note that an acute angulation (30–50°) is required for a thoracic epidural block, whereas only a slight cephalad orientation is usually required for cervical and lumbar epidural blocks.

ters are very resistant to kinking. The spiral or spring tip is associated with fewer, less intense paresthesias and may be associated with a lower incidence of inadvertent intravascular insertion.

Specific Technique for Epidural Anesthesia

Using the midline or paramedian approaches detailed previously, the epidural needle courses from the skin just through the ligamentum flavum. In epidural anesthesia the needle must stop short of piercing the dura. Two techniques make it possible to determine when the tip of the needle has entered the potential (epidural) space: the "loss of resistance" and "hanging drop" techniques.

The loss of resistance technique is preferred by most clinicians. The needle is advanced through the subcutaneous tissues with the stylet in place until the interspinous ligament is entered, as noted by an increase in tissue resistance. The stylet or introducer is removed and a glass syringe filled with approximately 2 mL of fluid or air is attached to the hub of the needle. If the tip of the needle is within the ligament, gentle attempts at injection are met with resistance and injection is not possible. The needle is then slowly advanced, millimeter by millimeter, with either continuous or rapidly repeating attempts at injection. As the tip of the needle just enters the epidural space there is a sudden loss of resistance and injection is easy.

Once the interspinous ligament has been entered and the stylet has been removed, the hanging drop technique requires that the hub of the needle be filled with solution so that a drop hangs from its outside opening. The needle is then slowly advanced deeper. As long as the tip of the needle remains within the ligamentous structures, the drop remains "hanging." However, as the tip of the needle enters the epidural space it

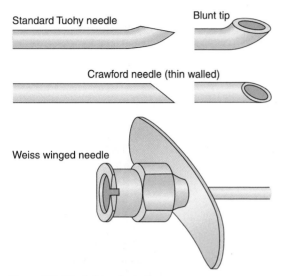

Figure 16–18. Epidural needles.

creates negative pressure and the drop of fluid is sucked into the needle. If the needle becomes plugged the drop will not be drawn into the hub of the needle and inadvertent dural puncture may occur. Some clinicians prefer to use this technique for the paramedian approach and for cervical epidurals.

Activating an Epidural

The quantity (volume and concentration) of local anesthetic needed for epidural anesthesia is very large compared with that needed for spinal anesthesia. Significant toxicity can occur if this amount is injected intrathecally or intravascularly. Safeguards against this include the epidural test dose and incremental dosing. This is true whether the injection is through the needle or through an epidural catheter.

A test dose is designed to detect both subarachnoid and intravascular injection. The classic test dose combines local anesthetic and epinephrine, typically 3 mL of 1.5% lidocaine with 1:200,000 epinephrine (0.005 mg/mL). The 45 mg of lidocaine, if injected intrathecally, will produce spinal anesthesia that should be rapidly apparent. Some clinicians have suggested use of lower doses of local anesthetic, as unintended injection of 45 mg of intrathecal lidocaine can be difficult to manage in areas such as labor rooms. The 15 μg dose of epinephrine, if injected intravascularly, should produce a noticeable increase in heart rate (20% or more) with or without hypertension. Unfortunately, epinephrine as a marker of intravenous injection is not ideal. False positives can occur (a uterine contraction causing pain or an increase in heart rate coincident to test dosing) as well as false negatives (patients taking β-blockers). A

25% or more increase in T-wave amplitude on the electrocardiograph (ECG) has been suggested to be a more reliable sign of intravascular injection. Both fentanyl and larger doses of local anesthetic without epinephrine have been advocated as intravenous injection test doses. Simply aspirating prior to injection is insufficient to avoid inadvertent intravenous injection; most experienced practitioners have encountered false-negative aspirations through both a needle and a catheter.

Incremental dosing is a very effective method of avoiding serious complications. If aspiration is negative, a fraction of the total intended local anesthetic dose is injected, typically 5 mL. This dose should be large enough for mild symptoms of intravascular injection to occur but small enough to avoid seizure or cardiovascular compromise. This is particularly important for labor epidurals that are to be used for cesarean section. If the initial labor epidural bolus was delivered through the needle and then the catheter was inserted, it may be erroneously assumed that the catheter is well positioned because the patient is still comfortable from the initial bolus. If the catheter was inserted intravascularly, or has since migrated intravascularly, systemic toxicity will likely result if the full anesthetic dose is injected. Catheters can migrate intrathecally or intravascularly from an initially correct epidural position anytime after initial placement. Some cases of "catheter migration" may represent delayed recognition of an improperly positioned catheter.

If a clinician uses an initial test dose, is diligent about aspirating prior to each injection, and always uses incremental dosing, significant systemic toxicity or inadvertent intrathecal injections are rare.

Factors Affecting Level of Block

Factors affecting the level of epidural anesthesia may not be as predictable as with spinal anesthesia. In adults, 1–2 mL of local anesthetic per segment to be blocked is a generally accepted guideline. For example, to achieve a T4 sensory level from an L4–L5 injection would require about 12–24 mL. For segmental or analgesic blocks, less volume is needed.

The dose required to achieve the same level of anesthesia decreases with age. This is probably a result of age-related decreases in the size or compliance of the epidural space. Although there is little correlation between body weight and epidural dosage requirements, patient height affects the extent of cephalad spread. Thus, shorter patients may require only 1 mL of local anesthetic per segment to be blocked, whereas taller patients generally require 2 mL per segment. Although less dramatic than with spinal anesthesia, spread of epidural local anesthetics tends to be partially affected by gravity. The lateral decubitus, Trendelenburg, and reverse Trendelenburg positions can be used to help achieve block-

Table 16–5. Agents for epidural anesthesia.

Agent	Concentration	Onset	Sensory Block	Motor Block
Chloroprocaine	2%	Fast	Analgesic	Mild to moderate
	3%	Fast	Dense	Dense
Lidocaine	≤ 1%	Intermediate	Analgesic	Minimal
	1.5%	Intermediate	Dense	Mild to moderate
	2%	Intermediate	Dense	Dense
Mepivacaine	1%	Intermediate	Analgesic	Minimal
	2–3%	Intermediate	Dense	Dense
Bupivacaine	≤ 0.25%	Slow	Analgesic	Minimal
	0.5%	Slow	Dense	Mild to moderate
	0.75%	Slow	Dense	Moderate to dense
Ropivacaine	0.2%	Slow	Analgesic	Minimal
	0.5%	Slow	Dense	Mild to moderate
	0.75–1.0%	Slow	Dense	Moderate to dense

ade in the desired dermatomes. Injection in the sitting position appears to deliver more local anesthetic to the larger L5–S1 and S2 nerve roots; patchy anesthesia or sparing of those dermatomes is sometimes encountered with lumbar epidural anesthesia.

Additives to the local anesthetic, particularly opioids, tend to have a greater effect on the quality of epidural anesthesia than on the duration of the block. Epinephrine in concentrations of 0.005 mg/mL prolongs the effect of epidural lidocaine, mepivacaine, and chloroprocaine more than that of bupivacaine, levobupivacaine, etidocaine, and ropivacaine. In addition to prolonging the duration and improving the quality of block, epinephrine decreases vascular absorption and peak systemic blood levels of epidurally administered local anesthetics. Phenylephrine generally is less effective than epinephrine as a vasoconstrictor for epidural anesthesia.

Epidural Anesthetic Agents

The epidural agent is chosen based on the desired clinical effect, whether it is to be used as a primary anesthetic, for supplementation of general anesthesia, or for analgesia. The anticipated duration of the procedure may call for a short- or long-acting single shot anesthetic or the insertion of a catheter (Table 16–5). Commonly used short- to intermediate-acting agents for surgical anesthesia include lidocaine, chloroprocaine, and mepivacaine. Long-acting agents include bupivacaine, levobupivacaine, and ropivacaine. Levobupivacaine, the S-enantiomer of bupivacaine, is less toxic than bupivicaine but is no longer available in the United States. Only preservative-free local anesthetic solutions or those specifically labeled for epidural or caudal use are employed.

Following the initial 1–2 mL per segment bolus (in fractionated doses), repeat doses delivered through an epidural catheter are either done on a fixed time interval, based on the practitioner's experience with the agent, or when the block demonstrates some degree of regression. Once some regression in sensory level has occurred, one-third to one-half the initial activation dose can generally safely be reinjected.

It should be noted that chloroprocaine, an ester with rapid onset, short duration, and extremely low toxicity, may interfere with the analgesic effects of epidural opioids. Previous chloroprocaine formulations with preservatives, specifically bisulfite and ethylenediaminetetraacetic acid (EDTA), proved to be problematic when inadvertently injected in a large volume intrathecally. Bisulfite preparations of chloroprocaine were believed to cause neurotoxicity, whereas EDTA formulations were associated with severe back pain (presumably due to localized hypocalcemia). Current preparations of chloroprocaine are preservative free and without these complications. Some experts believe the local anesthetics, when injected in very large doses intrathecally (see Lidocaine Toxicity below), may have been at least partly responsible for neurotoxicity.

Bupivacaine, an amide local anesthetic with a slow onset and long duration of action, has a high potential for systemic toxicity (see Chapter 14). Surgical anesthesia is obtained with a 0.5% or 0.75% formulation. The 0.75% concentration is not recommended for obstetric anesthesia. Its use in the past for cesarean section was associated with several reports of cardiac arrest resulting from inadvertent intravenous injection. The difficulty in resuscitation and the resultant high mortality rate result from the high protein binding and lipid solubility of bupivacaine, which causes the agent to accumulate in the cardiac conduction system leading to refractory reentrant arrhythmias. Very dilute concentrations of bupivacaine (eg, 0.0625%) are commonly combined with fentanyl and used for analgesia for labor and postoperative pain (see Chapters 18 and 43). The S-enantiomer of bupivacaine, levobupivacaine, appears to be primarily responsible for the local anesthetic action on nerve conduction but not the systemic toxic effects. Ropivacaine, a mepivacaine analogue introduced and marketed as a less toxic alternative to bupivacaine, is roughly equal to or slightly less than bupivacaine in potency, onset, duration, and quality of block. It may exhibit less motor block at lower concentrations while maintaining a good sensory block.

Local Anesthetic pH Adjustment

Local anesthetic solutions have a pH between 3.5 and 5.5 for chemical stability and bacteriostasis. Because they are weak bases, they exist primarily in the ionic form in commercial preparations. The onset of neural block depends on penetration of the lipid nerve cell membranes by the nonionic form of the local anesthetic (Chapter 14). Increasing the pH of the solutions increases the concentration of the nonionic form of the local anesthetic. Addition of sodium bicarbonate (1 mEq/10 mL of local anesthetic) immediately before injection may therefore accelerate the onset of the neural blockade. This approach is most useful for agents that can be adjusted to physiological pH, such as lidocaine, mepivacaine, and chloroprocaine. Sodium bicarbonate is usually not added to bupivacaine, which precipitates above a pH of 6.8.

Failed Epidural Blocks

Unlike spinal anesthesia, in which the end point is usually very clear (free flowing CSF) and the technique is associated with a very high success rate, epidural anesthesia is critically dependent on detection of a more subjective loss of resistance (or hanging drop). Also, the more variable anatomy of the epidural space and less predictable spread of local anesthetic in it make epidural anesthesia inherently less predictable.

Misplaced injections of local anesthetic can occur in a number of situations. In some young adults, the spinal ligaments are soft and either good resistance is never appreciated or a false loss of resistance is encountered. Similarly, entry into the paraspinous muscles during an off-center midline approach may cause a false loss of resistance. Other causes of failed epidural anesthesia (such as intrathecal, subdural, and intravenous injection) are discussed in the section of this chapter on complications.

Even if an adequate concentration and volume of an anesthetic were delivered into the epidural space, and sufficient time was allowed for the block to take effect, some epidural blocks are not successful. A unilateral block can occur if the medication is delivered through a catheter that has either exited the epidural space or coursed laterally. The chance of this occurring increases as the distance the catheter is threaded into the epidural space increases. When unilateral block occurs, the problem may be overcome by withdrawing the catheter 1–2 cm and reinjecting it with the patient turned with the unblocked side down. Segmental sparing, which may be due to septations within the epidural space, may also be corrected by injecting additional local anesthetic with the unblocked segment down. The large size of the L5, S1, and S2 nerve roots may prevent adequate penetration of local anesthetic and is thought to be responsible for sacral sparing. The latter is particularly a problem for surgery on the lower leg; in such cases, elevating the head of the bed and reinjecting the catheter can sometimes achieve a more intense block of these large nerve roots. Patients may complain of visceral pain despite a seemingly good epidural block. In some cases (eg, traction on the inguinal ligament and spermatic cord), a high thoracic sensory level may alleviate the pain; in other cases (traction on the peritoneum), intravenous supplementation with opioids or other agents may be necessary. Visceral afferent fibers that travel with the vagus nerve may be responsible.

■ CAUDAL ANESTHESIA

Caudal epidural anesthesia is one of the most commonly used regional techniques in pediatric patients. It may also be used in anorectal surgery in adults. The caudal space is the sacral portion of the epidural space. Caudal anesthesia involves needle and/or catheter penetration of the sacrococcygeal ligament covering the sacral hiatus that is created by the unfused S4 and S5 laminae. The hiatus may be felt as a groove or notch above the coccyx and between two bony prominences, the sacral cornua (Figure 16–3). Its anatomy is more easily appreciated in infants and children (Figure 16–19). The posterior superior iliac spines and the sacral hiatus define an equilateral triangle (Figure 16–12). Calcification of the sacrococcygeal ligament may make caudal anesthesia difficult or impossible in older adults. Within the sacral canal, the dural sac extends to the first sacral vertebra in adults and to about the third sacral vertebra in infants, making inadvertent intrathecal injection more common in infants.

In children, caudal anesthesia is typically combined with general anesthesia for intraoperative supplementation and postoperative analgesia. It is commonly used

Figure 16–19. Positioning an anesthetized child for caudal block and palpation for the sacral hiatus. An assistant gently helps flex the spine.

Sacral cornu

for procedures below the diaphragm, including urogenital, rectal, inguinal, and lower extremity surgery. Pediatric caudal blocks are most commonly performed after the induction of general anesthesia. The patient is placed in the lateral or prone position with one or both hips flexed, and the sacral hiatus is palpated. After sterile skin preparation, a needle or intravenous catheter (18–23 gauge) is advanced at a 45° angle cephalad until a pop is felt as the needle pierces the sacrococcygeal ligament. The angle of the needle is then flattened and advanced (Figure 16–20). Aspiration for blood and CSF is performed, and, if negative, injection can pro-

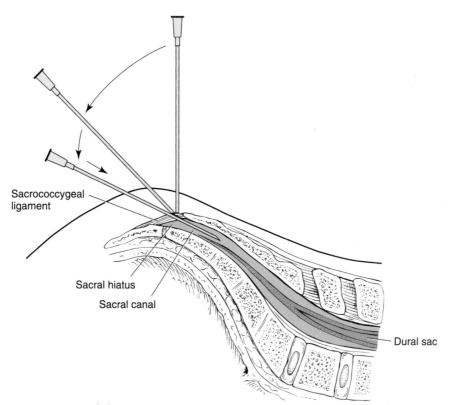

Sacrococcygeal ligament

Sacral hiatus

Sacral canal

Dural sac

Figure 16–20. Caudal block. Note the sacrococcygeal ligament is penetrated with the needle almost at 90° and then must be angled down and advanced to enter the sacral hiatus.

Figure 16–21. The prone jackknife position often used for anorectal surgery can also be used for caudal anesthesia in adults. (Reproduced, with permission, from Lambert DH, Covino BG: Hyperbaric, hypobaric, and isobaric spinal anesthesia. Res Staff Phys 1987;10:84.)

ceed. Some clinicians recommend test dosing as with other epidural techniques, although many simply rely on incremental dosing with frequent aspiration. Tachycardia (if epinephrine is used) and/or increasing size of the T waves on ECG may indicate intravascular injection. Clinical data have shown that the complication rate for "kiddie caudals" is very low. Complications include total spinal and intravenous injection causing seizure or cardiac arrest. Intraosseous injection has also been reported to cause systemic toxicity.

A dosage of 0.5–1.0 mL/kg of 0.125–0.25% bupivacaine (or ropivacaine) with or without epinephrine can be used. Opioids may also be added (eg, 50–70 µg/kg of morphine), although they are not recommended for outpatients because of the risk of delayed respiratory depression. The analgesic effects of the block extend for hours into the postoperative period. Pediatric outpatients can safely be discharged home even with mild residual motor block and without urinating, as most children will urinate within 8 h.

Repeated injections can be accomplished via repeating the needle injection or via a catheter left in place and covered with an occlusive dressing after being connected to extension tubing. Higher epidural anesthesia/analgesia can be accomplished with epidural catheters threaded cephalad into the lumbar or even thoracic epidural space from the caudal approach in infants and children. A technique has been described using a nerve stimulator to determine the level to which the catheter has been threaded. More commonly fluoroscopy is used. Smaller catheters are technically difficult to pass due to kinking. Catheters advanced into the thoracic epidural space have been used to achieve T2–T4 blocks for ex-premature infants undergoing inguinal hernia repair. This is achieved using chloroprocaine 1 mL/kg as an initial bolus and incremental doses of 0.3 mL/kg until the desired level is achieved.

For adults undergoing anorectal procedures, caudal anesthesia can provide dense sacral sensory blockade with limited cephalad spread. Furthermore, the injection can be given with the patient in the prone jackknife position, which is used for surgery (Figure 16–21). A dose of 15–20 mL of 1.5–2.0% lidocaine with or without epinephrine is usually effective. Fentanyl 50–100 µg may also be added. This technique should be avoided in patients with pilonidal cysts because the needle may pass through the cyst track and can potentially introduce bacteria into the caudal epidural space. Although no longer commonly used for obstetric analgesia, a caudal block can be useful for the second stage of labor in situations in which the epidural is not reaching the sacral nerves, or when repeated attempts at epidural blockade have been unsuccessful.

COMPLICATIONS OF NEURAXIAL BLOCKS

The complications of epidural, spinal, or caudal anesthetics range from the bothersome to the crippling and life-threatening (Table 16–6). Broadly, the complications can be thought of as those resulting from physiological excessive side effects, placement of the needle (or catheter), and drug toxicity.

A very large survey of regional anesthesia from France provides an indication of the relatively low incidence of serious complications from spinal and epidural anesthesia (Table 16–7). In contrast, the American Society of Anes-

Table 16–6. Complications of neuraxial anesthesia.

Adverse or exaggerated physiological responses
  Urinary retention
  High block
  Total spinal anesthesia
  Cardiac arrest
  Anterior spinal artery syndrome
  Horner's syndrome
Complications related to needle/catheter placement
  Trauma
    Backache
    Dural puncture/leak
      Postdural puncture headache
      Diplopia
      Tinnitus
  Neural injury
    Nerve root damage
    Spinal cord damage
    Cauda equina syndrome
  Bleeding
    Intraspinal/epidural hematoma
  Misplacement
    No effect/inadequate anesthesia
    Subdural block
    Inadvertent subarachnoid block[1]
    Inadvertent intravascular injection
  Catheter shearing/retention
  Inflammation
    Arachnoiditis
  Infection
    Meningitis
    Epidural abscess
Drug toxicity
  Systemic local anesthetic toxicity
  Transient neurological symptoms
  Cauda equina syndrome

[1]For epidural block only.

thesiologists (ASA) Closed Claims Project helps identify the most common causes of liability claims involving regional anesthesia in the operating room setting. In a 20-year period (1980–1999) regional anesthesia accounted for 18% of all liability claims. In the majority of these claims, the injuries were judged as temporary or nondisabling (64%). Serious injuries in the remaining claims included death (13%), permanent nerve injury (10%), permanent brain damage (8%), and other permanent injuries (4%). The majority of regional anesthesia claims involved either lumbar epidural anesthesia (42%) or spinal anesthesia (34%), and tended to occur mostly in obstetric patients. The latter may at least partly reflect the relatively higher use of neuraxial anesthesia compared to other regional techniques and its relatively very high utilization in obstetric patients. Of note is that caudal anesthesia was utilized in only 2% of claims.

Complications Associated with Adverse or Exaggerated Physiological Responses

A. HIGH NEURAL BLOCKADE

High levels of neural blockade can occur readily with either spinal or epidural anesthesia. Administration of an excessive dose, failure to reduce standard doses in selected patients (eg, the elderly, pregnant, obese, or very short), or unusual sensitivity or spread of local anesthetic may be responsible. Patients often complain of dyspnea and have numbness or weakness in the upper extremities. Nausea with or without vomiting often precedes hypotension. Once it is recognized patients should be reassured, oxygen supplementation may need to be increased, and bradycardia and hypotension should be corrected.

Spinal anesthesia ascending into the cervical levels causes severe hypotension, bradycardia, and respiratory insufficiency. Unconsciousness, apnea, and hypotension resulting from high levels of spinal anesthesia are referred to as a "high spinal" or "total spinal." It can also occur following attempted epidural/caudal anesthesia if there is inadvertent intrathecal injection (see below). Severe sustained hypotension with lower sensory blocks can also lead to apnea through medullary hypoperfusion. Anterior spinal artery syndrome (see Chapters 21 and 33) has been reported following neuraxial anesthesia, presumably due to prolonged severe hypotension together with an increase in intraspinal pressure.

Table 16–7. Incidence of serious complications from spinal and epidural anesthesia.[1]

Technique	Cardiac Arrest	Death	Seizure	Cauda Equina Syndrome	Paraplegia	Radiculopathy
Spinal (n = 40,640)	26	6	0	5	0	19
Epidural (n = 30,413)	3	0	4	0	1	5

[1]Data from Auroy Y, et al: Serious complications related to regional anesthesia, results of a prospective survey in France. Anesthesiology 1997;87:479.

Treatment of an excessively high neuraxial block involves maintaining an adequate airway and ventilation and supporting the circulation. When respiratory insufficiency becomes evident, in addition to supplemental oxygen, assisted ventilation, intubation, and mechanical ventilation may be necessary. Hypotension can be treated with rapid administration of intravenous fluids, a head-down position, and aggressive use of vasopressors. Epinephrine should be used early if ephedrine or phenylephrine is insufficient. Dopamine infusion may be helpful. Bradycardia should be treated early with atropine. Ephedrine or epinephrine can also increase heart rate. If respiratory and hemodynamic control can be readily achieved and maintained after high or total spinal anesthesia, surgery may proceed. Apnea is often transient, and unconsciousness may leave the patient amnestic without adverse recall.

B. Cardiac Arrest during Spinal Anesthesia

Examination of data from the ASA Closed Claim Project identified several cases of cardiac arrest during spinal anesthesia. Because many of the reported cases predated the routine use of pulse oximetry, many physicians believed oversedation and unrecognized hypoventilation and hypoxia were the causes. However, large prospective studies continue to report a relatively high incidence of cardiac arrest in patients having received a spinal anesthetic, perhaps as high as 1:1500. Many of the arrests were preceded by bradycardia and occurred in young healthy patients. A recent examination of this problem identified vagal responses and decreased preload as key factors and suggests that patients with high baseline vagal tone are at risk (see Chapter 46). Prophylactic volume expansion is recommended, as is early and aggressive vagolytic (atropine) treatment of bradycardia followed by ephedrine and epinephrine if necessary.

C. Urinary Retention

Local anesthetic block of S2–S4 root fibers decreases urinary bladder tone and inhibits the voiding reflex. Epidural opioids can also interfere with normal voiding. These effects are most pronounced in male patients. Urinary bladder catheterization should be used for all but the shortest acting blocks. If a catheter is not present postoperatively, close observation for voiding is necessary. Persistent bladder dysfunction can also be a manifestation of serious neural injury as discussed below.

Complications Associated with Needle or Catheter Insertion

A. Inadequate Anesthesia or Analgesia

As with other regional anesthesia techniques, neuraxial blocks are "blind" techniques that rely on indirect signs of correct needle placement. It is not surprising that they are associated with a small but significant failure rate that is usually inversely proportional to the clinician's experience. The end point for spinal anesthesia (CSF flow) is much more obvious than loss of resistance. Failure may still occur even when CSF is obtained during spinal anesthesia. Movement of the needle during injection, incomplete entry of the needle opening into the subarachnoid space, subdural injection, or loss of potency of the local anesthetic solution may be responsible. Commercially prepared tetracaine solutions may lose potency when stored for prolonged periods at high temperatures.

Causes for failed epidural blocks were discussed above (see Failed Epidural Blocks).

B. Intravascular Injection

Inadvertent intravascular injection of the local anesthetic for epidural and caudal anesthesia can produce very high serum levels. Extremely high levels of local anesthetics affect the central nervous system (seizure and unconsciousness) and the cardiovascular system (hypotension, arrhythmia, and cardiovascular collapse). Because the dosage of medication for spinal anesthesia is relatively small, this complication is seen primarily with epidural and caudal blocks. Local anesthetic may be injected directly into a vessel through a needle or later through a catheter that has entered a blood vessel (vein). The incidence of intravascular injection can be minimized by carefully aspirating the needle (or catheter) before every injection, using a test dose, always injecting local anesthetic in incremental doses, and close observation for early signs of intravascular injection (tinnitus, lingual sensations).

The local anesthetics vary in their toxicity (see Chapter 14). Chloroprocaine is the least toxic because it is broken down very rapidly; lidocaine, mepivacaine, levobupivacaine, and ropivacaine are intermediate in toxicity; and bupivacaine is most toxic.

C. Total Spinal Anesthesia

Total spinal anesthesia can occur following attempted epidural/caudal anesthesia if there is inadvertent intrathecal injection. Onset is usually rapid because the amount of anesthetic required for epidural and caudal anesthesia is 5–10 times that required for spinal anesthesia. Careful aspiration, use of a test dose, and incremental injection techniques during epidural and caudal anesthesia can help avoid this complication. In the event of an inadvertent large subarachnoid injection, particularly of lidocaine, consideration should be given to "subarachnoid lavage" by repeated withdrawal of 5 mL of CSF and replacement with preservative-free normal saline.

D. Subdural Injection

As with inadvertent intravascular injection and because of the larger amount of local anesthetic administered, inadvertent subdural injection of local anesthetic during attempted epidural anesthesia is much more serious than during attempted spinal anesthesia. A subdural injection of epidural doses of local anesthetic produces a clinical presentation similar to that of high spinal anesthesia, with the exception that the onset may be delayed for 15–30 min. The spinal subdural space is a potential space between the dura and the arachnoid containing a small amount of serous fluid. Unlike the epidural space, the subdural space extends intracranially, so that anesthetic injected into the spinal subdural space can ascend to higher levels than epidural medications. As with high spinal anesthesia, treatment is supportive and may require intubation, mechanical ventilation, and cardiovascular support. The effects generally last from one to several hours.

E. BACKACHE

As a needle passes through skin, subcutaneous tissues, muscle, and ligaments it causes varying degrees of tissue trauma. A localized inflammatory response with or without reflex muscle spasm may be responsible for postoperative backache. It should be noted that up to 25–30% of patients receiving only general anesthesia also complain of backache postoperatively and a significant percentage of the general population has chronic back pain. Postoperative back soreness or ache is usually mild and self-limited, although it may last for a number of weeks. If treatment is sought, acetaminophen, nonsteroidal antiinflammatory medication, and warm or cold compresses should suffice. Although backache is usually benign, it may be an important clinical sign of much more serious complications, such as epidural hematoma and abscess (see below).

F. POSTDURAL PUNCTURE HEADACHE

Any breach of the dura may result in a postdural puncture headache (PDPH). This may follow a diagnostic lumbar puncture, a myelogram, a spinal anesthetic, or an epidural "wet tap" in which the epidural needle passed through the epidural space and entered the subarachnoid space. Similarly, an epidural catheter might puncture the dura at any time and result in PDPH. An epidural wet tap is usually immediately recognized as CSF dripping from the needle or aspirated from an epidural catheter. However, PDPH can follow use of a seemingly uncomplicated epidural anesthetic and may be the result of just the tip of the needle scratching through the dura. Typically, PDPH is bilateral, frontal or retroorbital, and occipital and extends into the neck. It may be throbbing or constant and associated with photophobia and nausea. The hallmark of PDPH is its association with body position. The pain is aggravated by sitting or standing and relieved or decreased by lying down flat. The onset of headache is usually 12–72 h following the procedure; however, it may be seen almost immediately. Untreated, the pain may last weeks, and in rare instances has required surgical repair.

PDPH is believed to result from leakage of CSF from a dural defect and decreased intracranial pressure. Loss of CSF at a rate faster than it can be produced causes traction on structures supporting the brain, particularly the dura and tentorium. Increased traction on blood vessels also likely contributes to the pain. Traction on the cranial nerves may occasionally cause diplopia (usually the sixth cranial nerve) and tinnitus. The incidence of PDPH is strongly related to needle size, needle type, and patient population. The larger the needle, the greater the incidence of PDPH. Cutting-point needles are associated with a higher incidence of PDPH than pencil-point needles of the same gauge. A cutting needle introduced with the bevel parallel to the longitudinal fibers of the dura is said to separate these fibers rather than transecting them, therefore reducing the chance of PDPH. Factors that increase the risk of PDPH include young age, female sex, and pregnancy. The highest incidence, then, would be expected following an inadvertent wet tap with a large epidural needle in an obstetric patient (perhaps as high as 20–50%). The lowest incidence would be expected with an elderly male using a 27-gauge pencil-point needle (< 1%). Studies of obstetric patients undergoing spinal anesthesia for cesarean section with small-gauge pencil-point needles have shown rates as low as 3% or 4%.

Conservative treatment involves recumbent positioning, analgesics, intravenous or oral fluid administration, and caffeine. Keeping the patient supine will decrease the hydrostatic pressure driving fluid out the dural hole and minimizing the headache. Analgesic medication may range from acetaminophen to NSAIDs. Hydration and caffeine work to stimulate production of CSF. Caffeine further helps by vasoconstricting intracranial vessels. Stool softeners and soft diet are used to minimize Valsalva straining. Headache may persist for days despite conservative therapy.

An epidural blood patch is a very effective treatment for PDPH. It involves injecting 15–20 mL of autologous blood into the epidural space at, or one interspace below, the level of the dural puncture. It is believed to stop further leakage of CSF by either mass effect or coagulation. The effects may be immediate or may take some hours as CSF production slowly builds intracranial pressure. Approximately 90% of patients will respond to a single blood patch, and 90% of initial nonresponders will obtain relief from a second injection. Prophylactic blood patching has been advocated by injecting blood through an epidural catheter that was placed after a wet tap. However, not all patients will develop PDPH, and the tip of the catheter may be many levels away from the dural defect. Alternatively, a saline bolus can be injected through the epidural catheter but does not appear to be as effective as blood patching. Most practitioners either offer the epidural blood patch when PDPH becomes apparent or allow conservative therapy a trial of 12–24 h.

G. NEUROLOGICAL INJURY

Perhaps no complication is more perplexing or distressing than persistent neurological deficits following an apparently routine neuraxial block in which an epidural hematoma or abscess is ruled out. The nerve roots or spinal cord may be injured. The latter may be avoided if the neuraxial blockade is performed below L1 in adults and L3 in children. Postoperative peripheral neuropathies can be due to direct physical trauma to nerve roots. Although most resolve spontaneously, some are permanent. Some of these deficits have been associated with paresthesia from the needle or catheter or with complaints of pain during injection. Some studies have suggested that multiple attempts during a technically difficult block are also a risk factor. Any sustained paresthesia should alert the clinician to redirect the needle. Injections should be immediately stopped and the needle withdrawn if they are associated with pain. Direct injection into the spinal cord can cause paraplegia. Damage to the conus medullaris may cause isolated sacral dysfunction, including paralysis of the biceps femoris muscles; anesthesia in the posterior thigh, saddle area, or great toes; and loss of bowel or bladder function. Some animal studies suggest catheters can cause inflammation or even demyelination in nerve tissue.

It should be noted that not all neurological deficits occurring after a regional anesthetic are the result of the block. Surveys of complications have reported many instances of postoperative neurological deficits that were attributed to regional anesthesia when in fact only general anesthesia was used. Postpartum deficits including lateral femoral cutaneous neuropathy, foot drop, and paraplegia were recognized before the modern era of anesthesia and still occur in the absence of anesthetics. Less clear are the postanesthetic cases complicated by concurrent conditions such as atherosclerosis, diabetes mellitus, intervertebral disk disease, and spinal disorders.

H. SPINAL OR EPIDURAL HEMATOMA

Needle or catheter trauma to epidural veins often causes minor bleeding in the spinal canal although this is usually benign and self-limiting. A clinically significant spinal hematoma can occur following spinal or epidural anesthesia, particularly in the presence of abnormal coagulation or bleeding disorder. The incidence of such hematomas has been estimated to be about 1:150,000 for epidural blocks and 1:220,000 for spinal anesthetics. The vast majority of reported cases have occurred in patients with abnormal coagulation either secondary to disease or pharmacological therapies. Some have emphasized the association with a technically difficult or bloody block. It should be noted that many hemato-

mas have occurred immediately after the removal of an epidural catheter. Thus, insertion and removal of an epidural catheter are risk factors.

The pathological insult to the spinal cord and nerves is due to a mass effect compressing neural tissue and causing direct pressure injury and ischemia. The need for rapid diagnosis and intervention is paramount if permanent neurological sequelae are to be avoided. The onset of symptoms is typically more sudden compared with epidural abscess. **Symptoms include sharp back and leg pain with a progression to numbness and motor weakness and/or sphincter dysfunction.** When hematoma is suspected, neurological imaging (magnetic resonance imaging [MRI], computed tomography [CT], or myelography) must be obtained immediately and neurosurgical consultation should be requested. In many cases good neurological recovery has occurred in patients who have undergone surgical decompression within 8–12 h.

Neuraxial anesthesia is best avoided in patients with coagulopathy, significant thrombocytopenia, platelet dysfunction, or those who have received fibrinolytic/thrombolytic therapy.

I. MENINGITIS AND ARACHNOIDITIS

Infection of the subarachnoid space can follow neuraxial blocks as the result of contamination of the equipment or injected solutions, or as a result of organisms tracked in from the skin. Indwelling catheters may become colonized with organisms that then track deep, causing infection. Fortunately, these are rare occurrences.

Arachnoiditis, another reported rare complication of neuraxial anesthesia, may be infectious or noninfectious. Clinically, it is marked by pain and other neurological symptoms and on radiographic imaging is seen as a clumping of the nerve roots. Cases of arachnoiditis have been traced to detergent in a spinal procaine preparation. Lumbar arachnoiditis has been reported from subarachnoid steroid injection but is more commonly seen following spinal surgery or trauma. Prior to the use of disposable spinal needles, caustic cleaning solutions caused cases of chemical meningitis resulting in severe neurological dysfunction.

J. EPIDURAL ABSCESS

Spinal epidural abscess (EA) is a rare but potentially devastating complication of neuraxial anesthesia. The reported incidence varies widely from 1:6500 to 1:500,000 epidurals. Most cases in the literature are isolated case reports. Several prospective studies, including over 140,000 blocks, have failed to report one EA. EA can occur in patients who did not receive regional anesthesia; risk factors in such cases include back trauma, injecting drug use, and neurosurgical procedures. Most reported anesthesia-related cases involve epidural catheters. In one reported series, there was a mean of 5 days from catheter insertion to the development of symptoms, although presentation can be delayed for weeks.

There are four classic clinical stages of EA, although progression and time course can vary. Initially, symptoms include back or vertebral pain that is intensified by percussion over the spine. Second, nerve root or radicular pain develops. The third stage is marked by motor and/or sensory deficits or sphincter dysfunction. Paraplegia or paralysis marks the fourth stage. Ideally, the diagnosis is made in the early stages. Prognosis has consistently been shown to correlate to the degree of neurological dysfunction at the time the diagnosis is made. Back pain and fever after epidural anesthesia should alert the clinician to consider EA. Radicular pain or neurological deficit heightens the urgency to investigate. Once EA is suspected, the catheter should be removed (if still present) and the tip cultured. The injection site is examined for evidence of infection; if pus is expressed it is sent for culture. Blood cultures should be obtained. If suspicion is high and cultures have been obtained, anti-*Staphylococcus* coverage can be instituted, as the most common organisms causing EA are *Staphylococcus aureus* and *Staphylococcus epidermidis*. MRI or CT scanning should be performed to confirm or rule out the diagnosis. Early neurosurgical consultation is advisable. In addition to antibiotics, treatment of EA usually involves decompression (laminectomy), although percutaneous drainage with fluoroscopic or CT guidance has been reported. There are a few reports of patients with no neurological signs being treated with antibiotics alone.

Suggested strategies for guarding against the occurrence of EA include (1) minimizing catheter manipulations and maintaining a closed system when possible, (2) using a micropore (0.22-μm) bacterial filter, and (3) removing an epidural catheter after 96 h or at least changing the catheter, filter, and solution every 96 h. Although these interventions seem logical, they remain unproved. Sometimes the system can become disconnected and the clinician needs to decide whether to remove the catheter or try to reconnect it using aseptic techniques. No universal guidelines for performing an epidural exist; some practitioners use a cap and mask and thoroughly wash their hands prior to gloving as a minimum, in addition to sterile skin preparation and maintaining a sterile field.

K. Sheering of an Epidural Catheter

As with any catheter through the needle technique, there is a risk of the catheter sheering and breaking off inside tissues if it is withdrawn through the needle. If a catheter must be withdrawn before the needle is completely pulled out, both must be carefully withdrawn *together*. When a catheter breaks off deep within the epidural space many experts suggest leaving it alone and

carefully observing the patient. If, however, the breakage occurs in superficial tissues, particularly when part of the catheter is visible, bacteria can readily track along the catheter remnant and the catheter should be surgically removed.

Complications Associated with Drug Toxicity

A. Systemic Toxicity

Absorption of excessive amounts of local anesthetics can produce very high toxic serum levels (see Intravascular Injection). Excessive absorption from epidural or caudal blocks is rare if the maximum safe dosage of local anesthetic is not exceeded.

B. Transient Neurological Symptoms

First described in 1993, **transient neurological symptoms** (TNS), also referred to as transient radicular irritation, are characterized by back pain radiating to the legs without sensory or motor deficits, occurring after the resolution of spinal block and resolving spontaneously within several days. It is most commonly associated with hyperbaric lidocaine (incidence up to 11.9%), but has also been reported with tetracaine (1.6%), bupivacaine (1.3%), mepivacaine, prilocaine, procaine, and subarachnoid ropivacaine. There are also case reports of TNS following epidural anesthesia. The incidence of this syndrome is highest among outpatients (early ambulation) after surgery in the lithotomy position and lowest among inpatients in positions other than lithotomy. There is a paucity of reports of TNS following spinal lidocaine for cesarean section. The pathogenesis of TNS is believed to represent concentration-dependent neurotoxicity of local anesthetics.

C. Lidocaine Neurotoxicity

Cauda equina syndrome (CES) was associated with the use of continuous spinal catheters (prior to their withdrawal) and 5% lidocaine (see Spinal Catheters). CES is characterized by bowel and bladder dysfunction together with evidence of multiple nerve root injury. There is lower motor neuron type injury with paresis of the legs. Sensory deficits may be patchy, typically occurring in a peripheral nerve pattern. Pain may be similar to that of nerve root compromise. Animal studies suggest that pooling or "maldistribution" of hyperbaric solutions of lidocaine can lead to neurotoxicity of the nerve roots of the cauda equina. However, there are reports of CES occurring after uneventful single-shot lidocaine spinals. CES has also been reported following epidural anesthesia. Animal data suggest that the extent of histological evidence of neurotoxicity following repeat intrathecal injection is lidocaine = tetracaine > bupivacaine > ropivacaine.

A 56-year-old male presents for extracorporeal shock wave lithotripsy (ESWL) of a large kidney stone. The procedure involves immersing the patient in a water bath through which high-energy waves are focused onto the stone (see Chapter 33). The patient has a long history of spinal problems and has undergone fusion of the cervical spine (C3–C6) and laminectomy with fusion of the lower lumbar spine (L3–L5). On examination, he has no neck flexion or extension and has a Mallampati class IV airway (see Chapter 5).

What types of anesthesia are appropriate for this patient?

High-energy lithotripsy usually requires general or neuraxial anesthesia. A significant advantage of general anesthesia is that diaphragmatic excursion and secondary movement of the stone can be controlled by adjusting tidal volume and respiratory rate. Selection of the type of anesthesia as always should be based on patient preference after informed consent. This patient presents potential difficulties for both general and regional anesthesia. The limited excursion of the cervical spine together with the anatomy of a class IV airway makes difficulty in intubation and possibly ventilation almost certain. Induction of general anesthesia would be safest after the airway is secured with an awake fiberoptic intubation.

Regional anesthesia also presents a problem in that the patient has had previous back surgery in the lumbar area where neuraxial anesthesia is most commonly performed. Some clinicians consider prior back surgery to be a relative contraindication to neuraxial anesthesia. Postoperative distortion of the anatomy makes the block technically challenging and may increase the likelihood of a failure, inadvertent dural puncture during epidural anesthesia, paresthesias, and an unpredictable spread of the local anesthetics. Many clinicians believe that the neuraxial blockade can be safely done above or below the level of surgery. Indeed, lumbar laminectomy can facilitate spinal anesthesia at the level of the surgery.

If the patient chooses to have neuraxial anesthesia, would spinal or epidural anesthesia be more appropriate?

Many clinicians believe that epidural anesthesia is more appropriate for ESWL in a tub. Use of an epidural catheter may allow better control of the sensory level and duration of anesthesia. The associated sympathectomy and subsequent drop in blood pressure are more gradual than that following spinal anesthesia. Because the patient will be placed in a chair for the procedure, spinal anesthesia may be associated with a more marked degree of hypotension until the patient is placed in the tub (see Chapter 33). With either type of anesthesia, significant hypotension should be treated aggressively with intravenous fluids and vasoconstrictors; bradycardia should be treated with atropine. Placing the patient in a sitting position immediately after spinal anesthesia also increases the risk of a PDPH. If spinal anesthesia is elected, use of a small-gauge needle (25- gauge or less pencil-point needle) may help minimize the risk of PDPH.

After an explanation of the options, the patient appears to understand the risks of both types of anesthesia and desires epidural anesthesia. Placement of an epidural catheter is attempted at the L1–L2 interspace but inadvertent dural puncture occurs: What options are now available?

Options include injecting a spinal dose of local anesthetic through the epidural needle to induce spinal anesthesia, attempting epidural anesthesia at another level, attempting spinal anesthesia at a lower level, and abandoning regional anesthesia and proceeding with an awake fiberoptic intubation. If a spinal dose of local anesthetic is to be injected, the syringe and needle should be kept in place for a few moments to prevent significant back leakage of anesthetic through the large dural hole. Threading an epidural catheter through the needle into the subarachnoid space allows subsequent redosing, but above L1 it carries some risk of injury to the spinal cord (conus medullaris). Without radiographic confirmation, even experienced clinicians can misjudge the actual level of needle insertion by one to two spinal levels; thus the dural puncture site could be as high as the T11–T12 interspace. Even when a catheter is advanced in the subarachnoid space well below L2, it should not be advanced more than 2–3 cm to avoid injury to the cauda equina.

How might a dural puncture affect subsequent epidural or spinal anesthesia?

A potential hazard of epidural anesthesia at a level adjacent to a large dural puncture is the pos-

sibility that some local anesthetic might pass through the dural puncture into the subarachnoid space. This could result in a higher than expected level of sensory and motor blockade. Careful incremental injection of local anesthetic may help avoid this problem.

Conversely, a large dural puncture can theoretically diminish the effect of subsequent spinal anesthesia at an adjacent level. Because only a small amount is used, leakage of local anesthetic with CSF through dural puncture can theoretically limit the cephalad spread of the solution.

What can be done to prevent the occurrence of a spinal headache?

Studies suggest that successfully placing an epidural catheter after a wet tap at a different level decreases the incidence of PDPH by as much as 50%. Unfortunately, the same difficult anatomy that might have led to the dural puncture may increase the likelihood of a second inadvertent puncture. Observation is generally recommended. The management of PDPH was discussed earlier in this chapter.

SUGGESTED READING

Auroy Y, Narchi P, Messiah A, et al: Serious complications related to regional anesthesia: Results of a prospective survey in France. Anesthesiology 1997;87:479.

Ben-David B, Rawa R: Complications of neuraxial blockade. In: *Anesthesia Related Complications.* Gan TJ (editor). Anesth Clin North Am 2002;20:669.

Broadman LM, Hannallah RS, Norden JM, McGill WA: "Kiddie caudals": Experience with 1154 consecutive cases without complications. Anesth Analg 1987;66:S18.

Brookman CA, Rutledge ML: Epidural abscess: Case report and literature review. Reg Anesth Pain Med 2000;25:428.

Brown DL: *Atlas of Regional Anesthesia,* 2nd ed. W.B. Saunders, 1999.

Cousins MJ: *Neural Blockade in Clinical Anesthesia and Pain Management,* 3rd ed. Lippincott, Williams & Wilkins, 1998.

Dahlgren N, Tornebrandt K: Neurological complications after anaesthesia. A follow-up of 18,000 spinal and epidural anaesthetics performed over three years. Acta Anaesthesiol Scand 1995;39:872.

Ellis H, Feldman S, Harrop-Griffiths W: *Anatomy for Anaesthetists,* 8th ed. Blackwell Publishing, 2004.

Finucane BT: *Complications of Regional Anesthesia.* Churchill Livingstone, 1999.

Grass JA: The role of epidural anesthesia and analgesia in postoperative outcome. Anesth Clin North Am 2000;18:407.

Greene NM: *Physiology of Spinal Anesthesia,* 4th ed. Williams & Wilkins, 1993.

Khalil S, Campos C, Farag AM, et al: Caudal block in children. Anesthesiology 1999;91:1279.

Lee JA, Atkinson RS, Watt MJ: *Lumbar Puncture and Spinal Analgesia: Intradural and Extradural,* 5th ed. Churchill Livingstone, 1985.

Lee LA, Posner KL, Domino KB, et al: Injuries associated with regional anesthesia in the 1980s and 1990s: A closed claims analysis. Anesthesiology 2004;101:143.

Liu SS, McDonald SB: Current issues in spinal anesthesia. Anesthesiology 2001;94:888.

Mulroy MF: *Regional Anesthesia: An Illustrated Procedural Guide,* 3rd ed. Lippincott, Williams & Wilkins, 2002.

Munnur U, Suresh S: Backache, headache, and neurological deficit after regional anesthesia. In: *Issues in Obstetric Anesthesia.* Vadhera RB, Douglas MJ (editors). Anesth Clin North Am 2003;21:71.

Pollard JB: Cardiac arrest during spinal anesthesia: Common mechanisms and strategies for prevention. Anesth Analg 2001;92:252.

Raj PP: *Textbook of Regional Anesthesia.* Churchill Livingstone, 2002.

Rodgers A, Walker N, Schug S, et al: Reduction of postoperative mortality and morbidity with epidural or spinal anaesthesia: Results from overview of randomised trials. BMJ 2000;321:1493.

Sarubbi FA, Vasquez JE: Spinal epidural abscess associated with the use of temporary epidural catheters: Report of two cases and review. Clin Infect Dis 1997;25:1155.

Suresh S, Wheeler M: Practical pediatric regional anesthesia. In: *New concepts and Techniques in Pediatric Anesthesia.* Mason L, Kim M (editors). Anesth Clin North Am 2002;20:83.

Peripheral Nerve Blocks

17

KEY CONCEPTS

 The greatest immediate risk of nerve blocks is systemic toxicity from inadvertent intravascular injection. Delayed toxicity can follow the initial injection when rapid or excessive amounts of local anesthetics are absorbed systemically.

 Good surgical anesthesia is obtained only when local anesthetic is injected in close proximity to the nerve or nerves that are to be blocked.

 A perineural injection may produce a brief accentuation of the paresthesia, whereas an intraneural injection produces an intense, searing pain that serves as a warning to immediately terminate the injection and reposition the needle.

 Surgical anesthesia of the upper extremity and shoulder can be obtained following neural blockade of the brachial plexus (C5–T1) or its terminal branches at several sites.

 The interscalene approach is most optimal for procedures on the shoulder, arm, and forearm. Injection at the interscalene level tends to produce a block that is most intense at the C5–C7 dermatomes and least intense in the C8–T1 dermatomes.

 The axillary approach to the brachial plexus is most optimal for procedures from the elbow to the hand. This approach tends to produce the most intense block in the distribution of C7–T1 (ulnar nerve).

 Infraclavicular blocks provide good homogeneous anesthesia to the brachial plexus and can be used for procedures involving the hand, fore-arm, elbow, and upper arm and are quite conducive for placement of an indwelling catheter for postoperative analgesia.

 Intravenous regional anesthesia, also called a Bier block, can provide intense surgical anesthesia for short surgical procedures (< 45–60 min) on the forearm, hand, and even the leg.

 A femoral nerve block is very useful in numerous procedures involving the thigh and knee, such as skin grafting, knee arthroscopy, and patellar surgery, or as an adjunct to procedures distal to the knee that require anesthesia to the medial aspect of the lower leg (saphenous distribution).

 There has been a recent surge of interest in fascia iliaca blocks. Because it does not require a nerve stimulator, it can be performed very quickly, it is not very stimulating, and patients often do not require sedation. It is useful in procedures involving the hip, thigh, and knee.

 Blockade of the sciatic nerve is useful for many surgical procedures involving the hip, knee, or distal lower extremity. The nerve can be successfully blocked at numerous sites along its course.

 A popliteal nerve block is very useful for foot and ankle surgery and can result in complete anesthesia of the limb distal to the knee if a separate saphenous nerve block (terminal nerve of the femoral nerve) is also included.

(continued on next page)

(continued from previous page)

Paravertebral nerve blocks are being increasingly used as an effective technique for postoperative analgesia following mastectomy, inguinal hernia repair, and several procedures involving the chest and body wall.

Advancement in needle delivery devices, safer local anesthetics, and development of indwelling catheters for postoperative perineural infusion have led to a transformation in regional anesthesia; the focus has shifted from providing intraoperative regional anesthesia to providing intraoperative anesthesia and postoperative regional analgesia.

Fundamental to the success of regional anesthesia is the correct positioning of the needle tip in the perineural sheath, prior to injection of local anesthetic. In the past, this was accomplished either by eliciting a paresthesia with the needle tip or, in the case of an axillary nerve block, by using the transarterial approach. Either out of fear of persistent paresthesias or arterial injury, or because of advancement of the specialty and development of newer technologies, anesthesiologists today commonly employ a nerve stimulator to help define needle tip location. The use of nerve stimulators is not risk free, as morbidities have been reported with these devices, leaving providers in search of the optimal tool. Other technologies that are being studied are ultrasound, Doppler, and sensory nerve stimulation. Currently the best way to establish needle tip location is based on a motor response to nerve stimulation; a motor response at approximately 0.5 mA indicates that the needle is in the appropriate position and local anesthetic can be injected.

INDICATIONS

The choice of anesthesia is determined by patient comorbidities and by obtaining an informed consent that includes understanding all available options and their risks and benefits. Important considerations in discussing anesthetic choices include the suitability of the technique for the type of surgery, the surgeon's preference, the experience of the anesthesiologist, and the physiological and mental state of the patient.

The use of peripheral nerve blocks is increasing; they are being used as the primary and sole anesthetic technique to facilitate painless surgery, supplemented with monitored anesthesia care (moderate sedation) or with a "light" general anesthetic, with the airway protected with a laryngeal mask airway (LMA), or instituted preoperatively but primarily for postoperative analgesia.

Patient satisfaction is improved, there is less cognitive impairment with regional anesthesia compared to general anesthesia (particularly in elderly patients), and there is new evidence that peripheral nerve blocks (regional anesthesia) are less immunosuppressive than general anesthesia. Although peripheral nerve blocks are not risk free, they offer an excellent alternative for patients in whom postoperative nausea and vomiting are a problem, who are at risk for development of malignant hyperthermia, or who are hemodynamically compromised or too ill to tolerate general anesthesia.

The disadvantages of peripheral nerve blocks, although uncommon, include the toxicity of local anesthetics, chronic paresthesias and nerve damage, and, depending on the nerves being anesthetized (interscalene block, supraclavicular block, etc), respiratory failure due to phrenic nerve blockade, and seizures due to intraarterial injections.

When discussing the use of peripheral nerve blocks to facilitate a regional anesthetic compared to a general anesthetic, the risks and benefits of both techniques must be discussed with the patient so that the patient may make an informed choice.

CONTRAINDICATIONS

Most contraindications to peripheral nerve blockade using local anesthetics are relative, in that many patients are not good candidates for either regional or general anesthesia and, therefore, the physician must decide which is safest and advise the patient accordingly (Table 17–1).

Regional anesthetics require relatively cooperative patients and, therefore, pediatric patients, combative patients, and demented patients can present a challenge to the anesthesiologist. Many peripheral nerve blocks in pediatric patients are performed after general anesthesia is induced. In adult patients, however, there is some concern about performing peripheral nerve blocks in an anesthetized patient who cannot respond to an intraneuronal injection, placing the patient at increased risk

Roy A. Greengrass, MD

REGIONAL ANESTHESIA & CLINICAL PRACTICE

An 88-year-old male philanthropist is scheduled for repair of recurrent left inguinal hernia. He has a history of confusion with administration of any opioid. He has had previous urethral reconstruction surgery. An attending urologist is concerned that in the event of urinary retention urinary catheterization would be hazardous. What are the anesthetic options for this patient?

A 45-year-old man is scheduled for total shoulder arthroplasty for severe osteoarthritis of the shoulder. He has chronic pain for which he is on large-dose opioids. A recent minor ambulatory open-shoulder procedure under general anesthesia was associated with severe postoperative pain, which was not controlled with standard doses of intravenous opioids, necessitating hospitalization. What

are the anesthetic options for this patient's total shoulder arthroplasty?

General anesthesia is safe, efficient, and effective as attested by successful administration over the past 120 years. It is interesting, though, that the mechanisms of general anesthesia remain an enigma even today!

Coincident with the discovery of general anesthesia was the observation of side effects associated with its use including nausea and vomiting, urinary retention, and altered cognition, among others. Most general anesthetics are not analgesics and, in fact, have recently been determined to be antianalgesic in the early postoperative period.[1] In a review article analyzing postdischarge symptoms after outpatient surgery, it was determined that a significant number of patients experienced moderate to severe pain, particularly after orthopedic procedures. This pain experience interfered with activities of daily living and resulted in prolonged convalescence, significantly increasing secondary costs.[2]

A complication of ambulatory surgery, almost unique to general anesthesia and opioids, is nausea and vomiting. Nausea and vomiting are by far the most important determinants of prolonged postanesthetic care unit (PACU) stay in ambulatory anesthesia,[3] and have been described by patients as more debilitating than pain.

Regional anesthesia has been performed for over a century and, like general anesthesia, has a history of periods of decreased and increased popularity. Currently regional anesthesia is becoming increasingly utilized in clinical practice, particularly with the increased utilization of ambulatory surgery.

"Regional" anesthesia, as the name suggests, implies that the anesthetic is limited to the part of the

for an adverse event. Furthermore, in demented or combative patients, even if regional anesthesia can be induced, general anesthesia may also be required to ensure that the patient remains still for the surgical procedure. If general anesthesia is induced, it could be argued that if there is no reduction in postoperative pain as a result of using a peripheral nerve block, then additional risks should not be assumed by also using a regional anesthetic technique.

Bleeding diastasis induced with an anticoagulant or resulting from a genetic defect (hemophilia) or an acquired defect (disseminated intravascular coagula-

tion) increases the risks associated with regional anesthesia. A hematoma within a peripheral nerve sheath increases the risk of ischemic nerve damage and, in a circumferential extremity (ankle) field block, may lead to limb or digit ischemia.

Bloodstream infection is also a relative contraindication to regional anesthesia. Most anesthesiologists will perform a single-shot peripheral nerve block if indicated; however, if the patient is truly bacteremic, placement of a catheter for delivery of postoperative anesthesia/analgesia should be given careful consideration and should possibly be avoided, as these catheters body involved in the surgical procedure. Limiting the anesthetic to the site of surgery also limits the physiological side effects and stress associated with surgery. Regional anesthesia accords other advantages over general anesthesia, including the reduction of blood loss of 20–50% in many procedures, attenuation of the hypercoagulable state associated with surgery,[4] and less interference with immunocompetence.

Evidence-based medicine supporting the clinical advantages of regional anesthesia is accumulating. In a recent article comparing general anesthesia and infraclavicular peripheral nerve block for hand procedures, a significant number of patients who received regional anesthesia were able to bypass the recovery room. None of the patients who received regional anesthesia had to be treated for postoperative pain prior to discharge. Patients who received regional anesthesia ambulated earlier and were discharged earlier, resulting in significant cost savings and enhanced patient satisfaction compared to patients who received general anesthesia.[5]

Although studies showing advantages of regional anesthesia in terms of short-term outcome are attractive, the possibility of regional anesthesia enhancing long-term outcome is becoming an area of intense interest and investigation. General anesthesia and surgery act together to suppress immunocompetence and may enhance both susceptibility to infection and metastatic spread of tumors.[6,7] Regional anesthesia significantly improves immunocompetence by avoiding agents that have been shown to be immunosuppressive (general anesthetics, opioids), and also perhaps by the ability of the local anesthetics themselves to suppress the inflammatory response.[8]

It is hoped that this research will engender interest into more widespread application and investigation of regional anesthetic techniques.

Conduct of case 1: General anesthesia (autonomic effects) and central neuraxial anesthetics have a similar incidence of urinary retention following hernia surgery. Regional anesthetic techniques have one-tenth this incidence. The patient received paravertebral regional anesthesia for his herniorrhaphy and was discharged from the PACU after voiding. He had an uneventful convalescence.

Conduct of case 2: For total shoulder arthroplasty, the patient received continuous interscalene regional anesthesia allowing early discharge and convalescence at home utilizing an ambulatory local anesthetic infusion.

1. Zhang Y, Eger E, Dutton RC, Sonner JM: Inhaled anesthetics have hyperalgesic effects at 0.1 minimum alveolar anesthetic concentration. Anesth Analg 2000;91:462.

2. Wu CL, Berenholtz SM, Pronovost PJ, Fleisher LA: Systematic review and analysis of postdischarge symptoms after outpatient surgery. Anesthesiology 2002; 96:994.

3. Green G, Jonsson L: Nausea: The most important factor determining length of stay after ambulatory anaesthesia: A comparative study of isoflurane and/or propofol techniques. Acta Anaesthesiol Scand 1993;37:742.

4. Tuman KJ, McCarthy RJ, March PJ, et al: Effects of epidural anesthesia and analgesia on coagulation and outcome after major vascular surgery. Anesth Analg 1991;73:696.

5. Hadzic A, Arliss J, Kerimoglu B, et al: A comparison of infraclavicular nerve block versus general anesthesia for hand and wrist day-case surgeries. Anesthesiology 2004;101:127.

6. Tsuchiya Y, Sawada S, Yoshioka I, et al: Increased surgical stress promotes tumor metastasis. Surgery 2003;133: 547.

7. Matsuoka H, Kurosawa S, Horinouchi T, et al: Inhalation anesthetics induce apoptosis in normal peripheral lymphocytes in vitro. Anesthesiology 2001;95:1467.

8. Hollmann MW, Durieux ME: Local anesthetics and the inflammatory response. Anesthesiology 2000;93:858.

serve as a nidus for infection. All patients are at risk of local anesthetic toxicity if local anesthetics are injected into the intravascular space. Some blocks, however, require such a large volume of local anesthetic to be effective that if multiple nerves are to be blocked, the risk of local anesthetic toxicity is simply too great. Examples include bilateral axillary blocks for bilateral hand procedures and multiple thoracic intercostal nerve blocks for flail chest.

Finally, patients with a preexisting peripheral neuropathy may be at increased risk of permanent nerve damage, or if a defect is in a contralateral nerve, block-ade of an ipsilateral nerve may be of concern, eg, an interscalene block in a patient with contralateral phrenic nerve paralysis.

CHOICE OF ANESTHETIC

Local anesthetics are discussed elsewhere (see Chapter 14), but when performing a block, the anesthesiologist must weigh the toxicity of the agent to be used and the characteristics of individual local anesthetics such as time to onset and duration of action, degree of sensory versus motor block, and the cardiac toxicity of large

Table 17–1. Contraindications[1] to peripheral nerve blocks.

Uncooperative patient
Bleeding diathesis
Infection
Local anesthetic toxicity[2]
Peripheral neuropathy[3]

[1]These are relative contraindications.
[2]Toxicity should be expected if anesthetization of the requisite number of nerves requires too much local anesthetic (eg, bilateral axillary nerve blocks).
[3]If the patient has a contralateral phrenic nerve palsy, an ipsilateral interscalene block would be contraindicated.

volumes of local anesthetics delivered into the perineural sheath.

Placement of the Block

Because performing peripheral nerve blocks is time consuming and because operating room turnover time is critical, the procedure is often performed in the holding area or in a specially designed procedure room, ie, block room. Although regional anesthesia is relatively safe, patients undergoing a regional anesthetic must have adequate monitoring, meeting American Society of Anesthesiologists (ASA) guidelines, and must be in an environment that allows delivery of supplemental oxygen (nasal cannula or face mask) with necessary resuscitation equipment available.

The greatest immediate risk of nerve blocks is systemic toxicity from inadvertent intravascular injection. Delayed toxicity can follow the initial injection when rapid or excessive amounts of local anesthetics are absorbed systemically. Peak blood levels occur at various times after the block. A high index of suspicion is required to detect early signs of systemic toxicity. In addition to aspiration of the syringe, many clinicians always use a 3 mL test dose of local anesthetic with 1:200,000 (5 μg/mL) or 1:400,000 (2.5 μg/mL) epinephrine to detect intravascular placement of a needle or catheter. An abrupt increase in heart rate greater than 20% over baseline is generally indicative of an intravascular injection. Incremental dosing (5 mL injections at a time) with frequent intermittent aspiration helps minimize the risk of intravascular injection. The "immobile needle" technique is often used to prevent needle movement during injection: intravenous tubing is attached between the needle and syringe such that the needle can be easily stabilized in the correct position and is not readily displaced by injection. An assistant usually aspirates with the syringe and injects when asked to do so, allowing the operator to use one hand for palpation and the other to control the needle.

 Good surgical anesthesia is obtained only when local anesthetic is injected in close proximity to the nerve or nerves that are to be blocked. Common local anesthetic solutions that are used for surgical anesthesia include lidocaine 1.5–2%, mepivacaine 2%, bupivacaine 0.5%, levobupivacaine 0.5%, or ropivacaine 0.5%. More dilute solutions are used for postoperative analgesia. Injection techniques include use of a field block, reliance on fixed anatomic relationships, elicitation of paresthesias, and use of a nerve stimulator.

Premedication

Premedication with small doses of a benzodiazepine and/or opioid helps reduce anxiety and raise the pain threshold. The degree of sedation varies according to practitioner, but in general only light sedation is desirable when the elicitation of paresthesias is to be used for nerve localization. Use of a nerve stimulator allows deeper sedation. Supplemental oxygen should generally be administered to all patients via nasal cannula or face mask to reduce the incidence of hypoxemia following sedation.

Field Block

A single injection or multiple injections of a relatively large volume of local anesthetic in the general location of cutaneous nerves produces a field block. The superficial cervical plexus block is an example of a field block. Field blocks are also commonly used to supplement axillary brachial plexus and ankle blocks. Surgeons often use field blocks for minor, superficial operations. The technique may also be used to supplement patchy peripheral nerve blocks or when the level of a neuraxial block begins to recede. When a large volume of local anesthetic is to be injected, use of a dilute concentration and addition of epinephrine (1:200,000 [5 μg/mL] or 1:400,000 [2.5 μg/mL]) help reduce systemic absorption and the likelihood of systemic toxicity.

Fixed Anatomic Relationships

Some nerve block techniques rely on a constant anatomic relationship to locate correct needle position. High in the axilla, the brachial plexus is always in close association with the axillary artery in the axillary sheath. As described later, in the transarterial technique of a brachial plexus block, the artery is located and local anesthetic is injected just above and below it. Similarly, the musculocutaneous nerve can be blocked as it travels in the body of the coracobrachialis muscle; injection of coracobrachialis muscle can therefore be used to supplement axillary or interscalene brachial plexus anesthesia. Intercostal nerves travel in a neurovascular bundle on the undersurface of the inferior border of each rib. The nerve maintains an inferior position in the bundle; from superior to inferior the order is vein, artery, and nerve (VAN). Each intercostal nerve can therefore be blocked by an injection at the inferior border of the corresponding rib. Similarly, the femoral nerve has a constant position in a neurovascular bundle as it travels in the femoral canal. The femoral nerve is always lateral to the artery; from lateral to medial the order is nerve, artery, vein, empty space, and lymphatics (NAVEL).

ELICITATION OF PARESTHESIAS

When a needle makes direct contact with a sensory nerve, a paresthesia is elicited in its area of sensory distribution. With this technique, it is important to ascertain that the needle is making contact with the nerve rather than penetrating it, and that the injection is in proximity to the nerve (perineural) rather than within its substance (intraneural). The high pressures generated by a direct intraneural injection can cause hydrostatic (ischemic) injury to nerve fibers. A perineural injection may produce a brief accentuation of the paresthesia, whereas an intraneural injection produces an intense, searing pain that serves as a warning to immediately terminate the injection and reposition the needle. Pain intensity and duration help differentiate between accentuation and intraneural injection. Use of blunt bevel (B-bevel) needles appears to reduce the small incidence of nerve trauma associated with peripheral nerve blocks. B-bevel needles have a less blunt tip and smaller cutting edge than regular needles. This design helps push nerves aside upon contact, instead of piercing them. Many clinicians also believe that the blunt tip provides better feedback, allowing better appreciation of tissue planes and penetration of fascial compartments.

Nerve Stimulation

Low-level electrical current applied from the tip of a needle can elicit specific muscle contractions when the needle is in close proximity to a motor nerve. One lead of a low-output nerve stimulator is attached to a needle and the other lead is grounded elsewhere on the patient. Lower current is required when the negative lead is attached to the exploring needle. The special needles that are used are insulated and permit current flow only at the tip for precise localization of nerves, whereas the nerve stimulators used deliver a linear, constant current output of 0.1–6.0 mA. Muscle contractions occur and increase in intensity as the needle approaches the nerve and diminish when the needle moves away. Moreover, the evoked contractions require much less current as the needle approaches the nerve. Optimal positioning produces evoked contractions with 0.5 mA or less, but successful blocks can often be obtained with needle positions that produce contractions with as much as 1 mA. Characteristically, the evoked response rapidly diminishes (fades) after injection of 1–2 mL of local anesthetic. Transient augmentation may be observed before extinction of the motor response because the ionic anesthetic solutions transiently facilitate conduction of the current.

■ SOMATIC BLOCKADE OF THE UPPER EXTREMITY

Surgical anesthesia of the upper extremity and shoulder can be obtained following neural blockade of the brachial plexus (C5–T1) or its terminal branches at several sites (Figure 17–1). It may also be necessary to block additional nerves independently for shoulder surgery and for procedures in which use of a pneumatic upper arm tourniquet is planned. Some areas of the anterior shoulder are innervated by the superficial cervical plexus (C1–4). These nerve roots converge lateral to their respective transverse processes, and pass through the platysma at the posterior border of the sternocleidomastoid muscle where a field block can be used to supplement a brachial plexus block (Figure 17–2). **The medial brachial cutaneous (C8–T1) and intercostobrachial (T2) nerves must also be blocked separately to reliably prevent pain from an arm tourniquet.** They innervate the skin of the medial and posterior proximal upper arm (Figure 17–3). The medial brachial cutaneous nerve often leaves the sheath just below the clavicle and may therefore be missed with the axillary approach to the brachial plexus, whereas the intercostobrachial nerve does not travel in the sheath at all.

ANATOMY OF THE BRACHIAL PLEXUS

The brachial plexus is formed by the union of the anterior primary divisions (ventral rami) of the fifth through the eighth cervical nerves and the first thoracic nerves (see Figure 17–1). Contributions from C4 and T2 are often minor or absent. As the nerve roots leave the intervertebral foramina, they converge, forming trunks, divisions, cords, and then finally terminal nerves. Three distinct trunks are formed between the anterior and middle scalene muscles. Because they are vertically arranged, they are termed superior, middle, and inferior. The superior trunk is predominantly derived from C5–6, the middle trunk from C7, and the inferior trunk from C8–T1. As the trunks pass over the lateral border of the first rib and under the clavicle, each trunk divides into anterior and posterior divisions.

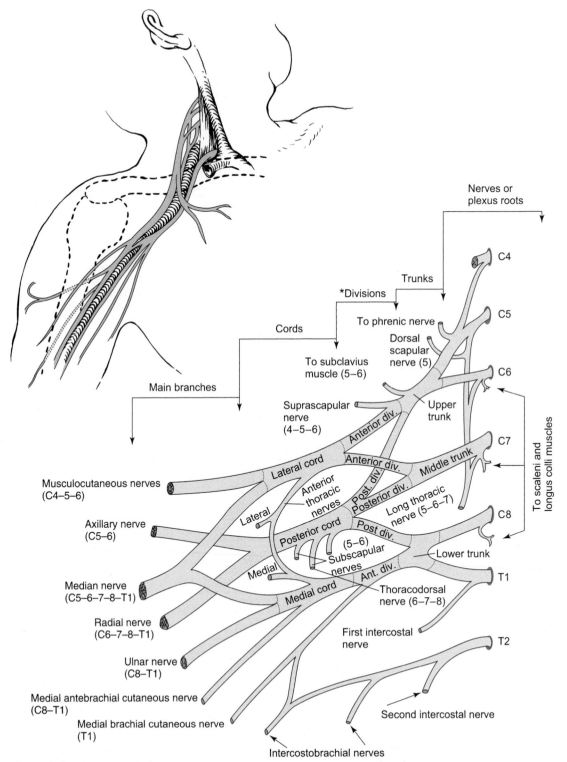

Figure 17–1. The brachial plexus. (Reproduced, with permission, from Waxman SG: *Correlative Neuroanatomy*, 24th ed. McGraw-Hill, 2000.)

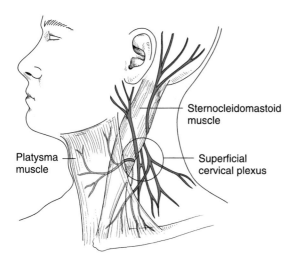

Figure 17–2. Superficial cervical plexus.

As the brachial plexus emerges below the clavicle, the fibers combine again to form three cords that are named according to their relationship to the axillary artery: lateral, medial, and posterior. The lateral cord is the union of the anterior divisions of the superior and middle trunks; the medial cord is the continuation of the anterior division of the inferior trunk; and the posterior cord is formed by the posterior division of all three trunks. At the lateral border of the pectoralis minor muscle, each cord gives off a large branch before terminating as a major terminal nerve. The lateral cord gives off the lateral branch of the median nerve and terminates as the musculocutaneous nerve; the medial cord gives off the medial branch of the median nerve and terminates as the ulnar nerve; and the posterior cord gives off the axillary nerve and terminates as the radial nerve.

TECHNIQUES FOR BRACHIAL PLEXUS BLOCK

A fascial sleeve that is derived from the prevertebral and scalene fascia encloses the brachial plexus. This sheath extends from the intervertebral foramina to the upper arm and serves as the anatomic basis for brachial plexus blocks. Injection into this sheath at any point allows local anesthetic to spread and block the C5–T1 nerve roots. The degree of neural blockade, however, may vary somewhat depending on the level of injection.

The interscalene approach is most optimal for procedures on the shoulder, arm, and forearm. Injection at the interscalene level tends to produce a block that is most intense at the C5–C7 dermatomes and least intense in the C8–T1 dermatomes.

The interscalene approach may therefore not provide optimal surgical anesthesia for procedures in the ulnar nerve distribution. In contrast, the axillary approach to the brachial plexus is most optimal for procedures from the elbow to the hand. This approach tends to produce the most intense block in the distribution of C7–T1 (ulnar nerve) but is usually inadequate for procedures on the shoulder and upper arm (C5–C6). The supraclavicular and infraclavicular approaches to the brachial plexus result in a more even distribution of local anesthetic and can be used for procedures on the arm, forearm, and hand.

Interscalene Brachial Plexus Block

A. ANATOMY

The cervical spinal nerves blend into trunks between the anterior and middle scalene muscles. This interscalene groove lies at the level of the cricoid cartilage and is a relatively easy place to enter the brachial plexus sheath to elicit a paresthesia or obtain an evoked motor response with a nerve stimulator.

B. TECHNIQUE

(Figure 17–4) Palpation of the interscalene groove is usually accomplished with the patient supine and the head rotated 30° or less to the contralateral side. The external jugular vein often crosses the interscalene groove at the level of the cricoid cartilage. The interscalene groove should not be confused with the groove between the sternocleidomastoid and the anterior scalene muscle, which lies more anterior. Having the patient lift and turn the head against resistance often helps delineate the anatomy. After injection of a skin

Figure 17–3. Intercostobrachial and medial brachial cutaneous nerve blocks.

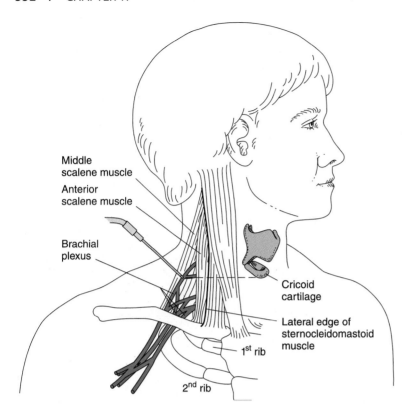

Middle
scalene muscle

Anterior
scalene muscle

Brachial
plexus

Cricoid
cartilage

Lateral edge of
sternocleidomastoid
muscle

1st rib

2nd rib

Figure 17–4. Interscalene approach to brachial plexus block.

wheal with a 25-gauge needle at the level of the cricoid cartilage, a 22-gauge, 1.5-in B-bevel needle is introduced nearly perpendicular to the skin and advanced in slightly medial and caudal directions until a paresthesia or evoked muscle contraction in the arm is elicited.

If a nerve stimulator is used, activity of the phrenic nerve suggests the needle is too "anterior," whereas stimulation of the trapezius muscle indicates the needle may be too "posterior." Motor activity of the arm, wrist, or hand should be elicited, but success has been reported with a response noted in the deltoid or pectoralis muscles, with subsequent local anesthetic injection. Some clinicians apply proximal pressure on the sheath to favor distal spread of local anesthetic. A total of 30–40 mL of local anesthetic solution is injected. For some surgical procedures such as total shoulder arthroplasty, catheters may be inserted and kept in place postoperatively for pain control. Such catheters are placed via an insulated stimulating Tuohy needle. Compared to needle insertion for a single-shot block, insertion should begin slightly more cephalad and advancement of the needle is more medial.

C. COMPLICATIONS

Interscalene blocks have a multitude of potential side effects. The proximity of the stellate ganglion, the phrenic nerve, and the recurrent laryngeal nerve to this location explains their high rate of incidental blockade. The phrenic nerve is commonly blocked, which may lead to respiratory failure in patients with inadequate pulmonary reserve. Patients may display a Horner's syndrome (myosis, ptosis, and anhidrosis), dyspnea, and hoarseness, respectively. The proximity of the vertebral artery to the injection site increases the risk of an intraarterial injection. Even a very small amount (1–3 mL) of local anesthetic injected into a vertebral artery can produce a seizure because the entire amount goes directly to the brain. Venous injection and rapid absorption can result in a slower onset of central nervous system toxicity. Inadvertent epidural, subarachnoid, or subdural injection can occur because of the close proximity of the cervical neural foramina and the presence of dural sleeves on nerve roots. Advancing the needle too far, particularly in a lateral direction, can result in puncture of the pleura and a pneumothorax.

Supraclavicular (Subclavian) Brachial Plexus Block

A. ANATOMY

At the lateral border of the anterior scalene muscle, the brachial plexus passes down between the first rib and clavicle to enter the axilla. The trunks are tightly oriented vertically on top of the first rib just posterior to

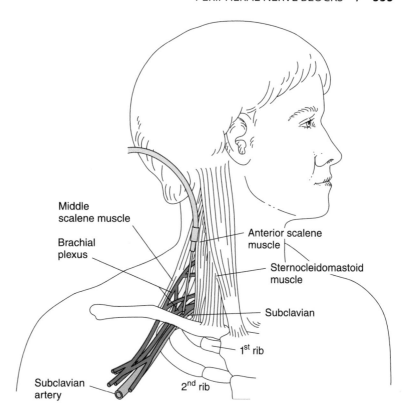

Middle
scalene muscle

Brachial
plexus

Anterior scalene
muscle

Sternocleidomastoid
muscle

Subclavian

1st rib

Subclavian
artery

2nd rib

Figure 17–5. Supraclavicular approach to brachial plexus block.

the subclavian artery. Because the plexus is so compacted here, blockade achieves excellent anesthesia of the entire arm, including the hand.

B. TECHNIQUE

(Figure 17–5) The patient is positioned supine with the head turned about 30° to the contralateral side. The interscalene groove is palpated at its most inferior point, which is just posterior to the subclavian artery pulse; the latter can be felt in a plane just medial to the midpoint of the clavicle. After a skin wheal with local anesthetic, a 22-gauge, 1.5-in needle is directed just above and posterior to the subclavian pulse and directed caudally at a very flat angle against the skin. The needle is advanced until a paresthesia is encountered or muscle contraction of the forearm is noted. If contraction is still observed or palpated with the stimulator voltage decreased to 0.5 mA, then 25–40 mL of local anesthetic is injected. If the rib is encountered without a paresthesia or if blood is encountered, the needle is withdrawn and the landmarks as well as the plane of the needle-insertion path are reevaluated.

Another technique is to identify and measure the width of the clavicular portion of the sternocleidomastoid muscle, double that width, and measure that distance from the medial head of the clavicle laterally along the clavicle. The terminal portion of the interscalene

groove should lie at this point, one fingerbreadth posterior to the clavicle. The needle should be reinserted posterior and lateral to the artery in a caudad (parallel to the floor) direction. The end points remain the same: (1) motor activity in the forearm or hand, (2) blood (redirect the needle more posterior and laterally), (3) bone (redirect and walk the needle in an anterior-to-posterior direction), and (4) no motor activity and the insertion depth of the needle is equal to the width of the clavicle (withdraw the needle and reassess the landmarks).

C. COMPLICATIONS

Although this is an excellent technique in experienced hands, a relatively high incidence of pneumothorax (1–6%) causes many clinicians to avoid this approach. Hemothorax has also been reported. As with the interscalene approach, Horner's syndrome and phrenic nerve block often occur.

Infraclavicular Brachial Plexus Block

A. ANATOMY

The brachial plexus continues beyond the first rib and enters the axilla. In this location, the trunks divide into six divisions and reform into three cords (lateral, medial, and posterior, so named because of their relationship to

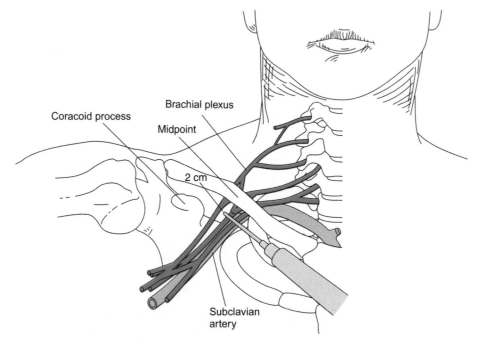

Figure 17–6. Infraclavicular block, classic approach.

the subclavian artery). The infraclavicular approach blocks the brachial plexus at the level of the cords.

B. Techniques

1. Classic approach—When performing this technique, the patient lies supine with the head slightly turned away from the side of the procedure. The operative limb is abducted to 90° and the axillary pulse is identified. The midpoint of the clavicle is identified and 2 cm caudal to this point a needle is inserted at a 45° angle and directed toward the axillary artery pulsation. With a 4-in, 21-gauge insulated nerve stimulator needle, motor activity in the hand is sought. Once identified, and after reducing the stimulation to < 0.5 mA, witnessing fade of motor activity after 1–2 mL of local anesthetic is injected and a negative aspiration of blood, 30–40 mL of local anesthetic is delivered (Figure 17–6).

2. Coracoid approach—In this approach the patient's arm can be in any position. The coracoid process is identified and marked. Two centimeters medial and 2 cm caudal from the coracoid process, the needle is inserted perpendicular to the floor (Figure 17–7). The end point again is to achieve satisfactory motor response with a 4-in 21-gauge insulated nerve stimulator. Once identified, and after reducing the stimulation to < 0.5 mA, witnessing fade of motor activity after injecting 1 mL of local anesthetic and a negative aspiration of

blood, 30–40 mL of local anesthetic is delivered. Accepting activity of the musculocutaneous nerve (ie, biceps or brachialis twitch) may result in an unsatisfactory block. In a significant percentage of patients, the musculocutaneous nerve splits early from the brachial plexus and delivery of the local anesthetic at that site will fail to adequately block the plexus.

C. Indications

Infraclavicular blocks provide good homogeneous anesthesia to the brachial plexus and can be used for procedures involving the hand, forearm, elbow, and upper arm and are quite conducive for placement of an indwelling catheter for postoperative analgesia.

D. Complications

Pneumothorax, hemothorax, and chylothorax (with a left-sided block) are possible and occur at a higher rate than with the supraclavicular approach.

Axillary Brachial Plexus Block

A. Anatomy

The subclavian artery becomes the axillary artery beneath the clavicle, where the trunks of the brachial plexus split into anterior and posterior divisions. At the lateral border of the pectoralis minor

Figure 17–7. Infraclavicular brachial plexus block, coracoid approach.

muscle, the cords form large terminal branches. **In the axilla, the musculocutaneous nerve has already left the sheath and lies within the coracobrachialis muscle** (Figure 17–8). Moreover, imaging studies suggest that the fascial sheath is multicompartmental and that fascial septa may be responsible for the "patchy" anesthesia observed in some patients. Fascial septa may result in incomplete spread of local anesthetic within the plexus sheath.

B. TECHNIQUES

Axillary block is most commonly performed by one of several techniques that use the axillary arterial pulse as a starting point (Table 17–2). The patient is positioned supine with the arm abducted, the elbow flexed at 90°, and externally rotated at the shoulder leaving the arm lying across the patient's head.

1. Transarterial technique—The pulse of the axillary artery is identified as high (proximal) in the axilla as possible. Using an "immobile needle" technique, a 22-gauge, 1.5-in needle is inserted until bright red blood is aspirated. The needle is then slightly advanced or withdrawn until blood aspiration ceases. Injection can be performed posteriorly, anteriorly, or in both locations in relation to the artery. A total of 40 mL of local anesthetic is usually injected; distal pressure on the sheath during the injection may promote better cephalad spread of the solution within the sheath. Some clinicians inject the entire quantity either anterior or posterior to the artery; clinicians who worry about septa in the sheath inject 20 mL anterior and 20 mL posterior to the artery.

2. Elicitation of paresthesia technique—With this technique, the needle is directed toward the axillary

artery to elicit a single, specific or multiple paresthesias. If the artery is entered, the needle is redirected until a paresthesia is obtained. Many practitioners try to elicit any paresthesia in the brachial plexus distribution, whereas others always try to specifically elicit paresthesias in the nerve distribution of the operative area before injection. Clinicians who are concerned about septations in the plexus sheath try to elicit paresthesias in the ulnar, median, and radial nerve distributions, injecting some

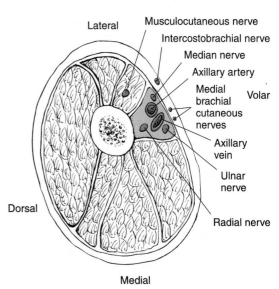

Figure 17–8. Axillary block, showing relationships of the nerves to the artery.

Table 17–2. Approaches to axillary block.

| Transarterial |
| Paresthesia |
| Nerve stimulator |
| Ultrasound |
| Perivascular infiltration |

local anesthetic at each site. Regardless of whether one or multiple paresthesias are elicited, a total of 40 mL of local anesthetic is usually injected.

3. Nerve stimulator technique—The axillary artery is "pinned" in a stabilized position. Each finger is positioned in parallel with the artery. It is important to understand the relationship between the axillary artery and the four nerves that are to be blocked. With the arm in the described position, as the axillary artery is palpated, the median nerve lies superior to the pulse.

The ulnar nerve lies inferior and the radial nerve inferior–posterior to the pulse. The musculocutaneous nerve is separate and deep within the coracobrachialis muscle, which is more superior in this position and, as a consequence, often is not blocked with this procedure. A good concept is to view the axillary artery as the "hub of a wheel" and the individual nerves radially surrounding it (Figure 17–9). Utilizing a nerve stimulator, a 2-in, 22-gauge insulated stimulating needle is inserted proximal to the operator's fingers and appropriate muscle twitches in the hand are sought. Once identified, and after reducing the stimulation to < 0.5 mA, witnessing fade of motor activity after 1 mL of local anesthetic is injected and a negative aspiration of blood, local anesthetic is delivered. Although some providers accept a single muscle contraction and deliver 40 mL of local anesthetic, many will pursue multiple nerve stimulations (ie, two or three nerves) and deliver divided doses of local anesthetic to increase the likelihood of a successful block.

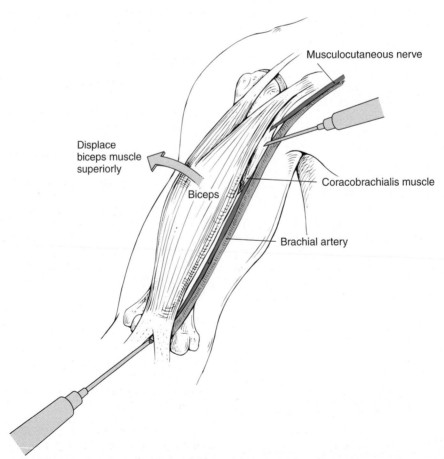

Figure 17–9. Musculocutaneous block, showing injection into the coracobrachialis.

A musculocutaneous block is essential to complete the anesthesia for the forearm and wrist and is commonly included when performing the axillary block. The musculocutaneous nerve is the terminal branch of the lateral cord and the most proximal of the major nerves to emerge from the brachial plexus. It innervates the biceps and brachialis muscles and distally terminates as the lateral antebrachial cutaneous nerve of the forearm, which supplies sensory input to the lateral aspect of the forearm and wrist. One of two approaches is commonly used to block this nerve. First, upon completion of the axillary block, the operator redirects the needle more superiorly and proximally, pierces the coracobrachialis muscle, and injects 5–10 mL of local anesthetic in a field block manner (Figure 17–9).

Alternatively, the block can be performed at the elbow as it courses superficially at the interepicondylar line at the elbow. The insertion of the biceps tendon is identified and the site is marked 1–2 cm laterally; a field block is performed with a 2-in 22-gauge needle injecting 5–10 mL of local anesthetic. After completion of the axillary and musculocutaneous blocks, the operator may quickly assess the adequacy of the blocks with a simple test of "pull-push-pin.-pin." The patient is asked to "pull" (flex) the arm (checks the musculocutaneous nerve), "push" the arm against a resistance (radial nerve), "pin." the thenar prominence (median nerve), and "pin." the fifth digit (ulnar nerve). This gives the operator a quick assessment of the quality of the block.

C. INDICATIONS

This is one of the most common approaches to the brachial plexus and, when used, provides an excellent block for procedures distal to the elbow.

D. COMPLICATIONS

The axillary approach to the brachial plexus is associated with a very low complication rate, providing intravascular injection is avoided. Although controversial, repeated elicitation of paresthesia at multiple sites may increase the incidence of postoperative neuropathies. Hematoma and infection are very rare.

Midhumeral Brachial Plexus Block

All four major nerves of the arm can be blocked separately at the level of the midhumerus. This relatively new technique uses a nerve stimulator to locate each nerve as it passes in the humeral canal. The success rate of this approach appears to be similar to the classic axillary block, but the onset of the blockade is slower.

PERIPHERAL NERVE BLOCKS OF THE ARM

Intercostobrachial & Medial Brachial Cutaneous Nerves

The intercostobrachial and the medial brachial nerves originate in the lower neck and upper thorax and become cutaneous on the medial upper arm. **Both must be blocked proximal to the axilla for shoulder surgery or for any upper extremity procedure that involves use of a pneumatic tourniquet.** The intercostobrachial nerve derives from the T2 somatic intercostal nerve, whereas the medial brachial cutaneous nerve derives from C8 and T1. Both become superficial and cutaneous at the pectoral ridge over the humeral head. They are easily blocked, with the arm abducted, by means of a linear injection (field block) from the deltoid prominence superiorly to the most inferior aspect of the medial upper arm (Figure 17–3). A total of 5 mL of local anesthesia is used.

Radial Nerve

An isolated radial nerve block is typically used to supplement an incomplete brachial plexus block that spares the radial distribution.

A. ANATOMY

The radial nerve—the terminal branch of the posterior cord of the brachial plexus—courses posterior to the humerus, innervating the triceps muscle, and enters the musculospiral groove of the humerus before it moves laterally at the elbow. Terminal sensory branches include the lateral cutaneous nerve of the arm and the posterior cutaneous nerve of the forearm. After exiting the musculospiral groove as it approaches the lateral epicondyle, it separates into superficial and deep branches. The deep branch remains close to the periosteum and innervates the postaxial extensor group of the forearm. The superficial branch comes close to the dermis and follows the radial artery to innervate the radial aspects of the dorsal wrist and the dorsal aspect of the lateral $3^{1}/_{2}$ digits.

B. TECHNIQUES

1. At the upper arm—(Figure 17–10) The radial nerve exits the musculospiral groove between the two heads of the triceps. Palpation of a line between this site and the lateral epicondyle often reveals a palpable nerve. Three to 4 cm proximal to the epicondyle, a 22-gauge needle is inserted toward the nerve and periosteum and once bone is contacted, the needle is withdrawn 0.5 cm, and 5 mL of local anesthetic is injected. Mild paresthesia is acceptable, but the intense paresthesia of intraneural injection must be avoided. At this level, localization with a nerve stimulator is possible with motor-evoked response of wrist extensors (wrist extension).

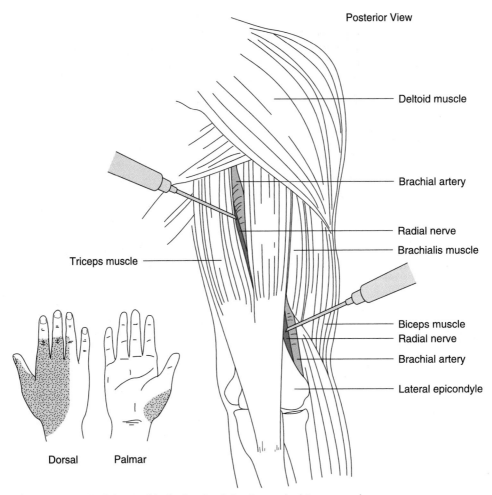

Figure 17–10. Radial nerve block, showing injection under biceps muscle.

2. At the elbow—(Figure 17–11) From the antecubital space, the lateral aspect of the biceps tendon is identified at the flexion crease. A 22-gauge, 1.5-in needle is inserted almost parallel to the forearm. It is directed just superficial to the radial head toward the lateral epicondyle until paresthesia is elicited or periosteum is encountered. With paresthesia, the needle is withdrawn slightly and injection then proceeds as long as intense paresthesia is not encountered. At the periosteum, the needle is withdrawn 1 cm, and 5 mL of local anesthetic is injected.

3. At the distal forearm—(Figure 17–12) At the level of the ulnar styloid, sensory branches to the lateral side of the thumb lie between the radial artery and the flexor carpi radialis tendon. One to 2 mL of local anesthetic deposited in this interval, deep to flexor carpi radialis tendon, will block this sensation. More proximally, dorsal branches are given off. In some persons, this is

palpable as the nerve moves from volar to dorsal. If palpable, 2–3 mL of local anesthetic as a directed field block can be given. If not palpable, a linear field block at the level of the ulnar styloid from the volar lateral edge of the radius to the mid forearm will anesthetize the dorsal aspect of the lateral $3^1/_2$ fingers.

C. COMPLICATIONS

Radial artery injection and intraneural injection may occur.

Median Nerve

Isolated median nerve block is performed usually as a supplement to a brachial plexus block.

A. ANATOMY

The median nerve is derived from the lateral and medial cords of the brachial plexus. It enters the arm

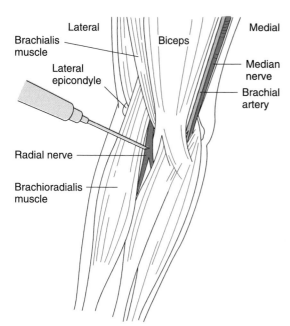

Figure 17–11. Radial nerve block in the antecubital space.

and runs just medial to the brachial artery. As it enters the antecubital space, it lies medial to the brachial artery near the insertion of the biceps tendon. Just distal to this, it gives off numerous motor branches to the wrist and finger flexors and follows the interosseous membrane to the wrist. At the level of the proximal wrist flexion crease, it lies directly behind the palmaris longus tendon in the carpal tunnel.

B. TECHNIQUES

1. At the elbow—(Figure 17–13) The brachial artery can be identified in the antecubital crease just medial to the biceps insertion. A 22-gauge, 1.5-in B-bevel needle is inserted just medial to the artery and directed toward the medial epicondyle until a paresthesia, motor-evoked response (wrist flexion), or periosteum is encountered. If periosteum is encountered, the needle is withdrawn 0.5–1 cm. Then 3–5 mL of anesthetic is injected.

2. At the wrist—(Figure 17–14) Asking the patient to flex the wrist against resistance can identify the palmaris longus tendon. It is marked at the proximal flexion crease. A 22- to 25-gauge, B-bevel needle is inserted just medial and deep to the palmaris longus, and 3–5 mL of anesthetic is injected.

C. COMPLICATIONS

Brachial artery injection or intraneural injection may occur.

Ulnar Nerve

An ulnar nerve block can also be used to supplement a patchy axillary or interscalene block or for minor surgical procedures in the distribution of the ulnar nerve.

A. ANATOMY

The ulnar nerve is the continuation of the medial cord of the brachial plexus and maintains a position medial to the axillary and brachial arteries in the upper arm. At the distal third of the humerus, the nerve moves more medially and passes under the arcuate ligament of the medial epicondyle. The nerve is frequently palpable just proximal to the medial epicondyle. In the mid forearm, the nerve lies between the flexor digitorum profundus and the flexor carpi ulnaris. At the wrist, it is lateral to the flexor carpi ulnaris tendon and medial to the ulnar artery.

TECHNIQUES

1. At the elbow—(Figure 17–15) A 22-gauge needle is inserted approximately one finger breadth proximal to the arcuate ligament and advanced until paresthesia or

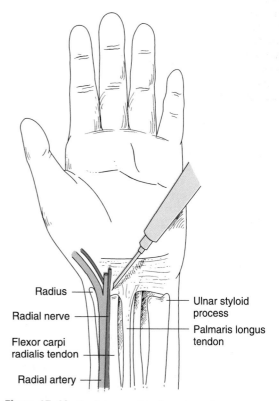

Figure 17–12. Radial nerve block at the wrist.

Lateral

Medial

Biceps

Brachial artery

Median nerve

Medial epicondyle

Bicipital aponeurosis

Flexors

Dorsal

Palmar

Figure 17–13. Median nerve block in the antecubital space.

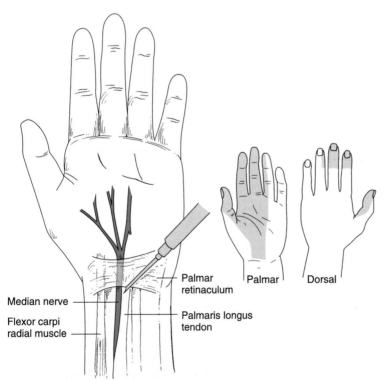

Palmar retinaculum

Palmar

Dorsal

Median nerve

Flexor carpi radial muscle

Palmaris longus tendon

Figure 17–14. Median nerve block at the wrist.

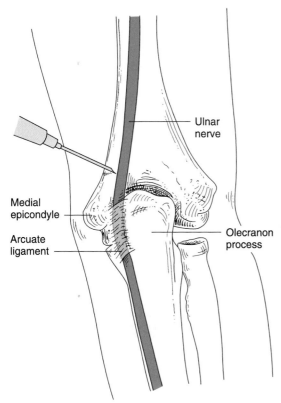

Figure 17–15. Ulnar nerve block at the elbow.

motor-evoked response is elicited (finger movement). Three to 5 mL of anesthetic is injected.

2. At the wrist—(Figure 17–16) A 22-gauge needle is directed just medial to the ulnar artery pulse, or immediately lateral to the flexor carpi ulnaris if no pulse is palpable. A total of 3–5 mL of anesthetic is injected.

C. Complications

Intraneural injection may occur at the elbow and intraneural or intraarterial injection at the wrist.

Digital Nerves

These nerve blocks are used for minor operations on the fingers and to supplement brachial plexus blocks.

A. Anatomy

Sensory innervation of each finger is provided by four small digital nerves that enter each digit at its base in each of the four corners.

B. Technique

(Figure 17–17) A 23- to 25-gauge needle is inserted at the medial and lateral aspects of the base of the selected

digit. A total of 2–3 mL of local anesthetic without epinephrine is injected on each side near the periosteum. Addition of a vasoconstrictor (epinephrine) can seriously compromise blood flow to the digit.

C. Complications

Nerve injury is the primary risk of a digital block. In summary, Table 17–3 outlines suggested blocks for specific-site, upper extremity surgery. These recommendations reflect the authors' bias of nerve root innervations of the sites, ease and risk of the blocks, and use of the block as an anesthetic versus use for postoperative pain control.

INTRAVENOUS REGIONAL ANESTHESIA OF THE ARM

 Intravenous regional anesthesia, also called a Bier block, can provide intense surgical anesthesia for short surgical procedures (< 45–60 min) on the forearm, hand, and even the leg. It is most commonly used for a carpal tunnel release. An intravenous catheter is usually inserted on the dorsum of the hand and a double pneumatic tourniquet is placed on the arm (Figure 17–18). The extremity is elevated and exsanguinated by tightly

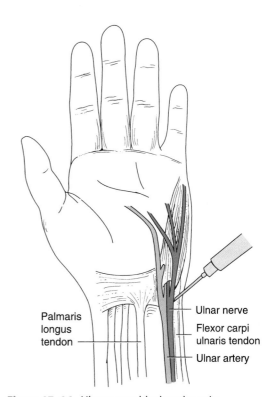

Figure 17–16. Ulnar nerve block at the wrist.

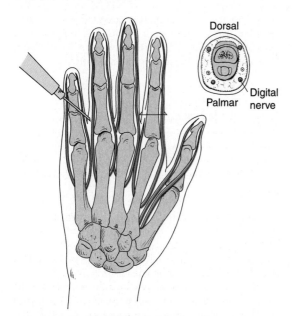

Figure 17–17. Digital block of the hand.

Figure 17–18. Intravenous regional anesthesia.

least 15–20 min to avoid a rapid intravenous systemic bolus of local anesthetic that can cause a seizure. Slow deflation may also provide a safety margin.

■ SOMATIC BLOCKADE OF THE LOWER EXTREMITY

ANATOMY

In performing lower extremity blocks, some familiarity with the lower extremity neuroanatomy is vital. The lumbar and the lumbosacral plexi are the major nerve distributions to the lower extremities. The lumbar plexus is derived from the ventral rami of L1–4, with some occasional contribution from T12 (Figure 17–19).

The lumbar plexus, primarily from L2 to L4, forms three major nerves that innervate the lower extremity: the lateral femoral cutaneous, femoral, and obturator nerves. These nerves predominantly supply motor and sensory innervation to the anterior portion of the lower extremity

wrapping an Eschmark elastic bandage from a distal to proximal direction. The upper (proximal) tourniquet is inflated, the Eschmark bandage is removed, and 0.5% lidocaine (25 mL for a forearm, 50 mL for an arm, and 100 mL for a thigh) is injected over 2–3 min through the catheter, which is removed at the end of the injection. Anesthesia is usually well established after 5–10 min. Patients often complain of tourniquet pain after 20–30 min. When this occurs, the lower (distal) tourniquet is inflated and then the proximal tourniquet is deflated. Patients usually tolerate the lower tourniquet for another 15–20 min because it is inflated over an anesthetized area. With very short procedures, the tourniquet must be left inflated for a total of at

Table 17–3. Appropriate blocks per site-specific procedures.

Procedure Site	Interscalene	Supraclavicular	Infraclavicular	Axillary[1]
Shoulder[2]	++	+[3]		
Arm[2]	+	++	+	
Elbow[2]		++	++	+
Forearm[2]		+	++	++
Hand[2]		+	+	++

[1]Include the musculocutaneous nerve.
[2]Consider including T1–2 blocks if the block is the anesthetic.
[3]Requires separate C3–4 block if the block is the anesthetic.

and the cutaneous sensory portion of the medial lower leg (saphenous nerve).

The lumbosacral plexus is derived from the nerve roots of L4–5 and S1–3 and primarily forms the sciatic nerve, which courses posteriorly and supplies both motor and sensory innervation to the posterior aspect of the lower extremity and foot, largely as its terminal branches into the tibial and the common peroneal nerves. Figure 17–20 is a simplified schematic of the global innervation of the lower extremity. Note that the posterior cutaneous nerve (S1–3) is highlighted but the sciatic nerve is not; it courses with the sciatic nerve as it emerges around the piriformis muscle and subsequently it too is blocked when a proximal sciatic nerve block is performed.

Spinal and epidural anesthesia are most often employed for regional anesthesia of the lower extremities. Peripheral nerve blocks in the lower extremity can also provide excellent surgical anesthesia for some procedures but require multiple injections and may be technically more challenging in some cases. Ankle block is the easiest and most commonly used lower extremity block; it is typically used for foot surgery.

Four major nerves innervate the lower extremities: the femoral (L2–4), obturator (L2–4), lateral femoral (L1–3), and sciatic nerves (L4–S3). The first three nerves are part of the lumbar plexus; they lie within the substance of the psoas muscle and emerge within a common fascial sheath that extends into the proximal thigh. The common peroneal and tibial nerves are continuations of the sciatic nerve in the lower leg.

Lumbar Plexus (Psoas) Block

A. ANATOMY

The lumbar plexus is derived from the ventral rami of the lumbar nerve roots. The plexus courses via the "psoas compartment" as defined by the fascia of the psoas muscle (which lies anterior to the plexus) and the fascia of the quadratus laborum (which lies posterior to the plexus).

B. TECHNIQUE

The patient should lie in a lateral decubitus position with the side to be blocked in the nondependent position. Both iliac crests are identified and a line is drawn connecting the crests. This line generally crosses the lumbar body of L4. The posterior superior iliac spine is identified and a line is drawn cephalad, parallel to the vertebral column. The intersection of the two lines indicates the most lateral location of the lumbar plexus. Generally, the insertion point is 4 cm from the midline or two-thirds the distance between the spinous processes of the lumbar vertebrae and this intersection (Figure 17–21).

A 4-in, 21-gauge insulated stimulating needle is advanced in a perpendicular plane at this insertion site. When the needle has entered the psoas compartment (70–90 mm), a quadriceps motor response is noted. After reducing the stimulation to < 0.5 mA, witnessing fade of motor

Figure 17–19. Lumbar plexus.

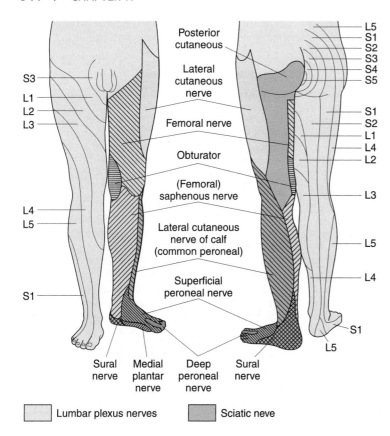

Figure 17–20. Innervation of the lower extremity.

Lumbar plexus nerves | **Sciatic neve**

activity after injection of 1 mL of local anesthetic and a negative aspiration of blood, 25–40 mL of local anesthetic is delivered. Early descriptions of this block employed a "loss of resistance" technique (similar to epidural placement) when the needle tip entered the psoas compartment.

C. INDICATIONS

A psoas block anesthetizes the lateral femoral cutaneous, femoral, and obturator nerves. This block is useful for procedures involving the knee, anterior thigh, and hip. Catheter placement and a continuous infusion administered for postoperative analgesia are common for patients recovering from total hip arthroplasty and occasionally total knee arthroplasty.

D. COMPLICATIONS

Local anesthetic toxicity and nerve damage from an intraneural injection or hematoma have been reported from this block.

Femoral Nerve & "Three-in-One" Block

A femoral nerve block can be used to provide anesthesia for the anterior thigh, knee, and a small part of the medial foot. It is typically used in conjunction with

other lower extremity blocks. It may also be used for postoperative pain relief following knee surgery.

A. ANATOMY

After passing through the psoas compartment, the femoral nerve enters the thigh lateral to the femoral artery just below the inguinal ligament. Distal to this point, motor branches to the quadriceps, sartorius, and pectineus mus-

Figure 17–21. Psoas block for anesthetizing the lumbar plexus. The site of entry is 4 cm lateral to the spinous processes on a line drawn between the iliac crests. PSIS, posterior superior iliac spine.

Anterior superior
iliac spine

Lateral femoral
cutaneous nerve

Femoral vein

Femoral artery

Femoral nerve

Genitofemoral nerve

Inguinal ligament

Pubic
symphysis

Figure 17–22. Femoral nerve block. The insertion site should be 1.5–2.0 cm lateral to the femoral pulse, 2 cm inferior to a line drawn between the pubic symphysis and the anterior superior iliac spine (which overlies the inguinal ligament).

cles arise as well as numerous sensory branches to the medial and anterior thigh. The nerve is encased in a sheath that extends from the psoas muscle to just below the inguinal ligament.

B. TECHNIQUE

(Figure 17–22) The inguinal ligament should first be identified (by drawing a line connecting the anterior superior iliac spine and the superior-lateral corner of the pubic tubercle). The operator approximates the midpoint along this line and palpates for the femoral pulse. Once the femoral pulse is identified, the insertion point for the femoral nerve block is located 2 cm lateral to the femoral artery pulse and 2 cm distal to the inguinal ligament line. With the nerve stimulator technique, a 2-in, 22-gauge stimulating needle is advanced seeking a quadriceps twitch or "patellar snap." Once identified, and after reducing the stimulation to < 0.5 mA, witnessing fade of motor activity after injection of 1 mL of local anesthetic and a negative aspiration of blood, 20–30 mL of local anesthetic is delivered.

C. INDICATIONS

 A femoral nerve block is very useful in numerous procedures involving the thigh and knee,

such as skin grafting, knee arthroscopy, and patellar surgery, or as an adjunct to procedures distal to the knee that require anesthesia to the medial aspect of the lower leg (saphenous distribution). An increasingly common practice in many centers is the insertion of an indwelling femoral catheter for continuous perineural infusion along with an accompanying sciatic nerve block for patients recovering from total knee arthroplasty.

This block is often referred to as Winnie's "3-in-1 block." As first described, placement of sufficient local anesthetic, directed proximally and with distal compression, blocked not only the femoral nerve, but the obturator and the lateral femoral cutaneous nerves as well, thus the "3-in-1." There have been many conflicting reports on the effectiveness of this approach as a true "3-in-1 block." Many practitioners view this as a femoral nerve only block with little ability to provide additional nerve coverage.

D. COMPLICATIONS

Careful aspiration and incremental dosing help avoid intravascular injection and systemic local anesthetic toxicity.

Figure 17–23. Fascia iliaca block.

Fascia Iliaca Block

A. ANATOMY

A fascia iliaca block takes advantage of the fact that the femoral nerve and, to a certain degree, the lateral femoral cutaneous, the obturator, and the genitofemoral nerves course posterior to the fascia iliaca and delivery of local anesthetic behind the fascia may result in a "compartment" block. The so-called "fascia iliaca compartment" is a potential space bordered anteriorly by the fascia iliaca (which is overlaid by the fascia lata) and posteriorly by the iliopsoas muscle.

B. TECHNIQUE

(Figure 17–23) In performing this block, the landmarks are similar to those used to identify the femoral nerve; a line is drawn from the anterior superior iliac spine and connected to the outer corner of the pubic tubercle. This line is then divided into thirds and the outer and middle third junction is identified. Two centimeters distal from this junction is the needle insertion site. In performing the block, it is preferable to use a B-bevel needle to accentuate the tactile sensation, as this block is not performed with a nerve stimulator. Commonly a 3.5-in, 22-gauge Whitacre spinal needle may be used (recognizing that other products are also available). As the needle is inserted, two "pops" will be felt. The first occurs as the needle passes through the fascia lata and the second as it passes through the fascia iliaca. Following negative aspiration of blood, approximately 25–30 mL of local anesthetic is injected.

C. INDICATIONS

There has been a recent surge of interest in fascia iliaca blocks. Because it does not require a nerve stimulator, it can be performed very quickly, it is not very stimulating, and patients often do not require sedation. It is useful in procedures involving the hip, thigh, and knee. A catheter for continuous infusion may be placed for analgesia in the postoperative period.

D. COMPLICATIONS

Some anesthesiologists have reservations regarding the block's consistency, reliability, and adequacy. Complications for this block are similar to those for other peripheral nerve blocks.

Lateral Femoral Cutaneous Block

A. ANATOMY

The lateral femoral cutaneous nerve (L2–3) departs from the lumbar plexus, transverses laterally from the psoas muscle, and courses anterolaterally along the iliacus muscle. It emerges inferior and medial to the anterior superior iliac spine to supply the cutaneous sensory innervation of the lateral thigh.

B. TECHNIQUE

(Figure 17–24) The block is performed via a field injection technique with 10–12 mL of local anesthetic at a mark approximately 2 cm distal and 2 cm medial to the anterior iliac spine. With insertion of a 2-in,

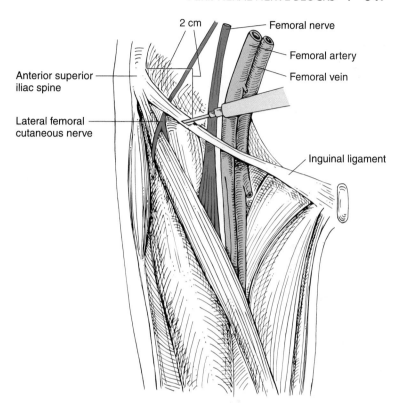

Figure 17–24. Lateral femoral cutaneous nerve block.

22-gauge needle, a "pop" may be felt as the needle passes through the fascia lata. This block is accomplished by repeatedly reinserting the needle while injecting local anesthetic above and below the fascia in a lateral to medial direction.

C. INDICATIONS

This nerve may be blocked concurrently with a femoral nerve block or a fascia iliaca block and certainly is included with a lumbar plexus block. For a skin or muscle biopsy or a harvest site for a skin graft from the lateral thigh, an isolated block of this nerve may be performed.

D. COMPLICATIONS

Complications with this block are few as the amount of local anesthetic injected is small, and the chance of intraneural injection unlikely, as would be for an intravascular injection.

Obturator Nerve Block

An obturator nerve block provides anesthesia to the medial thigh and muscle relaxation of the adductor muscles of the hip. It may be used for an adductor release procedure.

A. ANATOMY

The obturator nerve exits the pelvis and enters the medial thigh through the obturator foramen, which lies beneath the superior pubic ramus. It supplies sensation to the medial thigh and the hip joint and motor innervation to the adductor muscles of the thigh.

B. TECHNIQUE

(Figure 17–25) A 4-in, 21-gauge needle is inserted through a skin wheal 1.5 cm lateral and 1.5 cm inferior to the pubic tubercle. As the needle is advanced in a posterior direction toward the superior pubic ramus, small amounts of local anesthetic are injected to decrease patient discomfort. Upon contacting bone, the needle is redirected in a lateral and caudal direction another 2–4 cm to enter the obturator foramen. An adductor motor response should be elicited. Once identified, and after reducing the stimulation to < 0.5 mA, witnessing fade of motor activity after injection of 1 mL of local anesthetic and a negative aspiration of blood, 15–20 mL of local anesthetic is administered.

C. INDICATIONS

This block is commonly performed as a compliment to additional blocks performed for knee surgery (eg,

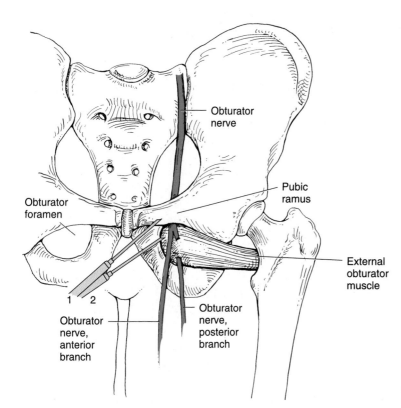

Figure 17–25. Obturator nerve block.

femoral and sciatic nerve blocks). Its role as an isolated block is limited, although it may be useful in the diagnosis of hip pain or to treat spasticity of the thigh adductors.

D. COMPLICATIONS

Careful aspiration and incremental dosing help avoid intravascular injection and systemic local anesthetic toxicity.

Sciatic Nerve Block

A. ANATOMY

The sciatic nerve originates from the lumbosacral trunk and is composed of nerve roots L4–5 and S1–3. It supplies sensory fibers to the posterior hip capsule as well as the knee. It provides motor activity to the hamstrings and to all the lower extremity muscles distal to the knee. It also provides all the sensory innervation to the lower extremity distal to the knee except along the anteromedial aspect, which is provided by the saphenous nerve.

B. TECHNIQUES

1. Classic or posterior approach—(Figure 17–26) The patient is placed in a lateral decubitus position (Sim's posi-

tion) with the operative extremity nondependent. Landmarks are the greater trochanter, the posterior superior iliac spine, and the sacral hiatus. A line is drawn from the greater trochanter to the posterior superior iliac spine and a second line is drawn from the greater trochanter to the sacral hiatus. The midpoint along the line of the greater trochanter–posterior superior iliac spine is marked and a perpendicular line is drawn caudad. The intersection of this line and the greater trochanter–sacral hiatus line (approximately 5 cm) is the insertion point for the block.

The operator advances a 4-in, 21-gauge insulated stimulating needle in a direction perpendicular to the skin. After encountering gluteal muscle stimulation, the needle is inserted further as a motor response is sought in the distal ankle, foot, or toes. Once identified, and after reducing the stimulation to < 0.5 mA, witnessing fade of motor activity after injection of 1 mL of local anesthetic and a negative aspiration of blood, 20–25 mL of local anesthetic is delivered. This approach readily accommodates placement of a perineural catheter for continuous infusion in the postoperative setting.

2. Lithotomy approach—(Figure 17–27) As the sciatic nerve courses from the pelvis to the leg, it characteristically travels between the ischial tuberosity and

Figure 17–26. Sciatic nerve block, posterior approach. PSIS, posterior superior iliac spine.

the greater trochanter. Taking advantage of this consistent course and the nerve's relatively superficial location, the patient is placed in a supine position with the hip and knee flexed (lithotomy position). In this position, the midpoint between the ischial tuberosity and the greater trochanter is identified and marked. A 4-in, 21-gauge insulated stimulating needle is inserted at the mark and advanced perpendicular to the skin. A motor response is sought in the distal ankle, foot, or toes. Once identified, and after reducing the stimulation to < 0.5 mA, witnessing fade of motor activity after injection of 1 mL of local anes-

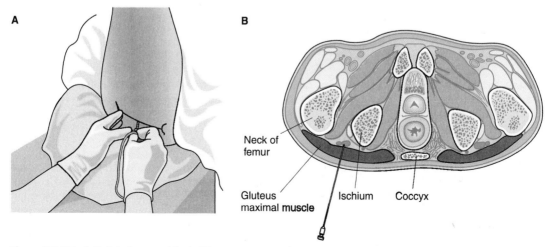

Figure 17–27. *A*, *B*: Sciatic nerve block, lithotomy approach.

Figure 17–28. Sciatic nerve block, anterior approach.

thetic and a negative aspiration of blood, 15–20 mL of local anesthetic is delivered.

3. Anterior approach—(Figure 17–28) The sciatic nerve can also be blocked using an anterior thigh approach. This approach minimizes patient movement, requires less preparation time (as it is often combined with the same preparation for a femoral block), and therefore theoretically can be placed more quickly. However, this approach is technically more challenging. Of all the procedures used to block the sciatic nerve, this involves the greatest distance the needle must travel to reach its target, thus making the time needed to perform this block, particularly for the inexperienced, much longer. To perform this block the patient is placed in a supine position with the legs in a slight internal rotation (this maneuver rotates the lesser trochanter posteriorly and out of the line of sight for needle passage). A common approach begins by identifying landmarks similar to those used for a femoral nerve block. The inguinal ligament is identified and marked (drawing a line between the anterior superior iliac spine and the pubic tubercle). A second line is drawn parallel to the inguinal ligament starting from the greater trochanter and going medially across the anterior thigh (this line connects the greater and the lesser trochanter). The inguinal ligament line is then divided into thirds. At the junction of the medial and middle thirds a perpendicular line is drawn that intersects the greater trochanter line at a right angle. At this point of intersection, a 4-in, 21-gauge insulated stimulating needle is inserted. As the needle is advanced, a motor response is sought in the distal ankle, foot, or toes. Once identified, and after reducing the stimulation to < 0.5 mA, witnessing fade of motor activity after injection

of 1 mL of local anesthetic and a negative aspiration of blood, 15–20 mL of local anesthetic is delivered.

C. INDICATIONS

 Blockade of the sciatic nerve is useful for many surgical procedures involving the hip, knee, or distal lower extremity. The nerve can be successfully blocked at numerous sites along its course.

D. COMPLICATIONS

Partial block due to an injection distal to the branching of the sciatic nerve and intraneural injection are the most frequent complications.

Popliteal Block

A. ANATOMY

The sciatic nerve divides into the tibial and common peroneal nerves, high in the popliteal fossa. The upper popliteal fossa is bounded laterally by the biceps femoris tendon and medially by the semitendinosus and semimembranosus tendons. Cephalad to the flexion crease of the knee, the popliteal artery is immediately lateral to the semitendinosus tendon. The popliteal vein is lateral to the artery, and the tibial and common peroneal nerves (within a sheath) are just lateral to the vein and medial to the biceps tendon, 4–6 cm deep to the skin. The tibial nerve continues deep behind the gastrocnemius muscle, whereas the common peroneal nerve leaves the popliteal fossa by passing between the head and neck of the fibula to supply to the lower leg.

B. TECHNIQUES

There are two main approaches for performing this block: the posterior approach and the lateral approach.

1. Posterior approach—(Figure 17–29) This is the traditional approach used to block the sciatic nerve at this level. The block is performed after placing the patient in the prone position. The popliteal fossa is identified as a triangle by outlining the borders of the biceps femoris laterally, the semitendinosus and semimembranosus medially, and the popliteal crease inferiorly. At the midpoint along the popliteal crease, a perpendicular line is drawn cephalad approximately 8–10 cm in length, bisecting the popliteal triangle. A mark is made 1 cm from the apex and 1 cm lateral for needle insertion. At this mark, a 2-in, 22-gauge insulated stimulating needle is inserted. As the needle is advanced, a motor response is sought in the distal ankle, foot, or toes. Once identified, and after reducing the stimulation to < 0.5 mA, witnessing fade of motor activity after injection of 1 mL of local anesthetic and a negative aspiration of blood, 30–40 mL of local anesthetic is delivered.

Figure 17–29. Landmarks for popliteal nerve block, posterior approach.

2. Lateral approach—(Figure 17–30) An advantage of this approach is that the patient remains supine for the procedure. The lateral approach is performed by palpating the intertendinous groove between the vastus lateralis and the biceps femoris muscles approximately 10–12 cm proximal to the superior notch of the patella. With a 4-in, 21-gauge insulated stimulating needle advanced at 30°, posteriorly angled, a motor response is sought in the distal ankle, foot, or toes. Once identified, and after reducing the stimulation to < 0.5 mA, witnessing fade of motor activity after injection of 1 mL of local anesthetic and a negative aspiration of blood, 30–40 mL of local anesthetic is injected.

C. INDICATIONS

A popliteal nerve block is very useful for foot and ankle surgery and can result in complete

Figure 17–30. Popliteal nerve block, lateral approach.

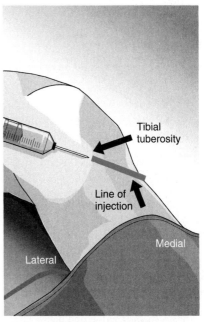

Figure 17–31. Saphenous nerve block.

anesthesia of the limb distal to the knee if a separate saphenous nerve block (terminal nerve of the femoral nerve) is also included. This block can accommodate placement of a catheter for continuous perineural infusion for postoperative analgesia and in an increasing number of ambulatory centers patients may be dismissed home with such infusions.

D. COMPLICATIONS

Intravascular or intraneural injections are possible.

Saphenous Nerve Block

A. ANATOMY

The saphenous nerve is the terminal extension of the femoral nerve and provides sensory innervation along the medial aspect of the lower leg between the knee and the medial malleolus.

B. TECHNIQUE

(Figure 17–31) Infiltrate subcutaneously 7–10 mL of local anesthetic starting from the tibial tuberosity and directed medially, completing the infiltration near the posterior aspect of the leg.

C. INDICATIONS

This is not commonly performed as an isolated block, but rather in conjunction with a popliteal block to complete the anesthesia for procedures done below the knee.

D. COMPLICATIONS

Complications are the same as for other field blocks.

Ankle Block

This is one of the more common peripheral nerve blocks, and is particularly helpful for foot surgery.

A. ANATOMY

Five nerves supply sensation to the foot. The saphenous nerve is a terminal branch of the femoral nerve and the only innervation of the foot not a part of the sciatic system. It supplies superficial sensation to the anteromedial foot and is most constantly located just anterior to the medial malleolus. The deep peroneal nerve runs in the anterior leg as a continuation of the common peroneal nerve; innervates toe extensors; enters the ankle between the flexor hallucis longus and the extensor digitorum longus tendons; and provides sensation to the medial half of the dorsal foot, particularly the first and second digits. The deep peroneal nerve has a constant location just lateral to the flexor hallucis longus at the level of the medial malleolus; the anterior tibial artery (which becomes the dorsalis pedis artery) lies between the nerve and this tendon. The superficial peroneal nerve, also a branch of the common peroneal nerve, descends toward the ankle in the lateral compartment, entering the ankle just lateral to the extensor digitorum longus and providing cutaneous sensation to the dorsum of the foot as well as all five toes. It is most con-

stantly located lateral to the extensor digitorum longus at the level of the lateral malleolus superficially. The posterior tibial nerve is a direct continuation of the tibial nerve and enters the foot posterior to the medial malleolus, branching into lateral and medial plantar nerves. It is constantly located behind the posterior tibial artery at the level of the medial malleolus, and is sensory to the heel, the medial sole, and part of the lateral sole of the foot. The sural nerve is the continuation of the tibial nerve and enters the foot between the Achilles tendon and the lateral malleolus to provide sensation to the lateral foot.

B. TECHNIQUE

A common approach to performing this block consists of administering local anesthetic in a ringlike field distribution about the ankle and directed at the five nerves innervating the foot (Figure 17–32A). The deep peroneal, superficial peroneal, and saphenous nerves can be blocked by infiltrating local anesthetic on a malleolar-level line across the anterior aspect of the foot. **The deep peroneal nerve is blocked by identifying the groove formed proximally by the extensor hallicus longus tendon and the extensor digitorum longus tendons.** Then 5–8 mL of local anesthetic is delivered at the apex of this groove as a field block with a 25-gauge needle inserted subcutaneously and then advanced to just contact the periosteum. From this insertion site, a subcutaneous infiltration with 5–8 mL of local anesthetic directed toward the lateral malleolus is used to block the superficial peroneal nerve. From the initial insertion site, redirecting the needle toward the medial malleolus, a subcutaneous infiltration with 5–8 mL of local anesthetic

A

Tibialis anterior tendon

Deep peroneal n.

Saphenous n.

Posterior tibial n.

Achilles tendon

Extensor hallucis longus tendon

Superficial peroneal n.

Tibia

Fibula

Sural n.

B

Figure 17–32. Ankle block. *A:* Anatomy. *B:* Posterior and anterior approaches to blocking nerves at ankle.

will block the saphenous nerve (Figure 17–32B). The tibial nerve travels posterior to the medial malleolus and lies adjacent to the posterior tibial artery. The block is performed by injecting 5–8 mL of local anesthetic in a fanlike manner posterior to the medial malleolus and at a right angle to the course direction of the nerve. The sural nerve subcutaneously courses posterior to the lateral malleolus. A field block performed posterior to the malleolus with 5–8 mL of local anesthetic will block this nerve.

C. INDICATIONS

This block is used for procedures on the distal foot.

D. COMPLICATIONS

Aggressive injection, particularly with excessively large volumes, may cause hydrostatic damage to small nerves, such as those within closed ligamentous spaces, like the tibial nerve.

■ SOMATIC BLOCKADE OF THE TRUNK

Superficial Cervical Plexus Block

The superficial cervical plexus block is performed for unilateral procedures on the neck, such as carotid endarterectomy. This block is also done as an adjunct to an interscalene block used for shoulder surgery, particularly with very anterior incisions.

A. ANATOMY

The cervical plexus is formed from the anterior rami of C1–4, which emerge from the platysma muscle posterior to the sternocleidomastoid muscle. It supplies sensation to the jaw, neck, the occiput posteriorly, and areas of the chest and shoulder close to the clavicle.

B. TECHNIQUE

(Figure 17–2) The patient is positioned supine with the neck slightly turned, and the posterior border of the sternocleidomastoid muscle is identified. A 22-gauge spinal needle is selected; the sternocleidomastoid is divided into thirds, and at the junction of the upper and middle thirds, a skin wheal is raised. The spinal needle is directed cephalad toward the mastoid along the posterior border of the sternocleidomastoid in a subcutaneous plane and injected with 2–3 mL of local anesthetic as the needle is withdrawn. Care is taken to avoid entering the external jugular vein. As the needle reaches the wheal, it is rotated 180° and directed subcutaneously caudad toward the clavicle

along the posterior border of the sternocleidomastoid. A similar amount of local anesthetic is injected as the needle is withdrawn.

C. COMPLICATIONS

Rapid systemic absorption and intravascular injection of local anesthetic are the most common complications.

Intercostal Block

Intercostal blocks are rarely employed as the sole anesthetic technique for surgery. **They are more commonly used as supplements to general anesthesia, for postoperative analgesia following thoracic and upper abdominal surgery, and for relief of pain associated with rib fractures, herpes zoster, and cancer.**

A. ANATOMY

The intercostal nerves arise from the dorsal and ventral rami of the thoracic spinal nerves. They exit from the spine at the intervertebral foramen and enter a groove on the underside of the corresponding rib, running with the intercostal artery and vein; the nerve is generally the most inferior structure in the neurovascular bundle. Branches are given off for sensation in the correct dermatome from the midline dorsally all the way to across the midline ventrally.

B. TECHNIQUE

(Figure 17–33) With the patient in the lateral decubitus or supine position, the level of each rib is palpated

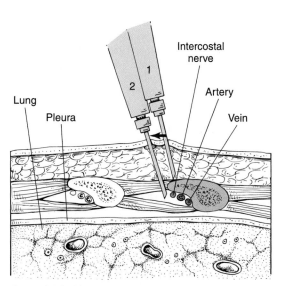

Figure 17–33. Intercostal block.

and marked in the mid and posterior axillary line. A skin wheal is raised over the inferior border at the selected ribs, and a 22- to 25-gauge needle is inserted down to the inferior edge of the rib and "walked-off" until it steps off the rib inferiorly. The needle is advanced 0.5 cm underneath the rib, and following a negative aspiration (for blood or air), 3–5 mL of local anesthetic is injected at each level.

C. COMPLICATIONS

Intercostal blocks result in the highest blood levels of local anesthetic per volume injected of any block in the body. Care must be taken to avoid toxic levels of local anesthetic. Careful aspiration may help prevent intravascular injection. The risk of pneumothorax is obvious, and any indication of entering the chest should be investigated with a chest radiograph.

Paravertebral Nerve Blocks

Initially described in the early 1900s, paravertebral blocks were popularized in the 1930s as a means to provide analgesia for labor. Although this approach was largely replaced with more effective alternate treatments for labor, today paravertebral nerve blocks are being increasingly used as an effective technique for postoperative analgesia following mastectomy, inguinal hernia repair, and several procedures involving the chest and body wall.

A. ANATOMY

Each spinal nerve emerges from the intervertebral foramina and divides into two rami: a larger anterior ramus, which innervates the muscles and skin over the anterolateral body wall and limbs, and a smaller posterior ramus, which reflects posteriorly and innervates the skin and muscles of the back and neck. The thoracic paravertebral space is defined posteriorly by the superior costotransverse ligament, anterolaterally by the parietal pleura, medially by the vertebrae and the intervertebral foramina, and inferiorly and superiorly by the heads of the ribs.

B. TECHNIQUE

(Figure 17–34) The paravertebral nerve block is performed first by having the patient placed in a sitting position, similar to that for a sitting epidural. The spinous processes are identified, starting with the most obvious lower cervical vertebra in the neck, C7 or "vertebra prominens." Each process is marked along its superior aspect. From the midpoint of the superior aspect of each spinous process, it is necessary to measure 2.5 cm laterally and mark these points. These are the insertion points for the blocks and because of the pronounced inferior

angulation of the thoracic spinous processes these marks generally overlie the transverse process of the next vertebrae below, ie, a mark across from the T4 spinous process overlies the transverse process of T5.

At each insertion point a 22-gauge Tuohy needle is advanced in a perpendicular fashion approximately 3 cm initially, seeking to contact the transverse process. If bone is encountered (transverse process), the needle is withdrawn and redirected caudad and advanced an additional 1 cm. A "pop" may be felt as the needle passes through the costotransverse ligament. Following a negative aspiration, 4 mL of local anesthetic is delivered. This step is repeated for each level being blocked. If bone is not encountered with the initial pass, the needle is withdrawn and redirected caudad and inserted the same distance (ie, 3 cm), again seeking contact with the transverse process. Failure to contact bone with this pass requires redirection of the needle in a cephalad angulation, again inserting it the same depth while searching for bone contact. Failure to contact bone after this three-pass sequence (midline, caudad, and cephalad at the same depth) necessitates repeating this sequence at an added depth of 1 cm. This three-pass sequence with the addition of 1 cm in depth may be repeated until contact with bone is achieved. Once bone contact is made, from that site and depth, the needle is withdrawn and redirected caudad and advanced an additional 1 cm to enter the paravertebral space. Subsequent levels are approximately similar in depth, except for the upper thoracic, which tends to lie deeper. Lumbar paravertebral blocks are performed in a similar fashion. However, the transverse processes are thinner than their thoracic counterparts; therefore, after making bone contact and redirecting the needle caudad, the needle is advanced only an additional 0.5 cm in depth.

C. INDICATIONS

Paravertebral nerve blocks require individual injections delivered at the various vertebral levels that correspond to the area of body wall to be anesthetized. For example, a simple mastectomy would require blocks at levels T3–6; for axillary node dissection, additional injections should be made at T1 and T2. For inguinal hernia repair, blocks should be performed at T10 through L1.

D. COMPLICATIONS

The most common complication of thoracic paravertebral block is pneumothorax, which is related to the number of levels and the experience of the operator. If air is aspirated, a chest radiograph is mandatory. Intravascular injection and failed block are other possible problems.

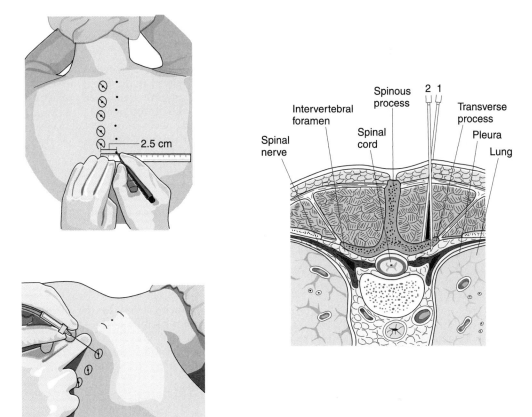

Figure 17–34. Thoracic paravertebral nerve block.

Inguinal Nerve Block

A. ANATOMY

The ilioinguinal and iliohypogastric nerves arise primarily from L1 but may derive fibers from T12. The iliohypogastric nerve splits into two branches prior to becoming cutaneous. The lateral branch is sensory to the lateral aspect of the buttock and hip. The anterior branch becomes superficial just medial to the anterior superior iliac spine, where it sends off a network of branches that innervates the lower abdomen. The ilioinguinal nerve follows the same course and exits the peritoneum to enter the inguinal canal, where it provides sensation to the scrotum, penis, and medial thigh in the male, or an equivalent area of the labia and mons pubis in the female. Both nerves pierce the transversalis abdominis and internal oblique muscles approximately 2 cm medial to the anterior superior iliac spine. The genitofemoral nerve is derived from L1 and L2. Its femoral branch travels with the femoral artery to provide cutaneous sensation just below the inguinal ligament, whereas its genital branch travels in the inguinal canal

to supply the scrotum in men and the labium majus in women.

B. TECHNIQUE

(Figure 17–35) A skin wheal is raised 2 cm medial to the upper aspect of the anterior superior iliac spine, and a 22-gauge, 3.5-in spinal needle is inserted perpendicular to the skin until it is just under the fascia, and 8–10 mL of anesthetic is injected fanwise to block both the ilioinguinal and iliohypogastric nerves. The genital branch of the genitofemoral nerve is blocked with 2–3 mL of local anesthetic injected just lateral to the pubic tubercle; the femoral branch can be anesthetized with 3–5 mL of local anesthetic injected subcutaneously just below the inguinal ligament.

C. INDICATIONS

Ilioinguinal and iliohypogastric blocks can be used for inguinal or genital operations, such as inguinal herniorrhaphy or orchiopexy, or for postoperative pain relief. Supplementation with a genitofemoral nerve block may be necessary.

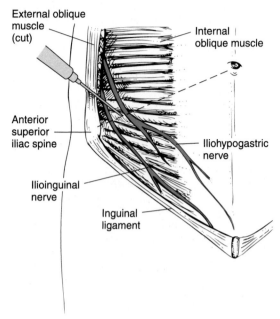

Figure 17–35. Ilioinguinal–iliohypogastric nerve block.

D. Complications

Patient discomfort and persistent paresthesia from intraneural injection are potential sequelae.

Penile Block

A. Anatomy

Innervation of the penis is derived from the pudendal nerve, which gives off the dorsal nerve of the penis bilaterally. It enters the penis deep to Buck's fascia and divides into dorsal and ventral branches. The genitofemoral and ilioinguinal nerves may additionally provide sensation to the base of the penis via subcutaneous branches.

B. Technique

(Figure 17–36) A fan-shaped (triangular) field block with 10–15 mL of local anesthetic injected at the base of the penis and 2–4 cm lateral to the base on both sides of the penis can block the sensory nerves without risk of vascular injury. If more profound block is necessary, or if extensive surgery is planned, the dorsal nerve is blocked just lateral to the base of the penis bilaterally with a 25-gauge, $^3/_4$- to 1-in needle just penetrating Buck's fascia at the 10:30 and 1:30 o'clock positions; 1 mL of local anesthetic is injected on each side, with care taken to avoid pressure. Epinephrine or other vasoconstrictors should be avoided to prevent end artery spasm and ischemic injury.

C. Indications

Penile block is performed for penile surgery or postoperative pain relief afterward.

Figure 17–36. Penile field block.

D. COMPLICATIONS

Careful aspiration is necessary to avoid intravascular injection. Injecting large volumes of local anesthetic or epinephrine-containing solutions may compromise blood flow to the penis.

SUMMARY

Regional anesthesia and peripheral nerve blocks have a long history in anesthesia. Over the past few decades, much effort and development have been centered on the advancement of general anesthesia, thus overshadowing interest in and applications of regional anesthesia. However, today there is a growing interest in regional techniques, particularly directed toward providing opioid-free postoperative analgesia. Although advancements in local anesthetics, types of needles, and development of peripheral catheters have all made this practice more common, it is knowledge of anatomy and recognition of possible benefits and adverse consequences, essential for the practitioner, that have truly advanced the practice.

CASE DISCUSSION:
DYSPNEA FOLLOWING
INTERSCALENE BLOCK

An anxious 54-year-old woman with a humeral fracture consents to regional anesthesia for open reduction and internal fixation. An interscalene block with 25 mL of 2% lidocaine with epinephrine (1:200,000) is administered using an "immobile needle" technique with incremental injection and careful aspiration. After 5 min, the patient notes numbness of the operative arm but starts to complain of increasing dyspnea.

What would appropriate management be?

Dyspnea following an interscalene block may be due to multiple causes that are often not immediately apparent. Familiarity with the complication of the block, a high index of suspicion, careful monitoring, and preparations for managing these complications can help avoid an adverse outcome. Immediate management should emphasize maintenance of adequate oxygenation and ventilation and maintaining hemodynamic stability. If not already present, full monitoring should be instituted (electrocardiogram, blood pressure readings every 2–3 min, and pulse oximetry), and supplemental oxygen should be given regardless of pulse oximetry readings to provide additional reserves should

apnea suddenly develop. Preparations should be made for induction of general anesthesia, tracheal intubation, controlled ventilation, and administration of vasopressors and atropine. Mental status and ventilatory exchange should also be followed carefully. Small amounts of midazolam (0.5 mg) may help alleviate anxiety but excessive sedation should be avoided until the cause of the dyspnea is determined.

What are the most likely causes?

Possible causes include anxiety, ipsilateral phrenic nerve block, pneumothorax, cervical epidural anesthesia, and a dural sleeve injection resulting in spinal anesthesia. Anxiety-related dyspnea is a diagnosis of exclusion. An immediate onset of dyspnea is suggestive of inadvertent spinal anesthesia. Other causes are typically more delayed in onset and become apparent only with time. Mental obtundation, apnea, hypotension, and bradycardia are characteristic of high spinal and inadvertent cervical epidural anesthesia. Pneumothorax and phrenic nerve block are usually asymptomatic but can decrease arterial oxygen saturation. A chest radiograph can help confirm the diagnosis. Clinical studies suggest that phrenic nerve block is an unavoidable complication of interscalene blocks; patients who are unusually anxious and those with preexisting pulmonary compromise are more likely to complain of dyspnea.

Why does inadvertent epidural or spinal injection cause apnea?

The relatively large volume of local anesthetic used for interscalene blocks can produce very high neuraxial anesthesia. Intrathecal injection at the cervical level results in total spinal anesthesia, whereas epidural injection results in bilateral blockade of the C3–5 nerve roots that innervate the diaphragm. A subdural injection at this level also has similar effects. Moreover, the sudden and profound sympathectomy associated with neuraxial anesthesia at this level can produce apnea from hypoperfusion of the brain stem.

How should an inadvertent epidural or spinal injection be managed?

Immediate ventilation with 100% oxygen should be instituted. Atropine 1–3 mg should be given to reverse bradycardia. Ephedrine 10–25 mg is administered for hypotension. If either the bradycardia or hypotension does not resolve immediately, 10–100 μg of epinephrine is administered. Rapid intubation of the trachea and controlled ventilation are usually necessary until spontaneous ventilation returns. Intravenous fluid administration also partially offsets the decreased venous return from the sympathectomy. Repeat administration or a continuous infusion of vasopressor may be necessary. The surgery should generally be postponed until the patient recovers and the neurological function can be assessed.

SUGGESTED READING

Capdevila X, Macaire P, Dadure C, et al: Continuous psoas compartment block for postoperative analgesia after total hip arthroplasty: New landmarks, technical guidelines, and clinical evaluation. Anesth Analg 2002;94:1606.

Hadzic A, Vloka J: *Peripheral Nerve Blocks: Principles and Practice.* McGraw-Hill, 2004.

Long T, Wass C, Burkle C: Perioperative interscalene blockade: An overview of its history and current clinical use. J Clin Anesth 2002;14:546.

Moore C, Sheppard D, Wildsmith J: Thigh rotation and the anterior approach to the sciatic nerve: A magnetic resonance imaging study. Reg Anesth Pain Med 2004;29:32.

Mulroy M: *Regional Anesthesia. An Illustrated Procedural Guide*, 3rd ed. Lippincott, Williams & Wilkins, 2002.

Raj P: *Textbook of Regional Anesthesia.* Churchill Livingstone, 2002.

Weltz C, Klein S, Arbo J, Greengrass R: Paravertebral block anesthesia for inguinal hernia repair. World J Surg 2003;27: 425.

Pain Management

18

KEY CONCEPTS

 Pain can be classified according to pathophysiology (eg, nociceptive or neuropathic pain), etiology (eg, postoperative or cancer pain), or the affected area (eg, headache or low back pain).

 Nociceptive pain is caused by activation or sensitization of peripheral nociceptors, specialized receptors that transduce noxious stimuli. Neuropathic pain is the result of injury or acquired abnormalities of peripheral or central neural structures.

 Acute pain can be defined as pain that is caused by noxious stimulation due to injury, a disease process, or the abnormal function of muscle or viscera. It is nearly always nociceptive.

 Chronic pain is defined as pain that persists beyond the usual course of an acute disease or after a reasonable time for healing to occur; this period can vary from 1 to 6 months. Chronic pain may be nociceptive, neuropathic, or mixed.

 Modulation of pain occurs peripherally at the nociceptor, in the spinal cord, or in supraspinal structures. This modulation can either inhibit (suppress) or facilitate (aggravate) pain.

 Moderate to severe acute pain, regardless of site, can affect nearly every organ function and may adversely influence postoperative morbidity and mortality.

 Neural blockade with local anesthetics can be useful in delineating pain mechanisms, but more importantly, it plays a major role in the management of patients with acute or chronic pain. The role of the sympathetic system and its pathways can be evaluated.

 Antidepressants are generally most useful in patients with neuropathic pain, eg, from postherpetic neuralgia and diabetic neuropathy. These agents demonstrate an analgesic effect that occurs at a dose lower than needed for their antidepressant action.

 Anticonvulsants have been found to be extremely useful in patients with neuropathic pain, particularly trigeminal neuralgia and diabetic neuropathy.

 Spinal cord stimulation is most effective for neuropathic pain. Proposed mechanisms include activation of descending modulating systems and inhibition of sympathetic outflow. Accepted indications include sympathetically mediated pain, spinal cord lesions with localized segmental pain, phantom limb pain, ischemic lower extremity pain due to peripheral vascular disease, and adhesive arachnoiditis.

 Studies show that patient-controlled analgesia (PCA) is a cost-effective technique that produces superior analgesia with very high patient satisfaction. Total drug consumption is less, compared with intramuscular injections. The routine use of a basal ("background") infusion is controversial.

(continued on next page)

(continued from previous page)

 The administration of local anesthetic–opioid mixtures neuraxially (particularly epidurally) is an excellent technique for managing postoperative pain following abdominal, pelvic, thoracic, or orthopedic procedures on the lower extremities. Patients often have better preservation of pulmonary function, are able to ambulate early, and benefit from early physical therapy. Patients may be at lower risk for postoperative venous thrombosis.

 The most serious side effect of epidural or intrathecal opioids is dose-dependent, delayed respiratory depression. Most cases of serious respiratory depression occur in patients receiving concomitant parenteral opioids or sedatives.

Elderly patients and those with sleep apnea appear to be particularly vulnerable and require reduced dosing.

 Physical dependence occurs in all patients on large doses of opioids for extended periods. A withdrawal phenomenon can be precipitated by the administration of opioid antagonists.

 Multiple triggers can induce sympathetically maintained pain, which is often overlooked or misdiagnosed. Patients often dramatically respond to sympathetic blocks. The likelihood of a cure is high (over 90%) if treatment is initiated within 1 month of symptoms and appears to decrease with time.

Pain—the most common symptom that brings patients to see a physician—nearly always manifests a pathological process. Any treatment plan must be directed at the underlying process as well as at controlling pain. Patients are generally referred for pain management by primary care practitioners or specialists once a diagnosis has been made and treatment of any underlying process has been initiated. Notable exceptions are patients with chronic pain in which the cause remains obscure after preliminary investigations; serious and life-threatening illnesses should, however, have been excluded.

The term "pain management" in a general sense applies to the entire discipline of anesthesiology, but its modern usage is restricted to management of pain outside the operating room. This type of practice may be broadly divided into acute and chronic pain management. The former primarily deals with patients recovering from surgery or with acute medical conditions in a hospital setting, whereas the latter includes diverse groups of patients in the outpatient setting. Unfortunately, this distinction is artificial because considerable overlap exists; a good example is the cancer patient who frequently requires short- and long-term pain management, both in and out of the hospital.

The practice of pain management is not just limited to anesthesiologists but includes other practitioners such as physicians (internists, oncologists, and neurologists) and nonphysicians (psychologists, chiropractors, acupuncturists, and hypnotists). Clearly, the most effective approach is multidisciplinary, in which the patient

is evaluated by one physician (the case manager) who conducts the initial examination and formulates a treatment plan, and the services and resources of other specialists are readily available. Moreover, the case manager and the various consultants meet regularly in formal case conferences to discuss patients. Single specialty pain clinics tend to be either syndrome or modality oriented. The former specialize in chronic back pain, headache, and temporomandibular joint dysfunction, whereas the latter offer nerve block, acupuncture, hypnosis, and biofeedback.

Anesthesiologists trained in pain management are in a unique position to coordinate multidisciplinary pain management centers because of broad training in dealing with a wide diversity of patients from surgical, obstetric, pediatric, and medical subspecialties, as well as expertise in clinical pharmacology and applied neuroanatomy, including the use of peripheral and central nerve blocks (see Chapters 16 and 17).

DEFINITIONS & CLASSIFICATION OF PAIN

Like other conscious sensations, normal pain perception depends on specialized neurons that function as receptors, detecting the stimulus, and then transducing and conducting it into the central nervous system. Sensation is often described as either protopathic (noxious) or epicritic (nonnoxious). Epicritic sensation (light touch, pressure, proprioception, and temperature discrimination) is characterized by low-threshold receptors and is generally conducted by large myelinated nerve fibers (see Table 16–1). In contrast, protopathic sensation (pain) is subserved by high-threshold receptors and conducted by smaller, lightly myelinated (Aδ) and unmyelinated (C) nerve fibers.

What Is Pain?

Pain is not just a sensory modality but is an experience. The International Association for the Study of Pain defines pain as "an unpleasant sensory and emotional experience associated with actual or potential tissue damage, or described in terms of such damage." This definition recognizes the interplay between the objective, physiological sensory aspects of pain and its subjective, emotional, and psychological components. The response to pain can be highly variable among persons as well as in the same person at different times.

The term "nociception," which is derived from *noci* (Latin for harm or injury), is used to describe the neural response only to traumatic or noxious stimuli. All nociception produces pain, but not all pain results from nociception. Many patients experience pain in the absence of noxious stimuli. It is therefore clinically useful to divide pain into one of two categories: (1) acute pain, which is primarily due to nociception, and (2) chronic pain, which may be due to nociception but in which psychological and behavioral factors often play a major role. Table 18–1 lists terms frequently used in describing pain.

Pain can also be classified according to pathophysiology (eg, nociceptive or neuropathic pain), etiology (eg, postoperative or cancer pain), or the affected area (eg, headache or low back pain). Such classifications are useful in the selection of treatment modalities and drug therapy. Nociceptive pain is caused by activation or sensitization of peripheral nociceptors, specialized receptors that transduce noxious stimuli. Neuropathic pain is the result of injury or acquired abnormalities of peripheral or central neural structures.

A. ACUTE PAIN

Acute pain can be defined as pain that is caused by noxious stimulation due to injury, a disease process, or the abnormal function of muscle or viscera. It is usually nociceptive. Nociceptive pain serves to detect, localize, and limit tissue damage. Four physiological processes are involved: transduction, transmission, modulation, and perception. This type of pain is typically associated with a neuroendocrine stress that is proportional to intensity. Its most common forms include posttraumatic, postoperative, and obstetric pain as well as pain associated with acute medical illnesses,

Table 18–1. Terms used in pain management.

Term	Description
Allodynia	Perception of an ordinarily nonnoxious stimulus as pain
Analgesia	Absence of pain perception
Anesthesia	Absence of all sensation
Anesthesia dolorosa	Pain in an area that lacks sensation
Dysesthesia	Unpleasant or abnormal sensation with or without a stimulus
Hypalgesia (hypoalgesia)	Diminished response to noxious stimulation (eg, pinprick)
Hyperalgesia	Increased response to noxious stimulation
Hyperesthesia	Increased response to mild stimulation
Hyperpathia	Presence of hyperesthesia, allodynia, and hyperalgesia usually associated with overreaction, and persistence of the sensation after the stimulus
Hypesthesia (hypoesthesia)	Reduced cutaneous sensation (eg, light touch, pressure, or temperature)
Neuralgia	Pain in the distribution of a nerve or a group of nerves
Paresthesia	Abnormal sensation perceived without an apparent stimulus
Radiculopathy	Functional abnormality of one or more nerve roots

such as myocardial infarction, pancreatitis, and renal calculi. Most forms of acute pain are self-limited or resolve with treatment in a few days or weeks. When the pain fails to resolve because of either abnormal healing or inadequate treatment, the pain becomes chronic (below). Two types of acute (nociceptive) pain—somatic and visceral—are differentiated based on origin and features.

1. Somatic pain—Somatic pain can be further classified as superficial or deep. Superficial somatic pain is due to nociceptive input arising from skin, subcutaneous tissues, and mucous membranes. It is characteristically well localized and described as a sharp, pricking, throbbing, or burning sensation.

Deep somatic pain arises from muscles, tendons, joints, or bones. In contrast to superficial somatic pain, it usually has a dull, aching quality and is less well-localized. An additional feature is that both the intensity

Table 18–2. Patterns of referred pain.

Location	Cutaneous Dermatome
Central diaphragm	C4
Lungs	T2–T6
Heart	T1–T4
Aorta	T1–L2
Esophagus	T3–T8
Pancreas and spleen	T5–T10
Stomach, liver, and gallbladder	T6–T9
Adrenals	T8–L1
Small intestine	T9–T11
Colon	T10–L1
Kidney, ovaries, and testes	T10–L1
Ureters	T10–T12
Uterus	T11–L2
Bladder and prostate	S2–S4
Urethra and rectum	S2–S4

and duration of the stimulus affect the degree of localization. For example, pain following brief minor trauma to the elbow joint is localized to the elbow, but severe or sustained trauma often causes pain in the whole arm.

2. Visceral pain—The visceral form of acute pain is due to a disease process or abnormal function of an internal organ or its covering (eg, parietal pleura, pericardium, or peritoneum). Four subtypes are described: (1) true localized visceral pain, (2) localized parietal pain, (3) referred visceral pain, and (4) referred parietal pain. True visceral pain is dull, diffuse, and usually midline. It is frequently associated with either abnormal sympathetic or parasympathetic activity causing nausea, vomiting, sweating, and changes in blood pressure and heart rate. Parietal pain is typically sharp and often described as a stabbing sensation that is either localized to the area around the organ or referred to a distant site (Table 18–2). The phenomenon of visceral or parietal pain referred to cutaneous areas results from patterns of embryological development and migration of tissues, and the convergence of visceral and somatic afferent input into the central nervous system. Thus, pain associated with disease processes involving the peritoneum or pleura over the central diaphragm is frequently referred to the neck and shoulder, whereas disease affecting the

parietal surfaces of the peripheral diaphragm is referred to the chest or upper abdominal wall.

B. CHRONIC PAIN

 Chronic pain is defined as pain that persists beyond the usual course of an acute disease or after a reasonable time for healing to occur; this period can vary from 1 to 6 months. Chronic pain may be nociceptive, neuropathic, or mixed. A distinguishing feature is that psychological mechanisms or environmental factors frequently play a major role. Patients with chronic pain often have an attenuated or absent neuroendocrine stress response and have prominent sleep and affective (mood) disturbances. Neuropathic pain is classically paroxysmal and lancinating, has a burning quality, and is associated with hyperpathia. When it is also associated with loss of sensory input (eg, amputation) into the central nervous system, it is termed "deafferentation pain." When the sympathetic system plays a major role, it is often termed "sympathetically maintained pain."

The most common forms of chronic pain include those associated with musculoskeletal disorders, chronic visceral disorders, lesions of peripheral nerves, nerve roots, or dorsal root ganglia (including diabetic neuropathy, causalgia, phantom limb pain, and postherpetic neuralgia), lesions of the central nervous system (stroke, spinal cord injury, and multiple sclerosis), and cancer pain. The pain of most musculoskeletal disorders (eg, rheumatoid arthritis and osteoarthritis) is primarily nociceptive, whereas pain associated with peripheral or central neural disorders is primarily neuropathic. The pain associated with some disorders, eg, cancer and chronic back pain (particularly after surgery), is often mixed. Some clinicians use the term "chronic benign pain" when pain does not result from cancer. This is to be discouraged, because pain is never benign from the patient's point of view, regardless of its cause.

■ ANATOMY & PHYSIOLOGY OF NOCICEPTION

PAIN PATHWAYS

To simplify for the sake of illustration, pain is conducted along three-neuron pathways that transmit noxious stimuli from the periphery to the cerebral cortex (Figure 18–1). Primary afferent neurons are located in the dorsal root ganglia, which lie in the vertebral foramina at each spinal cord level. Each neuron has a single axon that bifurcates, sending one end to the peripheral tissues it innervates and the other into the dorsal horn order neurons, which in turn send projections through the internal capsule and corona radiata to the postcentral gyrus of the cerebral cortex (Figure 18–2).

First-Order Neurons

The majority of first-order neurons send the proximal end of their axons into the spinal cord via the dorsal (sensory) spinal root at each cervical, thoracic, lumbar, and sacral level. Some unmyelinated afferent (C) fibers have been shown to enter the spinal cord via the ventral nerve (motor) root, accounting for observations that some patients continue to feel pain even after transection of the dorsal nerve root (rhizotomy) and report pain following ventral root stimulation. Once in the dorsal horn, in addition to synapsing with second-order neurons, the axons of first-order neurons may synapse with interneurons, sympathetic neurons, and ventral horn motor neurons.

Pain fibers originating from the head are carried by the trigeminal (V), facial (VII), glossopharyngeal (IX), and vagal (X) nerves. The gasserian ganglion contains the cell bodies of sensory fibers in the ophthalmic, maxillary, and mandibular divisions of the trigeminal nerve. Cell bodies of first-order afferent neurons of the facial nerve are located in the geniculate ganglion; those of the glossopharyngeal nerve lie in its superior and petrosal ganglia; and those of the vagal nerve are located in the jugular ganglion (somatic) and the ganglion nodosum (visceral). The proximal axonal processes of the first-order neurons in these ganglia reach the brain stem nuclei via their respective cranial nerves, where they synapse with second-order neurons in brain stem nuclei.

Second-Order Neurons

As afferent fibers enter the spinal cord, they segregate according to size, with large, myelinated fibers becoming medial, and small, unmyelinated fibers becoming lateral. Pain fibers may ascend or descend one to three spinal cord segments in Lissauer's tract before synapsing with second-order neurons in the gray matter of the ipsilateral dorsal horn. In many instances they communicate with second-order neurons through interneurons.

Spinal cord gray matter was divided by Rexed into 10 lamina (Figure 18–3 and Table 18–3). The first six lamina, which make up the dorsal horn, receive all afferent neural activity, and represent the principal site of modulation of pain by ascending and descending neural pathways. Second-order neurons are either nociceptive specific or wide dynamic range (WDR) neurons. Nociceptive-specific neurons serve only noxious stimuli, but WDR neurons also receive nonnoxious afferent input from Aβ, Aδ, and C fibers. Nociceptive-specific neurons are arranged somatotopically in lamina I and have discrete, somatic receptive fields; they are

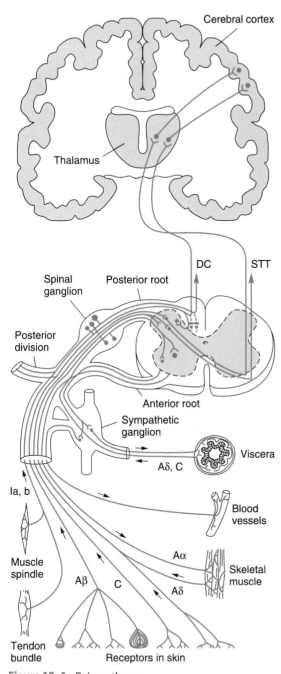

Figure 18–1. Pain pathways.

of the spinal cord. In the dorsal horn, the primary afferent neuron synapses with a second-order neuron whose axons cross the midline and ascend in the contralateral spinothalamic tract to reach the thalamus. Second-order neurons synapse in thalamic nuclei with third-

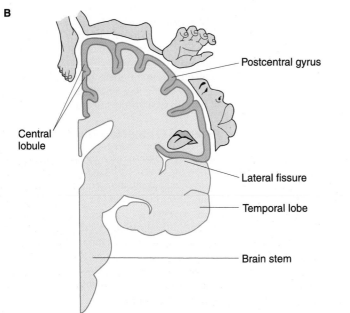

Figure 18–2. Lateral (**A**) and coronal (**B**) views of the brain show the location of the primary sensory cortex. Note the cortical representation of body parts, the sensory homunculus (**B**).

normally silent and respond only to high-threshold noxious stimulation, poorly encoding stimulus intensity. WDR neurons are the most prevalent cell type in the dorsal horn. Although they are found throughout the dorsal horn, WDR neurons are most abundant in lamina V. During repeated stimulation, WDR neurons characteristically increase their firing rate exponentially in a graded fashion ("wind-up"), even with the same

To dorsal columns

Mechanoreceptors — Aβ

Mechanoreceptors
Nociceptors   } — Aδ
Cold receptors

Nociceptors
Thermoreceptors   } — C
Mechanoreceptors

Figure 18–3. Rexed's spinal cord laminae. Note the termination of the different types of primary afferent neurons.

stimulus intensity. They also have large receptive fields compared with nociceptive-specific neurons.

Most nociceptive C fibers send collaterals to, or terminate on, second-order neurons in laminas I and II, and, to a lesser extent, in lamina V. In contrast, nociceptive Aδ fibers synapse mainly in laminas I and V, and, to a lesser degree, in lamina X. Lamina I responds primarily to noxious (nociceptive) stimuli from cutaneous and deep somatic tissues. Lamina II, also called the substantia gelatinosa, contains many interneurons and is believed to play a major role in processing and modulating nociceptive input from cutaneous nociceptors. It is also of special interest because it is believed to be a major site of action for opioids. Laminas III and IV receive primarily nonnociceptive sensory input. Laminas VIII and IX make up the anterior (motor) horn. Lamina VII is called the intermediolateral column and contains the cell bodies of preganglionic sympathetic neurons.

Visceral afferents terminate primarily in lamina V, and, to a lesser extent, in lamina I. These two lamina represent points of central convergence between somatic and visceral inputs. Lamina V responds to both noxious and nonnoxious sensory input and receives both visceral and somatic pain afferents. The phenomenon of convergence between visceral and somatic sensory input is manifested clinically as referred pain (Table 18–2). Compared with somatic fibers, visceral nociceptive fibers are fewer in number, more widely distributed, proportionately activate a larger number of spinal neurons, and are not organized somatotopically.

A. The Spinothalamic Tract

The axons of most second-order neurons cross the midline close to their level of origin (at the anterior commissure) to the contralateral side of the spinal cord before they form the spinothalamic tract and send their fibers to the thalamus, the reticular formation, the nucleus raphe magnus, and the periaqueductal gray. The spinothalamic tract, which is classically considered

Table 18–3. Spinal cord lamina.

Lamina	Predominant Function	Input	Name
I	Somatic nociception thermoreception	Aδ, C	Marginal layer
II	Somatic nociception thermoreception	C, Aδ	Substantia gelatinosa
III	Somatic mechanoreception	Aβ, Aδ	Nucleus proprius
IV	Mechanoreception	Aβ, Aδ	Nucleus proprius
V	Visceral and somatic nociception and mechanoreception	Aβ, Aδ, (C)	Nucleus proprius WDR neurons[1]
VI	Mechanoreception	Aβ	Nucleus proprius
VII	Sympathetic		Intermediolateral column
VIII		Aβ	Motor horn
IX	Motor	Aβ	Motor horn
X		Aβ	Central canal

[1]WDR, wide dynamic range.

the major pain pathway, lies anterolaterally in the white matter of the spinal cord (Figure 18–4). This ascending tract can be divided into a lateral and a medial tract. The lateral spinothalamic (neospinothalamic) tract projects mainly to the ventral posterolateral nucleus of the thalamus and carries discriminative aspects of pain, such as location, intensity, and duration. The medial spinothalamic (paleospinothalamic) tract projects to the medial thalamus and is responsible for mediating the autonomic and unpleasant emotional perceptions of pain. Some spinothalamic fibers also project to the periaqueductal gray and thus may be an important link between the ascending and descending pathways. Collateral fibers also project to the reticular activating system and the hypothalamus; these are likely responsible for the arousal response to pain.

B. Alternate Pain Pathways

As with epicritic sensation, pain fibers ascend diffusely, ipsilaterally, and contralaterally; hence, some patients continue to perceive pain following ablation of the contralateral spinothalamic tract. Thus, other ascending pain pathways are also important. The spinoreticular tract is thought to mediate arousal and autonomic responses to pain. The spinomesencephalic tract may be important in activating antinociceptive, descending pathways, because it has some projections to the periaqueductal gray. The spinohypothalamic and spinotelencephalic tracts activate the hypothalamus and evoke emotional behavior. The spinocervical tract ascends uncrossed to the lateral cervical nucleus, which relays the fibers to the contralateral thalamus; this tract is

likely a major alternative pathway for pain. Lastly, some fibers in the dorsal columns (which mainly carry light touch and proprioception) are responsive to pain; they ascend medially and ipsilaterally.

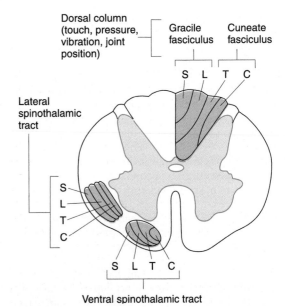

Figure 18–4. A cross section of the spinal cord showing the spinothalamic and other ascending sensory pathways. Note the spatial distribution of fibers from different spinal levels: cervical (C), thoracic (T), lumbar (L), and sacral (S).

C. INTEGRATION WITH THE SYMPATHETIC AND MOTOR SYSTEMS

Somatic and visceral afferents are fully integrated with the skeletal motor and sympathetic systems in the spinal cord, brain stem, and higher centers. Afferent dorsal horn neurons synapse both directly and indirectly with anterior horn motor neurons. These synapses are responsible for reflex muscle activity—whether normal or abnormal—that is associated with pain. In a similar fashion, synapses between afferent nociceptive neurons and sympathetic neurons in the intermediolateral column result in reflex sympathetically mediated vasoconstriction, smooth muscle spasm, and the release of catecholamines, both locally and from the adrenal medulla.

Third-Order Neurons

Third-order neurons are located in the thalamus and send fibers to somatosensory areas I and II in the postcentral gyrus of the parietal cortex and the superior wall of the sylvian fissure, respectively. Perception and discrete localization of pain take place in these cortical areas. Although most neurons from the lateral thalamic nuclei project to the primary somatosensory cortex, those from the intralaminar and medial nuclei project to the anterior cingulate gyrus and likely mediate the suffering and emotional components of pain.

PHYSIOLOGY OF NOCICEPTION

1. Nociceptors

Nociceptors are characterized by a high threshold for activation and encode the intensity of stimulation by increasing their discharge rates in a graded fashion. Following repeated stimulation, they characteristically display delayed adaptation, sensitization, and afterdischarges.

Noxious sensations can often be broken down into two components: a fast, sharp, and well-localized sensation ("first pain"), which is conducted with a short latency (0.1 s) by Aδ fibers (tested by pinprick); and a duller, slower onset, and often poorly localized sensation ("second pain"), which is conducted by C fibers. In contrast to epicritic sensation, which may be transduced by specialized end organs on the afferent neuron (eg, pacinian corpuscle for touch), protopathic sensation is transduced mainly by free nerve endings.

Most nociceptors are free nerve endings that sense heat and mechanical and chemical tissue damage. Types include (1) mechanonociceptors, which respond to pinch and pinprick, (2) silent nociceptors, which respond only in the presence of inflammation, and (3) polymodal mechanoheat nociceptors. The last are most prevalent and respond to excessive pressure, extremes of temperature (> 42°C and < 18°C), and alogens (pain-producing sub-stances). At least two nociceptor receptors (ion channels in nerve endings) have been identified, VR1 and VRL-1. Both respond to high temperatures. Alogens include bradykinin, histamine, serotonin (5-hydroxytryptamine or 5-HT), H$^+$, K$^+$, some prostaglandins, and possibly adenosine triphosphate. Capsaicin stimulates the VR1 receptor. Polymodal nociceptors are slow to adapt to strong pressure and display heat sensitization.

Cutaneous Nociceptors

Nociceptors are present in both somatic and visceral tissues. Primary afferent neurons reach tissues by traveling along spinal somatic, sympathetic, or parasympathetic nerves. Somatic nociceptors include those in skin (cutaneous) and deep tissues (muscle, tendons, fascia, and bone), whereas visceral nociceptors include those in internal organs. The cornea and tooth pulp are unique in that they are almost exclusively innervated by noci-ceptive Aδ and C fibers.

Deep Somatic Nociceptors

Deep somatic nociceptors are less sensitive to noxious stimuli than cutaneous nociceptors, but are easily sensitized by inflammation. The pain arising from them is characteristically dull and poorly localized. Specific nociceptors may exist in muscles and joint capsules; they respond to mechanical, thermal, and chemical stimuli.

Visceral Nociceptors

Visceral organs are generally insensitive tissues that mostly contain silent nociceptors. Some organs appear to have specific nociceptors, such as the heart, lung, testis, and bile ducts. Most other organs, such as the intestines, are innervated by polymodal nociceptors that respond to smooth muscle spasm, ischemia, and inflammation (alogens). These receptors generally do not respond to the cutting, burning, or crushing that occurs during surgery. A few organs, such as the brain, lack nociceptors altogether; however, the brain's meningeal coverings do contain nociceptors.

Like somatic nociceptors, those in the viscera are the free nerve endings of primary afferent neurons whose cell bodies lie in the dorsal horn. These afferent nerve fibers, however, frequently travel with efferent sympathetic nerve fibers to reach the viscera. Afferent activity from these neurons enters the spinal cord between T1 and L2. Nociceptive C fibers from the esophagus, larynx, and trachea travel with the vagus nerve to enter the nucleus solitarius in the brain stem. Afferent pain fibers from the bladder, prostate, rectum, cervix and urethra, and genitalia are transmitted into the spinal cord via parasympathetic nerves at the level of the S2–S4 nerve

Table 18–4. Major neurotransmitters mediating or modulating pain.

Neurotransmitter	Receptor[1]	Effect on Nociception
Substance P	NK–1	Excitatory
Calcitonin gene-related peptide		Excitatory
Glutamate	NMDA, AMPA, kainite, quisqualate	Excitatory
Aspartate	NMDA, AMPA, kainite, quisqualate	Excitatory
Adenosine triphosphate (ATP)	P_1, P_2	Excitatory
Somatostatin		Inhibitory
Acetylcholine	Muscarinic	Inhibitory
Enkephalins	μ, δ, κ	Inhibitory
β-Endorphin	μ, δ, κ	Inhibitory
Norepinephrine	α_2	Inhibitory
Adenosine	A_1	Inhibitory
Serotonin	$5\text{-}HT_1$ $(5\text{-}HT_3)$	Inhibitory
γ-Aminobutyric acid (GABA)	A, B	Inhibitory
Glycine		Inhibitory

[1]NMDA, *N*-methyl-D-aspartate; AMPA, 2-(aminomethyl)phenylacetic acid; 5-HT, 5-hydroxytryptamine.

roots. Though relatively few compared to somatic pain fibers, fibers from primary visceral afferent neurons enter the cord and synapse more diffusely with single fibers, often synapsing with multiple dermatomal levels and often crossing to the contralateral dorsal horn.

2. Chemical Mediators of Pain

Several neuropeptides and excitatory amino acids function as neurotransmitters for afferent neurons subserving pain (Table 18–4). Many if not most neurons contain more than one neurotransmitter, which is simultaneously coreleased. The most important of these peptides are substance P (sP) and calcitonin gene-related peptide (CGRP). Glutamate is the most important excitatory amino acid.

Substance P is an 11 amino acid peptide that is synthesized and released by first-order neurons both peripherally and in the dorsal horn. It is one of six tachykinin peptides that share a common amino acid carboxyl sequence. Substance P, which is also found in other parts of the nervous system and the intestines, facilitates transmission in pain pathways via NK-1 receptor activation. In the periphery, sP neurons send collaterals that are closely associated with blood vessels, sweat glands, hair follicles, and mast cells in the dermis. Substance P sensitizes nociceptors, degranulates hista-

mine from mast cells and 5-HT from platelets, and is a potent vasodilator and chemoattractant for leukocytes. Substance P–releasing neurons also innervate the viscera and send collateral fibers to paravertebral sympathetic ganglia; intense stimulation of viscera, therefore, can cause direct postganglionic sympathetic discharge.

Both opioid and α_2-adrenergic receptors have been described on or near the terminals of unmyelinated peripheral nerves. Although their physiological role is not clear, the latter may explain the observed analgesia of peripherally applied opioids, particularly in the presence of inflammation.

3. Modulation of Pain

Modulation of pain occurs peripherally at the nociceptor, in the spinal cord, or in supraspinal structures. This modulation can either inhibit (suppress) or facilitate (aggravate) pain.

Peripheral Modulation

Nociceptors and their neurons display sensitization following repeated stimulation. Sensitization may be manifested as an enhanced response to noxious stimulation or a newly acquired responsiveness to a wider range of stimuli, including nonnoxious stimuli.

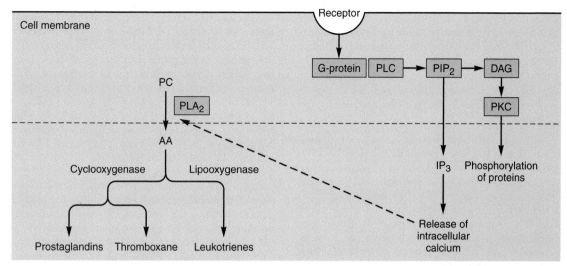

Figure 18–5. Phospholipase C (PLC) catalyzes the hydrolysis of phosphatidylinositol 4,5-bisphosphate (PIP_2) to produce inositol triphosphate (IP_3) and diacylglycerol (DAG). Protein kinase C (PKC) is also important. Phospholipase A_2 (PLA_2) catalyzes the conversion of phosphatidylcholine (PC) to arachadonic acid (AA).

A. PRIMARY HYPERALGESIA

Sensitization of nociceptors results in a decrease in threshold, an increase in the frequency response to the same stimulus intensity, a decrease in response latency, and spontaneous firing even after cessation of the stimulus (afterdischarges). Such sensitization commonly occurs with injury and following application of heat. Primary hyperalgesia is mediated by the release of alogens from damaged tissues. Histamine is released from mast cells, basophils, and platelets, whereas serotonin is released from mast cells and platelets. Bradykinin is released from tissues following activation of factor XII. Bradykinin activates free nerve endings via specific receptors (B1 and B2).

Prostaglandins are produced following tissue damage by the action of phospholipase A_2 on phospholipids released from cell membranes to form arachidonic acid (Figure 18–5). The cyclooxygenase (COX) pathway then converts the latter into endoperoxides, which in turn are transformed into prostacyclin and prostaglandin E_2 (PGE_2). PGE_2 directly activates free nerve endings, whereas prostacyclin potentiates the edema from bradykinin. The lipoxygenase pathway converts arachidonic acid into hydroperoxy compounds, which are subsequently converted into leukotrienes. The role of the latter is not well defined, but they appear to potentiate certain types of pain. Pharmacological agents such as acetylsalicylic acid (ASA, or aspirin), acetaminophen, and nonsteroidal antiinflammatory drugs (NSAIDs) produce analgesia by inhibition of COX. The analgesic effect of corticosteroids is likely the result of inhibition of prostaglandin production through blockade of phospholipase A_2 activation.

B. SECONDARY HYPERALGESIA

Neurogenic inflammation, also called secondary hyperalgesia, also plays an important role in peripheral sensitization following injury. It is manifested by the "triple response" of a red flush around the site of injury (flare), local tissue edema, and sensitization to noxious stimuli. Secondary hyperalgesia is primarily due to antidromic release of sP (and probably CGRP) from collateral axons of the primary afferent neuron. Substance P degranulates histamine and 5-HT, vasodilates blood vessels, causes tissue edema, and induces the formation of leukotrienes. The neural origin of this response is emphasized by the following: (1) it can be produced by antidromic stimulation of a sensory nerve, (2) it is not observed in denervated skin, and (3) it is diminished by injection of a local anesthetic such as lidocaine. The compound capsaicin, which is derived from the Hungarian red pepper, degranulates and depletes sP. When applied topically, capsaicin diminishes neurogenic inflammation and appears to be useful for some patients with postherpetic neuralgia.

Central Modulation

A. FACILITATION

At least three mechanisms are responsible for central sensitization in the spinal cord:

(1) Wind-up and sensitization of second-order neurons. WDR neurons increase their frequency of discharge with the same repetitive stimuli, and exhibit prolonged discharge, even after afferent C fiber input has stopped.

(2) Receptor field expansion. Dorsal horn neurons increase their receptive fields such that adjacent neurons become responsive to stimuli (whether noxious or not) to which they were previously unresponsive.

(3) Hyperexcitability of flexion reflexes. Enhancement of flexion reflexes is observed both ipsilaterally and contralaterally.

Neurochemical mediators of central sensitization include sP, CGRP, vasoactive intestinal peptide (VIP), cholecystokinin (CCK), angiotensin, and galanin, as well as the excitatory amino acids L-glutamate and L-aspartate. These substances trigger changes in membrane excitability by interacting with G protein–coupled membrane receptors on neurons, activating intracellular second messengers, which in turn phosphorylate substrate proteins. A common pathway is an increase in intracellular calcium concentration (Figure 18–5).

Glutamate and aspartate play an important role in wind-up, via activation of N-methyl-D-aspartate (NMDA) and non-NMDA receptor mechanisms. These amino acids are believed to be largely responsible for the induction and maintenance of central sensitization. Activation of NMDA receptors increases intracellular calcium concentration in spinal neurons and activates phospholipase C (PLC). Increased intracellular calcium concentration activates phospholipase A_2 (PLA$_2$), catalyzes the conversion of phosphatidylcholine (PC) to arachidonic acid (AA), and induces the formation of prostaglandins. Phospholipase C catalyzes the hydrolysis of phosphatidylinositol 4,5-bisphosphate (PIP$_2$) to produce inositol triphosphate (IP$_3$) and diacylglycerol (DAG), which functions as a second messenger; DAG, in turn, activates protein kinase C (PKC).

Activation of NMDA receptors also induces nitric oxide synthetase, resulting in the formation of nitric oxide. Both prostaglandins and nitric oxide facilitate the release of excitatory amino acids in the spinal cord. Thus, COX inhibitors such as ASA and NSAIDs also appear to have important analgesic actions in the spinal cord.

B. INHIBITION

Transmission of nociceptive input in the spinal cord can be inhibited by segmental activity in the cord itself, as well as descending neural activity from supraspinal centers.

1. Segmental inhibition—Activation of large afferent fibers subserving epicritic sensation inhibits WDR neuron and spinothalamic tract activity. Moreover, activation of noxious stimuli in noncontiguous parts of the body inhibits WDR neurons at other levels; ie, pain in one part of the body inhibits pain in other parts. These two observations support a "gate" theory for pain processing in the spinal cord.

Glycine and γ-aminobutyric acid (GABA) are amino acids that function as inhibitory neurotransmitters. They likely play an important role in segmental inhibition of pain in the spinal cord. Antagonism of glycine and GABA results in powerful facilitation of WDR neurons and produces allodynia and hyperesthesia. There are two subtypes of GABA receptors: GABA$_A$, of which muscimol is an agonist, and GABA$_B$, of which baclofen is an agonist. Segmental inhibition appears to be mediated by GABA$_B$ receptor activity, which increases K$^+$ conductance across the cell membrane. The GABA$_A$ receptor functions as a Cl$^-$ channel, which increases Cl$^-$ conductance across the cell membrane. Benzodiazepines potentiate this action. Activation of glycine receptors also increases Cl$^-$ conductance across neuronal cell membranes. Strychnine and tetanus toxoid are glycine receptor antagonists. The action of glycine is more complex than GABA, because the former also has a facilitatory (excitatory) effect on the NMDA receptor.

Adenosine also modulates nociceptive activity in the dorsal horn. At least two receptors are known: A$_1$, which inhibits adenylcyclase, and A$_2$, which stimulates adenylcyclase. The A$_1$ receptor mediates adenosine's antinociceptive action. Methylxanthines can reverse this effect through phosphodiesterase inhibition.

2. Supraspinal inhibition—Several supraspinal structures send fibers down the spinal cord to inhibit pain in the dorsal horn. Important sites of origin for these descending pathways include the periaqueductal gray, reticular formation, and nucleus raphe magnus (NRM). Stimulation of the periaqueductal gray area in midbrain produces widespread analgesia in humans. Axons from these tracts act presynaptically on primary afferent neurons and postsynaptically on second-order neurons (or interneurons). These pathways mediate their antinociceptive action via α$_2$-adrenergic, serotonergic, and opiate (μ, δ, and κ) receptor mechanisms. The role of monoamines in pain inhibition explains the analgesic action of antidepressants that block reuptake of catecholamines and serotonin. Activity at these receptors (which are also coupled to G proteins) activates secondary intracellular messenger, opening K$^+$ channels and inhibiting increases in intracellular calcium concentration.

Inhibitory adrenergic pathways originate primarily from the periaqueductal gray area and the reticular formation. Norepinephrine mediates this action via activation of presynaptic or postsynaptic α$_2$-receptors. At least part of the descending inhibition from the periaqueductal gray is relayed first to the NRM and medullary reticular formation; serotonergic fibers from the NRM then relay the inhibition to dorsal horn neurons via the dorsolateral funiculus.

The endogenous opiate system (primarily the NRM and reticular formation) acts via methionine enkephalin, leucine enkephalin, and β-endorphin, which are antagonized by naloxone. These opioids act presynaptically to hyperpolarize primary afferent neurons and inhibit the release of substance P; they also appear to cause some postsynaptic inhibition. In contrast, exogenous opioids may preferentially act postsynaptically on the second-order neurons or interneurons in the substantia gelatinosa.

4. Preemptive Analgesia

The importance of peripheral and central modulation in nociception has fostered the concept of "preemptive analgesia" in patients undergoing surgery. This type of management pharmacologically induces an effective analgesic state *prior* to the surgical trauma. This may involve infiltration of the wound with local anesthetic, central neural blockade, or the administration of effective doses of opioids, NSAIDs, or ketamine. Experimental evidence suggests that preemptive analgesia can effectively attenuate peripheral and central sensitization to pain. Although some studies have failed to demonstrate preemptive analgesia in humans, other studies have reported significant reductions in postoperative analgesic requirements in patients receiving preemptive analgesia.

PATHOPHYSIOLOGY OF CHRONIC PAIN

Chronic pain may be caused by a combination of peripheral, central, or psychological mechanisms. Sensitization of nociceptors plays a major role in the origin of pain associated with peripheral mechanisms, such as chronic musculoskeletal and visceral disorders.

Neuropathic pain involves peripheral–central and central neural mechanisms that are complex and generally associated with partial or complete lesions of peripheral nerves, dorsal root ganglia, nerve roots, or more central structures (Table 18–5). Peripheral mechanisms include spontaneous discharges; sensitization of receptors to mechanical, thermal, and chemical stimuli; and up-regulation of adrenergic receptors. Neural inflammation may also be present. Systemic administration of local anesthetics and anticonvulsants has been shown to suppress the spontaneous firing of sensitized or traumatized neurons. This observation is supported by the efficacy of agents such as lidocaine, mexiletine, and carbamazepine in many patients with neuropathic pain. Central mechanisms include loss of segmental inhibition, wind-up of WDR neurons, spontaneous discharges in deafferentated neurons, and reorganization of neural connections.

The sympathetic nervous system appears to play a major role in some patients with peripheral–central and central mechanisms. The efficacy of sympathetic nerve blocks in some patients supports the concept of sympa-

Table 18–5. Mechanisms of neuropathic pain.

Spontaneous self-sustaining neuronal activity in the primary afferent neuron (such as a neuroma).

Marked mechanosensitivity associated with chronic nerve compression.

Short-circuits between pain fibers and other types of fibers following demyelination, resulting in activation of nociceptive fibers by nonnoxious stimuli at the site of injury (ephaptic transmission).

Functional reorganization of receptive fields in dorsal horn neurons such that sensory input from surrounding intact nerves emphasizes or aggravates any input from the area of injury.

Spontaneous electrical activity in dorsal horn cells or thalamic nuclei.

Release of segmental inhibition in the spinal cord.

Loss of descending inhibitory influences that are dependent on normal sensory input.

Lesions of the thalamus or other supraspinal structures.

thetically maintained pain. Painful disorders that often respond to sympathetic blocks include reflex sympathetic dystrophy, deafferentation syndromes due to nerve avulsion or amputations, and postherpetic neuralgia (shingles). The simplistic theory of heightened sympathetic activity resulting in vasoconstriction, edema, and hyperalgesia fails to account for the warm and erythematous phase observed in some patients. Similarly, clinical and experimental observations do not satisfactorily support the theory of ephaptic transmission between pain fibers and demyelinated sympathetic fibers.

Psychological mechanisms or environmental factors are rarely the sole mechanisms for chronic pain, but are commonly associated with other mechanisms (Table 18–6). Patients with psychogenic pain typically experi-

Table 18–6. Psychological mechanisms or environmental factors associated with chronic pain.

Psychophysiological mechanisms in which emotional factors act as the initiating cause for somatic or visceral dysfunction (eg, tension headaches).

Learned or operant behavior in which chronic behavior patterns are rewarded (eg, by attention of a spouse) following an often minor injury.

Psychopathology due to psychiatric disorders such as major affective disorders (depression), schizophrenia, and somatization disorders (conversion hysteria) in which the patient has an abnormal preoccupation with bodily functions.

Pure psychogenic mechanisms (somatoform pain disorder), in which real suffering is experienced despite the absence of any nonciceptive input.

enced pain that was associated with great anxiety, fear of bodily harm, and loss of love early in life; later in life, anxiety is perceived as pain.

SYSTEMIC RESPONSES TO PAIN

Acute Pain

Acute pain is typically associated with a neuroendocrine stress response that is proportional to pain intensity. The pain pathways mediating the afferent limb of this response are discussed above. The efferent limb is mediated by the sympathetic nervous and endocrine systems. Sympathetic activation increases efferent sympathetic tone to all viscera and releases catecholamines from the adrenal medulla. The hormonal response results from increased sympathetic tone and hypothalamically mediated reflexes.

Minor or superficial operations are associated with little or no stress, whereas major upper abdominal and thoracic procedures produce major stress. Pain following abdominal and thoracic operations or trauma additionally has direct effects on respiratory function. Immobilization or bed rest due to pain in peripheral sites can also indirectly affect respiratory as well as hematological function. Moderate to severe acute pain, regardless of site, can affect nearly every organ function and may adversely influence postoperative morbidity and mortality. The latter suggests that effective management of postoperative pain is not only humane but is a very important aspect of postoperative care.

A. CARDIOVASCULAR EFFECTS

Cardiovascular effects are often prominent and include hypertension, tachycardia, enhanced myocardial irritability, and increased systemic vascular resistance. Cardiac output increases in most normal persons but may decrease in patients with compromised ventricular function. Because of the increase in myocardial oxygen demand, pain can aggravate or precipitate myocardial ischemia.

B. RESPIRATORY EFFECTS

An increase in total body oxygen consumption and carbon dioxide production necessitates a concomitant increase in minute ventilation. The latter increases the work of breathing, particularly in patients with underlying lung disease. Pain due to abdominal or thoracic incisions further compromises pulmonary function because of guarding (splinting). Decreased movement of the chest wall reduces tidal volume and functional residual capacity; this promotes atelectasis, intrapulmonary shunting, hypoxemia, and, less commonly, hypoventilation. Reductions in vital capacity impair coughing and the clearing of secretions. Regardless of the pain's location, prolonged bed rest or immobilization can produce similar changes in pulmonary function.

C. GASTROINTESTINAL AND URINARY EFFECTS

Enhanced sympathetic tone increases sphincter tone and decreases intestinal and urinary motility, promoting ileus and urinary retention, respectively. Hypersecretion of gastric acid can promote stress ulceration, and together with reduced motility, potentially predisposes patients to severe aspiration pneumonitis. Nausea, vomiting, and constipation are common. Abdominal distention further aggravates loss of lung volume and pulmonary dysfunction.

D. ENDOCRINE EFFECTS

The hormonal response to stress increases catabolic hormones (catecholamines, cortisol, and glucagon) and decreases anabolic hormones (insulin and testosterone). Patients develop a negative nitrogen balance, carbohydrate intolerance, and increased lipolysis. The increase in cortisol, together with increases in renin, aldosterone, angiotensin, and antidiuretic hormone, results in sodium retention, water retention, and secondary expansion of the extracellular space.

E. HEMATOLOGICAL EFFECTS

Stress-mediated increases in platelet adhesiveness, reduced fibrinolysis, and hypercoagulability have been reported.

F. IMMUNE EFFECTS

The stress response produces leukocytosis with lymphopenia and has been reported to depress the reticuloendothelial system. The latter predisposes patients to infection.

G. GENERAL SENSE OF WELL-BEING

The most common reaction to acute pain is anxiety. Sleep disturbances are also typical. When the duration of the pain becomes prolonged, depression is not unusual. Some patients react with anger that is frequently directed at the medical staff.

Chronic Pain

The neuroendocrine stress response is absent or attenuated in most patients with chronic pain. The stress response is generally observed only in patients with severe recurring pain due to peripheral (nociceptive) mechanisms and in patients with prominent central mechanisms such as pain associated with paraplegia. Sleep and affective disturbances, particularly depression, are often prominent. Many patients also experience significant changes in appetite (increase or decrease) and stresses on social relationships.

■ EVALUATING THE PATIENT WITH PAIN

The physician must first distinguish between acute and chronic pain. The management of acute pain is primarily therapeutic, whereas that of chronic pain additionally involves investigative measures. Thus, the patient with postoperative pain requires significantly less evaluation than the patient with a 10-year history of chronic low back pain who has sought multiple medical opinions and treatments. The former requires only a pertinent history and examination, including quantitative evaluation of pain severity, whereas the latter requires a careful history and physical examination, a review of prior medical evaluations and treatments, and thorough psychological and sociological evaluations.

The first evaluation is very important from both the physician and patient points of view. In addition to its diagnostic utility, this evaluation helps the physician demonstrate a sympathetic attitude to the patient. A written questionnaire can elicit valuable information about the nature of the pain, its onset and duration, and previous medication and treatments. Diagrams can be useful in defining patterns of radiation. The written questionnaire can help define the effect of the patient's pain on bodily functions, daily activities, and social interactions, and can offer insight about pain relief. The physical examination should emphasize the musculoskeletal and neurological systems. Imaging studies are often necessary and may include plain radiographs, computed tomography (CT), magnetic resonance imaging (MRI), or bone scans. These studies can often detect unsuspected trauma, tumors, or metabolic bone disease. MRI is particularly useful for soft tissue analysis and can show nerve compression.

PAIN MEASUREMENT

Reliable quantitation of pain severity helps determine therapeutic interventions and evaluate the efficacy of treatments. This is a challenge, however, because pain is a subjective experience that is influenced by psychological, cultural, and other variables. Clear definitions are necessary, because pain may be described in terms of tissue destruction or bodily or emotional reaction. Descriptive scales such as mild, moderate, and severe pain or verbal numerical scales are noncontinuous and generally unsatisfactory.

The numerical rating scale, faces rating scale, visual analog scale (VAS), and the McGill Pain Questionnaire (MPQ) are most commonly used. In the numerical scale, 0 corresponds to no pain and 10 designates the worst possible pain. The faces pain scale is more useful in patients with whom communication may be difficult. The patient is asked to point to various facial expressions ranging from a smiling face (no pain) to an extremely unhappy one that expresses the worst possible pain. The VAS is a 10-cm horizontal line labeled "no pain" at one end and "worst pain imaginable" on the other end. The patient is asked to mark on this line where the intensity of the pain lies. The distance from "no pain" to the patient's mark numerically quantitates the pain. The VAS is a simple, efficient, and minimally intrusive method that correlates well with other reliable methods.

The MPQ is a checklist of words describing symptoms. Unlike other pain rating methods that assume pain is unidimensional and describe intensity but not quality, the MPQ attempts to define the pain in three major dimensions: (1) sensory–discriminative (nociceptive pathways), (2) motivational–affective (reticular and limbic structures), and (3) cognitive–evaluative (cerebral cortex). It contains 20 sets of descriptive words that are divided into four major groups: (1) 10 sensory, (2) 5 affective, (3) 1 evaluative, and (4) 4 miscellaneous. The patient selects the sets that apply to his or her pain, and circles the words in each set that best describe the pain. The words in each class are given rank according to severity of pain. A pain rating index is derived based on the words chosen; scores may also be analyzed in each dimension (sensory, affective, evaluative, and miscellaneous). The MPQ is reliable and can be completed in 5–15 min. More importantly, the choice of descriptive words that characterize the pain correlates with pain syndromes and thus can be useful diagnostically. Unfortunately, high levels of anxiety and psychological disturbance can obscure the MPQ's discriminative capacity.

PSYCHOLOGICAL EVALUATION

Psychological evaluation is most useful whenever medical evaluation fails to reveal an apparent cause for pain, or when pain intensity is disproportionate to disease or injury. These types of evaluations help define the role of psychological or behavioral factors. The most commonly used tests are the Minnesota Multiphasic Personality Inventory (MMPI) and Beck Depression Inventory.

The MMPI consists of a 566-item true–false questionnaire that attempts to define the patient's personality on 10 clinical scales. Three validity scales serve to identify patients deliberately trying to hide traits or alter the results. It must be noted that cultural differences can affect scores. Moreover, the test is lengthy and some patients find its questions insulting. The MMPI is used primarily to confirm clinical impressions about the role of psychological factors; it cannot reliably distinguish between "organic" and "functional" pain.

Depression is very common in patients with chronic pain. It is often difficult to determine the contribution of depression to the suffering associated with pain. The

Table 18–7. Emotional and related disorders commonly associated with chronic pain.

Disorder	Brief Description
Somatization disorder	Physical symptoms of a medical condition that cannot be explained, resulting in involuntary distress and physical impairment.
Conversion disorder	Symptoms of voluntary motor or sensory deficits that suggest a medical condition; symptoms cannot be medically explained but are associated with psychological factors and are not intentionally feigned.
Hypochondriasis	Prolonged (> 6 months) preoccupation with the fear of having a serious illness despite adequate medical evaluation and reassurance.
Malingering	Intentional production of physical or psychological symptoms that is motivated by external incentives (eg, avoiding work or financial compensation).
Substance-related disorders	Habitual misuse of prescribed or illicit substances that often precedes and drives complaints of pain and drug-seeking behavior.

Beck Depression Inventory is a useful test for identifying patients with major depression.

Several tests have been developed to assess functional limitations or impairment (disability). These include the Multidimensional Pain Inventory (MPI), Medical Outcomes Survey 36-Item Short Form (SF-36), Pain Disability Index (PDI), and Oswestry Disability Questionnaire. These tests lack validity scales and largely reflect patient perception of disability.

Emotional disorders are commonly associated with complaints of chronic pain, and chronic pain often results in varying degrees of psychological distress. Determination of which came first is often difficult. In either case, both the pain and emotional distress need to be treated. Table 18–7 lists emotional disorders in which treatment should be primarily directed at the emotional disorder.

ELECTROMYOGRAPHY & NERVE CONDUCTION STUDIES

Electromyography and nerve conduction studies, which complement one another, are useful for confirming the diagnosis of entrapment syndromes, radicular syndromes, neural trauma, and polyneuropathies. They can often distinguish between neurogenic and myogenic disorders. Patterns of abnormalities can localize a lesion to the spinal cord, nerve root, limb plexus, or peripheral nerve. In addition, they may also be useful in excluding "organic" disorders when psychogenic pain or a "functional" syndrome is suspected.

Electromyography employs needle electrodes to record potentials in individual muscles. Muscle potentials are recorded first while the muscle is at rest and then as the patient is asked to move the muscle. Abnormal findings suggestive of denervation include persistent insertion potentials, the presence of positive sharp waves, fibrillary activity, or fasciculation potentials. A triphasic motor unit action potential is normally seen as the patient voluntarily moves the muscle. Abnormalities in muscles produce changes in amplitude and duration as well as polyphasic action potentials.

Peripheral nerve conduction studies employ supramaximal stimulations of motor or mixed sensorimotor nerve, whereas muscle potentials are recorded over the appropriate muscle. The time between the onset of the stimulation and the onset of the muscle potential (latency) is a measurement of the fastest conducting motor fibers in the nerve. The amplitude of the recorded potential indicates the number of functional motor units, whereas its duration reflects the range of conduction velocities in the nerve. Conduction velocity can be obtained by stimulating the nerve from two points and comparing the latencies. When a pure sensory nerve is evaluated, the nerve is stimulated while action potentials are recorded either proximally or distally (antidromic conduction).

Nerve conduction studies distinguish between mononeuropathies (due to trauma, compression, or entrapment) and polyneuropathies. The latter include systemic disorders that may produce abnormalities that are widespread and symmetrical or random (mononeuropathy multiplex). Moreover, the polyneuropathy may be due to axonal loss, demyelination, or both. Demyelination neuropathies slow nerve conduction, disperse action potentials, and prolong latencies. In contrast, axonal neuropathies decrease the amplitude of action potentials with preservation of nerve conduction velocities. Toxic, inherited, traumatic, and ischemic diseases typically cause axonal loss, whereas some inherited and most autoimmune diseases cause demyelination. Diabetic neuropathy frequently presents with mixed findings of both axonal loss and demyelination.

■ DIAGNOSTIC & THERAPEUTIC NEURAL BLOCKADE

 Neural blockade with local anesthetics can be useful in delineating pain mechanisms, but, more importantly, it plays a major role in the management of patients with acute or chronic pain. The role of the sympathetic system and its pathways can be evaluated. Pain relief following diagnostic neural blockade often carries favorable prognostic implications for a therapeutic series of blocks. Although the utility of differential neural blockade in differentiating between somatic and sympathetic mechanisms may be questionable, this technique can identify patients displaying a placebo response and those with psychogenic mechanisms. In selected patients, "permanent" neural blockade may be appropriate.

The efficacy of neural blockade is presumably due to interruption of afferent nociceptive activity. This is in addition to, or in combination with, blockade of afferent and efferent limbs of abnormal reflex activity (sympathetic and skeletal muscle). The pain relief frequently outlasts the known pharmacological duration of the agent employed by hours (or sometimes weeks). Selection of the type of block depends on the location of pain, its presumed mechanism, and the skills of the treating physician. Local anesthetic may be applied locally (infiltration), or at a peripheral nerve, somatic plexus, sympathetic ganglia, or nerve root. It can be applied centrally in the neuraxis. Spinal and epidural anesthesias are described in Chapters 16; somatic nerve blocks, which are commonly used for surgery, are described in Chapter 17.

SOMATIC BLOCKS

Trigeminal Nerve Blocks

A. INDICATIONS

The two principal indications are trigeminal neuralgia and intractable cancer pain in the face. Depending on the site of pain, these blocks may be performed on the gasserian ganglion itself, one of the major divisions (ophthalmic, maxillary, or mandibular), or one of their smaller branches.

B. ANATOMY

The rootlets of cranial nerve V arise from the brain stem and join one another to form a crescent-shaped sensory (gasserian) ganglion in Meckel's cave. Most of the ganglion is invested with a dural sleeve. The three subdivisions of the trigeminal nerve arise from the ganglia and exit the cranium separately. The ophthalmic division enters the orbit through the superior orbital fissure. The maxillary division exits the cranium via the foramen rotundum to enter the pterygopalatine fossa, where it divides into its various branches. The mandibular nerve exits through the foramen ovale, after which it divides into an anterior trunk, which is mainly motor to the muscles of mastication, and a posterior trunk, which further divides into the various sensory branches (Figure 18–6A).

C. TECHNIQUE

1. Gasserian ganglion block—To undertake this procedure (Figure 18–6B), radiographic guidance is mandatory. An anterolateral approach is most commonly employed. An 8- to 10-cm 22-gauge needle is inserted approximately 3 cm lateral to the angle of the mouth at the level of the upper second molar; it is advanced posteromedially and angled superiorly such that the needle is aligned with the pupil in the anterior plane and with the mid-zygomatic arch in the lateral plane. Without entering the mouth, the needle should pass between the mandibular ramus and the maxilla, and lateral to the pterygoid process to enter the cranium through the foramen ovale. After a negative aspiration for cerebrospinal fluid and blood, 2 mL of anesthetic is injected.

2. Blockade of the ophthalmic nerve and its branches—In this procedure, to avoid keratitis, the ophthalmic division itself is not blocked, so only the supraoptic branch is blocked in most cases (Figure 18–6C). The nerve is easily located and blocked with 2 mL of local anesthetic at the supraoptic notch, which is located on the supraoptic ridge above the pupil. The supratrochlear branch can also be blocked with 1 mL of local anesthetic at the superior medial corner of the orbital ridge.

3. Blockade of the maxillary nerve and its branches—With the patient's mouth slightly opened, an 8- to 10-cm 22-gauge needle is inserted between the zygomatic arch and the notch of the mandible (Figure 18–6D). After contact with the lateral pterygoid plate (at about 4-cm depth), the needle is partially withdrawn and angled slightly superiorly and anteriorly to pass into the pterygopalatine fossa. Anesthetic (4–6 mL) is injected once paresthesias are elicited. Both the maxillary nerve and the pterygopalatine ganglia are anesthetized by this technique. The pterygopalatine (sphenopalatine) ganglion (and anterior ethmoid nerves) can be anesthetized transmucosally with topical anesthetic applied through the nose; several cotton applicators soaked with local anesthetic (cocaine or lidocaine) are inserted along the medial wall of the nasal cavity into the area of the sphenopalatine recess.

The infraorbital branch passes through the infraorbital foramen, where it can be blocked with 2 mL of anesthetic. This foramen is approximately 1 cm below the orbit and is usually located with a needle inserted about 2 cm lateral to the nasal ala and directed superiorly, posteriorly, and slightly laterally.

4. Blockade of the mandibular nerve and its branches—This procedure is undertaken with the patient's mouth slightly opened (Figure 18–6E). An 8- to 10-cm 22-gauge needle is inserted between the zygo-

A. Blocks of the trigeminal nerve

B. Gasserian ganglion block

C. Supraorbital nerve block

Figure 18–6. Trigeminal nerve blocks.

(continued)

D. Maxillary nerve block

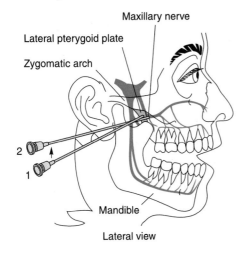

Maxillary nerve
Lateral pterygoid plate
Zygomatic arch
2
1
Mandible

Lateral view

E. Mandibular nerve block

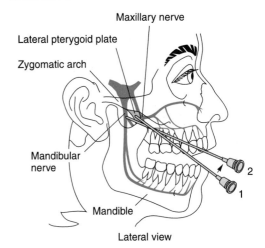

Maxillary nerve
Lateral pterygoid plate
Zygomatic arch
Mandibular nerve
2
1
Mandible

Lateral view

F. Lingual and inferior alveolar nerve block

Frontal view

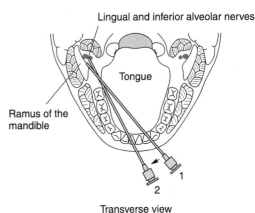

Lingual and inferior alveolar nerves
Tongue
Ramus of the mandible
1
2

Transverse view

Figure 18–6. (Continued)

matic arch and the mandibular notch. After contact with the lateral pterygoid plate, the needle is partially withdrawn and angled slightly superiorly and posteriorly toward the ear. Anesthetic (4–6 mL) is injected once paresthesias are elicited.

The lingual and inferior mandibular branches of the mandibular nerve may be blocked intraorally utilizing a 10-cm 22-gauge needle (Figure 18–6F). The patient is asked to open the mouth maximally and the coronoid notch is palpated with the index finger of the nonoperative hand. The needle is then introduced at the same level (approximately 1 cm above the surface of the last molar), medial to the finger but lateral to the pterygomandibular plicae (fold). It is advanced posteriorly 1.5–2 cm along the medial side of the mandibular ramus, making contact with the bone.

Both nerves are usually blocked following injection of 2–3 mL of local anesthetic.

The terminal portion of the inferior alveolar nerve may be blocked as it emerges from the mental foramen at the mid-mandible just beneath the corner of the mouth. Local anesthetic (2 mL) is injected once paresthesias are elicited or the needle is felt to enter the foramen.

D. Complications

Complications of a gasserian ganglion block include accidental intravascular injection, subarachnoid injection, Horner's syndrome, and motor block of the muscles of mastication. The potential for serious hemorrhage is greatest for blockade for the maxillary nerve. The facial nerve may be unintentionally blocked during blockade of the mandibular division.

Facial Nerve Block

A. INDICATIONS

Blockade of the facial nerve is occasionally indicated to relieve spastic contraction of the facial muscles and to treat herpes zoster affecting this nerve. This procedure is also used during certain eye surgery (see Chapter 38).

B. ANATOMY

The facial nerve exits the cranium through the stylomastoid foramen, where it can be blocked. A small sensory component supplies special sensation (taste) to the anterior two-thirds of the tongue and general sensation to the tympanic membrane, the external auditory meatus, soft palate, and part of the pharynx.

C. TECHNIQUE

The injection point is just anterior to the mastoid process, beneath the external auditory meatus, and at the midpoint of the mandibular ramus (see Chapter 38). The nerve is approximately 1–2 cm deep and is blocked with 2–3 mL of local anesthetic, just below the stylomastoid process.

D. COMPLICATIONS

If the needle is inserted too deeply past the level of the styloid bone, the glossopharyngeal and vagal nerves may also be blocked. Careful aspiration is necessary because of the proximity of the facial nerve to the carotid artery and the internal jugular vein.

Glossopharyngeal Block

A. INDICATIONS

Glossopharyngeal nerve block may be used for patients with pain due to malignant growths at the base of the tongue, the epiglottis, and palatine tonsils. It can also be used to distinguish glossopharyngeal neuralgia from trigeminal and geniculate neuralgia.

B. ANATOMY

The nerve exits from the cranium via the jugular foramen medial to the styloid process and courses anteromedially to supply the posterior third of the tongue, pharyngeal muscles, and mucosa. The vagus and spinal accessory nerves also exit the cranium via the jugular foramen and descend alongside the glossopharyngeal nerve; the carotid artery and internal jugular vein are closely associated structures.

C. TECHNIQUE

The block is performed with 2 mL of anesthetic using a 5-cm 22-gauge needle inserted just posterior to the angle of the mandible (Figure 18–7). The nerve is approximately 3–4 cm deep; use of a nerve stimulator facilitates correct placement of the needle. An alternative approach is from a point midway between the mas-

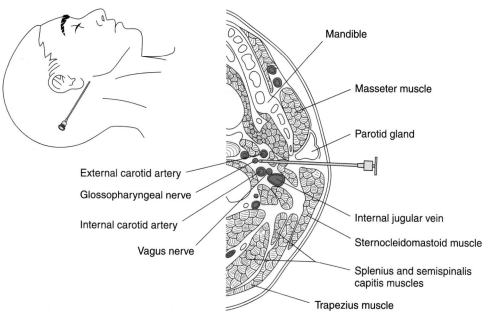

Figure 18–7. Glossopharyngeal nerve block.

toid process and the angle of the mandible and over the styloid process; the nerve is located just anterior to the styloid process.

D. COMPLICATIONS

Complications include dysphagia and vagal blockade resulting in ipsilateral vocal cord paralysis and tachycardia. Block of the accessory nerve and hypoglossal nerves causes ipsilateral paralysis of the trapezius muscle and the tongue, respectively. Careful aspiration is necessary to prevent intravascular injection.

Occipital Nerve Block

A. INDICATIONS

Occipital nerve block is useful diagnostically and therapeutically in patients with occipital headaches and neuralgias.

B. ANATOMY

The greater occipital nerve is derived from the dorsal primary rami of the C2 and C3 spinal nerves, whereas the lesser occipital nerve arises from the ventral rami of the same roots.

C. TECHNIQUE

The greater occipital nerve is blocked with 5 mL of anesthetic approximately 3 cm lateral to the occipital prominence at the level of the superior nuchal line (Figure 18–8); the nerve is just medial to the occipital artery, which is often palpable. The lesser occipital nerve is blocked with another 2–3 mL of anesthetic injected 2–3 cm more laterally along the nuchal ridge.

D. COMPLICATIONS

Rarely, intravascular injections may occur.

Phrenic Nerve Block

A. INDICATIONS

Blockade of the phrenic nerve may occasionally provide relief for pain arising from the central portion of the diaphragm. It can also be useful in patients with refractory hiccups (singultation).

B. ANATOMY

The phrenic nerve arises from the C3–C5 nerve roots at the lateral border of the anterior scalenus muscle.

C. TECHNIQUE

The nerve is blocked at a point 3 cm above the clavicle, just lateral to the posterior border of the sternocleidomastoid, and above the anterior scalene muscles. Anesthetic solution (5–10 mL) is injected.

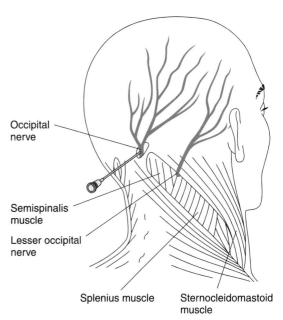

Figure 18–8. Occipital nerve blocks.

Labels: Occipital nerve; Semispinalis muscle; Lesser occipital nerve; Splenius muscle; Sternocleidomastoid muscle

D. COMPLICATIONS

In addition to serious intravascular injection, pulmonary compromise may occur in patients with preexisting lung disease or injury. Simultaneous bilateral phrenic nerve block should never be performed.

Suprascapular Nerve Block

A. INDICATIONS

This block is useful for painful conditions arising from the shoulder (most commonly arthritis and bursitis).

B. ANATOMY

The suprascapular nerve is the major sensory nerve of the shoulder joint. It arises from the brachial plexus (C4–C6) and passes over the upper border of the scapula in the suprascapular notch to enter the suprascapular fossa.

C. TECHNIQUE

The nerve is blocked with 5 mL of anesthetic solution at the supraspinal notch, which is located at the junction of the lateral and middle thirds of the superior scapular border (Figure 18–9). Correct placement of the needle is determined by paresthesia, or the use of a nerve stimulator.

D. COMPLICATIONS

Pneumothorax is possible if the needle is advanced too far anteriorly. Paralysis of the supraspinatus and infraspinatus muscles can be troublesome.

Figure 18–9. Suprascapular nerve block.

Cervical Paravertebral Nerve Block

A. INDICATIONS

Selective paravertebral blockade at the cervical level can be useful diagnostically and therapeutically for cancer patients with pain originating from the cervical spine or the shoulder.

B. ANATOMY

The cervical spinal nerves lie in the sulcus of the transverse process of their respective vertebral levels. The transverse processes can be palpated in most persons. Note that in contrast to thoracic and lumbar spinal nerves, cervical spinal nerves exit above their respective vertebral levels (see Chapter 16).

C. TECHNIQUE

The lateral approach is most commonly used to block C2–C7 (Figure 18–10). Patients are asked to turn their head to the opposite side while in a sitting position. A line is then drawn between the mastoid process and the Chassaignac's tubercle (the tubercle of the C6 transverse process). A series of 2-mL injections are made with a 5-cm 22-gauge needle along a second parallel line 0.5 cm posterior to the first line. Because the transverse process of C2 is usually difficult to palpate, the injection for this level is placed 1.5 cm beneath the mastoid process. The other transverse processes are usually interspaced 1.5 cm apart and are 2.5–3 cm deep. Fluoroscopy is useful in identifying vertebral levels during diagnostic blocks.

D. COMPLICATIONS

Unintentional intrathecal, subdural, or epidural anesthesia at this level rapidly causes respiratory paralysis and hypotension. Injection of even small volumes of local anesthetic into the vertebral artery causes unconsciousness and seizures. Other complications include Horner's syndrome, as well as blockade of the recurrent laryngeal and phrenic nerves.

Figure 18–10. Cervical paravertebral nerve block.

Thoracic Paravertebral Nerve Block

A. INDICATIONS

Unlike an intercostal nerve block, a thoracic paravertebral nerve block anesthetizes both the dorsal and ventral rami of spinal nerves (see Chapter 17). It is therefore useful in patients with pain originating from the thoracic spine, thoracic cage, or abdominal wall, including compression fractures, proximal rib fractures, and acute herpes zoster. This technique must be used for blockade of upper thoracic segments, because the scapula interferes with the intercostal technique at these levels.

B. ANATOMY

Each thoracic nerve root exits from the spinal canal just inferior to the transverse process of its corresponding spinal segment.

C. TECHNIQUE

This block may be performed with the patient prone or in the lateral position. A 5- to 8-cm 22-gauge spinal needle with an adjustable marker (bead or rubber stopper) is used. With the classic technique, the needle is inserted 4–5 cm lateral to the midline at the spinous process of the level above. The needle is directed anteriorly and medially using a 45° angle with the midsagittal plane, and advanced until it contacts the transverse process of the desired level. The needle is then partially withdrawn and redirected to pass just under the transverse process. The adjustable marker on the needle is used to mark the depth of the spinous process; when the needle is subsequently withdrawn and redirected, it should not be advanced more than 2 cm beyond this mark. Normally, 5 mL of local anesthetic is injected at each level.

An alternative technique that may decrease the risk of pneumothorax uses a more medial insertion point and a loss of resistance technique very similar to epidural anesthesia (see Chapter 17). The needle is inserted in a sagittal plane 1.5 cm lateral to the midline at the level of the spinous process above, and it is advanced until it contacts the lateral edge of the lamina of the level to be blocked. It is then withdrawn to a subcutaneous position and reinserted 0.5 cm more laterally but still in a sagittal plane; as the needle is advanced, it engages the superior costotransverse ligament, just lateral to the lamina and inferior to the transverse process. The correct position may be identified by loss of resistance to injection of saline when the needle penetrates the costotransverse ligament.

D. COMPLICATIONS

The most common complication of paravertebral block is pneumothorax; others include accidental subarachnoid, subdural, epidural, and intravascular injections. Sympathetic blockade and hypotension may be obtained if multiple segments are blocked or a large volume is injected at one level. A chest radiograph is mandatory afterward to rule out a pneumothorax.

Lumbar Paravertebral Somatic Nerve Block

A. INDICATIONS

Paravertebral block at this level is useful in evaluating pain due to disorders involving the lumbar spine or spinal nerves.

B. ANATOMY

The lumbar spinal nerves enter the psoas compartment as soon as they exit through the intervertebral foramina beneath the transverse processes. This compartment is formed by the psoas fascia anteriorly, the quadratus lumborum fascia posteriorly, and the vertebral bodies medially.

C. TECHNIQUE

The approach to lumbar spinal nerves is essentially the same as for thoracic paravertebral blockade (Figure 18–11). An 8-cm 22-gauge needle is usually used. Radiographic confirmation of the correct level is helpful. For diagnostic blocks, only 2 mL of local anesthetic is injected at any one level, because larger volumes block more than one level. Five milliliters of local anesthetic is used for therapeutic blocks, and yet even larger volumes (25 mL) at the level of L3 can produce complete somatic and sympathetic blockade of the lumbar nerves.

D. COMPLICATIONS

Complications are primarily those of unintentional subarachnoid, subdural, or epidural anesthesia.

Lumbar Medial Branch & Facet Blocks

A. INDICATIONS

These blocks may establish the contribution of lumbar facet (zygapophyseal) joint disease in back pain. Corticosteroids are commonly injected with the local anesthetic when the intraarticular technique is chosen.

B. ANATOMY

Each facet joint is innervated by the medial branches of the posterior primary division of the spinal nerves above and below the joint (Figure 18–12). Thus, every joint is supplied by two or more adjacent spinal nerves. Each medial branch crosses the upper border of the lower transverse process running in a groove between the root of the transverse process and the superior articular process.

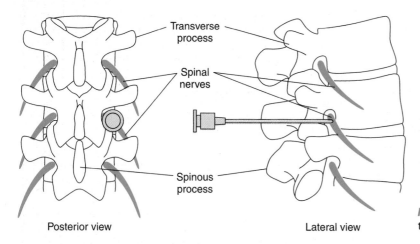

Figure 18–11. Lumbar paravertebral nerve blocks.

Posterior view

Lateral view

Transverse process

Spinal nerves

Spinous process

C. TECHNIQUE

These blocks should be performed under fluoroscopic guidance with the patient in a prone position (Figure 18–12). A 30° oblique posterior view facilitates visualization of the facet joints. A 6- to 8-cm 22-gauge needle is inserted 5–6 cm lateral to the spinous process of the desired level and directed medially toward the upper border of the root of the transverse process; 1–1.5 mL of local anesthetic is injected to block the medial branch of the posterior division of the spinal nerve.

Alternatively, local anesthetic with or without corticosteroid may be directly injected into the joint. Positioning the patient prone with slight obliquity (by placing a pillow beneath the anterior iliac crest on the affected side) facilitates identification of the joint space during fluoroscopy. Correct placement of the needle should be confirmed by injecting 0.5 mL of radiocontrast prior to injection of local anesthetic (2 mL).

D. COMPLICATIONS

Injection into a dural sleeve results in a subarachnoid block, whereas injection near the spinal nerve root results in sensory and motor blockade at that level. Because the joint normally has a 1–2 mL volume, larger injections can cause rupture of the joint capsule.

Trans-Sacral Nerve Block

A. INDICATIONS

This technique is useful in the diagnosis and treatment of pelvic and perineal pain. Blockade of the S1 spinal root can help define its role in back pain.

B. ANATOMY

The five paired sacral spinal nerves and one pair of coccygeal nerves descend in the sacral canal, forming the cauda equina. Each nerve then travels through its respective intervertebral foramen. The S5 and coccygeal nerves exit through the sacral hiatus.

C. TECHNIQUE

While the patient is prone, the sacral foramina are identified with a needle along a line drawn 1.5 cm medial to the posterior superior iliac spine and 1.5 cm lateral to the ipsilateral sacral cornu (Figure 18–13). Correct positioning requires entry of the needle into the posterior sacral foramen and usually produces paresthesias. The S1 nerve root is usually 1.5 cm above the level of the posterior superior iliac spine along this imaginary line. Two milliliters of local anesthetic is injected for diagnostic blocks and 5 mL is used for therapeutic blocks. Blockade of the S5 and coccygeal nerves can be accomplished by injection at the sacral hiatus (see Chapter 17).

D. COMPLICATIONS

Complications are rare but include nerve damage and intravascular injection.

Pudendal Nerve Block

A. INDICATIONS

Pudendal nerve block is useful in evaluating patients with perineal pain.

B. ANATOMY

The pudendal nerve arises from S2–S4 and courses between the sacrospinous and the sacrotuberous ligaments to reach the perineum.

C. TECHNIQUE

This block is usually performed transperineally in the lithotomy position (Figure 18–14). Injection of 5–10

A

Articular branches

Facet joints

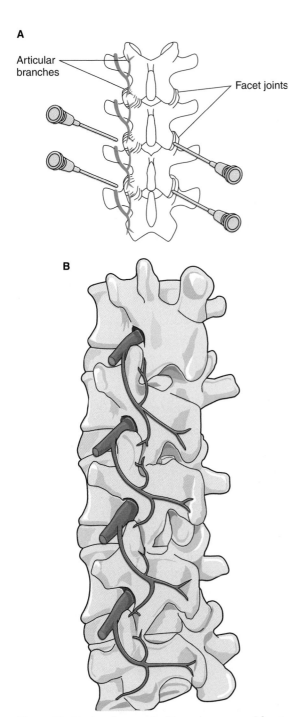

B

Figure 18–12. Lumbar medical branch nerve and facet blocks. *A:* Posterior view; *B:* 30° oblique posterior view.

mL of anesthetic is carried out percutaneously just posterior to the ischial spine at the attachment of the sacrospinous ligament. The ischial spine can be palpated transrectally or transvaginally. A special guide is typically used for a transvaginal approach (see Chapter 43).

D. COMPLICATIONS

Unintentional sciatic blockade and intravascular injection are common complications.

SYMPATHETIC BLOCKS

Sympathetic blockade can be accomplished by a variety of techniques including subarachnoid, epidural, as well as paravertebral blocks. Unfortunately, these approaches usually block both somatic and sympathetic fibers. Problems with differential spinal and epidural techniques are discussed below. The following techniques specifically block sympathetic fibers and can be used to define the role of the sympathetic system in a patient's pain and possibly provide long-term pain relief. The most common indications include reflex sympathetic dystrophy, visceral pain, acute herpetic neuralgia, postherpetic pain, and peripheral vascular disease. Isolated sympathetic blockade to a region is characterized by unaltered somatic sensation but loss of sympathetic tone as evidenced by increased cutaneous blood flow and temperature. Other tests include loss of the skin conductance (sympathogalvanic) and sweat response (ninhydrin, cobalt blue, or starch tests) following a painful stimulus.

Cervicothoracic (Stellate) Block

A. INDICATIONS

This block is often used in patients with head, neck, arm, and upper chest pain. It is commonly referred to as a stellate block but in reality usually blocks the upper thoracic as well as all cervical ganglia. Injection of large volumes of anesthetic (> 10 mL) often blocks down to the T5 ganglia. Stellate blocks may also be used for vasospastic disorders of the upper extremity.

B. ANATOMY

Sympathetic innervation of the head, neck, and most of the arm is derived from four cervical ganglia; the largest is the **stellate ganglion**. The latter usually represents a fusion of the lower cervical and first thoracic ganglia. Some sympathetic innervation of the arm (T1) as well as all innervation of the thoracic viscera are derived from the five upper thoracic ganglia. The sympathetic supply to the arm in some persons may also originate from T2–T3 via anatomically distinct nerves (Kuntz's nerves) that join the brachial plexus high in the axilla; these nerves may be missed by a stellate block but not

Posterior

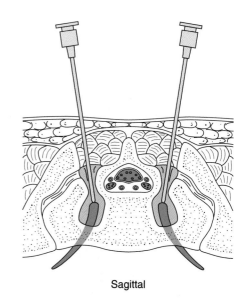

Sagittal

Figure 18–13. Trans-sacral nerve block.

an axillary block. The point of injection is at the level of the stellate, which lies posterior to the origin of the vertebral artery from the subclavian artery, anterior to the longus colli muscle and the first rib, anterolateral to the prevertebral fascia, and medial to the scalene muscles.

C. TECHNIQUE

The paratracheal technique is most commonly used (Figure 18–15). With the patient's head extended, a 4- to 5-cm 22-gauge needle is inserted at the medial edge of the sternocleidomastoid muscle just below the level of the cricoid cartilage at the level of the transverse process of C6 (Chassaignac's tubercle) or C7 (3–5 cm above the clavicle). The nonoperative hand should be used to retract the muscle together with the carotid sheath prior to needle insertion. The needle is advanced to the transverse process and withdrawn 2–3 mm prior to injection. Aspiration must be carried out in two planes before a 1-mL test dose is used to exclude unintentional intravascular injection (into the vertebral or subclavian arteries) or subarachnoid injection into a dural sleeve. A total of 10–15 mL of local anesthetic may be injected.

Correct placement of the needle is usually promptly followed by an increase in the skin temperature of the ipsilateral arm and the onset of Horner's syndrome. The latter consists of ipsilateral ptosis, meiosis, enophthalmos, nasal congestion, and anhidrosis of the neck and face.

D. COMPLICATIONS

In addition to intravascular and subarachnoid injection, other complications include hematoma, pneumothorax, epidural anesthesia, brachial plexus block, hoarse-

ness due to blockade of the recurrent laryngeal nerve, and, rarely, osteitis or mediastinitis following esophageal puncture.

Thoracic Sympathetic Chain Block

The thoracic sympathetic ganglia lie just lateral to the vertebral bodies and anterior to the spinal nerve roots,

Ischial spine

Figure 18–14. Pudendal nerve block.

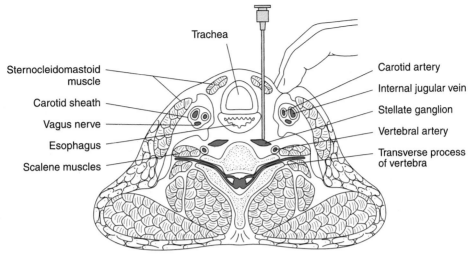

Figure 18–15. Stellate block.

but this block is generally not used because of a significant risk of pneumothorax.

Celiac Plexus Block

A. INDICATIONS

Celiac block is indicated in patients with pain arising from the abdominal viscera, particularly abdominal malignant growths. The technique usually also blocks the lumbar sympathetic chain.

B. ANATOMY

The celiac ganglia vary in number (1–5), form, and position. They are generally clustered at the level of the body of L1, posterior to the vena cava on the right, just lateral to the aorta on the left, and posterior to the pancreas.

C. TECHNIQUE

The patient is placed prone and a 15-cm 22-gauge needle is used to inject 15–20 mL of local anesthetic from the left side or bilaterally (Figure 18–16). Fluoroscopic or CT guidance with injection of radiocontrast increases the success rate, reduces the volume required, and decreases the incidence of complications. Each needle is inserted 3–8 cm from the midline at the inferior edge of the spinous process of L1; it is advanced under radiographic guidance toward the midline, making an approximately 10–45° angle. The needle passes under the edge of the twelfth rib and should be positioned anterior to the body of L1 in the lateral radiographic view and close to the midline overlying the same vertebral body in the anteroposterior view. When CT is used, the tip of the needle should come to lie anterolateral to the aorta at a level between the celiac and superior mesenteric arteries.

D. COMPLICATIONS

The most common complication is postural hypotension, which is largely due to blockade of the lumbar sympathetic chain. Intravascular injection into the vena cava is more likely to produce a severe systematic reaction than accidental intraaortic injection. Other less common complications include pneumothorax, retroperitoneal hemorrhage, injury to the kidneys or pancreas, sexual dysfunction, or, rarely, paraplegia (due to injury of a lumbar artery of Adamkiewicz).

Splanchnic Nerve Block

Although similar to celiac plexus block, this technique is preferred by a few clinicians because it is less likely to block the lumbar sympathetic chain and requires less anesthetic volume. Three groups of splanchnic nerves (greater, lesser, and least) arise from the lower seven thoracic sympathetic ganglia on each side and descend alongside the vertebral bodies to communicate with the celiac ganglia. The needle is inserted 6–7 cm from the midline at the lower end of the T11 spinous process, and advanced under fluoroscopic guidance to the anterolateral surface of T12. Ten milliliters of local anesthetic is injected on each side. The needle should maintain contact with the vertebral body at all times to avoid a pneumothorax. In addition to pneumothorax, complications may include hypotension and possible injuries to the azygos vein on the right or the hemiazygos vein and the thoracic duct on the left.

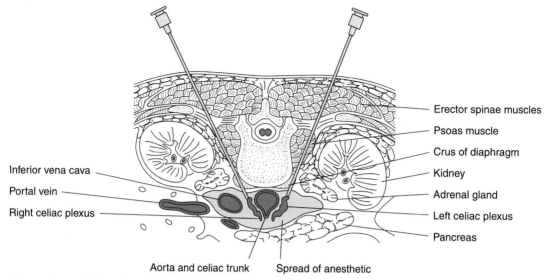

Figure 18–16. Celiac plexus block.

Lumbar Sympathetic Block

A. INDICATIONS

Lumbar sympathetic blockade may be indicated for painful conditions involving the pelvis or the lower extremities, and possibly in some patients with peripheral vascular disease.

B. ANATOMY

The lumbar sympathetic chain contains three to five ganglia and is a continuation of the thoracic chain; it also supplies sympathetic fibers to the pelvic plexus and ganglia. The lumbar sympathetic chain's ganglia lie in a more anteromedial position to the vertebral bodies than do the thoracic ganglia and are anterior to the psoas muscle and fascia. The lumbar chain is usually posterior to the vena cava on the right but is just lateral to the aorta on the left.

C. TECHNIQUE

A two-needle technique at the L2 and L4 levels is most commonly employed with the patient either prone or in a lateral position (Figure 18–17). The needle is inserted at the upper edge of the spinous process and is directed above or just lateral to the transverse process of the vertebrae (depending on the distance from the midline). Fluoroscopic guidance with injection of radiocontrast solution increases the success rate and may reduce complications.

D. COMPLICATIONS

Complications include intravascular injection (into the cava, aorta, or lumbar vessels), and somatic nerve block of the lumbar plexus.

Hypogastric Plexus Block

A. INDICATIONS

This procedure is indicated for pain that originates from the pelvis and that is unresponsive to lumbar or caudal epidural blocks. The hypogastric plexus contains visceral sensory fibers that bypass the lower spinal cord. This block is usually appropriate for patients with cancer of the cervix, uterus, bladder, prostate, or rectum. The block may also be effective in some women with chronic nonmalignant pelvic pain.

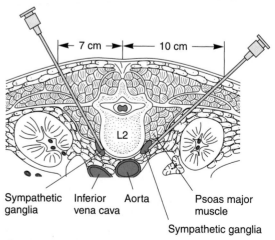

Figure 18–17. Lumbar sympathetic block.

B. ANATOMY

The hypogastric plexus not only contains postganglionic fibers derived from the lumbar sympathetic chain, but also visceral sensory fibers from the cervix, uterus, bladder, prostate, and rectum. The superior hypogastric plexus usually lies just to the left of the midline at the L5 vertebral body and beneath the bifurcation of the aorta. The fibers of this plexus divide into left and right branches and descend to the pelvic organs via the right and left inferior hypogastric and pelvic plexuses. The inferior hypogastric plexus additionally receives preganglionic parasympathetic fibers from S2–S4 spinal nerve roots.

C. TECHNIQUE

The patient is positioned prone, and a 15-cm needle is inserted approximately 7 cm lateral to the L4–L5 spinal interspace. The needle is directed medially and caudally at a 45° angle under fluoroscopic guidance so that it passes just over the transverse process of L5. In its final position, the needle should lie over the intervertebral disk between L5 and S1 and within 1 cm of the vertebral bodies in the anteroposterior view. Injection of radiocontrast dye confirms the correct position of the needle in the retroperitoneal space; 8–10 mL of local anesthetic is injected.

D. COMPLICATIONS

Complications include intravascular injection and transient bowel and bladder dysfunction.

Ganglion Impar Block

A. INDICATIONS

This block is effective in patients with visceral or sympathetically maintained pain in the perineal area.

B. ANATOMY

The ganglion impar (ganglion of Walther) is the most caudal part of the sympathetic trunks. The two lowest pelvic sympathetic ganglia often fuse forming one ganglion in the midline just anterior to the coccyx.

C. TECHNIQUE

The patient may be positioned in a lateral decubitus or lithotomy position. With the patient in a lateral decubitus position, a 22-gauge 8- to 10-cm curved needle is directed through the anococcygeal ligament upward into a position that is just anterior to the coccyx. Insertion of a finger in the rectum helps keep the needle in the midline and outside the rectal wall. An alternative approach utilizes a straight needle with the patient in the lithotomy position; a straight needle can be used in this position because the curvature of the coccyx is reduced. After con-

firmation of the correct position with radiocontrast dye, 4–6 mL of local anesthetic is injected.

D. COMPLICATIONS

No complications have been reported, but intravascular injection and transient bowel or bladder dysfunction are possible.

Intravenous Regional Sympathetic Blockade

A Bier block (see Chapter 17) utilizing guanethidine (20–40 mg) can selectively interrupt sympathetic innervation to an extremity. Ten milliliters of lidocaine 0.5% can also be added to prevent burning. A tourniquet is placed proximally on the extremity and usually left inflated for at least 20 min. Guanethidine causes depletion of norepinephrine and inhibits its reuptake at the terminals of postganglionic neurons. The selective sympathetic blockade lasts 3–7 days. Premature release of the tourniquet can result in hypotension, bradycardia, edema, diarrhea, and nausea. Reserpine (1–1.5 mg) and bretylium (5 mg/kg) can be used similarly. Intravenous regional sympathetic blockade is a safe alternative to standard sympathetic blocks in patients with hemostatic defects.

DIFFERENTIAL NEURAL BLOCKADE

Pharmacological or anatomic differential neural blockade has been advocated as a method of distinguishing somatic, sympathetic, and psychogenic pain mechanisms. The pharmacological approach relies on the differential sensitivity of nerve fibers to local anesthetics (see Chapter 14). Preganglionic sympathetic (B) fibers are reported to be most sensitive, closely followed by pain (C and Aδ), somatosensory (Aβ) fibers, and finally motor fibers (Aα). By using different concentrations of local anesthetic, it may be possible to selectively block certain types of fibers while preserving the function of others. Here the challenge is that the critical concentration needed to block sympathetic fibers can vary considerably between patients, and conduction block by local anesthetics is dependent not only on fiber size but the duration of contact and frequency of impulses conducted. Many clinicians have therefore abandoned the use of pharmacological differential neural blocks in favor of anatomic differential blockade.

Stellate ganglion blocks can be used to selectively block sympathetic fibers to the head, neck, and arm. Celiac plexus, hypogastric plexus, and lumbar paravertebral sympathetic blocks can be used for sympathetic blockade to the abdomen, pelvis, and leg, respectively. Selective nerve root, intercostal, cervical plexus, brachial plexus, or lumbosacral plexus blocks may be used for somatic nerve blockade.

Table 18–8. Solutions for differential epidural blockade.

Solution	Epidural[1]
Placebo	Saline
Sympatholytic	0.5% lidocaine
Somatic	1% lidocaine
All fibers	2% lidocaine

[1]Chloroprocaine may be used instead.

Differential epidural blockade may be used for thoracic pain when the techniques for sympathetic blockade carry a significant risk of pneumothorax (Table 18–8). After each epidural injection, the patient is evaluated for pain relief, signs of sympathetic blockade (a decrease in blood pressure), sensation to pinprick and light touch, and motor function. If the pain disappears after the saline injection, the patient either has psychogenic pain (usually a profound long-lasting effect) or is displaying a placebo effect (usually short-lasting). If pain relief coincides with isolated signs of sympathetic blockade, it is likely mediated by sympathetic fibers. If pain relief only follows somatosensory blockade, it is likely mediated by somatic fibers. Lastly, if the pain persists even after signs of motor blockade, the pain is either central (supraspinal) or psychogenic.

A serious disadvantage of the standard pharmacological differential technique is that it is very time consuming. Some clinicians therefore use a modified two-injection technique: a placebo injection followed by a maximally concentrated solution (2% chloroprocaine or 2% lidocaine epidurally). The patient is still evaluated after each injection, but the pain is correlated with the recovery of motor, sensory, and sympathetic function.

RADIOFREQUENCY ABLATION & CRYONEUROLYSIS

Percutaneous radiofrequency ablation relies on the heat produced by current flow from an active electrode that is incorporated at the tip of a special needle. The needle is positioned under fluoroscopy. Electrical stimulation (2 Hz for motor responses and 50 Hz for sensory responses) via the electrode and impedance measurement prior to ablation also help confirm correct positioning. Depending on the location of the block, the heating temperature generated at the electrode is precisely controlled (60–90°C for 1–3 min) to ablate the nerve without causing excessive tissue damage. Radiofrequency ablation is commonly used for trigeminal

rhizotomy and medial branch (facet) rhizotomy. It has also been used for dorsal root rhizotomy and lumbar sympathectomy. Pain relief usually lasts 3–12 months.

Cryoanalgesia can produce temporary neurolysis for weeks to months by freezing and thawing tissue. The temperature at the tip of a cryoprobe rapidly drops as gas (carbon dioxide or nitrous oxide) at a high pressure is allowed to expand. The probe tip, which can achieve temperatures of –50 to –70°C, is introduced via a 16- to 12-gauge catheter. Electrical stimulation (2–5 Hz for motor responses and 50–100 Hz for sensory responses) helps confirm correct positioning of the probe. Two or more 2-min cycles of freezing and thawing are usually administered. Cryoanalgesia is most commonly used to achieve long-term blockade of peripheral nerves. It may be particularly useful for postthoracotomy pain (see Chapter 24).

ALCOHOL & PHENOL NEUROLYTIC BLOCKS

Neurolytic blocks are indicated for patients with severe intractable cancer pain. They may occasionally be used in some patients with refractory neuralgia and rarely in patients with peripheral vascular disease. These blocks can be associated with considerable morbidity, so patients must be selected carefully. Moreover, the blocks are not permanent, because the original pain recurs or new (central) pain develops in a majority of patients within weeks to months. Temporary destruction of nerve fibers or ganglia can be accomplished by injection of alcohol or phenol. These agents are not selective, affecting visceral, sensory, and motor fibers equally. Ethyl alcohol (50–100%) causes extraction of membrane phospholipids and precipitation of lipoproteins in axons and Schwann cells, whereas phenol (6–12%) appears to coagulate proteins. Alcohol causes severe pain on injection. For peripheral nerve blocks, alcohol may be given undiluted, but for sympathetic blocks in which large volumes are injected, it is given in a 1:1 mixture with bupivacaine. Phenol is painless when injected either as an aqueous solution (6–8%) or in glycerol; a 12% phenol solution can be prepared in radiocontrast dye.

At least one diagnostic block with a local anesthetic solution should be used before considering any neurolytic technique. This serves to confirm the pain pathways involved and determine the potential efficacy of neurolytic blockade. Local anesthetic should again be injected immediately prior to the neurolytic agent. Moreover, fluoroscopy (or CT) with radiocontrast should be used whenever possible. Following injection of any neurolytic agent, the needle must be cleared with air or saline prior to withdrawal to prevent damage to superficial structures.

Neurolytic techniques are most commonly employed with celiac plexus, lumbar sympathetic chain, hypogastric plexus, and ganglion impar blocks in cancer patients but may be used for somatic or cranial nerves or even neural axial blocks. Many clinicians prefer alcohol for celiac plexus block but phenol for lumbar sympathetic blockade. With neurolytic subarachnoid techniques, very small amounts of the agent (0.1 mL) are injected, and the patient is carefully positioned such that the solution localizes to the appropriate level and is confined to the dorsal horn area. Alcohol is hypobaric, whereas phenol in glycerin is hyperbaric.

PHARMACOLOGICAL INTERVENTIONS

Pharmacological interventions in pain management include COX inhibitors, opioids, antidepressants, neuroleptic agents, anticonvulsants, corticosteroids, and systemic administration of local anesthetics. COX inhibitors are reviewed below in the discussion on postoperative pain management. Opioids, which are used primarily for acute moderate to severe pain and cancer pain, are discussed in Chapter 8 and below with cancer pain.

Antidepressants

These agents demonstrate an analgesic effect that occurs at a dose lower than needed for their antidepressant action. **Both actions are due to blockade of presynaptic reuptake of serotonin, norepinephrine, or both** (see Chapter 27). Older tricyclic agents appear to be more effective analgesics than selective serotonin reuptake inhibitors (SSRIs). In contrast, SSRIs appear to be more effective antidepressants. Antidepressants are generally most useful in patients with neuropathic pain, eg, from postherpetic neuralgia and diabetic neuropathy. They potentiate the action of opioids and frequently normalize sleep patterns.

Available agents differ in their side effects (Table 18–9), which include antimuscarinic effects, such as dry mouth (xerostomia), impaired visual accommodation, urinary retention, and constipation; antihistaminic effects (H_1 and H_2), such as sedation and increased gastric pH; α-adrenergic blockade resulting in orthostatic hypotension; and a quinidine-like effect, particularly with amitriptyline.

All agents undergo extensive first-pass hepatic metabolism and are highly protein bound. Most are highly lipophilic and have large volumes of distribution. Elimination half-lives vary between 1 and 4 days, and many have active metabolites.

Anticonvulsants

Anticonvulsants have been found to be extremely useful in patients with neuropathic pain, particularly trigeminal neuralgia and diabetic neuropathy. These agents block voltage-gated sodium channels and can suppress the spontaneous neural discharges that play a major role in these disorders. Gabapentin may offer additional unique beneficial effects. It has also been shown to be an effective adjuvant for postoperative pain. The most commonly employed agents are phenytoin, carbamazepine, valproic acid, clonazepam, and gabapentin (Table 18–10); see also Chapter 27). Lamotrigine and topiramate may also be effective. All are highly protein bound and have relatively long half-lives. Carbamazepine has a slow and unpredictable absorption, which requires monitoring of blood levels for optimal efficacy. Side effects are discussed in Chapter 27.

Neuroleptics

Some clinicians find neuroleptics useful in patients with refractory neuropathic pain. Neuroleptics may be most useful in patients with marked agitation or psychotic symptoms. The most commonly used agents are fluphenazine, haloperidol, chlorpromazine, and perphenazine. Their therapeutic action appears to be due to blockade of dopaminergic receptors in mesolimbic sites. Unfortunately, the same action in nigrostriatal pathways can produce undesirable extrapyramidal side effects, such as mask-like facies, a festinating gait, cogwheel rigidity, and bradykinesia. Some patients also develop acute dystonic reactions such as oculogyric crisis and torticollis. Long-term side effects include akathisia (extreme restlessness) and tardive dyskinesia (involuntary choreoathetoid movements of the tongue, lipsmacking, truncal instability). Like antidepressants, many of these drugs also have antihistaminic, antimuscarinic, and α-adrenergic–blocking effects.

Corticosteroids

Glucocorticoids are extensively used in pain management for their antiinflammatory and possibly analgesic actions. They may be given topically, orally, or parenterally (intravenously, subcutaneously, intrabursally, intraarticularly, epidurally). Table 18–11 lists the most commonly used agents, which differ in potency, relative glucocorticoid and mineralocorticoid activities, and duration. Large doses or prolonged administration result in significant side effects. Excess glucocorticoid activity can produce hypertension, hyperglycemia, increased susceptibility to infection, peptic ulcers, osteoporosis, aseptic necrosis of the femoral head, proximal myopathy, cataracts, and,

Table 18–9. Selected antidepressants.

Drug	Norepinephrine Reuptake Inhibition	Serotonin Reuptake Inhibition	Sedation	Antimuscarinic Activity	Orthostatic Hypotension	Half-Life (h)	Daily Dose (mg)
Amitriptyline (Elavil)	++	++++	High	High	Moderate	30–40	25–300
Bupropion (Wellbutrin)	+	+	Low	Low	Low	11–14	300–450
Citalopram (Celexa)	0	+++	Low	Low	Low	35	20–40
Clomipramine (Anaframil)	+++	+++	High	Moderate	Moderate	20–80	75–300
Desipramine (Norpramin)	+++	0	Low	Low	Low	12–50	50–300
Doxepine (Sinequan)	+	++	High	Nigh	Moderate	8–24	75–400
Escitalopram	0	+++	Low	Low	Low	27–32	10–20
Fluoxetine (Prozac)	0	+++	Low	Low	Low	160–200	20–80
Imipramine (Tofranil)	++	+++	Moderate	Moderate	High	6–20	75–400
Nefazodone (Serzone)	0	+	Low	Low	Low	2–4	300–600
Nortriptyline (Pamelor)	++	+++	Moderate	Moderate	Low	15–90	40–150
Paroxeline (Paxil)	0	+++	Low	Low	Low	31	20–40
Sertraline (Zoloft)	0	+++	Low	Low	Low	26	50–200
Trazodone (Desyrel)	0	++	High	Low	Moderate	3–9	150–400
Venlafaxine (Effexor)	+	+++	Low	Low	Low	5–11	75–375

rarely, psychosis. Patients can also develop the physical features characteristic of Cushing's syndrome (see Chapter 36). Excess mineralocorticoid activity causes sodium retention and hypokalemia, and can precipitate congestive heart failure.

Systemic Local Anesthetics

Local anesthetics (see Chapter 14) are occasionally used systemically in patients with neuropathic pain. They produce sedation and central analgesia; the anal-gesia frequently outlasts the pharmacokinetic profile of the local anesthetic and breaks the "pain cycle." Lidocaine, procaine, and chloroprocaine are the most commonly used agents. They are given either as a slow bolus or by continuous infusion. Lidocaine is given by infusion over 5–30 min for a total of 1–5 mg/kg. Procaine 200–400 mg can be given intravenously over the course of 1–2 h, whereas chloroprocaine (1% solution) is infused at a rate of 1 mg/kg/min for a total of 10–20 mg/kg. Monitoring should include the electrocardiogram (ECG), blood pressure, respirations, and

Table 18–10. Anticonvulsants possibly useful in pain management.

Anticonvulsant	Half-Life (h)	Daily Dose (mg)	Therapeutic Level[1] (μg/mL)
Carbamazepine (Tegratol)	10–20	200–1200	4–12
Clonazepam (Clonopin)	18–30	1–18	0.01–0.08
Gabapentin (Neurontin)	5–7	900–1800	> 2
Lamotrigine (Lamictal)	24	25–400	2–20
Phenytoin (Dilantin)	22	200–600	10–20
Topiramate (Topamax)	20–30	25–200	Unknown
Valproic acid (Depakene)	6–16	750–1250	50–100

[1]Efficacy in pain management may not correlate with blood level.

mental status; full resuscitation equipment should also be immediately available. Signs of toxicity such as tinnitus, slurring, excessive sedation, or nystagmus necessitate slowing or discontinuing the infusion.

Patients who do not respond to anticonvulsants but respond to intravenous local anesthetics may benefit from chronic oral antiarrhythmic therapy. Mexiletine (150–300 mg every 6–8 h) is the most commonly used agent and is generally well tolerated.

α₂-Adrenergic Agonists

The primary effect of α_2-adrenergic agonists is activation of descending inhibitory pathways in the dorsal horn. Epidural and intrathecal α_2-adrenergic agonists are particularly effective in neuropathic pain and opioid tolerance. Clonidine and other α_2-adrenergic agonists are reviewed in Chapter 15.

Botulinum Toxin

Botulinum toxin injections have been increasingly utilized in the treatment of painful conditions associated with skeletal muscle. Studies support the use of botulinum toxin in the treatment of conditions associated with involuntary muscle contraction (eg, focal dystonia and spasticity). Some clinicians have used the drug in the management of headaches and myofascial syndromes. Botulinum toxin blocks acetylcholine released at the synapse in motor nerve endings but not sensory nerve fibers. Proposed mechanisms of analgesia include improved local blood flow, relief of muscle spasms, and release of muscular compression of nerve fibers.

■ THERAPEUTIC ADJUNCTS

PSYCHOLOGICAL INTERVENTIONS

These techniques are most effective when employed by psychologists or psychiatrists. They include cognitive

Table 18–11. Selected corticosteroids.[1]

Drug	Routes Given[2]	Glucocorticoid Activity	Mineralocorticoid Activity	Equivalent Dose (mg)	Half-Life (h)
Hydrocortisone	O, I, T	1	1	20	8–12
Prednisone	O	4	0.8	5	12–36
Prednisolone	O, I	4	0.8	5	12–36
Methylprednisolone (Depo-Medrol, Solu-Medrol)	O, I, T	5	0.5	4	12–36
Triamcinolone (Aristocort)	O, I, T	5	0	4	12–36
Betamethasone (Celestone)	O, I, T	25	0	0.75	36–72
Dexamethasone (Decadron)	O, I, T	25	0	0.75	36–72

[1]Adapted from Goodman LS, Gilman AG: *The Pharmacologic Basis of Therapeutics*, 8th ed. Pergamon, 1990.
[2]O, oral; I, injectable; T, topical.

therapy, behavioral therapy, biofeedback and relaxation techniques, and hypnosis. Cognitive interventions are based on the assumption that a patient's attitude toward pain can influence the perception of pain. Maladaptive attitudes contribute to suffering and disability. The patient is taught skills for coping with the pain either individually or in group therapy. The most common techniques include attention diversion and imagery. Behavioral (operant) therapy is based on the premise that behavior in patients with chronic pain is determined by consequences of the behavior. Positive reinforcers (such as attention from a spouse) tend to aggravate the pain, whereas negative reinforcers reduce pain behavior. The therapist identifies "unhealthy" pain behavior and tries to manipulate reinforcers; this type of intervention requires the cooperation of family members and medical providers.

Relaxation techniques teach the patient to alter the arousal response and the increase in sympathetic tone associated with pain. The most commonly employed technique is a progressive muscle relaxation exercise. Biofeedback and hypnosis are closely related interventions. All forms of biofeedback are based on the principle that patients can be taught to control involuntary physiological parameters. Once proficient in the technique, the patient may be able to control physiological factors (eg, muscle tension) that aggravate pain, can induce a relaxation response, and can more effectively apply coping skills. The most commonly used physiological parameters are muscle tension (electromyographic biofeedback) and temperature (thermal biofeedback). The effectiveness of hypnosis varies considerably among individuals. Hypnotic techniques teach patients to alter pain perception by having them focus on other sensations, localize the pain to another site, and dissociate themselves from a painful experience through imagery. Patients with chronic headaches and musculoskeletal disorders appear to benefit most from these relaxation techniques.

PHYSICAL THERAPY

Heat and cold can provide pain relief by alleviating muscle spasm. In addition, heat decreases joint stiffness and increases blood flow and cold vasoconstricts and can reduce tissue edema. The analgesic action of heat and cold may also be at least partially explained by the gate theory of pain processing (above).

Superficial heating modalities include conductive (hot packs, paraffin baths, fluidotherapy), convective (hydrotherapy), and radiant (infrared) techniques. Techniques for application of deep heat include ultrasound as well as shortwave and microwave diathermy; these modalities are more effective for pain involving deep joints and muscles. Cold is most effective for pain

associated with acute injuries and edema. When applied selectively, cold can also relieve muscle spasm. Application may take the form of cold packs, ice massage, or vapocoolant sprays (ethyl chloride or fluoromethane).

Exercise should be part of any rehabilitation program for chronic pain. A graded exercise program prevents joint stiffness, muscle atrophy, and contractures, all of which can contribute to the patient's pain and functional disabilities.

ACUPUNCTURE

Acupuncture can be a useful adjunct for some patients with chronic pain, particularly pain associated with chronic musculoskeletal disorders and headaches. The technique involves insertion of needles into discrete anatomically defined points, called meridians. Stimulation of the needle after insertion takes the form of twirling or application of a mild electrical current. Insertion points appear to be unrelated to the conventional anatomy of the nervous system. Although the scientific literature concerning acupuncture's mechanism of action and role in pain management is conflicting, some studies suggest that acupuncture stimulates the release of endogenous opioids, because its effects can be antagonized by naloxone.

ELECTRICAL STIMULATION

Electrical stimulation of the nervous system can produce analgesia in patients with acute and chronic pain. Current may be applied transcutaneously, epidurally, or by electrodes implanted into the central nervous system.

Transcutaneous Stimulation

Transcutaneous electrical nerve stimulation (TENS) is thought to produce analgesia by stimulating large afferent fibers. It may have a role for patients with mild to moderate acute pain and those with chronic low back pain, arthritis, and neuropathic pain. The gate theory of pain processing suggests that the afferent input from large epicritic fibers competes with that from the smaller pain fibers. An alternative theory proposes that at high rates of stimulation, TENS causes conduction block in small afferent pain fibers. With conventional TENS, electrodes are applied to the same dermatome as the pain and are stimulated periodically by direct current from a generator (usually for 30 min several times a day). A current of 10–30 mA with a pulse width of 50–80 μs is applied at a frequency of 80–100 Hz. Some patients refractory to conventional TENS respond to low-frequency TENS (acupuncture-like TENS), which employs stimuli with a pulse width > 200 μs at frequencies < 10 Hz (for 5–15 min). Unlike conventional TENS, low-frequency stimulation is at least partly reversed by naloxone, suggesting a role for endogenous opioids.

Spinal Cord Stimulation (SCS)

This technique is also called dorsal column stimulation because it was thought to produce analgesia by directly stimulating large Aβ fibers in the dorsal columns of the spinal cord. **Proposed mechanisms include activation of descending modulating systems and inhibition of sympathetic outflow.** Spinal cord stimulation is most effective for neuropathic pain. Accepted indications include sympathetically mediated pain, spinal cord lesions with localized segmental pain, phantom limb pain, ischemic lower extremity pain due to peripheral vascular disease, and adhesive arachnoiditis. Patients with failed back surgery syndrome (FBSS), which is typically a mixed nociceptive–neuropathic disorder, also appear to benefit from SCS.

Temporary electrodes are initially placed epidurally and connected to an external generator to evaluate efficacy in a given patient for a 5- to 7-day trial. If a favorable response is obtained, a fully implantable system is placed; the permanent epidural electrodes are usually placed percutaneously, tunneled, and connected to a subcutaneous generator. Unfortunately, the efficacy of the technique decreases with time in some patients. Complications include infection, lead migration, and lead breakage.

Intracerebral Stimulation

Deep brain stimulation may be used for intractable cancer pain, and rarely for intractable neuropathic pain of nonmalignant origin. Electrodes are implanted stereotactically into the periaqueductal and periventricular gray areas for nociceptive pain (primarily cancer and chronic low back pain); for neuropathic pain, the electrodes are implanted into specific sensory thalamic nuclei. The most serious complications are intracranial hemorrhage and infection.

■ POSTOPERATIVE PAIN

The concept of "preemptive" analgesia (above) suggests that the best postoperative pain management begins preoperatively. Some studies suggest that anesthetic techniques can also reduce the neuroendocrine stress response to surgery and pain. Regional anesthetic techniques in which a catheter can be left in place also provide an excellent means for postoperative analgesia. Intercostal and epidural anesthesia can additionally improve respiratory function following thoracic and upper abdominal operations and encourage early ambulation. Epidural and possibly spinal anesthesia reduce the incidence of thromboembolism following hip surgery and attenuate the hypercoagulation state following vascular procedures.

Postoperative pain control is generally best managed by anesthesiologists, because they offer regional anesthetic techniques as well as pharmacological expertise in analgesics. Concerns over increased cost may be unjustified because some studies have demonstrated lower mortality and morbidity, as well as reduced hospital costs, with these techniques.

Postoperative analgesic modalities include oral or parenteral analgesics, peripheral nerve blocks, neuraxial blocks with local anesthetics, intraspinal opioids, as well as adjunctive techniques such as TENS and physical therapy. Selection of analgesic techniques is generally based on three factors: the patient, the procedure, and the setting (inpatient versus outpatient).

OUTPATIENTS

1. Oral Analgesics

Most patients who have mild to moderate pain following surgery can be managed with oral COX inhibitors, opioids, or a combination. Patients unable to resume an oral intake or with severe pain require inpatient admission regardless of the procedure.

Cyclooxygenase Inhibitors

Oral nonopioid analgesics include salicylates, acetaminophen, and NSAIDs (Table 18–12). These agents inhibit prostaglandin synthesis (COX) and have varying analgesic, antipyretic, and antiinflammatory properties. Acetaminophen lacks significant antiinflammatory activity. Analgesia is due to blockade of prostaglandin synthesis, which sensitizes and amplifies nociceptive input (above). Some types of pain, particularly pain that follows orthopedic and gynecological surgery, respond very well to these agents, suggesting an important role for prostaglandins. COX inhibitors likely have important peripheral and central nervous system actions. Their analgesic action is limited by side effects and toxicity at higher doses. At least two types of COX are recognized. COX-1 is constitutive and widespread throughout the body, but COX-2 is expressed primarily with inflammation. Selective COX-2 inhibitors, such as celecoxib, appear to have lower toxicity, particularly gastrointestinal side effects. Moreover, COX-2 inhibitors do not interfere with platelet aggregation. Unfortunately, some COX-2 inhibitors (rofecoxib and possibly others) appear to increase the risk of cardiovascular complications.

Table 18–12. Selected oral nonopioid analgesics.

Analgesic	Half-Life (h)	Onset (h)	Dose (mg)	Dosing Interval (h)	Maximum Daily Dosage (mg)
Salicylates					
Acetylsalicylic acid (aspirin)	2–3	0.5–1.0	500–1000	4	3600–6000
Diflunisal (Dolobid)	8–12	1–2	500–1000	8–12	1500
Choline magnesium trisalicylate (Trilisate)	8–12	1–2	500–1000	12	2000–3000
***p*-Aminophenols**					
Acetaminophen (Tylenol, others)	1–4	0.5	500–1000	4	1200–4000
Proprionic acids					
Ibuprofen (Motrin, others)	1.8–2.5	0.5	400	4–6	3200
Naproxen (Naprosyn)	12–15	1	250–500	12	1500
Naproxen sodium (Anaprox)	13	1–2	275–550	6–8	1375
Indoles					
Indomethacin (Indocin)	4	0.5	25–50	8–12	150–200
Ketorolac (Toradol)	4–6	0.5–1	10	4–6	40
COX-2 Inhibitors					
Celecoxib (Celebrex)	11	3	100–200	12	400

All these agents are well absorbed enterally. Food delays absorption but has no effect on bioavailability. Because most are highly protein bound (> 80%), these agents can displace other highly bound drugs such as warfarin. All undergo hepatic metabolism and are renally excreted. Dosages should therefore be reduced in patients with hepatic or renal impairment.

Acetaminophen has the fewest side effects but is a hepatotoxin at very high doses. Isoniazid, zidovudine, and barbiturates can potentiate acetaminophen toxicity. Aspirin and NSAIDs most commonly produce stomach upset, heartburn, nausea, and dyspepsia; some patients develop ulceration of the gastric mucosa, which appears to be due to inhibition of prostaglandin-mediated mucus and bicarbonate secretion. Other side effects include dizziness, headache, and drowsiness. With the exception of acetaminophen and COX-2 inhibitors, all other COX inhibitors induce platelet dysfunction. Aspirin irreversibly acetylates platelets, inhibiting platelet adhesiveness for 1–2 weeks, whereas the antiplatelet effect of NSAIDs is reversible and lasts about five elimination half-lives (24–96 h). This antiplatelet effect does not appear to appreciably increase the incidence of postoperative hemorrhage following most outpatient procedures. ASA and NSAIDs can exacerbate bronchospasm in patients with the triad of nasal polyps, rhinitis, and asthma. ASA should not be used in children with varicella or influenza infections because it may precipitate Reye's syndrome. Lastly, NSAIDs can cause acute renal insufficiency and renal papillary necrosis, particularly in patients with underlying renal dysfunction (see Chapter 31).

Opioids

Moderate postoperative pain should be treated with oral opioids either on an as-needed (PRN) basis or on a fixed schedule (Table 18–13). They are commonly combined with oral COX inhibitors; combination therapy enhances analgesia and decreases side effects. The most commonly used agents are codeine, oxycodone, and hydrocodone. These agents are well absorbed, but hepatic first-pass metabolism limits systemic delivery. Like other opioids (see Chapter 8), they undergo hepatic biotransformation and conjugation before renal elimination. Codeine is transformed by the liver into morphine. The side effects of orally administered opioids are similar to those of systemic opioids (see Chapter 8); when prescribed on a fixed schedule, stool softeners or laxatives may be indicated. Tramadol is a synthetic oral opioid that also blocks neuronal reuptake of norepinephrine and serotonin. It appears to have the same efficacy as the combination of codeine and acetaminophen but, unlike others, it is associated with significantly less respiratory depression and has little effect on gastric emptying.

Table 18–13. Oral opioids.

Opioid	Half-Life (h)	Onset (h)	Duration (h)	Relative Potency	Initial Dose (mg)	Dosing Interval (h)
Codeine	3	0.25–1.0	3–4	20	30–60	4
Hydromorphone (Dilaudid)	2–3	0.3–0.5	2–3	0.6	2–4	4
Hydrocodone[1] (Oxycontin)	1–3	0.5–1.0	3–6	3	5–7.5	4–6
Oxycodone[2]	2–3	0.5	3–6	3	5–10	6
Levorphanol (Levo-Dromoran)	12–16	1–2	6–8	0.4	4	6–8
Methadone (Dolophine)	15–30	0.5–1.0	4–6	1	20	6–8
Propoxyphene (Darvon)[3]	6–12	1–2	3–6	30	100	6
Tramadol (Ultram)	6–7	1–2	3–6	30	50	4–6
Morphine solution[4] (Roxanol)	2–4	0.5–1	4	1	10	3–4
Morphine controlled-release[4] (MS Contin)	2–4	1	8–12	1	15	8–12

[1]Preparations also contain acetaminophen (Vicodin, others).
[2]Preparations may contain acetaminphen (Percocet) or aspirin (Percodan).
[3]Some preparations contain acetaminophen (Darvocet).
[4]Used primarily for cancer pain.

2. Infiltration of Local Anesthetic

Direct infiltration of an incision or a field block with local anesthetic is an easy and safe method of achieving good postoperative pain relief. Ilioinguinal and femoral nerve blocks can be used for hernia repairs and scrotal procedures, and a penile block can be utilized with circumcision (see Chapter 17). A local-acting anesthetic such as bupivacaine should be used (see Chapter 14). The analgesia often outlasts the pharmacokinetic duration of the local anesthetic. It is preferable to administer the local anesthetic prior to the surgery to produce a preemptive analgesic effect (above).

Intraarticular injections of local anesthetics, opioids, or a combination thereof appear to be effective for many patients following arthroscopic procedures.

INPATIENTS

Most inpatients with moderate to severe postoperative pain require parenteral analgesics or neural blockade with local anesthetics during the first 1–6 days following surgery. Once the patient is able to resume an oral intake and pain intensity decreases, oral analgesics are initiated. Parenteral analgesics include NSAIDs (ketorolac), opioids, and ketamine (see Chapter 8). Ketorolac may be given intramuscularly or intravenously, whereas opioids can be given subcutaneously, intramuscularly, intravenously, or intraspinally. Transdermal opioid preparations are not recommended for postoperative pain because of an increased risk of respiratory depression.

1. Opioids

Opioid analgesia is achieved at a specific blood level for each patient for a given pain intensity. Patients with severe pain typically continue to report pain until the analgesic blood level reaches a certain concentration above which the patient experiences analgesia and the severity of pain rapidly diminishes. That point is referred to as the minimum effective analgesic concentration (MEAC). Small increases above this point produce a large increase in analgesia.

Subcutaneous & Intramuscular Injections

These two routes are least desirable because they are painful and produce unpredictable blood levels due to erratic absorption. Patient dissatisfaction is common because of delays in drug administration and incorrect dosing. Cycles of sedation, analgesia, and inadequate analgesia are common.

Intravenous Administration

Intravenous administration solves problems with unpredictable absorption but not necessarily those of correct dosing. An optimal balance between adequate analgesia, sedation, and respiratory depression can be achieved by frequent, intermittent, small doses of opioid (eg, morphine 1–2 mg). Regardless of the drug selected, because of drug redistribution (see Chapter 8), a short duration of action is observed until several doses have been given; adequate blood levels can then be maintained by a continuous infusion. Unfortunately, this technique is very labor intensive and requires close monitoring for respiratory depression. It must therefore be restricted to postanesthesia recovery, intensive care, and specialized oncology units.

Patient-Controlled Analgesia

Advances in computer technology have allowed the development of patient-controlled analgesia (PCA). By pushing a button, patients are able to self-administer precise doses of opioids intravenously (or intraspinally) on a PRN basis. The physician programs the infusion pump to deliver a specific dose, the minimum interval between doses (lockout period), and the maximum amount of opioid that can be administered in a given period (usually 1 or 4 h); a basal infusion can also be simultaneously delivered (Table 18–14). When PCA is first initiated, a loading dose of the opioid must be given by the medical staff in attendance, or, depending on the settings, the patient may be able to load himself or herself in the first hour. When an intravenous morphine PCA is used following major surgery, most adult patients require 2–3 mg/h in the first 24–48 h and 1–2 mg/h in the following 36–72 h.

 Studies show that PCA is a cost-effective technique that produces superior analgesia with very high patient satisfaction. Moreover, total drug consumption is less, compared with intramuscular injections. Patients additionally like the control that is given to them; they are able to adjust the analgesia according to their pain severity, which varies with activity and the time of day. PCA therefore requires the understanding and cooperation of the patient; this limits its use in very young or confused patients.

In addition to computerized drug-delivery safeguards, the inherent safety of PCA is based on the principle that if the patient becomes too sleepy, he or she will not be able to push the button that delivers the opioid. Others (such as family members or nurses) should therefore not push the button for the patient. The routine use of a basal ("background") infusion is controversial. Clinicians who advocate a basal infusion suggest it prevents the analgesic level from appreciably decreasing when patients sleep; presumably, patients are then less likely to awaken in severe pain. Other clinicians argue that because of highly variable pharmacokinetics among patients and the sometimes rapid decrease in analgesic requirements observed in postoperative patients, basal infusions are more likely to produce respiratory depression. Indeed factors associated with excessively respiratory depressions requiring administration of naloxone during PCA include a basal infusion, advanced age, and hypovolemia. Patients who benefit most from a continuous basal infusion are those requiring large amounts of opioid. Of the 24-h consumption, 30–50% can be given as a basal infusion. Thus, a patient who is consuming 60 mg of morphine per day can safely be given a basal infusion of 1–1.5 mg/h.

The most common side effects of opioids are nausea, vomiting, itching, and ileus (see Chapter 8). Nearly all opioid overdoses associated with PCA have been due to incorrect programming of parameters. Siphoning of a large amount of opioid into the patient's intravenous infusion (due to a crack in the delivery system) is a rare but potentially serious problem with older systems; in later systems, changes in mounting design and antisiphoning valves have mostly eliminated this problem. Mechanical malfunction of the PCA device has been reported, but appears to be very rare.

2. Peripheral Nerve Blocks

Intercostal, interpleural, brachial plexus, and femoral nerve blocks (see Chapter 17) can provide excellent postoperative analgesia. Catheter techniques allow intermittent or continuous infusions of local anesthetic (bupivacaine 0.125% or ropivacaine 0.125%), which can provide analgesia for 3–5 days postoperatively.

3. Central Neuraxial Blockade & Intraspinal Opioids

 The administration of local anesthetic–opioid mixtures neuraxially (particularly epidurally) is

Table 18–14. General guidelines for patient-controlled analgesia (PCA) orders for the average adult.

Opioid	Bolus Dose	Lockout (min)	Infusion Rate[1]
Morphine	1–3 mg	10–20	0–1 mg/h
Meperidine (Demerol)	10–15 mg	5–15	0–20 mg/h
Fentanyl (Sublimaze)	15–25 μg	10–20	0–50 μg/h
Hydromorphone (Dilaudid)	0.1–0.3 mg	10–20	0–0.5 mg/h

[1]The authors do not recommend continuous infusion for most patients.

Table 18–15. Epidural opioids.

Opioid	Relative Lipid Solubility	Dose	Onset (min)	Peak (min)	Duration (h)	Infusion Rate	PCA[1] Dose	PCA Lockout (min)
Morphine	1	2–5 mg	15–30	60–90	4–24	0.3–0.9 mg/h	0.2–0.3 mg	30
Fentanyl	600	50–100 μg	5–10	10–20	1–3	25–50 μg/h	20–30 μg	15
Hydromorphone	1.5	0.75–1.5 mg	10–15	20–30	6–18	0.1–0.2 mg/h	0.15 μg	30

[1]PCA, patient-controlled analgesia.

an excellent technique for managing postoperative pain following abdominal, pelvic, thoracic, or orthopedic procedures on the lower extremities. Patients often have better preservation of pulmonary function, are able to ambulate early, and benefit from early physical therapy. Moreover, patients may be at lower risk for postoperative venous thrombosis.

Single-shot neuraxial injections (subarachnoid or epidural) of local anesthetic, opioid, or a combination thereof may be useful in providing preemptive analgesia and analgesia on the day of surgery. These techniques, however, are most effective when a catheter is left in place for intermittent or continuous infusions. Epidural catheters are most commonly used because of reports of cauda equina syndrome with subarachnoid catheters (see Chapter 16).

Local Anesthetics

Local anesthetic solutions alone can provide excellent analgesia but produce sympathetic and motor blockade. The former can cause hypotension and the latter limits ambulation. Dilute local anesthetic solutions can provide excellent analgesia with little motor blockade (see Chapter 14). The most commonly used agents are bupivacaine and ropivacaine 0.125–0.25%. The infusion rate must be individualized for each patient, but generally depends on the level of the catheter tip relative to the dermatomes of the incision. With an optimally placed catheter, infusion rates of 5–10 mL/h generally produce satisfactory analgesia.

Opioids

The spinal analgesic action of opioids was discussed above (see also Table 18–15). Intrathecal morphine 0.2–0.4 mg can provide excellent analgesia for 4–24 h. Epidural morphine 3–5 mg is similarly effective and is more commonly employed. An extended-release liposomal formulation of morphine (DepoDur) can provide analgesia for up to 48 h. It has been approved only for lum-

bar epidural administration following hip arthroplasty (15 mg), lower abdominal surgery (10–15 mg), and cesarean section (10 mg). Whether given epidurally or intrathecally, opiate penetration into the spinal cord is both time and concentration dependent. Epidurally administered hydrophilic agents (such as morphine) produce analgesia at much lower blood levels than lipophilic agents (such as fentanyl). The latter may produce segmental effects and thus should generally be used only when the catheter tip is close to the incisional dermatome. Systemic blood levels of fentanyl during epidural infusion are nearly equivalent to those during intravenous administration. The efficacy of epidurally administered alfentanil and possibly sufentanil appears to be almost entirely due to systemic absorption.

Hydrophilic agents spread rostrally with time; thus, low lumbar morphine injections can provide good (although delayed) analgesia for thoracic and upper abdominal procedures. Important factors that influence dose requirements include the location of the catheter tip relative to the incision and the age of the patient. The closer the catheter tip is to the incision dermatome, the less opiate is required. Older patients generally require less opiate. When epidural morphine is used as the sole analgesic by continuous infusion (0.1 mg/mL), a 3–5 mg bolus is given initially followed by a 0.1–0.7 mg/h infusion. An intermittent bolus technique can be used, but continuous infusions may decrease side effects such as urinary retention and itching.

Fentanyl is the most commonly used lipophilic agent and is administered as a 3–10 μg/mL solution at 5–10 mL/h.

Local Anesthetic & Opioid Mixtures

Although intraspinal opioids alone can produce excellent analgesia, many patients experience significant dose-dependent side effects, particularly with lipid-soluble opioids. When dilute local anesthetic solutions are combined with opioids, significant synergy is observed. Bupivacaine 0.0625–0.125% (or ropivacaine 0.1–0.2%)

combined with morphine 0.1 mg/mL (or fentanyl 5 μg/mL) provides excellent analgesia with lower drug requirements and fewer side effects. Addition of even small doses of epinephrine (2 μg/mL) enhances and prolongs epidural analgesia and may reduce systemic absorption of lipophilic opioids (eg, fentanyl). Addition of small doses of clonidine similarly enhances and prolongs analgesia but also significantly increases the incidence of hypotension and bradycardia.

Contraindications

Contraindications include patient refusal, coagulopathy, or platelet abnormalities, and the presence of infection or tumor at the site of puncture (see Chapter 16). The presence of a systemic infection is only a relative contraindication unless bacteremia is documented. Placement of intraspinal catheters in patients to undergo heparinization intraoperatively is controversial because of the possibility of epidural hematoma. Available evidence suggests that the risk is very small when the catheter is placed atraumatically prior to heparinization and removed only after coagulation normalizes.

Side Effects of Intraspinal Opioids

The most serious side effect of epidural or intrathecal opioids is dose-dependent, delayed respiratory depression. Diffusion of the opiate into the cerebrospinal fluid and migration to the medullary respiratory center are thought to be responsible. Depression of the CO_2 response curve is typical (see Chapter 22); $PaCO_2$ values in the high 40s or low 50s are not unusual even in fully awake and alert patients. The incidence of respiratory depression is higher following intrathecal than after epidural administration. Early respiratory depression (within 1–2 h) can also be observed with epidural opioids and is thought to be due to systemic uptake of opioids via spinal blood vessels. The incidence of serious respiratory depression requiring naloxone is low (0.1%) with epidural opioids.

Most cases of serious respiratory depression occur in patients receiving concomitant parenteral opioids or sedatives. Elderly patients and those with sleep apnea appear to be particularly vulnerable and require reduced dosing. All patients require special monitoring, which is generally provided in intensive care or specially designated nursing units. Controversy exists concerning optimal monitoring. Pulse oximeters and apnea monitors may be used but are not adequate substitutes for close nursing observation. Changes in pulse oximetry readings may be late signs and apnea monitors produce high false-positive alarms. Excessive sedation appears to be a good clinical indicator of respiratory depression. Decreases in respiratory rate may also be helpful but not entirely reliable because airway obstruction can be

as lethal as apnea. Protocols should be established to allow the nursing staff to decrease or stop the opiate infusion, or even administer naloxone for severe respiratory depression. The amount of naloxone given should be based on the urgency of the clinical situation. Marked respiratory depression should be treated with large doses of naloxone (0.4 mg). A continuous naloxone infusion may be necessary because the half-life of naloxone is generally shorter than that of most opioids (see Chapter 8). Small doses of naloxone (0.04 mg increments) may reverse the respiratory depression but not the analgesia. Intravenous doxapram, 0.75–1 mg/kg followed by 1–2 mg/min, can also be used as a temporizing measure. The latter can reverse the respiratory depression without affecting analgesia.

Common side effects are itching, nausea, urinary retention, sedation, and ileus. Hydromorphone appears less likely than morphine to cause pruritus and nausea. The incidence of pruritus is up to 30%, whereas that of urinary retention is reported to be 40–100%. The same side effects are observed with parenteral opioids (see Chapter 8). The mechanism of the pruritus is poorly understood but is not related to histamine release. Small doses of naloxone (0.04 mg) have been reported to reverse pruritus without reversing the analgesia. Antihistamines such as diphenhydramine or hydroxyzine can also be used for itching but cause sedation. Nausea and vomiting may be treated with metoclopramide (5–10 mg), transdermal scopolamine, droperidol (0.625–1.25 mg), or ondansetron (4–6 mg). Urinary retention is generally not a problem, because many if not most patients have an indwelling urinary catheter for the first few days postoperatively.

Other Agents

Epidural butorphanol can also provide good analgesia (2–3 h duration) with little pruritus, but excessive sedation may be a side effect. Epidural clonidine has been shown to be an effective analgesic, but it can be associated with hypotension and bradycardia. Newer, more selective α₂-adrenergic agonists, such as dexmedetomidine, may prove to have fewer side effects.

■ CANCER PAIN

Approximately 19 million people worldwide experience cancer pain every year. Of these, 40–80% suffer from moderate to severe pain. Their pain may be due to the cancerous lesion itself, metastatic disease, complications such as neural compression or infections, treatment, or totally unrelated factors. The pain manager must therefore have a good understanding of the nature of the cancer, its stage, the presence of metastatic disease, and treatments.

Cancer pain can be managed with oral analgesics in most patients. The World Health Organization recommends a three-step approach: (1) nonopioid analgesics such as aspirin, acetaminophen, or NSAID for mild pain, (2) "weak" oral opioids (codeine and oxycodone) for moderate pain, and (3) stronger opioids (morphine and hydromorphone) for severe pain (Table 18–13). Parenteral therapy is necessary for refractory pain and when the patient cannot take medication orally or has poor enteral absorption. Regardless of the agent selected, in most instances drug therapy should be on a fixed time schedule rather than PRN. COX inhibitors and the less potent oral opioids are discussed above. Adjuvant drug therapy, particularly antidepressants, and other modalities should also be used liberally in cancer patients.

ORAL OPIOID THERAPY

Moderate to severe cancer pain is usually treated with an immediate-release morphine preparation (eg, liquid morphine, Roxanol, 10–30 mg every 1–4 h). These preparations have an effective half-life of 2–4 h. Once the patient's daily requirements are determined, the same dose can be given in the form of a sustained-release morphine preparation (MS Contin or Oramorph SR), which is dosed every 8–12 h. The immediate-release preparation is then used only for breakthrough pain (PRN). Oral transmucosal fentanyl lozenges (Actif, 200–1600 µg) can also be used for breakthrough pain. Excessive sedation can be treated with dextroamphetamine or methylphenidate 5 mg in the morning and the early afternoon. Most patients require a stool softener such as docusate sodium, senna, cascara, magnesium citrate, milk of magnesia, or lactulose. Nausea may be treated with transdermal scopolamine, oral meclizine, or metoclopramide.

Hydromorphone (Dilaudid) is an excellent alternative to morphine, particularly in elderly patients and those with impaired renal function. Methadone is reported to have a half-life of 15–30 h, but clinical duration is shorter and quite variable (usually 6–8 h). Patients who experience drug tolerance require escalating doses of opioid to maintain the same analgesic effect. Psychological tolerance, characterized by behavioral changes focusing on drug craving, is rare in cancer patients. Tolerance develops at different rates among persons and results in some desirable effects such as decreased sedation, nausea, and respiratory depression. Unfortunately, though, many patients continue to suffer from constipation. Physical dependence occurs in all patients on large doses of opioids for extended periods. A withdrawal phenomenon can be precipitated by the administration of opioid antagonists. Future concomitant use of peripheral opi-

oid antagonists that do not cross the blood–brain barrier, such as methylnaltrexone and alvimopan, may help reduce troublesome systemic side effects without significantly affecting analgesia.

TRANSDERMAL OPIOIDS

Transdermal fentanyl is an excellent alternative to sustained-release morphine preparations, particularly when oral medication is not possible. The currently available patches are constructed as a drug reservoir that is separated from the skin by a microporous rate-limiting membrane and an adhesive polymer. A very large quantity of fentanyl (10 mg) provides a large force for transdermal diffusion. The major obstacle to absorption is the stratum corneum. The transdermal route avoids hepatic first-pass metabolism. Transdermal fentanyl patches are available in 25, 50, 75, and 100 µg/h sizes that provide drug for 2–3 days. The largest patch is equivalent to 60 mg/d of intravenous morphine.

The major disadvantage of this route is its slow onset and the inability to rapidly change dosage in response to changing opioid requirements. Blood fentanyl levels rise and reach a plateau in 12–18 h, providing average concentrations of 1, 1.5, and 2 ng/mL for the 50, 75, and 100 patches, respectively. Large interpatient variability results in actual delivery rates ranging from 50 to 200 µg/h. The dermis acts as a secondary reservoir such that even after the patch is removed, fentanyl absorption continues for several hours.

PARENTERAL THERAPY

Severe uncontrolled cancer pain requires conversion from oral to parenteral or intraspinal opioids. When the character of the pain changes significantly, it is important to reevaluate the patient for disease progression. In many instances adjunctive treatments such as palliative surgery, radiation, or chemotherapy are helpful. Hormonal therapy should be used whenever possible. Surgery can debulk the tumor, alleviate compression, or fixate a fracture. Neurolytic techniques should also be considered whenever appropriate.

Parenteral opioid therapy is usually best accomplished by continuous intravenous infusion but can also be given subcutaneously through a butterfly needle. Modern portable infusion devices have PCA capability (above) allowing the patient to treat him or herself for breakthrough pain.

INTRASPINAL OPIOIDS

The use of intraspinal opioids is an excellent alternative for patients obtaining poor relief with other techniques or who experience excessive side effects. Epidural and subarachnoid opioids offer pain relief with substantially lower total doses of opioid and fewer side effects. Continuous infusion techniques reduce drug requirements (compared with intermittent boluses), minimize side effects, and decrease the likelihood of catheter occlusion. Myoclonic activity may be occasionally observed with intrathecal morphine or hydromorphone.

Epidural or intrathecal catheters can be placed percutaneously or implanted to provide long-term effective pain relief. Tunneling the catheter reduces the risk of infection. Epidural catheters can be attached to light-weight external pumps that can be worn by ambulatory patients. A temporary catheter must be inserted first to assess the potential efficacy of the technique. Correct placement of the permanent catheter should be confirmed by fluoroscopy and radiocontrast. Completely implantable intrathecal catheters with externally programmable pumps can also be used for continuous infusion; their major disadvantage is cost. The reservoir of the implanted pump is periodically refilled percutaneously; an additional injection port allows injection into the catheter directly. Implantable intrathecal systems are most appropriate for patients with a life expectancy of several months, whereas tunneled epidural catheters are appropriate for patients expected to live for only weeks. Formation of an inflammatory mass at the tip of the catheter can occur and may reduce efficacy.

The major problem with intraspinal opioids is tolerance. Generally a slow phenomenon, tolerance does develop rapidly in some patients. In such instances, adjuvant therapy must be used, including the intermittent use of local anesthetics or a mixture of opioids with local anesthetics (bupivacaine or ropivacaine 2–24 mg/d), intrathecal or epidural clonidine (2–4 μg/kg/h or 48–800 μg/d, respectively), or the GABA agonist baclofen intrathecally. Clonidine is particularly useful for neuropathic pain. In high doses, it is more likely to be associated with hypotension and bradycardia.

Complications include local skin infections and epidural abscess. Superficial infections can be reduced by the use of a silver-impregnated cuff close to the exit site. Other complications include hematoma, which may be immediate or delayed onset (days). The use of invasive spinal techniques can be complicated by increased intracranial pressure (from mass lesions) and coagulopathy. The risk–benefit ratio must be weighed carefully in terminal patients.

NEUROLYTIC TECHNIQUES

Neurolytic celiac plexus block is very effective for intraabdominal malignant growths, particularly in pancreatic cancer. Lumbar sympathetic, hypogastric plexus, or ganglion impar neurolytic blocks can also be used for malignant tumors of the pelvis. Neurolytic intercostal blocks can be helpful for patients with rib metastases. In patients with refractory pelvic pain, a neurolytic saddle block can provide pain relief; however, bowel and bladder dysfunction should be expected. Because of the significant morbidity associated with neurolytic blocks (loss of motor and somatic sensory function) these techniques should be utilized only after careful consideration of alternatives. Neurodestructive procedures, such as pituitary adenolysis and cordotomy, can be useful in terminal patients. Some centers additionally offer deep-brain stimulation.

■ SELECTED PAIN SYNDROMES

ENTRAPMENT SYNDROMES

Entrapment neuropathies are commonly overlooked entities that involve sensory, motor, or mixed nerves. Neural compression can occur wherever a nerve courses through an anatomically narrowed passage. Genetic factors and repetitive macrotrauma or microtrauma are likely involved; adjacent tenosynovitis is often responsible. Table 18–16 lists the most commonly recognized entrapment syndromes. When a sensory nerve is involved, patients complain of pain and numbness in its distribution distal to the site of entrapment; occasionally, a patient may complain of pain referred proximal to the site of entrapment. Entrapment of the sciatic nerve (the piriformis syndrome) can mimic a herniated intervertebral disease. Entrapment of a motor nerve produces weakness in the muscles it innervates. Even entrapments of "pure" motor nerves can produce a vague pain that may be mediated by afferent fibers from muscles and joints. The diagnosis can usually be confirmed by electromyography and nerve conduction studies. Neural blockade of the nerve with local anesthetic, with or without corticosteroid, may be diagnostic and can provide temporary pain relief. Treatment is generally symptomatic with oral analgesics and temporary immobilization, whenever appropriate. Development of reflex sympathetic dystrophy requires sympathetic blockade. Refractory symptoms require surgical decompression.

MYOFASCIAL PAIN

Myofascial syndromes are common disorders characterized by aching muscle pain, muscle spasm, stiffness, weakness, and, occasionally, autonomic dysfunction. Patients have discrete areas (trigger points) of marked tenderness in one or more muscles or the associated connective tissue. Palpation of the involved muscles may reveal tight, ropy bands over trigger points. Signs of autonomic dysfunction (vasoconstriction or piloerection) in the overlying muscles may be present. The pain characteristically radiates in a fixed pattern that does not follow dermatomes.

Table 18–16. Entrapment neuropathies.

Nerve	Entrapment Site	Location of Pain
Cranial nerves VII, IX, and X	Styloid process or stylohyoid ligament	Ipsilateral tonsil, base of tongue, temporomandibular joint, and ear (Eagle's syndrome)
Brachial plexus	Scalenus anticus muscle or a cervical rib	Ulnar side of arm and forearm (scalenus anticus syndrome)
Suprascapular nerve	Suprascapular notch	Posterior and lateral shoulder
Median nerve	Pronator teres muscle	Proximal forearm and palmar surface of the first three digits (pronator syndrome)
Median nerve	Carpal tunnel	Palmar surface of the first three digits (carpal tunnel syndrome)
Ulnar nerve	Cubital fossa (elbow)	Fourth and fifth digits of the hand (cubital tunnel syndrome)
Ulnar nerve	Guyon's canal (wrist)	Fourth and fifth digits of the hand
Lateral femoral cutaneous nerve	Anterior iliac spine under the inguinal ligament	Anterolateral thigh (meralgia paresthetica)
Obturator nerve	Obturator canal	Upper medial thigh
Saphenous nerve	Subsartorial tunnel (adductor canal)	Medial calf
Sciatic nerve	Sciatic notch	Buttock and leg (piriformis syndrome)
Common peroneal nerve	Fibular neck	Lateral distal leg and foot
Deep peroneal nerve	Anterior tarsal tunnel	Big toe or foot
Superficial peroneal nerve	Deep fascia above the ankle	Anterior ankle and dorsum of foot
Posterior tibial nerve	Posterior tarsal tunnel	Undersurface of foot (tarsal tunnel syndrome)
Interdigital nerve	Deep transverse tarsal ligament	Between toes and foot (Morton's neuroma)

Gross trauma or repetitive microtrauma is thought to play a major role in initiating myofascial syndromes. Trigger points develop following acute injury; stimulation of these active trigger points produces pain, and the ensuing muscle spasm sustains the pain. When the acute episode subsides, the trigger points become latent (tender, but not pain producing) only to be reactivated at a later time by subsequent stress. The pathophysiology is poorly understood, but the trigger points may represent areas of localized ischemia that develop as a result of muscle or vascular spasm.

The diagnosis of a myofascial syndrome is suggested by the character of the pain and palpation of discrete **trigger points** that reproduce it. Common syndromes produce trigger points in the levator scapulae, masseter, quadratus lumborum, and gluteus medius muscles. The latter two syndromes produce low back pain and should be considered in all patients with back pain; moreover, gluteal trigger points can mimic S1 radiculopathy.

Although myofascial pain can resolve spontaneously without sequelae, many patients continue to have latent trigger points. When trigger points are active, the treatment is directed at regaining muscle length and elasticity. Analgesia must be provided in the form of trigger point injections (1–3 mL) with a local anesthetic. Topical cooling with a vapocoolant, either an ethyl chloride or fluorocarbon (fluoromethane) spray, can also induce reflex muscle relaxation, and allows massage (stretch and spray) and ultrasound therapy. Ethyl chloride is preferable, because unlike fluorocarbons, it does not deplete the upper atmosphere's ozone layer. Physical therapy is important in maintaining a normal range of motion for affected muscles. Biofeedback may be helpful for some patients.

LOW BACK PAIN & RELATED SYNDROMES

Back pain is an extremely common complaint and a major cause of work disability worldwide. Lumbosacral strain, degenerative disk disease, and myofascial syndromes are the most common causes of low back pain. Many syndromes can also produce low back pain with or without associated leg pain. Causes can be congenital, traumatic, degenerative, inflammatory, infectious, metabolic, psychological, or cancerous. Moreover, back pain can be due to disease processes in the abdomen and pelvis, particularly those diseases affecting retroperitoneal structures (pancreas, kidneys, ureters, aorta, and tumors), the uterus and adnexa, prostate, and the rectosigmoid. Disorders of the hip can similarly mimic back disorders. A positive Patrick's sign helps identify pain due to hip disorder. This sign consists of pain in the hip while placing the ipsilateral heel on the contralateral knee and pressing the ipsilateral thigh. It is also referred to by an acronym, FABERE (sign), because the movement of the leg involves *f*lexion, *ab*duction, *e*xternal *r*otation, and *e*xtension.

1. Applied Anatomy of the Back

The back can be described as anterior or posterior. The anterior component consists of the cylindrical vertebral bodies that are interconnected by intervertebral disks and supported by anterior and posterior longitudinal ligaments. The posterior elements are bony arches that extend from each vertebral body, consisting of two pedicles, two transverse processes, two lamina, and a spinous process (see Chapter 16). The transverse and spinous processes provide points of attachment for the muscles that move and protect the spinal column. Adjacent vertebrae also articulate posteriorly by two gliding facet joints, allowing some motion.

Spinal structures are innervated by the sinuvertebral branches and posterior rami of spinal nerves. The sinuvertebral nerve arises before each spinal nerve divides into anterior and posterior rami, and reenters the intervertebral foramen to innervate the posterior longitudinal ligament, the posterior annulus fibrosus, periosteum, dura, and epidural vessels. Paraspinal structures are supplied by the posterior primary ramus. Each facet joint is innervated by the medial branch of the posterior primary rami of the spinal nerves above and below the joint.

As lumbar spinal nerve roots exit from the dural sac, they travel down 1–2 cm laterally before exiting through their respective intervertebral foramina; thus, the L5 nerve root leaves the dural sac at the level of the L4–L5 disk (where it is more likely to be compressed) but leaves the spinal canal beneath the L5 pedicle opposite the L5–S1 disk.

2. Paravertebral Muscle & Lumbosacral Joint Sprain/Strain

Approximately 80–90% of low back pain is due to sprain or strain associated with lifting heavy objects, falls, or sudden abnormal movements of the spine. The term "sprain" is generally used when the pain is related to a well-defined acute injury, whereas strain is used when the pain is more chronic and is likely related to repetitive minor injuries.

Injury to paravertebral muscles and ligaments results in reflex muscle spasm, which may or may not be associated with trigger points. The pain is usually dull and aching, and occasionally radiates down the buttocks or hips. Sprain is a self-limited benign process that resolves in 1–2 weeks. Symptomatic treatment consists of rest and oral analgesics.

The sacroiliac joint is particularly vulnerable to rotational injuries. Acute or chronic injury can cause slippage or subluxation of the joint. Pain originating from this joint is characteristically located along the posterior ilium and radiates down the hips and posterior thigh to the knees. The diagnosis is suggested by tenderness on palpation and compression of the joints. Pain relief following injection of the joint with local anesthetic (3 mL) is diagnostic and may be therapeutic. The role of intraarticular steroid injection is not well established.

3. Degenerative Disk Disease

Intervertebral disks bear at least one-third of the weight of the spinal column. Their central portion, which is called the nucleus pulposus, is composed of gelatinous material early in life. This material degenerates and becomes fibrotic with advancing age and following trauma. The nucleus pulposus is ringed by the annulus fibrosus, which is thinnest posteriorly and bounded superiorly and inferiorly by cartilaginous plates. Disk (diskogenic) pain may be due to one of two major mechanisms: (1) protrusion or extrusion of the nucleus pulposus posteriorly or (2) loss of disk height, resulting in the reactive formation of bony spurs (osteophytes) from the rims of the vertebral bodies above and below the disk. Degenerative disk disease most commonly affects the lumbar spine because it is subjected to the greatest motion and the posterior longitudinal ligament is thinnest at L2–L5.

Herniated Disk

Weakness and degeneration of the annulus fibrosus and posterior longitudinal ligament can cause herniation of the nucleus pulposus posteriorly into the spinal canal. Ninety percent of disk herniations occur at L5–S1 or L4–L5. Symptoms usually develop following flexion injuries and may be associated with (1) bulging, (2) protrusion, or (3) extrusion of the disk. Disk herniation usually occurs posterolaterally and thus often compresses adjacent nerve roots, producing pain that radiates along that dermatome (radiculopathy). The term "sciatica" is sometimes used because compression of the

Table 18–17. Lumbar disk radiculopathies.

	Disk Level		
	L3–L4 (L4 Nerve)	L4–L5 (L5 Nerve)	L5–S1 (S1 Nerve)
Pain distribution	Anterolateral thigh, antero-medial calf to the ankle	Lateral thigh, anterolateral calf, medial dorsum of foot, especially between the first and second toes	Gluteal region, posterior thigh, posterolateral calf, lateral dorsum and undersurface of the foot, particularly between fourth and fifth toes
Weakness	Quadriceps femoris	Dorsiflexion of the foot	Plantar flexion of foot
Reflex affected	Knee	None	Ankle

lower lumbar nerve roots produces pain along the sciatic nerve. When disk material is extruded through the annulus fibrosus and posterior longitudinal ligament, free fragments can become wedged in the spinal canal or the intervertebral foramina; the pain may also be due to a chemical reaction to the glycoproteins released from the degenerating disk. Less commonly a large disk bulges or large fragments extrude posterocentrally, compressing the cauda equina in the dural sac; in these instances patients can experience bilateral pain, urinary retention, or, less commonly, fecal incontinence.

The onset of disk pain is typically associated with heavy lifting. The pain is aggravated by bending, lifting, prolonged sitting, or anything that increases intra-abdominal pressure, such as sneezing, coughing, or straining. It is usually relieved by lying down. Numbness or weakness is indicative of radiculopathy (Table 18–17). Bulging of the disk through the posterior longitudinal ligament can also produce low back pain that radiates to the hips or buttocks. Straight leg-raising tests may be used to assess nerve root compression. With the patient supine and the knee fully extended, the leg on the affected side is raised and the angle at which the pain develops is noted; dorsiflexion of the ankle with the leg raised typically exacerbates the pain by further stretching the lumbosacral plexus. Pain while raising the contralateral leg is an even more reliable sign of nerve compression.

Plain radiographs of the lumbar spine are usually obtained in the anterior–posterior, lateral, and oblique views. Bone scans may be useful in older patients to exclude malignant growths. Although the most sensitive modality for detecting disk herniation is MRI, this technology does not always demonstrate bony detail as accurately as CT. Radiological findings should be carefully correlated with symptoms, because up to 30–40% of asymptomatic persons have abnormalities on CT or MRI. CT employing myelography is the most sensitive test for evaluating subtle neural compression. Discography may be considered when the pain pattern does not

match the clinical findings. The technique can provide three pieces of data: nucleogram, disk pressure measurement, and concordant pain. The nucleogram identifies the location and extent of disk disease and disruptions. Pain associated with a pressure of 15–50 psi is generally considered to be due to mechanical factors. Concordant pain is said to be present if the nucleogram injection reproduces the patient's pain.

The natural history is generally benign and the duration of pain is usually less than 2 months. Over 75% of patients treated nonsurgically, even those with radiculopathy, have complete or near complete pain relief. The goals of treatment should therefore be to alleviate the pain, rehabilitate the patient to return to work, and improve fitness. Acute back pain due to a herniated disk should be treated with complete bed rest for 3 days and with analgesics. The bed rest allows the acute injury to subside. NSAIDs are particularly useful. A short course of opioids may be indicated in patients with severe pain. After the acute symptoms subside, the patient should be sent to "back school" to improve back fitness. Physical therapy, including the application of cold or heat and massage, may also be helpful. Surgical decompression should be considered for patients with refractory pain, but a trial of epidural steroids should be considered first. For properly selected patients, laminectomy speeds recovery and reduces the incidence of recurrence.

When symptoms persist beyond 3 months, the pain may be considered chronic and therefore requires a multidisciplinary approach. Physical therapy becomes a very important component of rehabilitation. NSAIDs and antidepressants are also helpful. Back supports should be discouraged because they may weaken paraspinal muscles. When diskogenic pain persists beyond 6 months, intradiskal electrothermal therapy (IDET) may be considered for young patients (< 55 years) with a single affected disk. Other criteria include preserved disk height (> 50%), a posterior annular defect, and no spinal stenosis. The technique involves fluoroscopic, percutaneous placement of a special probe into the affected disk via a 17-gauge cannula. The probe is then twisted to the affected area and the disk material is heated. The heat causes the disk to shrink and may coagulate nerve endings (C fibers). Complications include nerve root injury (during insertion of the introducer needle), cauda equina, disk herniation, and catheter breakage.

Epidural Steroids

Epidural steroid injections are most effective for symptomatic relief of pain associated with nerve root compression (radiculopathy). Pathological studies often demonstrate inflammation following disk herniation. Clinical improvement appears to be correlated with the resolution of nerve root edema. Epidural steroid injections are clearly superior to local anesthetics alone. These injections are most effective when given within 2 weeks of the onset of pain but appear to be of little benefit in the absence of neural compression or irritation. Long-term studies have failed to show any persistent benefit after 3 months.

The two most commonly used agents are methylprednisolone acetate (40–80 mg) and triamcinolone diacetate (40–80 mg). The steroid may be injected with diluent (saline) or local anesthetic in volumes of 6–10 mL or 10–20 mL for lumbar and caudal injections, respectively. Simultaneous injection of opioids offers no added benefit. The epidural needle should be cleared of the steroid prior to its withdrawal to prevent formation of a fistula tract. Injection of local anesthetic along with the steroid can be helpful if the patient has significant muscle spasm, but it is associated with the risks of intrathecal, subdural, and intravascular complications (see Chapter 16). The local anesthetic provides immediate pain relief until the steroid's antiinflammatory effects take place, usually within 12–48 h. The pain is often transiently intensified following injection. Epidural steroid injections may be most effective when the injection is at the site of injury. Only a single injection is given if complete pain relief is achieved. If there is no initial response, a second injection may be given 2–4 weeks later. Larger or more frequent doses increase the risk of adrenal suppression and systemic side effects. Many pain practioners utilize fluoroscopy for epidural injection and confirm correct placement with radiocontrast (epidurogram). A transforaminal epidural steroid injection (selective nerve root block) is reported to be more effective than the standard translaminar epidural technique (Chapter 16). The needle is directed under fluoroscopic guidance into the foramen of the affected nerve root and contrast is injected to confirm entry into the epidural space prior to steroid injection.

Caudal injection may be preferable in patients with previous back surgery, because scarring and anatomic distortion often make lumbar epidural injections more difficult; unfortunately, the migration of the steroid to the site of injury may not be optimal. Subarachnoid steroid injections are not recommended because of the ethylene glycol preservative; this has been implicated in adhesive arachnoiditis following unintentional subarachnoid injections. Other reported complications include aseptic, cryptococcal, and tuberculous meningitis.

Spinal Stenosis

Degeneration of the nucleus pulposus reduces disk height and leads to osteophyte formation (spondylosis) at the rims of adjoining vertebral bodies and infolding of the spinal ligaments, leading to progressive narrowing of the intervertebral foramina and spinal canal. Neural compression can cause radiculopathy that mimics a herniated disk. Extensive osteophyte formation may compress multiple nerve roots and cause bilateral pain. When these growths encroach on the cauda equina, the term "spinal stenosis" is used.

Spinal stenosis is a disease of advancing age. The back pain usually radiates into both buttocks, thighs, and legs. It is characteristically worse with exercise and relieved by rest, particularly sitting with the spine flexed. The term "pseudoclaudication" is occasionally used. The diagnosis is suggested by the clinical presentation and is confirmed by MRI, CT, or both of the spine, with myelography. Electromyography and somatosensory evoked potentials can be useful in evaluating neurological compromise.

Conservative therapy and epidural steroids generally have a limited role. Patients with mild to moderate stenosis and radicular symptoms may benefit from epidural steroids. Severe symptoms are an indication for surgical decompression; the pseudoclaudication usually resolves but back pain may persist.

4. Facet Syndrome

Some patients complain of pain that is primarily related to degenerative changes in the facet (zygapophyseal) joints. The pain tends to be just off the midline and radiates down the back to the gluteal region, thigh, and knee; muscle spasm may also be present. Hyperextension and lateral rotation of the spine usually exacerbate the pain. The diagnosis may be suggested by oblique radiographs or CT of the spine, and is confirmed by pain relief following intraarticular injection of local anesthetic into affected joints or blockade of the medial branch of the posterior division (ramus) of the spinal nerves that innervate them. Long-term studies suggest medial branch nerve blocks are more effective than facet joint injections. Medial branch rhizotomy can provide long-term analgesia for facet joint disease in the lumbar (and cervical) spine.

5. Congenital Abnormalities

Congenital abnormalities of the back are often asymptomatic and remain occult. Abnormal spinal mechanics may make the patient prone to back pain and in some instances progressive deformities. Common anomalies include sacralization of L5 (the vertebral body is fused to the sacrum), lumbarization of S1 (it functions as a sixth lumbar vertebra), spondylolysis (a bony defect develops between the pedicle and the lamina), and spondylolisthesis (the vertebral body, pedicles, and superior facet joints slide anteriorly leaving the posterior elements behind—most commonly at L5). The diagnosis is made radiographically. Spinal fusion may be necessary in patients with progressive symptoms and spinal instability.

6. Tumors

Spinal tumors in patients younger than 50 years old are generally benign, whereas those in older patients are usually malignant. Breast, lung, prostate, renal, gastrointestinal, and thyroid carcinomas, lymphomas, and multiple myelomas frequently metastasize to the lumbar spine. The pain is usually constant and may be associated with localized tenderness over involved vertebrae. Bony destruction or neural or vascular compression produces the pain. Epidural or intradural tumors can present like a herniated disk and may rapidly progress to flaccid paralysis. The primary site may be asymptomatic or overlooked. The diagnosis is made radiographically or with a bone scan. Depending on the type of tumor, corticosteroids, radiation, or surgical decompression (with stabilization) may be indicated.

7. Infection

Bacterial infections of the spine usually affect the vertebral body, and can be due to pyogenic as well as tuberculous organisms. Patients, particularly those with spinal tuberculosis, present with chronic back pain without fever or leukocytosis. In contrast, those with epidural abscesses present acutely with pain, fever, and leukocytosis; urgent surgical evacuation and antibiotic therapy are necessary to prevent progression to flaccid paralysis.

8. Arthritides

Ankylosing spondylitis is a familial disorder that is associated with histocompatibility antigen HLA-B27. It typically presents as low back pain associated with early morning stiffness in a young man. The pain has an insidious onset and may initially improve with activity. After a few months to years, the pain gradually intensifies and is associated with progressive restricted movement of the spine. Diagnosis can be difficult early in the disease, but radiographic evidence of sacroiliitis is usually present. As the disease progresses, the spine develops a characteristic "bamboo-like" radiographic appearance. Some patients develop arthritis of the hips and shoulders as well as extraarticular inflammatory manifestations. Treatment is primarily directed at maintaining functional preservation of posture. NSAIDs, particularly indomethacin, are good analgesics and reduce the early morning stiffness.

Patients with Reiter's syndrome, psoriatic arthritis, or inflammatory bowel disease may also present with low back pain, but extraspinal manifestations are usually more prominent. Rheumatoid arthritis usually spares the spine except for the apophyseal joints of the cervical spine.

NEUROPATHIC PAIN

Neuropathic pain includes pain associated with diabetic neuropathy, causalgia, phantom limbs, postherpetic neuralgia, stroke, spinal cord injury, and multiple sclerosis. Cancer pain and chronic low back pain may have prominent neuropathic components. Neuropathic pain tends to be paroxysmal and sometimes lancinating with a burning quality, and is usually associated with hyperpathia. Mechanisms of neuropathic pain are reviewed earlier in the chapter.

Because of the often difficult nature of this type of pain, multiple treatment modalities may be necessary. Treatment may include anticonvulsants (eg, gabapentin), antidepressants (amitriptyline), antiarrhythmics (mexiletine), α_2-adrenergic agonists (clonidine), topical agents (lidocaine or capsaicin), and analgesics (NSAIDs and opioids). Spinal opioids may be very effective for some patients. Sympathetic blocks are effective in selected disorders (see below). Spinal cord stimulation may be effective for patients who do not tolerate or respond to other treatments.

Diabetic Neuropathy

Diabetic neuropathy is the most common type of neuropathic pain encountered in practice and is a major cause of morbidity. Its pathophysiology is poorly understood but it may be related to microangiopathy and chronic hyperglycemia resulting in abnormal activation of metabolic (polyol) pathways and glycation of proteins. Many diabetic neuropathy syndromes are recognized and more than one may be present in a given patient. They may be symmetric (generalized), focal, or multifocal, affecting peripheral (sensory or motor), cranial, or autonomic nerves.

The most common syndrome is peripheral polyneuropathy, which results in symmetric numbness ("stocking and glove" distribution), paresthesias, dysesthesias, and pain. The pain varies in intensity, is severe at times, and is often worst at night. Loss of proprioception may lead to gait disturbances and sensory deficits can lead to injuries. Isolated mononeuropathies affecting individual nerves may lead to wrist or foot drop or cranial nerve palsy. Mononeuropathies typically have a sudden onset and are reversible, lasting a few weeks. Radiculopathy, affecting the sensory dermatome, may also occur. Autonomic neuropathy typically affects the gastrointestinal track causing diarrhea, delayed gastric emptying, and esophageal motility. Orthostatic hypotension and other forms of autonomic dysfunction are common (Chapter 36).

Treatment of diabetic neuropathy is not only symptomatic but also directed at optimal glycemic control to help prevent or slow progression. Acetaminophen and NSAIDs are usually ineffective for moderate to severe pain. Treatment is primarily pharmacological, and can be difficult and frustrating. Patients can readily become tolerant of and addicted to opioids. Adjuvant drugs (see section above) therefore play a major role. The combination of an antiepileptic drug (eg, gabapentin) and a tricyclic antidepressant (amitriptyline) appears to be particularly effective. Tramadol may be a useful analgesic, with its unique mechanism, and a lower potential for abuse.

Sympathetically Maintained Pain

Sympathetically maintained pain refers to a group of neuropathic pain disorders in which the nervous system plays a prominent role. Multiple triggers can induce sympathetically maintained pain, which is often overlooked or misdiagnosed. The term "complex regional pain syndrome" (CRPS) is generally preferred for these and related pain syndromes. **The two most common syndromes are reflex sympathetic dystrophy (RSD or CRPS type I) and causalgia (CRPS type II).**

A. REFLEX SYMPATHETIC DYSTROPHY (CRPS TYPE I)

This form of sympathetically maintained pain typically affects the extremities and follows relatively minor trauma. Common preceding events include trauma (contusion, crush, or laceration), surgery, sprain, fracture, or dislocation. It may follow carpal tunnel release, palmar fasciotomy, or arthroplasties. The trauma is sometimes occult. Similar syndromes may be associated with burns, postherpetic neuralgia, multiple sclerosis, diabetic neuropathy, myocardial infarction, stroke, cancer, herniated intervertebral disks, and degenerative joint disease. Three phases can often be identified (Table 18–18). A technetium bone scan shows increased uptake in small joints during the acute phase; thermography reveals asymmetric hyperemission. Although the pain can resolve spontaneously, most patients typically progress to severe functional disabilities.

B. CAUSALGIA (CRPS TYPE II)

Causalgia, which means burning pain, typically follows high-velocity (eg, gunshot) injuries to large nerves. The pain frequently has an immediate onset and is associated with allodynia, hyperpathia, and vasomotor and sudomotor dysfunction. Anything that increases sympathetic tone, such as fear, anxiety, light, noise, or touch, exacerbates the pain. The syndrome has a variable progression that can range from days to months. Causalgia most commonly affects the brachial plexus, particularly the median nerve in the upper extremity, and the tibial division of the sciatic nerve in the lower extremity. Early in the course of the disease patients obtain dramatic pain relief from sympathetic blockade.

Treatment

Patients often dramatically respond to sympathetic blocks, but treatment must be multidisciplinary to

Table 18–18. Phases of reflex sympathetic dystrophy.

Characteristic	Phase		
	Acute	**Dystrophic**	**Atrophic**
Pain	Localized, severe, and burning	More diffuse, throbbing	Less severe; often involves other extremities
Extremity	Warm	Cold, cyanotic, and edematous; muscle wasting	Severe muscle atrophy; contractures
Skin	Dry and red	Sweaty	Glossy and atrophic
X-ray	Normal	Reveals osteoporosis	Reveals severe osteoporosis, and ankylosis of joints
Duration	1–3 months	3–6 months	Indefinite

avoid long-term functional and psychological disability. Physical therapy plays a central role. Some patients recover spontaneously; but without treatment, most patients progress to severe functional and irreversible disability. Sympathetic blocks and intravenous regional sympatholytic blockade are equally effective. These blocks should be continued until the response plateaus or a cure is achieved. The sympathetic blocks facilitate physical therapy, which usually consists of active movement without weights. Most patients require three to seven blocks. The likelihood of a cure is high (over 90%) if treatment is initiated within 1 month of symptoms and appears to decrease with time. Some patients benefit from TENS. Dorsal column (spinal cord) stimulation may be effective in some patients with longstanding symptoms. Oral α-adrenergic blockers, such as phenoxybenzamine or prazosin, clonidine, anticonvulsants, and antidepressants may also be beneficial. Surgical sympathectomy for chronic cases is often disappointing because of only transient relief.

ACUTE HERPES ZOSTER & POSTHERPATIC NEURALGIA

Acute herpes zoster represents a reactivation of the varicella-zoster virus. During the initial childhood infection (chickenpox), the virus infects dorsal root ganglia, where it remains latent until reactivation. The disease presents as a vesicular, dermatomal rash that is usually associated with severe pain. Dermatomes T3–L3 are most commonly affected. The pain often precedes the rash by 48–72 h; the rash usually lasts 1–2 weeks. Herpes zoster may occur at any age but is most common in elderly patients. It is typically a benign self-limited disorder in younger patients (< 50 years old). Treatment is primarily supportive consisting of oral analgesics and oral acyclovir, famciclovir, or *valacyclovir*. Antiviral therapy reduces the duration of the rash and speeds healing. Immunocompromised patients with disseminated infection require intravenous acyclovir therapy.

Older patients may continue to experience severe radicular pain, even after the rash resolves. The incidence of postherpetic neuralgia (PHN) is estimated to be 50% in patients older than 50 years of age. Moreover, PHN is often very difficult to treat. An oral course of corticosteroids during acute zoster may decrease the incidence of PHN but remains controversial. Corticosteroids may increase the likelihood of dissemination in immunocompromised patients. **Sympathetic blockade during acute herpes zoster can produce excellent analgesia and is also reported to decrease the incidence of PHN.** The latter suggests that PHN is sympathetically maintained. Studies suggest that when sympathetic blocks are initiated within 2 months of the rash, PHN resolves in up to 80% of patients. Once the neuralgia is well established, how-ever, the sympathetic blocks (like other treatments) are generally ineffective. Antidepressants, anticonvulsants, opioids, and TENS may be useful in some patients. Application of a transdermal lidocaine patch 5% (Lidoderm, 700 mg) over the most painful area may help some patients, presumably by decreasing peripheral sensitization of nerve endings and receptors.

HEADACHES

Headache is a common complaint that affects nearly all individuals at some time in their life. In the vast majority of cases, the headaches do not reflect a serious underlying disorder and are not of sufficient severity or frequency for the patient to seek medical attention. However, as with other complaints of pain, clinicians should always consider the possibility of a serious underlying disorder. The practitioner should therefore always solicit other associated symptoms or clinical findings that suggest serious underlying pathology. Table 18–19 lists important causes of headache. Disorders in which the primary complaint is headache are considered in the following discussion. As will become apparent, there is significant variability in clinical presentation and overlap in symptomatology among major headache syndromes, particularly between tension and migraine headaches. Postdural puncture headache is discussed in Chapter 16.

Tension Headaches

Tension headaches are classically described as tight bandlike pain or discomfort that is often associated with tightness in the neck muscles. The headache may be frontal, temporal, or occipital, being more often bilateral than unilateral. Pain intensity typically builds gradually and fluctuates, lasting hours to days. They may be associated with emotional stress or depression. Treatment is symptomatic with NSAIDs.

Migraine Headaches

Migraine headaches are typically described as throbbing or pounding and are often associated with photophobia, scotomata, nausea, vomiting, and localized transient neurological dysfunction (aura). The latter may be sensory, motor, visual, or olfactory. Classic migraines by definition are preceded by an aura, whereas common migraines are not. The pain is usually unilateral but can be bilateral with a frontotemporal location and lasts 4–72 h. Migraines primarily affect children (both sexes equally) and young adults (predominantly females). A family history is often present. Provocation by odors, certain foods (eg, red wine), menses, and sleep deprivation is common. Sleep characteristically relieves the headache. The mechanism

Table 18–19. Classification of headaches.

Classic headache syndromes
   Migraine
   Tension
   Cluster
Vascular disorders
   Temporal arteritis
   Stroke
   Venous thrombosis
Neuralgias
   Trigeminal
   Glossopharyngeal
   Occipital
Intracranial pathology
   Tumor
   Cerebrospinal fluid leak
   Pseudomotor cerebri
   Meningitis
   Aneurysm
Eye disorders
   Glaucoma
   Optic neuritis
Sinus disease
   Allergic
   Bacterial
Temporomandibular joint disease
Dental disorders
Drug-induced
   Acute ingestion
   Withdrawal (eg, caffeine and alcohol)
Systemic disorders
   Infections
      Viral (eg, influenza)
      Bacterial
      Fungal
   Metabolic
      Hypoglycemia
      Hypoxemia
      Hypercarbia
Trauma
Miscellaneous
   Cold stimulus (swallowing cold liquid)

is complex and may include vasomotor, autonomic (serotinergic brain stem systems), and trigeminal nucleus dysfunction. Treatment is both abortive (to terminate the attack) and prophylactic. Rapid abortive treatment includes oxygen, sumatriptan (6 mg subcutaneously), dihydroergotamine (1 mg intramuscularly or subcutaneously), intravenous lidocaine (100 mg), nasal butorphanol (1–2 mg), and sphenopalatine block. Other abortive options include zolmitriptan nasal spray, dihydroergotamine nasal spray, or an oral serotonin 5-$HT_{1B/1D}$-receptor agonist (almotriptan, frovatriptan, naratriptan, rizatriptan, eletriptan, or

sumatriptan). Prophylactic treatment may include β-adrenergic blockers, calcium channel blockers, valproic acid, and amitriptyline.

Cluster Headaches

Cluster headaches are classically unilateral and periorbital, occurring in clusters of one to three attacks a day over a 4- to 8-week period. The pain is described as a burning or drilling sensation that may awaken the patient from sleep. It lasts 30–120 min. Remissions for about a year at a time are common. Red eye, tearing, nasal stuffiness, and ptosis (Horner's syndrome) are classic findings. The headaches are typically episodic but can become chronic without remissions. Cluster headaches primarily affect males (90%). Abortive treatment includes oxygen and sphenopalatine block. Prophylactic treatment may include lithium and a short course of prednisone and verapamil.

Temporal Arteritis

Temporal arteritis is an inflammatory disorder of extracranial arteries. The headache can be bilateral or unilateral, dull and boring in quality, and located in the temporal area in at least 50% of patients. The pain develops over a few hours and may be lancinating at times, and worse at night and in cold weather. Scalp tenderness is usually present. Temporal arteritis is a relatively common disorder of older patients (> 55 years), with an incidence of about 1 in 10,000 per year with a slight female predominance. Polymyalgia rheumatica, fever, and weight loss are often also present. Early diagnosis is important because without treatment progression can lead to blindness through involvement of the ophthalmic artery. Corticosteroid treatment is highly effective. Temporal artery biopsy confirms the diagnosis.

Trigeminal Neuralgia

The pain of trigeminal neuralgia (tic douloureux) is classically unilateral, usually located in the V2 or V3 distribution of the trigeminal nerve. It has an electric shock quality lasting seconds up to 2 min at a time and is often provoked by contact with a discrete trigger area in the affected nerve branch. Facial muscle spasm may be present. It is a disease of middle-aged and elderly patients with a 2:1 female to male ratio. In at least some patients it may be due to irritation from tortuousity of blood vessels in the posterior fossa. The drug of choice for treatment is carbamazepine. Phenytoin or baclofen may be added, particularly if patients do not tolerate the required doses of carbamazepine. More invasive treatments for patients who do not tolerate drug therapy include glycerol injection or radiofrequency ablation of the gasserian ganglion and microsurgical decompression of the trigeminal nerve (Jannetta procedure).

CASE DISCUSSION: ANALGESIA FOLLOWING THORACOABDOMINAL SURGERY

An obese 21-year-old male is admitted to the recovery room following a right thoracoabdominal lymph node dissection for a testicular malignant growth. The incision extends from the eighth rib to the pubis and a right thoracostomy (chest tube) is present. He had consented to an epidural catheter for managing his pain postoperatively. Unfortunately, placement of the catheter prior to surgery proved to be very difficult because of his obesity, and could not be accomplished. He is extubated and awakens from anesthesia in severe pain and is noted to have shallow breathing at a rate of 35/min ("splinting"). A total of 10 mg of morphine sulfate is given intravenously before he stops complaining of pain and becomes very drowsy again.

While the patient was receiving 50% oxygen by face mask, an arterial blood reading is as follows: Pa_{O_2}, 58 mm Hg; Pa_{CO_2}, 53 mm Hg; pH, 7.25; and HCO_3^-, 21 mEq/L. The postoperative chest film reveals clear lung fields with diminished lung volumes.

Why is pain management very important in this patient?

The patient is at high risk for pulmonary complications because of his obesity and the extensive thoracoabdominal incision. He is unable to take deep breaths or cough effectively, and already has hypoxemia and respiratory acidosis. In fact, if his respiratory status cannot be improved promptly, endotracheal intubation and controlled mechanical ventilation should be considered. The chest film is very helpful in excluding residual right pneumothorax, significant hemothorax, or lobar atelectasis that could explain his marginal respiratory status. The most likely explanation of these findings is inadequate pain relief combined with opioid-induced respiratory depression. The hypoxemia is most likely due to microatelectasis and a low functional residual capacity (see Chapter 22), whereas the hypoventilation is due to splinting from incisional pain, the residual effects of intraoperative anesthetics (including opioids), and postoperative morphine. Clearly, satisfactory opioid analgesia could not be obtained in this patient without significant

respiratory depression and oversedation. Additional, more effective analgesic measures are indicated if postoperative mechanical ventilation is to be avoided.

What additional options are available to manage his pain more optimally?

Additional intravenous opioids would likely aggravate the respiratory depression and are to be avoided (unless the patient is reintubated). Intrathecal opioid administration may provide relatively rapid analgesia for the abdominal part of the incision but will require several hours for analgesia of its thoracic extension; the technique also predisposes to delayed respiratory depression. Moreover, performing a lumbar puncture in this setting is likely to be as difficult or more difficult than placing an epidural catheter preoperatively.

Intravenous ketorolac can offer additional analgesia without respiratory depression and can significantly reduce opioid requirements. The use of ketorolac immediately following such extensive surgical dissections, however, may be hazardous because of its antiplatelet effects and risk of postoperative hemorrhage.

Ketamine in low doses (10–20 mg/h) is a very potent analgesic and is not a respiratory depressant. In higher doses, it is more likely to cause excessive sedation and psychotomimetic effects. Although a ketamine infusion may be a reasonable option, concerns about oversedating this patient are justified.

Multiple intercostal blocks (see Chapter 17) can provide excellent analgesia for thoracic incisions and are indicated in this patient. Splinting can be abolished, and vital capacity and arterial blood gases often improve. Four to five milliliters of 0.25% bupivacaine can be injected at the appropriate dermatomal levels where the rib can be palpated. Moreover, because the patient already has a chest tube, the risk of a significant pneumothorax is minimal. A similarly effective technique that may be easier to perform in this obese patient is interpleural analgesia.

What is interpleural analgesia?

The technique can provide analgesia over the chest wall and upper abdomen. It involves placement of a catheter into a tissue plane within the chest wall such that a single injection of local anesthetic spreads to several intercostal nerves. The terms "intrapleural" and "interpleural" have been used interchangeably, but the latter is generally preferred.

What is the anatomic basis of interpleural analgesia?

The intercostal space posteriorly has three layers: the external intercostal muscle, the posterior intercostal membrane (which is the aponeurosis of the internal intercostal muscle), and the intercostalis intimus muscle (part of the transversus thoracis group of muscles, which is a continuation of the transversus abdominis). Intercostal nerves lie in between the posterior intercostal membrane and the intercostalis intimus muscle. Whereas the posterior intercostal membrane forms a complete barrier beneath the external intercostal muscle, the intercostalis intimus muscle is incomplete and freely allows fluid to pass into the subpleural space. Thus, interpleural analgesia can be accomplished by placing a catheter either deep to the internal intercostal muscle but superficial to the parietal pleura, or between the parietal and visceral layers of the pleura. In either case, the local anesthetic injected will diffuse to adjacent intercostal nerves. The number of nerves affected depends on the level of the catheter, the volume of anesthetic injected, and the effects of gravity. In some instances the local anesthetic may reach the paravertebral space.

How is interpleural anesthesia performed?

A single epidural catheter is most commonly inserted through a Tuohy needle at a level between T6 and T8. The needle is inserted at a point anywhere between 8 cm lateral to the posterior midline and the posterior axillary line. It is then "walked off" the inferior edge of the rib (see intercostal nerve block, Chapter 17) and advanced to a position either just deep to the posterior intercostal membrane just beneath a rib, or between the parietal and visceral space. In the first instance, a "pop" may be encountered as the needle pierces the posterior intercostal membrane. In the second instance, a loss of resistance technique (similar to that for epidural anesthesia) can be used to identify entry into the pleural cavity. The catheter is then advanced 3–6 cm past the tip of the needle and fixed in position as the needle is withdrawn. Local anesthetic (20–25 mL; usually 0.25% bupivacaine) is then injected. The mean duration of analgesia with bupivacaine is about 7 h (range 2–18 h). Peak plasma concentrations of the local anesthetic occur 15–20 min after injection. Adding epinephrine to the bupivacaine solution reduces and slightly delays the peak plasma concentration. Continuous infusions have also been employed at a rate of 0.125 mL/kg/h.

What are other indications for interpleural analgesia?

Interpleural analgesia is most effective in providing analgesia to patients with multiple rib fractures and those who have undergone open cholecystectomy. Postoperative analgesia is inconsistent following thoracotomy when multiple chest tubes are in place and a significant amount of blood is likely to be present in the chest; a significant amount of the local anesthetic may be lost through the chest. The technique can also be used for chest wall pain due to cancer, acute herpes zoster, and postherpetic neuralgia.

What are the hazards of interpleural anesthesia?

Pneumothorax is a significant risk if a chest tube is not already in place. Unilateral sympathetic block may be observed and can result in a Horner's syndrome. Chest wall hematoma has been reported. Systemic absorption is significant; high plasma concentrations of local anesthetics can be observed with continuous infusions, particularly after 2 days. Fortunately, clinical reports of systemic toxicity (seizures) are rare. Rarely, the local anesthetic can spread to the epidural space.

SUGGESTED READING

Abram SE: Treatment of lumbosacral radiculopathy with epidural steroids. Anesthesiology 1999;91:1937.

Aeschbach A, Mekhail NA: Common nerve blocks in chronic pain management. Anesth Clin North Am 2000;18:429.

Bridges D, Thompson SWN, Rice ASC: Mechanisms of neuropathic pain. Br J Anaesth 2001;87:12.

Brown DL: *Atlas of Regional Anesthesia,* 2nd ed. W.B. Saunders, 1999.

Christo PJ: Opioid effectiveness and side effects in chronic pain. Anesth Clin North Am 2003;21:699.

Cousins MJ: *Neural Blockade in Clinical Anesthesia and Pain Management,* 3rd ed. Lippincott, Williams & Wilkins, 1998.

Desborough JP: The stress response to trauma and surgery. Br J Anaesth 2000;85:109.

Dougherty PM, Staats PS: Intrathecal drug therapy for patients with chronic pain. Anesthesiology 1999;91:1891.

Finucane BT: *Complications of Regional Anesthesia.* Churchill Livingstone, 1999.

Hollmann MW, Durieux ME: Local anesthetics and the inflammatory response. Anesthesiology 2000;93:858.

Kamibayashi T, Maze M: Clinical uses of α_2-adrenergic agonists. Anesthesiology 2000;93:1345.

Kissin I: Preemptive analgesia. Anesthesiology 2000;93:1138.

Kohrs R, Durieux ME: Ketamine: Teaching an old drug new tricks. Anesth Analg 1998;87:1186.

Loeser JD, Butler SH, Chapman CR: *Bonica's Management of Pain.* Lippincott, Williams & Wilkins, 2001.

Macintyre PE, Ready LB: *Acute Pain Management: A Practical Guide,* 2nd ed. W.B. Saunders, 2001.

Morton NS: *Acute Paediatric Pain Management.* W.B. Saunders, 1998

Nguyen H, Garber JE, Hassenbusch SJ: Spinal analgesics. Anesth Clin North Am 2003;21:733.

Park GR, Fulton B, Senthuran S: *Management of Acute Pain.* Oxford University Press, 2000.

Peng PWH, Sandler AN: A review of the use of fentanyl analgesia in the management of acute pain in adults. Anesthesiology 1999;90:576.

Perkins FM, Kehlet H: Chronic pain as an outcome of surgery. Anesthesiology 2000;93:1123.

Practice Guidelines for Chronic Pain Management: A Report by the American Society of Anesthesiologists Task Force on Pain Management, Chronic Pain Section. Anesthesiology 1997; 86:995.

Raj PP: *Practical Management of Pain,* 3rd ed. Mosby, 2000.

Raj PP: Botulinum toxin therapy in pain management. Anesth Clin North Am 2003;21:715.

Raja SN, Grabow TS: Complex regional pain syndrome I (reflex sympathetic dystrophy). Anesthesiology 2002;96:1254.

Richardson J, Lönnqvist PA: Thoracic paravertebral block. Br J Anaesth 1998;81:230.

Slonimski M, Abram SE, Zuniga RE: Intrathecal baclofen in pain management. Reg Anesth Pain Med 2004;29:269.

Stanton-Hicks M: Complex regional pain syndrome. Anesth Clin North Am 2003;21:733.

Tarver JM, Rathmell JP, Alsofrom GF: Lumbar discography. Reg Anesth Pain Med 2001;26:263.

Tollison CD, Satterthwaite J: *Practical Pain Management,* 3rd ed. Lippincott, Williams & Wilkins, 2002.

Waldman SD: *Interventional Pain Management,* 2nd ed. W.B. Saunders, 2001.

Waldman SD: *Atlas of Uncommon Pain Syndromes.* W.B. Saunders, 2003.

Waldman SD: *Atlas of Interventional Pain Management,* 2nd ed. W.B. Saunders, 2004.

Wall PD, Melzack OC: *Textbook of Pain,* 4th ed. Churchill Livingstone, 2000.

Warfield C: *Principles & Practice of Pain Management,* 2nd ed. McGraw-Hill, 2001.

Wheatley RG, Schug SA, Watson D: Safety and efficacy of postoperative epidural analgesia. Br J Anaesth 2001;87:47.

SECTION IV
Physiology, Pathophysiology, & Anesthetic Management

Cardiovascular Physiology & Anesthesia

19

KEY CONCEPTS

 In contrast to action potentials in neurons, the spike in cardiac action potentials is followed by a plateau phase that lasts 0.2–0.3 s. Whereas the action potential for skeletal muscle and nerves is due to the abrupt opening of fast sodium channels in the cell membrane, in cardiac muscle it is due to the opening of both fast sodium channels (the spike) and slower calcium channels (the plateau).

 Halothane, enflurane, and isoflurane depress sinoatrial (SA) node automaticity. These agents appear to have only modest direct effects on the atrioventricular (AV) node, prolonging conduction time and increasing refractoriness. This combination of effects likely explains the frequent occurrence of junctional tachycardia when an anticholinergic is administered for sinus bradycardia during inhalation anesthesia; junctional pacemakers are accelerated more than those in the SA node.

 Studies suggest that all volatile anesthetics depress cardiac contractility by decreasing the entry of Ca^{2+} into cells during depolarization (affecting T- and L-type calcium channels), altering the kinetics of its release and uptake into the sarcoplasmic reticulum, and decreasing the sensitivity of contractile proteins to calcium.

 Because the normal cardiac index (CI) has a wide range, it is a relatively insensitive measurement of ventricular performance. Abnormalities in CI therefore usually reflect gross ventricular impairment.

 In the absence of hypoxia or severe anemia, measurement of mixed venous oxygen tension (or saturation) is the best determination of the adequacy of cardiac output.

 Because the atrial contribution to ventricular filling is important in maintaining low mean ventricular diastolic pressures, patients with reduced ventricular compliance are most affected by loss of a normally timed atrial systole.

 Cardiac output in patients with marked right or left ventricular impairment is very sensitive to acute increases in afterload.

 The ventricular ejection fraction, the fraction of the end-diastolic ventricular volume ejected, is the most commonly used clinical measurement of systolic function.

(continued on next page)

(continued from previous page)

 Left ventricular diastolic function can be assessed clinically by Doppler echocardiography on a transthoracic or transesophageal examination.

 Because the endocardium is subjected to the greatest intramural pressures during systole, it tends to be most vulnerable to ischemia during decreases in coronary perfusion pressure.

 The failing heart becomes increasingly dependent on circulating catecholamines. Abrupt withdrawal in sympathetic outflow or decreases in circulating catecholamine levels, such as can occur following induction of anesthesia, may lead to acute cardiac decompensation.

Anesthesiologists must have a thorough understanding of cardiovascular physiology both for its scientific significance in anesthesia and for its practical applications to modern patient management. This chapter reviews the physiology of the heart and the systemic circulation and the pathophysiology of heart failure. The pulmonary circulation and the physiology of blood and nutrient exchange are discussed in Chapters 22 and 28, respectively.

The circulatory system consists of the heart, the blood vessels, and the blood. Its function is to provide oxygen and nutrients to the tissues and to carry away the by-products of metabolism. The heart propels blood through two vascular systems arranged in series. In the pulmonary circulation, blood flows past the alveolar–capillary membrane, takes up oxygen, and eliminates CO_2. In the systemic circulation, oxygenated blood is pumped to metabolizing tissues, and the by-products of metabolism are taken up for elimination by the lungs, kidneys, or liver.

THE HEART

Although anatomically one organ, the heart can be functionally divided into right and left pumps, each consisting of an atrium and a ventricle. The atria serve as both conduits and priming pumps, whereas the ventricles act as the major pumping chambers. The right ventricle receives systemic venous (deoxygenated) blood and pumps it into the pulmonary circulation, whereas the left ventricle receives pulmonary venous (oxygenated) blood and pumps it into the systemic circulation. Four valves normally ensure unidirectional flow through each chamber. The normal pumping action of the heart is the result of a complex series of electrical and mechanical events.

The heart consists of specialized striated muscle in a connective tissue skeleton. Cardiac muscle can be divided into atrial, ventricular, and specialized pacemaker and conducting cells. The self-excitatory nature of cardiac muscle cells and their unique organization allow the heart to function as a highly efficient pump. Serial low-resistance connections (intercalated disks) between individual myocardial cells allow the rapid and orderly spread of electrical activity in each pumping chamber. Electrical activity readily spreads from one atrium to another and from one ventricle to another via specialized conduction pathways. The normal absence of direct connections between the atria and ventricles except through the atrioventricular (AV) node delays conduction and enables atrial contraction to prime the ventricle.

CARDIAC ACTION POTENTIALS

The myocardial cell membrane is normally permeable to K^+ but is relatively impermeable to Na^+. A membrane-bound Na^+–K^+-adenosine triphosphatase (ATPase) concentrates K^+ intracellularly in exchange for extrusion of Na^+ out of the cells (see Chapter 28). Intracellular Na^+ concentration is kept low, whereas intracellular K^+ concentration is kept high relative to the extracellular space. The relative impermeability of the membrane to calcium also maintains a high extracellular to cytoplasmic calcium gradient. Movement of K^+ out of the cell and down its concentration gradient results in a net loss of positive charges from inside the cell. An electrical potential is established across the cell membrane, with the inside of the cell negative with respect to the extracellular environment, because anions do not accompany K^+. Thus, the resting membrane potential represents the balance between two opposing forces: the movement of K^+ down its concentration gradient and the electrical attraction of the negatively charged intracellular space for the positively charged potassium ions.

The normal ventricular cell resting membrane potential is –80 to –90 mV. As with other excitable tissues (nerve and skeletal muscle), when the cell membrane potential becomes less negative and reaches a threshold value, a characteristic action potential (depolarization) develops (Figure 19–1 and Table 19–1). The action potential transiently raises the membrane potential of the myocardial cell to +20 mV. In contrast to action potentials in neurons (see Chapter 14), the spike in cardiac action potentials is followed by a plateau phase that lasts 0.2–0.3 s. Whereas the action potential for skeletal muscle and nerves is due to the abrupt opening of fast sodium channels in the cell membrane, in cardiac muscle it is due to the opening of both fast sodium channels (the spike) and slower calcium channels (the plateau). Depolarization is also accompanied by a transient decrease in potassium permeability. Subsequent restoration of normal potassium permeability and closure of sodium and calcium channels eventually restores the membrane potential to normal.

Following depolarization, the cells are typically refractory to subsequent normal depolarizing stimuli until phase 4. The effective refractory period is the minimum interval between two depolarizing impulses that are propagated. In fast-conducting myocardial cells, this period is generally closely correlated with the duration of the action potential. In contrast, the effective refractory period in slowly conducting myocardial cells can outlast the duration of the action potential.

Table 19–2 lists the multiple types of ion channels in cardiac muscle membrane. Some are activated by a change in cell membrane voltage, whereas others open only when bound by ligands. The voltage-gated fast Na^+ channel has an outer (m) gate that opens at –60 to –70 mV and an inner (h) gate that then closes at –30 mV. T-type (transient) voltage-gated calcium channels play a role in phase 0 of depolarization. During the plateau phase (phase 2), calcium inflow occurs through slow L-type (long-lasting), voltage-gated calcium channels. Three major types of K^+ channels are responsible for repolarization. The first results in a transient outward potassium current (I_{To}), the second is responsible for a short rectifying current (I_{Kr}), and the third produces a slowly acting rectifying current (I_{Ks}) that restores the cell membrane potential to normal.

INITIATION & CONDUCTION OF THE CARDIAC IMPULSE

The cardiac impulse normally originates in the sinoatrial (SA) node, a group of specialized pacemaker cells in the sulcus terminalis, posteriorly at the junction of the right atrium and the superior vena cava. These cells appear to have an outer membrane that leaks sodium (and possibly calcium). The slow influx of sodium, which results in a less negative, resting membrane potential (–50 to –60 mV), has three important consequences: constant inactivation of fast sodium channels, an action potential with a threshold of –40 mV that is primarily due to ion movement across the slow calcium channels, and regular spontaneous depolarizations. During each cycle, intracellular leakage of sodium causes the cell membrane to become progressively less negative; when the threshold potential is reached, calcium channels open, potassium permeability decreases, and an action potential develops. Restoration of normal potassium permeability returns the cells in the SA node to their normal resting membrane potential.

The impulse generated at the SA node is normally rapidly conducted across the atria and to the AV node. Specialized atrial fibers may speed up conduction to both the left atrium and the AV node. The AV node, which is located in the septal wall of the right atrium just anterior to the opening of the coronary sinus and above the insertion of the septal leaflet of the tricuspid valve, is actually made up of three distinct areas: an upper junctional (AN) region, a middle nodal (N) region, and a lower junctional (NH) region. Although the N region does not possess intrinsic spontaneous activity (automaticity), both junctional areas do. The normally slower rate of spontaneous depolarization in AV junctional areas (40–60 times/min) allows the faster SA node to control heart rate. Any factor that decreases the rate of SA node depolarization or increases the automaticity of AV junctional areas allows the junctional areas to function as the pacemaker for the heart.

Impulses from the SA node normally reach the AV node after about 0.04 s but leave after another 0.11 s. This delay is the result of the slowly conducting small myocardial fibers within the AV node, which depend on slow calcium channels for propagation of the action potential. In contrast, conduction of the impulse between adjoining cells in the atria and in the ventricles is due primarily to activation and inactivation of the fast sodium channels. The lower fibers of the AV node combine to form the common bundle of His. This specialized group of fibers passes into the interventricular septum before dividing into left and right branches to form the complex network of Purkinje fibers that depolarizes both ventricles. In sharp contrast to AV nodal tissue, His–Purkinje fibers have the fastest conduction velocities in the heart, resulting in nearly simultaneous depolarization of the entire endocardium of both ventricles (normally within 0.03 s). The spread of the impulse from the endocardium to the epicardium through ventricular muscle requires an additional 0.03 s. Thus, an impulse arising from the SA

A

B

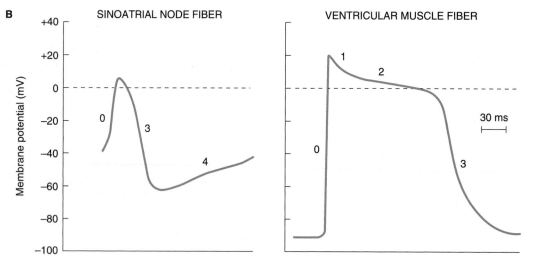

Figure 19–1. Cardiac action potentials. *A:* Note the characteristic action potentials of different parts of the heart. *B:* Pacemaker cells in the SA node lack the same distinct phases as atrial and ventricular muscle cells and display prominent spontaneous diastolic depolarization. See Table 19–1 for an explanation of the different phases of the action potential. (Modified and reproduced, with permission, from Ganong WF: *Review of Medical Physiology,* 20th ed. McGraw-Hill, 2001.)

Table 19–1. Cardiac action potential.

Phase	Name	Event	Cellular Ion Movement
0	Upstroke	Activation (opening) of fast Na$^+$ channels	Na$^+$ in and decreased permeability to K$^+$
1	Early rapid repolarization	Inactivation of Na$^+$ channel and transient increase in K$^+$ permeability	K$^+$ out (I_{T_o})
2	Plateau	Activation of slow Ca^{2+} channels	Ca^{2+} in
3	Final repolarization	Inactivation of Ca^{2+} channels and increased permeability to K$^+$	K$^+$ out
4	Resting potential	Normal permeability restored (atrial and ventricular cells)	K$^+$ out Na$^+$ in
	Diastolic repolarization	Intrinsic slow leakage of Ca^{2+} into cells that spontaneously depolarize	Ca^{2+} in

node normally requires less than 0.2 s to depolarize the entire heart.

Halothane, enflurane, and isoflurane depress SA node automaticity. These agents appear to have only modest direct effects on the AV node, prolonging conduction time and increasing refractoriness. This combination of effects likely explains the frequent occurrence of junctional tachycardia when an anticholinergic is administered for sinus bradycardia during inhalation anesthesia; junctional pacemakers are accelerated more than those in the SA node. The electrophysiological effects of volatile agents on Purkinje fibers and ventricular muscle are complex due to autonomic interactions. Both antiarrhythmic and arrhythmogenic properties are described. The former may be due to direct depression of Ca^{2+} influxes, whereas the latter generally involves potentiation of catecholamines (see Chapter 7). The arrhythmogenic effect requires activation of both α_1- and β-adrenergic receptors. Intravenous induction agents have limited electrophysiological effects in usual clinical doses. Opioids, particularly fentanyl and sufentanil, can depress cardiac conduction, increasing AV node conduction and refractory period and prolonging the duration of the Purkinje fiber action potential.

Local anesthetics have important electrophysiological effects on the heart at blood concentrations that are generally associated with systemic toxicity. In the case of lidocaine, electrophysiological effects at low blood concentrations can be therapeutic (see Chapter 47). At high blood concentrations, local anesthetics depress conduction by binding to fast sodium channels; at extremely high concentrations they also depress the SA node. The most potent local anesthetics—bupivacaine and, to lesser degrees, etidocaine and ropivacaine—

appear to have the greatest effects on the heart, particularly on Purkinje fibers and ventricular muscle. Bupivacaine binds inactivated fast sodium channels and dissociates from them slowly. It can cause profound sinus bradycardia and sinus node arrest as well as malignant ventricular arrhythmias.

Calcium channel blockers are organic compounds that block calcium influx through L-type but not T-type channels. Dihydropyridine blockers such as nifedipine simply plug the channel, whereas other agents such as verapamil and, to a lesser extent, diltiazem preferentially bind the channel in its depolarized inactivated state (use-dependent blockade).

Table 19–2. Cardiac ion channels.[1]

Voltage-gated channels
Na$^+$
T Ca^{2+}
L Ca^{2+}
K$^+$
  Transient outward
  Inward rectifying
  Slow (delayed) rectifying
Ligand-gated K$^+$ channels
Ca^{2+} activated
Na$^+$ activated
ATP sensitive[2]
Acetylcholine activated
Arachadonic acid activated

[1]From Ganong WF: *Review of Medical Physiology*, 21st ed. McGraw-Hill, 2003.
[2]ATP, adenosine triphosphate.

MECHANISM OF CONTRACTION

Myocardial cells contract as a result of the interaction of two overlapping, rigid contractile proteins, actin and myosin. These proteins are fixed in position within each cell during both contraction and relaxation. Dystrophin, a large intracellular protein, connects actin to the cell membrane (sarcolemma). Cell shortening occurs when the actin and myosin are allowed to fully interact and slide over one another (Figure 19–2). This interaction is normally prevented by two regulatory proteins, troponin and tropomyosin; troponin is composed of three subunits, troponin I, troponin C, and troponin T. Troponin is attached to actin at regular intervals, whereas tropomyosin lies within the center of the actin structure. An increase in intracellular calcium concentration (from about 10^{-7} to 10^{-5} mol/L) promotes contraction as calcium ions bind troponin C. The resulting conformational change in these regulatory proteins exposes the active sites on actin that allow interaction with myosin bridges (points of overlapping). The active site on myosin functions as a magnesium-dependent ATPase whose activity is enhanced by the increase in intracellular calcium concentration. A series of attachments and disengagements occur as each myosin bridge advances over successive active sites on actin. Adenosine triphosphate (ATP) is consumed during each attachment. Relaxation occurs as calcium is actively pumped back into the sarcoplasmic reticulum by a Ca^{2+}–Mg^{2+}-ATPase; the resulting drop in intracellular calcium concentration allows the troponin–tropomyosin complex to again prevent the interaction between actin and myosin.

Excitation–Contraction Coupling

The quantity of calcium required to initiate contraction exceeds that entering the cell through slow channels during phase 2. The small amount that does enter through slow channels triggers the release of much larger amounts of calcium stored intracellularly (calcium-dependent calcium release) within cisterns in the sarcoplasmic reticulum.

The action potential of muscle cells depolarizes their T systems, tubular extensions of the cell membrane that transverse the cell in close approximation to the muscle fibrils, via dihydropyridine receptors (voltage-gated Ca^{2+} channels). This initial increase in intracellular Ca^{2+} triggers an even greater calcium inflow across ryanodine receptors, a nonvoltage-dependent calcium channel, in the sarcoplasmic reticulum. The force of contraction is directly dependent on the magnitude of the initial calcium influx. During relaxation, when the slow channels close, a membrane-bound ATPase actively transports calcium back into the sarcoplasmic reticulum. Calcium is also extruded extracellularly by an exchange of intracellular calcium for extracellular sodium by an ATPase in the cell membrane. Thus, relaxation of the heart also requires ATP.

The quantity of intracellular Ca^{2+} available, its rate of delivery, and its rate of removal determine, respectively, the maximum tension developed, the rate of contraction, and the rate of relaxation. Sympathetic stimulation increases the force of contraction by raising intracellular calcium concentration via a β_1-adrenergic receptor-mediated increase in intracellular cyclic adenosine monophosphate (cAMP) (see Chapter 12), through the action of a stimulatory G protein (see Chapter 18). The increase in cAMP recruits additional open calcium channels. Moreover, adrenergic agonists enhance the rate of relaxation by enhancing calcium reuptake by the sarcoplasmic reticulum. Phosphodiesterase inhibitors, such as theophylline, amrinone, and milrinone, produce similar effects by preventing the breakdown of intracellular cAMP. Digitalis increases intracellular calcium concentration through inhibition of the membrane-bound Na$^+$–K$^+$-ATPase; the resulting small increase in intracellular Na$^+$ allows for a greater influx of Ca^{2+} via the Na$^+$–Ca^{2+} exchange mechanism. Glucagon enhances contractility by increasing intracellular cAMP levels via activation of a specific nonadrenergic receptor. In contrast, release of acetylcholine following vagal stimulation depresses contractility through increased cyclic guanosine monophosphate (cGMP) levels and inhibition of adenylyl cyclase; these effects are mediated by an inhibitory G protein. Acidosis blocks slow calcium channels and therefore also depresses cardiac contractility by unfavorably altering intracellular calcium kinetics.

Studies suggest that all volatile anesthetics depress cardiac contractility by decreasing the entry of Ca^{2+} into cells during depolarization (affecting T- and L-type calcium channels), altering the kinetics of its release and uptake into the sarcoplasmic reticulum, and decreasing the sensitivity of contractile proteins to calcium. Halothane and enflurane appear to depress contractility more than isoflurane, sevoflurane, and desflurane. Anesthetic-induced cardiac depression is potentiated by hypocalcemia, β-adrenergic blockade, and calcium channel blockers. Nitrous oxide also produces dose-dependent decreases in contractility by reducing the availability of intracellular Ca^{2+} during contraction. The mechanisms of direct cardiac depression from intravenous anesthetics are not well established but presumably involve similar actions. Of all the major intravenous induction agents, ketamine appears to have the least direct depressant effect on contractility. Local anesthetic agents also depress cardiac contractility by reducing calcium influx and release in a dose-dependent fashion. Bupivacaine, tetracaine, and ropivacaine cause greater depression than lidocaine and chloroprocaine.

Figure 19–2. Excitation–contraction coupling and the interaction between actin and myosin. **A:** Depolarization of the muscle cell membrane allows entry of calcium into the cell and release of calcium stored in the sarcoplasmic reticulum. **B:** The structure of the actin–myosin complex. **C:** Calcium binds troponin, allowing the interaction between actin and myosin. (Modified and reproduced, with permission, from Katz AM, Smith VE: Relaxation abnormalities. Part I: Mechanisms. Hosp Pract 1984;19:69; and from Braunwald E: *The Myocardium: Failure and Infarction.* HP Publishing, 1974.)

INNERVATION OF THE HEART

Parasympathetic fibers primarily innervate the atria and conducting tissues. Acetylcholine acts on specific cardiac muscarinic receptors (M_2) to produce negative chronotropic, dromotropic, and inotropic effects. In contrast, sympathetic fibers are more widely distributed throughout the heart. Cardiac sympathetic fibers originate in the thoracic spinal cord (T1–T4) and travel to the heart initially through the cervical ganglia (stellate) and then as the cardiac nerves. Norepinephrine release causes positive chronotropic, dromotropic, and inotropic effects primarily through activation of β_1-adrenergic receptors. β_2-Adrenergic receptors are fewer in number and are found primarily in the atria; activation increases heart rate and, to a lesser extent, contractility. α_1-Adrenergic receptors have a positive inotropic effect.

Cardiac autonomic innervation has an apparent *sidedness,* because the right sympathetic and right vagus nerves primarily affect the SA node, whereas the left sympathetic and vagus nerves principally affect the AV node. Vagal effects frequently have a very rapid onset and resolution, whereas sympathetic influences generally have a more gradual onset and dissipation. Sinus arrhythmia is a cyclic variation in heart rate that corresponds to respiration (increasing with inspiration and decreasing during expiration); it is due to cyclic changes in vagal tone.

THE CARDIAC CYCLE

The cardiac cycle can be defined by both electrical and mechanical events (Figure 19–3). *Systole* refers to contraction and *diastole* refers to relaxation. Most diastolic ventricular filling occurs passively before atrial contraction. Contraction of the atria normally contributes 20–30% of ventricular filling. **Three waves can generally be identified on atrial pressure tracings** (Figure 19–3). The *a* wave is due to atrial systole. The *c* wave coincides with ventricular contraction and is said to be caused by bulging of the AV valve into the atrium. The *v* wave is the result of pressure buildup from venous return before the AV valve opens again. The *x* descent is the decline in pressure between the *c* and *v* waves and is thought to be due to a pulling down of the atrium by ventricular contraction. Incompetence of the AV valve on either side of the heart abolishes the *x* descent on that side, resulting in a prominent *cv* wave. The *y* descent follows the *v* wave and represents the decline in atrial pressure as the AV valve opens. The notch in the aortic pressure tracing is referred to as the incisura and represents transient backflow of blood into the left ventricle just before aortic valve closure.

DETERMINANTS OF VENTRICULAR PERFORMANCE

Discussions of ventricular function usually refer to the left ventricle, but the same concepts apply to the right ventricle. Although the ventricles are often thought of as functioning separately, their interdependence has clearly been demonstrated. Moreover, factors affecting systolic and diastolic functions can be differentiated: Systolic function involves ventricular ejection, whereas diastolic function is related to ventricular filling.

Ventricular systolic function is most often equated with cardiac output, which can be defined as the volume of blood pumped by the heart per minute. Because the two ventricles function in series, their outputs are normally equal. Cardiac output (CO) is expressed by the following equation:

$$CO = SV \times HR$$

where SV is the stroke volume (the volume pumped per contraction) and HR is heart rate. To compensate for variations in body size, CO is often expressed in terms of total body surface area:

$$CI = \frac{CO}{BSA}$$

where CI is the cardiac index and BSA is total body surface area. BSA is usually obtained from nomograms based on height and weight (Figure 19–4). Normal CI is 2.5–4.2 $L/min/m^2$. Because the normal CI has a wide range, it is a relatively insensitive measurement of ventricular performance. Abnormalities in CI therefore usually reflect gross ventricular impairment. A more accurate assessment can be obtained if the response of the cardiac output to exercise is evaluated. Under these conditions, failure of the cardiac output to increase and keep up with oxygen consumption is reflected by a falling mixed venous oxygen saturation (see Chapter 22). A decrease in mixed venous oxygen saturation in response to increased demand usually reflects inadequate tissue perfusion. Thus, in the absence of hypoxia or severe anemia, measurement of mixed venous oxygen tension (or saturation) is the best determination of the adequacy of cardiac output.

1. Heart Rate

Cardiac output is generally directly proportional to heart rate (Figure 19–5). Heart rate is an intrinsic function of the SA node (spontaneous depolarization) but is modified by autonomic, humoral, and local factors. The normal intrinsic rate of the SA node in

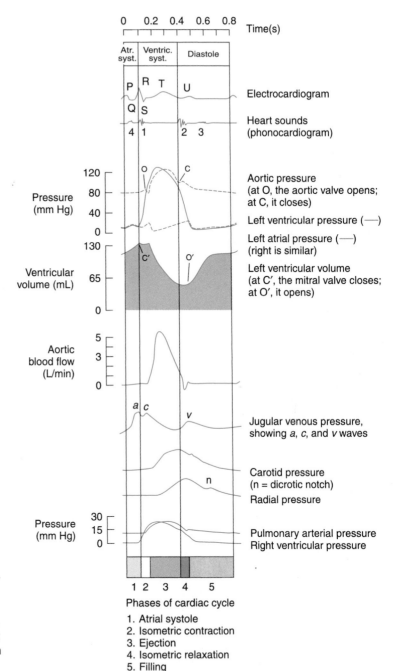

Figure 19–3. The normal cardiac cycle. Note the correspondence between electrical and mechanical events. (Modified and reproduced, with permission, from Ganong WF: *Review of Medical Physiology,* 20th ed. McGraw-Hill, 2001.)

young adults is about 90–100 beats/min, but it decreases with age based on the following formula:

Normal intrinsic heart rate = 118 beats/min

−(0.57 × age)

Enhanced vagal activity slows the heart rate via stimulation of M_2 cholinergic receptors, whereas enhanced sympathetic activity increases heart rate mainly through activation of β_1-adrenergic receptors and, to lesser extent, β_2-adrenergic receptors (see above).

Figure 19–4. Nomograms for calculating body surface area (BSA) in adult (**A**) and pediatric (**B**) patients. (From the formula of Du Bois and Du Bois: Arch Intern Med 1916;17:863. Copyright 1916, American Medical Association. Reprinted with permission.)

2. Stroke Volume

Stroke volume is normally determined by three major factors: preload, afterload, and contractility. This analysis is analogous to laboratory observations on skeletal muscle preparations. Preload is muscle length prior to contraction, whereas afterload is the tension against which the muscle must contract. Contractility is an intrinsic property of the muscle that is related to the force of contraction but is independent of both preload and afterload. Because the heart is a three-dimensional multichambered pump, both ventricular geometric form and valvular dysfunction can also affect stroke volume (Table 19–3).

Preload

Ventricular preload is end-diastolic volume, which is generally dependent on ventricular filling. The relationship

Figure 19–5. The relationship between heart rate and cardiac index. (Reproduced, with permission, from Wetsel RC: *Critical Care: State of the Art 1981*. Society of Critical Care Medicine, 1981.)

Table 19–3. Major factors affecting cardiac stroke volume.

Preload
Afterload
Contractility
Wall motion abnormalities
Valvular dysfunction

between cardiac output and left ventricular end-diastolic volume is known as Starling's law of the heart (Figure 19–6). Note that when the heart rate is constant, cardiac output is directly proportional to preload, until excessive end-diastolic volumes are reached. At that point cardiac output does not appreciably change—or may even decrease. Overdistention of either ventricle can lead to excessive dilatation and incompetence of the AV valves.

A. DETERMINANTS OF VENTRICULAR FILLING

Ventricular filling can be influenced by a variety of factors (Table 19–4), of which the most important is venous return. Because most of the other factors affecting venous return are usually fixed, venous tone is normally its major determinant. Increases in metabolic activity enhance venous tone, so that venous return to the heart increases as the volume of venous capacitance vessels decreases. Changes in blood volume and venous tone are important causes of intraoperative and postoperative changes in ventricular filling and cardiac output. Any factor that alters the normally small venous pressure gradient favoring blood return to the heart also affects cardiac filling. Such factors include changes in intrathoracic pressure (positive-pressure ventilation or thoracotomy), posture (positioning during surgery), and pericardial pressure (pericardial disease).

The most important determinant of right ventricular preload is venous return. **In the absence of significant pulmonary or right ventricular dysfunction, venous return is also the major determinant of left ventricular preload.** Normally, the end-diastolic volumes of both ventricles are similar.

Both heart rate and rhythm can also affect ventricular preload. Increases in heart rate are associated with proportionately greater reductions in diastole than systole. Ventricular filling therefore progressively becomes impaired at high heart rates (> 120 beats/min in adults). Absent (atrial fibrillation), ineffective (atrial flutter), or altered timing of atrial contraction (low atrial or junctional rhythms) can also reduce ventricular filling by 20–30%. Because the atrial contribution to ventricular filling is important in maintaining low mean ventricular diastolic pressures, patients with reduced ventricular compliance are most affected by the loss of a normally timed atrial systole.

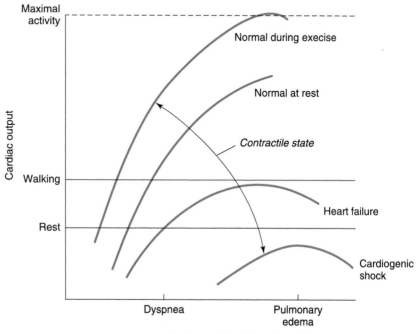

Figure 19–6. Starling's law of the heart.

Cardiac output

Maximal activity

Normal during execise

Normal at rest

Contractile state

Walking

Heart failure

Rest

Cardiogenic shock

Dyspnea

Pulmonary edema

Ventricular end-diastolic volume

Table 19–4. Factors affecting ventricular preload.

Venous return
Blood volume
Distribution of blood volume
   Posture
   Intrathoracic pressure
   Pericardial pressure
   Venous tone
Rhythm (atrial contraction)
Heart rate

B. Diastolic Function and Ventricular Compliance

Ventricular end-diastolic volume is difficult to measure clinically. Even imaging techniques such as two-dimensional transesophageal echocardiography (TEE), radionuclide imaging, and contrast ventriculography provide only approximations of the volume. **Left ventricular end-diastolic pressure (LVEDP) can be used as a measure of preload only if the relationship between ventricular volume and pressure (ventricular compliance) is constant.** Unfortunately, ventricular compliance is normally nonlinear (Figure 19–7). Moreover, because altered diastolic functions reduces ventricular compliance, the same LVEDP represents a decreased preload. Many factors are known to influence ventricular diastolic function and compliance. Nonetheless, measurement of LVEDP or other pressures approximating LVEDP (such as pulmonary capillary wedge pressure) remains the most common means of estimating left ventricular preload (see Chapter 6). Central venous pressure can be used as an index of both right as well as left ventricular preload in most normal individuals.

Factors affecting ventricular compliance can be separated into those related to the rate of relaxation (early diastolic compliance) and passive stiffness of the ventricles (late diastolic compliance). Hypertrophy, ischemia, and asynchrony reduce early compliance, whereas hypertrophy and fibrosis reduce late compliance. Extrinsic factors (such as pericardial disease, overdistention of the contralateral ventricle, increased airway or pleural pressure, tumors, and surgical compression) can also reduce ventricular compliance. Because of its normally thinner wall, the right ventricle is more compliant than the left.

Afterload

Afterload for the intact heart is commonly equated with either ventricular wall tension during systole or arterial impedance to ejection. Wall tension may be thought of as the pressure the ventricle must overcome to reduce its cavity. If the ventricle is assumed to be spherical, ventricular wall tension can be expressed by Laplace's law:

$$\text{Circumferential stress} = \frac{P \times R}{2 \times H}$$

where P is intraventricular pressure, R is the ventricular radius, and H is wall thickness. Although the normal ventricle is usually ellipsoidal, this relationship is still useful. The larger the ventricular radius, the greater the wall tension required to develop the same ventricular pressure. Conversely, an increase in wall thickness reduces ventricular wall tension.

Systolic intraventricular pressure is dependent on the force of ventricular contraction; the viscoelastic properties of the aorta, its proximal branches, and blood (viscosity and density); and **systemic vascular resistance (SVR).** Arteriolar tone is the primary determinant of SVR. Because viscoelastic properties are generally fixed in any given patient, left ventricular afterload is usually equated clinically with SVR, which is calculated by the following equation:

$$SVR = 80 \times \frac{MAP - CVP}{CO}$$

where MAP is mean arterial pressure in millimeters of mercury, CVP is central venous pressure in millimeters of mercury, and CO is cardiac output in liters per minute. Normal SVR is 900–1500 dyn · s cm^{-5}. Systolic blood pressure may also be used as an approximation of left ventricular afterload in the absence of chronic changes in the size, shape, or thickness of the ventricular wall or acute changes in systemic vascular

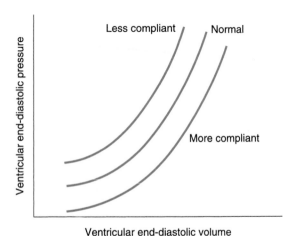

Figure 19–7. Normal and abnormal ventricular compliance.

resistance. Some clinicians prefer to use CI instead of CO in calculating a systemic vascular resistance index (SVRI), so that SVRI = SVR × BSA.

Right ventricular afterload is mainly dependent on pulmonary vascular resistance (PVR) and is expressed by the following equation:

$$PVR = 80 \times \frac{PAP - LAP}{CO}$$

where PAP is mean pulmonary artery pressure and LAP is left atrial pressure. In practice, pulmonary capillary wedge pressure (PCWP) is usually substituted as an approximation for LAP (see Chapter 6). Normal PVR is 50–150 dyn · s cm^{-5}.

Cardiac output is inversely related to afterload (Figure 19–8). Because of its thinner wall, the right ventricle is more sensitive to changes in afterload than the left ventricle. Cardiac output in patients with marked right or left ventricular impairment is very sensitive to acute increases in afterload. The latter is particularly true in the presence of myocardial depression (as often occurs during anesthesia).

Contractility

Cardiac contractility (inotropism) is the intrinsic ability of the myocardium to pump in the absence of changes in preload or afterload. Contractility is related to the rate of myocardial muscle shortening, which is in turn dependent on the intracellular calcium concentration during systole. Increases in heart rate can also enhance contractility under some conditions, perhaps because of the increased availability of intracellular calcium.

Contractility can be altered by neural, humoral, or pharmacological influences. Sympathetic nervous system activity normally has the most important effect on contractility. Sympathetic fibers innervate atrial and ventricular muscle as well as nodal tissues. In addition to its positive chronotropic effect, norepinephrine release also enhances contractility via β_1-receptor activation. α-Adrenergic receptors are also present in the myocardium but appear to have only minor positive inotropic and chronotropic effects. Sympathomimetic drugs and secretion of epinephrine from the adrenal glands similarly increase contractility via β_1-receptor activation.

Myocardial contractility is depressed by anoxia, acidosis, depletion of catecholamine stores within the heart, and loss of functioning muscle mass as a result of ischemia or infarction. Most anesthetics and antiarrhythmic agents are negative inotropes (ie, they decrease contractility).

Wall Motion Abnormalities

Regional wall motion abnormalities cause a breakdown of the analogy between the intact heart and

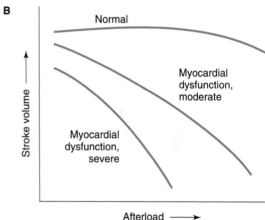

Figure 19–8. The relationship between cardiac output and afterload. **A:** The effect of increasing afterload on cardiac index. **B:** Note that patients with myocardial dysfunction become increasingly more sensitive to afterload.

skeletal muscle preparations. The abnormalities may be due to ischemia, scarring, hypertrophy, or altered conduction. When the ventricular cavity does not collapse symmetrically or fully, emptying becomes impaired. Hypokinesis (decreased contraction), akinesis (failure to contract), and dyskinesis (paradoxic bulging) during systole reflect increasing degrees of contraction abnormalities. Although contractility may be normal or even enhanced in some areas, abnormalities in other areas of the ventricle can impair emptying and reduce stroke volume. The severity of the impairment depends on the size and number of abnormally contracting areas.

Valvular Dysfunction

Valvular dysfunction can involve any one of the four valves in the heart and can lead to stenosis, regurgitation (incompetence), or both. Stenosis of an AV (tricuspid or mitral) valve reduces stroke volume primarily by decreasing ventricular preload, whereas stenosis of a semilunar (pulmonary or aortic) valve reduces stroke volume primarily by increasing ventricular afterload (see Chapter 20). In contrast, valvular regurgitation can reduce stroke volume without changes in preload, afterload, or contractility and without wall motion abnormalities. The effective stroke volume is reduced by the regurgitant volume with every contraction. When an AV valve is incompetent, a significant part of the ventricular end-diastolic volume can flow backward into the atrium during systole; the stroke volume is reduced by the regurgitant volume. Similarly, when a semilunar valve is incompetent, a fraction of end-diastolic volume returns backward into the ventricle during diastole.

ASSESSMENT OF VENTRICULAR FUNCTION

1. Ventricular Function Curves

Plotting cardiac output or stroke volume against preload is useful in evaluating pathological states and understanding drug therapy. Normal right and left ventricular function curves are shown in Figure 19–9.

Ventricular pressure–volume diagrams are even more useful because they dissociate contractility from both preload and afterload. Two points are identified on such diagrams: the end-systolic point (ESP) and the end-diastolic point (EDP) (Figure 19–10). ESP is reflective of systolic function, whereas EDP is more reflective of diastolic function. For any given contractile state, all ESPs are on the same line—ie, the relationship between end-systolic volume and end-systolic pressure is fixed.

2. Assessment of Systolic Function

The change in ventricular pressure over time during systole (*dP/dt*) is defined by the first derivative of the ventricular pressure curve and is often used as a measure of contractility. Contractility is directly proportional to *dP/dt*, but accurate measurement of this value requires a high-fidelity ventricular catheter. Although arterial pressure tracings are distorted due to properties of the vascular tree, the initial rate of rise in pressure (the slope) can serve as a rough approximation; the more proximal the catheter is in the arterial tree, the more accurate the extrapolation will be. The usefulness of *dP/dt* is also limited in that it may be affected by preload, afterload, and heart rate. Various correction factors have been used with only limited success.

Ejection Fraction

 The ventricular ejection fraction (EF), the fraction of the end-diastolic ventricular volume ejected, is the most commonly used clinical measurement of systolic function. EF can be calculated by the following equation:

$$EF = \frac{EDV - ESV}{EDV}$$

where EDV is left ventricular diastolic volume and ESV is end-systolic volume. Normal EF is approximately 0.67 ± 0.08. Measurements can be made preoperatively from cardiac catheterization, radionucleotide studies, or transthoracic or TEE. Pulmonary artery catheters with fast-response thermistors allow measurement of the right ventricular EF. Unfortunately, when pulmonary vascular resistance increases, decreases in right ventricular EF may reflect afterload rather than contractility.

3. Assessment of Diastolic Function

Left ventricular diastolic function can be assessed clinically by Doppler echocardiography on a transthoracic or transesophageal examination. Flow velocities are measured across the mitral valve during diastole. Three patterns of diastolic dysfunction are generally recognized based on isovolumetric relaxation time, the ratio of peak early diastolic flow (E) to peak atrial systolic flow (A), and the deceleration time (DT) of E (DT$_E$) (Figure 19–11).

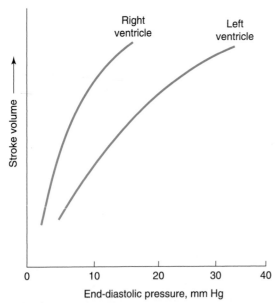

Figure 19–9. Function curves for the left and right ventricles.

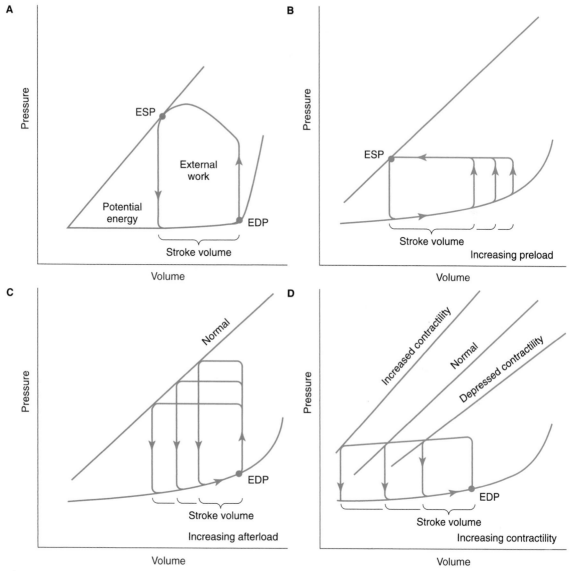

Figure 19–10. Ventricular pressure-volume diagrams. *A:* A single ventricular contraction. Note that stroke volume represents change in volume on the x-axis (difference between end-systolic volume and end-diastolic volume). Note also that the circumscribed area represents external work performed by the ventricle. *B:* Increasing preload with constant contractility and afterload. *C:* Increasing afterload with constant preload and contractility. *D:* Increasing contractility with constant preload and afterload. ESP, end-systolic point; EDP, end-diastolic point.

◼ SYSTEMIC CIRCULATION

The systemic vasculature can be divided functionally into arteries, arterioles, capillaries, and veins. Arteries are the high-pressure conduits that supply the various organs.

Arterioles are the small vessels that directly feed and control blood flow through each capillary bed. Capillaries are thin-walled vessels that allow the exchange of nutrients between blood and tissues (see Chapter 28). Veins return blood from capillary beds to the heart.

The distribution of blood between the various components of the circulatory system is shown in Table 19–5. Note that most of the blood volume is in the systemic

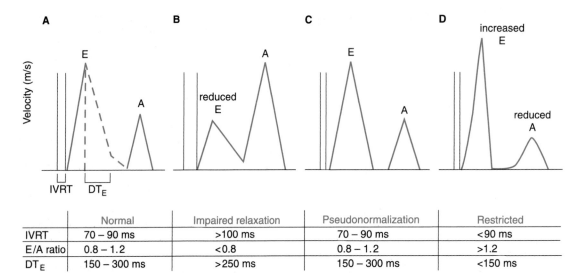

	Normal	Impaired relaxation	Pseudonormalization	Restricted
IVRT	70 – 90 ms	>100 ms	70 – 90 ms	<90 ms
E/A ratio	0.8 – 1.2	<0.8	0.8 – 1.2	>1.2
DT$_E$	150 – 300 ms	>250 ms	150 – 300 ms	<150 ms

Figure 19–11. Doppler echocardiography of diastolic flow across the mitral valve. ***A–D*** (from left to right) represents increasing severity of diastolic dysfunction. E, early diastolic flow; A, peak atrial systolic flow; IVRT, isovolumic relaxation time; DT$_E$, deceleration time of E.

circulation—specifically, within systemic veins. Changes in systemic venous tone allow these vessels to function as a reservoir for blood. Following significant blood or fluid losses, a sympathetically mediated increase in venous tone reduces the caliber of these vessels and shifts blood into other parts of the vascular system. Conversely, venodilation allows these vessels to accommodate increases in blood volume. Sympathetic control of venous tone is an important determinant of venous return to the heart. Loss of this tone following induction of anesthesia frequently contributes to hypotension.

A multiplicity of factors influences blood flow in the vascular tree. These include mechanisms of local and metabolic control, endothelium-derived factors, the autonomic nervous system, and circulating hormones.

AUTOREGULATION

Most tissue beds regulate their own blood flow (autoregulation). Arterioles generally dilate in response to reduced perfusion pressure or increased tissue demand. Conversely, arterioles constrict in response to increased pressure or reduced tissue demand. These phenomena are likely due to both an intrinsic response of vascular smooth muscle to stretch and the accumulation of vasodilatory metabolic by-products. The latter may include K^+, H^+, CO_2, adenosine, and lactate.

ENDOTHELIUM-DERIVED FACTORS

The vascular endothelium is active metabolically in elaborating or modifying substances that directly or indirectly play a major role in controlling blood pressure and flow. These include vasodilators (eg, nitric oxide, prostacyclin [PGI_2]), vasoconstrictors (endothelins, thromboxane A_2), anticoagulants (eg, thrombomodulin, protein C), fibrinolytics (tissue plasminogen activator), and factors that inhibit platelet aggregation (nitric oxide and PGI_2). Nitric oxide is synthesized from arginine by nitric oxide synthetase. This substance has a number of functions (see Chapter 13). In the circulation, it is a potent vasodilator that may be tonically secreted. It binds guanylate cyclase, increasing cGMP levels and producing vasodilation. Endothelially derived vasoconstrictors, endothelins, are released in response to thrombin and epinephrine.

AUTONOMIC CONTROL OF THE SYSTEMIC VASCULATURE

Although both the sympathetic and parasympathetic systems can exert important influences on the circulation,

Table 19–5. Normal distribution of blood volume.

Heart	7%
Pulmonary circulation	9%
Systemic circulation	
Arterial	15%
Capillary	5%
Venous	64%

autonomic control of the vasculature is primarily sympathetic. Sympathetic outflow to the circulation passes out of the spinal cord at all thoracic and the first two lumbar segments. These fibers reach blood vessels via specific autonomic nerves or by traveling along spinal nerves. Sympathetic fibers innervate all parts of the vasculature except for capillaries. Their principal function is to regulate vascular tone. Variations of arterial vascular tone serve to regulate blood pressure and the distribution of blood flow to the various organs, whereas variations in venous tone alter venous return to the heart.

The vasculature has sympathetic vasoconstrictor and vasodilator fibers, but the former are more important physiologically in most tissue beds. Sympathetic-induced vasoconstriction (via α_1-adrenergic receptors) can be potent in skeletal muscle, kidneys, gut, and skin; it is least active in the brain and heart. The most important vasodilatory fibers are those to skeletal muscle, mediating an increase in blood flow (via β_2-adrenergic receptors) in response to exercise. Vasodepressor (vasovagal) syncope, which can occur following intense emotional strain associated with high sympathetic tone, results from reflex activation of both vagal and sympathetic vasodilator fibers.

Vascular tone and autonomic influences on the heart are controlled by vasomotor centers in the reticular formation of the medulla and lower pons. Distinct vasoconstrictor and vasodilator areas have been identified. Vasoconstriction is mediated by the anterolateral areas of the lower pons and upper medulla. The adrenergic cells in this area project to the intermediolateral columns (see Chapter 18). They are also responsible for the adrenal secretion of catecholamines as well as the enhancement of cardiac automaticity and contractility. Vasodilatory areas, which are located in the lower medulla, are also adrenergic but function by projecting inhibitory fibers upward to the vasoconstrictor areas. Vasomotor output is modified by inputs from throughout the central nervous system, including the hypothalamus, cerebral cortex, and the other areas in the brain stem. Areas in the posterolateral medulla receive input from both the vagal and the glossopharyngeal nerves and play an important role in mediating a variety of circulatory reflexes. The sympathetic system normally maintains some tonic vasoconstriction on the vascular tree. Loss of this tone following induction of anesthesia or sympathectomy frequently contributes to perioperative hypotension.

ARTERIAL BLOOD PRESSURE

Systemic blood flow is pulsatile in large arteries because of the heart's cyclic activity; by the time blood reaches the systemic capillaries, flow is continuous (laminar). The mean pressure in large arteries, which is normally about 95 mm Hg, falls nearly to zero in the large systemic veins that return blood to the heart. The largest

pressure drop, nearly 50%, is across the arterioles, which account for the majority of SVR.

MAP is proportionate to the product of SVR × CO. This relationship is based on an analogy to Ohm's law as applied to the circulation:

$$MAP - CVP \approx SVR \times CO$$

Because CVP is normally very small compared with MAP, the former can usually be ignored. From this relationship, it is readily apparent that hypotension is the result of a decrease in SVR, CO, or both: To maintain arterial blood pressure, a decrease in one must be compensated by an increase in the other. MAP can be measured as the integrated mean of the arterial pressure waveform. Alternatively, MAP may be estimated by the following formula:

$$MAP = Diastolic\ pressure + \frac{Pulse\ pressure}{3}$$

where pulse pressure is the difference between systolic and diastolic blood pressure. Arterial pulse pressure is directly related to stroke volume but is inversely proportional to the compliance of the arterial tree. Thus, decreases in pulse pressure may be due to a decrease in stroke volume, an increase in SVR, or both.

Transmission of the arterial wave from large arteries to smaller vessels in the periphery is faster than the actual velocity of blood; the wave travels at a rate 15 times the velocity of blood in the aorta. Moreover, reflections of the propagating waves off arterial walls widen pulse pressure before the pulse wave is completely dampened in very small arteries (see Chapter 6).

Control of Arterial Blood Pressure

Arterial blood pressure is regulated by a series of immediate, intermediate, and long-term adjustments that involve complex neural, humoral, and renal mechanisms.

A. IMMEDIATE CONTROL

Minute-to-minute control of blood pressure is primarily the function of autonomic nervous system reflexes. Changes in blood pressure are sensed both centrally (in hypothalamic and brain stem areas) and peripherally by specialized sensors (baroreceptors). Decreases in arterial blood pressure enhance sympathetic tone, increase adrenal secretion of epinephrine, and suppress vagal activity. **The resulting systemic vasoconstriction, elevation in heart rate, and enhanced cardiac contractility increase blood pressure.** Conversely, hypertension decreases sympathetic outflow and enhances vagal tone.

Peripheral baroreceptors are located at the bifurcation of the common carotid arteries and the aortic arch.

Elevations in blood pressure increase baroreceptor discharge, inhibiting systemic vasoconstriction and enhancing vagal tone (**baroreceptor reflex**). Reductions in blood pressure decrease baroreceptor discharge, allowing vasoconstriction and reduction of vagal tone. Carotid baroreceptors send afferent signals to circulatory brain stem centers via Hering's nerve (a branch of the glossopharyngeal nerve), whereas aortic baroreceptor afferent signals travel along the vagus nerve. Of the two peripheral sensors, the carotid baroreceptor is physiologically more important and is primarily responsible for minimizing changes in blood pressure that are caused by acute events, such as a change in posture. Carotid baroreceptors sense MAP most effectively between pressures of 80 and 160 mm Hg. Adaptation to changes in acute blood pressure occurs over the course of 1–2 days, rendering this reflex ineffective for long-term blood pressure control. All volatile anesthetics depress the normal baroreceptor response, but isoflurane and desflurane appear to have the least effect. Cardiopulmonary stretch receptors located in the atria, left ventricle, and pulmonary circulation can cause a similar effect.

B. Intermediate Control

In the course of a few minutes, sustained decreases in arterial pressure together with enhanced sympathetic outflow activate the renin–angiotensin–aldosterone system (see Chapter 31), increase secretion of arginine vasopressin (AVP), and alter normal capillary fluid exchange (see Chapter 28). Both angiotensin II and AVP are potent arteriolar vasoconstrictors. Their immediate action is to increase SVR. In contrast to formation of angiotensin II, however, moderate to marked hypotension is required for enough AVP secretion to produce vasoconstriction. Angiotensin constricts arterioles via AT_1 receptors. AVP mediates vasoconstriction via V_1 receptors and exerts its antidiuretic effect via V_2 receptors.

Sustained changes in arterial blood pressure can also alter fluid exchange in tissues by their secondary effects on capillary pressures. Hypertension increases interstitial movement of intravascular fluid, whereas hypotension increases reabsorption of interstitial fluid. Such compensatory changes in intravascular volume can reduce fluctuations in blood pressure, particularly in the absence of adequate renal function (see below).

C. Long-Term Control

The effects of slower renal mechanisms become apparent within hours of sustained changes in arterial pressure. As a result, the kidneys alter total body sodium and water balance to restore blood pressure to normal. Hypotension results in sodium (and water) retention, whereas hypertension generally increases sodium excretion in normal individuals (see Chapter 28).

ANATOMY & PHYSIOLOGY OF THE CORONARY CIRCULATION

1. Anatomy

Myocardial blood supply is derived entirely from the right and left coronary arteries (Figure 19–12). Blood flows from epicardial to endocardial vessels. After perfusing the myocardium, blood returns to the right atrium via the coronary sinus and the anterior cardiac veins. A small amount of blood returns directly into the chambers of the heart by way of the thebesian veins.

The right coronary artery (RCA) normally supplies the right atrium, most of the right ventricle, and a variable portion of the left ventricle (inferior wall). In 85% of persons, the RCA gives rise to the posterior descending artery (PDA), which supplies the superior–posterior interventricular septum and inferior wall—a right dominant circulation; in the remaining 15% of persons, the PDA is a branch of the left coronary artery—a left dominant circulation.

The left coronary artery normally supplies the left atrium and most of the interventricular septum and left ventricle (septal, anterior, and lateral walls). After a short course the left main coronary artery bifurcates into the left anterior descending artery (LAD) and the circumflex artery (CX); the LAD supplies the septum and anterior wall and the CX supplies the lateral wall. In a left dominant circulation, the CX wraps around the AV groove and continues down as the PDA to also supply most of the posterior septum and inferior wall.

The arterial supply to the SA node may be derived from either the RCA (60% of individuals) or the LAD (the remaining 40%). The AV node is usually supplied by the RCA (85–90%) or, less frequently, by the CX (10–15%); the bundle of His has a dual blood supply derived from the PDA and LAD. The anterior papillary muscle of the mitral valve also has a dual blood supply that is fed by diagonal branches of the LAD and marginal branches of the CX. In contrast, the posterior papillary of the mitral valve is usually supplied only by the PDA and is therefore much more vulnerable to ischemic dysfunction.

2. Determinants of Coronary Perfusion

Coronary perfusion is unique in that it is intermittent rather than continuous, as it is in other organs. During contraction, intramyocardial pressures in the left ventricle approach systemic arterial pressure. The force of left ventricular contraction almost completely occludes the intramyocardial part of the coronary arteries; in fact, blood flow may transiently reverse in epicardial vessels. Even during the latter part of diastole, left ventricular pressure eventually exceeds venous (right atrial) pressure. **Thus, coronary perfusion pressure is usually**

A. RIGHT ANTERIOR OBLIQUE VIEW

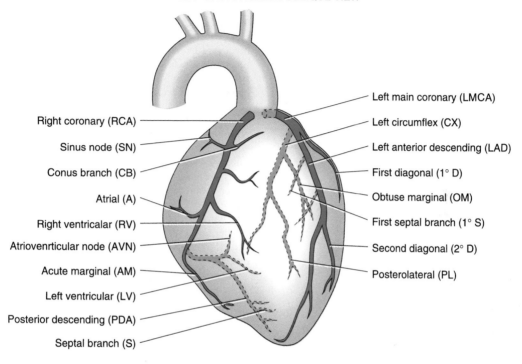

Left main coronary (LMCA)

Right coronary (RCA)

Left circumflex (CX)

Sinus node (SN)

Left anterior descending (LAD)

Conus branch (CB)

First diagonal (1° D)

Atrial (A)

Obtuse marginal (OM)

Right ventricalar (RV)

First septal branch (1° S)

Atriovenrticular node (AVN)

Second diagonal (2° D)

Acute marginal (AM)

Posterolateral (PL)

Left ventricular (LV)

Posterior descending (PDA)

Septal branch (S)

B. LEFT ANTERIOR OBLIQUE VIEW

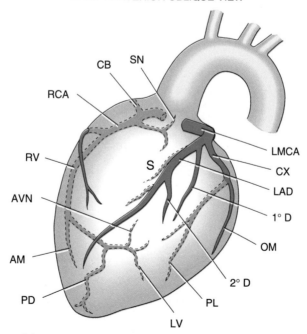

CB   SN

RCA

LMCA

RV

CX

LAD

S

AVN

1° D

OM

AM

2° D

PD

PL

LV

Figure 19–12. Anatomy of the coronary arteries in a patient with a right dominant circulation. *A:* Right anterior oblique view. *B:* Left anterior oblique view.

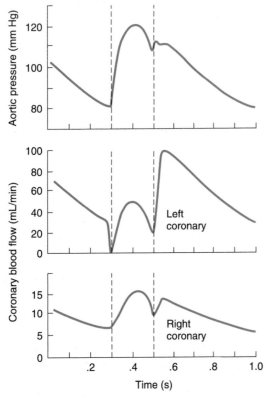

Figure 19–13. Coronary blood flow during the cardiac cycle. (Modified and reproduced, with permission, from Berne RM, Levy MD: *Cardiovascular Physiology*, 2nd ed. Mosby, 1972.)

Control of Coronary Blood Flow

Coronary blood flow normally parallels myocardial metabolic demand. In the average adult man, coronary blood flow is approximately 250 mL/min at rest. The myocardium regulates its own blood flow closely between perfusion pressures of 50 and 120 mm Hg. Beyond this range, blood flow becomes increasingly pressure dependent.

Under normal conditions, changes in blood flow are entirely due to variations in coronary arterial tone (resistance) in response to metabolic demand. Hypoxia—either directly, or indirectly through the release of adenosine—causes coronary vasodilation. Autonomic influences are generally weak. Both α_1- and β_2-adrenergic receptors are present in the coronary arteries. The α_1-receptors are primarily located on larger epicardial vessels, whereas the β_2-receptors are mainly found on the smaller intramuscular and subendocardial vessels. Sympathetic stimulation generally increases myocardial blood flow because of an increase in metabolic demand and a predominance of β_2-receptor activation. Parasympathetic effects on the coronary vasculature are generally minor and are weakly vasodilatory.

3. Myocardial Oxygen Balance

Myocardial oxygen demand is usually the most important determinant of myocardial blood flow. Relative contributions to oxygen requirements include basal requirements (20%), electrical activity (1%), volume work (15%), and pressure work (64%). The myocardium usually extracts 65% of the oxygen in arterial blood, compared with 25% in most other tissues (see Chapter 22). Coronary sinus oxygen saturation is

determined by the difference between aortic pressure and ventricular pressure, and the left ventricle is perfused almost entirely during diastole. In contrast, the right ventricle is perfused during both systole and diastole (Figure 19–13). Moreover, as a determinant of myocardial blood flow, arterial diastolic pressure is more important than mean arterial pressure:

$$\frac{\text{Coronary perfusion}}{\text{pressure}} = \frac{\text{Arterial}}{\text{diastolic} - \text{LVEDP}}_{\text{pressure}}$$

Decreases in aortic pressure or increases in ventricular end-diastolic pressure can reduce coronary perfusion pressure. Increases in heart rate also decrease coronary perfusion because of the disproportionately greater reduction in diastolic time as heart rate increases (Figure 19–14). Because it is subjected to the greatest intramural pressures during systole, the endocardium tends to be most vulnerable to ischemia during decreases in coronary perfusion pressure.

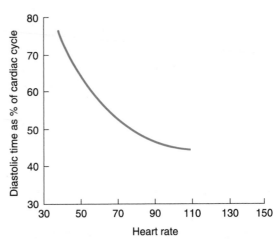

Figure 19–14. The relationship between diastolic time and heart rate.

Table 19–6. Factors affecting myocardial oxygen supply–demand balance.

Supply
Heart rate
Diastolic time
Coronary perfusion pressure
Aortic diastolic blood pressure
Ventricular end-diastolic pressure
Arterial oxygen content
Arterial oxygen tension
Hemoglobin concentration
Coronary vessel diameter
Demand
Basal requirements
Heart rate
Wall tension
Preload (ventricular radius)
Afterload
Contractility

usually 30%. Therefore, the myocardium (unlike other tissues) cannot compensate for reductions in blood flow by extracting more oxygen from hemoglobin. Any increases in myocardial metabolic demand must be met by an increase in coronary blood flow. Table 19–6 lists the most important factors in myocardial oxygen demand and supply. Note that the heart rate and, to a lesser extent, ventricular end-diastolic pressure are important determinants of both supply and demand.

Effects of Anesthetic Agents

Most volatile anesthetic agents are coronary vasodilators. Their effect on coronary blood flow is variable because of their direct vasodilating properties, reduction of myocardial metabolic requirements (and secondary decrease due to autoregulation), and effects on arterial blood pressure. Although the mechanism is not clear, it may involve activation of ATP-sensitive K$^+$ channels and stimulation of adenosine (A$_1$) receptors. Halothane and isoflurane appear to have the greatest effect; the former primarily affects large coronary vessels, whereas the latter affects mostly smaller vessels. Vasodilation due to desflurane appears to be primarily autonomically mediated, whereas sevoflurane appears to lack coronary vasodilating properties. Dose-dependent abolition of autoregulation may be greatest with isoflurane. Evidence that volatile anesthetics cause a coronary steal phenomenon in humans is lacking.

Volatile agents appear to exert beneficial effects in the setting of myocardial ischemia and infarction. They not only reduce myocardial oxygen requirements but appear to be protective against reperfusion injury; these effects may also be mediated by activation of ATP-

sensitive K$^+$ channels. Some evidence also suggests that volatile anesthetics enhance recovery of the "stunned" myocardium. Moreover, even though they decrease myocardial contractility, they can potentially be beneficial in patients with heart failure because they decrease preload and afterload.

■ THE PATHOPHYSIOLOGY OF HEART FAILURE

Systolic heart failure occurs when the heart is unable to pump a sufficient amount of blood to meet the body's metabolic requirements. Clinical manifestations usually reflect the effects of the low cardiac output on tissues (eg, fatigue, oxygen debt, acidosis), the damming-up of blood behind the failing ventricle (systemic or pulmonary venous congestion), or both. The left ventricle is most commonly involved, often with secondary involvement of the right ventricle. Isolated right ventricular failure can occur in the setting of advanced disease of the lung parenchyma or pulmonary vasculature. Left ventricular failure most commonly results from primary myocardial dysfunction (usually from coronary artery disease), but may also result from valvular dysfunction, arrhythmias, or pericardial disease.

Diastolic dysfunction can also cause symptoms of heart failure as a result of atrial hypertension (Figure 19–15). Common causes include hypertension, coronary artery disease, hypertrophic cardiomyopathy, and pericardial disease. Although diastolic dysfunction can cause symptoms of heart failure even in the presence of normal systolic function, systolic and diastolic dysfunction are commonly associated.

Cardiac output is reduced in most forms of heart failure. Inadequate oxygen delivery to tissues is reflected by a low mixed venous oxygen tension and an increase in the arteriovenous oxygen content difference (see Chapter 22). In compensated heart failure, the arteriovenous difference may be normal at rest, but it rapidly widens during stress or exercise.

Heart failure is less commonly associated with an elevated cardiac output. This form of heart failure is most often seen with sepsis and other hypermetabolic states, which are typically associated with a low SVR.

COMPENSATORY MECHANISMS

Major compensatory mechanisms generally present in patients with heart failure include increased preload, increased sympathetic tone, activation of the renin–angiotensin–aldosterone system, release of AVP, and ventricular hypertrophy. Although these mechanisms

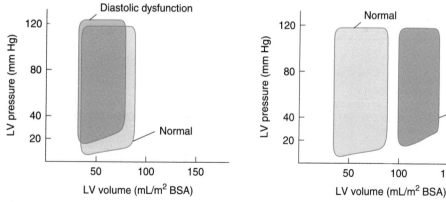

Figure 19–15. Ventricular pressure–volume relationships in isolated systolic and diastolic dysfunction. (Modified and reproduced, with permission, from Zile MR: Mod Concepts Cardiovasc Dis 1990;59:1.)

can initially compensate for mild to moderate cardiac dysfunction, with increasing severity of dysfunction they may actually contribute to the cardiac impairment.

Increased Preload

An increase in ventricular size not only reflects an inability to keep up with venous return but also serves to maximize stroke volume by moving the heart up the Starling curve (see Figure 19–6). Even when EF is reduced, an increase in ventricular end-diastolic volume can maintain a normal stroke volume. Worsening venous congestion caused by the damming-up of blood behind the failing ventricle and excessive ventricular dilatation can rapidly lead to clinical deterioration. Left ventricular failure results in pulmonary vascular congestion and progressive transudation of fluid, first into the pulmonary interstitium and then into alveoli (pulmonary edema). Right ventricular failure leads to systemic venous hypertension, which results in peripheral edema, hepatic congestion and dysfunction, and ascites. Dilatation of the annulus of either AV valve leads to valvular regurgitation, further impairing ventricular output.

Increased Sympathetic Tone

Sympathetic activation increases release of norepinephrine from nerve endings in the heart and the adrenal secretion of epinephrine into the circulation. Plasma catecholamine levels are generally directly proportional to the degree of left ventricular dysfunction. Although enhanced sympathetic outflow can initially maintain cardiac output by increasing heart rate and contractility, worsening ventricular function elicits increasing degrees of vasoconstriction in an effort to maintain arterial blood pressure. The associated increase in after-

load, however, reduces cardiac output and exacerbates the ventricular failure.

Chronic sympathetic activation in patients with heart failure eventually decreases the response of adrenergic receptors to catecholamines (down-regulation), the number of receptors, and cardiac catecholamine stores. Nonetheless, the failing heart becomes increasingly dependent on circulating catecholamines. Abrupt withdrawal in sympathetic outflow or decreases in circulating catecholamine levels, such as can occur following induction of anesthesia, may lead to acute cardiac decompensation. A reduced density of M_2 receptors also decreases parasympathetic influences on the heart.

Sympathetic activation tends to redistribute systemic blood flow output away from the skin, gut, kidneys, and skeletal muscle to the heart and brain. Decreased renal perfusion together with β_1-adrenergic activity at the juxtaglomerular apparatus activate the renin–angiotensin–aldosterone axis (see Chapter 28), which leads to sodium retention and interstitial edema. Moreover, vasoconstriction secondary to elevated angiotensin II levels increases left ventricular afterload and causes further deterioration of systolic function. The latter accounts for the efficacy of angiotensin-converting enzyme inhibitors in heart failure. Symptoms may also improve in some patients with careful, low-dose β-adrenergic blockade.

Circulating AVP levels are often twice normal levels in patients with severe heart failure. Elevations in AVP also increase ventricular afterload and are responsible for a defect in free water clearance that is commonly associated with hyponatremia (see Chapter 28).

Atrial natriuretic peptide is found predominantly in atrial tissue. This hormone is released in response to atrial distention and has salutary effects in heart failure.

It is a potent vasodilator and has properties that antagonize the effects of angiotensin, aldosterone, and AVP.

Ventricular Hypertrophy

Ventricular hypertrophy can occur with or without dilatation, depending on the type of stress imposed on the ventricle. When the heart is subjected to either pressure or volume overload, the initial response is to increase sarcomere length and optimally overlap actin and myosin. With time, ventricular muscle mass begins to increase in response to the abnormal stress.

In the volume-overloaded ventricle, the problem is an increase in diastolic wall stress. The increase in ventricular muscle mass is sufficient only to compensate for the increase in diameter: The ratio of the ventricular radius to wall thickness is unchanged. Sarcomeres replicate mainly in series, resulting in eccentric hypertrophy. Although ventricular EF remains depressed, the increase in end-diastolic volume can maintain normal at-rest stroke volume (and cardiac output).

The problem in a pressure-overloaded ventricle is an increase in systolic wall stress. Sarcomeres in this case mainly replicate in parallel, resulting in concentric hypertrophy: The hypertrophy is such that the ratio of myocardial wall thickness to ventricular radius increases. As can be seen from Laplace's law, systolic wall stress can then be normalized. Ventricular hypertrophy, particularly that caused by pressure overload, usually results in progressive diastolic dysfunction.

CASE DISCUSSION: A PATIENT WITH A SHORT P–R INTERVAL

A 38-year-old man is scheduled for endoscopic sinus surgery following a recent onset of headaches. He gives a history of having passed out at least once during one of these headaches. A preoperative electrocardiogram (ECG) is normal except for a P–R interval of 0.116 s with normal P-wave morphology.

What is the significance of the short P–R interval?

The P–R interval, which is measured from the beginning of atrial depolarization (P wave) to the beginning of ventricular depolarization (QRS complex), usually represents the time required for depolarization of both atria, the AV node, and the His–Purkinje system. Although the P–R interval can vary with heart rate, it is normally 0.12–0.2 s in duration. Abnormally short P–R intervals can be seen with either low atrial

(or upper AV junctional) rhythms or preexcitation phenomena. The two can usually be differentiated by P-wave morphology: With a low atrial rhythm, atrial depolarization is retrograde, resulting in an inverted P wave in leads II, III, and aVF; with preexcitation, the P wave is normal during sinus rhythm. If the pacemaker rhythm originates from a lower AV junctional focus, the P wave may be lost in the QRS complex or may follow the QRS.

What is preexcitation?

*Preexcitation usually refers to early depolarization of the ventricles by an abnormal conduction pathway from the atria. Rarely, more than one such pathway is present. The most common form of preexcitation is due to the presence of an accessory pathway (bundle of Kent) that connects one of the atria with one of the ventricles. This abnormal connection between the atria and ventricles allows electrical impulses to bypass the AV node (hence the term bypass tract). The ability to conduct impulses along the bypass tract can be quite variable and may be only intermittent or rate dependent. Bypass tracts can conduct in both directions, retrograde only (ventricle to atrium) or, rarely, anterograde only (atrium to ventricle). The name **Wolff–Parkinson–White (WPW) syndrome** is often applied to ventricular preexcitation associated with tachyarrhythmias.*

How does preexcitation shorten the P–R interval?

In patients with preexcitation, the normal cardiac impulse originating from the SA node is conducted simultaneously through the normal (AV nodal) and anomalous (bypass-tract) pathways. Because conduction is more rapid in the anomalous pathway than in the AV nodal pathway, the cardiac impulse rapidly reaches and depolarizes the area of the ventricles where the bypass tract ends. This early depolarization of the ventricle is reflected by a short P–R interval and a slurred initial deflection (δ wave) in the QRS complex. The spread of the anomalous impulse to the rest of the ventricle is delayed because it must be conducted by ordinary ventricular muscle, not by the much faster Purkinje system. The remainder of the ventricle is then depolarized by the normal impulse from the AV node as it catches up with the preexcitation front. Although the P–R interval is shortened, the resulting QRS is slightly prolonged and repre-

sents a fusion complex of normal and abnormal ventricular depolarizations.

The P–R interval in patients with preexcitation depends on relative conduction times between the AV nodal pathway and the bypass pathway. If conduction through the former is fast, preexcitation (and the δ wave) is less prominent, and QRS will be relatively normal. If conduction is delayed in the AV nodal pathway, preexcitation is more prominent, and more of the ventricle will be depolarized by the abnormally conducted impulse. When the AV nodal pathway is completely blocked, the entire ventricle is depolarized by the bypass pathway, resulting in a very short P–R interval, a very prominent δ wave, and a wide, bizarre QRS complex. Other factors that can affect the degree of preexcitation include interatrial conduction time, the distance of the atrial end of the bypass tract from the SA node, and autonomic tone. The P–R interval is often normal or only slightly shortened with a left lateral bypass tract (the most common location). Preexcitation may be more apparent at fast heart rates because conduction slows through the AV node with increasing heart rates. Secondary ST-segment and T-wave changes are also common because of abnormal ventricular repolarization.

What is the clinical significance of preexcitation?

Preexcitation occurs in approximately 0.3% of the general population. An estimated 20–50% of affected persons develop paroxysmal tachyarrhythmias, typically paroxysmal supraventricular tachycardia (PSVT). Although most patients are otherwise normal, preexcitation can be associated with other cardiac anomalies, including Ebstein's anomaly, mitral valve prolapse, and cardiomyopathies. Depending on its conductive properties, the bypass tract in some patients may predispose them to tachyarrhythmias and even sudden death. Tachyarrhythmias include PSVT, atrial fibrillation, and, less commonly, atrial flutter. Ventricular fibrillation can be precipitated by a critically timed premature atrial beat that travels down the bypass tract and catches the ventricle at a vulnerable period. Alternatively, very rapid conduction of impulses into the ventricles by the bypass tract during atrial fibrillation can rapidly lead to myocardial ischemia, hypoperfusion, and hypoxia and culminate in ventricular fibrillation.

Recognition of the preexcitation phenomenon is also important because its QRS morphology on the surface ECG can mimic bundle branch block, right ventricular hypertrophy, ischemia, myocardial infarction, and ventricular tachycardia (during atrial fibrillation).

What is the significance of the history of syncope in this patient?

This patient should be evaluated preoperatively by a cardiologist for possible electrophysiological studies, curative radiofrequency ablation of the bypass tract, and the need for perioperative drug therapy. Such studies can identify the location of the bypass tracts, reasonably predict the potential for malignant arrhythmias by programmed pacing, and assess the efficacy of antiarrhythmic therapy if curative ablation is not possible; ablation is reported to be curative in over 90% of patients. A history of syncope may be ominous because it may indicate the ability to conduct impulses very rapidly through the bypass tract, leading to systemic hypoperfusion and perhaps predisposing the patient to sudden death.

Patients with only occasional asymptomatic tachyarrhythmias generally do not require investigation or prophylactic drug therapy. Those with frequent episodes of tachyarrhythmias or arrhythmias associated with significant symptoms require drug therapy and close evaluation.

How do tachyarrhythmias generally develop?

Tachyarrhythmias develop as a result of either abnormal impulse formation or abnormal impulse propagation (reentry). Abnormal impulses result from enhanced automaticity, abnormal automaticity, or triggered activity. Usually, only cells of the SA node, specialized atrial conduction pathways, AV nodal junctional areas, and the His–Purkinje system depolarize spontaneously. Because diastolic repolarization (phase 4) is fastest in the SA node, other areas of automaticity are suppressed. Enhanced or abnormal automaticity in other areas, however, can usurp pacemaker function from the SA node and lead to tachyarrhythmias. Triggered activity is the result of either early afterdepolarizations (phase 2 or 3) or delayed afterdepolarizations (after phase 3). It consists of small-amplitude depolarizations that can follow action potentials under some conditions in atrial,

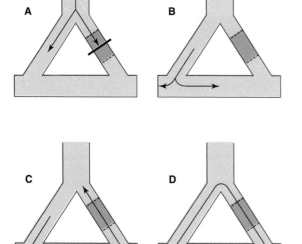

Figure 19–16. **A–D:** The mechanism of reentry. See text for description.

ventricular, and His–Purkinje tissue. If these after-depolarizations reach threshold potential, they can result in an extrasystole or repetitive sustained tachyarrhythmias. Factors that can promote the formation of abnormal impulses include increased catecholamine levels, electrolyte disorders (hyperkalemia, hypokalemia, and hypercalcemia), ischemia, hypoxia, mechanical stretch, and drug toxicity (particularly digoxin).

The most common mechanism for tachyarrhythmias is reentry. Four conditions are necessary to initiate and sustain reentry (Figure 19–16): (1) two areas in the myocardium that differ in conductivity or refractoriness and that can form a closed electrical loop; (2) unidirectional block in one pathway (Figure 19–16A and B); (3) slow conduction or sufficient length in the circuit to allow recovery of the conduction block in the first pathway (Figure 19–16C); and (4) excitation of the initially blocked pathway to complete the loop (Figure 19–16D). Reentry is usually precipitated by a premature cardiac impulse.

What is the mechanism of PSVT in patients with WPW syndrome?

If the bypass tract is refractory during anterograde conduction of a cardiac impulse, as during a critically timed atrial premature contraction (APC), and the impulse is conducted by the AV node, the same impulse can be conducted retrograde from the ventricle back into the atria via the bypass tract. The retrograde impulse can then depolarize the atrium and travel down the AV nodal pathway again, establishing a continuous repetitive circuit (circus movement). The impulse reciprocates between the atria and ventricles and conduction alternates between the AV nodal pathway and the bypass tract. The term concealed conduction is often applied because the absence of preexcitation during this arrhythmia results in a normal QRS that lacks a δ wave.

The circus movement less commonly involves anterograde conduction through the bypass tract and retrograde conduction through the AV nodal pathway. In such instances, the QRS has a δ wave and is completely abnormal; the arrhythmia can be mistaken for ventricular tachycardia.

What other mechanisms may be responsible for PSVT?

In addition to the WPW syndrome, PSVT can be caused by AV reentrant tachycardia, AV nodal reentrant tachycardia, and SA node and atrial reentrant tachycardias. Patients with AV reentrant tachycardia have an extranodal bypass tract similar to patients with WPW syndrome, but the bypass tract conducts only retrograde; preexcitation and a δ wave are absent. The PSVT may be initiated either by an APC or a ventricular premature contraction (VPC). A retrograde P wave is usually visible because atrial depolarization always follows ventricular depolarization.

Functional differences in conduction and refractoriness may occur within the AV node, SA node, or atria; a large bypass tract is not necessary. Thus the circus movement may occur on a smaller scale within the AV node, SA node, or atria, respectively. PSVT is always induced during AV nodal reentry by an APC with a prolonged P–R interval; a retrograde P wave is either absent or buried in the QRS complex. Another APC may terminate the arrhythmia.

PSVT associated with SA node or atrial reentry is always triggered by an APC. The P wave is usually visible and has a prolonged P–R interval. Its morphology is normal with SA nodal reentry and abnormal with atrial reentry.

How does atrial fibrillation in patients with WPW syndrome differ from the arrhythmia in other patients?

Atrial fibrillation can occur when a cardiac impulse is conducted rapidly retrograde up into the atria and arrives to find different parts of the atria out of phase in recovery from the impulse. Once atrial fibrillation is established, conduction into the ventricles most commonly occurs through the bypass tract only; because of the accessory pathway's ability to conduct very rapidly (unlike the AV nodal pathway), the ventricular rate is typically very rapid (180–300 beats/min). The majority of QRS complexes are bizarre, but periodic conduction of an impulse through the AV nodal pathway results in occasional normal-looking QRS complexes. Less commonly, impulses during atrial fibrillation are conducted mainly through the AV nodal pathway (resulting in mostly normal QRS complexes) or through both the bypass tract and the AV nodal pathway (resulting in a mixture of normal, fusion, and bizarre QRS complexes). As stated previously, atrial fibrillation in patients with WPW syndrome is a very dangerous arrhythmia.

What anesthetic agents can safely be used in patients with preexcitation?

*Few data are available comparing the use of different anesthetic agents or techniques in patients with preexcitation. Almost all the volatile and intravenous agents have been used with equal success. Volatile anesthetics increase antegrade refractoriness in both normal and accessory pathways (enflurane > isoflurane > halothane) and increase the coupling interval (a measure of the ability of an extrasystole to induce tachycardia). Propofol, opioids, and benzodiazepines appear to have little direct electrophysiological effects but can alter autonomic tone, generally reducing sympathetic outflow. Factors that tend to cause sympathetic stimulation and increased cardiac automaticity are undesirable. Premedication with a benzodiazepine helps reduce high sympathetic tone preoperatively. Agents that can increase sympathetic tone, such as ketamine and perhaps pancuronium in large bolus doses, should generally be avoided. Anticholinergics should be used cautiously; glycopyrrolate may be preferable to atropine (see Chapter 11). Endotracheal intubation should be carried out only after the patient is deeply anesthetized (see Chapter 20); pretreatment with a β-adrenergic blocker such as esmolol may be useful. Light anesthesia, hypercapnia, acidosis, and even transient hy-*poxia will activate the sympathetic system and are to be avoided. A deep extubation and good postoperative analgesia (without respiratory acidosis) may also help prevent the onset of arrhythmias. When patients with preexcitation are anesthetized for electrophysiological study and surgical ablation, opioids, propofol, and benzodiazepines may be the agents least likely to alter conduction characteristics.*

How are antiarrhythmic agents selected for tachyarrhythmias?

Most antiarrhythmic agents act by altering myocardial cell conduction (phase 0), repolarization (phase 3), or automaticity (phase 4). Prolongation of repolarization increases the refractoriness of cells. Many antiarrhythmic drugs also exert direct or indirect autonomic effects. Although antiarrhythmic agents are generally classified according to broad mechanisms of action or electrophysiological effects (Table 19–7), the most commonly used classification system is not perfect because some agents have more than one mechanism of action. Moreover, newer agents have very specific and unique actions; for example, dofetilide acts on the delayed rectifying potassium channels.

Selection of an antiarrhythmic agent generally depends on whether the arrhythmia is ventricular or supraventricular and whether acute control or chronic therapy is required. Intravenous agents are usually employed in the acute management of arrhythmias, whereas oral agents are reserved for chronic therapy (Table 19–8).

Which agents are most useful for tachyarrhythmias in patients with WPW syndrome?

Cardioversion (see Chapter 47) is the treatment of choice in hemodynamically compromised patients. Adenosine is the drug of choice for PSVT because of its short duration of action. Small doses of phenylephrine (100 μg) together with vagal maneuvers (carotid massage) help support arterial blood pressure and may terminate the arrhythmia. The most useful pharmacological agents are class Ia drugs, particularly procainamide. These agents increase the refractory period and decrease conduction in the accessory pathway. Moreover, class Ia drugs frequently terminate and can suppress the recurrence of PSVT and atrial fibrillation. Class Ic drugs and amiodarone are also useful because they slow conduction and prolong refractoriness in both the AV node and the accessory

Table 19–7. Classification of antiarrhythmic agents.[1]

Class	Mechanism of Action	Agents	Intravenous Loading Dose
I	Blocks fast sodium channels; decreases slope of phase 0 (V_{max})		
Ia	Moderate depression of V_{max}, prolongs APD	Quinidine[2–4] Procainamide (Pronestyl)[1,4] Disopyramide (Norpace)[1,4]	NR 5–10 mg/kg NA
Ib	Minimal effect on V_{max}, shorten APD	Lidocaine Phenytoin Tocainide (Tonocard) Mexiletine (Mexitil) Moricizine (Ethmozine)	1–2 mg/kg 5–15 mg/kg NA NA NA
Ic	Marked depression of V_{max}, minimal effect of APD	Flecainide (Tambacor) Propafenone (Rythmol)	NA NA
II	Blocks β-adrenergic receptors	Propranolol (Inderal) Esmolol (Brevibloc) Metoprolol (Lopressor)	1–3 mg 0.5 mg/kg 5–10 mg
III	Prolongs repolarization	Amiodarone (Cordarone)[5–7] Bretylium[8] Sotalol (Betapace)[9] Ibutilide (Corvert) Dofetilide (Tikosyn)	150 mg 5–10 mg/kg NA 1 mg NA
IV	Blocks slow calcium channels	Verapamil (Calan) Diltiazem (Cardizem)	2.5–10 mg 0.25–0.35 mg/kg
V	Various (miscellaneous agents)	Digoxin Adenosine (Adenocard)	0.5–0.75 mg 6–12 mg

[1]V_{max}, maximum velocity; APD, action potential duration; NR, not recommended; NA, not available for intravenous use.
[2]Also has antimuscarinic (vagolytic activity).
[3]Also blocks α-adrenergic receptors.
[4]Also prolongs repolarization.
[5]Also binds inactivated fast sodium channels.
[6]Also causes noncompetitive α- and β-adrenergic blockade.
[7]Also blocks slow calcium channels.
[8]Transiently releases catecholamine stores from nerve endings.
[9]Also has nonselective β-adrenergic blocking activity.

pathway. β-Adrenergic blocking agents may also be useful, particularly in controlling ventricular rate once these rhythms are established. Verapamil and digoxin are contraindicated during atrial fibrillation or flutter in these patients because they can dangerously accelerate the ventricular response. Both types of agents decrease conduction through the AV node, favoring conduction of impulses down the accessory pathway. The bypass tract is capable of conducting impulses into the ventricles much faster than the AV nodal pathway. Digoxin may also increase the ventricular response by shortening the refractory period and increasing conduction in accessory pathways. Although verapamil can terminate PSVT, its use in this setting may be hazardous because patients can subsequently develop atrial fibrillation or flutter. Moreover, atrial fibrillation may not be readily distinguishable from ventricular tachycardia in these patients if wide-QRS tachycardia develops. Procainamide may be preferable to lidocaine in such instances, because it is generally effective for both arrhythmias.

Table 19–8. Clinical pharmacological properties of antiarrhythmic drugs.[1]

Drug	Effect on SA Nodal Rate	Effect on AV Nodal Refractory Period	PR Interval	QRS Duration	QT Interval	Usefulness in Arrhythmias		Half-Life
						Supraventricular	Ventricular	
Adenosine	Little	↑↑↑	↑↑↑	0	0	++++	?	< 10 s
Amiodarone	↓↓[2]	↑↑	↑↑	↑	↑↑↑↑	+++	+++	(Weeks)
Bretylium	↑↓[3]	↑↓[3]	0	0	0	0	+	4 h
Diltiazem	↑↓	↑↑	↑	0	0	+++	−	4–8 h
Disopyramide	↑↓[2,4]	↑↓[4]	↑↓[4]	↑↑	↑↑	+	+++	6–8 h
Dofetilide	↓(?)	0	0	0	↑↑	++	None	7 h
Esmolol	↓↓	↑↑	↑↑	0	0	+	+	10 min
Flecainide	None	↑	↑	↑↑↑	0	+[5]	++++	20 h
Ibutilide	↓(?)	0	0	0	↑↑	++	?	6 h
Lidocaine	None[2]	None	0	0	0	None[6]	+++	1–2 h
Mexiletine	None[2]	None	0	0	0	None[7]	+++	12 h
Moricizine	None	None	↑	↑↑	0	None	+++	2–6 h[7]
Procainamide	↓[2]	↑↓[4]	↑↓[4]	↑↑	↑↑	+	+++	3–4 h
Propafenone	0	↑	↑	↑↑↑	0	+	+++	5–7 h
Propranolol	↓↓	↑↑	↑↑	0	0	+	+	8 h
Quinidine	↑↓[2,4]	↑↓[4]	↑↓[4]	↑↑	↑↑	+	+++	6 h
Sotalol	↓↓	↑↑	↑↑	0	↑↑↑	+++	+++	7 h
Tocainide	None[2]	None	0	0	0	None[6]	+++	12 h
Verapamil	↓↓	↑↑	↑↑	0	0	+++	−	7 h

[1]From Katzung BG: *Basic and Clinical Pharmacology*, 8th ed. McGraw-Hill, 2001.
[2]May suppress diseased sinus nodes.
[3]Initial stimulation by release of endogenous norepinephrine followed by depression.
[4]Anticholingergic effect and direct depressant action.
[5]Particularly in Wolff–Parkinson–White syndrome.
[6]May be effective in atrial arrhythmias caused by digitalis.
[7]Half-life of active metabolites is much longer.

SUGGESTED READING

Balser JR: The rational use of intravenous amiodarone in the perioperative period. Anesthesiology 1997;86:974.

Colson P, Ryckwaert F, Coriat P: Renin angiotensin system antagonists and anesthesia. Anesth Analg 1999;89:1143.

Ganong WF: *Review of Medical Physiology,* 21st ed. McGraw-Hill, 2003.

Gomez MN: Magnesium and cardiovascular disease. Anesthesiology 1998;89:222.

Jacobsohn E, Chorn R, O'Connor M: The role of the vasculature in regulating venous return and cardiac output: Historical and graphical approach. Can J Anaesth 1997;44:849.

Ross S, Foex P: Protective effects of anaesthetics in reversible and irreversible ischemia-reperfusion injury. Br J Anaesth 1999;82:622.

Van Gelder IC, Tuinenburg AE, Schoonderwoerd BS, et al: Pharmacologic versus direct-current electrical cardioversion of atrial flutter and fibrillation. Am J Cardiol 1999;84:147R.

Yost CS: Potassium channels. Basic aspects, functional roles and medical significance. Anesthesiology 1999;90:1186.

Anesthesia for Patients with Cardiovascular Disease

20

KEY CONCEPTS

 Cardiovascular complications account for 25–50% of deaths following noncardiac surgery. Perioperative myocardial infarction (MI), pulmonary edema, congestive heart failure (CHF), arrhythmias, and thromboembolism are most commonly seen in patients with preexisting cardiovascular disease.

The two most important preoperative risk factors are an unstable coronary syndrome and evidence of CHF. Generally accepted contraindications to elective noncardiac surgery include a myocardial infarction less than 1 month prior to surgery with evidence of persistent ischemic risk by symptoms or noninvasive testing, uncompensated heart failure, and severe aortic or mitral stenosis.

 Regardless of the level of preoperative blood pressure control, many patients with hypertension display an accentuated hypotensive response to induction of anesthesia, followed by an exaggerated hypertensive response to intubation. Hypertensive patients may display an exaggerated response to both endogenous catecholamines (from intubation or surgical stimulation) and exogenously administered sympathetic agonists.

 Patients with extensive (three-vessel or left main) coronary artery disease, a history of MI, or ventricular dysfunction are at greatest risk for cardiac complications. Perioperative risk following MI appears to be related to the amount of residual ischemia remaining (additional myocardium at risk of infarction).

 Holter monitoring, exercise electrocardiography, myocardial perfusion scans, and echocardiography are important in determining perioperative risk and the need for coronary angiography. But these tests are indicated only if their outcome would alter patient care.

 Sudden withdrawal of antianginal medication perioperatively—particularly β-blockers—can precipitate a sudden increase in ischemic episodes (rebound).

 The overwhelming priority in managing patients with ischemic heart disease is maintaining a favorable myocardial supply–demand relationship. Autonomic-mediated increases in heart rate and blood pressure should be controlled by deep anesthesia or adrenergic blockade, and excessive reductions in coronary perfusion pressure or arterial oxygen content are to be avoided.

 Intraoperative detection of ischemia depends on recognition of electrocardiographic changes, hemodynamic manifestations, or regional wall motion abnormalities on transesophageal echocardiography. Down-sloping and horizontal ST depression are of greater specificity for ischemia than up-sloping depression. New ST-segment elevations are rare during noncardiac surgery and are indicative of severe ischemia, vasospasm, or infarction.

(continued on next page)

(continued from previous page)

 The principal hemodynamic goals in managing mitral stenosis are to maintain a sinus rhythm (if present preoperatively) and to avoid tachycardia, large increases in cardiac output, and both hypovolemia and fluid overload by judicious fluid therapy.

 Anesthetic management should be tailored to the severity of mitral regurgitation as well as the underlying left ventricular function. Factors that exacerbate the regurgitation, such as slow heart rates (long systole) and acute increases in afterload, should be avoided. Excessive volume expansion can also worsen the regurgitation by dilating the left ventricle.

 Maintenance of normal sinus rhythm, heart rate, and intravascular volume is critical in patients with aortic stenosis. Loss of a normally timed atrial systole often leads to rapid deterioration, particularly when associated with tachycardia. Spinal and epidural anesthesia are contraindicated in patients with severe aortic stenosis.

 Bradycardia and increase in systemic vascular resistance (SVR) increase the regurgitant volume in patients with aortic regurgitation, whereas tachycardia can contribute to myocardial ischemia. Excessive myocardial depression should also be avoided. The compensatory increase in cardiac preload should be maintained, but overzealous fluid replacement can readily result in pulmonary edema.

 In patients with congenital heart disease, an increase in SVR relative to pulmonary vascular resistance (PVR) favors left-to-right shunting, whereas an increase in PVR relative to SVR favors right-to-left shunting.

 The presence of shunt flow between the right and left hearts, regardless of the direction of blood flow, mandates the meticulous exclusion of air bubbles or clot from intravenous fluids to prevent paradoxical embolism into the cerebral or coronary circulations.

 The goals of anesthetic management in patients with tetralogy of Fallot should be to maintain intravascular volume and SVR. Increases in PVR, such as might occur from acidosis or excessive airway pressures, should be avoided. The right-to-left shunting tends to slow the uptake of inhalation anesthetics; in contrast, it may accelerate the onset of intravenous agents.

The transplanted heart is totally denervated, so direct autonomic influences are absent. Moreover, the absence of reflex increases in heart rate can make patients particularly sensitive to rapid vasodilation. Indirect vasopressors such as ephedrine and dopamine are less effective than direct-acting agents because of the absence of catecholamine stores in myocardial neurons.

Cardiovascular diseases—particularly hypertensive, ischemic, and valvular heart disease—are the medical illnesses most frequently encountered in anesthetic practice and a major cause of perioperative morbidity and mortality. Management of patients with these diseases continues to challenge the ingenuity and resources of the anesthesiologist. The adrenergic response to surgical stimulation and the circulatory effects of anesthetic agents, endotracheal intubation, positive-pressure ventilation, blood loss, fluid shifts, and alterations in body temperature impose additional burdens on an often already compromised cardiovascular system. Most anesthetic agents cause cardiac depression, vasodilation, or both. Even anesthetics that have no direct circulatory effects may cause apparent circulatory depression in severely compromised patients who are dependent on chronically enhanced sympathetic activity. Interruption of this activity as a consequence of the anesthetized state can lead to acute circulatory decompensation.

Optimal anesthetic management of patients with cardiovascular disease requires a thorough knowledge of normal cardiac physiology (see Chapter 19), the circulatory effects of the various anesthetic agents (see Chapters 7–10), and the pathophysiology and treatment of these diseases. The same principles used in treating these diseases preoperatively should be applied intraoperatively. In most instances, the choice of anesthetic agent is not as important as how the agent is used and an understanding of the underlying pathophysiology.

Table 20–1. Clinical predictors of increased perioperative cardiovascular risk (myocardial infarction, heart failure, death).[1,2]

Major

Unstable coronary syndromes

    Acute or recent MI[3] with evidence of important ischemic risk by clinical symptoms or noninvasive study

    Unstable or severe[4] angina (Canadian class III and IV)[5]

Decompensated heart failure

Significant arrhythmias

    High-grade atrioventricular block

    Symptomatic ventricular arrhythmias in the presence of underlying heart disease

    Supraventricular arrhythmias with uncontrolled ventricular rate

Severe valvular disease

Intermediate

Mild angina pectoris (Canadian class I or II)

Previous MI by history or pathological Q waves

Compensated or prior heart failure

Diabetes mellitus (particularly insulin dependent)

Renal insufficiency

Minor

Advanced age

Abnormal ECG (left ventricular hypertrophy, left bundle-branch block, ST-T abnormalities)

Rhythm other than sinus (eg, atrial fibrillation)

Low functional capacity (eg, inability to climb one flight of stairs with a bag of groceries)

History of stroke

Uncontrolled systemic hypertension

---

[1]From ACC/AHA Guideline Update on Perioperative Cardiovascular Evaluation for Noncardiac Surgery.

[2]ECG, electrocardiogram; MI, myocardial infarction.

[3]The American College of Cardiology National Database Library defines recent MI as greater than 7 days but less than or equal to 1 month (30 days); acute MI is within 7 days.

[4]May include "stable" angina in patients who are unusually sedentary.

[5]Campeau L: Grading of angina pectoris. Circulation 1976;54:522.

■ CARDIAC RISK FACTORS

The prevalence of cardiovascular disease increases progressively with advancing age. Moreover, the number of patients over 65 years of age is expected to increase by 25–35% over the next two decades. Perioperative myocardial infarction (MI), pulmonary edema, congestive heart failure, arrhythmias, and thromboembolism are most commonly seen in patients with preexisting cardiovascular disease. Cardiovascular complications account for 25–50% of deaths following noncardiac surgery. The incidence of postoperative cardiogenic pulmonary edema is approximately 2% in all patients over 40 years, but it is 6% in patients with a history of heart failure and 16% in patients with poorly compensated heart failure. The relatively high prevalence of cardiovascular disorders in surgical patients has given rise to attempts to define *cardiac risk* or the likelihood of intraoperative or postoperative fatal or life-threatening cardiac complications.

An American College of Cardiology/American Heart Association Task Force Report has divided clinical markers of increased cardiovascular risk into major, intermediate, and minor predictors (Table 20–1). Major predictors mandate intensive management, intermediate predictors are markers of enhanced risk and require careful preoperative assessment, and minor predictors are recognized markers of cardiovascular disease that have not clearly been shown to independently increase perioperative risk. Patients with major predictors should undergo noninvasive cardiac evaluation and, when appropriate, as discussed later in the chapter, coronary angiography. The majority of patients with predictors of increased cardiovascular risk fall into the intermediate and minor categories. A simplified management scheme (Figure 20–1) calls for noninvasive cardiac testing if patients have two of the three clinical criteria in listed in Table 20–2.

The two most important preoperative risk factors are an unstable coronary syndrome and evidence of congestive heart failure. Identifying patients at greatest risk allows appropriate measures to be taken that may alter the outcome favorably. Indeed, some studies suggest that a lower complication rate is achieved when invasive monitoring and aggressive hemodynamic interventions (eg, vasodilators, adrenergic blockade) are employed for patients at high risk for cardiac complications. Generally accepted contraindications to elective noncardiac surgery include an MI less than 1 month prior to surgery with evidence of persistent ischemic risk by symptoms or noninvasive testing, uncompensated heart failure, and severe aortic or mitral stenosis.

The most important intraoperative risk factors appear to be the urgency of surgery and the operative site. Cardiac complications are two to five times more likely in patients undergoing emergency surgery. Table 20–3 lists the American College of Cardiology/American Heart Association Task Force cardiac risk stratification scheme for various noncardiac surgical procedures. The majority of cardiac complications are associated with major thoracic, abdominal, and vascular operations. Vascular operations, particularly infrainguinal

Figure 20–1. Management of patients with intermediate or minor predictors of increased perioperative cardiovascular risk. Note testing is indicated only if the result will impact patient care. *ETT, exercise tolerance testing. **In the presence of left bundle-branch block, vasodilator perfusion imaging is preferred. (From American College of Cardiology/American Heart Association [ACC/AHA] Guideline Update on Perioperative Cardiovascular Evaluation for Noncardiac Surgery.)

bypass procedures, represent particularly high-risk procedures because peripheral vascular disease and coronary artery disease (CAD) share common risk factors (eg, diabetes, history of smoking, hyperlipidemia, and advanced age); symptoms of CAD are obscured by limits to activity due to claudication and by the nature of the procedures, which may be prolonged and often associated with significant blood loss. Cardiovascular risks for carotid artery surgery appear to be less than for aortic and infrainguinal arterial bypass surgery. Although poorly controlled hypertension is not clearly established as a risk factor for postoperative complications, it is frequently associated with wide intraoperative swings in blood pressure. Interestingly, intraoperative hypertension has been more closely linked to cardiac morbidity than hypotension.

Although the superiority of regional anesthesia over general anesthesia for patients with cardiovascular dis-

ease might seem obvious, studies supporting this view are lacking. Moreover, the hemodynamic effects of spinal and epidural anesthesia (see Chapter 16) may be more detrimental than well-managed general anesthesia for some patients.

■ HYPERTENSION

Preoperative Considerations

Hypertension is a leading cause of death and disability in most Western societies and the most frequent preoperative abnormality in surgical patients, with an overall prevalence of 20–25%. Long-standing uncontrolled hypertension accelerates atherosclerosis and hyperten-

Table 20–2. Shortcut to noninvasive testing in preoperative patients if any two factors are present.[1,2]

---

1. Intermediate clinical predictors are present (Canadian class I or II angina, prior MI based on history or pathological Q waves, compensated or prior heart failure, or diabetes)
2. Poor functional capacity (less than 4 METs)
3. High surgical risk procedure (emergency major operations[3]; aortic repair or peripheral vascular surgery; prolonged surgical procedures with large fluid shifts or blood loss)

---

[1]Modified from ACC/AHA Guideline Update on Perioperative Cardiovascular Evaluation for Noncardiac Surgery.

[2]HF, heart failure; METs, metabolic equivalents; MI, myocardial infarction.

[3]Emergency major operations may require immediately proceeding to surgery without sufficient time for noninvasive testing or preoperative interventions.

Table 20–3. Cardiac risk[1] stratification for noncardiac surgical procedures.[2]

High (reported cardiac risk often greater than 5%)
  Emergent major operations, particularly in the elderly
  Aortic and other major vascular surgery
  Peripheral vascular surgery
  Anticipated prolonged surgical procedures associated with large fluid shifts and/or blood loss
Intermediate (reported cardiac risk generally less than 5%)
  Carotid endarterectomy
  Head and neck surgery
  Intraperitoneal and intrathoracic surgery
  Orthopedic surgery
  Prostate surgery
Low[3] (reported cardiac risk generally less than 1%)
  Endoscopic procedures
  Superficial procedure
  Cataract surgery
  Breast surgery

---

[1]Combined incidence of cardiac death and nonfatal myocardial infarction.

[2]ACC/AHA Guideline Update on Perioperative Cardiovascular Evaluation for Noncardiac Surgery.

[3]Do not generally require further preoperative cardiac testing.

sive organ damage. Hypertension is a major risk factor for cardiac, cerebral, renal, and vascular disease. **Complications include myocardial infarction, congestive heart failure, stroke, renal failure, peripheral occlusive disease, and aortic dissection.** The presence of left ventricular hypertrophy (LVH) in hypertensive patients may be an important predictor of cardiac mortality. Increased cardiac mortality has also been reported in patients with carotid bruits—even in the absence of symptoms.

Definitions

Blood pressure measurements are affected by many variables, including posture, time of day or night, emotional state, recent activity, and drug intake as well as the equipment and technique used. A diagnosis of hypertension cannot be made by one preoperative reading but requires confirmation by a history of consistently elevated measurements. Although preoperative anxiety or pain often produces some degree of hypertension even in normal patients, patients with a history of hypertension generally exhibit greater preoperative elevations in blood pressure.

Epidemiological studies demonstrate a direct and continuous correlation between both diastolic and systolic blood pressures and mortality rates. The definition of systemic hypertension is somewhat arbitrary but generally it is considered to be a consistently elevated diastolic blood pressure greater than 90–95 mm Hg or a systolic pressure greater than 140–160 mm Hg. A common classification scheme is listed in Table

20–4. Borderline hypertension is said to exist when the diastolic pressure is 85–89 mm Hg or the systolic pressure is 130–139 mm Hg. Even patients with borderline hypertension appear to be at some increased risk for cardiovascular complications. Accelerated, or severe, hypertension (stage 3) is defined as a recent, sustained, and progressive increase in blood pressure, usually with diastolic blood pressures in excess of

Table 20–4. Classification of blood pressure (adults).

Category of Blood Pressure	Systolic Pressure (mm Hg)	Diastolic Pressure (mm Hg)
Normal	< 130	< 85
High normal	130–139	85–89
Hypertension		
Stage 1/mild	140–159	90–99
Stage 2/moderate	160–179	100–109
Stage 3/severe	180–209	110–119
Stage 4/very severe	> 210	> 120

110–119 mm Hg; renal dysfunction is often present. Malignant hypertension is a true medical emergency characterized by severe hypertension (> 210/120 mm Hg) associated with papilledema and, frequently, encephalopathy.

Pathophysiology

Hypertension can be either idiopathic (essential) or, less commonly, secondary to other medical conditions such as renal disease, primary hyperaldosteronism, Cushing's syndrome, acromegaly, pheochromocytoma, pregnancy, or estrogen therapy. Essential hypertension accounts for 80–95% of cases and may be associated with an abnormal baseline elevation of cardiac output, systemic vascular resistance (SVR), or both. An evolving pattern is commonly seen over the course of the disease. Initially, cardiac output is elevated, but SVR appears to be in the normal range (in reality, it is inappropriately high). As the disease progresses, cardiac output returns to normal but SVR becomes abnormally high. Extracellular fluid volume and plasma renin activity (see Chapter 29) may be low, normal, or high. The chronic increase in cardiac afterload results in concentric LVH and altered diastolic function (see Chapter 19). Hypertension also alters cerebral autoregulation (see Chapter 25) so that normal cerebral blood flow is maintained in the face of high blood pressures; autoregulation limits may be in the range of mean blood pressures of 110–180 mm Hg.

The mechanisms responsible for the changes observed in hypertensive patients remain elusive but appear to involve vascular hypertrophy, hyperinsulinemia, abnormal increases in intracellular calcium, and increased intracellular sodium concentrations in vascular smooth muscle and renal tubular cells. The increased intracellular calcium presumably results in increased arteriolar tone, whereas the increased sodium concentration impairs renal excretion of sodium. Sympathetic nervous system overactivity and enhanced responses to sympathetic agonists are present in some patients. Hypertensive patients often display an exaggerated response to vasopressors. Overactivity of the renin–angiotensin–aldosterone system (see Chapter 29) appears to play an important role in patients with accelerated hypertension.

Long-Term Treatment

Drug therapy has been shown to reduce the progression of hypertension, and the incidence of stroke, congestive heart failure, CAD, and renal damage. Treatment also can reverse some of the concomitant pathophysiological changes, such as LVH and altered cerebral autoregulation.

Most patients with mild hypertension require only single-drug therapy, which may consist of a thiazide diuretic, angiotensin-converting enzyme (ACE) inhibitor, angiotensin-receptor blocker (ARB), β-adrenergic blocker, or calcium channel blocker. The Joint National Committee on Hypertension (USA) recommends low doses of a thiazide diuretic for most patients. However, concomitant illnesses should influence drug selection. An ACE inhibitor is considered an optimal first-line choice for patients with left ventricular dysfunction or heart failure, whereas an ACE inhibitor or ARB is considered an optimal initial single agent in the setting of hyperlipidemia, chronic kidney disease, or diabetes (particularly with nephropathy). A β-adrenergic blocker or, less commonly, a calcium channel blocker is used as a first-line agent for patients with CAD. ACE inhibitors, ARBs, and β-adrenergic blockers are generally less effective than diuretics and calcium channel blockers in black patients. Treatment guidelines recommend a diuretic with or without β-adrenergic blockade or a calcium channel blocker alone for elderly patients.

Patients with moderate to severe hypertension require a second or third drug. Diuretics are often used to supplement β-adrenergic blockers and ACE inhibitors when single-drug therapy is ineffective. ACE inhibitors have been shown to prolong survival in patients with congestive heart failure or left ventricular dysfunction. In addition, these agents appear to preserve renal function in patients with diabetes or with underlying renal disease. Familiarity with the names and mechanisms of action of commonly used antihypertensive agents is important for anesthesiologists (Table 20–5).

PREOPERATIVE MANAGEMENT

A recurring question in anesthetic practice is the degree of preoperative hypertension that is acceptable for patients scheduled for elective surgery. Except for optimally controlled patients, most hypertensive patients present to the operating room with some degree of hypertension. Although data suggest that even moderate preoperative hypertension (diastolic pressure < 90–110 mm Hg) is not clearly statistically associated with *postoperative* complications, other data indicate that the untreated or poorly controlled hypertensive patient is more apt to experience *intraoperative* episodes of myocardial ischemia, arrhythmias, or both hypertension and hypotension. Intraoperative adjustments in anesthetic depth and use of vasoactive drugs should reduce the incidence of postoperative complications referable to poor preoperative control of hypertension.

Although ideally patients should undergo elective surgery only when rendered normotensive, this is not always feasible or necessarily desirable because of altered

Table 20–5. Oral antihypertensive agents.

Category	Class	Subclass	Agent
Diuretics	Thiazide type		Chlorothiazide (Diuril)
			Chlorthalidone (Thalitone)
			Hydrochlorothiazide (Microzide)
			Indapamide (Lozol)
			Metolazone (Zaroxolyn)
	Potassium sparing		Spironolactone (Aldactone)
			Triamterene (Dyrenium)
			Amiloride (Midamor)
	Loop		Bumetanide (Bumex)
			Ethacrynic acid (Edecrin)
			Furosemide (Lasix)
			Torasemide (Demadex)
Sympatholytics	Adrenergic-receptor blockers	β	Acebutolol (Sectral)
			Atenolol (Tenormin)
			Betaxolol (Kerlone)
			Bisoprolol (Zebeta)
			Carteolol (Cartrol)
			Metoprolol (Lopressor)
			Nadolol (Corgard)
			Penbutolol (Levatol)
			Pindolol (Visken)
			Propranolol (Inderal)
			Timolol (Blocadren)
		α	α_1
			Doxazosin (Cardura)
			Prazosin (Minipress)
			Terazosin (Hytrin)
			$\alpha_1 + \alpha_2$
			Phenoxybenzamine (Dibenzyline)
		α and β	Labetalol (Trandate)
			Carvedilol (Coreg)
	Central α_2-agonists		Clonidine (Catapres)
			Guanabenz (Wytensin)
			Guanfacine (Tenex)
			Methyldopa (Aldomet)
	Postganglionic blockers	Guanadrel	Reserpine

(continued)

cerebral autoregulation. Excessive reductions in blood pressure can compromise cerebral perfusion. Moreover, the decision to delay or to proceed with surgery should be individualized, based on the severity of the preoperative blood pressure elevation; the likelihood of coexisting myocardial ischemia, ventricular dysfunction, or cerebrovascular or renal complications; and the surgical procedure (whether major surgically induced changes in cardiac preload or afterload are anticipated). In many instances, preoperative hypertension is due to the patient's noncompliance with the drug regimen. With rare exceptions, antihypertensive drug therapy should be continued up to the time of surgery. Some clinicians withhold ACE inhibitors on the morning of surgery because of their association with an increased incidence of intraoperative hypotension; however, withholding these agents increases the risk of marked perioperative hypertension and the need for parenteral antihyperten-

Table 20–5. Oral antihypertensive agents. (continued)

Category	Class	Subclass	Agent
Vasodilators	Calcium channel blockers	Benzothiazepine	Diltiazem[1] (Tiazac)
		Phenylalkylamines	Verapamil[1] (Calan SR)
		Dihydropyridines	Amlodipine (Norvasc) Felodipine (Plendil) Isradipine[1] (Dynacirc) Nicardipine[1] (Cardene) Nifedipine[1] (Procardia XL) Nisoldipine (Sular)
	ACE inhibitors[2]		Benazepril (Lotensin) Captopril (Capoten) Enalapril (Vasotec) Fosinopril (Monopril) Lisinopril (Zestril) Moexipril (Univasc) Perindopril (Aceon) Quinapril (Accupril) Ramipril (Altace) Trandopril (Mavik)
	Angiotensin-receptor antagonists		Candesartan (Atacand) Eprosartan (Tevetan) Irbesartan (Avapro) Losartan (Cozaar) Olmesartan (Benicar) Telmisartan (Micardis) Valsartan (Diovan)
	Direct vasodilators		Hydralazine (Apresoline) Minoxidil

[1]Extended realease.
[2]ACE, angiotensin-converting enzyme.

sive agents. Surgical procedures on patients with sustained preoperative diastolic blood pressures higher than 110 mm Hg—particularly those with evidence of end-organ damage—should be delayed until blood pressure is better controlled over the course of several days.

History

The preoperative history should inquire into the severity and duration of the hypertension, the drug therapy currently prescribed, and the presence or absence of hypertensive complications. Symptoms of myocardial ischemia, ventricular failure, impaired cerebral perfusion, or peripheral vascular disease should be elicited, as well as the patient's record of compliance with the drug regimen.

Questions should concern chest pains, exercise tolerance, shortness of breath (particularly at night), dependent edema, postural lightheadedness, syncope, amaurosis, and claudication. Adverse effects of current antihypertensive drug therapy (Table 20–6) should also be identified. Evaluating a history of a previous MI is dealt with below; stroke is discussed in Chapter 27.

Physical Examination & Laboratory Evaluation

Ophthalmoscopy is probably the most useful examination in hypertensive patients (other than sphygmomanometry), but unfortunately it is usually not done. Visible changes in the retinal vasculature usually par-

Table 20–6. Adverse effects of long-term antihypertensive therapy.

Class	Adverse Effects
Diuretics	
Thiazide	Hypokalemia, hyponatremia, hyperglycemia, hyperuricemia, hypomagnesemia, hyperlipidemia, hypercalcemia
Loop	Hypokalemia, hyperglycemia, hypocalcemia, hypomagnesemia, metabolic alkalosis
Potassium sparing	Hyperkalemia
Sympatholytics	
β-Adrenergic blockers	Bradycardia, conduction blockade, myocardial depression, enhanced bronchial tone, sedation, fatigue, depression
α-Adrenergic blockers	Postural hypertension, tachycardia, fluid retention
Central α$_2$-agonists	Postural hypotension, sedation, dry mouth, depression, decreased anesthetic requirements, bradycardia, rebound hypertension, positive Coombs test and hemolytic anemia (methyldopa), hepatitis (methyldopa)
Ganglionic blockers	Postural hypotension, diarrhea, fluid retention, depression (reserpine)
Vasodilators	
Calcium channels blockers	Cardiac depression, bradycardia, conduction blockade (verapamil, diltiazem), peripheral edema (nifedipine), tachycardia (nifedipine), enhanced neuromuscular nondepolarizing blockade
ACE inhibitors[1]	Cough, angioedema, reflex tachycardia, fluid retention, renal dysfunction, renal failure in bilateral renal artery stenosis, hyperkalemia, bone marrow depression (captopril)
Angiotensin-receptor antagonists	Hypotension, renal failure in bilateral renal artery stenosis, hyperkalemia
Direct vasodilators	Reflex tachycardia, fluid retention, headache, systemic lupus erythematosus-like syndrome (hydralazine), pleural or pericardial effusion (minoxidil)

[1]ACE, angiotensin-converting enzyme.

allel the severity and progression of arteriosclerosis and hypertensive damage in other organs. An S$_4$ cardiac gallop is common in patients with LVH. Other physical findings such as pulmonary rales and an S$_3$ cardiac gallop are late findings and indicate congestive heart failure. Blood pressure should be measured in both the supine and standing positions. Orthostatic changes can be due to volume depletion (see Chapter 29), excessive vasodilation, or sympatholytic drug therapy; preoperative fluid administration can prevent severe hypotension after induction of anesthesia in these patients. Although asymptomatic carotid bruits are usually hemodynamically insignificant (see Chapter 27), they are reflective of atherosclerotic vascular disease that may affect the coronary circulation. When a bruit is detected Doppler studies of the carotid arteries may be indicated to rule out hemodynamically significant blockages.

The electrocardiogram (ECG) is often normal, but in patients with a long history of hypertension it frequently shows evidence of ischemia, conduction abnormalities, an old infarction, or LVH or strain. A normal ECG does not necessarily exclude coronary artery disease or LVH. Similarly, a normal heart size on a chest radiograph does not necessarily exclude ventricular hypertrophy. Echocardiography is a more sensitive test of LVH and can be used to evaluate ventricular systolic and diastolic functions in patients with symptoms of heart failure (see Chapter 19). Chest radiographs are usually unremarkable but may show a boot-shaped heart (suggestive of LVH), frank cardiomegaly, or pulmonary vascular congestion.

Renal function is best evaluated by measurement of serum creatinine and blood urea nitrogen levels (see Chapter 32). Serum electrolyte levels should be determined in patients taking diuretics or digoxin or those with renal impairment. Mild to moderate hypokalemia is often seen in patients taking diuretics (3–3.5 mEq/L) but usually does not appear to affect outcome adversely. Potassium replacement should probably be undertaken only in patients who are symptomatic or who are also taking digoxin (see Chapter 28). Hypomagnesemia is also often present and may be an important cause of perioperative arrhythmias. Hyperkalemia may be encountered in patients—particularly those with impaired renal function (see Chapter 29)—who are taking potassium-sparing diuretics or ACE inhibitors.

Premedication

Premedication reduces preoperative anxiety and is highly desirable in hypertensive patients. Mild to moderate preoperative hypertension often resolves following administration of an anxiolytic agent, such as midazolam. Preoperative antihypertensive agents should be continued as close to schedule as possible and can be given with a small sip of water. As mentioned earlier in this chapter, some clinicians withhold ACE inhibitors because of concerns over an increased incidence of intraoperative hypotension. Central α_2-adrenergic agonists can be useful adjuncts for premedicating hypertensive patients; clonidine (0.2 mg) augments sedation, decreases the intraoperative anesthetic requirement, and reduces perioperative hypertension. Unfortunately, preoperative clonidine administration has been associated with profound intraoperative hypotension and bradycardia.

INTRAOPERATIVE MANAGEMENT

Objectives

The overall anesthetic plan for a hypertensive patient is to maintain an appropriate stable blood pressure range. Patients with borderline hypertension may be treated as normotensive patients. Those with long-standing or poorly controlled hypertension, however, have altered autoregulation of cerebral blood flow; higher than normal mean blood pressures may be required to maintain adequate cerebral blood flow. Because most patients with long-standing hypertension are assumed to have some element of CAD and cardiac hypertrophy, excessive blood pressure elevations are undesirable. Hypertension, particularly in association with tachycardia, can precipitate or exacerbate myocardial ischemia, ventricular dysfunction, or both. Arterial blood pressure should generally be kept within 10–20% of preoperative levels. If marked hypertension (> 180/120 mm Hg) is present preoperatively, arterial blood pressure should be maintained in the high-normal range (150–140/90–80 mm Hg).

Monitoring

Most hypertensive patients do not require special intraoperative monitors. Direct intraarterial pressure monitoring should be reserved for patients with wide swings in blood pressure and for those undergoing major surgical procedures associated with rapid or marked changes in cardiac preload or afterload. Electrocardiographic monitoring should focus on detecting signs of ischemia. Urinary output should generally be closely monitored with an indwelling urinary catheter in patients with renal impairment who are undergoing procedures expected to last more than 2 h. When invasive hemodynamic monitoring is used, reduced ventricular compliance (see Chap-

ter 19) is often apparent in patients with ventricular hypertrophy; higher pulmonary capillary wedge pressures (12–18 mm Hg) may be required to maintain adequate left ventricular end-diastolic volume and cardiac output.

Induction

Induction of anesthesia and endotracheal intubation are often a period of hemodynamic instability for hypertensive patients. Regardless of the level of preoperative blood pressure control, many patients with hypertension display an accentuated hypotensive response to induction of anesthesia, followed by an exaggerated hypertensive response to intubation. The hypotensive response at induction may reflect the additive circulatory depressant effects of anesthetic agents and antihypertensive agents (see Table 20–6). Many, if not most, antihypertensive agents and general anesthetics are vasodilators, cardiac depressants, or both. In addition, many hypertensive patients are already volume depleted. Sympatholytic agents also attenuate the normal protective circulatory reflexes (see Chapter 19), reducing sympathetic tone and enhancing vagal activity.

Up to 25% of patients may exhibit severe hypertension following endotracheal intubation. The duration of laryngoscopy, which bears some relationship to the degree of hypertension, should be as short as possible. Moreover, intubation should generally be performed under deep anesthesia (provided hypotension can be avoided). One of several techniques may be used before intubation to attenuate the hypertensive response:

- Deepening anesthesia with a potent volatile agent for 5–10 min.
- Administering a bolus of an opioid (fentanyl, 2.5–5 μg/kg; alfentanil, 15–25 μg/kg; sufentanil, 0.25–0.5 μg/kg; or remifentanil, 0.5–1 μg/kg).
- Administering lidocaine, 1.5 mg/kg intravenously or intratracheally.
- Achieving β-adrenergic blockade with esmolol, 0.3–1.5 mg/kg; propranolol, 1–3 mg; or labetalol, 5–20 mg.
- Using topical airway anesthesia (see Chapter 5).

Choice of Anesthetic Agents

A. INDUCTION AGENTS

The superiority of any one hypertensive agent or technique over another has not been clearly established. Even following regional anesthesia, hypertensive patients frequently have more exaggerated reductions in blood pressure than normotensive patients. Propofol, barbiturates, benzodiazepines, and etomidate are equally safe for inducing general anesthesia in most hypertensive patients. Ketamine by itself is contraindicated for elective procedures, because its sympathetic stimulation can precipitate marked hypertension (see Chapter 8); its sympathetic stimulating properties can be blunted or eliminated by the concomitant administration of a small dose of another agent, particularly a benzodiazepine or propofol.

B. Maintenance Agents

Anesthesia may be safely continued with volatile agents (alone or with nitrous oxide), a balanced technique (opioid + nitrous oxide + muscle relaxant), or totally intravenous techniques. Regardless of the primary maintenance technique, addition of a volatile agent or intravenous vasodilator generally allows more satisfactory intraoperative blood pressure control. The vasodilation and relatively rapid and reversible myocardial depression afforded by volatile agents allow titration of their effects against arterial blood pressure. Some clinicians believe that of the opioids, sufentanil may provide the greatest autonomic suppression and control over blood pressure.

C. Muscle Relaxants

With the possible exception of large boluses of pancuronium, any muscle relaxant (also called neuromuscular blocking agents) can be used routinely. Pancuronium-induced vagal blockade and neural release of catecholamines can exacerbate hypertension in poorly controlled patients. When pancuronium is given slowly in small increments, however, marked increases in heart rate or blood pressure are less likely. Moreover, pancuronium is useful in offsetting excessive vagal tone induced by opioids or surgical manipulations. Hypotension following large (intubating) doses of tubocurarine, metocurine, atracurium, or mivacurium (see Chapter 9) may be accentuated in hypertensive patients.

D. Vasopressors

Hypertensive patients may display an exaggerated response to both endogenous catecholamines (from intubation or surgical stimulation) and exogenously administered sympathetic agonists. If a vasopressor is necessary to treat excessive hypotension, a small dose of a direct-acting agent such as phenylephrine (25–50 μg) may be preferable to an indirect agent. Nonetheless, small doses of ephedrine (5–10 mg) are more appropriate when vagal tone is high. Patients taking sympatholytics preoperatively may exhibit a decreased response to vasopressors, particularly ephedrine; in rare instances small doses of epinephrine, 2–5 μg, may be necessary. Improper dosing of epinephrine in a hypertensive patient can cause significant cardiovascular morbidity.

Intraoperative Hypertension

Intraoperative hypertension not responding to an increase in anesthetic depth (particularly with a volatile agent) can be treated with a variety of parenteral agents (Table 20–7). Readily reversible causes—such as inade-

Table 20–7. Parenteral agents for the acute treatment of hypertension.

Agent	Dosage Range	Onset	Duration
Nitroprusside	0.5–10 μg/kg/min	30–60	1–5 min
Nitroglycerin	0.5–10 μg/kg/min	1 min	3–5 min
Esmolol	0.5 mg/kg over 1 min; 50–300 μg/kg/min	1 min	12–20 min
Labetalol	5–20 mg	1–2 min	4–8 h
Propranolol	1–3 mg	1–2 min	4–6 h
Trimethaphan	1–6 mg/min	1–3 min	10–30 min
Phentolamine	1–5 mg	1–10 min	20–40 min
Diazoxide	1–3 mg/kg slowly	2–10 min	4–6 h
Hydralazine	5–20 mg	5–20 min	4–8 h
Nifedipine (sublingual)	10 mg	5–10 min	4 h
Methyldopa	250–1000 mg	2–3 h	6–12 h
Nicardipine	0.25–0.5 mg 5–15 mg/h	1–5 min	3–4 h
Enalaprilat	0.625–1.25 mg	6–15 min	4–6 h
Fenoldopam	0.1–1.6 mg/kg/min	5 min	5 min

quate anesthetic depth, hypoxemia, or hypercapnia—should always be excluded before initiating antihypertensive therapy. Selection of a hypotensive agent (see Chapter 13) depends on the severity, acuteness, and cause of hypertension, the baseline ventricular function, the heart rate, and the presence of bronchospastic pulmonary disease. β-Adrenergic blockade alone or as a supplement is a good choice for a patient with good ventricular function and an elevated heart rate but is contraindicated in those with bronchospastic disease. Nicardipine may be preferable for patients with bronchospastic disease. Reflex tachycardia following sublingual nifedipine has been associated with myocardial ischemia and its antihypertensive effects have a delayed onset. Nitroprusside remains the most rapid and effective agent for the intraoperative treatment of moderate to severe hypertension. Nitroglycerin may be less effective but is also useful in treating or preventing myocardial ischemia. Fenoldopam is also a useful agent and may improve or maintain renal function. Hydralazine provides sustained blood pressure control but also has a delayed onset and can cause reflex tachycardia. The latter is not seen with labetalol because of combined α- and β-adrenergic blockade.

POSTOPERATIVE MANAGEMENT

Postoperative hypertension (see Chapter 48) is common and should be anticipated in patients who have poorly controlled hypertension. Close blood pressure monitoring should be continued in both the recovery room and the early postoperative period. In addition to myocardial ischemia and congestive heart failure, marked sustained elevations in blood pressure can contribute to the formation of wound hematomas and the disruption of vascular suture lines.

Hypertension in the recovery period is often multifactorial and enhanced by respiratory abnormalities, pain, volume overload, or bladder distention (see Chapter 48). Contributing causes should be corrected and parenteral antihypertensive agents given if necessary. Intravenous labetalol is particularly useful in controlling hypertension and tachycardia, whereas nicardipine is useful in controlling blood pressure in the setting of a slow heart rate, particularly if myocardial ischemia is suspected or bronchospasm is present. When the patient resumes oral intake, preoperative medications should be restarted.

ISCHEMIC HEART DISEASE

Preoperative Considerations

Myocardial ischemia is characterized by a metabolic oxygen demand that exceeds the oxygen supply (see Chapter 19). Ischemia can therefore result from a marked increase in myocardial metabolic demand, a reduction in myocardial oxygen delivery, or a combination of both. Common causes include severe hypertension or tachycardia (particularly in the presence of ventricular hypertrophy); coronary arterial vasospasm or anatomic obstruction; severe hypotension, hypoxemia, or anemia; and severe aortic stenosis or regurgitation.

By far the most common cause of myocardial ischemia is atherosclerosis of the coronary arteries. CAD is responsible for well over one-third of all deaths in Western societies and is a major cause of perioperative morbidity and mortality. The overall incidence of CAD in surgical patients is estimated to be between 5% and 10%. Major risk factors for CAD include hyperlipidemia, hypertension, diabetes, cigarette smoking, increasing age, male sex, and a positive family history. Other risk factors include obesity, a history of cerebrovascular or peripheral vascular disease, menopause, use of high-estrogen oral contraceptives (in women who smoke), a sedentary lifestyle, and perhaps a coronary-prone behavior pattern. By age 65 years, the incidence of CAD is close to 37% for men compared with 18% for women.

CAD may be clinically manifested by symptoms of myocardial necrosis (infarction), ischemia (usually angina), arrhythmias (including sudden death), or ventricular dysfunction (congestive heart failure). When symptoms of congestive heart failure predominate, the term ischemic cardiomyopathy is often used. Three major clinical syndromes are generally recognized: MI, unstable angina, and chronic stable angina. Acute MI is discussed in Chapter 49.

Unstable Angina

Unstable angina is defined as (1) an abrupt increase in severity, frequency (more than three episodes per day), or duration of anginal attacks (crescendo angina), (2) angina at rest, or (3) new onset of angina (within the past 2 months) with severe or frequent episodes (more than three per day). The anginal episodes are often not related to any apparent precipitating factors. Unstable angina may also occur following MI or be precipitated by noncardiac medical conditions (including severe anemia, fever, infections, thyrotoxicosis, hypoxemia, and emotional distress) in previously stable patients.

Unstable angina, particularly when it is associated with significant ST-segment changes at rest, usually reflects severe underlying coronary disease and frequently precedes MI. Plaque disruption with platelet aggregates or thrombi and vasospasm are frequent pathological correlates. Critical stenosis in one or more major coronary arteries is present in over 80% of patients. Patients with unstable angina require admission to a coronary care unit for evaluation and treatment. Anticoagulation with heparin is usually instituted, together with aspirin, intravenous nitroglycerin, β-blockers, and, possibly, calcium channel blockers. If the ischemia does not resolve within 24–48 h, the patient is evaluated by coronary angiography for angioplasty or emergency surgical revascularization.

Chronic Stable Angina

Chest pains are most often substernal, exertional, radiating to the neck or arm, and relieved by rest or nitroglycerin. Variations are common, including epigastric, back, or neck pain or transient shortness of breath from ventricular dysfunction (anginal equivalent). Nonexertional ischemia and silent (asymptomatic) ischemia are recognized as fairly common occurrences. Diabetics have a relatively high incidence of silent ischemia.

Symptoms are generally absent until the atherosclerotic lesions cause 50–75% occlusions in the coronary circulation. When a stenotic segment reaches 70% occlusion, maximum compensatory dilatation is usually present distally: blood flow is generally adequate at rest but becomes inadequate with increased metabolic demand. An extensive collateral blood supply allows some patients to remain relatively asymptomatic in spite of severe disease. Coronary vasospasm is also a cause of transient transmural ischemia in some patients; 90% of vasospastic episodes occur at preexisting stenotic lesions in epicardial vessels and are often precipitated by a variety of factors, including emotional upset and hyperventilation (Prinzmetal's angina). Coronary spasm is most often observed in patients who have angina with varying levels of activity or with emotional stress (variable-threshold); it is least common with classic exertional (fixed-threshold) angina.

The overall prognosis of patients with CAD is related to both the number and severity of coronary obstructions as well as ventricular function.

Treatment of Ischemic Heart Disease

The general approach in treating patients with ischemic heart disease is 5-fold:

- Correction of coronary risk factors in the hope of slowing disease progression.
- Modification of the patient's lifestyle to eliminate stress and improve exercise tolerance.
- Correction of complicating medical conditions that can exacerbate ischemia, such as hypertension, anemia, hypoxemia, thyrotoxicosis, fever, infection, or adverse drug effects.
- Pharmacological manipulation of the myocardial oxygen supply–demand relationship (see Chapter 19).
- Correction of coronary lesions by percutaneous coronary intervention or PCI (angioplasty with or without stenting, or atherectomy) or coronary artery bypass surgery.

The last three approaches are of direct relevance to anesthesiologists. The same principles should be applied in the care of these patients in both the operating room and the intensive care unit.

The most commonly used pharmacological agents are nitrates, β-blockers, and calcium channel blockers. These drugs also have potent circulatory effects, which are compared in Table 20–8. Any of these agents can be used for mild angina. Calcium channel blockers are the drugs of choice for patients with predominantly vasospastic angina, whereas β-adrenergic blocking agents are usually used in patients with exertional angina and adequate ventricular function. Nitrates are good agents for both types of angina.

Table 20–8. Comparison of antianginal agents.[1]

| | | | Calcium Channel Blockers | | |
| | | | Nifedipine Nicardipine | | |
Cardiac Parameter	Nitrates	*Verapamil*	*Nimodipine*	*Diltiazem*	β-Blockers
Preload	↓↓	—	—	—	—/↑
Afterload	↓	↓	↓↓	↓	—/↓
Contractility	—	↓↓	—	↓	↓↓↓
SA node automaticity	↑/—	↓↓	↑/—	↓↓	↓↓↓
AV conduction	—	↓↓↓	—	↓↓	↓↓↓
Vasodilation Coronary Systemic	↑ ↑↑	↑↑ ↑	↑↑↑ ↑↑	↑↑ ↑	—/↓ —/↓

[1]SA, sinoatrial; AV, atrioventricular; ↑, increases; —, no change; ↓, decreases.

A. Nitrates

Nitrates relax all vascular smooth muscle but have a much greater effect on venous than on arterial vessels. Decreasing venous tone and reducing venous return to the heart (cardiac preload) reduce wall tension and afterload. These effects tend to reduce myocardial oxygen demand. The prominent venodilation makes nitrates excellent agents when congestive heart failure is also present.

Perhaps equally important, nitrates dilate the coronary arteries. Even minor degrees of dilation at stenotic sites may be sufficient to increase blood flow, because flow is directly related to the fourth power of the radius. Nitrate-induced coronary vasodilation preferentially increases subendocardial blood flow in ischemic areas. This favorable redistribution of coronary blood flow to ischemic areas may be dependent on the presence of collaterals in the coronary circulation.

Nitrates can be used for both the treatment of acute ischemia and prophylaxis against frequent anginal episodes. Unlike β-blockers and calcium channel blockers, nitrates do not have a negative inotropic effect—a desirable feature in the presence of ventricular dysfunction. Intravenous nitroglycerin can also be used for controlled hypotensive anesthesia (see Chapter 13).

B. Calcium Channel Blockers

The effects and uses of the most commonly used calcium channel blockers are shown in Tables 20–8 and 20–9. Calcium channel blockers reduce myocardial oxygen demand by decreasing cardiac afterload and augment oxygen supply by increasing blood flow (coronary vasodilation). Verapamil and diltiazem also reduce demand by slowing the heart rate.

Nifedipine's potent effects on the systemic blood pressure may precipitate hypotension, reflex tachycardia, or both; its fast-onset preparations (eg, sublingual) have been associated with MI in some patients. Its tendency to decrease afterload generally offsets any negative inotropic effect. The slow-release form of nifedipine is associated with much less reflex tachycardia and is more suitable than other agents for patients with ventricular dysfunction. Amlodipine, which has a profile similar to nifedipine but almost no effect on heart rate, is also used in patients with ventricular dysfunction. In contrast, verapamil and diltiazem have greater effects on cardiac contractility and atrioventricular (AV) conduction and therefore should be used cautiously, if at all, in patients with ventricular dysfunction,

Table 20–9. Comparison of calcium channel blockers.

Agent	Route	Dosage[1]	Half-life	Angina	Hypertension	Cerebral Vasospasm	Supraventricular Tachycardia
Verapamil	PO	40–240 mg	5 h	+	+		+
	IV	5–15 mg	5 h	+			+
Nifedipine	PO	30–180 mg	2 h	+	+		
	SL	10 mg	2 h	+	+		
Diltiazem	PO	30–60 mg	4 h	+	+		+
	IV	0.25–0.35 mg/kg	4 h	+			+
Nicardipine	PO	60–120 mg	2–4 h	+	+		
	IV	0.25–0.5 mg/kg	2–4 h	+	+		
Nimodipine	PO	240 mg	2 h			+	
Bepridil[2]	PO	200–400 mg	24 h	+	+		
Isradipine	PO	2.5–5.0 mg	8 h		+		
Felodipine	PO	5–20 mg	9 h		+		
Amlodipine	PO	2.5–10 mg	30–50 h	+	+		

[1]Total oral dose per day divided into three doses unless otherwise stated.
[2]Also possesses antiarrhythmic properties.

conduction abnormalities, or bradyarrhythmias. Diltiazem appears to be better tolerated than verapamil in patients with impaired ventricular function. Nicardipine and nimodipine generally have the same effects as nifedipine; nimodipine is primarily used in preventing cerebral vasospasm following subarachnoid hemorrhage, whereas nicardipine is used as an intravenous arterial vasodilator.

Calcium channel blockers can have significant interactions with anesthetic agents. All agents appear to potentiate both depolarizing and nondepolarizing neuromuscular blocking agents and the circulatory effects of volatile agents. Verapamil may also modestly decrease anesthetic requirements. Both verapamil and diltiazem can potentiate depression of cardiac contractility and conduction in the AV node by volatile anesthetics. Nifedipine and similar agents can potentiate systemic vasodilation by volatile and intravenous agents.

C. β-ADRENERGIC BLOCKING AGENTS

These drugs decrease myocardial oxygen demand by reducing heart rate and contractility and, in some cases, afterload (via their antihypertensive effect). Optimal blockade results in a resting heart rate between 50 and 60 beats/min and prevents appreciable increases with exercise (< 20 beats/min increase during exercise). Available agents differ in receptor selectivity, intrinsic sympathomimetic (partial agonist) activity, and membrane-stabilizing properties (Table 20–10). Membrane stabilization, often described as a quinidine-like effect, results in antiarrhythmic activity. Agents with intrinsic sympathomimetic properties are better tolerated by patients with mild to moderate ventricular dysfunction. Low doses of β-blockers have been shown to be beneficial in some patients with compensated congestive heart failure. Nonselective β-receptor blockade is contraindicated in patients with significant ventricular dysfunction, conduction abnormalities, or bronchospastic disease. Blockade of β_2-adrenergic receptors also can mask hypoglycemic symptoms in awake diabetic patients, delay metabolic recovery from hypoglycemia, and impair the handling of large potassium loads (see Chapter 28). Nonselective blockers can also theoretically intensify coronary vasospasm in some patients and thus may be contraindicated

Table 20–10. Comparison of β-adrenergic blocking agents.

Agent	β_1-Receptor Selectivity	Half-life	Sympathomimetic	α-Receptor Blockade	Membrane Stabilizing
Acebutolol	+	2–4 h	+		+
Atenolol	++	5–9 h			
Betaxlol	++	14–22 h			
Esmolol	++	9 min			
Metoprolol	++	3–4 h			±
Bisoprolol	+	9–12 h			
Oxprenolol		1–2 h	+		+
Alprenolol		2–3 h	+		+
Pindolol		3–4 h	++		±
Penbutolol		5 h	+		+
Carteolol		6 h	+		
Labetalol		4–8 h		+	±
Propranolol		3–6 h			++
Timolol		3–5 h			
Sotalol[1]		5–13 h			
Nadolol		10–24 h			
Carvedilol		6–8 h		+	±

[1]Also possesses unique antiarrhythmic properties.l

in patients with predominantly vasospastic angina. Cardioselective (β_1-receptor-specific) agents must still be used cautiously in patients with reactive airways, because the selectivity of these agents tends to be dose dependent. Acebutolol may be most useful in patients with bronchospastic airway disease, because it has both β_1-selectivity and intrinsic sympathomimetic activity.

D. OTHER AGENTS

ACE inhibitors have been shown to prolong survival in patients with congestive heart failure or left ventricular dysfunction. Digoxin is beneficial for patients with atrial fibrillation who are capable of a rapid ventricular response and for patients with cardiomegaly, particularly if symptoms of heart failure are present. Chronic aspirin therapy appears to reduce coronary events even in patients with asymptomatic CAD. Antiarrhythmic therapy in patients with complex ventricular ectopy who have significant CAD and left ventricular dysfunction should be guided by an electrophysiological study. Patients with inducible sustained ventricular tachycardia or ventricular fibrillation are candidates for an automatic internal cardioverter-defibrillator (ICD). Treatment of ventricular ectopy (with the exception of sustained ventricular tachycardia) in patients with good ventricular function does not improve survival and may increase mortality. In contrast, ICDs have been shown to improve survival in patients with advanced cardiomyopathy (ejection fraction < 30%) even in the absence of demonstrable arrhythmias.

E. COMBINATION THERAPY

Moderate to severe angina frequently requires combination therapy with two or all three classes of agents. Patients with ventricular dysfunction may not tolerate the combined negative inotropic effect of a β-blocker and a calcium channel blocker together; an ACE inhibitor is better tolerated and appears to improve survival. Similarly, the additive effect of a β-blocker and a calcium channel blocker on the AV node may precipitate heart block in susceptible patients. The combination of amlodipine and a long-acting nitrate is generally well tolerated by patients with significant ventricular dysfunction but may cause excessive vasodilation in some patients.

PREOPERATIVE MANAGEMENT

The importance of ischemic heart disease—particularly a history of MI—as a risk factor for perioperative morbidity and mortality was discussed earlier in the chapter. Most studies confirm that perioperative outcome is related to both disease severity and ventricular function. Patients with extensive (three-vessel or left main) CAD, a recent history of MI, or ventricular dysfunction are at greatest risk for cardiac complications. The risk is the same whether the recent MI was transmural or subendocardial. Perioperative risk following MI appears to be related to the amount of residual ischemia remaining (additional myocardium at risk of infarction). Although the majority of perioperative MI events are reported to be non-Q wave infarctions, the mortality rates for a perioperative infarct in some older studies approached 50%. Figure 20–2 shows the American College of Cardiology/American Heart Association Task Force Guidelines for preoperative management of patients who have major clinical predictors of increased cardiovascular risk (Table 20–1). Studies have shown that preoperative testing of high-risk patients with surgical revascularization (coronary bypass), when appropriate prior to abdominal aortic surgery, improves short- and long-term survival. Similar data on preoperative PCI to reduce cardiovascular complications in high-risk patients are lacking. Moreover, surgical procedures must generally be delayed for a minimum of 2 weeks following PCI to prevent postsurgical bleeding while the patient is on antiplatelet therapy to prevent stent thrombosis.

Chronic stable (mild to moderate) angina does not appear to increase perioperative risk substantially. Similarly, a history of prior coronary artery bypass surgery or coronary angioplasty alone does not appear to substantially increase perioperative risk. A simplified management scheme for patients with intermediate and minor predictors of risk is presented in Table 20–2 and Figure 20–1. Preoperative β-receptor blockers have been shown to reduce perioperative mortality and the incidence of postoperative cardiovascular complications.

History

The history is of prime importance in patients with ischemic heart disease. Questions should encompass symptoms, current and past treatment, complications, and the results of previous evaluations. This information alone is usually enough to provide some estimate of disease severity and ventricular function.

The most important symptoms to elicit include chest pains, dyspnea, poor exercise tolerance, syncope, or near syncope. The relationship between symptoms and activity level should be established. Activity should be described in terms of everyday tasks such as walking or climbing stairs. The ability to do light work at home or climb one flight of stairs slowly corresponds to about 4 metabolic equivalents (METs) and is one of the important criteria in determining the need for noninvasive cardiac testing (Figure 20–1 and Table 20–2). Patients with severe disease may be relatively asymptomatic because of a very sedentary lifestyle. Diabetic patients are particularly prone to silent ischemia (Chapter 36). The patient's description of chest pains may suggest a major role for vasospasm (variable-threshold

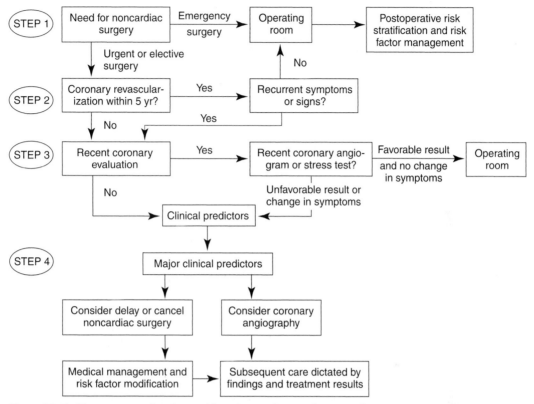

Figure 20–2. Management of patients with major predictors of increased perioperative cardiovascular risk. Note testing is indicated only if the result will impact patient care. (From ACC/AHA Guideline Update on Perioperative Cardiovascular Evaluation for Noncardiac Surgery.)

angina). Easy fatigability or shortness of breath suggests compromised ventricular function.

A history of unstable angina or MI should include the time of its occurrence and whether it was complicated by arrhythmias, conduction disturbances, or heart failure. Patients with prior anterior infarctions tend to have more severe disease than those with prior inferior infarctions. Localization of the areas of ischemia is invaluable in deciding which electrocardiographic leads to monitor intraoperatively. Arrhythmias and conduction abnormalities are more common in patients with previous infarction and those with poor ventricular function. This latter group of patients often have ICDs.

Physical Examination & Routine Laboratory Evaluation

Evaluation of patients with CAD is similar to that of patients with hypertension; indeed, both diseases are often simultaneously present in the same patient. Laboratory evaluation for patients who have a history com-

patible with recent unstable angina and are undergoing emergency procedures should also include serum cardiac enzymes. Serum levels of cardiac-specific troponins (T or I), creatine kinase (MB isoenzyme), and lactate dehydrogenase (type 1 isoenzyme) are useful in excluding MI. Serum digoxin and other antiarrhythmic levels may also be useful in excluding drug toxicity.

The baseline ECG is normal in 25–50% of patients with CAD but no prior MI. A very straight ST-segment has been associated with underlying CAD; the normal ST-segment gradually slopes away from the QRS complex and into the T wave. Electrocardiographic evidence of ischemia often becomes apparent only during chest pain. The most common baseline abnormalities are nonspecific ST-segment and T-wave changes. Prior infarction is often manifested by Q waves or loss of R waves in the leads closest to the infarct. First-degree AV block, bundle-branch block, or hemiblock may be present. Persistent ST-segment elevation following MI is often indicative of a left ventricular aneurysm. A long rate-corrected QT interval ($QT_c > 0.44$ s) may reflect the underlying ischemia, drug toxicity (usually class Ia antiarrhythmic agents, antidepressants, or phenothiazines), electrolyte abnormalities (hypokalemia or hypomagnesemia), autonomic dysfunction, mitral valve prolapse, or, less commonly, a congenital abnormality. Patients with a long QT interval are at risk for developing ventricular arrhythmias—particularly polymorphic ventricular tachycardia (torsade de pointes), which can lead to ventricular fibrillation. The long QT interval reflects nonuniform prolongation of ventricular repolarization and predisposes patients to reentry phenomena (see Chapter 19). Elective surgery should be postponed until drug toxicity and electrolyte imbalances are excluded. In contrast to polymorphic ventricular arrhythmias with a normal QT interval, which respond to conventional antiarrhythmics (see Chapters 19 and 47), polymorphic tachyarrhythmias with a long QT interval generally respond best to pacing or magnesium. Patients with congenital prolongation generally respond to β-adrenergic blocking agents. Left stellate ganglion blockade (see Chapter 18) is also effective and suggests that autonomic imbalance plays an important role in this group of patients.

The chest film is a useful screening test in excluding cardiomegaly or pulmonary vascular congestion secondary to ventricular dysfunction. Rarely, calcification of the coronaries, aorta, or the aortic valve may be seen.

Specialized Studies

When used as screening tests for the general population, noninvasive stress tests have a low predictability in normal patients but are sufficiently reliable in patients with suspected coronary disease (Bayes' theorem). Correct preoperative interpretation of these tests is important, particularly in patients in whom CAD is suspected. Holter monitoring, exercise electrocardiography, myocardial perfusion scans, and echocardiography are important in determining perioperative risk and the need for coronary angiography. But these tests are indicated only if their outcome would alter patient care.

A. Holter Monitoring

Continuous ambulatory electrocardiographic (Holter) monitoring is useful in evaluating arrhythmias, antiarrhythmic drug therapy, and the severity and frequency of ischemic episodes. Silent (asymptomatic) ischemic episodes are frequent findings in patients with CAD. Moreover, the preoperative occurrence of frequent ischemic episodes on Holter monitoring correlates well with intraoperative and postoperative ischemia. Holter monitoring may be a good screening test because it has an excellent negative predictive value for postoperative cardiac complications.

B. Exercise Electrocardiography

The usefulness of this test is limited in patients with baseline ST-segment abnormalities and those who are unable to increase their heart rate (> 85% of maximal predicted) because of fatigue, dyspnea, or drug therapy. Overall sensitivity is 65% and specificity is 90%. The test is most sensitive (85%) in patients with three-vessel or left main CAD. Disease that is limited to the left circumflex artery may also be missed because ischemia in its distribution may not be evident on the standard surface ECG. A normal test does not necessarily exclude CAD but suggests that severe disease is not likely. The degree of ST-segment depression, its severity and configuration, the time of onset in the test, and the time required for resolution are important findings. A myocardial ischemic response at low levels of exercise is associated with a significantly increased risk of perioperative complications and long-term cardiac events. Other significant findings include changes in blood pressure and the occurrence of arrhythmias. Exercise-induced ventricular ectopy frequently indicates severe CAD associated with ventricular dysfunction. The ischemia presumably leads to electrical instability in myocardial cells. Factors associated with severe multivessel disease are listed in Table 20–11.

C. Myocardial Perfusion Scans

Myocardial perfusion imaging using thallium-201 or technetium-99m is used in evaluating patients who cannot exercise (eg, peripheral vascular disease) or who have underlying ECG abnormalities that preclude interpretation during exercise (eg, left bundle-branch block). If the patient cannot exercise, images are obtained before and after injection of an intravenous coronary dilator, eg, dipyridamole or adenosine, to produce a hyperemic response similar to exercise. Myocardial perfusion studies following exercise or injection of dipyridamole or adenosine have a high sensitivity but only fairly good specificity for detecting CAD. They are best for detect-

Table 20–11. Factors associated with severe multivessel disease during exercise electrocardiography.

More than 2 mm horizontal or down-sloping ST depression
Early onset of ST depression with low workload
Persistence of ST depression after exercise for 5 min or longer
Sustained decrease (≥ 10 mm Hg) in systolic blood pressure during exercise
Failure to reach a maximum heart rate greater than 70% of predicted
Frequent or complex ventricular dysrhythmias at a low heart rate

ing two- or three-vessel disease. These scans can locate and quantitate areas of ischemia or scarring and differentiate between the two. Perfusion defects that fill in on the redistribution phase represent ischemia, not previous infarction. The negative predictive value of a normal perfusion scan is approximately 99%.

D. ECHOCARDIOGRAPHY

This technique provides information about both regional and global ventricular function, and may be carried out at rest, following exercise, or with administration of dobutamine. Detectable regional wall motion abnormalities and the derived left ventricular ejection fraction correlate well with angiographic findings. Moreover, dobutamine stress echocardiography appears to be a reliable predictor of adverse cardiac complications in patients who cannot exercise. New or worsening wall motion abnormalities following dobutamine infusion are indicative of significant ischemia. Patients with an ejection fraction less than 50% tend to have more severe disease and increased perioperative morbidity. Dobutamine stress echocardiography, however, may not be reliable in patients with left bundle-branch block because septal motion may be abnormal even in the absence of left anterior descending CAD in some patients.

E. CORONARY ANGIOGRAPHY

Coronary angiography remains the gold standard in evaluating CAD and is associated with an acceptably low complication rate (< 1%). Nonetheless, coronary angiography should be performed only to determine if the patient may benefit from percutaneous coronary angioplasty or coronary artery bypass grafting prior to noncardiac surgery. The location and severity of occlusions can be defined, and coronary vasospasm may also be observed on angiography. In evaluating fixed stenotic lesions, occlusions greater than 50–75% are generally considered significant. Estimates of the percentage of occlusion can be misleading (particularly when between 40% and 80%) because of differences among observers and the typical assumption that occlusions are concentric when they are often eccentric. The severity of disease is often expressed according to the number of major coronary vessels affected (one-, two-, or three-vessel disease). Significant stenosis of the left main coronary artery is ominous because it affects almost the entire left ventricle. Moreover, even 50–75% occlusions in the left main artery can be hemodynamically significant.

Ventriculography and measurement of intracardiac pressures also provide important information. The most important measurement is the ejection fraction. Indicators of significant ventricular dysfunction include an ejection fraction less than 0.5%, a left ventricular end-diastolic pressure greater than 18 mm Hg after injection of contrast, a cardiac index less than 2.2 L/min/m², and marked or multiple wall motion abnormalities.

Premedication

Allaying fear, anxiety, and pain preoperatively are desirable goals in patients with CAD. Satisfactory premedication prevents sympathetic activation, which adversely affects the myocardial oxygen supply–demand balance. Overmedication is equally detrimental, however, and should be avoided because it may result in hypoxemia, respiratory acidosis, and hypotension. A benzodiazepine, alone or in combination with a opioid, is most commonly used (see Chapter 8). Excellent results can also be obtained by a combination of morphine, 0.1–0.15 mg/kg, and scopolamine, 0.2–0.4 mg, intramuscularly. Concomitant administration of oxygen via nasal cannula helps avoid hypoxemia following premedication. Patients with poor ventricular function and with coexistent lung disease should receive reduced doses. Preoperative medications should generally be continued until the time of surgery. They may be given orally with a small sip of water, intramuscularly, intravenously, sublingually, or transdermally. Sudden withdrawal of antianginal medication perioperatively—particularly β-blockers—can precipitate a sudden increase in ischemic episodes (rebound). Moreover, prophylactic β-adrenergic blockade has been shown to reduce the incidence of intraoperative and postoperative ischemic episodes and appears to be superior to prophylaxis with a calcium channel blocker alone. Many clinicians prophylactically administer nitrates intravenously or transdermally to patients with CAD in the perioperative period. Although this practice may be theoretically advantageous, its efficacy in patients not previously on long-term nitrate therapy and without evidence of ongoing ischemia is not well established. Transdermal absorption of nitroglycerin may be erratic in the perioperative period, whereas intravenous administration can significantly decrease cardiac preload, which can readily cause hypotension if not compensated with intravenous fluids.

INTRAOPERATIVE MANAGEMENT

The intraoperative period is regularly associated with factors and events that can adversely affect the myocardial oxygen demand–supply relationship. Activation of the sympathetic system plays a major role. Hypertension and enhanced contractility increase myocardial oxygen demand, whereas tachycardia increases demand and reduces supply (see Chapter 19). Although myocardial ischemia is commonly associated with tachycardia, it can occur in the absence of any apparent hemodynamic derangement.

Objectives

⑦ The overwhelming priority in managing patients with ischemic heart disease is maintaining a favorable myocardial supply–demand relationship. Autonomic-mediated increases in heart rate and blood pressure should be controlled by deep anesthesia or adrenergic blockade, and excessive reductions in coronary perfusion pressure (see Chapter 19) or arterial oxygen content are to be avoided. Although exact limits are not predictable, diastolic arterial pressure should generally be maintained at 50 mm Hg or above. Higher diastolic pressures may be preferable in patients with high-grade coronary occlusions. Excessive increases—such as those caused by fluid overload—in left ventricular end-diastolic pressure should be avoided because they increase ventricular wall tension (afterload) and can reduce subendocardial perfusion (see Chapter 19). Adequate blood hemoglobin concentrations (> 9–10 mg/dL) and arterial oxygen tensions (> 60 mm Hg) should generally be maintained.

Monitoring

Intraarterial pressure monitoring is advisable for all patients with severe CAD and with major or multiple cardiac risk factors (see Table 20–1). Central venous or pulmonary artery pressure should be monitored during prolonged or complicated procedures involving large fluid shifts or blood loss (see Chapter 6). Monitoring of pulmonary artery pressure may be desirable for patients with significant ventricular dysfunction (ejection fraction < 40–50%). Transesophageal echocardiography (TEE) can provide valuable information, both qualitative and quantitative, on contractility and ventricular chamber size (preload). It is important to note that although clinical experience might suggest otherwise, neither pulmonary artery pressure monitoring nor TEE monitoring has clearly been shown to improve outcome in most clinical studies.

⑧ Intraoperative detection of ischemia depends on recognition of electrocardiographic changes, hemodynamic manifestations, or regional wall motion abnormalities on TEE. Doppler TEE also allows detection of the onset of mitral regurgitation caused by ischemic papillary muscle dysfunction.

A. ELECTROCARDIOGRAPHY

Early ischemic changes are subtle and can often be overlooked. They involve changes in T wave morphology, including inversion, tenting, or both (Figure 20–3). More obvious ischemia may be seen in the form of progressive ST-segment depression. Downsloping and horizontal ST depression are of greater specificity for ischemia than up-sloping depression. New ST-segment elevations are rare during noncardiac surgery and are indicative of severe ischemia, vasospasm, or infarction. It should be noted that an isolated minor ST elevation in the mid-precordial leads (V_3 and V_4) can be a normal variant in young patients. Ischemia may also present as an unexplained intraoperative atrial or ventricular arrhythmia or the onset of a new conduction abnormality. The sensitivity of the ECG in detecting ischemia is related to the number of leads monitored. Studies suggest that the V_5, V_4, II, V_2, and V_3 leads (in decreasing sensitivity) are most useful. Ideally, at least two leads should be monitored simultaneously. Usually, lead II is monitored for inferior wall ischemia and arrhythmias and V_5 for anterior wall ischemia. An esophageal lead may also be useful in patients with posterior wall ischemia. When only one channel can be monitored, a modified V_5 lead provides the highest sensitivity (see Chapter 6).

B. HEMODYNAMIC MONITORING

The most common hemodynamic abnormalities observed during ischemic episodes are hypertension and tachycardia. They are almost always a cause rather than the result of ischemia. Hypotension is a late and ominous manifestation of progressive ventricular dysfunction. The most sensitive hemodynamic correlates are derived from pulmonary artery pressure monitoring. Ischemia is frequently, but not always, associated with an abrupt increase in pulmonary capillary wedge pressure. The sudden appearance of a prominent v wave on the wedge waveform is usually indicative of acute mitral regurgitation from ischemic papillary muscle dysfunction or acute left ventricular dilatation.

C. TRANSESOPHAGEAL ECHOCARDIOGRAPHY

TEE can be extremely helpful in detecting both global and regional cardiac dysfunction as well as valvular function in selected patients. Moreover, detection of new regional wall motion abnormalities is a rapid and more sensitive indicator of myocardial ischemia than the ECG. In animal studies in which coronary blood flow is gradually reduced, regional wall motion abnormalities develop before the ECG changes. Although the occurrence of new intraoperative abnormalities correlates with postoperative MIs in some studies, not all such abnormalities are necessarily ischemic. Both regional and global abnormalities can be caused by changes in heart rate, altered conduction, preload, afterload, or drug-induced changes in contractility. Decreased systolic wall thickening may be a more reliable index for ischemia than endocardial wall motion alone. Unfortunately, TEE requires expen-

Figure 20–3. Electrocardiographic signs of ischemia. Patterns of ischemia and injury. (Modified and reproduced, with permission, from Schamroth L: *The 12 Lead Electrocardiogram.* Blackwell, 1989.)

sive equipment and considerable familiarity with the technique to make correct—and rapid—interpretations intraoperatively.

Internal Cardioverter-Defibrillator Management

Increasing numbers of patients with a CAD and automatic ICDs are presenting for surgery. Patients usually have an advanced cardiomyopathy and/or a history of symptomatic ventricular tachycardia or fibrillation. ICDs, which can act as a pacemaker as well as a defibrillator, present a problem because of the use of surgical electrocautery. The latter can cause (1) ICD firing because the device may interpret it as ventricular fibrillation, (2) inhibition of pacemaker function due to cautery artifact, (3) increased pacing rate due to activation of a rate-responsive sensor, and (4) temporary or permanent resetting to a back-up or reset mode. Use of

bipolar cautery, placement of the grounding pad far from the ICD device, and limiting use of the cautery to only short bursts help reduce the likelihood of problems but does not eliminate them.

ICD devices should have the defibrillator function programmed off immediately before surgery and reprogrammed back on immediately afterward. External defibrillation pads should be applied and attached to an external machine intraoperatively. Careful monitoring of the arterial pulse with pulse oximetry or an arterial waveform is necessary to ensure the pacemaker is not inhibited and there is arterial perfusion during ECG artifact from surgical cautery. The manufacturer should be contacted to determine the best method for managing the device (eg, reprogramming or applying a magnet) prior to surgery. A large number of ICD models are in use. However, most suspend their antitachycardia function in response to a magnet and their behavior varies according to the model.

Choice of Anesthesia

A. Regional Anesthesia

Although studies documenting the superiority of regional over general anesthesia are lacking, regional anesthesia is often a good choice for procedures involving the extremities, the perineum, and possibly the lower abdomen. Precipitous decreases in blood pressure following spinal or epidural anesthesia should be rapidly treated with small doses (25–50 µg) of phenylephrine or a similar agent to preserve coronary perfusion pressure until sufficient intravenous fluid can be given. Small doses of ephedrine (5–10 mg) may be preferable in the presence of bradycardia. Marked hypotension can usually be avoided by prior volume loading (see Chapter 16). Hypotension not responding to phenylephrine or ephedrine may be treated with epinephrine (2–10 µg).

Patients with compensated congestive heart failure usually tolerate the sympathectomy surprisingly well and may not need preoperative volume loading. Patchy or incomplete surgical anesthesia or excessive sedation during regional anesthesia defeats the purpose of selecting a regional technique, unnecessarily stresses the patient, and may precipitate myocardial ischemia. Conversion of the regional anesthetic to a general anesthetic is appropriate in such instances and corrects the often-associated hypertension, tachycardia, hypoxia, or hypercapnia.

B. General Anesthesia

1. Induction—The same general principles that apply to patients with hypertension also apply to most patients with ischemic heart disease. Many, if not most, patients with CAD have hypertension. The induction technique for patients with moderate to severe CAD (three-vessel disease, left main disease, or ejection fractions < 40%) requires some modification. The induction should have minimal hemodynamic effects, produce reliable loss of consciousness, and provide sufficient depth of anesthesia to prevent a vasopressor response to intubation (if intubation is required); however, in many cases, mild to moderate hypertension is better tolerated than hypotension. Regardless of the agent used, these objectives are most consistently achieved by a slow controlled technique. Induction with small incremental doses of the selected agent usually avoids the precipitous decreases in blood pressure that can be seen following a large bolus. Titration of the induction agent—first against loss of consciousness and then to an acceptable decrease in blood pressure—allows individual variations in response. Moreover, sufficient anesthetic depth for endotracheal intubation can be achieved with less cardiovascular depression than that caused by the bolus technique.

Administration of a muscle relaxant (as soon as the eyelid reflex is lost) and controlled ventilation ensure generally adequate oxygenation throughout induction. Hypercarbia is often associated with hypertension. Endotracheal intubation is performed once sufficient anesthetic depth is reached or arterial blood pressure reaches its lowest acceptable limit. Blood pressure, heart rate, and the ECG should be repeatedly assessed with each step during induction.

2. Choice of agents

a. Induction agents—Selection of a specific agent is not critical for most patients. Propofol, barbiturates, etomidate, benzodiazepines, opioids, and various combinations of these drugs are often used. Ketamine by itself is relatively contraindicated because its indirect sympathomimetic effects can adversely affect the myocardial oxygen demand–supply balance. When combined with a benzodiazepine or propofol, however, ketamine does not appreciably increase sympathetic activity and results in relatively stable hemodynamics with minimal myocardial depression. The combination of a benzodiazepine and ketamine may be most useful in patients with poor ventricular function (ejection fraction < 30%).

High-dose opioid anesthesia had previously been used widely for patients with significant ventricular dysfunction. With the exception of meperidine (in large doses), opioids alone are generally associated with minimal or no cardiac depression. Combining them with other intravenous agents (particularly benzodiazepines), however, often results in significant, dose-dependent cardiac depression. Apparent cardiac depression may also occur with pure high-dose opioid inductions (see Chapter 21); this likely represents withdrawal of an elevated baseline sympathetic tone. Patients with poor ventricular function often rely on an elevated sympathetic tone to maintain their cardiac output (see Chapter 19) and may decompensate even with pure high-dose opioid anesthesia. Moreover, opioids used as sole agents may not be complete anesthetics because of an unacceptably high incidence of intraoperative awareness (recall) and hypertension (see Chapter 21); the prolonged respiratory depression following this technique is also unsuitable for most noncardiac operations. Most clinicians always use small supplemental doses of an intravenous agent or volatile anesthetic with a primarily opioid-based anesthetic.

Control of the adrenergic response to endotracheal intubation has been discussed in the section on hypertension.

b. Maintenance agents—Patients are generally managed with an opioid-volatile anesthetic technique. Patients with ejection fractions less than 40% may be very sensitive to the depressant effects of the potent volatile agents or large boluses of opioids. Nitrous oxide, particularly in the presence of opioids, can also produce significant cardiac depression.

The effects of the potent volatile agents on the coronary circulation are discussed in Chapter 19. All volatile agents generally have a favorable effect on myocardial oxygen balance, reducing demand more than supply. Isoflurane dilates intramyocardial arteries more than the larger epicardial vessels but there is little evidence that isoflurane causes an intracoronary steal phenomenon in clinical practice.

Detection of intraoperative ischemia should prompt a search for precipitating factors and initiation of interventions to correct it. Oxygenation and the hematocrit (or hemoglobin) should be checked and hemodynamic abnormalities (hypotension, hypertension, or tachycardia) corrected. Hematocrits less than 28% have been associated with perioperative ischemia and postoperative complications, particularly in patients undergoing vascular surgery. Failure to identify a cause or to reverse the ischemic manifestations may indicate that intravenous nitroglycerin should be started. Nitroglycerin optimally requires insertion of an arterial line and, in some patients (those with moderate to severe ventricular impairment), a pulmonary artery catheter. Nitroglycerin paste may be used if intravenous nitroglycerin cannot be used, but it is associated with a delayed onset and variable absorption.

c. Muscle relaxants—Lack of significant circulatory side effects generally makes rocuronium, vecuronium, pipecuronium, and doxacurium good muscle relaxants for patients with ischemic heart disease. Severe bradycardia has been reported with vecuronium (and atracurium) on rare occasions, but in nearly all instances it has been associated with concomitant administration of a synthetic opioid. When used properly, other muscle relaxants (see Chapter 9) can also be safely administered to patients with CAD. Moreover, their circulatory side effects can be used to balance the side effects of other anesthetic agents—eg, the vagolytic properties of pancuronium can counteract the vagotonic effects of potent opioids (see Chapter 8). Atracurium in doses less than 0.4 mg/kg and mivacurium, in doses up to 0.15 mg/kg, given slowly also generally have minimal hemodynamic effects. The circulatory effects of succinylcholine are primarily due to stimulation of autonomic ganglia and cardiac muscarinic receptors and can result in variable effects on heart rate and blood pressure (see Chapter 9). Its net effect is influenced by preexisting relative sympathetic and parasympathetic tone, premedication with an anticholinergic, and β-adrenergic blockade. Bradycardia may be seen following administration of succinylcholine in patients taking β-adrenergic blocking agents.

Reversal of muscle paralysis with standard agents does not appear to have any detrimental effects in patients with CAD. Use of glycopyrrolate instead of atropine may decrease the likelihood of transient tachycardia (see Chapter 10).

POSTOPERATIVE MANAGEMENT

Recovery from anesthesia and the immediate postoperative period can continue to stress the myocardium. The patient should receive supplemental oxygen until adequate oxygenation is established. Shivering usually resolves following administration of meperidine, 20–30 mg intravenously; other reported treatments include clonidine, 75 μg, or butorphanol, 1–2 mg intravenously. Hypothermia should be corrected with a forced-air surface warmer. Postoperative pain should be controlled with generous analgesics or a regional anesthetic technique (see Chapter 18). If there is a suspicion of fluid overload or the patient has a history of poor ventricular function, a postoperative chest film is useful. Pulmonary congestion can be rapidly treated with furosemide, 20–40 mg intravenously, or intravenous vasodilator therapy (usually nitroglycerin).

The greatest risk to these patients postoperatively is unrecognized ischemia. Although the majority of perioperative Q-wave MIs occur within the first 3 days following surgery (usually after 24–48 h), a significant number of non-Q-wave infarctions present in the first 24 h. Because fewer than 50% patients have chest pain, routine postoperative 12-lead ECGs may be necessary to detect such events. A common presentation is unexplained hypotension. Other presentations include congestive heart failure and altered mental status. Nearly all patients experiencing this complication are older than 50 years. The diagnosis is usually based on electrocardiographic findings and cardiac enzyme or, less commonly, radionuclide studies. Transthoracic or TEE may also be invaluable.

■ VALVULAR HEART DISEASE

1. General Evaluation of Patients

Regardless of the lesion or its cause, preoperative evaluation should be primarily concerned with determining the severity of the lesion and its hemodynamic significance, residual ventricular function, and the presence of secondary effects on pulmonary, renal, and hepatic function. Concomitant CAD should not be overlooked, particularly in older patients and those with known risk factors (see above). Myocardial ischemia may also occur in the absence of significant coronary occlusion in patients with severe aortic stenosis or regurgitation.

Table 20–12. Modified New York Association functional classification of heart disease.

Class	Description
I	Asymptomatic except during severe exertion
II	Symptomatic with moderate activity
III	Symptomatic with minimal activity
IV	Symptomatic at rest

History

The preanesthesia history should focus on symptoms related to ventricular function and should be correlated with laboratory data. Questions should concern exercise tolerance, fatigability, and pedal edema and shortness of breath in general (dyspnea), when lying flat (orthopnea), or at night (paroxysmal nocturnal dyspnea). The New York Heart Association functional classification of heart disease (Table 20–12) is useful for grading the clinical severity of heart failure, comparing patients, and estimating prognosis. Patients should also be questioned about chest pains and neurological symptoms. Some valvular lesions are associated with thromboembolic phenomena. Prior procedures such as valvotomy or valve replacement and their effects should also be well documented.

A review of medications should evaluate efficacy and exclude serious side effects. Commonly used agents include digoxin, diuretics, vasodilators, ACE inhibitors, antiarrhythmics, and anticoagulants. Digoxin is generally most effective for controlling the ventricular rate in patients with atrial fibrillation. The ventricular rate should be less than 80–90 beats/min at rest and should not exceed 120 beats/min with stress or exercise. Signs of digoxin toxicity are primarily cardiac (arrhythmias), gastrointestinal (nausea or vomiting), neurological (confusion), or visual (altered color perception or scotomas). Arrhythmias caused by digoxin arise from a combination of enhanced automaticity and decreased conduction in specialized cells in the atria, ventricles, and AV and sinoatrial (SA) nodes. Preoperative vasodilator therapy may be used to decrease preload, afterload, or both. Excessive vasodilation worsens exercise tolerance and is often first manifested as postural hypotension.

Physical Examination

The most important signs to search for on physical examination are those of congestive heart failure. Left-sided (S_3 gallop or pulmonary rales) as well as right-sided signs (jugular venous distention, hepatojugular reflux, hepatosplenomegaly, or pedal edema) may be present. Auscultatory findings may confirm the valvular dysfunction (Table 20–13), but echocardiographic studies are generally more reliable. Neurological deficits, which are usually secondary to embolic phenomena, should be documented.

Laboratory Evaluation

In addition to the laboratory studies discussed for patients with hypertension and CAD, liver function tests (see Chapter 34) are useful in assessing hepatic dysfunction caused by passive hepatic congestion in patients with severe or chronic right-sided failure. Arte-

Table 20–13. Effects of diagnostic maneuvers on heart murmurs (variable effects omitted).[1]

Maneuver	Systolic Murmurs							Diastolic Murmurs			
	PS	TR	HCM	MVP	MR	VSD	AS	PR	TS	AR	MS
Inspiration	↑	↑						↑	↑		
Valsalva	↑		↑	↑			↓	↑			↓
Standing			↑	↑	↓						
Squatting or handgrip			↓	↓	↑	↑	↓			↑	↑
Leg elevation		↑	↓	↓			↑		↑		
Transient arterial occlusion					↑	↑				↑	
Amyl nitrite inhalation	↑	↑	↑	↑	↓	↓	↑	↑	↑	↓	↑

[1]↑, increases; ↓, decreases; PS, pulmonary stenosis; TR, tricuspid regurgitation; HCM, hypertrophic cardiomyopathy; MVP, mitral valve prolapse; MR, mitral regurgitation; VSD, ventricular septal defect; AS, aortic stenosis; PR, pulmonary regurgitation; TS, tricuspid stenosis; AR, aortic regurgitation; MS, mitral stenosis.

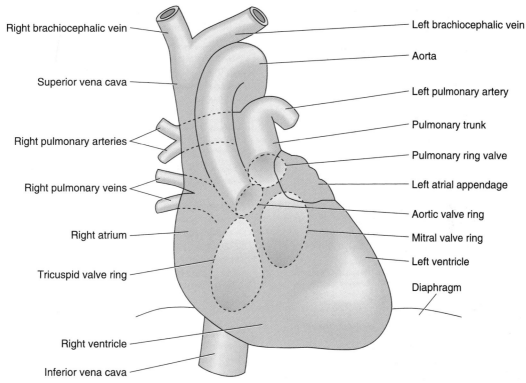

Figure 20–4. Radiological localization of cardiac chambers and structures on the front chest film.

rial blood gases should be measured in patients with significant pulmonary symptoms. Reversal of anticoagulants should be documented with a prothrombin time and partial thromboplastin time prior to surgery.

Electrocardiographic findings are generally nonspecific. They may include T-wave or ST-segment changes, arrhythmias, conduction abnormalities, or QRS-axis deviation reflecting ventricular hypertrophy. A prolonged P–R interval may suggest digoxin toxicity. Arrhythmias associated with digoxin toxicity include (in order of decreasing frequency) ventricular ectopy, paroxysmal atrial tachycardia with 2:1 AV block, AV block alone, marked sinus bradycardia, low atrial or AV junctional rhythms, and AV dissociation.

The chest film is invaluable in assessing cardiac size and pulmonary vascular congestion. Specific cardiac chamber enlargement may be apparent (Figure 20–4).

Special Studies

Echocardiography, radionuclide angiography, and cardiac catheterization provide important diagnostic and prognostic information about valvular lesions. More than one valvular lesion is often found. In many instances, noninvasive studies obviate the need for cardiac catheterization. Information from these studies is best reviewed with a cardiologist. The following questions must be answered:

- Which valvular abnormality is most important hemodynamically?
- What is the severity of that lesion?
- What degree of ventricular impairment is present?
- What is the hemodynamic significance of other identified abnormalities?
- Is there any evidence of CAD?

2. Premedication

Premedication with standard doses of any of the commonly used agents (see Chapter 8) is desirable and well tolerated in patients with normal or near-normal ventricular function. Patients with poor ventricular function, on the other hand, tend to be very sensitive to most agents, and premedication doses should be reduced in proportion to the severity of ventricular impairment. Patients should generally receive their usual medications on the morning of surgery. Supplemental oxygen may be desirable in patients with pulmonary hypertension or underlying pulmonary disease.

Table 20–14. Cardiac conditions associated with endocarditis.[1]

High-risk category
    Prosthetic cardiac valves, including bioprosthetic and
        homograft valves
    Previous bacterial endocarditis
    Complex cyanotic congenital heart disease (eg, single-
        ventricle states, transposition of the great arteries,
        tetralogy of Fallot)
    Surgically constructed systemic pulmonary shunts or
        conduits
Moderate-risk category
    Most other congenital cardiac malformations (other
        than above and below)
    Acquired valvar dysfunction (eg, rheumatic heart disease)
    Hypertrophic cardiomyopathy
    Mitral valve prolapse with valvar regurgitation and/or
        thickened leaflets
Negligible-risk category (no greater risk than the general
    population)
    Isolated secundum atrial septal defect
    Surgical repair of atrial septal defect, ventricular septal
        defect, or patent ductus arteriosus (without residua
        beyond 6 months)
    Previous coronary artery bypass graft surgery
    Mitral valve prolapse without valvar regurgitation
    Physiological, functional, or innocent heart murmurs
    Previous Kawasaki disease without valvar dysfunction
    Previous rheumatic fever without valvar dysfunction
    Cardiac pacemakers (intravascular epicardial) and
        implanted defibrillators

[1]Adapted from AHA Guidelines.

Antibiotic Prophylaxis

The risk of endocarditis varies according to the abnormality (Table 20–14). The risk of infective endocarditis in patients with valvular heart disease following bacteremic events—including dental, oropharyngeal or nasopharyngeal, gastrointestinal, or genitourinary surgery or any incision and drainage (I & D)—is well established. Prophylaxis should generally follow the general guidelines recommended by the American Heart Association (Table 20–15).

Anticoagulation Management

Patients who are receiving anticoagulants can generally have their drug regimen interrupted for 1–3 days perioperatively without danger. The incidence of thromboembolic complications increases with a prior history of embolism and the presence of a thrombus, atrial fibrillation, or a prosthetic mechanical valve. The risk of thromboembolism is highest with a caged-ball

Table 20–15. Prophylactic regimens for various procedures.[1]

For dental, oral, respiratory tract, or esophageal procedures[2]
  I. Standard general prophylaxis for patients at risk:
    Amoxicillin: adults, 2.0 g (children, 50 mg/kg) given orally
      1 h before procedure
  II. Unable to take oral medications:
    Ampicillin: Adults, 2.0 g (children, 50 mg/kg) given IM or IV
      within 30 min before procedure
  III. Amoxicillin/ampicillin/penicillin allergic patients:
    Clindamycin: adults, 600 mg (children, 20 mg/kg) given
      orally 1 h before procedure or
    Cephalexin[3] or Cefadroxil[3]: adults, 2.0 g (children, 50 mg/kg)
      orally 1 h before procedure or
    Azithromycin or Clarithromycin: adults, 500 mg (children,
      15 mg/kg) orally 1 h before procedure
  IV. Amoxicillin/ampicillin/penicillin allergic patients unable to take oral medications:
    Clindamycin: adults, 600 mg (children, 20 mg/kg) IV within
      30 min before procedure or
    Cefazolin[3]: adults, 1.0 g (children, 25 mg/kg) IM or IV
      within 30 min before procedure

For genitourinary/gastrointestinal procedures:
  I. High-risk patients:
    Ampicillin plus gentamicin: ampicillin (adults, 2.0 g; children, 50 mg/kg) plus gentamicin 1.5 mg/kg (for both adults and children, not to exceed 120 mg) IM or IV within 30 min before starting procedure; 6 h later, ampicillin (adults, 1.0 g; children, 25 mg/kg) IM or IV, or amoxicillin (adults, 1.0 g; children, 25 mg/kg) orally
  II. High-risk patients allergic to ampicillin/amoxicillin:
    Vancomycin plus gentamicin: vancomycin (adults, 1.0 g; children, 20 mg/kg) IV over 1–2 h plus gentamicin 1.5 mg/kg (for both adults and children, not to exceed 120 mg) IM or IV; complete injection/infusion within 30 min before starting procedure
  III. Moderate-risk patients:
    Amoxicillin: adults, 2.0 g (children, 50 mg/kg) orally 1 h before procedure or
    Ampicillin: adults, 2.0 g (children, 50 mg/kg) IM or IV within 30 min before starting procedure
  IV. Moderate-risk patients allergic to ampicillin/amoxicillin:
    Vancomycin: adults, 1.0 g (children 20 mg/kg) IV over 1–2 h; complete infusion within 30 min of starting the procedure

[1]Based on AHA Guidelines.
[2]Follow-up dose no longer recommended. Total children's dose should not exceed adult dose.
[3]Cephalosporins should not be used in patients with immediate-type hypersensitivity reaction to penicillins.

mechanical (Starr–Edwards) prosthesis, particularly in the mitral or tricuspid position; intermediate for tiltingdisc (St. Jude) valves; and lowest for bioprostheses (porcine or bovine tissue valves). Most patients can safely have their warfarin stopped 3 days prior to surgery and restarted 2–3 days postoperatively. If the thromboembolic risk is deemed high, anticoagulation can be stopped the day before surgery and reversed with vitamin K or fresh frozen plasma; intravenous heparin therapy can then be initiated 12–24 h postoperatively once surgical hemostasis is believed to be adequate.

3. Specific Valvular Disorders

MITRAL STENOSIS

Preoperative Considerations

Mitral stenosis almost always occurs as a delayed complication of acute rheumatic fever. Two-thirds of patients with mitral stenosis are female. The stenotic process is estimated to begin after a minimum of 2 years following the acute disease and results from progressive fusion and calcification of the valve leaflets. Symptoms generally develop after 20–30 years, when the mitral valve orifice is reduced from its normal 4–6 cm^2 opening to less than 2 cm^2. Less than 50% of patients have isolated mitral stenosis; the remaining patients also have mitral regurgitation and up to 25% also have rheumatic involvement of the aortic valve (stenosis or regurgitation).

Pathophysiology

The rheumatic process causes the valve leaflets to thicken, calcify, and become funnel shaped; annular calcification may also be present. The mitral commissures fuse, the chordae tendinae fuse and shorten, and the valve cusps become rigid; as a result, the valve leaflets typically display bowing or doming during diastole on echocardiography.

Significant restriction of blood flow through the mitral valve results in a transvalvular pressure gradient that depends on cardiac output, heart rate (diastolic time), and the presence or absence of a normal atrial kick. Increases in either cardiac output or heart rate (decreased diastolic time) necessitate higher flows across the valve and result in higher transvalvular pressure gradients. The left atrium is often markedly dilated and promotes supraventricular tachycardias, particularly atrial fibrillation. Blood flow stasis in the atrium promotes the formation of thrombi, usually in the left atrial appendage. Loss of normal atrial systole (which is usually responsible for 20–30% of ventricular filling) necessitates even higher diastolic flow across the valve to maintain the same cardiac output and increases the transvalvular gradient.

Acute elevations in left atrial pressure are rapidly transmitted back to the pulmonary capillaries. If mean pulmonary capillary pressure acutely rises above 25 mm Hg, transudation of capillary fluid results in pulmonary edema. Chronic elevations in pulmonary capillary pressure are partially compensated by increases in pulmonary lymph flow but eventually result in pulmonary vascular changes leading to irreversible increases in pulmonary vascular resistance (PVR) and pulmonary hypertension. Reduced lung compliance and a secondary increase in the work of breathing contribute to chronic dyspnea. Right ventricular failure is frequently precipitated by acute or chronic elevations in right ventricular afterload. Marked dilatation of the right ventricle can result in tricuspid or pulmonary valve regurgitation.

Embolic events are common in patients with mitral stenosis and atrial fibrillation. Dislodgment of clots from the left atrium results in systemic emboli, most commonly to the cerebral circulation. Patients also have an increased incidence of pulmonary emboli, pulmonary infarction, hemoptysis, and recurrent bronchitis. Hemoptysis most commonly results from rupture of pulmonary–bronchial venous communications. Chest pain occurs in 10–15% of patients with mitral stenosis, even in the absence of coronary atherosclerosis; its etiology often remains unexplained but may be emboli in the coronary circulation or acute right ventricular pressure overload. Patients may develop hoarseness as a result of compression of the left recurrent laryngeal nerve by the enlarged left atrium.

Left ventricular function is normal in the majority of patients with pure mitral stenosis (Figure 20–5), but

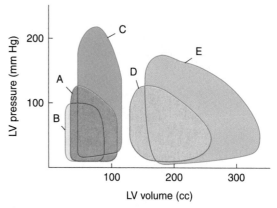

Figure 20–5. Pressure–volume loops in patients with valvular heart disease. A, normal; B, mitral stenosis; C, aortic stenosis; D, mitral regurgitation (chronic); E, aortic regurgitation (chronic). LV, left ventricular. (Reproduced, with permission, from Jackson JM, Thomas SJ, Lowenstein E: Anesthetic management of patients with valvular heart disease. Semin Anesth 1982;1:239.)

impaired left ventricular function may be encountered in up to 25% of patients and presumably represents residual damage from rheumatic myocarditis or coexistent hypertensive or ischemic heart disease.

Calculating Mitral Valve Area & Transvalvular Gradient

The relationship between cardiac output, valvular area, and the transvalvular gradient can be expressed by the Gorlin equation:

$$\text{Valve area} = \frac{\text{Flow across valve}}{K \times \sqrt{\text{Mean transvalvular gradient}}}$$

where K is a hydraulic-pressure constant. When mitral valvular flow is expressed as mL/s, pressure as mm Hg, and valve area as cm^2, $K = 38$. Mitral valve flow (MVF) can be estimated as follows:

$$\text{MVF} = \frac{\text{Cardiac output}}{\text{Diastolic filling period} \times \text{heart rate}}$$

Two-dimensional and Doppler echocardiography can be used to estimate both the pressure drop across a stenotic valve and the valve area. Based on the assumption that the velocity of blood flow is much greater distal than proximal to an obstruction, the Bernoulli equation can be simplified:

$$\Delta P = 4V^2$$

where ΔP is the pressure gradient (mm Hg) and V is blood flow velocity (m/s) distal to the obstruction. Valve orifice can be estimated from the time it takes for the initial peak pressure gradient to fall to one-half its original value, the pressure half-time ($T_{1/2}$). This relationship is approximated by

$$A = \frac{220}{T_{1/2}}$$

where A is valve orifice (cm^2) and $T_{1/2}$ is the time from peak flow velocity (V_{max}) to $V_{max}\sqrt{2}$ ($V_{max}/1.4$). This relationship is based on the observation that $T_{1/2}$ remains relatively constant for a given orifice over a wide range of flows. A pressure half-time of 220 ms corresponds to a mitral valve area of 1 cm^2. Valve area can also be estimated by planimetry in a short-axis view of the left ventricle (see Chapter 21). In the absence of significant mitral regurgitation, mitral valve area (MVA) can additionally be derived from the continuity equation (see section on aortic stenosis):

$$\text{MVA} = \text{SV}_{mv} / \text{VTI}_{\text{MS–jet}}$$

where SV_{mv} is stroke volume (transmitral) and $\text{VTI}_{\text{MS-jet}}$ is the velocity time integral of the Doppler signal of the mitral stenosis jet; stroke volume can be calculated from measuring the cross-sectional area and Doppler velocity time integral in the left ventricular outflow tract (see section on aortic stenosis).

Mitral valve areas less than 1 cm^2 are typically associated with transvalvular gradients of 20 mm Hg at rest and dyspnea with minimal exertion; a mitral valve area less than 1 cm^2 is often referred to as critical mitral stenosis. Patients with valve areas between 1.5 and 2.0 cm^2 are generally asymptomatic or have only mild symptoms with exertion. When the mitral valve area is between 1 and 1.5 cm^2, most patients are symptomatic with mild to moderate exertion. Although cardiac output may be normal at rest, it fails to increase appropriately during exertion because of decreased left ventricular preload.

Treatment

The time from onset of symptoms to incapacitation averages 5–10 years. At that stage, most patients die within 2–5 years. Surgical correction (open valvuloplasty) is therefore usually undertaken once significant symptoms develop. Recurrent mitral stenosis following valvuloplasty is usually managed with valve replacement. Percutaneous transseptal balloon valvuloplasty may be used in selected young or pregnant patients as well as older patients who are poor surgical candidates. Medical management is primarily supportive and includes limitation of physical activity, sodium restriction, and diuretics. Digoxin is useful only in patients with atrial fibrillation and a rapid ventricular response. Small doses of a β-adrenergic blocking drug may also be useful in controlling heart rate in patients with mild to moderate symptoms. Patients with a history of emboli and those at high risk (older than 40 years; a large atrium with chronic atrial fibrillation) are usually anticoagulated.

Anesthetic Management

A. OBJECTIVES

The principal hemodynamic goals are to maintain a sinus rhythm (if present preoperatively) and to avoid tachycardia, large increases in cardiac output, and both hypovolemia and fluid overload by judicious fluid therapy.

B. MONITORING

Full hemodynamic monitoring (of direct intraarterial pressure and pulmonary artery pressure) is generally indicated for all major surgical procedures, particularly those associated with large fluid shifts. Overzealous fluid replacement readily precipitates pulmonary edema in patients with severe disease. Pulmonary artery pressures should be monitored closely. Pulmonary capillary wedge pressure measurements in the presence of mitral stenosis reflect the transvalvular gradient and not necessarily left ventricular end-diastolic pressure. Prominent *a* waves and a decreased *y* descent are typically present on the pulmonary capillary wedge pressure waveform in patients who are in sinus rhythm. A prominent *cv* wave on the central venous pressure waveform is usually indicative of secondary tricuspid regurgitation. The ECG typically shows a notched P wave in patients who are in sinus rhythm.

C. Choice of Agents

Patients may be very sensitive to the vasodilating effects of spinal and epidural anesthesia. Epidural is preferable to spinal anesthesia because of the more gradual onset of sympathetic blockade. Ketamine by itself is generally a poor induction agent for general anesthesia because of its sympathetic stimulation. Similarly, pancuronium-induced tachycardia is to be avoided. In considering the type of agent to use, an opioid may be a better choice than a volatile agent. The latter can produce undesirable vasodilation or precipitate junctional rhythm with loss of an effective atrial kick. Of the volatile agents, halothane may be the most suitable because it decreases heart rate and is the least vasodilating, but other volatile agents have been used safely. Nitrous oxide should be used cautiously, as it can acutely increase PVR in some patients.

Intraoperative tachycardia may be controlled by deepening anesthesia with an opioid (excluding meperidine) or β-blocker (esmolol or propranolol). In the presence of atrial fibrillation, ventricular rate may be controlled with diltiazem or digoxin. Verapamil may be less desirable because of the associated vasodilation. **Marked hemodynamic deterioration from sudden supraventricular tachycardia necessitates cardioversion. Phenylephrine is preferred over ephedrine as a vasopressor because the former lacks β-adrenergic agonist activity.** Treatment of acute hypertension or afterload reduction with potent vasodilators should be undertaken only with full hemodynamic monitoring.

MITRAL REGURGITATION

Preoperative Considerations

Mitral regurgitation can develop acutely or insidiously as a result of a large number of disorders. Chronic mitral regurgitation is usually the result of rheumatic fever (often with concomitant mitral stenosis); congenital or developmental abnormalities of the valve apparatus; or dilation, destruction, or calci-

fication of the mitral annulus. Acute mitral regurgitation is usually due to myocardial ischemia or infarction (papillary muscle dysfunction or rupture of a chorda tendinea), infective endocarditis, or chest trauma.

Pathophysiology

The principal derangement is a reduction in forward stroke volume due to backward flow of blood into the left atrium during systole. The left ventricle compensates by dilating and increasing end-diastolic volume (Figure 20–5). Regurgitation through the mitral valve reduces left ventricular afterload, which often initially enhances contractility. End-systolic volume thus remains normal but eventually increases as the disease progresses. By increasing end-diastolic volume, the volume-overloaded left ventricle can maintain a normal cardiac output even as ejection fraction decreases. With time, patients with chronic mitral regurgitation eventually develop eccentric left ventricular hypertrophy (see Chapter 19) and progressive impairment in contractility, as reflected by a decrease in ejection fraction (< 50%). In patients with severe mitral regurgitation, the regurgitant volume may exceed the forward stroke volume.

The regurgitant volume passing through the mitral valve is dependent on the size of the mitral valve orifice (which can vary with ventricular cavity size), the heart rate (systolic time), and the left ventricular–left atrial pressure gradient during systole. The last factor is affected by the relative resistances of the two outflow paths from the left ventricle, namely, SVR and left atrial compliance. Thus, a decrease in SVR or an increase in mean left atrial pressure will reduce the regurgitant volume. Atrial compliance also determines the predominant clinical manifestations. Patients with normal or reduced atrial compliance (acute mitral regurgitation) have primarily pulmonary vascular congestion and edema. Patients with increased atrial compliance (long-standing mitral regurgitation resulting in a large dilated left atrium) primarily show signs of a low cardiac output. Most patients are between the two extremes and exhibit symptoms of both pulmonary congestion and low cardiac output. Patients with a regurgitant fraction less than 30% of the total stroke volume generally have mild symptoms. Regurgitant fractions of 30–60% generally cause moderate symptoms, whereas fractions greater than 60% are associated with severe disease.

Echocardiography, particularly TEE, is extremely useful in delineating the underlying pathophysiology of mitral regurgitation as well as in guiding treatment. Mitral valve leaflet motion is often described as normal, excessive (prolapsing), or restrictive (Figure 20–6). Excessive motion or prolapse is defined by systolic

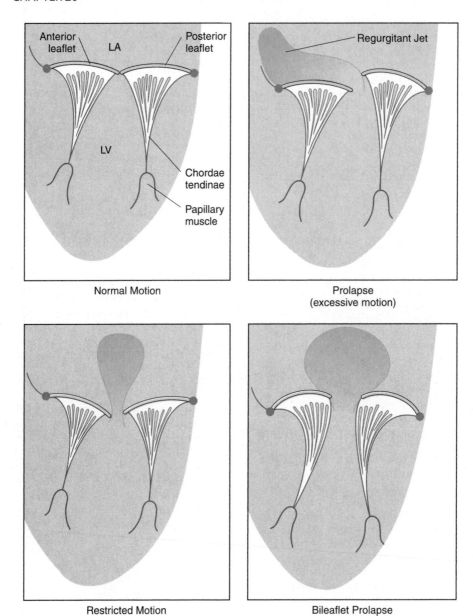

Figure 20–6. Classification of mitral valve leaflet motion (as seen from transesophageal echocardiography). Note that with prolapse, the free edge of the leaflet(s) extends beyond the plane of the mitral annulus producing an eccentric jet. With restricted motion, the leaflets fail to coapt resulting in a central jet.

movement of a leaflet beyond the plane of the mitral valve and into the left atrium (see the section below on mitral valve prolapse). **Eccentric regurgitant jets on color-flow Doppler echocardiography are typical of a prolapsing valve, whereas central jets are more typical of regurgitation with normal or restricted valve motion.**

Calculating Regurgitant Fraction

To calculate regurgitant fraction (RF), forward stroke volume (SV) and the regurgitant stroke volume (RSV) must be measured. Although they can both be estimated by catheterization data, pulsed Doppler echocardiography provides reasonably acute calculations. Stroke volume is measured at the left ventricular outflow tract (LVOT) and at the mitral valve (MV), where

$$\text{Stroke volume} = \text{cross-sectional area } (A) \times (\text{TVI})$$

and cross-sectional area (A) can be approximated as,

$$A = 0.785 \times (\text{diameter})^2$$

The time velocity integral (TVI) is the area of velocity versus the time signal obtained with pulsed Doppler (see Chapter 21). Thus,

$$RSV_{\text{mitral regurgitation}} = (A_{MV} \times VTI_{MV})$$
$$- (A_{LVOT} \times TVI_{LVOT}),$$

and

$$RF = RSV/SV$$

An RSV greater than 65 mL usually correlates with severe mitral regurgitation.

Treatment

Medical treatment includes digoxin, diuretics, and vasodilators—including ACE inhibitors. Afterload reduction is beneficial in most patients and may even be lifesaving in patients with acute mitral regurgitation. Reduction of SVR increases forward SV and decreases the regurgitant volume. Surgical treatment is usually reserved for patients with moderate to severe symptoms. Surgical valvuloplasty is performed whenever possible to avoid the problems associated with valve replacement (eg, thromboembolism, hemorrhage, and prosthetic failure).

Anesthetic Management

A. OBJECTIVES

 Anesthetic management should be tailored to the severity of mitral regurgitation as well as the underlying left ventricular function. Factors that exacerbate the regurgitation, such as slow heart rates (long systole) and acute increases in afterload, should be avoided. Bradycardia can increase the regurgitant volume by increasing left ventricular end-diastolic volume and acutely dilating the mitral annulus. The heart rate should ideally be kept between 80 and 100 beats/min. Acute increases in left ventricular afterload, such as following endotracheal intubation and surgical stimulation, should be treated rapidly but without excessive myocardial depression. Excessive volume expansion can also worsen the regurgitation by dilating the left ventricle.

B. MONITORING

Monitors are based on the severity of ventricular dysfunction as well as the procedure. Pulmonary artery pressure monitoring is extremely useful in patients with symptomatic disease. Intraoperative afterload reduction with a vasodilator requires full hemodynamic monitoring. Mitral regurgitation may be recognized on the pulmonary artery wedge waveform as a large v wave and a rapid y descent (Figure 20–7). The height of the v wave is inversely related to atrial and pulmonary vascular compliance but is directly proportional to pulmonary blood flow and the regurgitant volume; thus the v wave may not be prominent in patients with chronic mitral regurgitation except during acute deterioration. Very large v waves are often apparent on the pulmonary

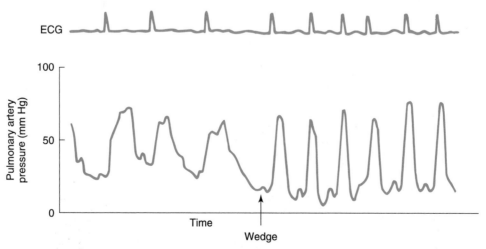

Figure 20–7. The pulmonary capillary wedge waveform in mitral regurgitation, demonstrating a large v wave.

Table 20–16. Echocardiographic assessment of regurgitant lesions by color-flow Doppler.

Grade	Description	Criterion
0	None	No regurgitation into receiving chamber
1+	Mild	Regurgitant flow limited to area immediately near valve
2+	Mild to moderate	Regurgitant flow occupies up to one-third of receiving chamber
3+	Moderate to severe	Regurgitant flow occupies up to two-thirds of receiving chamber
4+	Severe	Regurgitant flow occupies most of receiving chamber and flow reversal is present[1]

[1]For atrioventricular valves flow reversal occurs proximally in the veins filling the atrium; for semilunar valves flow reversal occurs distally in the great vessels.

artery pressure waveform even without wedging the catheter. Color-flow Doppler TEE can be invaluable in quantitating the severity of the regurgitation and guiding therapeutic interventions in patients with severe mitral regurgitation (Table 20–16). By definition, blood flow reverses in the pulmonary veins during systole with severe mitral regurgitation.

C. Choice of Agents

Patients with relatively well-preserved ventricular function tend to do well with most anesthetic techniques. Spinal and epidural anesthesia are well tolerated, provided bradycardia is avoided. Patients with moderate to severe ventricular impairment are often very sensitive to the depressant effects of volatile agents. A primarily opioid-based anesthetic may be more suitable for those patients—again, provided bradycardia is avoided. The selection of pancuronium as a muscle relaxant with an opioid-based anesthetic may be useful in this regard.

MITRAL VALVE PROLAPSE

Preoperative Considerations

Mitral valve prolapse is classically characterized by a midsystolic click with or without a late apical systolic murmur on auscultation. It is a relatively common abnormality that is present in up to 5% of the general population, being most common in women (up to 15%). The diagnosis is based on auscultatory findings and is confirmed by echocardiography, which shows systolic prolapse of mitral valve leaflets into the left atrium. Patients with the murmur often have some element of mitral regurgitation. The posterior mitral leaflet is more commonly affected than the anterior leaflet. The mitral annulus may also be dilated. Pathologically, most patients have redundancy or some myxomatous degeneration of the valve leaflets. Most cases of mitral valve prolapse are sporadic or familial, affecting other-

wise normal persons. A high incidence of mitral valve prolapse is found in patients with connective tissue disorders (particularly Marfan syndrome).

The overwhelming majority of patients with mitral valve prolapse are asymptomatic, but in a small percentage the myxomatous degeneration is progressive. Manifestations, when they occur, can include chest pains, arrhythmias, embolic events, florid mitral regurgitation, infective endocarditis and, rarely, sudden death. The diagnosis can be made preoperatively by auscultation of the characteristic click but must be confirmed by echocardiography. The prolapse is accentuated by maneuvers that decrease ventricular volume (preload). The ECG is usually normal but in some patients often shows inverted or biphasic T waves or ST-segment changes inferiorly. Both atrial and ventricular arrhythmias are common. Although bradyarrhythmias are also reported, paroxysmal supraventricular tachycardia is the most commonly encountered sustained arrhythmia. An increased incidence of abnormal AV bypass tracts (see Chapter 19) is reported in patients with mitral valve prolapse.

Most patients have a normal life span. About 15% develop progressive mitral regurgitation. A smaller percentage develop embolic phenomena or infective endocarditis. Patients with both a click and a systolic murmur appear to be at greater risk for developing complications. Anticoagulation or antiplatelet agents may be used for patients with a history of emboli, whereas β-adrenergic blocking drugs are commonly employed for arrhythmias.

Anesthetic Management

The management of these patients is based on their clinical course. Most patients are asymptomatic and, except for antibiotic prophylaxis, do not require special care. Patients with a systolic murmur appear to be at greatest risk for infective endocarditis. Ventricular arrhythmias may occur intraoperatively, particularly following sympathetic stimulation, and will generally respond to lidocaine or β-adrenergic blocking agents. Relatively deep anesthesia with a volatile agent usually decreases the likelihood of intraoperative arrhythmias. Mitral regurgitation caused by prolapse is generally exacerbated by decreases in ventricular size. Hypovolemia and factors that increase ventricular emptying—such as increased sympathetic tone or decreased afterload—should therefore be avoided. Vasopressors with pure α-adrenergic agonist activity (such as phenylephrine) may be preferable to those that are primarily β-adrenergic agonists (ephedrine).

AORTIC STENOSIS

Preoperative Considerations

Valvular aortic stenosis is the most common cause of obstruction to left ventricular outflow. Left ventricular outflow obstruction is less commonly due to hypertrophic cardiomyopathy, discrete congenital subvalvular stenosis, or, rarely, supravalvular stenosis. Valvular aortic stenosis is nearly always congenital, rheumatic, or degenerative. Abnormalities in the number of cusps (most commonly a bicuspid valve) or in their architecture produce turbulence that traumatizes the valve and eventually leads to stenosis. Rheumatic aortic stenosis is rarely isolated; it is more commonly associated with aortic regurgitation or mitral valve disease. In the most common degenerative form, calcific aortic stenosis, wear and tear results in the buildup of calcium deposits on normal cusps, preventing them from opening completely.

Pathophysiology

In contrast to acute obstruction of left ventricular outflow, which rapidly dilates the ventricle and reduces SV (see Chapter 21), obstruction caused by valvular aortic stenosis is almost always gradual, allowing the ventricle, at least initially, to compensate and maintain SV. Concentric ventricular hypertrophy enables the left ventricle to maintain SV by generating a significant transvalvular gradient and to reduce ventricular wall stress (Figure 20–5).

Critical aortic stenosis is said to exist when the aortic valve orifice is reduced to 0.5–0.7 cm^2 (normal is 2.5–3.5 cm^2). With this degree of stenosis, patients generally have a transvalvular gradient of approximately 50 mm Hg at rest (with a normal cardiac output) and are unable to increase cardiac output appreciably. Moreover, further increases in the transvalvular gradient do not significantly increase SV. Aortic valve areas between 0.7 and 0.9 cm^2 are generally associated with mild to moderate symptoms. With long-standing aortic steno-

sis, myocardial contractility progressively deteriorates and further compromises left ventricular function. Most patients with aortic stenosis have a long latency period of 30–60 years (depending on the cause) before significant symptoms develop.

Classically, patients with advanced aortic stenosis have the triad of dyspnea on exertion, angina, and orthostatic or exertional syncope. A prominent feature of aortic stenosis is a decrease in left ventricular compliance as a result of hypertrophy (see Chapter 19). Diastolic dysfunction is the result of an increase in ventricular muscle mass, fibrosis, or myocardial ischemia. In contrast to left ventricular end-diastolic volume, which remains normal until very late in the disease, left ventricular end-diastolic pressure is elevated early. The decreased diastolic pressure gradient between the left atrium and left ventricle impairs ventricular filling, which becomes quite dependent on a normal atrial contraction. Loss of atrial systole can precipitate congestive heart failure or hypotension in patients with aortic stenosis. Cardiac output may be normal in symptomatic patients at rest, but characteristically, it does not appropriately increase with exertion. Patients may experience angina even in the absence of CAD. Myocardial oxygen demand increases because of ventricular hypertrophy, whereas myocardial oxygen supply decreases as a result of the marked compression of intramyocardial coronary vessels caused by high intracavitary systolic pressures (up to 300 mm Hg). Exertional syncope or near-syncope is thought to be due to an inability to tolerate the vasodilation in muscle tissue during exertion. Arrhythmias leading to severe hypoperfusion may also account for syncope and sudden death in some patients. Calcium emboli may occasionally result in neurological complications.

Calculating Aortic Valve Area & Transvalvular Gradient

As with mitral stenosis, valve area can be derived from catheterization data because the transvalvular gradient is proportionate to cardiac output. Using the Gorlin equation:

$$\text{Valve area} = \frac{\text{Flow across valve}}{K \times \sqrt{\text{mean transvalvular gradient}}}$$

Aortic valve flow is expressed as mL/s, pressure as mm Hg, and valve area as cm^2; $K = 44$. Aortic valve flow can be derived as follows:

$$\text{Aortic valve flow} = \frac{\text{Cardiac output}}{\text{Systolic ejection period} \times \text{heart rate}}$$

As with mitral stenosis, the pressure gradient across the aortic valve can be determined noninvasively using continuous wave Doppler echocardiography:

$$\Delta P = 4V^2$$

where ΔP is the peak pressure gradient (mm Hg) and V is peak blood flow velocity (m/s) distal to the obstruction. Peak velocities greater than 4.5 m/s are usually indicative of severe stenosis. Moreover, if the area proximal to the stenosis (LVOT) can be measured, the continuity equation can then be applied to estimate valve area. Either TVIs or maximum velocities can be used:

$$A_2 = \frac{A_1 V_1}{V_2}$$

where A_2 is valve area, A_1 is the cross-sectional area of the LVOT, V_1 is maximum blood flow velocity in LVOT, and V_2 is maximum flow velocity through the aortic valve. The presence of aortic regurgitation does not affect the accuracy of this calculation.

Treatment

Once significant symptoms develop, most patients, without surgical treatment, die within 2–5 years. Patients with congestive heart failure are treated with digoxin, sodium restriction, and small doses of diuretics. Percutaneous balloon valvuloplasty is generally used for younger patients with congenital aortic stenosis; it can also be used for elderly patients with calcific aortic stenosis who are poor candidates for aortic valve replacement. Its efficacy for the latter group is short-lived, however, and restenosis usually occurs within 6–12 months.

Anesthetic Management

A. OBJECTIVES

Maintenance of normal sinus rhythm, heart rate, and intravascular volume is critical in patients with aortic stenosis. Loss of a normally timed atrial systole often leads to rapid deterioration, particularly when associated with tachycardia. The combination of the two (atrial fibrillation) seriously impairs ventricular filling and necessitates immediate cardioversion. The reduced ventricular compliance also makes the patient very sensitive to abrupt changes in intravascular volume. Many patients behave as though they have a fixed SV in spite of adequate hydration; under these conditions, cardiac output becomes very rate dependent. Bradycardia (< 50 beats/min) is therefore poorly tolerated. Heart rates between 60 and 90 beats/min are optimal in most patients.

B. MONITORING

Close monitoring of the ECG and blood pressure is crucial. Monitoring for ischemia is complicated by baseline ST-segment and T-wave abnormalities. Intraarterial pressure monitoring is desirable in patients with severe aortic stenosis, as many of these patients do not tolerate even brief episodes of hypotension. Pulmonary artery catheterization is also useful, but data should be interpreted carefully; a higher than normal pulmonary capillary wedge pressure is often required to maintain adequate left ventricular end-diastolic volume and cardiac output. Prominent *a* waves are often visible on the pulmonary artery wedge pressure waveform. Vasodilators should generally be employed only when a pulmonary artery catheter is in place, because patients are often very sensitive to these agents. TEE can be useful in these patients for monitoring ischemia, ventricular preload, contractility, valvular function, and the effects of therapeutic interventions.

C. CHOICE OF AGENTS

Patients with mild to moderate aortic stenosis (generally asymptomatic) may tolerate spinal or epidural anesthesia. These techniques should be employed very cautiously, however, because hypotension readily occurs as a result of reductions in preload, afterload, or both. Epidural anesthesia is preferable to spinal anesthesia because of its slower onset of hypotension, which allows more aggressive correction. Spinal and epidural anesthesia are contraindicated in patients with severe aortic stenosis.

The selection of general anesthetic agents is most critical in patients with symptomatic (moderate to severe) aortic stenosis. In these patients, a primarily opioid-based anesthetic technique generally results in minimal cardiac depression; suitable nonopioid induction agents include etomidate and the combination of ketamine and a benzodiazepine. If a volatile agent is used, the concentration should be carefully controlled to avoid excessive myocardial depression, vasodilation, or loss of normal atrial systole. Tachycardia and hypertension, which can precipitate ischemia, should be treated by increasing anesthetic depth. If a β-adrenergic blocking agent is used, esmolol may be preferable because of its short half-life. Most patients with aortic stenosis are extremely sensitive to vasodilators. Moreover, because of an already precarious myocardial oxygen demand–supply balance, they tolerate even mild degrees of hypotension poorly. Hypotension should generally be treated with small doses (25–50 μg) of phenylephrine. Intraoperative supraventricular tachycardias with hemodynamic compromise should be treated with immediate synchronized cardioversion. Frequent ventricular ectopy (which often reflects ischemia) is usually poorly tolerated hemodynamically and should be treated with intravenous lidocaine. Amiodarone is generally effective for both supraventricular and ventricular arrhythmias.

HYPERTROPHIC CARDIOMYOPATHY

Preoperative Considerations

Hypertrophic cardiomyopathy can be hereditary (usually with variable penetrance) or may occur sporadically. It has been referred to by many other names: idiopathic hypertrophic subaortic stenosis, asymmetric septal hypertrophy, hypertrophic obstructive cardiomyopathy, and muscular subaortic stenosis. It is characterized by heterogeneous left ventricular hypertrophy with no obvious cause. The hypertrophied muscle typically displays abnormal cellular architecture.

Affected patients characteristically display *diastolic dysfunction* that is reflected by elevated left ventricular end-diastolic pressures in spite of often hyperdynamic ventricular function. The diastolic stiffness is presumably due to the abnormal hypertrophied muscle, which tends to be located in the upper interventricular septum below the aortic valve; rarely, only the ventricular apex is involved. In about 25% of patients, the hypertrophy results in dynamic obstruction of left ventricular outflow during systole. Obstruction is the result of narrowing in the subaortic area caused by a systolic anterior motion (SAM) of the anterior mitral valve leaflet against the hypertrophied septum. SAM may be at least partly due to a Venturi effect drawing in the anterior leaflet during rapid ejection of the hypertrophied ventricle. In contrast to fixed obstruction (valvular aortic stenosis), the resulting obstruction (and pressure gradient) is dynamic and peaks in mid-to-late systole. Moreover, the degree of obstruction can vary from beat to beat. Factors that tend to worsen the obstruction include enhanced contractility, decreased ventricular volume, and decreased left ventricular afterload. Mitral regurgitation secondary to SAM is due to failure of mitral leaflets to normally coapt in late systole usually resulting in a posteriorly directed regurgitant jet. Anatomic studies also suggest that most patients have abnormalities of the mitral valve; the mitral leaflets, particularly the anterior one, are frequently longer than normal.

Most patients are asymptomatic. Patients who are symptomatic generally complain of dyspnea on exertion, but they may also have fatigue, syncope, near-syncope, or angina. Symptoms do not necessarily correlate with the presence or severity of dynamic left ventricular outflow obstruction. Sudden cardiac death is often the first manifestation of the disorder in patients younger than 30 years and is the most common cause of death. Both supraventricular and ventricular arrhythmias are common. Patients with obstruction have a characteristic harsh systolic murmur (see Table 20–13). The ECG typically shows left ventricular hypertrophy and deep, broad Q waves. The diagnosis can be confirmed by echocardiography. Even asymptomatic patients may show myocardial perfusion defects on thallium-201 scans. The peak pressure gradient can be measured with Doppler echocardiography by determining peak velocity in the LVOT (see the section above on aortic stenosis).

Treatment is with β-adrenergic and calcium channel blocking agents. Both agents decrease contractility and can prevent increases in the subaortic pressure gradient in patients with obstruction. Calcium channel blockers may also improve diastolic compliance (relaxation). Amiodarone is generally effective for both supraventricular and ventricular arrhythmias. Nitrates, digoxin, and diuretics are avoided because they can worsen left ventricular obstruction. Surgical myomectomy/myotomy is reserved for patients with moderate to severe symptoms; TEE is an invaluable aid for such resections.

Anesthetic Management

Preoperative evaluation of patients with hypertrophic cardiomyopathy should focus on evaluating the potential for significant dynamic obstruction, malignant arrhythmias, and myocardial ischemia. The results of echocardiography (or angiography) and Holter monitoring should ideally be reviewed with a cardiologist. Anesthetic goals should be to minimize sympathetic activation, expand intravascular volume to avoid hypovolemia, and minimize decreases in left ventricular afterload.

Monitoring requirements are dictated by the severity of obstruction and the surgical procedure. Full hemodynamic monitoring is generally desirable to guide fluid therapy in the presence of abnormal ventricular compliance. The arterial pressure waveform in patients with obstruction may be bifid (bisferiens pulse): The initial rapid peak represents early unobstructed ventricular ejection, whereas the subsequent decrease and second peak are the result of dynamic obstruction.

In patients with significant obstruction, some degree of myocardial depression is usually desirable and can be achieved by the use of volatile anesthetic agents, particularly halothane and enflurane. β-Adrenergic agents are also useful in counteracting the effects of sympathetic activation and decreasing obstruction. Regional anesthesia may exacerbate left ventricular outflow obstruction by decreasing both cardiac preload and afterload. **Phenylephrine and other pure α-adrenergic agonists are ideal vasopressors in these patients because they do not augment contractility but increase SVR (ventricular afterload).**

AORTIC REGURGITATION

Preoperative Considerations

Aortic regurgitation usually develops slowly and is progressive (chronic), but it can also develop quickly (acute). Chronic aortic regurgitation may be caused by abnormalities of the aortic valve, the aortic root, or both. Abnormalities in the valve are usually congenital (bicuspid valve) or due to rheumatic fever. Diseases affecting the ascending aorta cause regurgitation by dilating the aortic annulus; they include syphilis, annuloaortic ectasia, cystic medial necrosis (with or without Marfan syndrome), ankylosing spondylitis, rheumatoid and psoriatic arthritis, and a variety of other connective tissue disorders. Acute aortic insufficiency most commonly follows infective endocarditis, trauma, or aortic dissection.

Pathophysiology

Regardless of the cause, aortic regurgitation produces volume overload of the left ventricle (Figure 20–5). The effective forward SV is reduced because of backward (regurgitant) flow of blood into the left ventricle during diastole. Systemic arterial diastolic pressure and SVR are typically low. The decrease in cardiac afterload helps facilitate ventricular ejection. Total SV is the sum of the effective stroke volume and the regurgitant volume. The regurgitant volume depends on the heart rate (diastolic time) and the diastolic pressure gradient across the aortic valve (diastolic aortic pressure minus left ventricular end-diastolic pressure). Slow heart rates increase regurgitation because of the associated disproportionate increase in diastolic time (see Chapter 19), whereas increases in diastolic arterial pressure favor regurgitant volume by increasing the pressure gradient for backward flow.

With chronic aortic regurgitation, the left ventricle progressively dilates and undergoes eccentric hypertrophy. Patients with severe aortic regurgitation have the largest end-diastolic volumes of any heart disease; the massively dilated heart is often referred to as cor bovinum. The resulting increase in end-diastolic volume maintains an effective SV because end-systolic volume is unchanged. Any increase in the regurgitant volume is compensated by an increase in end-diastolic volume. Left ventricular end-diastolic pressure is usually normal or only slightly elevated, because ventricular compliance initially increases. Eventually, as ventricular function deteriorates, the ejection fraction declines, and impaired ventricular emptying is manifested as gradual increases in left ventricular end-diastolic pressure and end-systolic volume.

Sudden incompetence of the aortic valve does not allow compensatory dilation or hypertrophy of the left ventricle. Effective SV rapidly declines because the normal-sized ventricle is unable to accommodate a sudden large regurgitant volume. The sudden rise in left ventricular end-diastolic pressure is transmitted back to the pulmonary circulation and causes acute pulmonary congestion.

Acute aortic regurgitation typically presents as the sudden onset of pulmonary edema and hypotension, whereas chronic regurgitation usually presents insidiously as congestive heart failure. Symptoms are generally minimal (in the chronic form) when the regurgitant volume remains under 40% of SV but become severe when it exceeds 60%. Angina can occur even in the absence of coronary disease. The myocardial oxygen demand is increased from muscle hypertrophy and dilatation, whereas the myocardial blood supply is reduced by low diastolic pressures in the aorta as a result of the regurgitation.

Calculating Regurgitant Fraction & Other Measurements of Severity

As with mitral regurgitation, RSV and RF for aortic regurgitation can be estimated by pulsed Doppler echocardiography. Stroke volume is measured at the left ventricular outflow tract (LVOT) and at the mitral valve (MV).

Thus,

$$RSV_{\text{aortic regurgitation}} = (A_{LVOT} \times TVI_{LVOT}) - (A_{MV} \times VTI_{MV})$$

and

$$RF = RSV/SV$$

Pressure half-time ($T_{1/2}$, see the section on mitral stenosis above) of the regurgitant jet is another useful echocardiographic parameter for clinically assessing the severity of aortic regurgitation. The shorter the half-time the more severe the regurgitation; severe regurgitation rapidly raises left ventricular diastolic pressure and results in more rapid pressure equilibration. Unfortunately, $T_{1/2}$ is affected not only by the regurgitant orifice area but also by aortic and ventricular pressure. An aortic regurgitation jet with a $T_{1/2}$ less than 240 ms is associated with severe regurgitation.

Treatment

Most patients with chronic aortic regurgitation remain asymptomatic for 10–20 years. Once significant symptoms develop, the expected survival time is about 5 years without valve replacement. Digitalis, diuretics, and afterload reduction, particularly with ACE inhibitors, generally benefit patients with advanced chronic aortic regurgitation. The decrease in arterial blood pressure reduces the diastolic gradient for regurgitation. Patients with chronic aortic regurgitation should be operated on before irreversible ventricular dysfunction occurs.

Patients with acute aortic regurgitation typically require intravenous inotropic (dopamine or dobutamine) and vasodilator (nitroprusside) therapy. Early surgery is indicated for patients with acute aortic regurgitation: medical management alone is associated with a high mortality rate.

Anesthetic Management

A. OBJECTIVES

The heart rate should be maintained toward the upper limits of normal (80–100 beats/min). Bradycardia and increases in SVR increase the regurgitant volume in patients with aortic regurgitation, whereas tachycardia can contribute to myocardial ischemia. Excessive myocardial depression should also be avoided. The compensatory increase in cardiac preload should be maintained, but overzealous fluid replacement can readily result in pulmonary edema.

B. MONITORING

Full hemodynamic monitoring should generally be employed for all patients with acute aortic regurgitation and those with severe chronic regurgitation. Premature closure of the mitral valve often occurs during acute aortic regurgitation and may cause pulmonary capillary wedge pressure to give a falsely high estimate of left ventricular end-diastolic pressure. The appearance of a large *v* wave suggests mitral regurgitation secondary to dilation of the left ventricle. The arterial pressure wave in patients with aortic regurgitation characteristically has a very wide pulse pressure. A bisferiens pulse may also be present in some patients and is thought to result from the rapid ejection of a large SV. Color-flow Doppler TEE can be invaluable in quantitating the severity of the regurgitation and guiding therapeutic interventions (see Table 20–16). By definition, some reversal of blood flow is present in the aorta during all of diastole (holodiastolic) with severe aortic regurgitation; moreover, the further down the aorta holodiastolic flow reversal is detected, the more severe the regurgitation.

C. CHOICE OF AGENTS

Most patients tolerate spinal and epidural anesthesia, provided intravascular volume is maintained. When general anesthesia is required, isoflurane and desflurane may be ideal because of the associated vasodilation. A primarily opioid-based general anesthetic technique is more suitable for patients with depressed ventricular function. Pancuronium is a good choice as a muscle relaxant with the latter technique because it often prevents bradycardia. Intraoperative afterload reduction with nitroprusside optimally requires full hemodynamic monitoring. Ephedrine is generally the preferred vasopressor for the treatment of hypotension. Small doses of phenylephrine (25–50 μg) can be used when the hypotension is clearly due to excessive vasodilation, however. Large doses of phenylephrine can increase SVR (and arterial diastolic pressure) and may exacerbate the regurgitation.

TRICUSPID REGURGITATION

Preoperative Considerations

Up to 70–90% of patients have mild tricuspid regurgitation on echocardiography; the regurgitant volume in these cases is almost always insignificant. Clinically significant tricuspid regurgitation, however, is most commonly due to dilation of the right ventricle from the pulmonary hypertension that is associated with chronic left ventricular failure. Tricuspid regurgitation can also follow infective endocarditis (usually in injecting drug abusers), rheumatic fever, carcinoid syndrome, or chest trauma or may be due to Ebstein's anomaly (downward displacement of the valve because of abnormal attachment of the valve leaflets).

Pathophysiology

Chronic left ventricular failure often leads to sustained increases in pulmonary vascular pressures. The chronic increase in afterload causes progressive dilation of the thin-walled right ventricle, and excessive dilation of the tricuspid annulus eventually results in regurgitation. An increase in end-diastolic volume allows the right ventricle to compensate for the regurgitant volume and maintain an effective forward flow. Because the right atrium and the vena cava are compliant and can usually accommodate the volume overload, mean right atrial and central venous pressures are generally only slightly elevated. Acute or marked elevations in pulmonary artery pressures increase the regurgitant volume and are reflected by an increase in central venous pressure. Moreover, sudden marked increases in right ventricular afterload sharply reduce the effective right ventricular output, reduce left ventricular preload, and can precipitate systemic hypotension.

Chronic venous hypertension leads to passive congestion of the liver and progressive hepatic dysfunction, which can eventually result in cardiac cirrhosis. Severe right ventricular failure with underloading of the left heart may also produce right-to-left shunting through an incompletely closed (or probe-patent) foramen ovale, which can result in marked hypoxemia.

Calculating Regurgitant Volume & Pulmonary Artery Pressure

To calculate the regurgitant volume, stroke volume is calculated at the tricuspid valve and at another (unaffected) site such as the LVOT or mitral valve (see the section above on mitral regurgitation):

$$RSV_{tricuspid\ regurgitation} = (A_{TV} \times VTI_{TV})$$
$$-(A_{LVOT} \times TVI_{LVOT})$$

where A_{TV} is the area of tricuspid valve and VTI_{TV} is the time velocity integral of flow across the tricuspid valve. With severe tricuspid regurgitation the normal systolic inflow into the right atrium is reversed and the reversal of flow is also observed in the hepatic veins.

Systolic pulmonary artery pressure (PAS) can be estimated from the peak velocity of the regurgitant:

$$\Delta P = 4 \times V^2$$

where ΔP is the systolic pressure gradient (mm Hg) between the right ventricle and right atrium and V is peak blood flow velocity (m/s) of the regurgitant jet. If the central venous pressure (CVP) is known or assumed, then

$$PAS = CVP + \Delta P$$

Treatment

Tricuspid regurgitation is generally well tolerated by most patients. In the absence of pulmonary hypertension, many even tolerate complete surgical excision of the tricuspid valve. Because the underlying disorder is generally more important than the tricuspid regurgitation itself, treatment is aimed at the underlying disease process. With moderate to severe regurgitation, tricuspid annuloplasty may be performed in conjunction with replacement of another valve.

Anesthetic Management

A. OBJECTIVES

Hemodynamic goals should be directed primarily toward the underlying disorder. Hypovolemia and factors that increase right ventricular afterload, such as hypoxia and acidosis, should be avoided to maintain effective right ventricular SV and left ventricular preload. Positive end-expiratory pressure and high mean airway pressures may also be undesirable during mechanical ventilation because they reduce venous return and increase right ventricular afterload.

B. MONITORING

In these patients, monitoring of both central venous and pulmonary artery pressures is useful. The latter is not always possible, as a large regurgitant flow may make passage of a pulmonary artery catheter across the tricuspid valve difficult. CVP is extremely useful in following right ventricular function, whereas pulmonary artery pressures allow measurement of its afterload and left ventricular preload. Increasing CVPs imply worsening right ventricular dysfunction. The x descent is absent and a prominent cv wave is usually present on the CVP waveform. Thermodilution cardiac output measurements are falsely elevated because of the tricuspid regurgitation. Color-flow Doppler TEE is useful in evaluating the severity of the regurgitation and other associated abnormalities.

C. CHOICE OF AGENTS

The selection of anesthetic agents should be based on the underlying disorder. Most patients tolerate spinal and epidural anesthesia well. Coagulopathy secondary to hepatic dysfunction should be excluded prior to any regional technique. During general anesthesia, nitrous oxide may exacerbate the pulmonary hypertension and should be administered cautiously, if at all.

■ CONGENITAL HEART DISEASE

Preoperative Considerations

Congenital heart disease encompasses a seemingly endless list of abnormalities that may be detected in infancy, early childhood, or, less commonly, adulthood. The incidence of congenital heart disease in all live births approaches 1%. The natural history of some defects is such that patients often survive to adulthood (Table 20–17). Moreover, the number of surviving adults with congenital heart disease appears to be

Table 20–17. Common congenital heart defects in which patients typically survive to adulthood without treatment.

Bicuspid aortic valve
Coarctation of the aorta
Pulmonic valve stenosis
Ostium secundum atrial septal defect
Ventricular septal defect
Patent ductus arteriosus

Table 20–18. Classification of congenital heart disease.

Lesions causing outflow obstruction
  Left ventricle
    Coarctation of the aorta
    Aortic stenosis
  Right ventricle
    Pulmonic valve stenosis
Lesions causing left-to-right shunting
  Ventricular septal defect
  Patent ductus arteriosus
  Atrial septal defect
  Endocardial cushion defect
  Partial anomalous pulmonary venous return
Lesions causing right-to-left shunting
  With decreased pulmonary blood flow
    Tetralogy of Fallot
    Pulmonary atresia
    Tricuspid atresia
  With increased pulmonary blood flow
    Transposition of the great vessels
    Truncus arteriosus
    Single ventricle
    Double-outlet right ventricle
    Total anomalous pulmonary venous return
    Hypoplastic left heart

---

steadily increasing, possibly as a result of advances in medical treatment. An increasing number of patients with congenital heart disease may therefore be encountered during noncardiac surgery and obstetric deliveries.

The complex nature and varying pathophysiology of congenital heart defects make classification difficult. A commonly used scheme is presented in Table 20–18. Most patients present with cyanosis, congestive heart failure, or an asymptomatic abnormality. Cyanosis is typically the result of an abnormal intracardiac communication that allows unoxygenated blood to reach the systemic arterial circulation (right-to-left shunting). Congestive heart failure is most prominent with defects that either obstruct left ventricular outflow or markedly increase pulmonary blood flow. The latter is usually due to an abnormal intracardiac communication that returns oxygenated blood to the right heart (left-to-right shunting). Whereas right-to-left shunts generally decrease pulmonary blood flow, some complex lesions increase pulmonary blood flow—even in the presence of right-to-left shunting. In many cases, more than one lesion is present. In fact, survival with some anomalies (eg, transposition, total anomalous venous return, pulmonary atresia) depends on the simultaneous presence of another shunting lesion (eg, patent ductus arteriosus, patent foramen ovale, ventricular septal defect). Chronic

hypoxemia in patients with cyanotic heart disease typically results in erythrocytosis. This increase in red cell mass, which is due to enhanced erythropoietin secretion from the kidneys, serves to restore tissue oxygen concentration to normal. Unfortunately, blood viscosity can also rise to the point at which it may interfere with oxygen delivery. Moreover, iron deficiency exacerbates the hyperviscosity by making red cells more rigid and less deformable in the microcirculation. When tissue oxygenation is restored to normal, the hematocrit is stable (usually < 65%), and symptoms of the hyperviscosity syndrome are absent, the patient is said to have compensated erythrocytosis. Patients with compensated erythrocytosis do not establish this equilibrium; they have symptoms of hyperviscosity and may be at risk for thrombotic complications, particularly stroke. The last is aggravated by dehydration and iron deficiency. Children younger than 4 years appear to be at greatest risk for stroke. Factors that may lead to stroke in adults are excessive phlebotomy and aspirin or anticoagulation therapy. Phlebotomy is generally not recommended if symptoms of hyperviscosity are absent and the hematocrit is < 65%.

Coagulation abnormalities are common in patients with cyanotic heart disease. Platelet counts tend to be low-normal, and many patients have subtle or overt defects in the coagulation cascade. Phlebotomy may improve hemostasis in some patients. Hyperuricemia often occurs because of increased urate reabsorption secondary to renal hypoperfusion. Gouty arthritis is uncommon, but the hyperuricemia can result in progressive renal impairment.

Preoperative Doppler echocardiography is invaluable in helping define the anatomy of the defect(s), confirm or exclude the existence of other lesions or complications, their physiological significance, and the effects of any therapeutic interventions.

Anesthetic Management

This population of patients includes four groups: those who have undergone corrective cardiac surgery and require no further operations, those who have had only palliative surgery, those who have not yet undergone any cardiac surgery, and those whose conditions are inoperable and may be awaiting cardiac transplantation. Although the management of the first group of patients may be the same as for normal patients (except for consideration of prophylactic antibiotic therapy, see Table 20–15), the care of others requires familiarity with the complex pathophysiology of these defects. Even patients who have had corrective surgery may be prone to development of perioperative problems (Table 20–19). Some surgical procedures eliminate the risk of endocarditis whereas others increase the risk through the use of pros-

Table 20–19. Common problems in survivors of surgery for congenital heart defects.

Arrhythmias
Hypoxemia
Pulmonary hypertension
Existing shunts
Paradoxical embolism
Bacterial endocarditis

thetic valves or conduits or the creation of new shunts. Patients with ostium secundum atrial septal defects and those with mild pulmonic stenosis appear to have the lowest risk.

The management of patients for cardiac surgery and during obstetric delivery is discussed in Chapters 21 and 43, respectively. The general management of the pediatric patient is discussed in Chapter 44.

For the purpose of anesthetic management, congenital heart defects may be divided into obstructive lesions, predominantly left-to-right shunts, or predominantly right-to-left shunts (see Table 20–18). In reality, shunts can also be bidirectional and may reverse under certain conditions.

1. Obstructive Lesions

Congenital aortic stenosis has already been discussed above (see the section on aortic stenosis) and coarctation of the aorta is discussed in Chapter 21.

Pulmonic Stenosis

Pulmonary valve stenosis obstructs right ventricular outflow and causes concentric right ventricular hypertrophy. Severe obstruction presents in the neonatal period, whereas lesser degrees of obstruction may go undetected until adulthood. The valve is usually deformed, and is either bicuspid or tricuspid. Valve leaflets are often partially fused and display systolic doming on echocardiography. The right ventricle undergoes hypertrophy and poststenotic dilation of the pulmonary artery is often present. Symptoms are those of right ventricular heart failure (see Chapter 19). Symptomatic patients readily develop fatigue, dyspnea, and peripheral cyanosis with exertion as a result of the limited pulmonary blood flow and increased oxygen extraction by tissues. With severe stenosis, the pulmonic valve gradient exceeds 60–80 mm Hg, depending on the age of the patient. Right-to-left shunting may also occur in the presence of a patent foramen ovale or atrial septal defect. Cardiac output is very dependent on an elevated heart rate, but excessive increases in the latter can compromise ventricular fill-

ing. Percutaneous balloon valvuloplasty is generally considered the initial treatment of choice for most patients with symptomatic pulmonic stenosis. Anesthetic management for patients undergoing surgery should maintain a normal or slightly high heart rate, augment preload, and avoid factors that increase PVR (see Chapter 22).

2. Predominantly Left-to-Right (Simple) Shunts

Simple shunts are isolated abnormal communications between the right and left sides of the heart. Because pressures are normally higher on the left side, blood usually flows across from left to right, and blood flow through the right heart and the lungs increases. Depending on the size and location of the communication, the right ventricle may also be subjected to the higher left-sided pressures, resulting in both pressure and volume overload. Right ventricular afterload is normally 5% that of the left ventricle, so even small left-to-right pressure gradients can produce large increases in pulmonary blood flow. The ratio of pulmonary to systemic blood flow can be calculated from oxygen saturations at the time of catheterization by the following equation:

$$\frac{\dot{Q}_P}{\dot{Q}_S} = \frac{Ca_{O_2} - C\bar{v}_{O_2}}{Cpv_{O_2} - Cpa_{O_2}}$$

where Ca_{O_2} is systemic arterial blood flow, $C\bar{v}_{O_2}$ is mixed venous blood flow, Cpv_{O_2} is the oxygen content of pulmonary venous blood (ie, in pulmonary veins), and Cpa_{O_2} is the oxygen content of pulmonary artery blood.

A ratio greater than 1 usually indicates a left-to-right shunt, whereas a ratio less than 1 indicates a right-to-left shunt. A ratio of 1 indicates either no shunting or a bidirectional shunt of opposing magnitudes.

Large increases in pulmonary blood flow produce pulmonary vascular congestion and increase extravascular lung water. The latter interferes with gas exchange, decreases lung compliance, and increases the work of breathing. Left atrial distention also compresses the left bronchus, whereas distention of pulmonary vessels compresses smaller bronchi.

Over the course of several years, chronic increases in pulmonary blood flow produce vascular changes that irreversibly increase PVR. Elevation of right ventricular afterload produces hypertrophy and progressively raises right-sided cardiac pressures. With advanced disease, the pressures within the right heart can exceed those within the left heart. Under these conditions, the intracardiac shunt reverses and becomes a right-to-left shunt (Eisenmenger syndrome).

When a communication is small, shunt flow depends primarily on the size of the communication (restrictive shunt). When the communication is large (nonrestrictive shunt), shunt flow depends on the relative balance between PVR and SVR. An increase in SVR relative to PVR favors left-to-right shunting, whereas an increase in PVR relative to SVR favors right-to-left shunting. Common chamber lesions (eg, single atrium, single ventricle, truncus arteriosus) represent the extreme form of nonrestrictive shunts; shunt flow with these lesions is bidirectional and totally dependent on relative changes in the ventricular afterload.

The presence of shunt flow between the right and left hearts, regardless of the direction of blood flow, mandates the meticulous exclusion of air bubbles or clot from intravenous fluids to prevent paradoxical embolism into the cerebral or coronary circulations.

Atrial Septal Defects

Ostium secundum atrial septal defects (ASDs) are the most common type and usually occur as isolated lesions in the area of the fossa ovalis. The defect is sometimes associated with partial anomalous pulmonary venous return, most commonly of the right upper pulmonary vein. A secundum ASD may result in single or multiple (fenestrated) openings between the atria. The less common sinus venosus, and ostium primum ASDs are typically associated with other cardiac abnormalities. Sinus venosus defects are located in the upper interatrial septum close to the superior vena cava; one or more of the right pulmonary veins often abnormally drains into the superior vena cava. In contrast, ostium primum ASDs are located in the lower interatrial septum and overlie the mitral and tricuspid valves; most patients also have cleft in the anterior leaflet of the mitral valve and some have an abnormal septal leaflet in the tricuspid valve.

Most children with ASDs are minimally symptomatic; some have recurrent pulmonary infections. Congestive heart failure and pulmonary hypertension are more commonly encountered in adults with ASDs. Patients with ostium primum defects often have large shunts and may also develop significant mitral regurgitation. In the absence of heart failure, anesthetic responses to inhalation and intravenous agents are generally not significantly altered in patients with ASDs. Increases in SVR should be avoided because they may worsen the left-to-right shunting.

Ventricular Septal Defects

Ventricular septal defect (VSD) is the most common congenital heart defect, accounting for up to 25–35% of congenital heart disease. The defect is most fre-

quently in the membranous part of the interventricular septum (membranous or infracristal VSD) in a posterior position and anterior to the septal leaflet of the tricuspid valve. Muscular VSDs are the next most frequent type and are located in the mid or apical portion of the interventricular septum, where there may be a single defect or multiple openings (resembling Swiss cheese). Defects in the subpulmonary (supracristal) septum are often associated with aortic regurgitation because the right coronary cusp can prolapse into the VSD. Septal defects at the ventricular inlet are usually similar in development and location to AV septal defects (see the following section).

The resulting functional abnormality of a VSD is dependent on the size of the defect, PVR, and the presence or absence of other abnormalities. Small VSDs, particularly of the muscular type, often close during childhood. Restrictive defects are associated with only small left-to-right shunts (pulmonary–systemic blood flow ratios less than 1.75:1). Large defects produce large left-to-right shunts (shunts larger than 2:1) that vary directly with SVR and indirectly with PVR. Recurrent pulmonary infections and congestive heart failure are common with pulmonary–systemic flow ratios of 3–5:1. Patients with small VSDs are treated medically and followed by electrocardiography (for signs of right ventricular hypertrophy) and by echocardiography. Surgical closure is usually undertaken for patients with large VSDs before pulmonary vascular disease and Eisenmenger physiology develop. As with atrial defects, in the absence of heart failure, anesthetic responses to inhalation and intravenous agents are generally not significantly altered. Similarly, increases in SVR worsen the left-to-right shunting. When right-to-left shunting is present, abrupt increases in PVR or decreases in SVR are poorly tolerated.

Atrioventricular Septal Defects

Endocardial cushion (AV canal) defects produce contiguous atrial and ventricular septal defects often with very abnormal AV valves. This is a common lesion in patients with Down syndrome (see Chapter 44). The defect can produce large shunts both at the atrial and ventricular levels. Mitral and tricuspid regurgitation exacerbate the volume overload on the ventricles. Initially, shunting is predominately left to right; however, with increasing pulmonary hypertension, Eisenmenger syndrome with obvious cyanosis develops.

Patent Ductus Arteriosus

Persistence of the communication between the main pulmonary artery and the aorta can produce restrictive or nonrestrictive left-to-right shunts. This abnormality is commonly responsible for the cardiopulmonary deterioration of premature infants, and occasionally presents later in life. Anesthetic goals should be similar to atrial and ventricular septal defects.

Partial Anomalous Venous Return

This defect is present when one or more pulmonary veins drains into the right side of the heart; the anomalous veins are usually from the right lung. Possible anomalous entry sites include the right atrium, the superior or inferior vena cava, and the coronary sinus. The resulting abnormality produces a variable amount of left-to-right shunting. The clinical course and prognosis are usually excellent and similar to that of a secundum ASD. A very large coronary sinus on TEE suggests anomalous drainage into the coronary sinus, which may complicate the management of cardioplegia during cardiac surgery (see Chapter 21).

3. Predominantly Right-to-Left (Complex) Shunts

Lesions within this group (some also called **mixing lesions**) often produce both ventricular outflow obstruction and shunting. The obstruction favors shunt flow toward the unobstructed side. When the obstruction is relatively mild, the amount of shunting is affected by the ratio of SVR to PVR, but increasing degrees of obstruction fix the direction and magnitude of the shunt. Atresia of any one of the cardiac valves represents the extreme form of obstruction. Shunting occurs proximal to the atretic valve and is completely fixed; survival depends on another distal shunt (usually a patent ductus arteriosus [PDA], patent foramen ovale, ASD, or VSD), where blood flows in the opposite direction. This group of defects may also be divided according to whether they increase or decrease pulmonary blood flow (see Table 20–18).

Tetralogy of Fallot

This tetralogy classically includes right ventricular obstruction, right ventricular hypertrophy, and a VSD with an overriding aorta. Right ventricular obstruction in most patients is due to infundibular stenosis, which is due to hypertrophy of the subpulmonic muscle (crista ventricularis). At least 20–25% of patients also have pulmonic stenosis, and a small percentage have some element of supravalvular obstruction. The pulmonic valve is often bicuspid or less commonly atretic. Infundibular obstruction may be increased by sympathetic tone and is therefore dynamic; this obstruction is likely responsible for the hypercyanotic spells observed in very young patients. **The combination of right ventricular obstruction and a VSD results in ejection of unoxygenated right ventricular blood as** well as oxygenated left ventricular blood into the aorta. The right-to-left shunting across the VSD has both fixed and variable components. The fixed component is determined by the severity of the right ventricular obstruction, whereas the variable component depends on SVR and PVR.

Neonates with severe right ventricular obstruction may deteriorate quickly as pulmonary blood flow decreases when a PDA starts to close. Intravenous prostaglandin E_1 (0.05–0.2 µg/kg/min) is used to prevent ductal closure in such instances. Surgical palliation with a left-to-right systemic shunt or complete correction is then usually undertaken. For the former, a modified Blalock–Taussig (left subclavian-pulmonary artery) shunt is most often used to increase pulmonary blood flow. In this procedure, a synthetic graft is anastomosed between a subclavian artery and an ipsilateral pulmonary artery. Complete correction involves closure of the VSD, removal of obstructing infundibular muscle, and pulmonic valvulotomy or valvuloplasty, when necessary.

The goals of anesthetic management in patients with tetralogy of Fallot should be to maintain intravascular volume and SVR. Increases in PVR, such as might occur from acidosis or excessive airway pressures, should be avoided. **Ketamine (intramuscular or intravenous) is a commonly used induction agent because it maintains or increases SVR and therefore does not aggravate the right-to-left shunting.** Patients with milder degrees of shunting generally tolerate inhalation induction with halothane. The right-to-left shunting tends to slow the uptake of inhalation anesthetics (see Chapter 7); in contrast, it may accelerate the onset of intravenous agents. Oxygenation often improves following induction of anesthesia. Muscle relaxants that release histamine should be avoided. Hypercyanotic spells may be treated with intravenous fluid and phenylephrine (5 µg/kg). Propranolol (0.1 µg/kg) may also be effective in relieving infundibular spasm. Sodium bicarbonate, to correct the resulting metabolic acidosis, may also be helpful when the hypoxemia is severe and prolonged.

Tricuspid Atresia

With tricuspid atresia, blood can flow out of the right atrium only via a patent foramen ovale (or an ASD). Moreover, a PDA (or VSD) is necessary for blood to flow from the left ventricle into the pulmonary circulation. Cyanosis is usually evident at birth and its severity depends on the amount of pulmonary blood flow that is achieved. Early survival is dependent on prostaglandin E_1 infusion with or without a percutaneous, Rashkind balloon atrial septostomy. Severe cyanosis requires a modified Blalock–Taussig shunt early in life. The preferred surgical management is a modified Fontan procedure, in which the right atrium is anastomosed to the right pulmonary artery. In some centers a superior vena cava to the main pulmonary artery (bidirectional Glenn) shunt may be employed before or instead of a Fontan procedure. With both procedures, blood from the systemic veins flows to the left atrium entirely as a result of a pressure gradient. Success of the procedure depends on a high systemic venous pressure and maintaining both low PVR and a low left atrial pressure. Heart transplantation may be necessary for a failed Fontan procedure.

Transposition of the Great Arteries

In patients with transposition of the great arteries (TGA), pulmonary and systemic venous return flow normally back to the right and left atrium, respectively, but the aorta arises from the right ventricle and the pulmonary artery arises from the left ventricle. Thus, deoxygenated blood returns back into the systemic circulation and oxygenated blood returns back to the lungs. Survival is possible only through mixing of oxygenated and deoxygenated blood across the foramen ovale and a PDA. The presence of a VSD increases mixing and reduces the level of hypoxemia. Prostaglandin E_1 infusion is usually necessary. Rashkind septostomy may be necessary if surgical correction is delayed. Corrective surgical treatment involves an arterial switch procedure in which the aorta is divided and reanastomosed to the left ventricle and the pulmonary artery is divided and reanastomosed to the right ventricle. The coronary arteries must also be reimplanted into the old pulmonary artery root. A VSD, if present, is closed. Less commonly, an atrial switch (Senning) procedure may be carried out if an arterial switch is not possible. In this latter procedure, an intraatrial baffle is created from the atrial wall and blood from the pulmonary veins flows across an ASD to the right ventricle, from where it is ejected into the systemic circulation.

Transposition of the great vessels may occur with a VSD and pulmonic stenosis. This combination of defects mimics tetralogy of Fallot; however, the obstruction affects the left ventricle not the right ventricle. Corrective surgery involves patch closure of the VSD, directing left ventricular outflow into the aorta, ligation of the proximal pulmonary artery, and connecting the right ventricular outflow to the pulmonary artery with a valved conduit (Rastelli procedure).

Total Anomalous Venous Return

The absence of a direct connection between the pulmonary veins and the left atrium results in total anomalous venous return. Mixing of deoxygenated and oxygenated blood occurs at or before the right atrial level because the pulmonary veins usually drain into the superior or inferior vena cava, coronary sinus, or ductus venosus. Blood usually reaches the left atrium via the foramen ovale or an ASD. Obstruction of the pulmonary venous return, which may occur when the blood drains into the ductus venous and it begins to close, results in severe pulmonary congestion. Surgical correction involves reanastomosing the common pulmonary venous trunk directly into the left atrium and closure of any ASD.

Truncus Arteriosus

With a truncus arteriosus defect, a single arterial trunk supplies the pulmonary and systemic circulation. The truncus always overrides a VSD, allowing both ventricles to eject into it. As PVR gradually decreases after birth, pulmonary blood flow increases greatly resulting in heart failure. If left untreated, PVR increases and cyanosis develops again along with Eisenmenger physiology. Surgical correction closes the VSD, separates the pulmonary artery from the truncus, and connects the right ventricle to the pulmonary artery with a conduit (Rastelli repair).

Hypoplastic Left Heart Syndrome

This syndrome describes a group of defects characterized by marked underdevelopment of the left ventricle. It is often associated with other major noncardiac congenital anomalies. The right ventricle is the main pumping chamber for both systemic and pulmonary circulations. It ejects normally into the pulmonary artery and all (or nearly all) blood flow entering the aorta is usually derived from a PDA. Surgical treatment options are either palliation with the very complicated Norwood procedure or cardiac transplantation. The Norwood procedure is typically carried out in three stages.

■ THE PATIENT WITH A TRANSPLANTED HEART

Preoperative Considerations

The number of patients with cardiac transplants is increasing because of both the increasing frequency of transplantation and improved survival rates. These patients may present to the operating room early in the postoperative period for mediastinal exploration or retransplantation, or they may appear later for incision and drainage of infections, orthopedic surgery, or unrelated procedures.

The transplanted heart is totally denervated, so direct autonomic influences are absent. Cardiac impulse formation and conduction are normal, but the absence of vagal influences causes a relatively high resting heart rate (100–120 beats/min). Although sympathetic fibers are similarly interrupted, the response to circulating catecholamines is normal or even enhanced because of denervation sensitivity (increased receptor density). Partial reinnervation may occur in some patients after some time. Cardiac output tends to be low-normal and increases relatively slowly in response to exercise because the response is dependent on an increase in circulating catecholamines. Because the Starling relationship between end-diastolic volume and cardiac output (see Chapter 19) is normal, the transplanted heart is also often said to be preload dependent. Coronary autoregulation is preserved.

Preoperative evaluation should focus on evaluating the functional status of the transplanted organ and detecting complications of immunosuppression. The highest incidence of rejection occurs within the first 3 months; thereafter rejection rates are about one per patient-year. Rejection may be heralded by arrhythmias (in the first 6 months) or decreased exercise tolerance from a progressive deterioration of myocardial performance. Periodic echocardiographic evaluations are commonly used to monitor for rejection, but the most reliable technique is endomyocardial biopsy. Accelerated atherosclerosis in the graft is a very common and serious problem that limits the life of the transplant. Moreover, myocardial ischemia and infarction are almost always silent because of the denervation. Because of this, patients must undergo periodic evaluations, including angiography, for coronary atherosclerosis.

Immunosuppressive therapy usually includes cyclosporine, azathioprine, and prednisone. Important side effects include nephrotoxicity, bone marrow suppression, hepatotoxicity, opportunistic infections, and osteoporosis. Hypertension and fluid retention are common and typically require treatment with a diuretic and an ACE inhibitor. Stress doses of corticosteroids are needed when patients undergo major procedures (see Chapter 36).

Anesthetic Management

Almost all anesthetic techniques, including regional anesthesia, have been used successfully for transplanted patients. The preload-dependent function of the graft makes maintenance of a normal or high cardiac preload desirable. Moreover, the absence of reflex increases in heart rate can make patients particularly sensitive to rapid vasodilation. Indirect vasopressors such as ephedrine and dopamine are less effective than direct-acting agents because of the absence of catecholamine stores in myocardial neurons (see Chapter 12). Isoproterenol or dilute epinephrine (10 µg/mL) should be readily available to increase the heart rate if necessary. Bradycardia secondary to opioids and cholinesterase inhibitors is absent. Similarly, increases in heart rate are not seen following anticholinergics, pancuronium, or meperidine. An anticholinergic must still be given to reverse muscle relaxants to block the noncardiac muscarinic effects of acetylcholine.

Careful electrocardiographic monitoring for ischemia is necessary. The ECG usually demonstrates two sets of P waves, one representing the recipient's own SA node (which is left intact) and the other representing the donor's SA node. The recipient's SA node may still be affected by autonomic influences, but it does not affect cardiac function. Direct arterial, central venous, and pulmonary artery pressure monitoring should be used for major operations; strict asepsis should be observed during placement.

CASE DISCUSSION: HIP FRACTURE IN AN ELDERLY WOMAN WHO FELL

A 71-year-old woman presents for open reduction and internal fixation of a left hip fracture. She gives a history of two episodes of lightheadedness several days prior to her fall today. When questioned about her fall, she can only recall standing in her bathroom while brushing her teeth and then awakening on the floor with hip pain. The preoperative ECG shows a sinus rhythm with a P–R interval of 220 ms and a right bundle-branch block (RBBB) pattern.

Why should the anesthesiologist be concerned about a history of syncope?

A history of syncope in elderly patients should always raise the possibility of arrhythmias and underlying organic heart disease. Although arrhythmias can occur in the absence of organic heart disease, the two are commonly related. Cardiac syncope usually results from an abrupt arrhythmia that suddenly compromises cardiac output and impairs cerebral perfusion. Lightheadedness, presyncope, may reflect lesser degrees of cerebral impairment. Both bradyarrhythmias and tachyarrhythmias (see Chapter 19) can produce syncope. Table 20–20 lists other cardiac and noncardiac causes of syncope.

How do bradyarrhythmias commonly arise?

Bradyarrhythmias may arise from either SA node dysfunction or abnormal AV conduction of the cardiac impulse. A delay or block of the impulse can occur anywhere between the SA node and the distal His-Purkinje system (see Chapter 19). Reversible abnormalities may be due to abnormal vagal tone, electrolyte abnormalities, drug toxicity, hypothermia, or myocardial ischemia. Irreversible abnormalities, which initially may be only intermittent before they become permanent, reflect either isolated conduction system abnormalities or underlying heart disease (most commonly hypertensive, coronary artery, or valvular heart disease).

What is the pathophysiology of sinus node dysfunction?

Patients with sinus node dysfunction may have a normal baseline 12-lead ECG but abrupt pauses in SA node activity (sinus arrest) or intermittent block of conduction of the SA impulse to the surrounding tissue (exit block). Symptoms are usually present when pauses are prolonged (> 3 s) or the effective ventricular rate is less than 40 beats/min. Patients may experience intermittent dizziness, syncope, confusion, fatigue, or shortness of breath. Symptomatic SA node dysfunction, or sick sinus syndrome, is often unmasked by β-adrenergic blocking agents, calcium channel blockers, digoxin, or quinidine. The term tachycardia–bradycardia syndrome is often used when patients experience paroxysmal tachyarrhythmias (usually atrial flutter or fibrillation) followed by sinus pauses or bradycardia. The latter, bradycardia, probably represents failure of the SA node to recover normal automaticity following suppression by the tachyarrhythmia. The diagnosis must be based on electrocardiographic recordings made during symptoms (Holter monitoring) or after provocative tests (carotid baroreceptor stimulation or rapid atrial pacing).

How are AV conduction abnormalities manifested on the surface 12-lead ECG?

AV conduction abnormalities are usually manifested by abnormal ventricular depolarization (bundle-branch block), prolongation of the P–R interval (first-degree AV block), failure of some atrial impulses to depolarize the ventricles

Table 20–20. Causes of syncope.

Cardiac
 Arrhythmias
  Tachyarrhythmias (usually > 180 beats/min)
  Bradyarrhythmias (usually < 40 beats/min)
 Impairment of left ventricular ejection
  Aortic stenosis
  Hypertrophic cardiomyopathy
  Massive myocardial infarction
  Atrial myxoma
 Impairment of right ventricular output
  Tetralogy of Fallot
  Primary pulmonary hypertension
  Pulmonary embolism
  Pulmonic valve stenosis
 Biventricular impairment
  Cardiac tamponade
  Massive myocardial infarction
Noncardiac
 Accentuated reflexes
  Vasodepressor reflex (ie, vasovagal syncope)
  Carotid sinus hypersensitivity
  Neuralgias
 Postural hypotension
  Hypovolemia
  Sympathectomy
  Autonomic dysfunction
 Sustained Valsalva maneuver
 Cerebrovascular disease
 Seizures
 Metabolic
  Hypoxia
  Marked hypocapnia
  Hypoglycemia

(second-degree AV block), or AV dissociation (third-degree AV block; also called complete heart block).

What determines the significance of these conduction abnormalities?

The significance of a conduction system abnormality depends on its location, its likelihood for progression to complete heart block, and the likelihood that a more distal pacemaker site will be able to maintain a stable and adequate escape rhythm (> 40 beats/min). The His bundle is normally the lowest area in the conduction system that can maintain a stable rhythm (usually 40–60 beats/min). When conduction fails anywhere above it, a normal His bundle can take over the pacemaker function of the heart and maintain a normal QRS complex unless a distal intraventricular conduc-

tion defect is present. When the escape rhythm arises farther down the His-Purkinje system, the rhythm is usually slower (< 40 beats/min) and is often unstable; it results in a wide QRS complex.

What is the significance of isolated bundle-branch block with a normal P–R interval?

A conduction delay or block in the right bundle-branch results in a typical RBBB QRS pattern on the surface ECG (M-shape or rSR' in V_1) and may represent a congenital abnormality or underlying organic heart disease. In contrast, a delay or block in the main left bundle-branch results in a left bundle-branch block (LBBB) QRS pattern (wide R with a delayed upstroke in V_5) and nearly always represents underlying heart disease. The term hemiblock is often used if only one of the two fascicles of the left bundle-branch is blocked (left anterior or left posterior hemiblock). When the P–R interval is normal—and in the absence of an acute MI—a conduction block in either the left or right bundle rarely leads to complete heart block.

Can the site of AV block always be determined from a 12-lead ECG?

No. A first-degree AV block (P–R interval > 200 ms) can reflect abnormal conduction anywhere between the atria and the distal His-Purkinje system. Mobitz type I second-degree AV block, which is characterized by progressive lengthening of the P–R interval before a P wave is not conducted (a QRS does not follow the P wave), is usually due to a block in the AV node itself, and can be caused by digitalis toxicity or myocardial ischemia; progression to third-degree AV block is uncommon.

In patients with Mobitz type II second-degree AV block, atrial impulses are periodically not conducted into the ventricle without progressive prolongation of the P–R interval. The conduction block is nearly always in or below the His bundle and frequently progresses to complete (third-degree) AV block, particularly following an acute anteroseptal MI. The QRS is typically wide.

In patients with third-degree AV block, the atrial rate and ventricular depolarization rates are independent (AV dissociation) because atrial impulses completely fail to reach the ventricles. If the site of the block is in the AV node, a stable His bundle rhythm will result in a normal QRS complex and the ventricular rate will often increase following administration of atropine. If the block involves the His bundle, the origin of the ventricular rhythm is more distal, resulting in wide QRS com-

plexes. A wide QRS complex does not necessarily exclude a normal His bundle, as it may represent a more distal block in one of the bundle branches.

Can AV dissociation occur in the absence of AV block?

Yes. AV dissociation is common during anesthesia with volatile agents in the absence of AV block and results from sinus bradycardia or an accelerated AV junctional rhythm. During isorhythmic dissociation, the atria and ventricles beat independently at nearly the same rate. The P wave often just precedes or follows the QRS complex, and their relationship is generally maintained. In contrast, interference AV dissociation results from a junctional rhythm that is faster than the sinus rate—such that sinus impulses always find the AV node refractory.

How do bifascicular and trifascicular blocks present?

A bifascicular block exists when two of the three major His bundle-branches (right, left anterior, or left posterior) are partially or completely blocked. If one fascicle is completely blocked and the others are only partially blocked, a bundle-branch block pattern will be associated with either first-degree or second-degree AV block. If all three are affected, a trifascicular block is said to exist. A delay or partial block in all three fascicles results in either a prolonged P–R interval (first-degree AV block) or alternating LBBB and RBBB. Complete block in all three fascicles results in third-degree AV block.

What is the significance of the electrocardiographic findings in this patient?

The electrocardiographic findings (first-degree AV block plus RBBB) suggest a bifascicular block. Extensive disease of the conduction system is likely. Moreover, the patient's syncopal and near-syncopal episodes suggest that she may be at risk for life-threatening bradyarrhythmias (third-degree AV block). Intracardiac electrocardiographic recordings would be necessary to confirm the site of the conduction delay.

What is appropriate management for this patient?

Cardiological evaluation is required because of the symptomatic bifascicular block. One of two approaches can be recommended, depending on the urgency of the surgery. If the surgery is truly emergent, a temporary transvenous pacing catheter is indicated prior to induction of general or regional anesthesia. If the surgery can be postponed 24–48 h (as in this case), continuous electrocardiographic monitoring, serial 12-lead ECGs, and measurements of cardiac isoenzymes are required to exclude myocardial ischemia or infarction and to try to record findings during symptoms. Moreover, a brief intracardiac His bundle study may be useful in determining the need for a permanent pacemaker if a clinical diagnosis of symptomatic bradycardia cannot be made. If the HV interval is greater than 100 ms, the patient needs a pacemaker prior to surgery (see above). If the HV interval is normal or 60–100 ms, permanent pacing may not necessarily be indicated, but central (internal jugular) venous access and ready access to pacing equipment are still advisable because of the history of syncope.

What are general perioperative indications for temporary pacing?

Suggested indications include the following: any documented symptomatic bradyarrhythmia; a new bundle-branch block, second-degree (type II) AV block, or third-degree AV block associated with MI; bifascicular block in a comatose patient (controversial); and refractory supraventricular tachyarrhythmias.

The first three indications generally require ventricular pacing, whereas the fourth requires atrial pacing electrodes and a programmable rapid atrial pulse generator.

How can temporary cardiac pacing be established?

Pacing can be established by transvenous, transcutaneous, epicardial, or transesophageal electrodes. The most reliable method is generally via a transvenous pacing electrode in the form of a pacing wire or a balloon-tipped pacing catheter. A pacing wire should always be positioned fluoroscopically, but a flow-directed pacing catheter can also be placed in the right ventricle under pressure monitoring. A pacing wire must be used when blood flow has ceased. If the patient has a rhythm, intracardiac electrocardiographic recording showing ST-segment elevation when the electrode comes in contact with the right ventricular endocardium confirms placement

of either type of electrode. Specially designed pulmonary artery catheters have an extra port for passage of a right ventricular pacing wire. These catheters are particularly useful in patients with LBBB, who can develop complete heart block during catheter placement. Transcutaneous ventricular pacing is also possible via large stimulating adhesive pads placed on the chest and should be used whenever transvenous pacing is not readily available. Epicardial electrodes are usually used during cardiac surgery. Pacing the left atrium via an esophageal electrode is a simple, relatively noninvasive technique, but it is useful only for symptomatic sinus bradycardias and for terminating some supraventricular tachyarrhythmias.

Once positioned, the pacing electrodes are attached to an electrical pulse generator that periodically delivers an impulse at a set rate and magnitude. Most pacemaker generators can also sense the heart's spontaneous (usually ventricular) electrical activity: when activity is detected, the generator suppresses its next impulse. By altering the generator's sensing threshold, the pacemaker generator can function in a fixed (asynchronous) mode or in a demand mode (by increasing sensitivity). The lowest current through the electrode that can depolarize the myocardium is called the threshold current (usually < 2 mA for transvenous electrodes). An LBBB pattern is observed when the pacing electrode is within the right ventricle, because the right ventricle is depolarized directly, whereas the left ventricle is depolarized (later) by conduction across the myocardium, not the normal conducting system.

What is AV sequential pacing?

Ventricular pacing often reduces cardiac output because the atrial contribution to ventricular filling is lost. When the AV conducting system is diseased, atrial contraction can still be maintained by sequential stimulation by separate atrial and ventricular electrodes. The P–R interval can be varied by adjusting the delay between the atrial and ventricular impulses (usually set at 150–200 ms).

How are pacemakers classified?

Pacemakers are categorized by a five-letter code, according to the chambers paced, chambers sensed, response to sensing, programmability, and arrhythmia function (Table 20–21). The two most commonly used pacing modes are VVI and DDD (the last two letters are frequently omitted).

Table 20–21. Classification of pacemakers.

Chamber-Paced	Chamber-Sensed	Response to Sensing	Programmability	Antitachyarrhythmia Function
O = none	O = none	O = none	O = none	O = none
A = atrium	A = atrium	T = triggered	P = simple	P = pacing
V = ventricle	V = ventricle	I = inhibited	M = multiprogrammable	S = shock
D = dual (atrium and ventricle)	D = dual (atrium and ventricle)	D = dual (triggered and inhibited)	C = communicating	D = dual (pacing and shock)
			R = rate modulation	

If a pacemaker is placed in this patient, how can its function be evaluated?

If the patient's underlying rhythm is slower than the rate of a demand pacemaker, pacing spikes should be seen on the ECG. The spike rate should be identical to the programmed (permanent pacemaker—usually 72/min) or set (temporary) pacemaker rate; a slower rate may indicate a low battery. Every pacing spike should be followed by a QRS complex (100% capture). Moreover, every impulse should be followed by a palpable arterial pulse. If the patient has a temporary pacemaker, the escape rhythm can be established by temporarily slowing the pacing rate or decreasing the current output.

When the patient's heart rate is faster than the set pacemaker rate, pacing spikes should not be observed if the generator is sensing properly. In this instance, ventricular capture cannot be evaluated unless the pacemaker rate increases or the spontaneous heart rate decreases. The latter may be accomplished by transiently increasing vagal tone (Valsalva maneuver or carotid stimulation). Fortunately, when the battery is low, sensing is generally affected before pacing output decreases. A chest radiograph is useful in excluding fracture or displacement of pacing leads. If pacemaker malfunction is suspected, cardiological consultation is essential.

What intraoperative conditions may cause the pacemaker to malfunction?

Electrical interference from surgical electrocautery units can be interpreted as myocardial electrical activity and can suppress the pacemaker generator. *Problems with electrocautery may be minimized by limiting its use to short bursts, limiting its power output, placing its* grounding plate as far from the pacemaker generator as possible, and using bipolar cautery. Moreover, continuous monitoring of an arterial pulse wave (pressure, plethysmogram, or oximetry signal) is mandatory to ensure continuous perfusion during electrocautery. Accentuated myopotentials associated with succinylcholine-induced fasciculations or postoperative shivering can similarly suppress the pacemaker generator.

Both hypokalemia and hyperkalemia can alter the pacing electrodes' threshold for depolarizing the myocardium and can result in failure of the pacing impulse to depolarize the ventricle. Myocardial ischemia, infarction, or scarring can also increase the electrodes' threshold and cause failure of ventricular capture.

What are appropriate measures if a pacemaker fails intraoperatively?

If a temporary pacemaker fails intraoperatively, the inspired oxygen concentration should be increased to 100%. All connections and the generator battery should be checked. Most units have a battery-level indicator and a light that flashes with every impulse. The generator should be set into the asynchronous mode, and the ventricular output should be set on maximum. Failure of a temporary transvenous electrode to capture the ventricle is usually due to displacement of the electrode away from the ventricular endocardium; careful slow advancement of the catheter or wire while pacing often results in capture. Pharmacological management (atropine, isoproterenol, or epinephrine) may be useful until the problem is resolved. If an adequate arterial blood pressure cannot be maintained with adrenergic agonists, cardiopulmonary resuscitation should be instituted until another pacing electrode is placed or a new generator box is obtained.

If a permanent pacemaker malfunctions (as with electrocautery), it should generally be converted to an asynchronous mode. Some units will automatically reprogram themselves to the asynchronous mode if malfunction is detected. Other pacemaker units must be reprogrammed by placing either an external magnet or, preferably, a programming device over the generator. The effect of an external magnet on some pacemakers—particularly during electrocautery—may be unpredictable and should generally be determined prior to surgery.

Which anesthetic agents are appropriate for patients with pacemakers?

All anesthetic agents have been safely used in patients who already have pacemakers. Even volatile agents appear to have no effect on pacing electrode thresholds. Local anesthesia with light intravenous sedation is usually used for placement of permanent pacemakers.

When permanent transvenous pacemaker leads are placed, how is their function assessed?

The function of the permanent leads in their final position is analyzed by an external testing device that measures voltage threshold, lead impedance, and the amplitude of the sensed potentials. With an initial voltage output of 5 mV and a pulse duration of 0.5 ms, the pacing rate is increased until 100% capture occurs. At that point, the voltage output is slowly decreased to determine the minimum voltage that results in

100% capture (voltage threshold). The ventricular voltage threshold should be ≤ 0.8 mV and the atrial voltage threshold should be ≤ 1.5 mV. Lead impedance should be 250–1000 Ω at a nominal output of 5 V. The amplitude of the sensed potentials is usually > 6 mV and > 2 mV for ventricular and atrial electrodes, respectively.

SUGGESTED READING

Amar D: Perioperative atrial tachyarrhythmias. Anesthesiology 2002;97:1618.

Atlee JL, Bernstein AD: Cardiac rhythm management devices (part I). Indications, device selection, and function. Anesthesiology 2001;95:1265.

Atlee JL, Bernstein AD: Cardiac rhythm management devices (Part II). Perioperative management. Anesthesiology 2001;95:1492.

Braunwald E, Zipes DP, Libby P: *Heart Disease*, 6th ed. W.B. Saunders, 2001.

Chassot PG, Delabays A, Spahn DR: Preoperative evaluation of patients with, or at risk of, CAD undergoing non-cardiac surgery. Br J Anaesth 2002;89:747.

Eagle KA, Berger PB, Calkins H, et al: ACC/AHA guideline update for perioperative cardiovascular evaluation for noncardiac surgery—Executive summary. Anesth Analg 2002;94:1052.

Howell SJ, Sear JW, Foex P: Hypertension, hypertensive heart disease and perioperative cardiac risk. Br J Anaesth 2004;92:570.

Kaplan JA, Reich DL, Kronstadt SN: *Cardiac Anesthesia*, 4th ed. W.B. Saunders, 1999.

Lake CL: *Pediatric Cardiac Anesthesia*, 3rd ed. McGraw-Hill, 1998.

Otto CM: *Valvular Heart Disease*, 2nd ed. W.B. Saunders, 2003.

Otto CM: *Textbook of Clinical Echocardiography*, 3rd ed. W.B. Saunders, 2004.

Park KW: Preoperative cardiac evaluation. Anesth Clin North Am 2004;22:199.

Anesthesia for Cardiovascular Surgery

KEY CONCEPTS

 Cardiopulmonary bypass (CPB) diverts venous blood away from the heart, adds oxygen, removes CO_2, and returns the blood to a large artery (usually the aorta). As a result, nearly all blood flow through the heart and most of the flow through the lungs cease.

 The fluid level in the reservoir of the CPB machine is critical: If the reservoir is allowed to empty, air can enter the main pump and cause a fatal air embolism.

 Initiation of CPB is associated with a marked increase in stress hormones and a variable systemic inflammatory response.

 Establishing the adequacy of cardiac reserve should be based on exercise (activity) tolerance, measurements of myocardial contractility such as ejection fraction, the severity and location of coronary stenoses, ventricular wall motion abnormalities, cardiac end-diastolic pressures, cardiac output, and valvular areas and gradients.

 Blood should be available for immediate transfusion if the patient has already had a midline sternotomy (a "redo"); in these cases, the right ventricle or coronary grafts may be adherent to the sternum and may be inadvertently entered during the repeat sternotomy.

 In general, pulmonary artery catheterization should be used in patients with compromised ventricular function (ejection fraction < 40–50%) or pulmonary hypertension and in those undergoing complicated procedures.

 Transesophageal echocardiography (TEE) provides valuable information about cardiac anatomy and function during surgery. Two-dimensional, multiplane TEE can detect regional and global ventricular abnormalities, chamber dimensions, valvular anatomy, and the presence of intracardiac air.

 Anesthetic dose requirements are extremely variable and generally are inversely related to ventricular function. Severely compromised patients should be given anesthetic agents in small doses, slowly, and in increments.

 Anticoagulation must be established before CPB to prevent acute disseminated intravascular coagulation and formation of clots in the CPB pump.

 Aprotinin therapy should be considered for patients who are undergoing a repeat operation; who refuse blood products, such as Jehovah's Witnesses; who are at high risk for postoperative bleeding because of recent administration of glycoprotein IIb/IIIa inhibitors (abciximab, eptifibatide, or tirofiban); who have preexisting coagulopathy; and who are undergoing long and complicated procedures involving the heart or aorta.

Hypotension from impaired ventricular filling often occurs during manipulation of the venae cavae and the heart.

(continued on next page)

(continued from previous page)

 Hypothermia (< 34°C) itself is usually anesthetic, but failure to give anesthetic agents, particularly during rewarming on CPB, frequently results in light anesthesia that may result in awareness and recall.

 Protamine administration can result in a number of adverse hemodynamic effects, which appear to be either immune or idiosyncratic nonimmune reactions. Although protamine given slowly (5–10 min) usually has minimal effects, hypotension from acute systemic vasodilation, myocardial depression, and marked pulmonary hypertension may be encountered.

 Persistent bleeding following bypass may be due to inadequate surgical control of bleeding sites, inadequate reversal of heparin, reheparinization, thrombocytopenia, platelet dysfunction, hypothermia, undiagnosed preoperative hemostatic defects, or newly acquired defects. If oozing continues despite adequate surgical hemostasis and the activated clotting time (ACT) is normal or the heparin–protamine titration assay shows no residual heparin, thrombocytopenia or platelet dysfunction is most likely.

 Chest tube drainage in the first 2 h of more than 250–300 mL/h (10 mL/kg/h)—in the absence of a hemostatic defect—is excessive and often requires surgical reexploration. Intrathoracic bleeding at a site not adequately drained causes cardiac tamponade, which necessitates immediate reopening of the chest.

 Factors known to increase pulmonary vascular resistance (PVR) such as acidosis, hypercapnia, hypoxia, enhanced sympathetic tone, and high mean airway pressures are to be avoided for patients with right-to-left shunting; hyperventilation (hypocapnia) with 100% oxygen is usually effective in lowering PVR. Conversely, patients with left-to-right shunting benefit from systemic vasodilation and increases in PVR, although specific hemodynamic manipulation is generally not attempted.

 Induction of general anesthesia in patients with cardiac tamponade can precipitate severe hypotension and cardiac arrest. The anesthetic technique should maintain a high sympathetic tone until the tamponade is relieved. Cardiac depression, vasodilation, and slowing of the heart rates should be avoided. Ketamine is the induction and maintenance agent of choice until the tamponade is relieved.

 The sudden increase in left ventricular afterload after application of the aortic cross-clamp during aortic surgery may precipitate acute left ventricular failure and myocardial ischemia, particularly in patients with underlying ventricular dysfunction or coronary disease. The period of greatest hemodynamic instability follows the release of the aortic cross-clamp; the abrupt decrease in afterload together with bleeding and the release of vasodilating acid metabolites from the ischemic lower body can precipitate severe systemic hypotension.

 The emphasis of anesthetic management during carotid surgery is on maintaining adequate cerebral perfusion without stressing the heart. Regardless of the anesthetic agents selected, mean arterial blood pressure should be maintained at—or slightly above—the patient's usual range.

Anesthesia for cardiovascular surgery requires a precise understanding of circulatory physiology, pharmacology, and pathophysiology as well as a thorough familiarity with cardiopulmonary bypass (CPB), transesophageal echocardiography (TEE), myocardial preservation, and surgical techniques. Because surgical manipulations often have a profound impact on circulatory function, the anesthesiologist must follow the progress of the surgery intently and anticipate problems associated with each step.

This chapter presents an overview of cardiovascular anesthesia and the principles, techniques, and physiol-

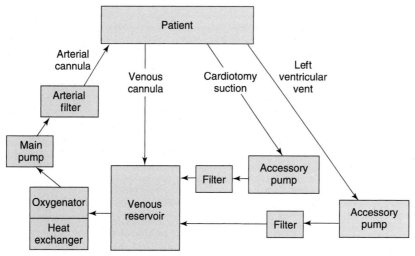

Figure 21–1. The basic design of cardiopulmonary bypass machines.

ogy of CPB. Surgery on the aorta, the carotid arteries, and the pericardium presents problems that also require special anesthetic considerations.

■ CARDIOPULMONARY BYPASS

CPB is a technique that diverts venous blood away from the heart, adds oxygen, removes CO_2, and returns the blood to a large artery (usually the aorta). As a result, nearly all blood flow through the heart and most of the flow through the lungs cease. When CPB is fully established, the extracorporeal circuit is in series with the systemic circulation and provides both artificial ventilation and perfusion. Unfortunately, this technique is entirely non-physiological, because arterial pressure is typically below normal and blood flow is usually nonpulsatile. To minimize organ damage during this stressful period, systemic hypothermia (20–32°C) is usually employed. Topical hypothermia (an ice-slush solution) and cardioplegia (a chemical solution for arresting myocardial electrical activity) are also used to protect the heart.

The operation of the CPB machine is a complex task requiring the uninterrupted attention of a perfusionist—a highly specialized technician. Optimal results with CPB require close cooperation and communication between the surgeon, anesthesiologist, and perfusionist.

BASIC CIRCUIT

The CPB machine has five basic components: a venous reservoir, an oxygenator, a heat exchanger, a main pump, and an arterial filter (Figure 21–1). Modern machines use a single disposable unit with the reservoir, oxygenator, and heat exchanger built in. Most machines also have separate accessory pumps that can be used for blood salvage (cardiotomy suction), venting (draining) the left ventricle, and cardioplegia. A number of other filters, alarms, and in-line pressure, oxygen-saturation, and temperature monitors are also typically used.

Prior to use, the CPB circuit must be primed with fluid (1200–1800 mL for adults) that is devoid of bubbles. A balanced salt solution, such as Plasma-Lyte A, is generally used, but other components are frequently added, including colloid (albumin or hetastarch), mannitol (for renal protection), heparin (500–5000 units), bicarbonate, and potassium (if cardioplegia will not be used). ε-Aminocaproic acid or aprotinin may also be added. At the onset of bypass, hemodilution usually decreases the hematocrit to about 22–25% in most patients. Blood is used as a priming solution for small pediatric and severely anemic adult patients to prevent severe hemodilution.

Reservoir

The reservoir of the CPB machine receives blood from the patient via one or two venous cannulas in the right atrium or the superior and inferior vena cava. Blood flows to the reservoir by gravity drainage. Because venous pressure is normally low, the driving force is directly proportional to the difference in height between the patient and the reservoir but inversely proportional to the resistance of the cannulas and tubing. Priming the machine creates a siphon effect. Entrainment of air can produce an air lock that may prevent blood flow. In some cases (eg, use of an unusually small venous cannula) assisted venous drainage may be required; a regulated vacuum together with a hard shell venous reservoir or centrifugal pump (see below) is used in such instances. The fluid level in the reservoir is critical: If the reservoir is allowed to empty, air can enter the main pump and cause a fatal air embolism. A low reservoir level alarm is typically present.

Oxygenator

Blood is drained by gravity from the bottom of the venous reservoir into the oxygenator, which contains a blood–gas interface that allows blood to equilibrate with the gas mixture (primarily oxygen). A volatile anesthetic is also frequently added at the oxygenator gas inlet. The blood–gas interface in a modern, membrane-type oxygenator is a very thin, gas-permeable silicone membrane. Arterial oxygenation is generally inversely related to the thickness of the blood film in contact with the membrane, whereas arterial CO_2 tension during CPB is dependent on total gas flow. Because the inspired oxygen concentration can be varied, a membrane oxygenator allows independent control of PaO_2 and $PaCO_2$.

Heat Exchanger

Blood from the oxygenator enters the heat exchanger. The blood is then either cooled or warmed, depending on the temperature of the water flowing through the exchanger (4–42°C); heat transfer occurs by conduction. Because gas solubility decreases as blood temperature rises, a filter is built into the unit to catch any bubbles that may form during rewarming.

Main Pump

Modern CPB machines use either an electrically driven double-arm roller (positive displacement) or a centrifugal pump to propel blood through the CPB circuit.

A. ROLLER PUMPS

Roller pumps produce flow by compressing large-bore tubing in the main pumping chamber as the heads turn. Subtotal occlusion of the tubing prevents excessive red cell trauma. The constant speed of the rollers pumps blood regardless of the resistance encountered, and produces a continuous nonpulsatile flow. Flow is directly proportional to the number of revolutions per minute. In some pumps, an emergency back-up battery provides power in case of an electrical power failure. All roller pumps have a hand crank to allow manual pumping.

B. CENTRIFUGAL PUMPS

Centrifugal pumps consist of a series of cones in a plastic housing. As the cones spin, the centrifugal forces created propel the blood from the centrally located inlet to the periphery. In contrast to roller pumps, blood flow with centrifugal pumps is pressure sensitive and must be monitored by an electromagnetic flowmeter. Increases in distal pressure will decrease flow and must be compensated for by increasing the pump speed. Because these pumps are nonocclusive, they are less traumatic to blood than roller pumps. Unlike roller pumps, which are placed after the oxygenator (Figure 21–1), centrifugal pumps are normally between the venous reservoir and the oxygenator.

C. PULSATILE FLOW

Pulsatile blood flow is possible with some roller pumps. Pulsations can be produced by instantaneous variations in the rate of rotation of the roller heads; they can also be added after flow is generated. Pulsatile flow is not available with centrifugal pumps. Although the matter is controversial, some clinicians believe that pulsatile flow improves tissue perfusion, enhances oxygen extraction, attenuates the release of stress hormones, and results in lower systemic vascular resistances (SVRs) during CPB. These observations are supported by experimental studies suggesting improved renal and cerebral blood flow during pulsatile perfusion in animals.

Arterial Filter

Particulate matter (eg, thrombi, fat globules, calcium, tissue debris) enters the CPB circuit with alarming regularity. Although filters are often used at other locations, a final, in-line, arterial filter (27–40 μm) is mandatory to prevent systemic embolism. Once filtered, the propelled blood returns to the patient, usually via a cannula in the ascending aorta. A normally functioning aortic valve prevents blood from entering the left ventricle.

The filter is always constructed with a (normally clamped) bypass limb in case it becomes clogged or develops high resistance. For the same reason, arterial inflow pressure is measured before the filter. The filter is also designed to trap air, which can be bled out through a built-in stopcock.

Accessory Pumps & Devices

A. CARDIOTOMY SUCTION

The cardiotomy suction pump aspirates blood from the surgical field during CPB and returns it to the main pump reservoir. A cell-saver suction device may also be used, but blood is then returned to a separate reservoir. At the end of the procedure, the cell-saver blood is centrifuged, washed, and returned to the patient. Excessive suction pressure contributes to red cell trauma. Moreover, excessive use of cell-saver suction (instead of cardiotomy suction) during bypass depletes CPB circuit volume. The high negative pressure of ordinary wall suction produces excessive red cell trauma and precludes blood salvage from that source.

B. LEFT VENTRICULAR VENT

With time, even after institution of total bypass, blood reaccumulates in the left ventricle as a result of residual pulmonary flow from the bronchial arteries (which arise directly from the aorta or the intercostal arteries) or thebesian vessels (see Chapter 19) or as a result of aortic regurgitation. Aortic regurgitation can occur as a result of either structural valvular abnormalities or surgical manipulation of the heart (functional). Distention of the left ventricle compromises myocardial preservation (see below) and requires decompression (venting). In most centers, this is accomplished by a catheter inserted into the left ventricle via the right superior pulmonary vein and left atrium. Venting is less commonly accomplished through a catheter in the left ventricular apex or through the aortic valve. The blood aspirated by the vent pump normally passes through a filter and is returned to the venous reservoir.

C. CARDIOPLEGIA PUMP

Cardioplegia is most often administered via an accessory pump on the CPB machine. This technique allows optimal control over the infusion pressure, rate, and temperature (see below). A separate heat exchanger ensures control of the temperature of the cardioplegia solution. Alternatively, cardioplegia may be infused from a cold intravenous fluid bag given under pressure or by gravity.

D. ULTRAFILTER

Ultrafiltration can be used during CPB to increase the patient's hematocrit without transfusion. Hemultrafilters consist of hollow capillary fibers that can function as membranes, allowing separation of the aqueous phase of blood from its cellular and proteinaceous elements. Blood can be diverted to pass through the fibers either from the arterial side of the main pump or from the venous reservoir using an accessory pump. Hydrostatic pressure forces water and electrolytes across the fiber membrane. Effluents of up to 40 mL/min may be removed.

SYSTEMIC HYPOTHERMIA

Intentional hypothermia is routinely used following the initiation of CPB. Core body temperature is usually reduced to 20–32°C. Metabolic oxygen requirements are generally halved with each reduction of 10°C in body temperature. At the end of the surgical procedure, rewarming via the heat exchanger restores normal body temperature.

Profound hypothermia to temperatures of 15–18°C allows total circulatory arrest for complex repairs for up to 60 min. During that time, both the heart and the CPB machine are stopped.

The adverse effects of hypothermia are platelet dysfunction; potentiation of citrate toxicity, which leads to reduction in serum ionized calcium; reversible coagulopathy; and depression of myocardial contractility.

MYOCARDIAL PRESERVATION

Optimal results in cardiac surgery not only require a rapid and perfect surgical repair of the pathology with minimal physical trauma to the heart but also prevention of myocardial damage and maintenance of normal cellular integrity and function during CPB. Nearly all patients sustain some myocardial damage during cardiac surgery. With proper preservation techniques, however, most of the damage is usually reversible. Although myocardial injury can be related to the anesthetic or surgical technique, it most commonly appears to be related to suboptimal myocardial preservation during CPB. A common denominator in most instances is an imbalance between myocardial oxygen demand and supply, resulting in cell ischemia, injury, or death. Additionally, reperfusion injury may play a major role. Reperfusion following a period of ischemia can result in generation of excess oxygen-derived free radicals, intracellular calcium overload, abnormal endothelial–leukocyte interactions, and myocardial cellular edema. Patients at greatest risk are those in the New York Heart Association (NYHA) functional class IV (see Table 20–12) and those who have ventricular hypertrophy or severe coronary artery disease. Inadequate myocardial preservation is usually manifested at the end of bypass as a persistently low cardiac output, electrocardiographic signs of myocardial ischemia, or cardiac arrhythmias. Myocardial stunning, resulting from ischemia and reperfusion injury, produces systolic and/or diastolic dysfunction but is reversible with time. In contrast to myocardial necrosis, the injury is irreversible.

Aortic cross-clamping during CPB completely abolishes coronary blood flow. Although estimates of a safe cross-clamping period are not valid because of differing vulnerabilities among patients, CPB times longer than 120 min are generally considered undesirable. Myocardial ischemia during bypass can also occur before and after release of the cross-clamp. Low arterial pressures, coronary embolism (from thrombi, platelets, air, fat, or calcium), reperfusion injury, coronary or graft vasospasm, and excessive surgical manipulation of the heart—causing compression or distortion of the coronary vessels—are all contributory. Areas of myocardium distal to a high-grade coronary obstruction are at greatest risk.

Ischemia causes depletion of high-energy phosphate compounds and an accumulation of intracellular calcium. The latter, through its action on contractile proteins, further depletes energy supplies (see Chapter 19). Maintenance of normal cellular integrity and function during CPB depends on reducing energy expenditure and preserving the availability of high-energy phosphate compounds. When coronary blood flow ceases, creatine phosphate and anaerobic metabolism become the principal sources of cellular energy; fatty acid oxidation is impaired. Unfortunately, these energy stores rapidly become depleted, and the progressive acidosis that develops limits glycolysis. Although measures directed at increasing or replenishing energy substrates in the form of glucose or glutamate infusions are used, the emphasis of myocardial preservation has been on reducing cellular energy requirements to minimal levels. This is accomplished by systemic and topical cardiac hypothermia (ice slush) and the use of potassium cardioplegia (below). The former reduces basal metabolic oxygen consumption and the latter abolishes the energy expenditure associated with both electrical and mechanical activity. Myocardial temperature can be monitored directly; 10–15°C is usually considered desirable.

Ventricular fibrillation and distention are important causes of myocardial damage. Fibrillation can double myocardial oxygen consumption, whereas distention not only increases oxygen demand but also reduces oxygen supply by interfering with subendocardial blood flow. The combination of the two is particularly detrimental. Other factors that might contribute to myocardial damage include the use of inotropes and excessive administration of calcium. In open heart procedures, deairing of cardiac chambers and venting before and during initial cardiac ejection are critically important in preventing coronary embolism (and strokes—see below). Deairing of grafts during coronary bypass procedures is similarly important. Depending on their amount and the location of coronary emboli, even small air bubbles can cause varying degrees of ventricular dysfunction at the end of CPB. To some extent, air emboli may be preferentially directed into the right coronary ostium because of its higher position in the aortic root.

Potassium Cardioplegia

The most widely used method of arresting myocardial electrical activity is the administration of potassium-rich crystalloid or blood. Following initiation of CPB, induction of hypothermia, and aortic cross-clamping, the coronary circulation is perfused intermittently with cold cardioplegia. The resulting increase in extracellular potassium concentration reduces the transmembrane potential (less negative inside). The latter progressively interferes with the normal sodium current during depolarization, decreasing the rate of rise, amplitude, and conduction velocity of subsequent action potentials (see Chapter 19). Eventually, the sodium channels are completely inactivated, action potentials are abolished, and the heart is arrested in diastole. Usually, cold cardioplegia must be repeated several times (about every 30 min) because of gradual washout and rewarming of the myocardium. Washout occurs as a result of the persistence of noncollateral coronary blood flow derived from pericardial vessels, which are branches of intercostal arteries. Moreover, multiple doses of cardioplegia solutions may improve myocardial preservation by preventing the excessive build-up of metabolites that inhibit anaerobic metabolism. Preferential warming of the posterior ventricular wall can also occur as a result of direct contact with warmer blood in the descending aorta.

Although the exact composition varies from center to center, the essential element of cardioplegia is the same: potassium 10–40 mEq/L. Potassium concentration is kept below 40 mEq/L, because higher levels can be associated with a paradoxic increase in myocardial energy requirements and excessive potassium loads. Sodium concentration in cardioplegia solutions is usually less than in plasma (< 140 mEq/L) because ischemia tends to increase intracellular sodium content. A small amount of calcium (0.7–1.2 mmol/L) is needed to maintain cellular integrity, whereas magnesium (1.5–15 mmol/L) is usually added to control excessive intracellular influxes of calcium. A buffer—most commonly bicarbonate—is necessary to prevent excessive build-up of acid metabolites; in fact, alkalotic perfusates are reported to produce better myocardial preservation. Alternative buffers include histidine and tromethamine (also known as THAM). Other components may include hypertonic agents to control cellular edema (mannitol), procaine, lidocaine, or glucocorticoids (for their membrane-stabilizing effect). Energy substrates are provided as glucose, glutamate, or aspartate. The question of whether to use crystalloid or blood as a vehicle for achieving cardioplegia remains somewhat controversial. Evidence suggests that at least some groups of high-risk patients may do better with blood cardioplegia. Certainly, oxygenated blood cardioplegia has the added benefit of delivering more oxygen than crystalloid cardioplegia.

Because cardioplegia may not reach areas distal to high-grade coronary obstructions (the areas that need it most), many surgeons also administer cardioplegia retrogradely through a coronary sinus catheter. Some centers have reported that the combination of antegrade and retrograde cardioplegia is superior to either technique alone. Others have suggested that continuous warm blood cardioplegia is superior to intermittent hypothermic cardioplegia for myocardial preservation, but the absence of a bloodless field complicates surgery. Moreover, warm cardiac surgery raises additional concerns about loss of the potentially protective effects of hypothermia, particularly on cerebral function.

As discussed previously, when ischemic damage to the myocardium is prolonged, reperfusion of the myocardium can be associated with extensive cell injury, rapid accumulation of intracellular calcium, and potentially irreversible cellular necrosis. Depletion of endogenous free radical scavengers during CPB may allow an accumulation of deleterious oxygen-derived free radicals; free radical scavengers, such as with mannitol therapy, may help decrease reperfusion injury. Several steps may help limit reperfusion injury before unclamping of the aorta. Just prior to reperfusion, the heart may be arrested by a low potassium cardioplegia that serves to wash out accumulated metabolic byproducts. Alternatively, a "hot shot" or warm blood cardioplegia is administered to wash out byproducts and replenish metabolic substrates. Hypercalcemia should be avoided. Reperfusion pressures should be controlled closely because of altered coronary autoregulation. Aortic pressure is reduced just prior to clamp release; it is then brought up initially to about 40 mm Hg before gradually being increased and maintained at about 70 mm Hg. To further minimize metabolic requirement, the heart should be in an empty and beating state for an additional 5–10 min before weaning the patient from CPB. Acidosis and hypoxia should be corrected.

Excessive cardioplegia can result in an absence of electrical activity, atrioventricular conduction block, or a poorly contractile heart at the end of bypass. Persistent systemic hyperkalemia may also result. Although calcium administration partially offsets these effects, excessive calcium can enhance myocardial damage. Myocardial performance generally improves with time as the contents of the cardioplegia are cleared from the heart.

PHYSIOLOGICAL EFFECTS OF CARDIOPULMONARY BYPASS

Hormonal, Humoral, & Immunological Responses

 Initiation of CPB is associated with a marked increase in stress hormones and a variable systemic inflammatory response. Elevated levels of catecholamines, cortisol, arginine vasopressin, and angiotensin are observed. This phenomenon is at least partly due to decreased metabolism secondary to hypothermia and exclusion of the pulmonary circulation, where many of these substances are normally broken down. Anesthetic agents may only partially suppress the hormonal stress response to CPB.

Multiple humoral systems are also activated, including complement, coagulation, fibrinolysis, and the kallikrein system. Contact of blood with the internal surfaces of the CPB system activates complement via the alternate pathway (C3) as well as the classic pathway through activation of Hageman factor (XII); the latter also activates the coagulation cascade, platelets, plasminogen, and kallikrein. Mechanical trauma also appears to activate platelets and leukocytes. Increased amounts of oxygen-derived free radicals are generated. A systemic inflammatory response syndrome similar to that seen with sepsis and trauma can develop (see Chapter 49). When this response is intense or prolonged, patients can develop the same complications, including generalized edema, the acute respiratory distress syndrome, coagulopathy, and acute renal failure.

CPB also alters and depletes glycoprotein receptors on the surface of platelets. The resulting platelet dysfunction increases perioperative bleeding and potentiates other coagulation abnormalities (activation of plasminogen and the inflammatory response described above).

Animal and clinical research has demonstrated that the inflammatory response to CPB can be modulated by various therapies. Aprotinin possesses potent anti-inflammatory properties and has been shown to reduce the incidence of pulmonary and central nervous system complications following CPB. Leukocyte depletion reduces inflammation and may similarly reduce complications. Leukocyte-depleted blood cardioplegia has been shown to improve myocardial preservation in some studies. Hemofiltration (ultrafiltration) during CPB, which presumably removes inflammatory cytokines, appears beneficial in pediatric patients. Administration of free radical scavengers such as high-dose vitamins C and E and mannitol has improved outcome in some studies. Other studies suggest that cyclooxygenase-2 inhibitors and pentoxifylline may also offer some benefit. Systemic corticosteroids before and during CPB can modulate the inflammatory response during CPB but improved outcome is not well established.

Altered Pharmacokinetics

Plasma and serum concentrations of most drugs acutely decrease at the onset of CPB but the unbound fraction may remain unaltered for some drugs. The effects of CPB are complex because of the sudden increase in volume of distribution with hemodilution, decreased protein binding, and changes in perfusion and redistribution between peripheral and central compartments. Some drugs, such as opioids, also bind CPB components. Heparin potentially alters protein binding by releasing and activating lipoprotein lipase, which hydrolyzes plasma triglycerides into free fatty acids; the latter can competitively inhibit drug binding to plasma proteins. With the possible exception of propofol, constant infusion of a drug during CPB generally causes progressively higher blood levels as a result of reduced hepatic and renal perfusion (reduced elimination) and hypothermia (reduced metabolism). Alterations in α_1-acid glycoprotein, which increases after CPB, can also affect drug binding in the postoperative period.

◼ ANESTHETIC MANAGEMENT OF CARDIAC SURGERY

ADULTS

The preoperative evaluation and anesthetic management of common cardiovascular diseases are discussed in Chapter 20. The same principles apply whether these patients are undergoing cardiac or noncardiac surgery. An important distinction is that patients undergoing cardiac procedures generally have more advanced disease, and the importance of establishing the adequacy of cardiac reserve cannot be overemphasized. This information should be based on exercise (activity) tolerance, measurements of myocardial contractility such as ejection fraction, the severity and location of coronary stenoses, ventricular wall motion abnormalities, cardiac end-diastolic pressures, cardiac output, and valvular areas and gradients (see Chapter 20). Fortunately, unlike noncardiac surgery, cardiac surgery improves cardiac function in the majority of patients. Preoperative evaluation should also focus on pulmonary, neurological, and renal function, as impairment of these organ systems predisposes patients to postoperative complications.

1. Preinduction Period

Premedication

The prospect of heart surgery is frightening. Relatively heavy premedication is generally desirable, particularly for patients with coronary artery disease with good left ventricular function (see Chapter 20). Conversely, light premedication is more appropriate in frail patients with valvular disease or ischemic cardiomyopathy, who are often physiologically dependent on enhanced sympathetic tone. Habitus, age, and physiological status should be considered in selecting agents and doses.

Benzodiazepine sedative-hypnotics (midazolam, 2–10 mg intramuscularly; diazepam, 5–10 mg orally; or lorazepam, 2–4 mg orally), alone or in combination with an opioid (morphine, 4–10 mg intramuscularly or hydromorphone, 1–2 mg intramuscularly), are commonly used. The dose of a benzodiazepine should generally be halved when the drug is combined with an opioid. Alternatively, the time-honored combination of intramuscular morphine, 0.1–0.15 mg/kg, and scopolamine, 0.2–0.3 mg, also provides excellent sedation, analgesia, and amnesia. Again doses should be reduced in patients with poor cardiac reserve and those with underlying pulmonary disease. Scopolamine should generally be avoided in patients older than 70 years because it is associated with a high incidence of confusion in this group. Supplemental oxygen (5 L/min via nasal cannula) is useful in avoiding hypoxemia following premedication.

Preparation

Formulation of a clear anesthetic plan and adequate preparations are essential for cardiac anesthesia. Many patients are critically ill, and there is little time intraoperatively to debate the merits of one technique over another or to search for drugs and equipment. At the same time, the anesthetic plan should not be too rigid; if problems are encountered with one technique, the anesthesiologist should be ready to change to another without delay. Organization and meticulous attention to detail are crucial in dealing with intraoperative problems. The anesthesia machine, monitors, infusion pumps, and blood warmer should all be checked before the patient arrives. Drugs—including anesthetic and vasoactive agents—should be immediately available. Many clinicians prepare one vasodilator and one inotropic infusion solution for use before the start of the procedure.

Venous Access

Cardiac surgery is commonly associated with large and rapid fluid shifts, often with the need for multiple drug infusions. Ideally, two large-bore (16-gauge or larger) intravenous catheters should be placed. One of these should be in a large central vein, usually the internal jugular vein, although the subclavian and external jugular veins are suitable alternatives. Entry into the superior vena cava is not always possible with the external jugular vein; nonetheless, it serves as a good site for an extra peripheral intravenous line. Central venous cannulations may be accomplished while the patient is awake but sedated or after induction of anesthesia. Small doses of midazolam (1–2 mg) with or without an opioid can be used for sedation. Supplemental oxygen via face mask helps avoid hypoxemia during catheterization.

Drug infusions should ideally be given into a central catheter, preferably directly into the catheter or into the injection port closest to the catheter (to minimize dead space). Multilumen central venous and pulmonary artery catheters facilitate multiple drug infusions and allow simultaneous measurement of vascular pressures. One intravenous port should be dedicated for drug infusions and nothing else, and another port should be used for drug and fluid boluses. The side port of the introducer sheath used for a pulmonary catheter can be used for drug infusions but serves better as a fluid bolus line when a large-bore introducer (9F) is used.

Blood should be available for immediate transfusion if the patient has already had a midline sternotomy (a "redo"); in these cases, the right ventricle or coronary grafts may be adherent to the sternum and may be inadvertently entered during the repeat sternotomy.

Monitoring

In addition to all basic monitoring, arterial cannulation is generally performed prior to induction of anesthesia, as the induction period represents a time of major hemodynamic stress. Depending on the patient, central venous cannulation may be done before or after induction of anesthesia.

A. ELECTROCARDIOGRAPHY

The electrocardiogram (ECG) is continuously monitored with two leads, usually leads II and V_5. Baseline tracings of all leads may be recorded on paper for further reference. The advent of monitors with computerized ST-segment analysis and the use of additional monitoring leads (V_4, aVF, and V_{4R}) have greatly improved detection of ischemic episodes.

B. ARTERIAL BLOOD PRESSURE

Arterial blood pressure should generally be directly monitored by catheterization of the radial artery in the nondominant hand. Radial arterial catheters, particularly on the left side, may occasionally give falsely low readings following sternal retraction as a result of compression of the subclavian artery between the clavicle

and the first rib. The radial artery on the side of a brachial artery cutdown (for cardiac catheterization) should not be used, because its use is associated with a high incidence of arterial thrombosis and wave distortion. Other useful catheterization sites include the ulnar, brachial, femoral, and axillary arteries. A backup manual or automatic blood pressure cuff should also be placed on the opposite side for comparison with direct measurements.

C. CENTRAL VENOUS AND PULMONARY ARTERY PRESSURE

Central venous pressure should be monitored in all patients. The decision on whether to use a pulmonary artery catheter is based on the patient, the procedure, and the preferences of the surgical team. Routine use of a pulmonary artery catheter is controversial. Left ventricular filling pressures can be measured with a left atrial pressure line inserted by the surgeon during bypass. In general, pulmonary artery catheterization should be used in patients with compromised ventricular function (ejection fraction < 40–50%) or pulmonary hypertension and in those undergoing complicated procedures. The most useful data are pulmonary artery pressures, the wedge pressure, and thermodilution cardiac outputs (see Chapter 6). Specialized catheters provide extra infusion ports, continuous measurements of mixed venous oxygen saturation and cardiac output, and the capability for right ventricular or atrioventricular sequential pacing.

The internal jugular vein is the preferred approach for central venous cannulation (see Chapter 6). Catheters placed through the subclavian or external jugular veins, particularly on the left side, may be prone to kinking following sternal retraction (above).

Pulmonary artery catheters often migrate distally during CPB and may spontaneously wedge without balloon inflation. Inflation of the balloon under these conditions can rupture a pulmonary artery and cause lethal pulmonary hemorrhage. When a pulmonary artery catheter is used, it should be routinely pulled back slightly (2–3 cm) during CPB and the balloon subsequently inflated slowly. If the catheter wedges with less than 1.5 mL of air in the balloon, it should be pulled back farther.

D. URINARY OUTPUT

Once the patient is asleep, an indwelling urinary catheter is placed to monitor the hourly output. Bladder temperature is often monitored but may be affected by low urinary flow. The sudden appearance of red urine may indicate excessive red hemolysis caused by CPB or a transfusion reaction.

E. TEMPERATURE

Multiple temperature monitors are usually placed once the patient is anesthetized. Bladder or rectal, esophageal, and pulmonary artery (blood) temperatures are usually simultaneously monitored. Because of the heterogeneity of readings during cooling and rewarming, bladder and rectal readings are generally taken to represent an average body temperature, whereas esophageal and, to a lesser extent, pulmonary artery values represent core temperature. Nasopharyngeal and tympanic probes may be most reflective of brain temperature. Myocardial temperature is often measured directly during CPB.

F. LABORATORY PARAMETERS

Intraoperative laboratory monitoring is mandatory during cardiac surgery. Blood gases, hematocrit, serum potassium, ionized calcium, and glucose measurements should be immediately available. Serum magnesium measurements may also be useful. The **activated clotting time (ACT)** is used to monitor anticoagulation; some centers also use heparin assays. The role of thromboelastography is not well defined during CPB.

G. SURGICAL FIELD

One of the most important intraoperative monitors is the surgical field. Once the sternum is opened, lung expansion can be seen through the pleura. When the pericardium is opened, the heart (primarily the right ventricle) is visible, so that cardiac rhythm, volume, and contractility can often be judged visually. Blood loss and surgical maneuvers must be closely watched and related to changes in hemodynamics and rhythm.

H. TRANSESOPHAGEAL ECHOCARDIOGRAPHY

TEE provides extremely valuable information about cardiac anatomy and function during surgery. Two-dimensional, multiplane TEE can detect regional and global ventricular abnormalities, chamber dimensions, valvular anatomy, and the presence of intracardiac air. It can also be helpful in confirming cannulation of the coronary sinus for cardioplegia. Multiple views can be obtained from the upper esophagus, mid esophagus, and transgastric positions in the transverse, sagittal, and in-between planes (Figure 21–2). The two most

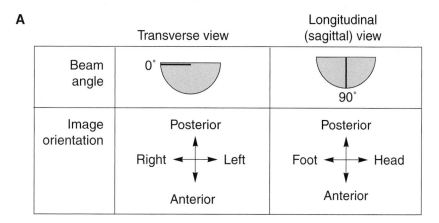

Figure 21–2. Useful views during transesophageal echocardiography. **A:** The relationship between the angle of the ultrasound beam and image orientation relative to the patient. **B–D:** Echocardiographic views from the upper mid-esophagus, lower mid-esophagus, and transgastric position (**C**). Note that different views can be obtained in each position as the tip of the probe is tilted either upward (anteflexion) or backward (retroflexion) and the angle of the beam is changed from 0° to 180°. The angle of the beam is shown in the upper left hand corner of each image. The probe is also rotated clockwise or counterclockwise to optimize viewing of the various structures. AO, aorta; AV, aortic valve; CS, coronary sinus; IVC, inferior vena cava; LA, left atrium; LAA, left atrial appendage; LUPV, left upper pulmonary vein; LV, left ventricle; LVOT, left ventricular outflow tract; MPA, main pulmonary artery; MV, mitral valve; PA, pulmonary artery; RA, right atrium; RPA, right pulmonary artery; RV, right ventricle; SVC, superior vena cava.

(continued)

Figure 21–2. (Continued)

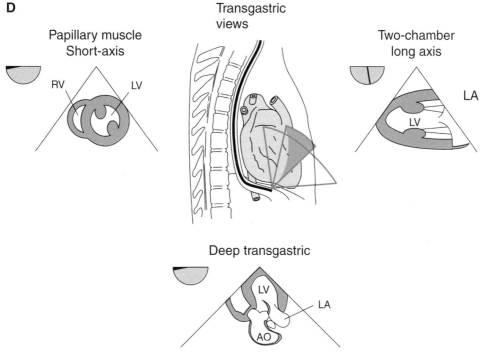

Figure 21–2. (Continued)

commonly used views for monitoring during cardiac surgery are the four-chamber view (Figure 21–3) and the transgastric (short-axis) view (Figure 21–4). The advent of live three-dimensional echocardiography offers great promise for better visualization of complex anatomic features, assessment of valvular function, and assessment of regional/global function.

The following represent the most important applications of intraoperative TEE.

1. Assessing ventricular function—Ventricular function can be assessed by global systolic function, determined by ejection fraction and left ventricular end-diastolic volume; diastolic function (ie, looking for

Figure 21–3. Transesophageal echocardiogram of the mid-esophageal four-chamber view, showing the right and left atria and ventricles.

Figure 21–4. Transesophageal echocardiogram at the lower esophageal/transgastric level looking up at the left ventricle at the level of the papillary muscles.

PROFILES IN ANESTHETIC PRACTICE

Daniel M. Thys, MD

ECHOCARDIOGRAPHY IS AN ESSENTIAL SKILL FOR THE CARDIOVASCULAR ANESTHESIOLOGIST

Intraoperative echocardiography (IOE) is widely used because it is perceived to provide information that significantly influences clinical management and improves patient outcome. Although there is limited scientific evidence to substantiate such a perception, recent guidelines have documented the usefulness of IOE in adult and pediatric cardiac surgery.[1] Although none of the quoted literature withstands rigorous scientific scrutiny, it confirms the clinical opinion that IOE provides new information on cardiac pathology in a significant number of patients (12.8–38.6%) and that the new information results in frequent management changes (4.4–14.6%). Most physicians who care for cardiac surgical patients believe these benefits to be real and have adopted the technique in their clinical practice. An additional factor in favor of IOE is that its risks are low. Kallmeyer et al reported no mortality and a morbidity of only 0.2% in a case series of 7200 cardiac surgical patients.[2]

The development of intraoperative echocardiography has been an enormous blessing for anesthesiology in general and cardiovascular anesthesiology more specifically. From mere facilitators of disease management, anesthesiologists have become active participants in the planning, performance, and evaluation of cardiac surgical interventions. The cardiac surgeons have grown accustomed to the skillful inter-

pretation of echocardiograms by anesthesiologists. Surgeons rely upon cardiovascular anesthesiologists to provide them with accurate information on the patients' cardiac lesions and function. After carrying out the surgery, they expect the anesthesiologists to evaluate the quality and completeness of the surgical intervention. In acquiring the skills necessary to become proficient echocardiographers, anesthesiologists have dramatically broadened the scope of anesthesiology and have added significant value to the services that the specialty provides.

With such new activities have also come new challenges and responsibilities. One of the greatest challenges has been the development of training criteria and processes for IOE. In a recent survey of all active members of the Society of Cardiovascular Anesthesiologists (SCA) residing in the United States or Puerto Rico, Morewood et al documented that 94% of respondents practiced at institutions that use IOE.[3] Furthermore, 72% of anesthesiologists working at such institutions responded that they personally employed transesophageal echocardiography (TEE) during anesthetic care. Of the anesthesiologists using TEE, about 70% had undergone training after completion of their residency or fellowship. Most described their training as "self-taught" (22%), "by others on the job" (27%), and/or consisting of "short courses" (35%). A minority of individuals had obtained experience with TEE during residency (12%) or fellowship (17%).

Problems with education in echocardiography have been recognized since the earliest days of the technology. In an editorial in 1974, Harvey Feigenbaum described the growing demands from clinicians for echocardiographic information, yet deplored the paucity of adequately trained echocardiographers.[4] Over the years, professional organizations of many countries have published recommendations and guidelines concerning training in echocardiography. The principal themes of these recommendations are the following:

1. The comprehensive evaluation of a patient with heart disease involves the use of several, related diagnostic techniques such as M-mode, two-dimensional, and Doppler echocardiography. Under certain circumstances, these techniques may need to be supplemented with specialized examinations such as contrast echocardiography, stress echocardiography, or invasive echocardiography. All of these techniques are re-

lated, are usually complementary, and together define the field of echocardiography. Physicians who take responsibility for the performance and interpretation of echocardiography should, therefore, have a clear understanding of the fundamental principles of, and practical experience with, all of these techniques.

2. Physicians who take responsibility for the performance and interpretation of echocardiography should have a broad background knowledge that spans the physical principles of echocardiography, echocardiographic instrumentation, the experience needed to recognize normal and abnormal information, and experience with other cardiac diagnostic techniques.

3. Physicians training in echocardiography ideally should spend a specified period of time in an active echocardiographic laboratory, working under the direction of an experienced echocardiographer who has achieved an advanced level of training.

4. Techniques in echocardiography evolve rapidly and, therefore, physicians responsible for the performance and interpretation of echocardiographic examinations should maintain active and ongoing continuing education in the field.

More recently, the American Society of Echocardiography and the Society of Cardiovascular Anesthesiologists jointly developed training guidelines that are specific for intraoperative echocardiography.[5] Like prior published guidelines, these guidelines recognize different levels (basic and advanced) of expertise in echocardiography and make level-specific recommendations for training. They also state that regardless of the level of expertise, all practitioners, even experts, must recognize that timely consultation during perioperative echocardiography may be necessary because of constraints of time or experience.

The essential components of basic training include independent work, supervised activities, and assessment programs. Through a structured independent reading and study program, trainees must acquire an understanding of the principles of ultrasound and indications for perioperative echocardiography. This independent work should be supplemented by regularly scheduled didactics such as lectures and seminars designed to reinforce the most important aspects of perioperative echocardiography. Under appropriate supervision the trainee learns to place the TEE probe, operate the ultrasonograph, and perform a TEE examination. Subsequently, some clinical work should be performed with progressively more independence. However, a practi-

tioner with advanced training must review every examination performed by the trainee with him or her. For basic training, the task force recommends study of 150 complete examinations under appropriate supervision. These examinations must include the full spectrum of commonly encountered perioperative diagnoses, and at least 50 comprehensive intraoperative TEE examinations personally performed, interpreted, and reported by the trainee. The trainee must be taught how to convey and document the results of the examination effectively. Periodic formal and informal evaluations of the trainee's progress should be conducted during training. Trainees should keep a log of examinations performed and reviewed to document the depth and breadth of their training.

For advanced practice, the comprehensiveness of training is paramount. The essential components include independent work, supervised activities, and assessment programs. The task force recommends study of 300 complete examinations under appropriate supervision. These examinations must include a wide spectrum of cardiac diagnoses and at least 150 comprehensive intraoperative TEE examinations personally performed, interpreted, and reported by the trainee. The trainee must develop the skills to convey and document the results of the examinations effectively and independently. Periodic formal and informal evaluations of the trainee's progress should be conducted during training. The experience and case numbers acquired during basic training may be counted for advanced training provided the basic training was completed in an advanced training environment.

1. Cheitlin MD, Armstrong WF, Aurigemma GP, et al: ACC/AHA/ASE 2003 guideline update for the clinical application of echocardiography—summary article: a report of the American College of Cardiology/American Heart Association Task Force on Practice Guidelines (ACC/AHA/ASE Committee to Update the 1997 Guidelines for the Clinical Application of Echocardiography). J Am Coll Cardiol 2003;42(5):954.

2. Kallmeyer IJ, Collard CD, Fox JA, et al: The safety of intraoperative transesophageal echocardiography: a case series of 7,200 cardiac surgical patients. Anesth Analg 2001;92:1126.

3. Morewood GH, Gallagher ME, Gaughan JP, Conlay LA: Current practice patterns for perioperative transesophageal echocardiography in the United States. Anesthesiology 2001;95:1507.

4. Feigenbaum H: Editorial: educational problems in echocardiography. Am J Cardiol 1974;34:741.

5. Cahalan MK, Abel M, Goldman M, et al: American Society of Echocardiography and Society of Cardiovascular Anesthesiologists task force guidelines for training in perioperative echocardiography. Anesth Analg 2002;94:1384.

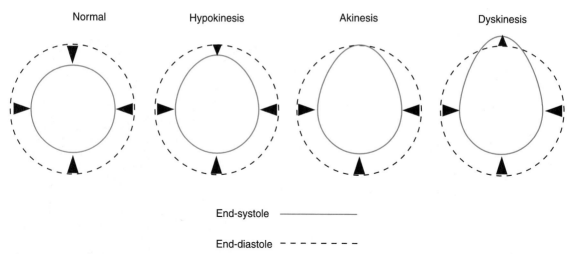

Normal   Hypokinesis   Akinesis   Dyskinesis

End-systole ————

End-diastole – – – – – – –

Figure 21–5. Classification of regional wall motion abnormalities.

abnormal relaxation and restrictive diastolic patterns by checking mitral flow velocity); and regional systolic function, by assessing wall motion and thickening abnormalities. Regional wall abnormalities following myocardial ischemia often appear before ECG changes.

Regional wall motion abnormalities can be classified into three categories based on severity (Figure 21–5): hypokinesis (reduced wall motion), akinesis (no wall motion), and dyskinesis (paradoxical wall motion). The left ventricular myocardium is supplied by three major

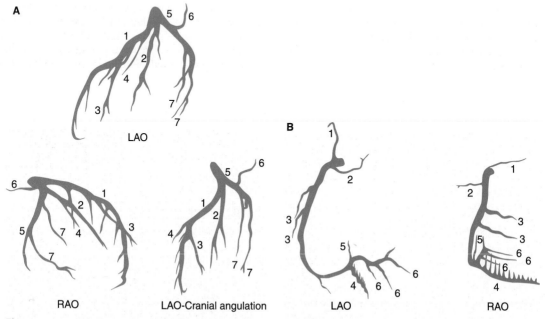

Figure 21–6. Standard angiographic views of the left (*A*) and right (*B*) coronary arteries. Note the left main coronary artery quickly divides into the left anterior descending and the left circumflex arteries. *A:* (1) Left anterior descending artery with septal branches; (2) ramus medianus; (3) diagonal artery; (4) first septal branch; (5) left circumflex artery; (6) left atrial circumflex artery; (7) obtuse marginal artery. *B:* (1) Conus artery; (2) SA node artery; (3) acute marginal artery; (4) posterior descending artery with septal branches; (5) AV node artery; (6) posterior left ventricular artery.

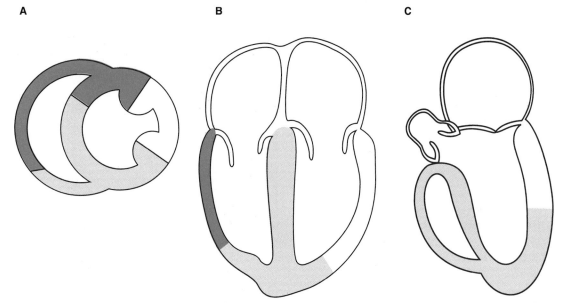

Figure 21–7. Coronary artery supply of the left and right ventricles in three views: the short-axis view (***A***), the four-chamber view (***B***), and the three-chamber view (***C***). Dark green, RCA; light green, LAD; white, CX.

arteries: the left anterior descending artery, the left circumflex artery, and the right coronary artery (Figure 21–6). The areas of distribution of these arteries on echocardiographic views are shown in Figure 21–7. The ventricular short-axis mid view at the mid-papillary muscle level contains all three blood supplies from the major coronary arteries (see Figure 21–4).

2. Assessing valvular function—Valvular morphology can be assessed by multiplane TEE. Pressure gradients, stenotic valve area, severity of stenosis, and severity of valvular regurgitation can be assessed reliably by Doppler echocardiography and color-flow imaging (Figure 21–8). Colors are usually adjusted so that flow toward the probe is red and flow in the opposite direc-

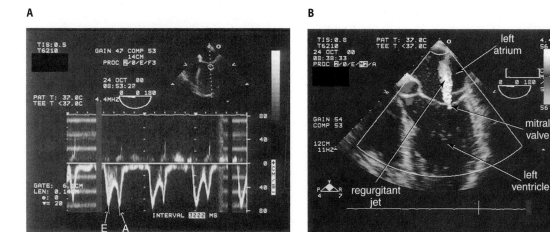

Figure 21–8. Transesophageal echocardiography Doppler and color-flow imaging. Pulse-wave Doppler recording of mitral valve inflow showing two phases, E (early filling) and A (atrial filling) (***A***). Color-flow imaging demonstrates backward flow (regurgitant jet) across the mitral valve during systole (mitral regurgitation) (***B***).

A

B

Figure 21–9. Two views of the aortic valve. Between 40° and 60°, all three leaflets are usually visualized (**A**). Between 110° and 130°, the left ventricular outflow, aortic valve, and ascending aorta are clearly visualized (**B**).

tion is blue. TEE also can detect prosthetic valve dysfunction, such as obstruction, regurgitation, and endocarditis. The TEE images in the upper mid-esophagus at 40–60° and 110–130° are most useful for examining the aortic valve and ascending aorta (Figure 21–9). The valve annular diameter can also be estimated with reasonable accuracy. Doppler flow across the aortic valve must be measured looking up from the transgastric view (Figure 21–10). The anatomic features of the mitral valve relevant to TEE are shown in Figure 21–11. The mitral valve is examined from the mid-esophageal position, looking at the mitral valve apparatus with and without color in the 0° through 150° views (Figure 21–12). TEE is an invaluable aid in mitral valve repair surgery. The commissural view (at about 60°) is particularly helpful because it cuts across many scallops of the mitral valve.

3. Examination for residual air—Air is introduced into the heart during all open-heart procedures. Residual amounts of air often remain even after the best deairing maneuvers. TEE is very helpful in detecting residual air, so that additional surgical maneuvers can be undertaken to help avoid cerebral or coronary embolism.

4. Assessment of other cardiac structures and abnormalities—TEE can also detect congenital heart diseases such as a patent foramen ovale, atrial septal defect, and ventricular septal defect; pericardial diseases such as pericardial tamponade and constrictive pericarditis; and cardiac tumors. Doppler color-flow imaging helps delineate abnormal intracardiac blood flows and shunts. TEE is used to assess the extent of myomectomy in patients with hypertrophic cardiomyopa-

thy (idiopathic hypertrophic subaortic stenosis). Upper, mid, and lower esophageal views are extremely valuable in diagnosing aortic disease processes such as aortic dissection, aortic aneurysm, and atheroma (Figure 21–13). The extent of dissections in the ascending and descending aorta can be accurately assessed; airway structures prevent adequate visualization of the aortic arch. The presence of protruding atheroma in the ascending aorta significantly increases the risk of postoperative stroke and may prompt the use of an alternate arterial cannulation site.

Figure 21–10. Transesophageal echocardiographic recording of continuous-wave Doppler from the transgastric view looking up at the aortic valve, demonstrating severe aortic stenosis. Peak velocity of 409 cm/s indicates a gradient of 66.9 mm Hg.

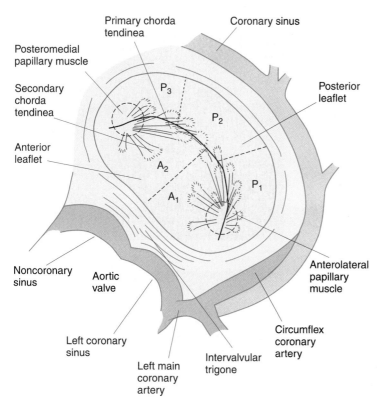

Figure 21–11. The anatomy of the mitral valve and its anatomic relationships to the aortic valve and left circumflex coronary artery. The posterior leaflet has three scallops, P_1, P_2, and P_3. The anterior leaflet is usually divided into A_1 and A_2 regions; in some classifications the anterior leaflet is divided into three areas (A_1, A_2, A_3), corresponding to the opposing corresponding areas of the posterior leaflet.

I. Electroencephalography

Computer-processed electroencephalographic (EEG) recordings can be useful in assessing anesthetic depth during cardiac surgery and, perhaps more importantly, ensuring complete electrical silence prior to circulatory arrest. However, the usefulness of these recordings in detecting neurological insults during CPB is limited by the combined effects of anesthetic agents, hypothermia, and hemodilution. Progressive hypothermia is typically associated with electroencephalographic slowing, burst suppression, and, finally, an isoelectric recording. Moreover, most strokes during CPB are due to small emboli and are not likely to be detected on the EEG. Artifacts from the CPB roller pump may be seen on the raw EEG but can usually be identified as such by computer processing.

J. Transcranial Doppler (TCD)

This modality provides noninvasive measurements of blood flow velocity in the basal arteries of the brain (usually the middle cerebral artery) through the temporal bone. Although studies have not shown that these flow velocities correlate reliably with other measurements of cerebral blood flow, TCD appears to be useful for detecting cerebral emboli. Preliminary evidence suggests that emboli detected by TCD are often associated with postoperative neuropsychological changes.

Induction of Anesthesia

Cardiac operations usually require general anesthesia, endotracheal intubation, and controlled ventilation. Some European centers use high thoracic epidural anesthesia together with light general endotracheal anesthesia for cardiac surgery; in some instances only thoracic epidural anesthesia is used for patients undergoing coronary bypass without CPB. Concerns about the risk of spinal hematoma formation following heparinization and the associated medical–legal consequences have limited the use of neuraxial anesthesia for cardiac surgery in the United States. Some U.S. centers use a single preoperative intrathecal morphine injection to provide postoperative analgesia.

For elective procedures, induction of general anesthesia should generally be performed in a slow, smooth, controlled fashion often referred to as a cardiac induction. The principles are discussed in Chapter 20. Selection of anesthetic agents is generally less important than the way they are used. Indeed, studies have failed to show clear differences in long-term out-

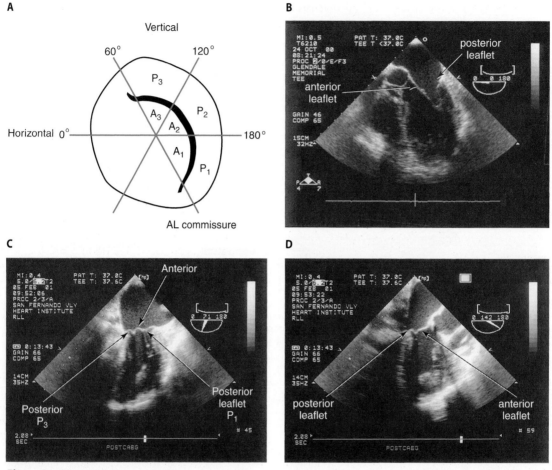

A

Vertical

60° 120°

P_3

A_3 P_2

A_2

Horizontal 0° 180°

A_1

P_1

AL commissure

B

posterior leaflet

anterior leaflet

C

Anterior

Posterior leaflet P_1

Posterior P_3

D

posterior leaflet

anterior leaflet

Figure 21–12. Multiplane imaging cuts across different segments of the mitral valve apparatus between 0° and 180° (***A***). Images of the mitral valve at 0°, 71°, and 142° (***B, C,*** and ***D,*** respectively).

come with various anesthetic techniques. It should be emphasized that anesthetic dose requirements are extremely variable and generally are inversely related to ventricular function. Severely compromised patients should be given anesthetic agents in small doses, slowly, and in increments. A series of challenges may be used to judge when anesthetic depth will allow intubation without a marked vasopressor response or excessive hypotension. Blood pressure and heart rate are continuously evaluated following unconsciousness (loss of the eyelid reflex), insertion of a nasal or oral airway, urinary catheterization, and intubation. A sudden increase in heart rate or blood pressure indicates light anesthesia and the need for more anesthetic prior to the next challenge, whereas a decrease or no change suggests that the patient is ready for the subsequent stimulus. Muscle relaxant is given as soon as consciousness is lost.

Reductions in blood pressure greater than 20% generally call for administration of a vasopressor (see below). The period following intubation is often characterized by a gradual decrease in blood pressure resulting from the anesthetized state (often associated with vasodilation and decreased sympathetic tone) and a lack of surgical stimulation. Patients are often volume depleted from preoperative fasting or diuretic therapy and usually respond to fluid boluses. Colloid boluses are, in most cases, more effective than crystalloid boluses in rapidly expanding intravascular volume (see Chapter 29). In the absence of bleeding, the administration of large amounts of intravenous fluids prior to the bypass accentuates the hemodilution associated with CPB (below). Small doses of phenylephrine (25–50 µg) or ephedrine (5–10 mg) may be necessary to avoid excessive hypotension. Following intubation and controlled ventilation, hemodynamic measurements are

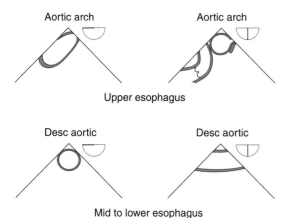

Figure 21–13. Upper esophageal TEE views of the aortic arch and descending aorta. The ascending aorta can be visualized in the upper mid-esophagus at 110–130° with anteflexion at the aortic valve level (see Figures 21–2B and 21–9B).

usually repeated; the baseline ACT (normal < 130 s), arterial blood gases, hematocrit, serum potassium, and glucose concentrations are measured.

Choice of Anesthetic Agents

Anesthetic techniques for cardiac surgery have evolved over the years: from primarily volatile inhalation anesthesia, to high-dose opioid infusions, to total intravenous anesthesia, and more recently to mixed intravenous/volatile anesthesia. Combined neuraxial/light general anesthesia techniques are primarily limited to some European centers.

A. HIGH-DOSE OPIOID ANESTHESIA

This technique was originally developed to circumvent the myocardial depression associated with older volatile anesthetics, such as halothane and enflurane. But pure high-dose opioid anesthesia (eg, fentanyl 50–100 μg/kg or sufentanil 15–25 μg/kg) produces prolonged postoperative respiratory depression (12–24 h), results in an unacceptably high incidence of patient awareness (recall) during surgery, and/or often fails to control the hypertensive response to stimulation in many patients with good left ventricular function. Other undesirable effects include rigidity during induction, postoperative ileus, and possible impairment of immunity. Moreover, simultaneous administration of benzodiazepines can produce hypotension and myocardial depression in some patients. Patients anesthetized with sufentanil generally regain consciousness sooner and can be extubated earlier than those anesthetized with fentanyl.

B. TOTAL INTRAVENOUS ANESTHESIA (TIVA)

The drive for cost containment in cardiac surgery was a major impetus for development of total intravenous techniques with short-acting agents. Although the drugs may be costlier, large economic benefits resulted from early extubation, decreased intensive care unit stays, and early hospital discharge ("fast-track" management). One technique employs infusions of propofol, 0.5–1.5 mg/kg followed by 25–100 μg/kg/min, and remifentanil, 0–1 μg/kg bolus followed by 0.25–1 μg/kg/min. Target controlled infusion (TCI) employs software and hardware (computerized infusion pump) to deliver a drug and achieve a set blood concentration based on pharmacokinetic modeling. For propofol the clinician sets only the patient's age and weight, and the desired blood concentration. During cardiac surgery, this technique can be used for propofol with a target concentration of 1.5–2 μg/mL. Because of the very short half-life of remifentanil, intravenous morphine has to be given at the end of the surgery to provide postoperative analgesia. Alternatively, preoperative intrathecal morphine (8 μg/kg mg) may be administered.

C. MIXED INTRAVENOUS/INHALATION ANESTHESIA

Renewed interest in volatile agents came about following studies demonstrating the protective effects of volatile agents on ischemic myocardium, and the availability of volatile inhalation anesthetics that produce less myocardial depression than older agents and that are rapidly eliminated (eg, desflurane and sevoflurane), and an emphasis on fast-track management. Selection of anesthetic agents is oriented to hemodynamic stability as well as early extubation (1–6 h). Propofol (0.5–1.5 mg/kg) or etomidate (0.1–0.3 mg/kg) is most commonly used for induction. Alternate induction agents include thiopental 1–2 mg/kg and midazolam 0.05 mg/kg. Opioids are given in small doses together with a volatile agent (0.5–1.5 minimum alveolar concentration [MAC]) for maintenance anesthesia and to blunt the sympathetic response to stimulation. The opioid may be given in small intermittent boluses, by continuous infusion, or both (Table 21–1). To facilitate fast-track management, total doses of fentanyl and sufentanil should generally not exceed 15 and 5 μg/kg, respectively. Some clinicians also administer a low-dose infusion of propofol (25–50 μg/kg/min) for maintenance. The major advantage of a volatile agent and intravenous infusion of remifentanil (or propofol) is the ability to change the anesthetic concentration and depth rapidly. Isoflurane, sevoflurane, and desflurane are the most commonly used volatile anesthetics. Early reports of isoflurane inducing intracoronary steal have not been substantiated and it remains a commonly used volatile agent. Nitrous oxide is generally not used because of its

Table 21-1. Doses of opioid boluses and infusions during cardiac surgery.

Opioid	Loading Dose (μg/kg)	Maintenance Infusion	Boluses (μg/kg)
Fentanyl	1–2	1–3 μg/kg/h	0.5–1
Sufentanil	0.25–0.5	0.25–0.75 μg/kg/h	0.125–0.25
Remifentanil	0.5–1	0.1–1 μg/kg/min	0.25–1

tendency to expand any intravascular air bubbles that may form during CPB.

D. OTHER TECHNIQUES

The combination of ketamine with midazolam for induction and maintenance of anesthesia is a particularly useful technique in frail patients with hemodynamic compromise. It is associated with relatively stable hemodynamics, good amnesia and analgesia, minimal postoperative respiratory depression, and rare (if any) psychotomimetic side effects. Ketamine and midazolam have similar pharmacokinetic profiles, are compatible in solution, and may be mixed together in the same syringe or infusion bag in a 20:1 ratio. For induction, ketamine, 1–2 mg/kg, with midazolam, 0.05–0.1 mg/kg, is given as a slow intravenous bolus. Anesthesia can then be maintained by infusion of ketamine, 1.3–1.5 mg/kg/h, and midazolam, 0.065–0.075 mg/kg/h. Significant hypertension following intubation or surgical stimulation requires supplementation with small doses of propofol during induction and a volatile agent during maintenance. Small doses of an opioid may also be administered but may cause hypotension in frail patients. The combination of ketamine and diazepam also results in stable hemodynamics with minimal side effects, but is associated with a more prolonged emergence.

E. MUSCLE RELAXANTS

Muscle relaxation is necessary for intubation, to facilitate sternal retraction, and to prevent patient movement and shivering. Unless airway difficulties are expected, intubation is usually performed with a nondepolarizing muscle relaxant. The choice of muscle relaxant is based primarily on the desired hemodynamic response. Ideally, in most instances, the agent should be devoid of significant circulatory effects. Rocuronium and vecuronium are most commonly used. Vecuronium, however, has been reported to markedly enhance opioid-induced bradycardia. Pancuronium may be a good choice in patients with marked bradycardia because of its vagolytic effects. Succinylcholine should be considered for endotracheal intubation if the potential for a difficult airway exists (see Chapter 5). Judi-

cious dosing and use of a nerve stimulator allow "fast-tracking" with any of these agents.

2. Prebypass Period

Following induction and intubation, the anesthetic course is typically characterized by an initial period of minimal stimulation (skin preparation and draping) that is frequently associated with hypotension, followed by discrete periods of intense stimulation that can produce tachycardia and hypertension. These periods of stimulation include the skin incision, sternotomy and sternal retraction, opening the pericardium, and, sometimes, aortic dissection. The anesthetic agent should be adjusted appropriately in anticipation of these events.

Accentuated vagal responses resulting in marked bradycardia and hypotension may occur during sternal retraction or opening of the pericardium. This response may be more pronounced in patients who have been taking β-adrenergic blocking agents, diltiazem, or verapamil. Deeply anesthetized patients frequently have a progressive decline in cardiac output after the chest is opened. The reduction in cardiac output is probably due to decreased venous return as the normally negative intrathoracic pressure becomes atmospheric. Intravenous fluid administration at least partially reverses this effect.

Myocardial ischemia in the prebypass period is often but not always associated with hemodynamic perturbations such as tachycardia, hypertension, or hypotension. Although controversial, prophylactic infusion of nitroglycerin (1–2 μg/kg/min) intraoperatively may reduce the incidence of ischemic episodes.

Anticoagulation

Anticoagulation must be established prior to CPB to prevent acute disseminated intravascular coagulation and formation of clots in the CPB pump. Moreover, the adequacy of anticoagulation must be confirmed with determination of the ACT. An ACT longer than 400–450 s is considered safe at most centers. Heparin, 300–400 U/kg, is usually given while the aortic pursestring sutures are placed during cannulation. Many surgeons prefer to administer the heparin themselves directly into the right atrium. If heparin is administered by the anesthesiologist, it should be given through a central line, and the ACT should be measured after 3–5 min. If the ACT is less than 400 s, additional heparin, 100 U/kg, is given. When aprotinin is used, a kaolin-ACT rather than celite-ACT should be used to guide heparin therapy. If kaolin-ACTs are not available, heparin therapy should be given as a fixed-dose regimen based on the patient's weight and the duration of CPB. Heparin concentration assays (see Reversal of Anticoagulation, below) measure heparin levels and not necessarily effect; these assays are therefore not reliable for measuring the degree of anticoagulation but can be used as an adjunct when celite-ACTs are used during aprotinin therapy. A whole blood heparin concentration of 3–4 U/mL is usually sufficient for CPB. The high-dose thrombin time (HiTT) is unaffected by aprotinin but is more complicated to perform than a kaolin-ACT. HiTT cannot provide a preheparin control and does not provide an index for the adequacy of reversal with protamine (see below).

Resistance to heparin is occasionally encountered; most patients have antithrombin III deficiency (acquired or congenital). Antithrombin III is a circulating serine protease that irreversibly binds and inactivates thrombin (as well as the activated forms of factors X, XI, XII, and XIII). When heparin complexes with antithrombin III, the anticoagulant activity of antithrombin III is enhanced 1000-fold. Patients with antithrombin III deficiency will achieve adequate anticoagulation following infusion of 2 U of fresh frozen plasma, antithrombin III concentrate, or synthetic antithrombin III. Alternatively, recombinant human antithrombin III may be administered.

Patients with a history of heparin-induced thrombocytopenia (HIT) require special consideration. These patients produce heparin-dependent antibodies that agglutinate platelets and produce thrombocytopenia with or without thromboembolic phenomena. If the history of HIT is remote and antibodies can no longer be demonstrated, heparin may safely be used but only for CPB. When significant antibody titers are detected, plasmapheresis may be used to eliminate them transiently, allowing normal heparinization. Alternative anticoagulants include hirudin, bivalirudin, ancrod, and possibly argatroban, but experience with them is limited. Inactivation of platelets prior to heparinization with aspirin, dipyridamole, or iloprost, a prostacyclin analogue, has also been used in emergency cardiac surgery for patients with HIT.

Bleeding Prophylaxis

Bleeding prophylaxis with antifibrinolytic agents may be initiated before or after anticoagulation. Some clinicians prefer to administer antifibrinolytic agents after heparinization to reduce the possible incidence of

thrombotic complications; delayed administration may reduce their efficacy. Aprotinin therapy should be considered for patients who are undergoing a repeat operation; who refuse blood products (such as Jehovah's Witnesses); who are at high risk for postoperative bleeding because of recent administration of glycoprotein IIb/IIIa inhibitors (abciximab [RheoPro], eptifibatide [Integrilin], or tirofiban [Aggrastat]); who have preexisting coagulopathy; and who are undergoing long and complicated procedures involving the heart or aorta. The antiplatelet effect of abciximab typically lasts 24–48 h whereas that of eptifibatide and tirofiban are 2–4 and 4–8 h, respectively. The combination of aspirin and the ADP receptor antagonist clopidogrel (Plavix) is also associated with excessive bleeding. Although its exact mechanism is not known, aprotinin is an inhibitor of serine proteases, such as plasmin, kallikrein, and trypsin. Its most important action, however, may be to preserve platelet function (adhesiveness and aggregation). Aprotinin therapy is highly effective in reducing perioperative blood loss and transfusion requirements (by 40–80%). It also appears to blunt the intense inflammatory response associated with CPB. Serious allergic reactions, including anaphylaxis (< 0.5%), may be encountered with aprotinin. Reactions are more likely to occur upon repeat exposure. A test dose of 1.4 mg (10,000 KIU) is given prior to a loading dose of 280 mg (2 million KIU) over 20–30 min via a central venous catheter. The drug is then infused at 70 mg/h (500,000 KIU/h) for the duration of the surgery. The CPB pump is also primed 280 mg (2 million KIU). The celite-ACT should not be used because it is artificially prolonged by aprotinin in the presence of heparin; the latter can potentially lead to inadequate coagulation during CPB. The kaolin-ACT is affected less by aprotinin therapy; it appears that the kaolin activator adsorbs aprotinin from blood.

Although possibly less effective, ε-aminocaproic acid 5–10 g followed by 1 g/h or tranexamic acid 10 mg/kg followed by 1 mg/kg/h can be used instead of aprotinin. ε-Aminocaproic acid and tranexamic acid do not affect the ACT and are less likely to induce allergic reactions. Unlike aprotinin, they do not appear to preserve platelet function. Intraoperative collection of platelet-rich plasma by pheresis prior to CPB is employed by some centers; reinfusion following bypass may decrease bleeding and reduce transfusion requirements.

Cannulation

Cannulation for CPB is a critical time. *After heparinization,* aortic cannulation is usually done first because of the hemodynamic problems frequently associated with venous cannulation. Moreover, rapid fluid infusions can be given through the aortic cannula if necessary. The ascending aorta is most frequently used. The small opening of most arterial cannulas produces a jet stream that, if not positioned properly, can cause aortic dissection or preferential flow of blood to the innominate artery during CPB. Reduction of systemic arterial pressure (to 90–100 mm Hg systolic) facilitates placement of the aortic cannula. Bubbles should be completely removed from the arterial cannula, and backflow of blood into the arterial line must be demonstrated before bypass is initiated. Failure to remove all the bubbles results in air emboli, usually into the coronary or cerebral circulations, whereas failure to enter the aorta properly results in aortic dissection. Some clinicians advocate temporary compression of the carotid arteries during aortic cannulation to decrease the likelihood of cerebral emboli.

One or two venous cannulas are placed in the right atrium, usually through the right atrial appendage. One cannula is usually adequate for most coronary artery bypass and aortic valve operations. The single cannula used often has two ports (two-stage) such that when it is properly positioned, one is in the right atrium and the other is in the inferior vena cava.

Separate caval cannulas are used for open-heart procedures. Hypotension from impaired ventricular filling often occurs during manipulation of the venae cavae and the heart. Venous cannulation also frequently precipitates atrial or, less commonly, ventricular arrhythmias. Premature atrial contractions and transient bursts of a supraventricular tachycardia are common. Sustained paroxysmal atrial tachycardia or atrial fibrillation frequently leads to hemodynamic deterioration, which must be treated pharmacologically, electrically, or by immediate anticoagulation and initiation of bypass. Malpositioning of the venous cannulas can interfere with venous return or impede venous drainage from the head and neck (superior vena cava syndrome). Upon initiation of CPB, the former is manifested as poor venous return to the reservoir, whereas the latter produces edema of the head and neck. Under these circumstances, central venous pressure increases only if the tip of the catheter is high in the vena cava.

3. Bypass Period

Initiation

Once the cannulas are properly placed and secured, the ACT is acceptable, and the perfusionist is ready, CPB is initiated. The clamps placed across cannulas during insertion are removed (venous first, then arterial), and the main CPB pump is started. Establishing the adequacy of venous return to the pump reservoir is critical. Normally, the reservoir level rises and CPB pump flow is gradually increased. If venous return is poor, as shown by a decreasing reservoir level, the pump prime will quickly empty and air can enter the pump circuit. The cannulas should be checked for proper placement

and for forgotten clamps, kinks, or an air lock. Under these circumstances, pump flow should be slowed until the problem is resolved. Adding volume (blood or colloid) to the reservoir may be necessary. With full CPB, the heart should gradually empty; failure to do so or progressive distention implies malpositioning of the venous cannula or aortic regurgitation. In the latter instance, immediate aortic cross-clamping and cardioplegia are necessary.

Flow & Pressure

Systemic arterial pressure is closely monitored as pump flow is gradually increased to 2–2.5 L/min/m². At the onset of CPB, systemic arterial pressure usually decreases abruptly. Initial mean systemic arterial (radial) pressures of 30–40 mm Hg are not unusual. This decrease is usually attributed to abrupt hemodilution, which reduces blood viscosity and effectively lowers SVR. The effect is partially compensated by subsequent hypothermia, which tends to raise blood viscosity again.

Persistent and excessive decreases (< 30 mm Hg) should prompt a search for unrecognized aortic dissection. If dissection is present, CPB must be temporarily stopped until the aorta is recannulated distally. Other possible causes include poor venous return, pump malfunction, or pressure-transducer error. Factitious hypertension can occur when the right radial artery is used for monitoring and the aortic cannula is directed toward the innominate artery.

The relationship between pump flow, SVR, and mean systemic arterial blood pressure may be conceptualized as follows:

$$\text{Mean arterial pressure} = \text{Pump flow} \times \text{SVR}$$

Consequently, with a constant SVR, mean arterial pressure is proportional to pump flow. Similarly, at any given pump flow, mean arterial pressure is proportional to SVR. The general conduct of CPB should be such as to maintain both adequate arterial pressures and blood flows by manipulating pump flow and SVR. Although some controversy still surrounds this issue, most centers strive for blood flows of 2–2.5 L/min/m² (50–60 mL/kg/min) and mean arterial pressures between 50 and 80 mm Hg. Flow requirements are generally proportional to core body temperature. Evidence also suggests that during deep hypothermia (20–25°C), mean blood pressures as low as 30 mm Hg may still provide adequate cerebral blood flow. SVR can be increased with phenylephrine.

High systemic arterial pressures (> 150 mm Hg) are also deleterious and may promote aortic dissection or cerebral hemorrhage. Generally, when mean arterial pressure exceeds 100 mm Hg, hypertension is said to exist and is treated by decreasing pump flow or adding isoflurane to the oxygenator inflow gas. If the hypertension is refractory to these maneuvers or if pump flow is already low, a vasodilator, such as nitroprusside, is used.

Monitoring

Additional monitoring during CPB includes the pump flow rate, venous reservoir level, arterial inflow line pressure (see above), blood (perfusate and venous) and myocardial temperatures, and in-line (arterial and venous) oxygen saturations. In-line pH, CO_2 tension, and oxygen tension sensors are also available. Blood gas tensions and pH should be confirmed by direct measurements (see below). In the absence of hypoxemia, low venous oxygen saturations (< 70%), a progressive metabolic acidosis, or low urinary output are indicative of inadequate flow rates.

During bypass, arterial inflow line pressure is almost always higher than the systemic arterial pressure recorded from a radial artery or even an aortic catheter.

The difference in pressure represents the pressure drop across the arterial filter, the arterial tubing, and the narrow opening of the aortic cannula. Nonetheless, monitoring this pressure is important in detecting problems with an arterial inflow line. Inflow pressures should remain below 300 mm Hg; higher pressures may indicate a clogged arterial filter, obstruction of the arterial tubing or cannula, or aortic dissection.

Serial ACT, hematocrit, and potassium measurements are necessary during CPB. Blood glucose should also generally be checked at least once even in patients without a history of diabetes. The ACT is measured immediately after bypass and then every 20–30 min thereafter. Cooling generally increases the half-life of heparin and prolongs its effect. A heparin dose–response curve is often used to facilitate calculation of subsequent heparin doses and protamine reversal (Figure 21–14). Although the relationship does not always conform to a linear function,

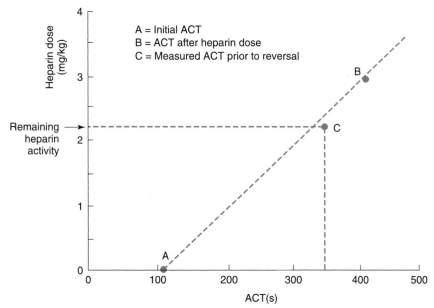

Figure 21–14. Heparin dose–response curve. Activated clotting time (ACT) in seconds versus total heparin dose in milligrams per kilogram.
1. Plot the initial ACT on the *x*-axis.
2. Plot the ACT after heparinization.
3. Draw the line defined by these two points.
4. If additional anticoagulation is needed, find the desired ACT on that line. The amount of additional heparin needed is the difference on the *y*-axis between the present ACT and the desired ACT.
5. If the third point does not lie on the original line, a new line is drawn originating from the baseline ACT and passing midway between the other two points.
6. For reversal of anticoagulation, the protamine dose is based on the remaining heparin activity, estimated to be the heparin dose corresponding to the latest ACT on the dose–response line.

it remains clinically useful. The hematocrit is usually kept between 20% and 25%. Red cell transfusions into the pump reservoir may be necessary. Marked increases in serum potassium concentrations (secondary to cardioplegia) are usually treated with furosemide.

Hypothermia & Cardioplegia

Moderate (26–32°C) or deep (20–25°C) hypothermia is used routinely for most procedures. The lower the temperature, the longer the time necessary for cooling and rewarming. Low temperatures, however, allow lower CPB flows. At a temperature of 20°C, flows as low as 1.2 L/min/m² may be adequate.

Ventricular fibrillation often occurs as the heart is cooled below 28–29°C. Cardioplegia should be established immediately, as fibrillation rapidly consumes high-energy phosphates and jeopardizes myocardial preservation. Cardioplegia is achieved by cross-clamping the ascending aorta proximal to the aortic inflow cannula and infusing cardioplegia solution through a small catheter proximal to the cross-clamp; alternatively, it can be given directly into the coronary ostia if the aorta is opened. Many surgeons routinely employ retrograde cardioplegia via a catheter in the coronary sinus (see above). During aortocoronary bypass grafting, cardioplegia solution may also be given through the graft if the surgeon elects to do the distal anastomosis first.

Ventilation

Ventilation of the lungs is usually continued until adequate pump flows are reached and the heart stops ejecting blood. Following institution of full CPB, ventricular ejection continues briefly until the left ventricular volume reaches a critically low level. Discontinuing ventilation prematurely causes any remaining pulmonary blood flow to act as a right-to-left shunt that can promote hypoxemia (see Chapter 22). The importance of this mechanism depends on the relative ratio of remaining pulmonary blood flow to pump flow. At some centers, once ventilation is stopped, oxygen flow is continued in the anesthesia circuit with a small amount of positive end-expiratory pressure (5 cm H_2O) to prevent postoperative pulmonary dysfunction. Most centers stop all gas flow or continue a low flow of oxygen (1–2 L/min) in the anesthesia circuit. Ventilation is resumed at the conclusion of CPB when the heart begins to eject blood.

Management of Respiratory Gases

There is some controversy about whether to use corrected or uncorrected arterial blood gas tensions during hypothermic CPB. The controversy stems from the fact that the solubility of a gas increases with hypothermia. As a result, although total content does not change (in a closed system), the partial pressure of the gas will decrease as blood temperature drops. The problem is most significant for arterial CO_2 tension because of its effect on arterial pH and cerebral blood flow. As the temperature decreases, the plasma bicarbonate concentration does not change, but the decrease in arterial CO_2 tension tends to increase pH and make blood alkalotic (by normothermic definitions). Blood with a CO_2 tension of 40 mm Hg and a pH of 7.40 at 37°C, when cooled to 25°C, will have a CO_2 tension of about 23 mm Hg and a pH of 7.60.

Normally—regardless of the patient's temperature—blood samples are heated to 37°C in blood gas analyzers before gas tensions are measured. If a temperature-corrected reading is desired, a table or a program in the blood gas machine can be used to estimate gas tension and pH at the patient's temperature. The practice of temperature correcting gas tensions and maintaining a "normal" CO_2 tension of 40 mm Hg and a pH of 7.40 during hypothermia is referred to as **pH-stat management** and has come into question. During hypothermic CPB, pH-stat management, which may require adding CO_2 to the oxygenator gas inflow, increases total blood CO_2 content. Under these conditions, cerebral blood flow becomes more dependent on CO_2 tension and mean arterial blood pressure than on oxygen consumption (see Chapter 25).

The use of uncorrected gas tensions during hypothermia—**α-stat management**—is more common. The basis of this approach is that preservation of normal protein function depends on maintaining a constant state of intracellular electroneutrality (the balance of charges on proteins). At physiological pH, these charges are primarily located on the imidazole rings of histidine residues (referred to as α residues). Moreover, as temperature decreases, K_w—the dissociation constant for water—also decreases (pK_w increases). Therefore, at lower temperatures, the electroneutrality of aqueous solutions, where $[H^+] = [OH^-]$, corresponds to a lower $[H^+]$ (a higher pH). Hypothermic alkalosis thus does not necessarily reflect $[OH^-]$ > $[H^+]$ but rather an absolute decrease in $[H^+]$. Hypothermic CPB with α-stat management usually does not require addition of CO_2 to the oxygenator: the total CO_2 content of blood and the electroneutrality are unchanged. In contrast to pH-stat management, α-stat management appears to preserve cerebral autoregulation of blood flow and may improve myocardial preservation. Despite the theoretical and observed differences, comparisons between the two techniques fail to reveal appreciable differences in patient outcome.

Anesthesia

Hypothermia (< 34°C) itself is usually anesthetic, but failure to give anesthetic agents, particularly during rewarming on CPB, frequently results in light anesthesia that may result in awareness and recall. Hypertension often develops and, if muscle paralysis is also allowed to wear off, the patient may begin to move. Additional doses of muscle relaxants and anesthetic agents may be necessary during CPB. Low concentrations of a volatile agent (isoflurane) via the oxygenator are frequently used. The volatile agent, however, should generally be discontinued just prior to termination of bypass to avoid residual myocardial depression. Patients with poor left ventricular function may be very sensitive to the combined residual effects of cardioplegia and a volatile agent. If a maintenance anesthetic infusion is not used during CPB, additional doses of an opioid or small doses of a benzodiazepine are preferable for these patients. Many clinicians routinely administer a benzodiazepine (eg, midazolam, 5–10 mg intravenously) or scopolamine (0.2–0.4 mg) when rewarming is initiated. Alternatively, a propofol, opioid, or ketamine–midazolam infusion may be continued throughout CPB. Sweating during rewarming is common and does not necessarily reflect light anesthesia but rather a hypothalamic response to perfusion with blood that is often at 39°C.

Cerebral Protection

Neurological complications following CPB may be as high as 40–80%. Fortunately, in most instances, they consist of transient neuropsychiatric dysfunction (ranging from subtle cognitive and intellectual changes to delirium and organic brain syndromes). More serious complications such as strokes are less common (2–6%). Factors that have been associated with neurological sequelae include intracardiac (valvular) procedures, advanced age, and preexisting cerebrovascular disease.

During open-heart procedures, deairing of cardiac chambers, a head-down position, and venting before and during initial cardiac ejection are critically important in preventing emboli. TEE may help detect residual air and the need for further deairing procedures. During coronary bypass procedures, minimizing the amount of aortic manipulation, the number of aortic clampings, and the use of sutureless proximal anastomotic devices may help reduce atheromatous emboli. Palpation of the aorta, TEE, and/or epiaortic echocardiography can help identify high-risk patients and guide management. Epiaortic echocardiography is the most sensitive and specific technique.

Although embolic phenomena appear responsible for most neurological deficits, the contribution of cerebral hypoperfusion remains unclear. Although somewhat controversial, prophylactic thiopental infusions (completely suppressing electroencephalographic activity) immediately prior to and during intracardiac (open ventricle) procedures have been reported to decrease the incidence and severity of neurological deficits. This technique, however, increases the need for inotropic support upon termination of CPB. Prior to circulatory arrest with very deep hypothermia, in addition to thiopental, corticosteroid (methylprednisolone 30 mg/kg) and mannitol (0.5 g/kg) are also usually administered; phenytoin (10–15 mg/kg) may also be used to prevent seizures. The head is also covered with ice bags (avoiding the eyes). Data suggest high-dose aprotinin therapy may decrease perioperative stroke, possibly because of its antiinflammatory effects. Animal studies suggest that magnesium may also be beneficial. Studies have not shown a beneficial effect for calcium channel blockers, and the roles of N-methyl-D-aspartate (NMDA) antagonists (remacemide) and lazaroids (tirilazad) remain largely investigational. Animal studies and some clinical data suggest preoperative erythropoietin therapy may provide neuroprotective effects against a variety of potential brain injuries. Suggested mechanisms include promotion of cell survival signaling cascades, attenuation of intracellular calcium and nitric oxide production, and antioxidative and antiinflammatory actions.

4. Termination of CPB

Discontinuation of bypass is accomplished by a series of necessary procedures and conditions:
1. Rewarming must be completed.
2. Air must be evacuated from the heart and any bypass grafts.
3. The aortic cross-clamp must be removed.
4. Lung ventilation must be resumed.

The surgeon's decision about when to rewarm is critical; adequate rewarming requires time, but rewarming too soon removes the protective effects of hypothermia. Rapid rewarming often results in large temperature gradients between well-perfused organs and peripheral vasoconstricted tissues; subsequent equilibration following separation from CPB decreases core temperature again. Infusion of a vasodilator drug (nitroprusside or nitroglycerin) by allowing higher pump flows often speeds the rewarming process and decreases large temperature gradients. Allowing some pulsatile flow (ventricular ejection) may also speed rewarming. Excessively rapid rewarming, however, can result in the formation of gas bubbles in the bloodstream as the solubility of gases rapidly decreases. If the heart fibrillates during rewarming, defibrillation (5–10 J) may be necessary. Administration of lidocaine 100–200 mg and magnesium sulfate 1–2 g prior to removal of aortic cross-clamping may decrease the likelihood of fibrillation. Many clinicians advocate a head-down position while intracardiac air is being evacuated to decrease the likelihood of cerebral emboli. Lung inflation facilitates expulsion of (left-sided) intracardiac air by squeezing pulmonary vessels and returning blood into the left heart. TEE is extremely useful in detecting residual intracardiac air. Reinflation of the lungs requires temporarily higher than normal airway pressure and should generally be done with direct visualization (or through the pleura) because overzealous lung expansion can interfere with internal mammary artery grafts.

General guidelines for separation from CPB include the following:

- The core body temperature should be at least 37°C.
- A stable rhythm (preferably sinus) must be present. Atrioventricular pacing may be necessary and confers the benefit of a properly timed atrial systole. Persistence of atrioventricular block should prompt measurement of serum potassium concentration. If hyperkalemia is present, it can be treated with calcium, $NaHCO_3$, furosemide, or glucose and insulin (see Chapter 28).
- The heart rate must be adequate (generally 80–100 beats/min). Slow heart rates are generally more of a problem than rapid ones and are best treated by pacing. Inotropic agents are useful in increasing heart rate. Supraventricular tachycardias generally require cardioversion.
- Laboratory values must be within acceptable limits. Significant acidosis (pH < 7.20), hypocalcemia (ionized), and hyperkalemia (> 5.5 mEq/L) should be treated; the hematocrit should be at least 22–25%. When CPB reservoir volume and flow are adequate, ultrafiltration may be used to increase the hematocrit (see above).
- Adequate ventilation with 100% oxygen must have been resumed.
- All monitors should be rechecked for proper function and recalibrated if necessary.

Weaning from CPB

Discontinuation of CPB should be gradual as systemic arterial pressure, ventricular volumes and filling pressures, and cardiac output (if available) are assessed. Central aortic pressure is often measured directly and should be correlated with the radial artery pressure and cuff pressure (if necessary). A reversal of the normal systolic pressure gradient, with aortic pressure becoming higher than radial pressure (see Chapter 6) between these two sites, is often seen. Central aortic root pressure can also be estimated by palpation by the surgeon.

Ventricular volume and contractility can be estimated visually, whereas filling pressures are measured directly by central venous, pulmonary artery, or left atrial catheters. Cardiac output is measured by thermodilution. TEE also provides invaluable information about chamber volumes, contractility, and valvular function.

Weaning is accomplished by releasing any tapes around the vena cava and progressively clamping the venous return line (tubing). As the beating heart fills, ventricular ejection resumes. Pump flow is gradually decreased as arterial pressure rises. Once the venous line is completely occluded and systolic arterial pressure is judged to be adequate (> 80–90 mm Hg), pump flow is stopped and the patient is evaluated. **Most patients fall into one of four groups when coming off bypass (Table 21–2).** Patients with good ventricular function are usually quick to develop good blood pressure and cardiac output and can be separated from CPB immediately. Hyperdynamic patients can also be rapidly weaned. These patients emerge from CPB with a very low SVR, demonstrating good contractility and adequate volume, but have low arterial pressure; their hematocrit is usually very low (< 22%). The diagnosis is confirmed by measuring cardiac output. Ultrafiltration (off CPB) or red blood cell transfusions increase arterial blood pressure.

Hypovolemic patients are a mixed group that includes both patients with normal ventricular function and those with varying degrees of impairment. Those with preserved myocardial function quickly respond to 100-mL aliquots of pump blood infused via the aortic cannula. Blood pressure and cardiac output rise with each bolus, and the increase becomes progressively more sustained. Most of these patients maintain good blood pressure and cardiac output with a left ventricular filling pressure below 10–15 mm Hg. Ventricular impairment should be suspected in hypovolemic patients whose filling pressures rise during volume infusion without appreciable changes in blood pressure or cardiac output or in those who require filling pressures above 10–15 mm Hg.

Patients with pump failure emerge from CPB with a sluggish, poorly contracting heart that progressively distends. In such cases, CPB is reinstituted while inotropic therapy is initiated. If SVR is high, afterload reduction with nitroprusside or an inodilator (eg, milrinone) can be tried. The patient should be evaluated for unrecognized ischemia (kinked graft or coronary vasospasm), valvular dysfunction, shunting, or right ventricular failure (the distention is primarily right sided). TEE may facilitate the diagnosis in these cases. If inotropes and afterload reduction fail, **intraaortic balloon pump** (IABP) is initiated before another attempt is made to wean the patient. The efficacy of IABP is critically dependent on proper timing of inflation and deflation of the balloon (Figure 21–15). **The balloon is ideally**

Table 21–2. Post-CPB hemodynamic subgroups.[1]

	Group I: Vigorous	Group II: Hypovolemic	Group IIIA: LV Pump Failure	Group IIIB: RV Pump Failure	Group IV: Vasodilated (Hyperdynamic)
Blood pressure	Normal	Low	Low	Low	Low
Central venous pressure	Normal	Low	Normal or high	High	Normal or low
Pulmonary artery pressure	Normal	Low	High	Normal or high	Normal or low
Pulmonary wedge pressure	Normal	Low	High	Normal or low	Normal or low
Cardiac output	Normal	Low	Low	Low	High
Systemic vascular resistance	Normal	Normal or high	High	Normal or high	Low
Treatment	None	Volume	Inotrope; reduce afterload, IABP, LVAD	Pulmonary vaso-dilator; RVAD	Increase hematocrit

[1]CPB, cardiopulmonary bypass; LV, left ventricular; RV, right ventricular; IABP, intraaortic balloon pump; LVAD, left ventricular assist device; RVAD, right ventricular assist device.

inflated just after the dicrotic notch to augment diastolic blood pressure and coronary flow. Early inflation can increase afterload and exacerbate aortic regurgitation, whereas late inflation reduces diastolic augmentation. Maximum deflation should be timed just prior to left ventricular ejection to decrease its afterload. Early deflation makes diastolic augmentation and afterload reduction less effective. Use of partial bypass, in the form of a left or right ventricular assist device (LVAD or RVAD, respectively), may be necessary for patients with refractory pump failure. If myocardial stunning is a major contributor or there are areas of hibernating myocardium that decrease the potential for recovery, a delayed improvement in contractile function may allow complete weaning after only 12–48 h in some patients. Circulatory assist devices, such as the Abiomed and HeartMate, can be used as a bridge to cardiac transplantation; the former can be used for several days whereas the latter device can be left in place for up to several months.

Many clinicians believe that inotropes should not routinely be used in patients coming off CPB because they increase myocardial oxygen demand. The routine use of calcium similarly may worsen ischemic injury and may contribute to coronary spasm (particularly in patients who were taking calcium channel blockers

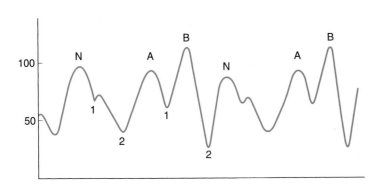

Figure 21–15. A central arterial waveform during 1:2 intraaortic balloon pump counterpulsation. Ideally the balloon, which is positioned in the descending aorta just distal to the left subclavian artery, should inflate at the dicrotic notch and be completely deflated just as the left ventricle begins to eject. Note the lower end-diastolic pressures after balloon augmentation and slightly lower systolic pressure in the following beat. N, nonaugmented beat; A, augmented beat; B, balloon augmentation.

Table 21–3. Vasopressors and inotropic agents.[1]

	Bolus	Infusion	Adrenergic Activity			Phosphodiesterase Inhibition
			α	β	Indirect	
Epinephrine	2–10 μg	1–2 μg/min	+	+++	0	0
		2–10 μg/min	++	+++	0	0
		>10 μg/min (0.01–0.1 μg/kg/min)	+++	++	0	0
Norepinephrine		1–16 μg/min (0.01–0.1 μg/kg/min)	+++	++	0	0
Isoproterenol	1–4 μg	1–5 μg/min (0.01–0.1 μg/kg/min)	0	+++	0	0
Dobutamine		2–20 μg/kg/min	0	++	0	0
Dopamine		2–10 μg/kg/min	+	++	+	0
		10–20 μg/kg/min	++	++	+	0
		>20 μg/kg/min	+++	++	+	0
Ephedrine	5–25 mg		+	++	+	0
Metaraminol	50–100 μg	40–400 μg/min	+++	++	+	0
Phenylephrine	50–200 μg	10–50 μg/min	+++	0	0	0
Amrinone	0.5–1.5 mg/kg	5–10 μg/kg/min	0	0	0	++
Milrinone	50 μg/kg	0.375–0.75 μg/kg/min	0	0	0	++
T₃		0.12 μg/kg/min	0	0	0	0
Arginine vasopressin		2–8 U/h	0	0	0	0

[1]+, mild activity; ++, moderate activity; +++, marked activity.

preoperatively). Commonly used inotropes and vasopressors are listed in Table 21–3. Dopamine and dobutamine are the most commonly used agents. Dobutamine, unlike dopamine, does not increase filling pressures and may be associated with less tachycardia; unfortunately, cardiac output often increases without significant changes in blood pressure. On the other hand, dopamine specifically improves renal blood flow (in low doses; see Chapter 12) and is often more effective in raising blood pressure than in raising cardiac output. Clinically, epinephrine is the most potent inotrope and is usually effective in increasing both cardiac output and systemic blood pressure when others agents have failed. In lower doses, it has predominantly β-agonist activity. Amrinone and milrinone, both selective phosphodiesterase type III inhibitors, are inotropes with significant arterial and venodilator properties; milrinone may be less likely than amrinone to decrease the platelet count. Unlike other inotropes, these two inodilators may not appreciably increase myocardial oxygen consumption because they decrease left ventricular afterload and do not directly increase heart rate. The combination of an inodilator and a β-adrenergic agonist results in synergistic inotropic effects. Norepinephrine is useful for increasing SVR, but high doses compromise renal blood flow. Some clinicians use norepinephrine in combination with phosphodiesterase inhibitors to prevent excessive reductions in systemic arterial pressure. Arginine vasopressin may be used in patients with refractory hypotension, a low SVR, and resistance to norepinephrine. Inhaled nitric oxide and prostaglandin E_1 may also be helpful for refractory pulmonary hypertension and right ventricular failure (Table 21–4); nitric oxide has the added advantage of not decreasing systemic arterial pressure. The role of nesiritide, a human B-type natriuretic peptide, is not clear following CPB. Similarly, the role of additional inotropic support in the form of thyroid hormone (T_3)

Table 21–4. Vasodilators.

Fenoldopam	0.03–0.6 μg/kg/min
Nesiritide	2 μg/kg bolus plus 0.1 μg/kg/min
Nitroglycerin	0.5–10 μg/kg/min
Nitroprusside	0.5–10 μg/kg/min
Nitric oxide	10–60 ppm (inhaled)
Nicardipine	2.5–10 mg/h
Prostaglandin E$_1$	0.01–0.2 μg/kg/min

and glucose–insulin–potassium infusions is not well defined.

5. Postbypass Period

During the postbypass period, bleeding is controlled, bypass cannulas are removed, anticoagulation is reversed, and the chest is closed. Systolic arterial pressure is generally maintained at 90–110 mm Hg to minimize bleeding. Checking for bleeding, particularly from the posterior surface of the heart, requires lifting the heart, which can cause severe hypotension. If it does, the surgeon should be informed of the extent and duration of the hypotension. Atrial cannulas are removed before the aortic cannula in case the latter must be used to rapidly administer volume to the patient. Most patients need additional blood volume subsequent to termination of bypass. Administration of blood, colloids, and crystalloid fluid is guided by filling pressures and the postbypass hematocrit. A final hematocrit of 25–30% is generally desirable. Blood remaining in the CPB reservoir can be transfused via the aortic cannula (if still in place) or processed by a cell saver device and given intravenously. Frequent ventricular ectopy may reflect electrolyte disturbances or residual ischemia and should be treated with lidocaine, procainamide, or amiodarone; hypokalemia or hypomagnesemia should be corrected. Ventricular arrhythmias in this setting can rapidly deteriorate into ventricular tachycardia and fibrillation.

Reversal of Anticoagulation

Once hemostasis is judged acceptable and the patient continues to remain stable, heparin activity is reversed with protamine. **Protamine** is a highly positively charged protein that binds and effectively inactivates heparin (a highly negatively charged polysaccharide). Heparin–protamine complexes are then removed by the reticuloendothelial system. Several protamine dosing

techniques of varying sophistication can be used, but all are empiric and should be checked for adequacy by repeating the ACT 3–5 min after reversal. Additional increments of protamine may be necessary.

The simplest technique bases the protamine dose on the amount of heparin initially required to produce the desired ACT; the protamine is then given in a ratio of 1–1.3 mg of protamine per 100 U of heparin. Another approach calculates the protamine dose based on the heparin dose–response curve (Figure 21–14). Automated heparin–protamine titration assays effectively measure residual heparin concentration and can also be used to calculate the protamine dose. This methodology is based on the observation that when protamine is given in excess it has anticoagulant activity (1/100 that of heparin). Premeasured amounts of protamine are therefore added in varying quantities to several wells, each containing a blood sample. The well whose protamine concentration best matches the heparin concentration will clot first. Clotting will be prolonged in wells containing either too much or too little protamine. The protamine dose can then be estimated by multiplying the concentration in the tube that clots first by the patient's calculated blood volume. Supplemental protamine (50–100 mg) should be considered after administration of unwashed blood remaining in the pump reservoir after CPB as that blood contains heparin.

Protamine administration can result in a number of adverse hemodynamic effects, which appear to be either immune or idiosyncratic nonimmune reactions (see Chapter 46). Although protamine given slowly (5–10 min) usually has minimal effects, hypotension from acute systemic vasodilation, myocardial depression, and marked pulmonary hypertension may be encountered. Diabetics previously maintained on protamine-containing insulin may be at increased risk for allergic reactions.

Persistent Bleeding

Persistent bleeding following bypass often follows long bypass periods (> 2 h) and in most instances is due to multifactorial causes. Inadequate surgical control of bleeding sites, inadequate reversal of heparin, reheparinization, thrombocytopenia, platelet dysfunction, hypothermia, undiagnosed preoperative hemostatic defects, or newly acquired defects may be responsible. The absence of clot formation may be noted. The ACT should return to baseline following administration of protamine; additional doses of protamine (25–50 mg) may be necessary. Reheparinization (heparin rebound) after apparent adequate reversal may be explained by a redistribution either of protamine to peripheral compartments or of peripherally bound heparin to the central compartment. Hypothermia (< 35°C) accentuates hemostatic defects and should be corrected. The administration of platelets and coagulation factors should generally be guided by additional coagulation studies, but empiric therapy may be necessary when such tests are not readily available as well as following massive transfusion (see Chapter 29).

If oozing continues despite adequate surgical hemostasis and the ACT is normal or the heparin–protamine titration assay shows no residual heparin, thrombocytopenia or platelet dysfunction is most likely. Both defects are recognized complications of CPB. Platelet transfusion may be necessary and should be given to maintain the platelet count above $100,000/\mu L$. Significant depletion of coagulation factors, particularly factors V and VIII, during CPB is less commonly responsible for bleeding but should be treated with fresh frozen plasma; both the prothrombin time and partial thromboplastin time are usually prolonged in such instances. Hypofibrinogenemia (fibrinogen level < 100 mg/dL or a prolonged thrombin time without residual heparin) should be treated with cryoprecipitate. The role of aprotinin for prophylaxis against excessive bleeding has already been discussed above. Desmopressin (DDAVP), $0.3\,\mu g/kg$ (intravenously over 20 min), can increase the activity of factors VIII and XII and the von Willebrand factor by releasing them from the vascular endothelium. DDAVP may be effective in reversing qualitative platelet defects in some patients but is not recommended for routine use. Accelerated fibrinolysis may occasionally be encountered following CPB and should be treated with ε-aminocaproic acid (5 g followed by 1 g/h) or tranexamic acid (10 mg/kg), if not already being given; the diagnosis should be confirmed by elevated fibrin degradation products (> –32 mg/mL), or evidence of clot lysis on thromboelastography.

Anesthesia

Unless a continuous intravenous infusion technique is used, additional anesthetic agents are necessary following CPB; the choice is often determined by the hemodynamic response of the patient following CPB. Unstable patients usually receive small amounts of an opioid, benzodiazepine, or scopolamine, whereas hyperdynamic patients tolerate anesthetic doses of a volatile agent. Hypertension not responding to boluses of a narcotic or the addition of a volatile agent should be treated with nitroglycerin or nitroprusside (Table 21–4). Fenoldopam may also be used and has the added benefit of increasing renal blood flow and possibly improving creatinine clearance in the early postoperative period.

Even if a volatile agent is used following CPB, an opioid is usually given to provide sedation during transfer to the intensive care unit and analgesia during emergence.

Transportation

Transporting patients from the operating room to the intensive care unit (ICU) is a hazardous process that is complicated by the possibilities of a complete monitoring blackout, overdosing with or interruption of drug infusions, and hemodynamic instability en route. Portable monitoring equipment, infusion pumps, and a full oxygen cylinder with a self-inflating bag for ventilation should be readied prior to the end of the operation. Minimum monitoring during transportation includes the ECG, arterial blood pressure, and pulse oximetry. An extra pressure channel for central pressures is also desirable. An endotracheal tube, laryngoscope, succinylcholine, and emergency resuscitation drugs should also accompany the patient. Upon arrival in the ICU, the patient should be attached to the ventilator, breath sounds should be checked, and an orderly transfer of monitors and infusions (one at a time) should follow. The ICU staff should be given a brief summary of the procedure, intraoperative problems, current drug therapy, and any expected difficulties.

6. Postoperative Period

Depending on the patient, the type of surgery, and local practices, most patients remain on mechanical ventilation for 2–12 h postoperatively. Sedation may be accomplished by small doses of morphine (2–3 mg) or a propofol infusion (20–30 μg/kg/min). The emphasis in the first few postoperative hours should be on maintaining hemodynamic stability and monitoring for excessive postoperative bleeding. Chest tube drainage in the first 2 h of more than 250–300 mL/h (10 mL/kg/h)—in the absence of a hemostatic defect—is excessive and often requires surgical reexploration. Subsequent drainage that exceeds 100 mL/h is also worrisome. Intrathoracic bleeding at a site not adequately drained causes cardiac tamponade, which necessitates immediate reopening of the chest.

Hypertension that is unresponsive to analgesics or sedation is a common postoperative problem and should generally be treated aggressively so as not to exacerbate bleeding or myocardial ischemia. Nitroprusside or nitroglycerin is generally used. Longer-acting agents or β-blockade may be suitable for patients with good ventricular function.

Fluid replacement should be guided by filling pressures. Most patients continue to require volume for several hours following operation. Hypokalemia and hypomagnesemia (from intraoperative diuretics) often develop and require replacement therapies.

Extubation should be considered only when muscle paralysis has worn off and the patient is hemodynamically stable. Caution should be exercised in obese and elderly patients and those with underlying pulmonary

Figure 21–16. Schematic illustration of the Octopus retractor for off-pump coronary artery bypass surgery.

disease. Thoracic procedures are typically associated with marked decreases in functional residual capacity and postoperative diaphragmatic dysfunction (see Chapter 23). Most patients can be extubated by the following morning.

■ OFF-PUMP CORONARY ARTERY BYPASS SURGERY

The development of advanced epicardial stabilizing devices, such as the Octopus (Figure 21–16), has allowed coronary artery bypass grafting without the use of CPB, also known as off-pump coronary artery bypass (OPCAB). This type of retractor uses suction to stabilize and lift the anastomotic site rather than compress it down, which allows for greater hemodynamic stability. β-Adrenergic blockade is not required to slow the heart rate as with older OPCAB techniques. Full or half (CPB) dose heparinization is usually given and the CPB machine is usually primed and immediately available if needed.

Intravenous fluid loading together with intermittent or low-dose infusion of a vasopressor may be necessary during the distal anastomosis. In contrast, a vasodilator is usually required to reduce the systolic pressure to 90–100 mm Hg during partial clamping of the aorta for the proximal anastomosis. Intravenous nitroglycerin is the generally preferred antihypertensive agent because of its ability to ameliorate myocardial ischemia.

Although OPCAB was initially developed for one- or two-vessel bypass grafting on patients with good left ventricular function, careful application of the technique has allowed it to be used routinely for multigraft surgery, redo operations, and patients with compromised left ventricular function. Some surgeons may use an intraluminal flowthrough device (shunt) to maintain coronary blood flow during most of distal anastomosis. Myocardial preconditioning, brief periods of coronary occlusion prior to the more prolonged occlusion, has been shown to reduce areas of necrosis following prolonged periods of ischemia in animal studies, but the technique has found limited us for OPCAB. Moreover, it has been demonstrated that volatile anesthetic agents provide myocardial protection during prolonged periods of ischemia. Maintenance of anesthesia with a volatile agent may therefore by desirable. Although controversial, long-term graft patency may be similar to procedures done with CPB in selected patients. Patients with extensive coronary disease, particularly those with poor target vessels, may not be good candidates. OPCAB does not decrease the incidence of postoperative neurological complications, though the need for transfusion may reduced.

PEDIATRIC PATIENTS

Cardiovascular function in young children differs from that in adults (see Chapter 44). The Starling relationship (see Chapter 19) plateaus early. Stroke volume is relatively fixed, so that cardiac output is primarily dependent on heart rate. The relatively immature hearts of neonates and infants often poorly tolerate pressure or volume overload. Furthermore, the functions of both ventricles are more interdependent, so that failure of one ventricle often precipitates failure of the other (**biventricular heart failure**). Transition of the neonate from the fetal to the adult circulation is discussed in Chapter 42.

Preoperative Evaluation

The complex nature of these lesions and their operative repair require close communication among the anesthesiologist, cardiologist, and surgeon. The full hemodynamic significance of the lesion and the surgical plan must be clear preoperatively. Moreover, the patient's condition must be optimized to the maximum extent possible. Congestive heart failure and pulmonary infections should be controlled. Prostaglandin E_1 infusion ($0.05–0.1$ µg/kg/min) is used preoperatively to prevent closure of the ductus arteriosus in patients dependent on ductal flow for survival. Indications for operation include severe hypoxemia, excessive increases in pulmonary blood flow, refractory congestive heart failure, severe left ventricular obstruction, and preservation of ventricular function.

Assessment of disease severity relies on both clinical and laboratory evaluation. Deterioration in infants is manifested by increasing tachypnea, cyanosis, or sweating, particularly during feeding. Older children may complain of easy fatigability. Body weight is generally a good indication of overall disease severity. Signs of congestive heart failure include tachycardia, an S_3 gallop, weak pulses, tachypnea, pulmonary rales, bronchospasm, and hepatomegaly. Cyanosis may be noted, but hypoxemia is best assessed by measurements of arterial blood gas and the hematocrit. In the absence of iron deficiency, the degree of polycythemia is directly related to the severity and duration of hypoxemia. Clubbing of the fingers is frequently noted in children with cyanotic defects. The evaluation should also search for other congenital abnormalities, which are present in up to 30% of patients with congenital heart disease.

The results of echocardiography, heart catheterization, electrocardiography, and chest radiography should be reviewed. Laboratory evaluation should include a complete blood cell count, platelet count, coagulation studies, electrolytes, blood urea nitrogen, and serum creatinine. Ionized calcium and glucose determinations are also useful in neonates and critically ill children.

Preinduction Period

A. FASTING

Fasting requirements vary according to the patient's age (see Chapter 44). Patients younger than 1 year should

have their last feeding 4 h prior to surgery and may be given clear liquids until 2 h prior to surgery. Patients between 1 and 2 years of age should have their last feeding 6 h prior to surgery and may receive clear liquids up to 4 h before induction. Patients older than 2 years can generally fast for 8 h. A preoperative intravenous infusion that provides maintenance fluid requirements should be used in patients susceptible to dehydration or with severe polycythemia and when excessive delays occur prior to surgery.

B. PREMEDICATION

Premedication varies according to age and cardiac and pulmonary reserves. Atropine, 0.02 mg/kg intramuscularly (minimum dose: 0.15 mg), is usually given to all pediatric cardiac patients to counteract enhanced vagal tone. Neonates and infants under 6 months of age are given only atropine. Sedation is desirable in older patients, particularly those with cyanotic lesions (tetralogy of Fallot), as agitation and crying worsen right-to-left shunting. Some clinicians additionally administer pentobarbital, 2 mg/kg intramuscularly or 2–4 mg/kg orally, to patients 6 months to 1 year of age. Patients older than 1 year are usually given morphine, 0.1 mg/kg, and pentobarbital, 2–3 mg/kg, intramuscularly in addition to atropine. Alternatively, midazolam can be used orally (0.5–0.6 mg/kg) or intramuscularly (0.08 mg/kg).

Induction of Anesthesia

A. HEMODYNAMIC ANESTHETIC GOALS

1. Obstructive lesions—Anesthetic management should strive to avoid hypovolemia, bradycardia, tachycardia, and myocardial depression. The optimal heart rate should be selected according to age (see Chapter 44); slow rates decrease cardiac output, whereas fast rates can impair ventricular filling. Some cardiac depression may be desirable in hyperdynamic patients with coarctation of the aorta.

2. Shunts—A favorable ratio of pulmonary vascular resistance (PVR) to SVR should be maintained in the presence of shunting. Factors known to increase PVR such as acidosis, hypercapnia, hypoxia, enhanced sympathetic tone, and high mean airway pressures are to be avoided for patients with right-to-left shunting; hyperventilation (hypocapnia) with 100% oxygen is usually effective in lowering PVR. Specific pulmonary vasodilators are not available; alprostadil (prostaglandin E_1) or nitroglycerin may be tried but they often cause systemic hypotension. Systemic vasodilation also worsens right-to-left shunting and should be avoided; phenylephrine may be used to raise SVR. Inhaled nitric oxide has no effect on systemic arterial pressure. Conversely, patients with left-to-right shunting benefit from systemic vasodilation and increases in PVR, although specific hemodynamic manipulation is generally not attempted.

B. Monitoring

Standard intraoperative monitors are generally used until the patient is anesthetized. A large discrepancy between end-tidal and arterial CO_2 tensions should be anticipated in patients with large right-to-left shunts because of increased dead space. Following induction, intraarterial and central venous pressure monitoring are employed for thoracotomies and all procedures employing CPB. A 20- or 22-gauge catheter is used to enter the radial artery; 24-gauge catheters may be more appropriate for small neonates and premature infants. A cutdown may be necessary in some instances. The internal or external jugular vein is generally used for central venous cannulation; if unsuccessful, the central venous catheter may be placed intraoperatively by the surgeon. Pulmonary artery catheterization is much less commonly used in pediatric patients; 7F catheters may be used for patients weighing more than 25 kg, whereas patients weighing 7–25 kg require a 5F catheter.

TEE can be invaluable in pediatric patients, particularly for assessing the surgical repair following CPB. It is generally most useful in patients over 12 kg because the probes required for smaller patients have less resolution. Probes are available for patients as small as 3 kg. Intraoperative epicardial echocardiography is commonly used either in addition to or instead of TEE.

C. Venous Access

Venous access is desirable but not always necessary for induction. The use of EMLA (eutectic [easily melted] mixture of local anesthetic) cream (see Chapter 14) can greatly facilitate placement of a venous cannula prior to induction. Agitation and crying are particularly undesirable in patients with cyanotic lesions because they can increase right-to-left shunting. Intravenous access can be established after induction but before intubation in most patients. Subsequently, at least two intravenous fluid infusions are required; one is typically via a central venous catheter. Extreme caution is necessary to avoid even the smallest air bubbles. Shunting lesions allow the passage of venous air into the arterial circulation; paradoxical embolism can occur through the foramen ovale even in patients without obvious right-to-left shunting (see Chapter 26). Aspiration prior to each injection prevents dislodgment of any trapped air at the injection port.

D. Route of Induction

In premature infants and young neonates, the trachea is usually intubated while the patient is awake and after adequate preoxygenation. In older patients, inhalation, intravenous, or intramuscular induction is necessary prior to intubation. To a major extent, the effect of premedication and the presence of venous access determine the induction technique. Intubation is facilitated by a nondepolarizing agent (rocuronium, 1.2 mg/kg, or pancuronium, 0.1 mg/kg) or, less commonly, succinylcholine, 1.5–2 mg/kg (see Chapter 44). Pancuronium's vagolytic effects are particularly useful in pediatric patients.

1. Intravenous—Thiopental (3–5 mg/kg), propofol (2–3 mg/kg), ketamine (1–2 mg/kg), fentanyl (25–50 μg/kg), or sufentanil (5–15 μg/kg) can be used for intravenous induction. High-dose opioids may be suitable for very small and critically ill patients when postoperative ventilation is planned. The onset of intravenous agents may be more rapid in patients with right-to-left shunting; drug boluses should be given slowly to avoid transiently high arterial blood levels. In contrast, recirculation in patients with large left-to-right shunts dilutes arterial blood concentration and can delay the onset of intravenous agents.

2. Intramuscular—Ketamine, 4–10 mg/kg, is most commonly used, and onset of anesthesia is within 5 min. Preoperative atropine helps prevent excessive secretions. Ketamine is a good choice for agitated and uncooperative patients as well as patients with decreased cardiac reserve. Its safety with cyanotic lesions is well established. Ketamine does not appear to increase PVR in children.

3. Inhalation—Halothane is the most commonly used volatile agent. The technique is the same as for noncardiac surgery (see Chapter 44), except that the concentration is increased slowly to avoid excessive cardiac depression. Halothane and sevoflurane are most suitable for patients with good cardiac reserve. The safety of halothane in patients with cyanotic heart disease and good cardiac reserve is also well established; systemic arterial vasodilation is generally minimal. Halothane induction should not be used in very young patients and those with low cardiac outputs. Nitrous oxide is typically used with inhalation inductions; its concentration should be limited to 50% in patients with cyanotic lesions. Nitrous oxide does not appear to increase PVR in pediatric patients. The uptake of inhalation agents, particularly less soluble agents such as nitrous oxide, may be slowed in patients with right-to-left shunts; in contrast, no significant effect on uptake is generally observed with left-to-right shunting.

Maintenance Anesthesia

Following induction, opioids or inhalation anesthetics are used for maintenance. Fentanyl and sufentanil are the most commonly used intravenous agents and halothane, isoflurane, sevoflurane, and nitrous oxide are the most commonly used inhalation agents. The choice of agent should be modified according to the patient's hemodynamic response. Isoflurane and sevoflurane may be more suitable than halothane in some cases; in equivalent anesthetic doses, they cause less myocardial depression, less slowing of the heart rate, and more vasodilation than halothane. Nitrous oxide can cause cardiac depression in patients with poor cardiac reserve. Moreover, it should probably be discontinued in all patients well before bypass to decrease the likelihood of expansion of intravascular air bubbles (see above).

Cardiopulmonary Bypass

The circuit and technique used are the same as for adults. Because the smallest circuit volume used is still about three times their blood volume, blood is used to prime the machine for neonates and infants to prevent excessive hemodilution. CPB may be complicated by intracardiac and extracardiac shunts and a very compliant arterial system (in very young patients); both tend to lower mean arterial pressure (20–50 mm Hg) and can impair systemic perfusion. Shunts should be controlled as much as possible at the start of bypass. High flow rates (up to 200 mL/kg/min) may be necessary to ensure adequate perfusion in very young patients. Some evidence suggests that pH-stat management during CPB may be associated with better neurological outcome in children. Weaning from CPB is generally not a problem in pediatric patients if the surgical repair is adequate; primary pump failure is unusual. Difficulty in weaning should prompt the surgeon to check the repair and search for undiagnosed lesions. Intraoperative echocardiography, together with measurement of the pressure and oxygen saturation within the various chambers, usually reveals the problem. Inotropic support may be provided by any of the agents used for adults. Calcium chloride is useful in critically ill young patients, who often have impaired calcium homeostasis; ionized calcium measurements are invaluable in such cases. Close monitoring of glucose is required because both hyperglycemia and hypoglycemia may be observed. Dopamine and epinephrine are the most commonly used inotropes in pediatric patients. Addition of a phosphodiesterase inhibitor is also useful when PVR or SVR is increased. Hypocapnia, systemic alkalosis, and a high inspired oxygen concentration should also be used to decrease PVR in patients with pulmonary hypertension (see Chapter 22); additional pharmacological adjuncts may include prostaglandin E_1 (0.05–0.1 µg/kg/min) or prostacyclin (1–40 µg/kg/min). Inhalation nitric oxide may also be helpful for refractory pulmonary hypertension.

Children appear to have a very intense inflammatory response during CPB that may be related to their blood being exposed to very large artificial surfaces relative to their size. Corticosteroids are often given to suppress this response. Many centers use modified ultrafiltration after weaning from CPB to not only partially correct the hemodilution but remove inflammatory vasoactive substances (cytokines); the technique takes blood from the aortic cannula and venous reservoir, passes it through an ultrafilter, and returns it to the right atrium.

Surgical correction of complex congenital lesions sometimes requires complete circulatory arrest under deep hypothermia (hypothermic circulatory arrest). Following institution of CPB, cooling is accomplished by a combination of surface cooling and a cold perfusate. At a core temperature of 15°C, up to 60 min of complete circulatory arrest may be safe. Ice packing around the head is used for surface cooling of the brain. Pharmacological brain protection is also usually attempted with methylprednisolone, 30 mg/kg; mannitol, 0.5 g/kg; and phenytoin, 10 mg/kg. Following the repair, CPB flow is restarted and rewarming takes place.

Postbypass Period

Because of the large priming volumes used (often 200–300% of the patient's blood volume), hemostatic defects from dilution of clotting factors and platelets are commonly seen after CPB in infants; in addition to heparin reversal, administration of fresh frozen plasma and platelets is often necessary. The use of fresh whole blood transfusions instead of packed red blood cells may decrease the need for platelets and clotting factors.

All patients younger than 6 months should generally remain intubated, as should all other patients undergoing extensive or complicated procedures. Extubation may be considered for older, relatively healthy patients undergoing simple procedures such as closure of a small patent ductus or atrial septal defect or repair of a coarctation.

■ CARDIAC TRANSPLANTATION

Preoperative Considerations

Cardiac transplantation is the treatment of choice for patients with end-stage heart disease who are unlikely to survive the next 6–12 months. The procedure is generally associated with 80–90% postoperative survival at 1 year and 60–90% survival at 5 years. Moreover, transplantation significantly improves the quality of life and many, if not most, patients are able to resume a relatively normal lifestyle. Unfortunately, the number of cardiac transplants performed is limited by the supply of donor hearts, which are obtained from brain-dead patients (see Chapter 49), most commonly following head trauma.

Patients with intractable heart failure have an ejection fraction of less than 20% and fall into NYHA functional class IV (see Chapter 20). For most patients, the primary diagnosis is either a cardiomyopathy or coronary artery disease. Others may have a severe congenital lesion, a prior transplantation, or valvular heart disease. Medical therapy has usually consisted of diuretics, vasodilators, and even oral inotropes; oral anticoagulation with warfarin may also be necessary. Patients may become dependent on intravenous dopamine or dobutamine while awaiting transplantation. Intraaortic balloon counterpulsation, an LVAD, or even a total mechanical heart may also be necessary.

Transplant candidates must not have suffered extensive end-organ damage or have other major systemic illnesses. Reversible renal and hepatic dysfunction are common because of chronic hypoperfusion and venous congestion. PVR must be normal or at least responsive to oxygen or vasodilators. Irreversible pulmonary vascular disease is usually associated with a PVR of more than 6–8 Wood units (1 Wood unit = 80 $dyn \cdot s \cdot cm^{-5}$), and is a contraindication to orthotopic cardiac transplantation because right ventricular failure is a major cause of early postoperative mortality. Patients with long-standing pulmonary hypertension may, however, be candidates for combined heart–lung transplantation.

Tissue cross-matching is generally not performed. Donor–recipient compatibility is based on size, ABO blood-group typing, and cytomegalovirus serology. Donor organs from patients with hepatitis B or C or HIV infection are excluded.

ANESTHETIC MANAGEMENT

Proper timing and coordination are necessary between the donor organ retrieval team and the transplant center. Premature induction of anesthesia unnecessarily prolongs CPB, whereas delaying induction jeopardizes graft function by prolonging the period of ischemia.

Patients may receive little advance warning of the availability of a suitable organ. Many—if not most—will have eaten a recent meal and should be considered to have a full stomach. Oral cyclosporine must be given preoperatively. Administration of a clear antacid (sodium citrate), a histamine H_2-receptor blocker, and metoclopramide should be considered. Patients are typically very sensitive to premedication, which may be best administered intravenously and judiciously.

Monitoring is similar to that used for other cardiac procedures and is generally established prior to induction. Strict asepsis should be observed during invasive procedures. Use of the right internal jugular vein for central access does not appear to compromise its future use for postoperative endomyocardial biopsies. A pulmonary artery catheter is routinely used in many centers. Placement is often complicated by tricuspid regurgitation, a tendency to coil in the right ventricle, and ventricular irritability.

Unfortunately, patients usually do not tolerate a rapid-sequence induction. Slight head-up positioning and maintenance of cricoid pressure during induction may decrease the risk of aspiration. The principal objective of anesthetic management is to maintain organ perfusion until the patient is on CPB. Induction may be carried out with small doses of opioids (fentanyl, 5–10 µg/kg) with or without etomidate (0.2–0.3 mg/kg). A low-dose ketamine–midazolam technique (above) may also be suitable. Succinylcholine, 1.5 mg/kg, or rocuronium, 1 mg/kg, can be used to intubate the trachea rapidly. Many clinicians prefer pancuronium (0.1 mg/kg) because it counteracts any opioid-induced bradycardia. Additional boluses or an infusion of an opioid are usually used for maintenance of anesthesia. A TEE probe is placed following induction, and an intravenous infusion of azathioprine is given. Hypotension following induction is relatively common and requires the judicious use of inotropes, vasopressors, and fluids.

Sternotomy and cannulation for CPB typically require 1–2 h and are complicated by prior cardiac operations. Aprotinin can be used to decrease postoperative bleeding. CPB is initiated following cannulation of the aorta and both cavae. If a pulmonary artery catheter was placed, it must be completely withdrawn from the heart and placed into the introducer sheath. It must remain in its sterile, protective sheath if it is to be refloated again into the pulmonary artery following CPB. The recipient's heart is then excised, allowing the posterior wall of both atria (with the caval and pulmonary vein openings) to remain. The atria of the donor heart are anastomosed to the recipient's atrial remnants (left side first). The aorta and then the pulmonary artery are anastomosed end to end. The heart is then flushed with saline and intracardiac air is evacuated. Methylprednisolone is given before the aortic cross-clamp is released.

Inotropic support (isoproterenol) is usually started prior to separation from CPB. Prolonged graft ischemia may result in transient myocardial depression. Slow junctional rhythms are common and may require epicardial pacing. Although the transplanted heart is totally denervated and direct autonomic influences are absent, its response to circulating catecholamines is usually normal (see Chapter 20). The pulmonary artery catheter can be refloated into position after CPB and is used in conjunction with TEE to evaluate the patient. The most common post-CPB problem is right ventricular failure from pulmonary hypertension, which should be treated with hyperventilation, prostaglandin

E_1 (0.025–0.2 µg/kg/min), nitric oxide (10–60 ppm), and an RVAD, if necessary. Bleeding is a common problem because of extensive suture lines and preoperative hemostatic defects.

Patients remain intubated as with other major cardiac operations. The postoperative course is frequently complicated by acute rejection, renal and hepatic dysfunction, and infections.

PERICARDIAL DISEASE

The parietal pericardium is a fairly stiff fibrous membrane surrounding the heart. The negative pericardial pressure following cardiac systole helps promote diastolic ventricular filling. The pericardium encompasses a relatively fixed intrapericardial volume that includes the pericardial sac, the pericardial fluid (20–50 mL in adults), the heart, and blood. As a result, the pericardium normally limits acute dilatation of the ventricles and promotes diastolic coupling of the two ventricles (distention of one ventricle interferes with filling of the other). The latter effect is also due to the interventricular septal wall they share. Moreover, diseases affecting the pericardium or pericardial fluid volume can seriously impair ventricular function.

1. Cardiac Tamponade

Preoperative Considerations

Cardiac tamponade exists when an increase in pericardial pressure impairs diastolic filling of the heart. Cardiac filling is ultimately related to the diastolic transmural (distending) pressure across each chamber. The transmural pressure across a chamber is the pressure within the chamber minus the pericardial pressure. Consequently, any increase in pericardial pressure relative to the pressure within the chamber reduces filling. Although pericardial pressure is applied equally to each chamber, the thin-walled atria and the right ventricle appear to be most affected.

Pericardial pressure is normally similar to pleural pressure (see Chapter 22), varying with respiration between –4 and +4 mm Hg. Elevations in pericardial pressure are most commonly due to increases in pericardial fluid volume (as a consequence of effusions or bleeding). The magnitude of the increase depends on the rate of fluid accumulation; sudden increases exceeding 100–200 mL precipitously increase pericardial pressure, whereas very slow accumulations up to 1000 mL allow the pericardium to stretch with minimal increases in pericardial pressure.

The principal hemodynamic feature of cardiac tamponade is a decrease in cardiac output from a reduced stroke volume with an increase in central venous pressure. In the absence of severe left ventricular dysfunction, equalization of diastolic pressure occurs throughout the heart (right atrial pressure [RAP] = right ventricular end-diastolic pressure [RVEDP] = left atrial pressure [LAP] = left ventricular end-diastolic pressure [LVEDP]).

The central venous pressure waveform (see Chapter 19) is characteristic in cardiac tamponade. Impairment of both diastolic filling and atrial emptying abolishes the *y* descent; the *x* descent (systolic atrial filling) is normal or even accentuated. Reflex sympathetic activation is a prominent compensatory response in cardiac tamponade. Increases in heart rate and contractility help maintain cardiac output. Arterial vasoconstriction (increased SVR) supports systemic blood pressure, whereas venoconstriction augments the venous return to the heart. Because stroke volume remains relatively fixed, cardiac output becomes primarily dependent on heart rate.

Acute cardiac tamponade usually presents as sudden hypotension, tachycardia, and tachypnea. Physical signs include jugular venous distention, inability to lie flat, a narrowed arterial pulse pressure, and muffled heart sounds. A friction rub may be audible. A prominent pulsus paradoxus (a cyclic inspiratory decrease in systolic blood pressure of more than 10 mm Hg) is typically present. The latter actually represents an exaggeration of a normal phenomenon related to inspiratory decreases in intrathoracic pressure. Each decrease augments venous return and increases right ventricular end-diastolic volume (preload) but reduces left ventricular end-diastolic volume. The latter is probably due to a right ventricular distention and rightward shift of the interventricular septum. A marked pulsus paradoxus may also be seen with severe airway obstruction and right ventricular infarction. The heart may be normal or enlarged on a chest radiograph. Electrocardiographic signs are generally nonspecific and are often limited to decreased voltage in all leads and nonspecific ST-segment and T-wave abnormalities. Electrical alternans (a cyclic alteration in magnitude of the P waves, QRS complex, and T waves) may be seen with large pericardial effusions and is thought to be due to pendular swinging of the heart within the pericardium. Generalized ST-segment elevation may also be seen in two or three limb leads as well as V_2 to V_6 in the early phase of pericarditis. Echocardiography is invaluable in diagnosing pericardial effusions and cardiac tamponade and as an aid to pericardiocentesis. Two-dimensional echocardiography is particularly accurate in estimating effusion size. Signs of tamponade include diastolic compression or collapse of the right atrium and right ventricle, leftward displacement of the ventricular septum, and an exaggerated increase in right ventricular size with a reciprocal decrease in left ventricular size during inspiration.

Large pericardial effusions may develop slowly without overt signs of tamponade. Some patients may have "low-pressure tamponade" in which pericardial pressure is only slightly elevated and central venous pressure is normal. These patients may complain of weakness or dyspnea on exertion.

Pericardial effusions may be due to viral, bacterial, or fungal infections; malignancies or surgery; trauma; uremia; myocardial infarction; aortic dissection; hypersensitivity or autoimmune disorders; drugs; or myxedema.

Anesthetic Considerations

Cardiac tamponade requires expeditious evacuation of the pericardial fluid, either surgically or by pericardiocentesis. The latter is associated with a significant risk of lacerating the heart or coronary arteries and of pneumothorax. Traumatic postoperative (following thoracotomy) cardiac tamponade is always treated surgically (a second thoracotomy), whereas tamponade from other causes may be treated by either route. Surgical treatment is also often undertaken for large recurrent pericardial effusions (infectious, malignant, autoimmune, uremic, or radiation induced) to prevent tamponade. Simple drainage of pericardial fluid may be achieved through a subxiphoid approach, whereas drainage combined with pericardial biopsy or pericardiectomy may be performed via a left anterior thoracotomy or median sternotomy. Drainage and biopsies can also be accomplished through left-sided thoracoscopy (see Chapter 24).

The anesthetic approach must be tailored to the clinical setting. For the still intubated postoperative cardiac patient in extremis, the chest may be reopened immediately in the intensive care unit without the benefit of anesthesia (at least initially). For awake conscious patients undergoing left thoracotomy or median sternotomy, general anesthesia and endotracheal intubation are necessary. Local anesthesia may be used for patients undergoing simple drainage through a subxiphoid approach. Premedication with atropine has been recommended to prevent reflex bradycardia during pericardial manipulation. Small doses of ketamine also provide excellent supplemental analgesia.

(17) Induction of general anesthesia in patients with cardiac tamponade can precipitate severe hypotension and cardiac arrest. Pericardiocentesis or subxiphoid drainage under local anesthesia prior to induction is often advisable. Removal of even a small volume of fluid may be sufficient to greatly improve cardiac output and allow safe induction of general anesthesia.

Large-bore intravenous access is mandatory. Monitoring of intraarterial and central venous pressures is desirable, but placement of these monitors should not delay pericardial drainage if the patient is unstable. The anesthetic technique should maintain a high sympathetic tone until the tamponade is relieved. Cardiac depression, vasodilation, and slowing of the heart rates should be avoided. Similarly, increases in mean airway pressures can seriously jeopardize venous return. Awake intubation with maintenance of spontaneous ventilation is theoretically desirable, but coughing, straining, hypoxemia, and respiratory acidosis are equally detrimental and should be avoided. Thoracoscopy generally requires one-lung anesthesia (see Chapter 24).

Ketamine is the induction and maintenance agent of choice until the tamponade is relieved. The circulatory effects of pancuronium also make it the muscle relaxant of choice, but succinylcholine can be used initially for intubation. Small doses of epinephrine (5–10 μg) may be useful as a temporary inotrope and chronotrope. Generous intravenous fluid administration is useful in maintaining venous return.

2. Constrictive Pericarditis

Preoperative Considerations

Constrictive pericarditis may develop as a sequela of acute or recurrent pericarditis. Pathologically, the pericardium is thickened, fibrotic, and often calcified. The parietal pericardium is typically adherent to the heart, often obliterating the pericardial space. The very stiff pericardium limits diastolic filling of the heart, allowing it to fill only to a fixed volume. In contrast to acute cardiac tamponade, diastolic filling does occur, but to a limited extent; in fact, filling during early diastole is typically accentuated and manifested by a prominent *y* descent on the central venous pressure waveform.

Patients with constrictive pericarditis display jugular venous distention, hepatomegaly, and often ascites. Abnormal liver function may be present. In contrast to acute tamponade, constrictive pericarditis prevents respiratory fluctuations in pericardial pressure; because venous return to the heart does not increase during inspiration, a pulsus paradoxus is uncommon. In fact, venous pressure does not fall or may paradoxically rise during inspiration (Kussmaul's sign). The heart may be large or small on a chest radiograph, which often reveals pericardial calcification. Low QRS voltage and diffuse T-wave abnormalities are usually present on the ECG. Atrial fibrillation and conduction blocks may be present. Echocardiography may be helpful in making the diagnosis but confirmation requires computed tomography or magnetic resonance imaging.

Anesthetic Considerations

Pericardiectomy is usually reserved for patients with moderate to severe disease. The procedure is usually performed through a median sternotomy. It is complicated by the necessity for extensive manipulations of the heart that interfere with cardiac filling and ejection, induce frequent arrhythmias, and risk cardiac perforation. CPB facilitates management, but the need for heparinization increases blood loss. The pericardium is generally dissected away from the left ventricle first; freeing the right ventricle first has occasionally resulted in pulmonary edema.

Selection of anesthetic agents is generally not as critical as avoiding excessive cardiac depression, vasodilation, and bradycardia. Cardiac output is generally very rate dependent. Adequate large-bore intravenous access and direct arterial and central venous pressure monitoring are mandatory. Antiarrhythmic therapy (generally lidocaine) is often necessary. Although cardiac function usually improves immediately following pericardiectomy, some patients display a persistently low cardiac output and require temporary postoperative inotropic support.

■ ANESTHETIC MANAGEMENT OF VASCULAR SURGERY

ANESTHESIA FOR SURGERY ON THE AORTA

Preoperative Considerations

Surgery on the aorta represents one of the greatest challenges for anesthesiologists. Regardless of which part of the vessel is involved, the procedure is complicated by the need to cross-clamp the aorta and by the potential for large intraoperative blood losses. Aortic cross-clamping without CPB acutely increases left ventricular afterload and severely compromises organ perfusion distal to the point of occlusion. Severe hypertension, myocardial ischemia, left ventricular failure, or aortic valve regurgitation may be precipitated. Interruption of blood flow to the spinal cord and kidneys can produce paraplegia and renal failure, respectively. Moreover, emergency aortic surgery is frequently necessary in critically ill patients who are acutely hypovolemic and have a high incidence of coexistent cardiac, renal, and pulmonary disease; hypertension; and diabetes.

Indications for aortic surgery include aortic dissections, aneurysms, occlusive disease, trauma, and coarctation. Lesions of the ascending aorta lie between the aortic valve and the innominate artery, whereas lesions of the aortic arch lie between the innominate and left subclavian arteries. Disease distal to the left subclavian artery but above the diaphragm involves the descending thoracic aorta; lesions below the diaphragm involve the abdominal aorta.

SPECIFIC LESIONS OF THE AORTA

Aortic Dissection

In an aortic dissection an intimal tear allows blood to be forced into the aortic wall (the media) or hemorrhage in the aortic media extends and disrupts the aortic intima. In either case, a primary degenerative process called medial cystic necrosis is necessary for dissection to occur. Propagation of the dissection is thought to occur as a result of hemodynamic shear forces acting on the intimal tear; indeed, hypertension is a common finding in patients with aortic dissection. Patients with hereditary connective tissue defects such as Marfan syndrome and Ehlers–Danlos syndrome eventually develop medial cystic necrosis and are at risk for aortic dissection. Dissection can also occur from hemorrhage into an atheromatous plaque or at the cannulation site following cardiac surgery.

Dissection along the aortic media may occlude the opening of any artery arising directly from the aorta; may extend into the aortic root, producing incompetence of the aortic valve; or may rupture into the pericardium or pleura, producing cardiac tamponade or hemothorax, respectively. TEE plays an important role in diagnosing aortic dissections. Dissections are most commonly of the proximal type (Stanford type A, De Bakey types I and II) involving the ascending aorta. Type II dissections do not extend beyond the innominate artery. Distal dissections (Stanford type B, De Bakey type III) originate beyond the left subclavian artery and propagate only distally. Proximal dissections are nearly always treated surgically, whereas distal dissections may be treated medically. In either case, from the time the diagnosis is suspected, measures to reduce systolic blood pressure (usually to 90–120 mm Hg) and aortic wall stress are initiated. This usually includes intravenous nitroprusside and β-adrenergic blockade (esmolol). The latter is important in reducing the shear forces related to the rate of rise of aortic pressure (dP/dt); dP/dt may actually rise with nitroprusside alone. Alternatively, trimethaphan or labetalol can be used (see Chapter 13).

Aortic Aneurysms

Aneurysms most commonly involve the abdominal aorta but may involve any part of the aorta. The vast majority of aortic aneurysms are due to atherosclerosis; medial cystic necrosis is also an important cause of thoracic aortic aneurysms. Syphilitic aneurysms characteristically involve the ascending aorta. Other etiologies include rheumatoid arthritis, spondyloarthropathies, and trauma. Dilatation of the aortic root often produces aortic regurgitation. Expanding aneurysms of the upper thoracic aorta can also cause tracheal or bronchial compression or deviation, hemoptysis, and superior vena cava syndrome. Compression of the left recurrent laryngeal nerve produces hoarseness and left vocal cord paralysis. Distortion of the normal anatomy may also complicate endotracheal or endobronchial intubation or cannulation of the internal jugular and subclavian veins.

The greatest danger from aneurysms is rupture and exsanguination. A pseudoaneurysm forms when the intima and media are ruptured and only adventia or blood clot forms the outer layer. Acute expansion (from leaking), manifested as sudden severe pain, may herald rupture. The likelihood of catastrophic rupture is related to size. The data are least equivocal for abdominal aortic aneurysms; rupture occurs in 50% of patients within 1 year when an aneurysm is 6 cm or more in diameter. The normal aorta in adults varies from 2 to 3 cm in width (it is wider cephalad). Elective resection is generally performed in most patients with aneurysms greater than 4 cm. A prosthetic graft is usually used, and the aneurysm may be completely excised or left in place around the graft. The operative mortality rate is about 2–5% in good-risk patients and exceeds 50% if leaking or rupture has already occurred.

Occlusive Disease of the Aorta

Thromboembolic obliteration of the aorta is most commonly atherosclerotic in origin and occurs at the aortic bifurcation (Leriche's syndrome). Occlusion results from a combination of atherosclerotic plaque and thrombosis. The atherosclerotic process is usually generalized and affects other parts of the arterial system, including the cerebral and coronary arteries (see Chapters 20 and 27). Surgical treatment consists of an aorto-bifemoral bypass with a synthetic graft; proximal thromboendarterectomy may also be necessary.

Aortic Trauma

Aortic trauma may be penetrating or nonpenetrating. Both types of injuries can result in massive hemorrhage and require immediate operation. Whereas penetrating injuries are usually obvious, blunt aortic trauma may be easily overlooked if not suspected and sought. Nonpenetrating aortic trauma typically results from sudden high-speed decelerations such as those caused by automobile accidents and falls. The injury can vary from a partial tear to a complete aortic transection. Because the aortic arch is relatively fixed whereas the descending aorta is relatively mobile, the shear forces are greatest and the site of injury most common just distal to the subclavian artery (aortic isthmus). The most consistent finding is a wide mediastinum on a chest film.

Coarctation of the Aorta

This lesion is usually considered to be a congenital heart defect. Two types are generally recognized and are classified according to the position of the narrowed segment relative to the position of the ductus arteriosus. In the preductal (infantile) type, the narrowing occurs proximal to the opening of the ductus. This lesion, which is often associated with other congenital heart defects, is recognized in infancy because of a marked difference in perfusion between the upper and lower halves of the body; the lower half is cyanotic. Perfusion to the upper body is derived from the aorta, whereas perfusion to the lower body is primarily from the pulmonary artery. Postductal coarctation of the aorta may not be recognized until adulthood. The symptoms and hemodynamic significance of this lesion depend on the severity of the narrowing and the extent of collateral circulation that develops to the lower body (internal mammary, subscapular, and lateral thoracic to intercostal arteries). Hypertension in the upper body, with or without left ventricular failure, is usually present.

ANESTHETIC MANAGEMENT

Surgery on the Ascending Aorta

Surgery on the ascending aorta routinely uses median sternotomy and cardiopulmonary bypass. The conduct of anesthesia is similar to that for cardiac operations involving CPB, but the intraoperative course may be complicated by aortic regurgitation, long aortic cross-clamp times, and large intraoperative blood losses; TEE monitoring is extremely useful. Blood loss can be reduced by administration of aprotinin (discussed earlier). Concomitant aortic valve replacement and coronary reimplantation are often necessary (Bentall procedure). The left radial artery should be used to monitor arterial blood pressure, because clamping of the innominate artery may be necessary during the procedure; the femoral and dorsalis pedis arteries are suitable alternatives. Nitroprusside for precise blood pressure control is generally used. β-Adrenergic blockade (esmolol) should also be employed in the presence of an aortic dissection. Bradycardia worsens aortic regurgitation and should be avoided (see Chapter 20). The arterial inflow cannula for CPB is placed in a femoral artery for patients with dissections. In the event that sternotomy may rupture an aneurysm, prior establishment of partial CPB (using the femoral artery and femoral vein) should be considered.

Surgery Involving the Aortic Arch

These procedures are usually performed through a median sternotomy with deep hypothermic circulatory arrest (following institution of CPB). Additional considerations focus on achieving optimal cerebral protection with systemic and topical hypothermia (above). Hypothermia to 15°C, thiopental infusion to maintain a flat EEG, methylprednisolone or dexamethasone, mannitol, and phenytoin are also commonly used. The necessarily long rewarming periods probably contribute to the large intraoperative blood loss commonly observed after CPB.

Surgery Involving the Descending Thoracic Aorta

Surgery limited to the descending thoracic aorta is typically performed through a left thoracotomy without CPB; a thoracoabdominal incision is necessary for lesions that also involve the abdominal aorta. One-lung anesthesia (see Chapter 24) greatly facilitates surgical exposure and reduces pulmonary trauma from retractors. Correct positioning of the endobronchial tube may be difficult because of distortion of the anatomy; a flexible pediatric fiberoptic bronchoscope can be invaluable in this case. A right-sided double-lumen tube or a regular endotracheal tube with a bronchial blocker may be necessary.

The aorta must be cross-clamped above and below the lesion. Acute hypertension develops above the clamp, with hypotension below. Arterial blood pressure should be monitored from the right radial artery, as clamping of the left subclavian artery may be necessary. The sudden increase in left ventricular afterload after application of the aortic cross-clamp during aortic surgery may precipitate acute left ventricular failure and myocardial ischemia, particularly in patients with underlying ventricular dysfunction or coronary disease; it can also exacerbate preexisting aortic regurgitation. Cardiac output falls and left ventricular end-diastolic pressure and volume rise. The magnitude of these changes is inversely related to ventricular function. Moreover, these effects become less pronounced as the clamp is applied more distally. A nitroprusside infusion is almost always needed to prevent excessive increases in blood pressure and decreases in cardiac output. In patients with good ventricular function, increasing anesthetic depth just prior to cross-clamping may also be helpful.

A major problem in management during these procedures is excessive intraoperative bleeding. Prophylaxis with aprotinin may be helpful. A blood scavenging device (cell saver) for autotransfusion is routinely used. Adequate venous access and intraoperative monitoring are critical. Multiple large-bore (14-gauge) intravenous catheters (pref-erably with two blood warmers) are mandatory. Pulmonary artery catheterization is invaluable for guiding intraoperative fluid replacement and following cardiac function, particularly in conjunction with TEE. The latter is additionally a very useful monitor for myocardial ischemia (see Chapter 20). The period of greatest hemodynamic instability follows the release of the aortic cross-clamp (release hypotension); the abrupt decrease in afterload together with bleeding and the release of vasodilating acid metabolites from the ischemic lower body can precipitate severe systemic hypotension and less commonly hyperkalemia. Decreasing anesthetic depth, volume loading, and partial or slow release of the cross-clamp are helpful in avoiding severe hypotension. A small dose of a vasopressor may be necessary. Sodium bicarbonate should be used for persistent severe metabolic acidosis (pH < 7.20) in association with hypotension. Calcium chloride may be necessary following massive transfusion of citrated blood products (see Chapter 29).

A. PARAPLEGIA

A major complication of clamping the thoracic aorta is spinal cord ischemia and paraplegia. The incidence of transient postoperative deficits and postoperative paraplegia are 11% and 6%, respectively. Higher rates are associated with cross-clamping periods longer than 30 min, extensive surgical dissections, and emergency procedures. The classic deficit is an anterior spinal artery syndrome with loss of motor function and pinprick sensation but preservation of vibration and proprioception. Anatomic variations in spinal cord blood supply are responsible for the unpredictable occurrence of deficits. The spinal cord receives its blood supply from the vertebral arteries and from the thoracic and abdominal aorta. One anterior and two posterior arteries descend along the cord. Intercostal arteries feed the anterior and posterior arteries in the upper thoracic aorta; in the lower thoracic and lumbar cord the anterior spinal artery is supplied by the thoracolumbar artery of Adamkiewicz. This artery has a variable origin from the aorta, arising between T5 and T8 in 15%, between T9 and T12 in 60%, and between L1 and L2 in 25% of individuals; it nearly always arises on the left side. It may be damaged during surgical dissection or occluded by the aortic cross-clamping. Monitoring motor and somatosensory evoked potentials (SSEP; see Chapters 6 and 25) may be useful in preventing paraplegia.

Use of a temporary heparin-coated shunt or partial CPB with hypothermia maintains distal perfusion and decreases the incidence of paraplegia, hypertension, and ventricular failure. Partial CPB is generally not used because heparinization increases blood loss. Using a heparin-coated shunt may preclude the need for heparinization. It is usually positioned proximally in the ascending aorta, left subclavian artery, or left ventricular apex and distally in a common femoral artery. Other therapeutic measures that may be protective of the spinal cord include methylprednisolone, mild hypothermia, mannitol, and drainage of cerebrospinal fluid (CSF); magnesium is also protective in some animal models. The efficacy of mannitol appears to be related to its ability to lower CSF pressure by decreasing its production. Spinal cord perfusion pressure is mean arterial blood pressure minus CSF pressure; the rise in CSF pressure following experimental cross-clamping of the aorta may explain how mannitol can increase spinal cord perfusion pressure. Drainage of CSF via a lumbar catheter may have a similar mechanism.

The use of nitroprusside to control the hypertensive response to cross-clamping may be a contributing factor in spinal cord ischemia, as its hypotensive actions also occur distal to the cross-clamp. Excessive reduction in blood pressure above the cross-clamp should therefore be avoided to prevent excessive hypotension below it.

B. RENAL FAILURE

An increased incidence of renal failure following aortic surgery is reported after emergency procedures, prolonged cross-clamping periods, and prolonged hypotension, particularly in patients with preexisting renal disease. Infusion of mannitol (0.5 g/kg) prior to cross-clamping may decrease the incidence of renal failure. Low (renal)-dose dopamine is not as effective but may be used as an adjunct for a persistently low urinary output after the cross-clamp is released. Fenoldopam infusion appears to preserve renal blood flow and may help reduce postoperative renal impairment. Maintenance of adequate cardiac function (preload, contractility, and systemic perfusion pressure) is also mandatory.

Surgery on the Abdominal Aorta

Either an anterior transperitoneal or an anterolateral retroperitoneal approach can be used to access the abdominal aorta. Depending on the location of the lesion, the cross-clamp can be applied to the supraceliac, suprarenal, or infrarenal aorta. Heparinization prior to occlusion is necessary. Intraarterial blood pressure can be monitored from either upper extremity. In general, the farther distally the clamp is applied, the less the effect on left ventricular afterload. In fact, occlusion of the infrarenal aorta in patients with good ventricular function frequently results in minimal hemodynamic changes. In contrast, release of the clamp frequently produces hypotension; the same techniques to prevent release hypotension (see above) should be used. The large incision and extensive retroperitoneal surgical dissection significantly increase fluid requirements (up to 10–12 mL/kg/h) beyond intraoperative blood loss. A combination of colloid and crystalloid fluids is gener-

ally used (see Chapter 29). Fluid replacement should be guided by monitoring central venous or pulmonary artery pressure, using the latter for all patients with ventricular dysfunction or significant coronary artery disease. TEE should also be considered for this group of patients.

Renal prophylaxis with mannitol should be considered, particularly in patients with preexisting renal impairment. Clamping of the infrarenal aorta has been shown to significantly decrease renal blood flow, which may contribute to postoperative renal failure. The decrease in renal blood flow is not prevented by epidural anesthesia or blockade of the renin–angiotensin system.

Some centers use continuous epidural anesthesia—in addition to general anesthesia—for abdominal aortic surgery. This combined technique decreases the general anesthetic requirement and appears to suppress the release of stress hormones. It also provides an excellent route for administering postoperative epidural analgesia. Unfortunately, systemic heparinization during surgery introduces the risk of paraplegia secondary to an epidural hematoma. Some studies suggest that careful placement of the epidural catheter prior to heparinization—and removal only when coagulation function is normal—lowers the risk of an epidural hematoma.

Postoperative Considerations

Most patients undergoing surgery on the ascending aorta, the arch, or the thoracic aorta should remain intubated and ventilated for 2–24 h postoperatively. As with cardiac surgery, the initial emphasis in their postoperative care should be on maintaining hemodynamic stability and monitoring for postoperative bleeding. Patients undergoing abdominal aortic surgery are often extubated at the end of the procedure. All patients typically continue to require a marked increase in maintenance fluids for several hours postoperatively.

ANESTHESIA FOR CAROTID ARTERY SURGERY

Preoperative Considerations

Ischemic cerebrovascular disease accounts for 80% of strokes; the remaining 20% are due to hemorrhage (see Chapter 27). Ischemic strokes are usually the result of either thrombosis or embolism in one of the blood vessels supplying the brain; vasospasm can also be responsible (see Chapter 26). By convention, a stroke is defined as a neurological deficit that lasts more than 24 h; its pathological correlate is typically focal infarction of brain. Transient ischemic attacks (TIAs), on the other hand, are neurological deficits that resolve within 24 h; they may be due to a low-flow state at a tightly stenotic lesion or to emboli that arise from an extracranial vessel or the heart. When a stroke results in progressive worsening of signs and symptoms, it is frequently termed a stroke in evolution. A second distinction is also often made between complete and incomplete strokes, based on whether the territory involved is completely affected or additional brain remains at risk for focal ischemia (for example, hemiplegia versus hemiparesis). These distinctions are potentially important in the treatment of stroke.

The origin of the internal carotid artery is the most common site of atherosclerosis leading to TIA or stroke. The mechanism may be embolization of platelet-fibrin or plaque material, stenosis, or complete occlusion. The last may be the result of thrombosis or hemorrhage into a plaque. Symptoms depend on the adequacy of collateral circulation (see Chapter 25). The majority of thrombotic strokes are preceded by TIAs or by a minor stroke that later evolves into a major stroke. Emboli distal to areas of collateral blood flow are more likely to produce symptoms. Small emboli in the ophthalmic branches can cause transient monocular blindness (amaurosis fugax). Larger emboli usually enter the middle cerebral artery, producing contralateral motor and sensory deficits that primarily affect the arm and face. Aphasia also develops if the dominant hemisphere is affected. Emboli in the anterior cerebral artery territory typically result in contralateral motor and sensory deficits that are worse in the leg.

Indications for carotid endarterectomy include TIAs associated with ipsilateral severe carotid stenosis (> 70% occlusion), severe ipsilateral stenosis in a patient with a minor (incomplete) stroke, and 30–70% occlusion in a patient with ipsilateral symptoms (usually an ulcerated plaque). Some surgeons also advocate carotid endarterectomy for asymptomatic but significantly stenotic lesions (> 60%). Operative mortality is 1–4% and is primarily due to cardiac complications (myocardial infarction). Perioperative morbidity is 4–10% and is principally neurological; it is highest in patients with preexisting neurological deficits. Studies suggest that age greater than 75 years, symptomatic lesions, uncontrolled hypertension, angina, carotid thrombus, and occlusions near the carotid siphon increase operative risk.

Preoperative Anesthetic Evaluation & Management

Most patients undergoing carotid endarterectomy are elderly and hypertensive, with generalized arteriosclerosis. A significant number are also diabetic. Preoperative evaluation and management should focus on defining preexisting neurological deficits as well as optimizing the patient's clinical status in terms of coexisting diseases. Although most postoperative neurological deficits appear to be related to surgical technique, uncontrolled preoperative hypertension increases the incidence of new deficits following surgery. Uncontrolled hyperglycemia can also increase morbidity by enhancing ischemic cerebral injury (see Chapter 25).

With the possible exception of diuretics, patients should receive their usual medications on schedule until the time of surgery. Blood pressure and the plasma-glucose concentration should be well controlled preoperatively. Angina should be stable and controlled, and signs of overt congestive heart failure should be absent. Premedication is tailored to each patient's needs. Alleviation of anxiety to prevent hypertension and tachycardia is desirable. Because most patients are elderly, enhanced sensitivity to premedication should be expected.

General Anesthesia

The emphasis of anesthetic management during carotid surgery is on maintaining adequate cerebral perfusion without stressing the heart. Traditionally, this is accomplished by close regulation of arterial blood pressure and avoidance of tachycardia. Monitoring of intraarterial pressure is therefore mandatory. Electrocardiographic monitoring should include the V5 lead to detect ischemia. Continuous computerized ST-segment analysis is desirable. Additional hemodynamic monitoring should be based primarily on underlying cardiac function, as carotid endarterectomy is not usually associated with significant blood loss or fluid shifts.

Regardless of the anesthetic agents selected, mean arterial blood pressure should be maintained at—or slightly above—the patient's usual range. Thiopental, propofol, and etomidate are the most popular choices for induction because of their favorable cerebral effects, reducing cerebral metabolic rate proportionately more than cerebral blood flow (see Chapter 25). Propofol and etomidate appear to lack the same protective effects as thiopental in focal ischemia, but propofol allows more rapid awakening. Small doses of an opioid or β-adrenergic blocker can be used to blunt the hypertensive response to endotracheal intubation (see Chapter 20). Isoflurane may be the volatile agent of choice because it appears to provide the greatest protection against cerebral ischemia (see Chapter 25). Desflurane qualitatively has similar cerebral effects but may not be as effective as isoflurane; however, desflurane is very useful in accelerating awakening and allowing immediate neurological assessment in the operating room. Some clinicians also use remifentanil as the opioid for the same reasons.

Intraoperative hypertension is common and usually necessitates the use of an intravenous vasodilator. Nitroglycerin is usually a good choice for mild to moderate hypertension because of its beneficial effects on the coronary circulation. Marked hypertension requires a more potent agent, such as nitroprusside. β-Adrenergic blockade facilitates management of the hypertension and prevents tachycardia, but should be used cautiously. Intravenous nicardipine (see Chapter 20) may be a good alternative because of its possible protective effect in focal ischemia. Hypotension should be treated with judicious amounts of intravenous fluid and/or vasopressors. Some clinicians consider phenylephrine the vasopressor of choice; if selected, it should be administered in 25-μg increments to prevent excessive hypertension.

Pronounced or sustained reflex bradycardia or heart block caused by manipulation of the carotid baroreceptor should be treated with atropine. To prevent this response, some surgeons infiltrate the area of the carotid sinus with lidocaine, but the infiltration itself can induce bradycardia. Arterial CO_2 tension should be routinely measured because end-tidal measurements are not sufficiently reliable (see Chapter 6). Hypercapnia can induce intracerebral steal (see Chapter 25) whereas excessive hypocapnia decreases cerebral perfusion. Ventilation should be adjusted to maintain normocapnia. Intravenous fluids should generally consist of glucose-free solutions because of the potentially adverse effects of hyperglycemia. Heparin (5000–7500 units intravenously) is necessary prior to occlusion of the carotid artery. Some clinicians also routinely administer thiopental, 4–6 mg/kg, just prior to carotid cross-clamping for cerebral protection, but the routine use of a shunt (see below) may obviate the need. Protamine, 50–150 mg, is usually given for reversal prior to skin closure.

Although rapid emergence from anesthesia is desirable because it allows immediate neurological assessment, it frequently results in hypertension and tachycardia requiring a vasodilator, β-adrenergic blocker, or combined α- and β-adrenergic blocker. **Postoperative hypertension may be related to surgical denervation of the ipsilateral carotid baroreceptor. Denervation of the carotid body blunts the ventilatory response to hypoxemia.** Following extubation, patients should be observed closely for the development of a wound hematoma, which can rapidly compromise the airway. Transient postoperative hoarseness and ipsilateral deviation of the tongue may be noted; they are due to surgical retraction of the recurrent laryngeal and hypoglossal nerves, respectively.

Monitoring Cerebral Function

Unless regional anesthesia is used (see below), indirect methods must be relied upon to assess the adequacy of cerebral perfusion during carotid cross-clamping. Many surgeons routinely use a shunt, but this practice may increase the incidence of postoperative neurological deficits; shunt insertion can dislodge emboli. Carotid stump pressure distal to the cross-clamp, EEG, and SSEPs have been used by some centers to determine the need for a shunt; a distal stump pressure < 50 mm Hg has traditionally been used as an indication for a shunt. Electrophysiological signs of ischemia after cross-clamping dictate the use of a shunt; changes lasting more than 10 min may be associated with a new postoperative neurological deficit. Although multichannel recordings and computer processing can enhance the sensitivity of the EEG, neither EEG nor SSEP monitoring is sufficiently sensitive or specific to reliably predict the need for shunting or the occurrence of postoperative deficits. Other techniques, including measurements of regional cerebral blood flow with radioactive xenon-133, transcranial Doppler measurement of middle cerebral artery flow velocity, cerebral oximetry, jugular venous oxygen saturation, and transconjunctival oxygen tension, are also not sufficiently reliable.

Regional Anesthesia

Carotid surgery may be performed under regional anesthesia. Superficial and deep cervical plexus blocks (see Chapter 17) effectively block the C2–C4 nerves and allow the patient to remain comfortably awake during surgery. The principal advantage of regional anesthesia is that the patient can be examined intraoperatively; thus, the need for a temporary shunt can be assessed and any new neurological deficits diagnosed during surgery. In fact, intraoperative neurological examination may be the most reliable method for assessing the adequacy of cerebral perfusion during carotid cross-clamping. The examination minimally consists of level of consciousness, speech, and contralateral handgrip. Some studies also suggest that when compared with general anesthesia, regional anesthesia results in more stable hemodynamics but outcomes appear similar. Unfortunately, regional anesthesia requires the full cooperation of the patient. Moreover, the airway is not secured, and access to it is difficult once the operation begins. Cervical plexus block and the surgery itself may result in ipsilateral phrenic nerve paralysis; it usually is well tolerated and transient.

CASE DISCUSSION:
A PATIENT FOR CARDIOVERSION

A 55-year-old man with new-onset atrial fibrillation is scheduled for elective cardioversion.

What are the indications for an elective cardioversion?

Direct current (DC) cardioversion may be used to terminate supraventricular and ventricular tachyarrhythmias caused by reentry. It is not effective for arrhythmias from enhanced automa-

ticity (multifocal atrial tachycardia) or triggered activity (digitalis toxicity). By simultaneously depolarizing the entire myocardium and possibly prolonging the refractory period, DC cardioversion can terminate atrial fibrillation and flutter, atrioventricular nodal reentry, reciprocating tachycardias from preexcitation syndromes, and ventricular tachycardia or fibrillation.

Specific indications for patients with atrial fibrillation include symptomatic fibrillation of less than 12 months duration, a history of embolism, recent onset, and no response to medications. Patients with long-standing fibrillation, a large atrium, chronic obstructive lung disease, congestive heart failure, or mitral regurgitation have a high recurrence rate. A TEE is usually performed to rule out a left atrial blood clot prior to cardioversion. Such clots are typically located in the left atrial appendage.

Emergency cardioversion is indicated for any tachyarrhythmia associated with significant hypotension, congestive heart failure, or angina (see Chapter 19).

How is cardioversion performed?

Although usually performed by cardiologists, the need for immediate cardioversion may arise in the operating room, intensive care unit, or during cardiopulmonary resuscitation (see Chapter 47). Anesthesiologists must therefore be familiar with the technique. Following heavy sedation or light general anesthesia, DC shock is applied by either self-adhesive pads or 8- to 13-cm paddles. Larger paddles help reduce any shock-induced myocardial necrosis by distributing the current over a wider area. The energy output should be kept at the minimally effective level to prevent myocardial damage. Placement of the electrodes can be anterolateral or anteroposterior. In the first position, one electrode is placed on the right second intercostal space next to the sternum and the other is placed on the left fifth intercostal space in the midclavicular line. When pads are used for the anteroposterior technique, one is placed anteriorly over the ventricular apex in the fifth intercostal space and the other underneath the patient in the left infrascapular region.

For supraventricular tachycardias, with the notable exception of atrial fibrillation, energy levels of 25–50 J can successfully reestablish normal sinus rhythm. Synchronized shocks should be used for all tachyarrhythmias except ventricular fibrillation. Synchronization times the delivery so that it is given during the QRS complex. If the shock occurs in the ST segment or the T wave (un-synchronized), it can precipitate a more serious arrhythmia, including ventricular fibrillation. All medical personnel should stand clear of the patient and the bed during the shock.

Atrial fibrillation usually requires a minimum of 50–100 J. Hemodynamically stable ventricular tachycardia can often be terminated with 25–50 J, but ventricular fibrillation and unstable ventricular tachycardia require 200–400 J (see Chapter 47). Regardless of the arrhythmia, a higher energy level is necessary when the first shock is ineffective. If ventricular arrhythmias develop following the initial shock, lidocaine should be given prior to the next one.

The cardiologist wants to do the cardioversion in the recovery room. Is this an appropriate place for cardioversion?

Elective cardioversion can be performed in any setting in which full provisions for cardiopulmonary resuscitation, including cardiac pacing capabilities, are immediately available. A physician skilled in airway management should be in attendance. Cardioversions are most commonly performed in an intensive care unit, emergency room, recovery room, or cardiac catheterization suite.

How would you evaluate this patient?

The patient should be evaluated and treated as though he were receiving a general anesthetic in the operating room. Patients should fast for 6–8 h prior to the procedure to decrease the risk of aspiration; airway reflexes will be depressed by sedatives and anesthetic agents. A 12-lead ECG is performed immediately before the procedure to confirm that the arrhythmia is still present; another one is performed immediately afterward to confirm the new rhythm. Preoperative laboratory values should be within normal limits because metabolic disorders, particularly electrolyte and acid–base abnormalities, may contribute to the arrhythmia; if not corrected preoperatively, they can reinitiate the tachycardia following cardioversion. Withholding digitalis in a patient without evidence of toxicity is not necessary. Quinidine or another antiarrhythmic is often started in patients with atrial fibrillation 1–2 days prior to the procedure to help maintain normal sinus rhythm. Patients may also be anticoagulated with warfarin for 1–2 weeks prior to cardioversion. A TEE may be performed immediately before to rule out an atrial thrombus.

What are the minimum monitors and anesthetic equipment required?

Minimum monitoring consists of the ECG, blood pressure, and pulse oximetry. A precordial stethoscope is useful for monitoring breath sounds. It is essential to monitor the patient's level of consciousness; maintaining continuous verbal contact with the patient may the best method.

In addition to a DC defibrillator capable of delivering up to 400 J (synchronized or unsynchronized) and transcutaneous pacing, the minimum equipment should include the following:

- *Reliable intravenous access.*
- *A functional bag-mask device capable of delivering 100% oxygen (see Chapter 3).*
- *An oxygen source from a wall outlet or a full tank.*
- *An airway kit with oral and nasal airways and appropriate laryngoscopes and endotracheal tubes.*
- *A functional suction apparatus.*
- *An anesthetic drug kit that includes at least one sedative-hypnotic as well as succinylcholine.*
- *A crash cart that includes all necessary drugs and equipment for cardiopulmonary resuscitation (see Chapter 47).*

What anesthetic techniques would be appropriate?

Premedication is not necessary. Only very brief (1–2 min) amnesia or light general anesthesia is required. A short-acting barbiturate (methohexital), propofol, etomidate, or a benzodiazepine (eg, midazolam, diazepam) can be used. Following preoxygenation with 60–100% oxygen for 3–5 min, the sedative-hypnotic is given in small increments (eg, propofol, 50 mg or methohexital, 20 mg) every 2–3 min (if necessary) while maintaining verbal contact with the patient. The shock is delivered when the patient is no longer able to respond verbally; some clinicians use loss of the eyelid reflex as an end point. The shock usually arouses the patient. Transient airway obstruction or apnea may be observed, particularly if more than one shock is necessary.

What are the complications of cardioversion?

Complications include transient myocardial depression, postshock arrhythmias, and arterial embolism. Arrhythmias are usually due to inadequate synchronization, but even a properly timed cardioversion can occasionally result in ventricular fibrillation. Most arrhythmias are transient and resolve spontaneously. Although patients may develop ST-segment elevation, serum creatine phosphokinase levels (MB fraction) are usually normal. Embolism may be responsible for delayed awakening.

How should the patient be cared for following cardioversion?

Although recovery of consciousness is usually very rapid, patients should be treated like others receiving general anesthesia (see Chapter 48). Recovery also specifically includes monitoring for both recurrence of the arrhythmia and signs of cerebral embolism.

SUGGESTED READING

Arrowsmith JE, Grocott HP, Reves JG, Newman MF: Central nervous system complications of cardiac surgery. Br J Anaesth 2000;84:378.

Beique FA, Joffe D, Tousignant G, Konstadt S: Echocardiography-based assessment and management of atherosclerotic disease of the thoracic aorta. J Cardiothorac Vasc Anesth 1998;12:206.

Chassot P-G, van der Linden P, Zaugg M, et al: Off-pump coronary artery bypass surgery: physiology and anaesthetic management. Br J Anaesth 2004;92:400.

Comunale ME, Van Cott EM: Heparin-induced thrombocytopenia. Int Anesthesiol Clin 2004;42:27.

Cook DJ: Changing temperature management for cardiopulmonary bypass. Anesth Analg 1999;88:1254.

Davies LK: Cardiopulmonary bypass in infants and children: How is it different? J Cardiothorac Vasc Anesth 1999;13:330.

Estafanous FG, Barash PG, Reves JG: *Cardiac Anesthesia: Principles and Clinical Practice,* 2nd ed. Lippincott, 2001.

Gomez MN: Magnesium and cardiovascular disease. Anesthesiology 1998;89:222.

Gravlee G: *Cardiopulmonary Bypass.* Lippincott, Williams & Wilkins, 2000.

Grocott HP, Nussmeier NA: Neuroprotection in cardiac surgery. Anesth Clin North Am 2003;21:487.

Hensley FA, Martin DE, Gravlee GP: *A Practical Approach to Cardiac Anesthesia,* 3rd ed. Lippincott, Williams & Wilkins, 2003.

Higgens TL: Quantifying risk and assessing outcome in cardiac surgery. J Cardiothorac Vasc Anesth 1998;12:330.

Hirsch DJ, Cooper JR: Cardiac failure and left ventricular assist devices. Anesth Clin North Am 2003;21:625.

Kam PCA, Egan MK: Platelet glycoprotein IIb/IIIa antagonists. Pharmacology and clinical developments. Anesthesiology 2002;96:1237.

Kaplan JA, Reich DL, Kronstadt SN: *Cardiac Anesthesia,* 4th ed. W.B. Saunders, 1999.

Kaplan JA, Lake CL, Murray MJ: *Vascular Anesthesia,* 2nd ed. Churchill Livingstone, 2004.

Kohrs R, Durieux M: Ketamine: teaching an old drug new tricks. Anesth Analg 1998;87:1186.

Kronstadt SN, Sherman SK, Oka Y: *Clinical Transesophageal Echocardiography,* 2nd ed. Lippincott, Williams & Wilkins, 2003.

Laffy JG, Boylan JF, Cheng DCH: The systemic inflammatory response to cardiac surgery. Anesthesiology 2002;97:215.

Lake CL: *Pediatric Cardiac Anesthesia,* 4th ed. Lippincott, Williams & Wilkins, 2004.

Ling E, Arellano R: Systematic overview of the evidence supporting the use of cerebrospinal fluid drainage in the thoracoabdominal aneurysm surgery for prevention of paraplegia. Anesthesiology 2000;93:1115.

Martlew VJ: Perioperative management of patients with coagulation disorders. Br J Anaesth 2000;85:446.

Maslow, A, Schwartz, C: Cardiopulmonary bypass-associated coagulopathies and prophylactic therapy. Int Anesthesiol Clin 2004;42:103.

Mets B: Anesthesia for left ventricular assist device placement. J Cardiothorac Vasc Anesth 2000;14:316.

Myles PS, Daly DJ, Djaiani G, et al: A systematic review of the safety and effectiveness of fast-track cardiac anesthesia. Anesthesiology 2003;99:982.

Nanda NC, Domanski MJ: *Atlas of Transesophageal Echocardiography.* Williams & Wilkins, 1998.

Otto CM: *Valvular Heart Disease,* 2nd ed. W.B. Saunders, 2003.

Otto CM: *Textbook of Clinical Echocardiography,* 3rd ed. W.B. Saunders, 2004.

Park, KW: Protamine and protamine reactions. Int Anesthesiol Clin 2004;42:135.

Pintar T, Collard CD: The systemic inflammatory response to cardiopulmonary bypass. Anesth Clin North Am 2003;21:453.

Poortmanns G, Schupfer G, Roosens C, Poelaert J: Transesophageal echocardiographic evaluation of left ventricular function. J Cardiothorac Vasc Anesth 1999;14:588.

Pravinkumar E, Webster NR: HIT/HITT and alternative anticoagulation: current concepts. Br J Anaesth 2003;90:676.

Priebe HJ: Triggers of perioperative myocardial ischaemia and infarction. Br J Anaesth 2004;93:9.

Pua HL, Bissonnette B: Cerebral physiology in paediatric cardiopulmonary bypass. Can J Anaesth 1998;45:960.

Shanewise JS, Ramsay JG: Off-pump coronary surgery: how do the anesthetic considerations differ? Anesth Clin North Am 2003;21:613.

Sherman SK: Perioperative myocardial ischemia reperfusion injury. Anesth Clin North Am 2003;21:465.

Shine TSJ, Murray MJ: Intraoperative management of aortic aneurysm surgery. Anesth Clin North Am 2004;22:289.

Shore-Lesserson L: Monitoring anticoagulation and hemostasis in cardiac surgery. Anesth Clin North Am 2003;21:511.

Slaughter TF, Greenberg CS: Heparin-associated thrombocytopenia and thrombosis. Anesthesiology 1997;87:667.

Stayer SA, Andropoulos DB, Russell IA: Anesthetic management of the adult patient with congenital heart disease. Anesth Clin North Am 2003;21:653.

Steudel W, Hurford WE, Zapol WM: Inhaled nitric oxide: basic biology and clinical application. Anesthesiology 1999;91:1090.

Stoneham MD, Knighton JD: Regional anaesthesia for carotid endarterectomy. Br J Anaesth 1999;82:910.

Stump DA, Jones TJ, Rorie KD: Neurophysiologic monitoring and outcomes in cardiovascular surgery. J Cardiothorac Vasc Anesth 1999;13:600.

Tempe DK, Siddiquie RA: Awareness during cardiac surgery. J Cardiothorac Vasc Anesth 1999;13:214.

Thys D: *Textbook of Cardiothoracic Anesthesia.* McGraw-Hill, 2001.

Willens HJ, Kessler KM: Transesophageal echocardiography in the diagnosis of diseases of the thoracic aorta: Part II—Atherosclerotic and traumatic diseases of the aorta. Chest 2000;117:233.

Yastrebov K: Intraoperative management: carotid endarterectomies. Anesth Clin North Am 2004;22:265.

Youngberg JA, Lake CL, Roizen MF, Wilson RS: *Cardiac, Vascular, and Thoracic Anesthesia.* Churchill Livingstone, 2000.

Zaugg M, Schaub MC, Foëx P: Myocardial injury and its prevention in the perioperative setting. Br J Anaesth 2004;93:21.

Respiratory Physiology: The Effects of Anesthesia

22

KEY CONCEPTS

 1 General anesthesia typically reduces both $\dot{V}_{O_2}$ and $\dot{V}_{CO_2}$ by about 15%. Additional reductions are often seen as a result of hypothermia. The greatest reductions are in cerebral and cardiac O_2 consumption.

 2 At end-expiration, intrapleural pressure normally averages about –5 cm H_2O and because alveolar pressure is 0 (no flow), transpulmonary pressure is +5 cm H_2O.

3 The lung volume at the end of a normal exhalation is called functional residual capacity (FRC). At this volume, the inward elastic recoil of the lung approximates the outward elastic recoil of the chest (including resting diaphragmatic tone).

 4 Closing capacity is normally well below FRC, but it rises steadily with age. This increase is probably responsible for the normal age-related decline in arterial O_2 tension.

5 Whereas both forced expiratory volume in 1 s (FEV_1) and forced vital capacity (FVC) are effort dependent, forced midexpiratory flow ($FEF_{25-75\%}$) is effort independent and may be a more reliable measure of obstruction.

 6 Induction of anesthesia consistently produces an additional 15–20% reduction in FRC (400 mL in most patients) beyond what occurs with the supine position alone.

 7 Local factors are more important than the autonomic system in influencing pulmonary vascular tone. Hypoxia is a powerful stimulus for pulmonary vasoconstriction (the opposite of its systemic effect).

 8 Because alveolar ventilation ($\dot{V}_A$) is normally about 4 L/min and pulmonary capillary perfusion ($\dot{Q}$) is 5 L/min, the overall $\dot{V}/\dot{Q}$ ratio is about 0.8.

 9 Shunting denotes the process whereby desaturated, mixed venous blood from the right heart returns to the left heart without being resaturated with O_2 in the lungs. The overall effect of shunting is to decrease (dilute) arterial O_2 content; this type of shunt is referred to as right-to-left.

 10 General anesthesia commonly increases venous admixture to 5–10%, probably as a result of atelectasis and airway collapse in dependent areas of the lung.

 11 Note that large increases in Pa_{CO_2} (> 75 mm Hg) readily produce hypoxia (Pa_{O_2} < 60 mm Hg) at room air but not at high inspired O_2 concentrations.

 12 The binding of O_2 to hemoglobin appears to be the principal rate-limiting factor in the transfer of O_2 from alveolar gas to blood.

 13 The greater the shunt, the less likely the possibility that an increase in the fraction of inspired oxygen (F_{IO_2}) will prevent hypoxemia.

(continued on next page)

(continued from previous page)

 A rightward shift in the oxygen–hemoglobin dissociation curve lowers O_2 affinity, displaces O_2 from hemoglobin, and makes more O_2 available to tissues; a leftward shift increases hemoglobin's affinity for O_2, reducing its availability to tissues.

 Bicarbonate represents the largest fraction of CO_2 in blood.

 Central chemoreceptors are thought to lie on the anterolateral surface of the medulla and

respond primarily to changes in cerebrospinal fluid $[H^+]$. This mechanism is effective in regulating $Paco_2$, because the blood–brain barrier is permeable to dissolved CO_2 but not to bicarbonate ions.

 With increasing depth of anesthesia, the slope of the $Paco_2$/minute ventilation curve decreases and the apneic threshold increases.

The importance of pulmonary physiology to anesthetic practice is obvious. The most commonly used anesthetics—the inhalation agents—depend on the lungs for uptake and elimination. The most important side effects of both inhalation and intravenously administered anesthetics are primarily respiratory. Moreover, muscle paralysis, unusual positioning during surgery, and techniques such as one-lung anesthesia and cardiopulmonary bypass profoundly alter normal pulmonary physiology.

Much of modern anesthetic practice is based on a thorough understanding of pulmonary physiology and may be considered applied pulmonary physiology. This chapter reviews the basic pulmonary concepts necessary for understanding and applying anesthetic techniques. Although the pulmonary effects of each of the various anesthetic agents are discussed elsewhere in the book, this chapter also reviews the overall effects of general anesthesia on lung function.

CELLULAR RESPIRATION

The principal function of the lungs is to allow gas exchange between blood and inspired air. This need arises as a direct result of cellular aerobic metabolism, which creates a constant demand for uptake of oxygen (O_2) and elimination of carbon dioxide (CO_2).

1. Aerobic Metabolism

Normally, nearly all human cells derive energy aerobically (ie, by using O_2). Carbohydrates, fats, and proteins are metabolized to two-carbon fragments (acetyl-coenzyme A [acetyl-CoA]) that enter the citric acid cycle within mitochondria (see Chapter 34). As the acetyl-CoA is metabolized to CO_2, energy is derived

and stored in nicotine adenine dinucleotide (NAD), flavin adenine dinucleotide (FAD), and guanosine triphosphate (GTP). That energy is subsequently transferred to adenosine triphosphate (ATP) through a process called oxidative phosphorylation. Oxidative phosphorylation accounts for more than 90% of total body O_2 consumption and involves a series of enzyme-mediated (cytochrome) electron transfers that are coupled to ATP formation. In the last step, molecular O_2 is reduced to water.

For glucose, an important cellular fuel, the overall reaction is as follows:

$$C_6H_{12}O_6 + 6\,O_2 \rightarrow 6\,CO_2 + 6\,H_2O + Energy$$

The energy generated (approximately 1200 kJ/mol of glucose) is actually stored in the third phosphate bond on ATP:

$$Energy + ADP + P \rightarrow ATP$$

For every molecule of glucose oxidized, up to a total of 38 molecules of ATP can be produced. Once formed, the energy stored in ATP can be used for ion pumps, muscle contraction, protein synthesis, or cellular secretion; in the process, the adenosine diphosphate (ADP) is regenerated:

$$ATP \rightarrow ADP + P + Energy$$

Cells maintain a ratio of ATP to ADP of 10:1.

Note: ATP cannot be stored but must be continually formed requiring a constant supply of metabolic substrates and O_2.

The ratio of total CO_2 production ($\dot{V}CO_2$) to O_2 consumption ($\dot{V}O_2$) is referred to as the respiratory quotient (RQ) and is generally indicative of the primary type of fuel being utilized. The respiratory quotients for carbohydrates, lipids, and proteins are 1.0, 0.7, and 0.8, respectively. $\dot{V}CO_2$ is normally about 200 mL/min, whereas $\dot{V}O_2$ is approximately 250 mL/min. Because proteins are generally not used as a primary fuel source, the normal respiratory quotient of 0.8 probably reflects utilization of a combination of both fats and carbohydrates. An RQ of > 1 is seen with lipogenesis (overfeeding), and an RQ of 0.7 implies lipolysis (fasting or starvation). Oxygen consumption can also be estimated based on a patient's weight in kilograms (see Chapter 7):

$$\dot{V}O_2 = 10\,(weight)^{3/4}$$

2. Anaerobic Metabolism

Compared with aerobic metabolism, anaerobic metabolism produces a very limited amount of ATP. In the absence of O_2, ATP can be produced only from the conversion of glucose to pyruvate to lactic acid. The anaerobic metabolism of each molecule of glucose yields a net of only two ATP molecules (61 kJ) (compared with 38 ATP molecules formed aerobically). Moreover, the progressive lactic acidosis that develops severely limits the activity of the enzymes involved. When O_2 tension is restored to normal, lactate is reconverted to pyruvate and aerobic metabolism is resumed.

3. Effects of Anesthesia on Cell Metabolism

General anesthesia typically reduces both $\dot{V}O_2$ and $\dot{V}CO_2$ by about 15%. Additional reductions are often seen as a result of hypothermia (see Chapter 21). The greatest reductions are in cerebral and cardiac O_2 consumption.

FUNCTIONAL RESPIRATORY ANATOMY

1. Rib Cage & Muscles of Respiration

The rib cage contains the two lungs, each surrounded by its own pleura. The apex of the chest is small, allowing only for entry of the trachea, esophagus, and blood vessels, whereas the base is formed by the diaphragm. Contraction of the diaphragm—the principal pulmonary muscle—causes the base of the thoracic cavity to descend 1.5–7 cm and its contents (the lungs) to expand. Diaphragmatic movement normally accounts for 75% of the change in chest volume. Accessory pulmonary muscles also increase chest volume (and lung expansion) by their action on the ribs. Each rib (except for the last two) articulates posteriorly with a vertebra and is angulated downward as it attaches anteriorly to the sternum. Upward and outward rib movement expands the chest.

During normal breathing, the diaphragm and, to a lesser extent, the external intercostal muscles are responsible for inspiration; expiration is generally passive. With increasing effort, the sternocleidomastoid, scalene, and pectoralis muscles can be recruited during inspiration. The sternocleidomastoids assist in elevating the rib cage, whereas the scalene muscles prevent inward displacement of the upper ribs during inspiration. The pectoralis muscles can assist chest expansion when the arms are placed on a fixed support. Expiration is normally passive in the supine position but becomes active in the upright position and with increased effort. Exhalation is facilitated by muscles—including the abdominal muscles (rectus abdominis, external and internal oblique, and transversus) and perhaps the internal intercostals—aiding the downward movement of the ribs.

Although not usually considered pulmonary muscles, some pharyngeal muscles are important in maintaining the patency of the airway (see Chapter 5). Tonic and reflex inspiratory activity in the genioglossus keeps the tongue away from the posterior pharyngeal wall. Tonic activity in the levator palati, tensor palati, palatopharyngeus, and palatoglossus prevents the soft palate from falling back against the posterior pharynx, particularly in the supine position.

2. Tracheobronchial Tree

Humidification and filtering of inspired air are functions of the upper airway (nose, mouth, and pharynx). The function of the tracheobronchial tree is to conduct gas flow to and from the alveoli. Dichotomous division (each branch dividing into two smaller branches), starting with the trachea and ending in alveolar sacs, is estimated to involve 23 divisions, or generations (Figure 22–1). With each generation, the number of airways is approximately doubled. Each alveolar sac contains, on average, 17 alveoli. An estimated 300 million alveoli provide an enormous membrane (50–100 m^2) for gas exchange in the average adult.

With each successive division, the mucosal epithelium and supporting structures of the airways gradually change. The mucosa makes a gradual transition from ciliated columnar to cuboidal and finally to flat alveolar epithelium. Gas exchange can occur only across the flat epithelium, which begins to appear on pulmonary bronchioles (generations 17–19). The wall of the airway gradually loses its cartilaginous support (at the bronchioles) and then its smooth muscle. Loss of cartilaginous support causes the patency of smaller airways to become dependent on radial traction by the elastic recoil of the surrounding tissue; as a corollary, airway diameter becomes dependent on total lung volume (see below).

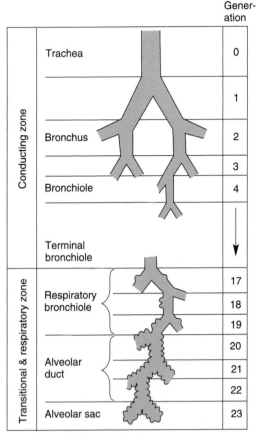

Gener-
ation

Figure 22–1. Dichotomous division of the airways. (Reproduced, with permission, from Guyton AC: *Textbook of Medical Physiology,* 7th ed. W.B. Saunders, 1986.)

Cilia on the columnar and cuboidal epithelium normally beat in a synchronized fashion such that the mucus produced by the secretory glands lining the airway (and any associated bacteria or debris) moves up toward the mouth.

Alveoli

Alveolar size is a function of both gravity and lung volume. The average diameter of an alveolus is thought to be 0.05–0.33 mm. In the upright position, the largest alveoli are at the pulmonary apex, whereas the smallest tend to be at the base. With inspiration, discrepancies in alveolar size diminish.

Each alveolus is in close contact with a network of pulmonary capillaries. The walls of each alveolus are asymmetrically arranged (Figure 22–2). On the thin side, where gas exchange occurs, the alveolar epithelium

and capillary endothelium are separated only by their respective cellular and basement membranes; on the thick side, where fluid and solute exchange occurs, the pulmonary interstitial space separates alveolar epithelium from capillary endothelium. The pulmonary interstitial space contains mainly elastin, collagen, and perhaps nerve fibers. Gas exchange occurs primarily on the thin side of the alveolocapillary membrane, which is less than 0.4 μm thick. The thick side (1–2 μm) provides structural support for the alveolus.

The pulmonary epithelium contains at least two cell types. Type I pneumocytes are flat and form tight (1-nm) junctions with one another. These tight junctions are important in preventing the passage of large oncotically active molecules such as albumin into the alveolus. Type II pneumocytes, which are more numerous than type I pneumocytes (but because of their shape occupy less than 10% of the alveolar space), are round cells that contain prominent cytoplasmic inclusions (lamellar bodies). These inclusions contain surfactant, an important substance necessary for normal pulmonary mechanics (see below). Unlike type I cells, type II pneumocytes are capable of cell division and can produce type I pneumocytes if the latter are destroyed. They are also resistant to O_2 toxicity.

Other cell types present in the lower airways include pulmonary alveolar macrophages, mast cells, lymphocytes, and APUD (amino precursor uptake and decarboxylation) cells. Neutrophils are also typically present in smokers and in patients with acute lung injury.

3. Pulmonary Circulation & Lymphatics

The lungs are supplied by two circulations, pulmonary and bronchial. The bronchial circulation arises from the left heart and sustains the metabolic needs of the tracheobronchial tree down to the level of the pulmonary bronchioles. Below that level, lung tissue is supported by a combination of the alveolar gas and the pulmonary circulation.

The pulmonary circulation normally receives the total output of the right heart via the pulmonary artery, which divides into right and left branches to supply each lung. Deoxygenated blood passes through the pulmonary capillaries, where O_2 is taken up and CO_2 is eliminated. The oxygenated blood is then returned to the left heart by four main pulmonary veins (two from each lung). Although flows through the systemic and pulmonary circulations are equal, the lower pulmonary vascular resistance results in pulmonary vascular pressures one-sixth as great as those in the systemic circulation; as a result, both pulmonary arteries and veins normally have thinner walls with less smooth muscle.

There are connections between the bronchial and the pulmonary circulations. Direct pulmonary arteriovenous communications, bypassing the pulmonary capillaries, are normally insignificant but may become

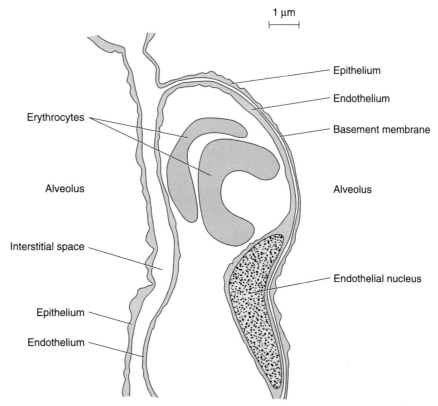

Figure 22–2. The pulmonary interstitial space, with a capillary passing between the two alveoli. The capillary is incorporated into the thin (gas-exchanging) side of the alveolus on the right. The interstitial space is incorporated into the thick side of the alveolus on the left. (Redrawn and reproduced, with permission, from Nunn JF: *Applied Physiology*, 4th ed. Butterworth, 1993.)

important in certain pathological states. The importance of the bronchial circulation in contributing to the normal venous admixture is discussed below.

Pulmonary Capillaries

Pulmonary capillaries are incorporated into the walls of alveoli. The average diameter of these capillaries (about 10 μm) is barely enough to allow passage of a single red cell. Because each capillary network supplies more than one alveolus, blood may pass through several alveoli before reaching the pulmonary veins. Because of the relatively low pressure in the pulmonary circulation, the amount of blood flowing through a given capillary network is affected by both gravity and alveolar size. Large alveoli have a smaller capillary cross-sectional area and consequently increased resistance to blood flow. In the upright position, apical capillaries tend to have reduced flows, whereas basal capillaries have higher flows.

The pulmonary capillary endothelium has relatively large junctions, 5 nm wide, allowing the passage of large molecules such as albumin. As a result, pulmonary interstitial fluid is relatively rich in albumin. Circulating macrophages and neutrophils are able to pass through the endothelium as well as the smaller alveolar epithelial junctions with relative ease. Pulmonary macrophages are commonly seen in the interstitial space and inside alveoli; they serve to prevent bacterial infection and to scavenge foreign particles.

Pulmonary Lymphatics

Lymphatic channels in the lung originate in the interstitial spaces of large septa. Because of the large endothelial junctions, pulmonary lymph has a relatively high protein content, and total pulmonary lymph flow is normally as much as 20 mL/h. Large lymphatic vessels travel upward alongside the airways, forming the tracheobronchial chain of lymph nodes. Lymphatic drainage channels from both lungs communicate along the trachea. Fluid from the left lung drains primarily into the thoracic duct, whereas fluid from the right lung empties into the right lymphatic duct.

4. Innervation

The diaphragm is innervated by the phrenic nerves, which arise from the C3–C5 nerve roots. Unilateral phrenic nerve block or palsy only modestly reduces most indices of pulmonary function (about 25%). Although bilateral phrenic nerve palsies produce more severe impairment, accessory muscle activity may maintain adequate ventilation in some patients. Intercostal muscles are innervated by their respective thoracic nerve roots. Cervical cord injuries above C5 are incompatible with spontaneous ventilation because both phrenic and intercostal nerves are affected.

The vagus nerves provide sensory innervation to the tracheobronchial tree. Both sympathetic and parasympathetic autonomic innervation of bronchial smooth muscle and secretory glands is present. Vagal activity mediates bronchoconstriction and increases bronchial secretions via muscarinic receptors. Sympathetic activity (T1–T4) mediates bronchodilation and also decreases secretions via β_2-receptors. α_1-Adrenergic receptor stimulation decreases secretions but may cause bronchoconstriction. A nonadrenergic, noncholinergic bronchodilator system is also present; vasoactive intestinal peptide is its putative neurotransmitter. The nerve supply of the larynx is reviewed in Chapter 5.

Both α- and β-adrenergic receptors are present in the pulmonary vasculature but the sympathetic system normally has little effect on pulmonary vascular tone. α_1-Activity causes vasoconstriction; β_2-activity mediates vasodilation. Parasympathetic vasodilatory activity appears to be mediated via the release of nitric oxide.

BASIC MECHANISM OF BREATHING

The periodic exchange of alveolar gas with the fresh gas from the upper airway reoxygenates desaturated blood and eliminates CO_2. This exchange is brought about by small cyclic pressure gradients established within the airways. During spontaneous ventilation, these gradients are secondary to variations in intrathoracic pressure; during mechanical ventilation they are produced by intermittent positive pressure in the upper airway.

Spontaneous Ventilation

Normal pressure variations during spontaneous breathing are shown in Figure 22–3. The pressure within alveoli is always greater than the surrounding (intrathoracic) pressure unless the alveoli are collapsed. Alveolar pressure is normally atmospheric (zero for reference) at end-inspiration

and end-expiration. By convention in pulmonary physiology, pleural pressure is used as a measure of intrathoracic pressure. Although it may not be entirely correct to refer to the pressure in a potential space, the concept allows the calculation of transpulmonary pressure. Transpulmonary pressure, or $P_{transpulmonary}$, is then defined as follows:

$$P_{transpulmonary} = P_{alveolar} - P_{intrapleural}$$

At end-expiration, intrapleural pressure normally averages about –5 cm H_2O and because alveolar pressure is 0 (no flow), transpulmonary pressure is +5 cm H_2O.

Diaphragmatic and intercostal muscle activation during inspiration expands the chest and decreases intrapleural pressure from –5 cm H_2O to –8 or 9 cm H_2O. As a result, alveolar pressure also decreases (between –3 and –4 cm H_2O), and an alveolar-upper airway gradient is established; gas flows from the upper airway into alveoli. At end-inspiration (when gas inflow has ceased), alveolar pressure returns to zero, but intrapleural pressure remains decreased; the new transpulmonary pressure (5 cm H_2O) sustains lung expansion.

During expiration, diaphragmatic relaxation returns intrapleural pressure to –5 cm H_2O. Now the transpulmonary pressure does not support the new lung volume, and the elastic recoil of the lung causes a reversal of the previous alveolar–upper airway gradient; gas flows out of alveoli, and original lung volume is restored.

Mechanical Ventilation

Most forms of mechanical ventilation intermittently apply positive airway pressure at the upper airway. During inspiration, gas flows into alveoli until alveolar pressure reaches that in the upper airway. During the expiratory phase of the ventilator, the positive airway pressure is removed or decreased; the gradient reverses, allowing gas flow out of alveoli.

Effects of Anesthesia on Respiratory Pattern

The effects of anesthesia on breathing are complex and relate to both changes in position and anesthetic agents. When a patient is placed supine from an upright or sitting position, the proportion of breathing from rib cage excursion decreases; abdominal breathing predominates. The diaphragm's higher position in the chest (about 4 cm) allows it to contract more effectively than when the patient is upright. Similarly, in the lateral decubitus position, ventilation favors the dependent lung because the dependent hemidiaphragm takes a higher position in the chest (see Chapter 24).

Regardless of the agent used, light anesthesia often results in irregular breathing patterns; breath holding is

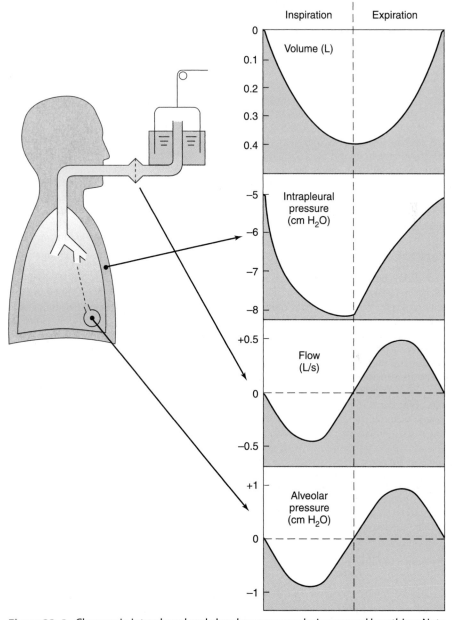

Figure 22–3. Changes in intrapleural and alveolar pressures during normal breathing. Note that at maximal tidal volume, flow is zero and alveolar pressure is atmospheric. (Adapted from West JB: *Respiratory Physiology—The Essentials,* 3rd ed. Williams & Wilkins, 1985.)

common. Breaths become regular with deeper levels of anesthesia. Inhalation agents generally produce rapid, shallow breaths, whereas nitrous–opioid techniques result in slow, deep breaths.

Interestingly, induction of anesthesia often activates expiratory muscles; expiration becomes active. The latter

regularly necessitates paralysis during abdominal surgery. At 1.2 minimum alveolar concentration (MAC), inhalation agents increase respiratory rate and decrease tidal volume (VT). The absolute volumes displaced by both the thorax and diaphragm both decrease under anesthesia, but the ratio remains the same (ie, the thoracic and diaphragmatic contributions to V_T remain the same). At deeper levels of anesthesia, muscle activity is depressed, but if there is any rebreathing of CO_2, muscle activity in all muscle groups is increased.

MECHANICS OF VENTILATION

The movement of the lungs is passive and determined by the impedance of the respiratory system, which can be divided into the elastic resistance of tissues and the gas–liquid interface, and nonelastic resistance to gas flow. The former governs lung volume and the associated pressures under static conditions (no gas flow). The latter relates to frictional resistance to airflow and tissue deformation. The work necessary to overcome elastic resistance is stored as potential energy, but the work necessary to overcome nonelastic resistance is lost as heat.

1. Elastic Resistance

Both the lungs and the chest have elastic properties. The chest has a tendency to expand outward, whereas the lungs have a tendency to collapse. When the chest is exposed to atmospheric pressure (open pneumothorax), it usually expands about 1 L in adults. In contrast, when the lung is exposed to atmospheric pressure, it collapses completely and all the gas within it is expelled. The recoil properties of the chest are due to structural components that resist deformation and probably include chest wall muscle tone. The elastic recoil of the lungs is due to their high content of elastin fibers and, even more important, the surface tension forces acting at the air–fluid interface in alveoli.

Surface Tension Forces

The gas–fluid interface lining the alveoli causes them to behave as bubbles. Surface tension forces tend to reduce the area of the interface and favor alveolar collapse. Laplace's law can be used to quantify these forces:

$$\text{Pressure} = \frac{2 \times \text{Surface tension}}{\text{Radius}}$$

The pressure derived from the equation is that within the alveolus. Alveolar collapse is therefore directly proportional to surface tension but inversely proportional to alveolar size. Collapse is more likely when surface tension increases or alveolar size decreases. **Fortunately, pulmonary surfactant decreases alveolar surface tension.** Moreover, the ability of the surfactant to lower surface tension is directly proportional to its concentration within the alveolus. As alveoli become smaller, the surfactant within becomes more concentrated, and surface tension is more effectively reduced. Conversely, when alveoli are overdistended, surfactant becomes less concentrated, and surface tension increases. The net effect is to stabilize alveoli; small alveoli are prevented from getting smaller, whereas large alveoli are prevented from getting larger.

Compliance

Elastic recoil is usually measured in terms of compliance (C), which is defined as the change in volume divided by the change in distending pressure. Compliance measurements can be obtained for either the chest, the lung, or both together (Figure 22–4). In the supine position, chest wall compliance (CW) is reduced because of the weight of the abdominal contents against the diaphragm. Measurements are usually obtained under static conditions, ie, at equilibrium. (Dynamic lung compliance [Cdyn,L], which is measured during rhythmic breathing, is also dependent on airway resistance.) **Lung compliance (CL)** is defined as

$$C_L = \frac{\text{Change in lung volume}}{\text{Change in transpulmonary pressure}}$$

CL is normally 150–200 mL/cm H_2O. A variety of factors, including lung volume, pulmonary blood volume, extravascular lung water, and pathological processes such as inflammation and fibrosis (see Chapter 23), affect CL.

$$\frac{\text{Chest wall}}{\text{compliance (CW)}} = \frac{\text{Change in chest volume}}{\text{Change in transthoracic pressure}}$$

where transthoracic pressure equals atmospheric pressure minus intrapleural pressure.

Normal chest wall compliance is 200 mL/cm H_2O. Total compliance (lung and chest wall together) is 100 mL/cm H_2O and is expressed by the following equation:

$$\frac{1}{C_{total}} = \frac{1}{CW} + \frac{1}{CL}$$

2. Lung Volumes

Lung volumes are important parameters in respiratory physiology and clinical practice (Table 22–1 and Figure 22–5). The sum of all the named lung volumes equals the maximum to which the lung can be inflated. Lung capacities are clinically useful measurements that represent a combination of two or more volumes.

Functional Residual Capacity

The lung volume at the end of a normal exhalation is called functional residual capacity (FRC). At this volume, the inward elastic recoil of the lung approximates the outward elastic recoil of the chest (including resting diaphragmatic tone). Thus, the elastic properties of both chest and lung define the point from which normal breathing takes place. Functional residual capacity can be measured by nitrogen wash-out or helium

Figure 22–4. The pressure–volume relationship for the chest wall, lung, and both together in the upright (**A**) and supine (**B**) positions. (Modified and reproduced, with permission, from Scurr C, Feldman S: *Scientific Foundations of Anesthesia.* Heinemann, 1982.)

wash-in technique or by body plethysmography. Factors known to alter the FRC include the following:

- **Body habitus:** FRC is directly proportional to height. Obesity, however, can markedly decrease FRC (primarily as a result of reduced chest compliance).

- **Sex:** FRC is reduced by about 10% in females compared with males.
- **Posture:** FRC decreases as a patient is moved from an upright to a supine or prone position. This is the result of reduced chest compliance as the abdominal

Table 22–1. Lung volumes and capacities.

Measurement	Definition	Average Adult Values (mL)
Tidal volume (V_T)	Each normal breath	500
Inspiratory reserve volume (IRV)	Maximal additional volume that can be inspired above V_T	3000
Expiratory reserve volume (ERV)	Maximal volume that can be expired below V_T	1100
Residual volume (RV)	Volume remaining after maximal exhalation	1200
Total lung capacity (TLC)	RV + ERV + V_T + IRV	5800
Functional residual capacity (FRC)	RV + ERV	2300

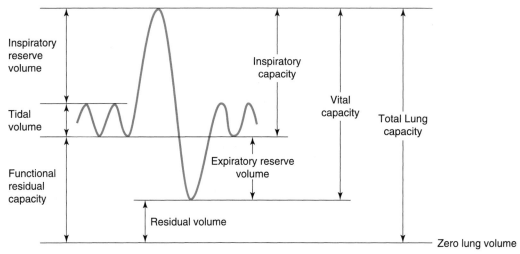

Figure 22–5. Spirogram showing static lung volumes. (Reproduced, with permission, from Nunn JF: *Applied Respiratory Physiology,* 5th ed. Lumb A [editor]. Butterworth-Heinemann, 2000.)

contents push up against the diaphragm. The greatest change occurs between 0 and 60° of inclination. No further decrease is observed with a head-down position of up to 30°.

- **Lung disease:** Decreased compliance of the lung, chest, or both is characteristic of restrictive pulmonary disorders (see Chapter 23), all of which are necessarily associated with a low FRC.
- **Diaphragmatic tone:** This normally contributes to FRC.

Closing Capacity

As described above (see the section on Functional Respiratory Anatomy), small airways lacking cartilaginous support depend on radial traction caused by the elastic recoil of surrounding tissue to keep them open; patency of these airways, particularly in basal areas of the lung, is highly dependent on lung volume. The volume at which these airways begin to close in dependent parts of the lung is called the **closing capacity.** At lower lung volumes, alveoli in dependent areas continue to be perfused but are no longer ventilated; **intrapulmonary shunting** of deoxygenated blood promotes hypoxemia (see below).

Closing capacity is usually measured using a tracer gas (xenon-133), which is inhaled near residual volume and then exhaled from total lung capacity.

Closing capacity is normally well below FRC (Figure 22–6), but it rises steadily with age (Figure 22–7). This increase is probably responsible for the normal age-related decline in arterial O_2 tension. At an average age of 44 years, closing capacity equals FRC in the supine position; by age 66, closing capacity equals or

exceeds FRC in the upright position in most individuals. Unlike FRC, closing capacity is unaffected by posture.

Vital Capacity

Vital capacity (VC) is the maximum volume of gas that can be exhaled following maximal inspiration. In addition to body habitus, VC is also dependent on respiratory muscle strength and chest–lung compliance. Normal VC is about 60–70 mL/kg.

3. Nonelastic Resistances

Airway Resistance to Gas Flow

Gas flow in the lung is a mixture of laminar and turbulent flow. Laminar flow can be thought of as consisting of concentric cylinders of gas flowing at different velocities; velocity is highest in the center and decreases toward the periphery. During laminar flow,

$$\text{Flow} = \frac{\text{Pressure gradient}}{\text{Raw}}$$

where Raw is airway resistance.

$$\text{Raw} = \frac{8 \times \text{Length} \times \text{Gas viscosity}}{\pi \times (\text{Radius})^4}$$

Turbulent flow is characterized by random movement of the gas molecules down the air passages. Mathematical description of turbulent flow is considerably more complex:

$$\text{Pressure gradient} \approx \text{Flow}^2 \times \frac{\text{Gas density}}{\text{Radius}^5}$$

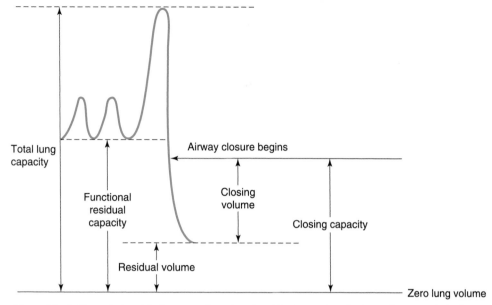

Figure 22–6. The relationship between functional residual capacity, closing volume, and closing capacity. (Reproduced, with permission, from Nunn JF: *Applied Respiratory Physiology,* 5th ed. Lumb A [editor]. Butterworth-Heinemann, 2000.)

Resistance is not constant but increases in proportion to gas flow. Moreover, resistance is directly proportional to gas density and inversely proportional to the fifth power of the radius. As a result, turbulent gas flow is extremely sensitive to airway caliber.

Turbulence generally occurs at high gas flows, at sharp angles or branching points, and in response to abrupt changes in airway diameter. Whether turbu-lent or laminar flow occurs can be predicted by the Reynolds number, which is arrived at by the following equation.

$$\text{Reynolds number} = \frac{\text{Linear velocity} \times \text{Diameter} \times \text{Gas density}}{\text{Gas viscosity}}$$

Figure 22–7. The effect of age on closing capacity and its relationship to functional residual capacity (FRC). Note that FRC does not change. (Reproduced, with permission, from Nunn JF: *Applied Respiratory Physiology,* 5th ed. Lumb A [editor]. Butterworth-Heinemann, 2000.)

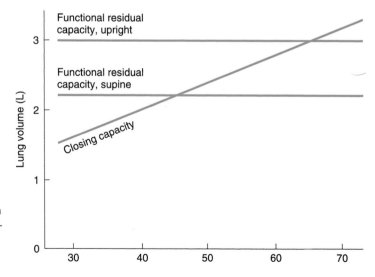

Table 22–2. Physical properties of several gas mixtures.[1]

Mixture	Viscosity[2]	Density[2]	Density/Viscosity[2]
Oxygen (100%)	1.11	1.11	1.00
N_2O/O_2	0.89	1.41	1.49
Helium/O_2 (80:20)	1.08	0.33	0.31

[1]Reproduced, with permission, from Nunn JF: *Applied Respiratory Physiology*, 5th ed. Lumb A (editor). Butterworth-Heineman, 2000.
[2]Viscosities and densities are expressed relative to air.

A low Reynolds number (< 1000) is associated with laminar flow, whereas a high value (> 1500) produces turbulent flow. Laminar flow normally occurs only distal to small bronchioles (< 1 mm). Flow in larger airways is probably turbulent. Of the gases used clinically, only helium has a significantly lower density-to-viscosity ratio, making it useful clinically during severe turbulent flow (as caused by upper airway obstruction). A helium–O_2 mixture not only is less likely to cause turbulent flow but also reduces airway resistance when turbulent flow is present (Table 22–2).

Normal total airway resistance is about 0.5–2 cm $H_2O/L/s$, with the largest contribution coming from medium-sized bronchi (before the seventh generation). Resistance in large bronchi is low because of their large diameters, whereas resistance in small bronchi is low because of their large total cross-sectional area. The most important causes of increased airway resistance include bronchospasm, secretions, and mucosal edema (see Chapter 23), as well as volume-related and flow-related airway collapse.

A. VOLUME-RELATED AIRWAY COLLAPSE

At low lung volumes, loss of radial traction increases the contribution of small airways to total resistance;

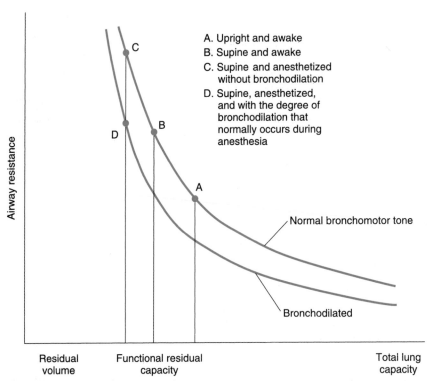

A. Upright and awake
B. Supine and awake
C. Supine and anesthetized without bronchodilation
D. Supine, anesthetized, and with the degree of bronchodilation that normally occurs during anesthesia

Normal bronchomotor tone

Bronchodilated

Residual volume

Functional residual capacity

Total lung capacity

Figure 22–8. The relationship between airway resistance and lung volume. (Modified and reproduced, with permission, from Nunn JF: *Applied Respiratory Physiology*, 5th ed. Lumb A [editor]. Butterworth-Heinemann, 2000.)

airway resistance becomes inversely proportional to lung volume (Figure 22–8). Increasing lung volume up to normal with positive end-expiratory pressure (PEEP) can reduce airway resistance.

B. FLOW-RELATED AIRWAY COLLAPSE

During forced exhalation, reversal of the normal transmural airway pressure can cause collapse of these airways (dynamic airway compression). Two contributing factors are responsible: generation of a positive pleural

pressure and a large pressure drop across intrathoracic airways as a result of increased airway resistance. The latter is in turn due to high (turbulent) gas flow and the reduced lung volume. The terminal portion of the flow/volume curve is therefore termed effort independent (Figure 22–9).

The point along the airways where dynamic compression occurs is called the equal pressure point. It is normally beyond the eleventh to thirteenth generation of bronchioles where cartilaginous support is absent

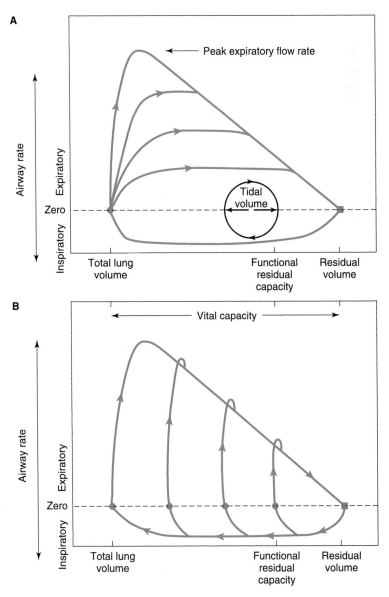

Figure 22–9. Gas flow (**A**) during forced exhalation from total lung capacity with varying effort and (**B**) with maximal effort from different lung volumes. Note that regardless of initial lung volume or effort, terminal expiratory flows are effort independent. (Reproduced, with permission, from Nunn JF: *Applied Respiratory Physiology,* 5th ed. Lumb A [editor]. Butterworth-Heinemann, 2000.)

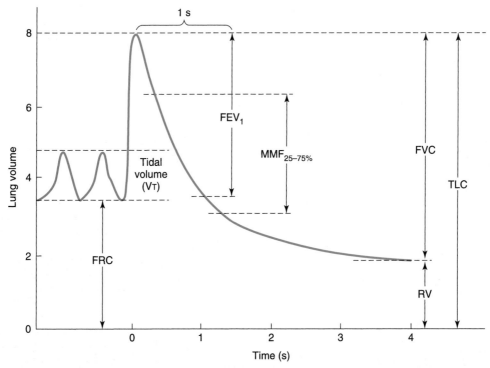

Figure 22–10. The normal forced exhalation curve. FEF$_{25-75\%}$ is also called the maximum midexpiratory flow rate (MMF$_{25-75\%}$). FRC, functional residual capacity; FEV$_1$, forced expiratory volume in 1 s; FVC, forced vital capacity; RV, residual volume; TLC, total lung capacity.

(see above). The equal pressure point moves toward smaller airways as lung volume decreases. Emphysema or asthma predisposes patients to dynamic airway compression. Emphysema destroys the elastic tissues that normally support smaller airways. In patients with asthma, bronchoconstriction and mucosal edema intensify airway collapse and promote reversal of transmural pressure gradients across airways. Patients may terminate exhalation prematurely or purse their lips to increase expiratory resistance at the mouth; both maneuvers help prevent reversal of transmural pressure gradients and lessen the trapping of air. Premature termination of exhalation also increases FRC above normal (auto-PEEP).

C. FORCED VITAL CAPACITY

Measuring vital capacity as an exhalation that is as hard and as rapid as possible (Figure 22–10) provides important information about airway resistance. The ratio of the forced expiratory volume in 1 s (FEV$_1$) to the total forced vital capacity (FVC) is proportional to the degree of airway obstruction. Normally, FEV$_1$/FVC is $\geq$ 80%. Whereas both FEV$_1$ and FVC are effort dependent, forced midexpiratory flow

(FEF$_{25-75\%}$) is effort independent and may be a more reliable measurement of obstruction.

Tissue Resistance

This component of nonelastic resistance is generally underestimated and often overlooked, but may account for up to half of total airway resistance. It appears to be primarily due to viscoelastic (frictional) resistance of tissues to gas flow.

4. Work of Breathing

Because expiration is normally entirely passive, both the inspiratory and the expiratory work of breathing is performed by the inspiratory muscles (primarily the diaphragm). Three factors must be overcome during ventilation: the elastic recoil of the chest and lung, frictional resistance to gas flow in the airways, and tissue frictional resistance.

Respiratory work can be expressed as the product of volume and pressure (Figure 22–11). During inhalation, both inspiratory airway resistance and pulmonary elastic recoil must be overcome; nearly 50% of the

Figure 22–11. The work of breathing and its components during inspiration. (Reproduced, with permission, from Guyton AC: *Textbook of Medical Physiology,* 7th ed. W.B. Saunders, 1986.)

energy expended is stored pulmonary elastic recoil. During exhalation, the stored potential energy is released and overcomes expiratory airway resistance. Increases in either inspiratory or expiratory resistance are compensated by increased inspiratory muscle effort. When expiratory resistance increases, the normal compensatory response is to increase lung volume such that V_T breathing occurs at an abnormally high FRC. The greater elastic recoil energy stored at a higher lung volume overcomes the added expiratory resistance. Excessive amounts of expiratory resistance also activate expiratory muscles (see above).

Respiratory muscles normally account for only 2–3% of O_2 consumption but operate at about 10% efficiency. Ninety percent of the work is dissipated as heat (due to elastic and airflow resistance). In pathological conditions that increase the load on the diaphragm, muscle efficiency usually progressively decreases and contraction may become uncoordinated with increasing ventilatory effort; moreover, a point is reached whereby any increase in O_2 uptake (because of augmented ventilation) is consumed by the pulmonary muscles themselves.

The work required to overcome elastic resistance increases as V_T increases, whereas the work required to overcome airflow resistance increases as respiratory rate (and, necessarily, expiratory flow) increases. Faced with either condition, patients minimize the work of breathing by altering respiratory rate and V_T (Figure 22–12). Patients with reduced compliance tend to have rapid, shallow breaths, whereas those with increased airflow resistance have a slow, deep breathing pattern.

5. Effects of Anesthesia on Pulmonary Mechanics

Effects on Lung Volumes & Compliance

Induction of anesthesia consistently produces an additional 15–20% reduction in FRC (400 mL in most patients) beyond what occurs with the supine position alone. This decrease in FRC has commonly been thought to be due to a cephalad shift of the diaphragm secondary to loss of muscle tone. We now know that the mechanisms are far more complex; only the dependent (dorsal) part of the diaphragm in the supine position moves cephalad. Other factors are likely due to a change in intrathoracic volume secondary to increased blood volume in the lung and changes in chest wall shape (Figure 22–13). The higher position of the dorsal diaphragm and changes in the thoracic cavity itself decrease lung volume. This decrease in FRC is not related to anesthetic depth and may persist for several hours after anesthesia. Steep head-down (Trendelenburg) position (> 30°) may reduce FRC even further as intrathoracic blood volume increases. In contrast, induction of anesthesia in the sitting position appears to have little effect on FRC. Muscle paralysis does not appear to change FRC significantly when the patient is already anesthetized.

The effects of anesthesia on closing capacity are more variable. Both FRC and closing capacity, however, are generally reduced to the same extent under anesthesia. Thus, the risk of increased intrapulmonary shunting under anesthesia is similar to that in the conscious state; it is greatest in the elderly, in obese patients, and in those with underlying pulmonary disease.

Effects on Airway Resistance

The reduction in FRC associated with general anesthesia would be expected to increase airway resistance. Increases in resistance are not usually observed, however, because of the bronchodilating properties of the volatile inhalation anesthetics. Increased airway resistance is more commonly due to pathological factors (posterior displacement of the tongue; laryngospasm; bronchoconstriction; or secretions, blood, or tumor in the airway) or equipment problems (small tracheal tubes or connectors, malfunction of valves, or obstruction of the breathing circuit).

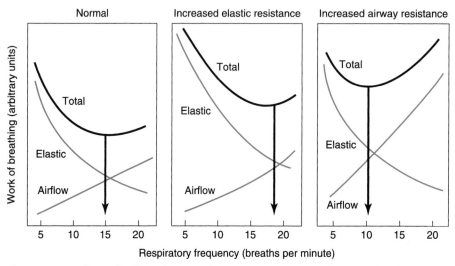

Figure 22–12. The work of breathing in relation to respiratory rate for normal individuals, patients with increased elastic resistance, and patients with increased airway resistance. (Reproduced, with permission, from Nunn JF: *Applied Respiratory Physiology,* 5th ed. Lumb A [editor]. Butterworth-Heinemann, 2000.)

Effects on the Work of Breathing

Increases in the work of breathing under anesthesia are most often secondary to reduced lung and chest wall compliance and, less commonly, increases in airway resistance (see above). The problems of increased work of breathing are usually circumvented by controlled mechanical ventilation.

VENTILATION/PERFUSION RELATIONSHIPS

1. Ventilation

Ventilation is usually measured as the sum of all exhaled gas volumes in 1 min (minute ventilation, or $\dot{V}$). If V_T is constant,

Minute ventilation = Respiratory rate × Tidal volume

For the average adult at rest, minute ventilation is about 5 L/min.

Not all the inspired gas mixture reaches alveoli; some of it remains in the airways and is exhaled without being exchanged with alveolar gases. That part of the V_T not participating in alveolar gas exchange is known as dead space (V_D). Alveolar ventilation ($\dot{V}_A$) is the volume of inspired gases actually taking part in gas exchange in 1 min.

$$\dot{V}_A = \text{Respiratory rate} \times V_T - V_D$$

Dead space is actually composed of gases in nonrespiratory airways (anatomic dead space) as well as in alveoli that are not perfused (alveolar dead space). The sum of the two is referred to as physiological dead space. In the upright position, dead space is normally about 150 mL for most adults (approximately 2 mL/kg) and is nearly all anatomic. The weight of an individual in pounds is roughly equivalent to dead space in milliliters. Dead space can be affected by a variety of factors (Table 22–3).

Because V_T in the average adult is approximately 450 mL (6 mL/kg), V_D/V_T is normally 33%. This ratio can be derived by the Bohr equation:

$$\frac{V_D}{V_T} = \frac{P_{ACO_2} - P_{ECO_2}}{P_{ACO_2}}$$

where P_{ACO_2} is the alveolar CO_2 tension and P_{ECO_2} is the mixed expired CO_2 tension. This equation is useful clinically if arterial CO_2 tension (P_{aCO_2}) is used to approximate the alveolar concentration and the CO_2 tension in expired air gases is the average measured over several minutes.

Distribution of Ventilation

Regardless of body position, alveolar ventilation is unevenly distributed in the lungs. The right lung receives more ventilation than the left one (53% versus 47%), and lower (dependent) areas of both lungs tend to be better ventilated than do the upper areas because of a gravitationally induced gradient in intrapleural

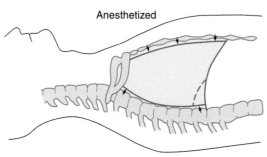

Figure 22–13. With induction of anesthesia in the supine position, the abdominal contents exert cephalad pressure on the diaphragm. At end-expiration, the dorsal portion of the diaphragm is more cephalad and the ventral portion is more caudal than when awake, the thoracic spine is more lordotic, and the rib cage moves inward, all secondary to loss of motor tone.

pressure (and necessarily transpulmonary pressure). Pleural pressure decreases about 1 cm H_2O (becomes less negative) per 3 cm decrease in lung height. This difference places alveoli from different areas at different points on the pulmonary compliance curve (Figure 22–14). Because of a higher transpulmonary pressure, alveoli in upper lung areas are near-maximally inflated and relatively noncompliant, and they undergo little more expansion during inspiration. In contrast, the smaller alveoli in dependent areas have a lower transpulmonary pressure, are more compliant, and undergo greater expansion during inspiration.

Airway resistance can also contribute to regional differences in pulmonary ventilation. Final alveolar inspiratory volume is solely dependent on compliance only if inspiratory time is unlimited. In reality, inspiratory time is necessarily limited by the respiratory rate and the time necessary for expiration; consequently, an excessively short inspiratory time will prevent alveoli from reaching the expected change in volume. Moreover, alveolar filling follows an exponential function that is dependent on both compliance and airway resis-

tance. Therefore, even with a normal inspiratory time, abnormalities in either compliance or resistance can prevent complete alveolar filling.

Time Constants

Lung inflation can be described mathematically by the time constant, τ.

$$\tau = \text{Total compliance} \times \text{Airway resistance}$$

Regional variations in resistance or compliance not only interfere with alveolar filling but can cause asynchrony in alveolar filling during inspiration; some alveolar units may continue to fill as others empty.

Variations in time constants within the normal lung can be demonstrated in normal individuals breathing spontaneously during abnormally high respiratory rates. Rapid shallow breathing reverses the normal distribution of ventilation, preferentially favoring upper (nondependent) areas of the lung over the lower areas.

2. Pulmonary Perfusion

Of the approximately 5 L/min of blood flowing through the lungs, only about 70–100 mL at any one time is within the pulmonary capillaries undergoing gas exchange. At the alveolar–capillary membrane, this small volume forms a 50–100 m^2 sheet of blood approximately one red cell thick. Moreover, to ensure optimal gas exchange, each capillary perfuses more than one alveolus.

Table 22–3. Factors affecting dead space.

Factor	Effect
Posture	
Upright	↑
Supine	↓
Position of airway	
Neck extension	↑
Neck flexion	↓
Age	↑
Artificial airway	↓
Positive-pressure ventilation	↑
Drugs—anticholinergic	↑
Pulmonary perfusion	
Pulmonary emboli	↑
Hypotension	↑
Pulmonary vascular disease	
Emphysema	↑

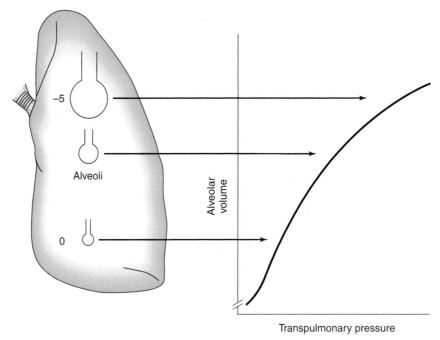

Figure 22-14. The effect of gravity on alveolar compliance in the upright position.

Although capillary volume remains relatively constant, total pulmonary blood volume can vary between 500 mL and 1000 mL. Large increases in either cardiac output or blood volume are tolerated with little change in pressure as a result of passive dilation of open vessels and perhaps some recruitment of collapsed pulmonary vessels. Small increases in pulmonary blood volume normally occur during cardiac systole and with each normal (spontaneous) inspiration. A shift in posture from supine to erect decreases pulmonary blood volume (up to 27%); Trendelenburg positioning has the opposite effect. Changes in systemic capacitance also influence pulmonary blood volume: systemic venoconstriction shifts blood from the systemic to the pulmonary circulation, whereas vasodilation causes a pulmonary-to-systemic redistribution. In this way, the lung acts as a reservoir for the systemic circulation.

Local factors are more important than the autonomic system in influencing pulmonary vascular tone (above). Hypoxia is a powerful stimulus for pulmonary vasoconstriction (the opposite of its systemic effect). Both pulmonary arterial (mixed venous) and alveolar hypoxia induce vasoconstriction, but the latter is a more powerful stimulus. This response appears to be due to either the direct effect of hypoxia on the pulmonary vasculature or increased production of leukotrienes relative to vasodilatory prostaglandins. Inhibition of nitric oxide production may also play a role. Hypoxic pulmonary vasoconstriction is an important physiological mechanism in reducing intrapulmonary shunting and preventing hypoxemia (see below). Hyperoxia has little effect on the pulmonary circulation in normal individuals. Hypercapnia and acidosis have a constrictor effect, whereas hypocapnia causes pulmonary vasodilation, the opposite of what occurs in the systemic circulation.

Distribution of Pulmonary Perfusion

Pulmonary blood flow is also not uniform. Regardless of body position, lower (dependent) portions of the lung receive greater blood flow than upper (nondependent) areas. This pattern is the result of a gravitational gradient of 1 cm H_2O/cm lung height. The normally low pressures in the pulmonary circulation (see Chapter 19) allow gravity to exert a significant influence on blood flow.

For simplification, each lung can be divided into three zones, based on alveolar (PA), arterial (Pa), and venous (Pv) pressures (Figure 22–15). Zone 1 is the upper zone and represents alveolar dead space because alveolar pressure continually occludes the pulmonary capillaries. In the middle zone (zone 2), pulmonary capillary flow is intermittent and varies during respiration according to the arterial–alveolar pressure gradient. Pulmonary capillary flow is continuous in zone 3 and is proportional to the arterial–venous pressure gradient.

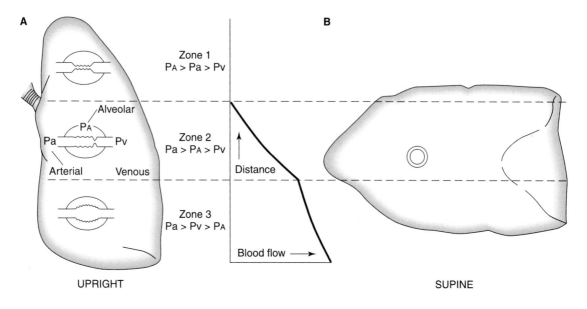

Figure 22–15. The three-zone model of the lung. *A:* Upright position. *B:* Supine position.

Ventilation/Perfusion Ratios

Because alveolar ventilation ($\dot{V}A$) is normally about 4 L/min and pulmonary capillary perfusion ($\dot{Q}$) is 5 L/min, the overall $\dot{V}/\dot{Q}$ ratio is about 0.8. $\dot{V}/\dot{Q}$ for individual lung units (each alveolus and its capillary) can range from 0 (no ventilation) to infinity (no perfusion); the former is referred to as intrapulmonary shunt, whereas the latter constitutes alveolar dead space. $\dot{V}/\dot{Q}$ normally ranges between 0.3 and 3.0; the majority of lung areas are close to 1.0 (Figure 22–16A). Because perfusion increases at a greater rate than ventilation, nondependent (apical) areas tend to have higher $\dot{V}/\dot{Q}$ ratios than do dependent (basal) areas (Figure 22–16B).

The importance of $\dot{V}/\dot{Q}$ ratios relates to the efficiency with which lung units resaturate venous blood with O_2 and eliminate CO_2. **Pulmonary venous blood (the effluent) from areas with low $\dot{V}/\dot{Q}$ ratios has a low O_2 tension and high CO_2 tension—similar to systemic mixed venous blood.** Blood from these units tends to depress arterial O_2 tension and elevate arterial CO_2 tension. Their effect on arterial O_2 tension is much more profound than that on CO_2 tension; in fact, arterial CO_2 tension often decreases from a hypoxemia-induced reflex increase in alveolar ventilation. An appreciable compensatory increase in O_2 uptake cannot take place in remaining areas where $\dot{V}/\dot{Q}$ is normal, because pulmonary end-capillary blood is usually already maximally saturated with O_2 (see below).

3. Shunts

Shunting denotes the process whereby desaturated, mixed venous blood from the right heart returns to the left heart without being resaturated with O_2 in the lungs (Figure 22–17). The overall effect of shunting is to decrease (dilute) arterial O_2 content; this type of shunt is referred to as right-to-left. Left-to-right shunts (in the absence of pulmonary congestion), however, do not produce hypoxemia.

Intrapulmonary shunts are often classified as absolute or relative. Absolute shunt refers to anatomic shunts and lung units where $\dot{V}/\dot{Q}$ is zero. A relative shunt is an area of the lung with a low but finite $\dot{V}/\dot{Q}$ ratio. Clinically, hypoxemia from a relative shunt can usually be partially corrected by increasing the inspired O_2 concentration; hypoxemia caused by an absolute shunt cannot.

Venous Admixture

Venous admixture refers to a concept rather than an actual physiological entity. **Venous admixture** is the amount of mixed venous blood that would have to be mixed with pulmonary end-capillary blood to account for the difference in O_2 tension between arterial and pulmonary end-capillary blood. Pulmonary end-capillary blood is considered to have the same concentrations as alveolar gas. Venous admixture ($\dot{Q}S$) is usually expressed as a fraction of total cardiac output ($\dot{Q}T$). The equation

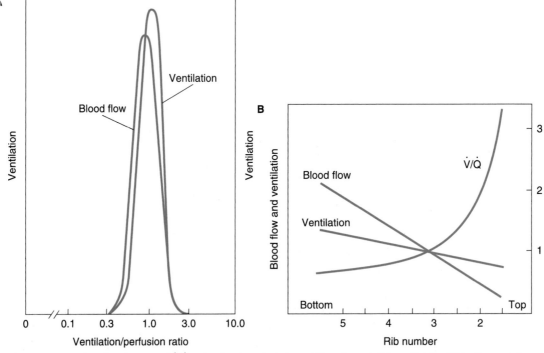

Figure 22–16. The distribution of V̇/Q̇ ratios for the whole lung (**A**) and according to height (**B**) in the upright position. Note that blood flow increases more rapidly than ventilation in dependent areas. (Reproduced, with permission, from West JB: *Ventilation/Blood Flow and Gas Exchange,* 3rd ed. Blackwell, 1977.)

for $\dot{Q}s/\dot{Q}T$ may be derived with the law for the conservation of mass for O_2 across the pulmonary bed:

$$\dot{Q}T \times Ca_{O_2} = (\dot{Q}s \times C\bar{v}_{O_2}) + (\dot{Q}c' \times Cc'_{O_2})$$

where

$\dot{Q}c'$ = Blood flow across normally ventilated pulmonary capillaries

$\dot{Q}T = \dot{Q}c' + \dot{Q}s$

Cc'_{O_2} = oxygen content of ideal pulmonary end-capillary blood

Ca_{O_2} = arterial oxygen content

$C\bar{v}_{O_2}$ = mixed venous content

The simplified equation is

$$\dot{Q}s/\dot{Q}T = \frac{Cc'_{O_2} - Ca_{O_2}}{Cc'_{O_2} - C\bar{v}_{O_2}}$$

The formula for calculating the O_2 content of blood is given below.

$\dot{Q}s/\dot{Q}T$ can be calculated clinically by obtaining mixed venous and arterial blood gas measurements;

the former requires a pulmonary artery catheter. The alveolar gas equation is used to derive pulmonary end-capillary O_2 tension. Pulmonary capillary blood is usually assumed to be 100% saturated for an $FIO_2 \geq 0.21$.

The calculated venous admixture assumes that all shunting is intrapulmonary and is due to absolute shunts (V̇/Q̇ = 0). In reality, neither is ever the case; nonetheless, the concept is useful clinically. Normal $\dot{Q}s/\dot{Q}T$ is primarily due to communication between deep bronchial veins and pulmonary veins, the thebesian circulation in the heart, and areas of low but finite V̇/Q̇ in the lungs (Figure 22–18). The venous admixture in normal individuals (physiologic shunt) is typically less than 5%.

4. Effects of Anesthesia on Gas Exchange

Abnormalities in gas exchange during anesthesia are common. They include increased dead space, hypoventilation, and increased intrapulmonary shunting. There is increased scatter of V̇/Q̇ ratios. Increases in alveolar dead space are most commonly seen during controlled ventilation, but may also occur during spontaneous ventilation. General anesthesia commonly increases venous admixture to 5–10%, probably as a result of atelectasis and airway collapse in dependent areas of the

Figure 22–17. A three-compartment model of gas exchange in the lungs, showing dead space ventilation, normal alveolar–capillary exchange, and shunting (venous admixture). (Modified and reproduced, with permission, from Nunn JF: *Applied Respiratory Physiology*, 5th ed. Lumb A [editor]. Butterworth-Heinemann, 2000.)

lung. Inhalation agents, including nitrous oxide, also can inhibit **hypoxic pulmonary vasoconstriction** in high doses; for volatile agents, the ED_{50} is about 2 MAC. Elderly patients appear to have the largest increases in $\dot{Q}s/\dot{Q}T$. Inspired O_2 tensions of 30–40% usually prevent hypoxemia suggesting anesthesia increases relative shunt. PEEP is often effective in reducing venous admixture and preventing hypoxemia during general anesthesia as long as cardiac output is maintained (see Chapter 49). Prolonged administration of high inspired O_2 concentrations (> 50%) may be associated with increases in absolute shunt. In these instances, complete collapse of alveoli with previously low $\dot{V}/\dot{Q}$ ratios is thought to occur once all the O_2 within is absorbed (absorption atelectasis).

ALVEOLAR, ARTERIAL, & VENOUS GAS TENSIONS

When dealing with gas mixtures, each gas is considered to contribute separately to total gas pressure, and its partial pressure is directly proportional to its concentration. Air has an O_2 concentration of approximately 21%; therefore, if the barometric pressure is 760 mm Hg (sea level), the partial pressure of oxygen (PO_2) in air is normally 159.6 mm Hg:

$$760 \text{ mm Hg} \times 0.21 = 159.6 \text{ mm Hg}$$

In its general form, the equation may be written as follows:

$$PIO_2 = PB \times FIO_2$$

where PB = barometric pressure and FIO_2 = the fraction of inspired oxygen.

Two general rules can also be used:

- Partial pressure in millimeters of mercury approximates the percentage × 7.
- Partial pressure in kilopascals is approximately the same as the percentage.

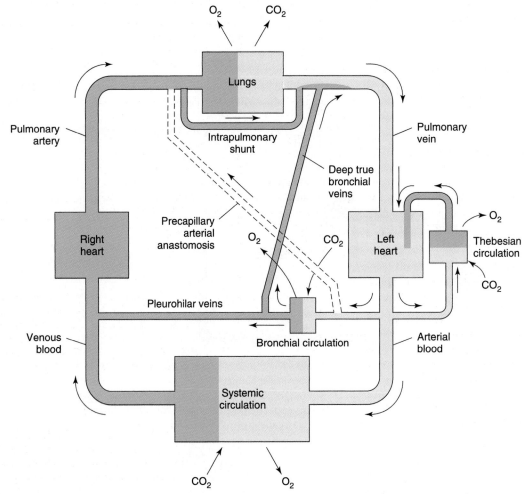

Figure 22–18. Components of the normal venous admixture. (Reproduced, with permission, from Nunn JF: *Applied Respiratory Physiology,* 5th ed. Lumb A [editor]. Butterworth-Heinemann, 2000.)

1. Oxygen

Alveolar Oxygen Tension

With every breath, the inspired gas mixture is humidified at 37°C in the upper airway. The inspired tension of oxygen (PIO_2) is therefore reduced by the added water vapor. Water vapor pressure is dependent only on temperature, being 47 mm Hg at 37°C. In humidified air, the normal partial pressure of O_2 at sea level is 149.7 mm Hg:

$$(760 - 47) \times 0.21 = 149.7 \text{ mm Hg}$$

The general equation is

$$PIO_2 = (PB - PH_2O) \times FIO_2$$

where PH_2O = the vapor pressure of water at body temperature.

In alveoli, the inspired gases are mixed with residual alveolar gas from previous breaths, O_2 is taken up, and CO_2 is added. The final alveolar oxygen tension (PAO_2) is therefore dependent on all these factors and can be estimated by the following equation:

$$PAO_2 = PIO_2 - \frac{PaCO_2}{RQ}$$

where $PaCO_2$ = arterial CO_2 tension and RQ = respiratory quotient.

RQ is usually not measured. Note that large increases in $PaCO_2$ (> 75 mm Hg) readily produce hypoxia (PaO_2 < 60 mm Hg) at room air but not at high inspired O_2 concentrations.

A yet simpler method of approximating PAO_2 in millimeters of mercury is to multiply the percentage of inspired O_2 concentration by 6. Thus, at 40%, PAO_2 is 6×40, or 240 mm Hg.

Pulmonary End-Capillary Oxygen Tension

For all practical purposes, pulmonary end-capillary oxygen tension ($Pc'O_2$) may be considered identical to PAO_2; the PAO_2–$Pc'O_2$ gradient is normally minute. $Pc'O_2$ is dependent on the rate of O_2 diffusion across the alveolar–capillary membrane as well as on pulmonary capillary blood volume and transit time. The large capillary surface area in alveoli and the 0.4–0.5 μm thickness of the alveolar–capillary membrane greatly facilitate O_2 diffusion. Enhanced O_2 binding to hemoglobin at saturations above 80% also augments O_2 diffusion (see below). Capillary transit time can be estimated by dividing pulmonary capillary blood volume by cardiac output (pulmonary blood flow); thus, normal capillary transit time is 70 mL ÷ 5000 mL/min (0.8 s). Maximum $Pc'O_2$ is usually attained after only 0.3 s, providing a large safety margin.

The binding of O_2 to hemoglobin appears to be the principal rate-limiting factor in the transfer of O_2 from alveolar gas to blood. Therefore, pulmonary diffusing capacity reflects not only the capacity and permeability of the alveolar–capillary membrane but also pulmonary blood flow. Moreover, O_2 uptake is normally limited by pulmonary blood flow, not O_2 diffusion across the alveolar–capillary membrane; the latter may become significant during exercise in normal individuals at high altitudes and in patients with extensive destruction of the alveolar–capillary membrane.

O_2 transfer across the alveolar–capillary membrane is expressed as oxygen diffusing capacity (DLO_2):

$$DLO_2 = \frac{\text{Oxygen uptake}}{PAO_2 - Pc'O_2}$$

Because $Pc'O_2$ cannot be measured accurately, measurement of carbon monoxide diffusion capacity ($DLCO$) is used instead to assess gas transfer across the alveolar–capillary membrane. Because carbon monoxide has a very high affinity for hemoglobin, there is little or no CO in pulmonary capillary blood so that even when it is administered at low concentration, $Pc'CO$ can be considered zero. Therefore,

$$DLCO = \frac{\text{Carbon monoxide uptake}}{PACO}$$

Reductions in $DLCO$ imply an impediment in gas transfer across the alveolar–capillary membrane. Such impediments may be due to abnormal $\dot{V}/\dot{Q}$ ratios, extensive destruction of the gas alveolar–capillary membrane, or very short capillary transit times. Abnormalities are accentuated by increases in O_2 consumption and cardiac output, such as occurs during exercise.

Table 22–4. Mechanisms of hypoxemia.

Low alveolar oxygen tension
Low inspired oxygen tension
Low fractional inspired concentration
High altitude
Alveolar hypoventilation
Third gas effect (diffusion hypoxia)
Increased oxygen consumption
Increased alveolar–arterial gradient
Right-to-left shunting
Increased areas of low $\dot{V}/\dot{Q}^1$ ratios
Low mixed venous oxygen tension
Decreased cardiac output
Increased oxygen consumption
Decreased hemoglobin concentration

[1] $\dot{V}/\dot{Q}$, ventilation/perfusion.

Arterial Oxygen Tension

PaO_2 cannot be calculated like PAO_2 but must be measured at room air. The alveolar-to-arterial O_2 partial pressure gradient (A–a gradient) is normally less than 15 mm Hg, but progressively increases with age up to 20–30 mm Hg. Arterial O_2 tension can be approximated by the following formula (in mm Hg):

$$PaO_2 = 102 - \frac{Age}{3}$$

The range is 60–100 mm Hg (8–13 kPa). Decreases are probably the result of a progressive increase in closing capacity relative to FRC (see above). Table 22–4 lists the mechanisms of hypoxemia ($PaO_2 < 60$ mm Hg).

The most common mechanism for hypoxemia is an increased alveolar–arterial gradient. The A–a gradient for O_2 depends on the amount of right-to-left shunting, the amount of $\dot{V}/\dot{Q}$ scatter, and the mixed venous oxygen tension (see below). The last depends on cardiac output, O_2 consumption, and hemoglobin concentration.

The A–a gradient for O_2 is directly proportional to shunt but inversely proportional to mixed venous O_2 tension. The effect of each variable on PaO_2 (and consequently the A–a gradient) can be determined only when the other variables are held constant. Figure 22–19 shows the effect of different degrees of shunting on PaO_2. It should also be noted that the greater the shunt, the less likely the possibility that an increase in FIO_2 will prevent hypoxemia. Moreover, isoshunt lines appear to be most useful for O_2 concentrations between 35% and 100%. Lower O_2 concentrations require modification of isoshunt lines to account for the effect of $\dot{V}/\dot{Q}$ scatter.

Figure 22–19. Isoshunt curves showing the effect of varying amounts of shunt on PaO₂. Note that there is little benefit in increasing inspired oxygen concentration in patients with very large shunts. (Modified and reproduced, with permission, from Benatar SR, Hewlett AM, Nunn JF: The use of isoshunt lines for control of oxygen therapy. Br J Anaesth 1973;45: 711.)

The effect of cardiac output on the A–a gradient (Figure 22–20) is due not only to its secondary effects on mixed venous O_2 tension (see Chapter 19), but also to a direct relationship between cardiac output and intrapulmonary shunting. As can be seen, a low cardiac output tends to accentuate the effect of shunt on PaO_2. A reduction in venous admixture is usually observed with low cardiac outputs secondary to accentuated pulmonary vasoconstriction from a lower mixed venous O_2 tension. On the other hand, high cardiac outputs can increase venous admixture by elevating mixed venous O_2 tension; the latter inhibits hypoxic pulmonary vasoconstriction.

O_2 consumption and hemoglobin concentration can also affect PaO_2 through their secondary effects on mixed venous O_2 tension (below). High O_2 consumption rates and low hemoglobin concentrations can increase the A–a gradient and depress PaO_2.

Mixed Venous Oxygen Tension

Normal mixed venous oxygen tension ($P\bar{v}O_2$) is about 40 mm Hg and represents the overall balance between O_2 consumption and O_2 delivery (Table 22–5; see below). A true mixed venous blood sample contains venous drainage from the superior vena cava, the inferior vena cava, and the heart; it must therefore be obtained from a pulmonary artery catheter (see Chapter 6).

2. Carbon Dioxide

Carbon dioxide is a by-product of aerobic metabolism in mitochondria. There are therefore small continuous gradients for CO_2 tension from mitochondria to cell cytoplasm, extracellular fluid, venous blood, and alveoli, where the CO_2 is finally eliminated.

Mixed Venous Carbon Dioxide Tension

Normal mixed venous CO_2 tension ($P\bar{v}CO_2$) is about 46 mm Hg and is the end result of mixing of blood from tissues of varying metabolic activity. Venous CO_2 tension is lower in tissues with low metabolic activity (eg, skin) but higher in blood from those with relatively high activity (eg, heart).

Alveolar Carbon Dioxide Tension

Alveolar CO_2 tension ($PACO_2$) is generally considered to represent the balance between total CO_2 production ($\dot{V}CO_2$) and alveolar ventilation (elimination):

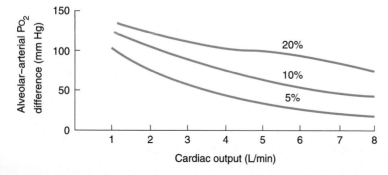

Figure 22–20. The effect of cardiac output on the alveolar–arterial PO₂ difference with varying degrees of shunting. ($\dot{V}O_2 = 200$ mL/min and $PaO_2 = 180$ mm Hg.). (Modified and reproduced, with permission, from Nunn JF: *Applied Respiratory Physiology*, 5th ed. Lumb A [editor]. Butterworth-Heinemann, 2000.)

Table 22–5. Alterations in mixed venous oxygen tension (and saturation).

Decreased $P\bar{v}O_2$
  Increased O_2 consumption
    Fever
    Shivering
    Exercise
    Malignant hyperthermia
    Thyroid storm
  Decreased O_2 delivery
    Hypoxia
    Decreased cardiac output
    Decreased hemoglobin concentration
    Abnormal hemoglobin
Increased $P\bar{v}O_2$
  Left-to-right shunting
  High cardiac output
  Impaired tissue uptake
    Cyanide poisoning
  Decreased oxygen consumption
    Hypothermia
  Combined mechanisms
    Sepsis
  Sampling error
    Wedged pulmonary artery catheter

$$\text{Paco}_2 = \frac{\dot{V}\text{CO}_2}{\dot{V}_A}$$

where $\dot{V}_A$ is alveolar ventilation (Figure 22–21). In reality, $PACO_2$ is related to CO_2 elimination rather than production. Although the two are equal in a steady state, an imbalance occurs during periods of acute hypoventilation or hypoperfusion and the excess CO_2 increases total body CO_2 content. Clinically, $PACO_2$ is more dependent on alveolar ventilation than is $\dot{V}CO_2$, because CO_2 output does not vary appreciably under most circumstances. Moreover, the body's large capacity to store CO_2 (see below) buffers acute changes in $\dot{V}CO_2$.

Pulmonary End-Capillary Carbon Dioxide Tension

Pulmonary end-capillary CO_2 tension ($Pc'CO_2$) is virtually identical to $PACO_2$ for the same reasons as those discussed in the section about O_2. In addition, the diffusion rate for CO_2 across the alveolar–capillary membrane is 20 times that of O_2.

Arterial Carbon Dioxide Tension

Arterial CO_2 tension ($PACO_2$), which is readily measurable, is identical to $Pc'CO_2$ and, necessarily, $PACO_2$. Normal $PACO_2$ is 38 ± 4 mm Hg (5.1 ± 0.5 kPa); in practice, 40 mm Hg is usually considered normal.

Although low $\dot{V}/\dot{Q}$ ratios tend to increase $PACO_2$ whereas high $\dot{V}/\dot{Q}$ ratios tend to decrease it (in contrast to the case for O_2 [see above]), significant arterial-to-alveolar gradients for CO_2 develop only in the presence of marked $\dot{V}/\dot{Q}$ abnormalities (> 30% venous admixture); even then the gradient is relatively small (2–3 mm Hg). Moreover, small increases in the gradient appreciably increase CO_2 output into alveoli with relatively normal $\dot{V}/\dot{Q}$. Even moderate to severe disturbances usually fail to appreciably alter arterial CO_2 because of a reflex increase in ventilation from concomitant hypoxemia.

End-Tidal Carbon Dioxide Tension

Because end-tidal gas is primarily alveolar gas and $PACO_2$ is virtually identical to $PACO_2$, end-tidal CO_2 tension ($PETCO_2$) is used clinically as an estimate of $PACO_2$. The $PACO_2$–$PETCO_2$ gradient is normally less than 5 mm Hg and represents dilution of alveolar gas with CO_2-free gas from nonperfused alveoli (alveolar dead space).

TRANSPORT OF RESPIRATORY GASES IN BLOOD

1. Oxygen

O_2 is carried in blood in two forms: dissolved in solution and in reversible association with hemoglobin.

Dissolved Oxygen

The amount of O_2 dissolved in blood can be derived from **Henry's law,** which states that the concentration

Figure 22–21. The effect of alveolar ventilation on alveolar PCO_2 at two rates of CO_2 production. (Modified and reproduced, with permission, from Nunn JF: *Applied Respiratory Physiology,* 5th ed. Lumb A [editor]. Butterworth-Heinemann, 2000.)

Figure 22–22. The normal adult hemoglobin–oxygen dissociation curve. (Modified, with permission, from West JB: *Respiratory Physiology—The Essentials,* 3rd ed. Williams & Wilkins, 1985.)

of any gas in solution is proportional to its partial pressure. The mathematical expression is as follows:

$$\text{Gas concentration} = \alpha \times \text{Partial pressure}$$

where α = the gas solubility coefficient for a given solution at a given temperature.

The solubility coefficient for O_2 at normal body temperature is 0.003 mL/dL per mm Hg. Even with a PaO_2 of 100 mm Hg, the maximum amount of O_2 dissolved in blood is very small (0.3 mL/dL) compared with that bound to hemoglobin.

Hemoglobin

Hemoglobin is a complex molecule consisting of four heme and four protein subunits. Heme is an iron–porphyrin compound that is an essential part of the O_2-binding sites; only the divalent form (+2 charge) of iron can bind O_2. The normal hemoglobin molecule (hemoglobin A_1) consists of two α and two β chains (subunits); the four subunits are held together by weak bonds between the amino acid residues. Each gram of hemoglobin can theoretically carry up to 1.39 mL of O_2.

Hemoglobin Dissociation Curve

Each hemoglobin molecule binds up to four O_2 molecules. The complex interaction between the hemoglobin subunits results in nonlinear (an elongated **S** shape)

binding with O_2 (Figure 22–22). Hemoglobin saturation is the amount of O_2 bound as a percentage of its total O_2-binding capacity. Four separate chemical reactions are involved in binding each of the four O_2 molecules. The change in molecular conformation induced by the binding of the first three molecules greatly accelerates binding of the fourth O_2 molecule. The last reaction is responsible for the accelerated binding between 25% and 100% saturation. At about 90% saturation, the decrease in available O_2 receptors flattens the curve until full saturation is reached.

Factors Influencing the Hemoglobin Dissociation Curve

Clinically important factors altering O_2 binding include hydrogen ion concentration, CO_2 tension, temperature, and 2,3-diphosphoglycerate (2,3-DPG) concentration. Their effect on hemoglobin–O_2 interaction can be expressed by P_{50}, the O_2 tension at which hemoglobin is 50% saturated (Figure 22–23). Each factor shifts the dissociation curve either to the right (increasing P_{50}) or to the left (decreasing P_{50}). A rightward shift in the oxygen–hemoglobin dissociation curve lowers O_2 affinity, displaces O_2 from hemoglobin, and makes more O_2 available to tissues; a leftward shift increases hemoglobin's affinity for O_2, reducing its availability to tissues. The normal P_{50} in adults is 26.6 mm Hg (3.4 kPa).

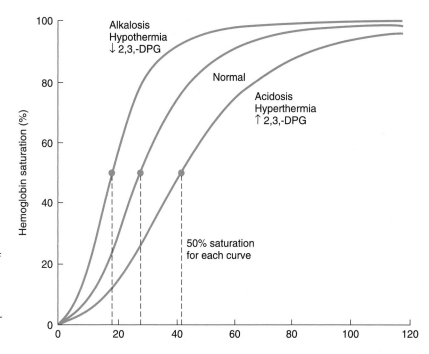

Figure 22–23. The effects of changes in acid–base status, body temperature, and 2,3-DPG concentration on the hemoglobin–oxygen dissociation curve.

An increase in blood hydrogen ion concentration reduces O_2 binding to hemoglobin (Bohr effect). Because of the shape of the **hemoglobin dissociation curve,** the effect is more important in venous blood than arterial blood (Figure 22–23); the net result is facilitation of O_2 release to tissue with little impairment in O_2 uptake (unless severe hypoxia is present).

The influence of CO_2 tension on hemoglobin's affinity for O_2 is important physiologically and is secondary to the associated rise in hydrogen ion concentration when CO_2 tension increases. The high CO_2 content of venous capillary blood, by decreasing hemoglobin's affinity for O_2, facilitates the release of O_2 to tissues; conversely, the lower CO_2 content in pulmonary capillaries increases hemoglobin's affinity for O_2 again, facilitating O_2 uptake from alveoli.

2,3-DPG is a by-product of glycolysis (the Rapoport–Luebering shunt) and accumulates during anaerobic metabolism. Although its effects on hemoglobin under these conditions are theoretically beneficial, its physiological importance normally appears minor. 2,3-DPG levels may, however, play an important compensatory role in patients with chronic anemia and may significantly affect the O_2-carrying capacity of blood transfusions.

Abnormal Ligands & Abnormal Forms of Hemoglobins

Carbon monoxide, cyanide, nitric acid, and ammonia can combine with hemoglobin at O_2-binding sites.

They can displace O_2 and shift the saturation curve to the left. Carbon monoxide is particularly potent, having 200–300 times the affinity of O_2 for hemoglobin, combining with it to form carboxyhemoglobin. Carbon monoxide decreases hemoglobin's O_2-carrying capacity and impairs the release of O_2 to tissues.

Methemoglobin results when the iron in heme is oxidized to its trivalent (+3) form. Nitrates, nitrites, sulfonamides, and other drugs can rarely result in significant methemoglobinemia. Methemoglobin cannot combine with O_2 unless reconverted by the enzyme methemoglobin reductase; methemoglobin also shifts the normal hemoglobin saturation curve to the left. Methemoglobinemia, like carbon monoxide poisoning, therefore decreases the O_2-carrying capacity as well as impairing the release of O_2. Reduction of methemoglobin to normal hemoglobin is facilitated by such agents as methylene blue or ascorbic acid.

Abnormal hemoglobins can also result from variations in the protein subunit composition. Each variant has its own O_2-saturation characteristics. These include fetal hemoglobin, hemoglobin A_2, and sickle hemoglobin (see Chapter 29).

Oxygen Content

The total O_2 content of blood is the sum of that in solution plus that carried by hemoglobin. In reality, O_2 binding to hemoglobin never achieves the theoretical maximum (see above) but is closer to 1.31 mL O_2/dL blood per mm Hg. Total O_2 content is expressed by the following equation:

$$O_2 \text{ content} = ([0.003 \text{ mL } O_2 /\text{dL blood per mm Hg}] \times Po_2) + (So_2 \times Hb \times 1.31 \text{ mL } /\text{dL blood})$$

where Hb is hemoglobin concentration in g/dL blood and So_2 is hemoglobin saturation at the given Po_2.

Using the above formula and a hemoglobin of 15 g/dL, the normal O_2 content for both arterial and mixed venous blood and the arteriovenous difference can be calculated:

$$Cao_2 = (0.003 \times 100) + (0.975 \times 15 \times 1.39)$$
$$= 19.5 \text{ mL/dL blood}$$
$$C\bar{v}o_2 = (0.003 \times 40) + (0.75 \times 15 \times 1.31)$$
$$= 14.8 \text{ mL/dL blood}$$
$$(Cao_2 - C\bar{v}o_2) = 4.7 \text{ mL/dL blood}$$

Oxygen Transport

O_2 transport is dependent on both respiratory and circulatory function (see Chapter 19). Total O_2 delivery ($\dot{D}o_2$) to tissues is the product of arterial O_2 content and cardiac output:

$$\dot{D}o_2 = Cao_2 \times \dot{Q}T$$

Note that arterial O_2 content is dependent on Pao_2 as well as hemoglobin concentration. **As a result, deficiencies in O_2 delivery may be due to a low Pao_2, a low hemoglobin concentration, or an inadequate cardiac output.** Normal O_2 delivery can be calculated as follows:

$$O_2 \text{ delivery} = 20 \text{ mL } O_2/\text{dL blood} \times 50 \text{ dL per blood/min}$$
$$= 1000 \text{ mL } O_2/\text{min}$$

The Fick equation expresses the relationship between O_2 consumption, O_2 content, and cardiac output:

$$O_2 \text{ consumption} = \dot{V}o_2 = \dot{Q}T \times (Cao_2 - C\bar{v}o_2)$$

Rearranging the equation:

$$Cao_2 = \frac{\dot{V}o_2}{\dot{Q}T} + C\bar{v}o_2$$

Consequently, the arteriovenous difference is a good measure of the overall adequacy of O_2 delivery.

With a normal O_2 consumption of approximately 250 mL/min and a cardiac output of 5000 mL/min, the normal arteriovenous difference by this equation again is calculated to be about 5 mL O_2/dL blood. Note that the normal extraction fraction for $O_2 [(Cao_2 - C\bar{v}o_2)/Cao_2]$ is 5 mL ÷ 20 mL, or 25%; thus, the body normally con-

sumes only 25% of the O_2 carried on hemoglobin. When O_2 demand exceeds supply, the extraction fraction exceeds 25%. Conversely, if O_2 supply exceeds demand, the extraction fraction falls below 25%.

When $\dot{D}o_2$ is even moderately reduced, $\dot{V}o_2$ usually remains normal because of increased O_2 extraction (mixed venous O_2 saturation decreases); $\dot{V}o_2$ remains independent of delivery. With further reductions in $\dot{D}o_2$, however, a critical point is reached beyond which $\dot{V}o_2$ becomes directly proportional to $\dot{D}o_2$. **This state of supply-dependent O_2 is typically associated with progressive lactic acidosis caused by cellular hypoxia.**

Oxygen Stores

The concept of O_2 stores is important in anesthesia. When the normal flux of O_2 is interrupted by apnea, existing O_2 stores are consumed by cellular metabolism; if stores are depleted, hypoxia and eventual cell death follow. Theoretically, normal O_2 stores in adults are about 1500 mL. This amount includes the O_2 remaining in the lungs, that bound to hemoglobin (and myoglobin), and that dissolved in body fluids. Unfortunately, the high affinity of hemoglobin for O_2 (the affinity of myoglobin is even higher) and the very limited quantity of O_2 in solution restrict the availability of these stores. The O_2 contained within the lungs at FRC (initial lung volume during apnea), therefore, becomes the most important source of O_2. Of that volume, however, probably only 80% is usable.

Apnea in a patient previously breathing room air leaves approximately 480 mL of O_2 in the lungs. (If $Fio_2 = 0.21$ and FRC = 2300 mL, O_2 content = $Fio_2 \times$ FRC.) The metabolic activity of tissues rapidly depletes this reservoir (presumably at a rate equivalent to $\dot{V}o_2$); severe hypoxemia usually occurs within 90 s. The onset of hypoxemia can be delayed by increasing the Fio_2 prior to the apnea. Following ventilation with 100% O_2, FRC contains about 2300 mL of O_2; this delays hypoxemia following apnea for 4–5 min. This concept is the basis for preoxygenation prior to induction of anesthesia (see Chapter 5).

2. Carbon Dioxide

Carbon dioxide is transported in blood in three forms: dissolved in solution, as bicarbonate, and with proteins in the form of carbamino compounds (Table 22–6). The sum of all three forms is the total CO_2 content of blood (routinely reported with electrolyte measurements).

Dissolved Carbon Dioxide

Carbon dioxide is more soluble in blood than O_2, with a solubility coefficient of 0.031 mmol/L/mm Hg (0.067 mL/dL/mm Hg) at 37°C.

Table 22–6. Contributions to carbon dioxide transport in 1 L of whole blood.[1,2]

Form	Plasma	Erythrocytes	Combined	Contribution (%)
Mixed venous whole blood				
Dissolved CO_2	0.76	0.51	1.27	5.5
Bicarbonate	14.41	5.92	20.33	87.2
Carbamino CO_2	Negligible	1.70	1.70	7.3
Total CO_2	15.17	8.13	23.30	
Arterial whole blood				
Dissolved CO_2	0.66	0.44	1.10	5.1
Bicarbonate	13.42	5.88	19.30	89.9
Carbamino CO_2	Negligible	1.10	1.10	5.1
Total CO_2	14.08	7.42	21.50	

[1]Modified, with permission, from Nunn JF: *Applied Respiratory Physiology,* 5th ed. Lumb A (editor). Butterworth-Heinemann, 2000.
[2]Values are expressed in millimoles, except where indicated otherwise.

Bicarbonate

In aqueous solutions, CO_2 slowly combines with water to form carbonic acid and bicarbonate, according to the following reaction:

$$H_2O + CO_2 \leftrightarrow H_2CO_3 \leftrightarrow H^+ + HCO_3^-$$

In plasma, although less than 1% of the dissolved CO_2 undergoes this reaction, the presence of the enzyme **carbonic anhydrase** within erythrocytes and endothelium greatly accelerates the reaction. As a result, bicarbonate represents the largest fraction of the CO_2 in blood (see Table 22–6). Administration of acetazolamide, a carbonic anhydrase inhibitor, can impair CO_2 transport between tissues and alveoli.

On the venous side of systemic capillaries, CO_2 enters red blood cells and is converted to bicarbonate, which diffuses out of red cells into plasma; chloride ions move from plasma into red cells to maintain electrical balance. In the pulmonary capillaries, the reverse occurs: chloride ions move out of red cells as bicarbonate ions reenter them for conversion back to CO_2, which diffuses out into alveoli. This sequence is referred to as the chloride or Hamburger shift.

Carbamino Compounds

Carbon dioxide can react with amino groups on proteins as shown by the following equation:

$$R\text{-}NH_2 + CO_2 \rightarrow RNH - CO_2^- + H^+$$

At physiological pH, only a small amount of CO_2 is carried in this form, mainly as carbamino-hemoglobin. Deoxygenated hemoglobin (deoxyhemoglobin) has a greater affinity (3.5 times) for CO_2 than does oxyhemoglobin. As a result, venous blood carries more CO_2 than arterial blood does (Haldane effect; see Table 22–6). PCO_2 normally has little effect on the fraction of CO_2 carried as carbamino-hemoglobin.

Effects of Hemoglobin Buffering on Carbon Dioxide Transport

The buffering action of hemoglobin (see Chapter 30) also accounts for part of the Haldane effect. Hemoglobin can act as a buffer at physiological pH because of its high content of histidine. Moreover, the acid–base behavior of hemoglobin is influenced by its oxygenation state:

$$H^+ + HbO_2 \rightarrow HbH^+ + O_2$$

Removal of O_2 from hemoglobin in tissue capillaries causes the hemoglobin molecule to behave more like a base; by taking up hydrogen ions, hemoglobin shifts the CO_2–bicarbonate equilibrium in favor of greater bicarbonate formation:

$$CO_2 + H_2O + HbO_2 \rightarrow HbH^+ + HCO_3^- + O_2$$

As a direct result, deoxyhemoglobin also increases the amount of CO_2 that is carried in venous blood as bicarbonate. As CO_2 is taken up from tissue and con-

Table 22–7. Carbon dioxide content of plasma (mmol/L).[1,2]

	Arterial	Venous
Dissolved CO_2	1.2	1.4
Bicarbonate	24.4	26.2
Carbamino CO_2	Negligible	Negligible
Total CO_2	25.6	27.6

[1]Modified, with permission, from Nunn JF: *Applied Respiratory Physiology,* 5th ed. Lumb A (editor). Butterworth-Heinemann, 2000.
[2]Values are expressed in millimoles, except where indicated otherwise.

verted to bicarbonate, the total CO_2 content of blood increases (see Table 22–6).

In the lungs, the reverse is true. Oxygenation of hemoglobin favors its action as an acid, and the release of hydrogen ions shifts the equilibrium in favor of greater CO_2 formation:

$$O_2 + HCO_3^- + HbH^+ \rightarrow H_2O + CO_2 + HbO_2$$

Bicarbonate concentration decreases as CO_2 is formed and eliminated, so that the total CO_2 content of blood decreases in the lungs. Note that there is a difference between CO_2 content (concentration per liter) of whole blood (see Table 22–6) and plasma (Table 22–7).

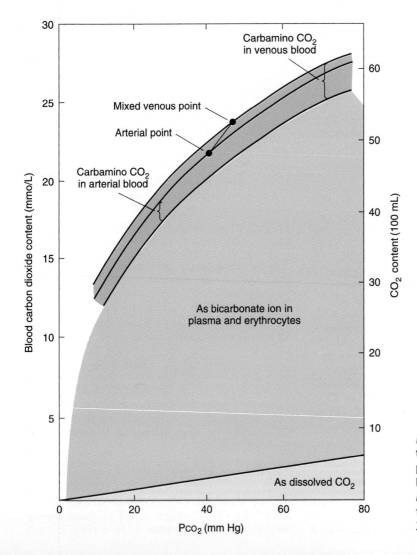

Figure 22–24. The CO_2 dissociation curve for whole blood. (Reproduced, with permission, from Nunn JF: *Applied Respiratory Physiology,* 5th ed. Lumb A [editor]. Butterworth-Heinemann, 2000.)

Carbon Dioxide Dissociation Curve

A CO_2 dissociation curve can be constructed by plotting the total CO_2 content of blood against PCO_2. The contribution of each form of CO_2 can also be quantified in this manner (Figure 22–24).

Carbon Dioxide Stores

Carbon dioxide stores in the body are large (approximately 120 L in adults) and primarily in the form of dissolved CO_2 and bicarbonate. When an imbalance occurs between production and elimination, establishing a new CO_2 equilibrium requires 20–30 min (compared with less than 4–5 min for O_2; see above). Carbon dioxide is stored in the rapid-, intermediate-, and slow-equilibrating compartments. Because of the larger capacity of the intermediate and slow compartments, the rate of rise in arterial CO_2 tension is generally slower than its fall following acute changes in ventilation.

CONTROL OF BREATHING

Spontaneous ventilation is the result of rhythmic neural activity in respiratory centers within the brain stem. This activity regulates pulmonary muscles to maintain normal tensions of O_2 and CO_2 in the body. The basic neuronal activity is modified by inputs from other areas in the brain, volutional and autonomic, as well as various central and peripheral receptors (sensors).

1. Central Respiratory Centers

The basic breathing rhythm originates in the medulla. Two medullary groups of neurons are generally recognized: a dorsal respiratory group, which is primarily active during inspiration; and a ventral respiratory group, which is active during expiration. Although not firmly established, the origin of the basic rhythm is due to either intrinsic spontaneous discharge activity in the dorsal group or reciprocating activity between the dorsal and ventral groups. The close association of the dorsal respiratory group of neurons with the tractus solitarius may explain reflex changes in breathing from vagal or glossopharyngeal nerve stimulation.

Two pontine areas influence the dorsal (inspiratory) medullary center. A lower pontine (apneustic) center is excitatory, whereas an upper pontine (pneumotaxic) center is inhibitory. The pontine centers appear to fine-tune respiratory rate and rhythm.

2. Central Sensors

The most important of these sensors are chemoreceptors that respond to changes in hydrogen ion concentration. Central chemoreceptors are thought to lie on the anterolateral surface of the medulla and respond primarily to changes in cerebrospinal fluid (CSF) [H^+]. This mechanism is effective in regulating $PaCO_2$, because the blood–brain barrier (see Chapter 25) is permeable to dissolved CO_2 but not to bicarbonate ions. Acute changes in $PaCO_2$ but not in arterial [HCO_3^-] are reflected in CSF; thus, a change in CO_2 must result in a change in [H^+]:

$$CO_2 + H_2O \leftrightarrow H^+ + HCO_3^-$$

Over the course of a few days, CSF [HCO_3^-] can compensate to match any change in arterial [HCO_3^-].

Increases in $PaCO_2$ elevate CSF hydrogen ion concentration and activate the chemoreceptors. Secondary stimulation of the adjacent respiratory medullary centers increases alveolar ventilation (Figure 22–25) and reduces $PaCO_2$ back to normal. Conversely, decreases in CSF hydrogen ion concentration secondary to reductions in $PaCO_2$ reduce alveolar ventilation and elevate $PaCO_2$. Note that the relationship between $PaCO_2$ and minute volume is nearly linear. Also note that very high arterial $PaCO_2$ tensions depress the ventilatory response (CO_2

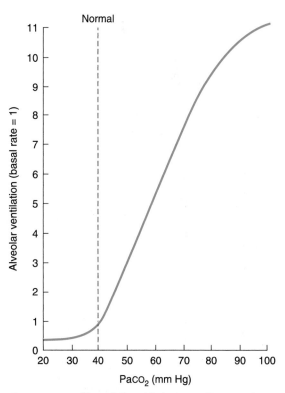

Figure 22–25. The relationship between $PaCO_2$ and minute ventilation. (Reproduced, with permission, from Guyton AC: *Textbook of Medical Physiology*, 7th ed. W.B. Saunders, 1986.)

Figure 22–26. The relationship between PaO$_2$ and minute ventilation at rest and with a normal PaO$_2$. (Reproduced, with permission, from Nunn JF: *Applied Respiratory Physiology*, 5th ed. Lumb A [editor]. Butterworth-Heinemann, 2000.)

narcosis). The PaCO$_2$ at which ventilation is zero (*x*-intercept) is known as the apneic threshold. Spontaneous respirations are typically absent under anesthesia when PaCO$_2$ falls below the apneic threshold. (In the awake state, cortical influences prevent apnea, so apneic thresholds are not ordinarily seen.) In contrast to peripheral chemoreceptors (see below), central chemoreceptor activity is depressed by hypoxia.

3. Peripheral Sensors

Peripheral Chemoreceptors

Peripheral chemoreceptors include the carotid bodies (at the bifurcation of the common carotid arteries) and the aortic bodies (surrounding the aortic arch). The carotid bodies are the principal peripheral chemoreceptors in humans and are sensitive to changes in PaO$_2$, PaCO$_2$, pH, and arterial perfusion pressure. They interact with central respiratory centers via the glossopharyngeal nerves, producing reflex increases in alveolar ventilation in response to reductions in PaO$_2$, arterial perfusion, or elevations in [H$^+$] and PaCO$_2$. Peripheral chemoreceptors are also stimulated by cyanide, doxapram, and large doses of nicotine. In contrast to central chemoreceptors, which respond primarily to PaCO$_2$ (really [H$^+$]), the carotid bodies are most sensitive to PaO$_2$ (Figure 22–26). Note that receptor activity does not appreciably increase until PaO$_2$ decreases below 50 mm Hg. Cells of the carotid body (glomus cells) are

thought to be primarily dopaminergic neurons. Antidopaminergic drugs (such as phenothiazines), most commonly used anesthetics, and bilateral carotid surgery abolish the peripheral ventilatory response to hypoxemia.

Lung Receptors

Impulses from these receptors are carried centrally by the vagus nerve. Stretch receptors are distributed in the smooth muscle of airways; they are responsible for inhibition of inspiration when the lung is inflated to excessive volumes (Hering–Breuer inflation reflex) and shortening of exhalation when the lung is deflated (deflation reflex). Stretch receptors normally play a minor role in humans. In fact, bilateral vagal nerve blocks have a minimal effect on the normal respiratory pattern.

Irritant receptors in the tracheobronchial mucosa react to noxious gases, smoke, dust, and cold gases; activation produces reflex increases in respiratory rate, bronchoconstriction, and coughing. J (juxtacapillary) receptors are located in the interstitial space within alveolar walls; these receptors induce dyspnea in response to expansion of interstitial space volume and various chemical mediators following tissue damage.

Other Receptors

These include various muscle and joint receptors on pulmonary muscles and the chest wall. Input from these sources is probably important during exercise and in pathological conditions associated with decreased lung or chest compliance.

4. Effects of Anesthesia on the Control of Breathing

The most important effect of most general anesthetics on breathing is a tendency to promote hypoventilation. The mechanism is probably dual: central depression of the chemoreceptor and depression of external intercostal muscle activity. The magnitude of the hypoventilation is generally proportional to anesthetic depth. With increasing depth of anesthesia, the slope of the PaCO$_2$/ minute ventilation curve decreases and the apneic threshold increases (Figure 22–27). This effect is at least partially reversed by surgical stimulation.

The peripheral response to hypoxemia is even more sensitive to anesthetics than the central CO$_2$ response and is nearly abolished by even subanesthetic doses of most inhalation agents (including nitrous oxide) and many intravenous agents. Anesthetic agents may also impair the peripheral stimulatory response of doxapram, but its central actions

Figure 22–27. The effect of volatile agents (halothane) on the P_{ETCO_2}–ventilation response curve (see text). (Modified and reproduced, with permission, from Nunn JF: *Applied Respiratory Physiology,* 5th ed. Lumb A [editor]. Butterworth-Heinemann, 2000.)

appear to be preserved (see Chapter 15). The respiratory effects of individual agents are discussed in Chapters 7 and 8.

NONRESPIRATORY FUNCTIONS OF THE LUNG

Filtration & Reservoir Function

A. FILTRATION

The unique in-series position of the pulmonary capillaries within the circulation allows them to act as a filter for debris in the bloodstream. The lungs' high content of heparin and plasminogen activator facilitates the breakdown of entrapped fibrin debris. Although pulmonary capillaries have an average diameter of 7 μm, larger particles have been shown to pass through to the left heart.

B. RESERVOIR FUNCTION

The role of the pulmonary circulation as a reservoir for the systemic circulation was discussed above.

Metabolism

The lungs are metabolically very active organs. In addition to surfactant synthesis, pneumocytes account for a major portion of extrahepatic mixed-function oxidation. Neutrophils and macrophages in the lung produce O_2-derived free radicals in response to infection (and systemic inflammatory responses; see Chapter 49). The pulmonary endothelium metabolizes a variety of vasoactive compounds, including norepinephrine, serotonin, bradykinin, and a variety of prostaglandins and leukotrienes. Histamine and epinephrine are generally not metabolized in the lungs; in fact the lungs can be a major site of histamine synthesis and release during allergic reactions.

The lungs are also responsible for converting angiotensin I to its physiologically active form, angiotensin II. The enzyme responsible, angiotensin-converting enzyme, is bound on the surface of the pulmonary endothelium.

CASE DISCUSSION: UNILATERALLY DIMINISHED BREATH SOUNDS DURING GENERAL ANESTHESIA

A 67-year-old man with carcinoma is undergoing colon resection under general anesthesia. His history includes an old anterior myocardial infarction and compensated congestive heart failure. Arterial and pulmonary artery catheters are placed preoperatively for monitoring during surgery. Following a smooth thiopental–fentanyl induction and an atraumatic intubation with succinylcholine, anesthesia is maintained with 60% nitrous oxide in O_2, isoflurane, and vecuronium. One-half hour into the operation, the surgeon asks for the Trendelenburg position to facilitate surgical exposure. The pulse oximeter, which had been reading 99% saturation, suddenly drops and remains at 93%. The pulse oximeter's signal strength and waveform are unchanged. Auscultation of the lungs reveals diminished breath sounds over the left lung.

What is the most likely explanation?

Unilaterally diminished breath sounds under anesthesia are most commonly caused by inadvertent placement or migration of the tracheal tube into one of the two main bronchi. As a result, only one lung is ventilated. Other causes of unilaterally diminished breath sounds (such as pneumothorax, a large mucus plug, lobar atelectasis, or an undiagnosed mediastinal mass) are less easily diagnosed but are fortunately less common during anesthesia.

The Trendelenburg (head-down) position typically causes the tip of the tracheal tube to advance 1–2 cm relative to the carina. In this case, the tube was apparently placed just above the carina with the patient in the supine position but migrated into the right bronchus when the Trendelenburg position was imposed. The diagnosis is confirmed by drawing the tube back 1–2 cm at a time as the chest is auscultated. Breath sounds will become equal again when the tip of the tube reenters the trachea. Following initial placement, tracheal tubes should be routinely checked for correct positioning by auscultating the chest, ascertaining depth of tube insertion by the markings on the tube (normally 20–24 cm at the teeth for an adult), and feeling for the cuff in the suprasternal notch. Tube position can also be quickly confirmed with a flexible fiberoptic bronchoscope.

Are tracheal tubes just as likely to enter either main bronchus?

In most cases of unintentional bronchial intubation, the tracheal tube enters the right bronchus because the latter diverges away from the trachea at a less acute angle than does the left bronchus (see Chapter 24).

Why did hemoglobin saturation decrease?

Failure to ventilate one lung as it continues to be perfused creates a large intrapulmonary shunt. Venous admixture increases and tends to depress Pa_{O_2} and hemoglobin saturation.

Does a saturation of 93% exclude bronchial intubation?

No; if both lungs continued to have equal blood flow, venous admixture should have theoretically increased to 50%, resulting in severe hypoxemia and very low hemoglobin saturation. Fortunately, hypoxic pulmonary vasoconstriction is a powerful compensatory response that tends to reduce flow to the hypoxic lung and reduces the expected venous

admixture. In fact, if the patient has been receiving a higher inspired O_2 concentration (50–100%), the drop in arterial tension may not be detectable by the pulse oximeter due to the characteristics of the normal hemoglobin saturation curve. For example, bronchial intubation in a patient inspiring 50% O_2 might drop Pa_{O_2} from 250 mm Hg to 95 mm Hg; the resulting change in pulse oximeter readings (100–99 to 98–97) would hardly be noticeable.

Arterial and mixed venous blood gas tensions are obtained with the following results:

$Pa_{O_2} = 69$ mm Hg; $Pa_{CO_2} = 42$ mm Hg; $Sa_{O_2} = 93\%$; $P\bar{v}_{O_2} = 40$ mm Hg; and $S\bar{v}_{O_2} = 75\%$. Hemoglobin concentration is 15 g/dL.

What is the calculated venous admixture?

In this case, $Pc'_{O_2} = Pa_{O_2} = ([760 - 47] \times 0.4) - 42 = 243$ mm Hg. Therefore, $Cc'_{O_2} = (15 \times 1.31 \times 1.0) + (243 \times 0.003) = 20.4$ mL/dL.
$Ca_{O_2} = (15 \times 1.31 \times 0.93) + (69 \times 0.003) = 18.5$ mL/dL
$C\bar{v}_{O_2} = (15 \times 1.31 \times 0.75) + (40 \times 0.003) = 14.8$ mL/dL
$\dot{Q}s/\dot{Q}T = (20.4 - 18.5)/(20.4 - 14.8) = 34\%$

How does bronchial intubation affect arterial and end-tidal CO_2 tensions?

Pa_{CO_2} is typically not appreciably altered as long as the same minute ventilation is maintained (see One-Lung Anesthesia, Chapter 24). Clinically, the Pa_{CO_2}–PET_{CO_2} gradient often widens, possibly because of increased alveolar dead space (overdistension of the ventilated lung). Thus, PET_{CO_2} may decrease or remain unchanged.

SUGGESTED READING

Ganong WF: *Review of Medical Physiology,* 20th ed. McGraw-Hill, 2001.

Guyton AC: *Textbook of Medical Physiology,* 10th ed. W.B. Saunders, 2000.

Nunn JF: *Applied Respiratory Physiology,* 5th ed. Lumb A (editor). Butterworth-Heinemann, 2000.

Warner DO: Diaphragm function during anesthesia: Still crazy after all these years. Anesthesiology 2002;97:295. An excellent, brief discussion of the effects of anesthetics on the diaphragm.

West JB: *Respiratory Physiology—The Essentials,* 6th ed. Lippincott, Williams & Wilkins, 2000.

Anesthesia for Patients with Respiratory Disease

23

KEY CONCEPTS

1. In a patient with an acute asthma attack, a normal or high $PaCO_2$ indicates that the patient can no longer maintain the work of breathing and is often a sign of impending respiratory failure. A pulsus paradoxus and electrocardiographic signs of right ventricular strain (ST-segment changes, right-axis deviation, and right bundle branch block) are also indicative of severe airway obstruction.

2. Asthmatic patients with active bronchospasm presenting for emergency surgery should be treated aggressively whenever possible. Supplemental oxygen, aerosolized β_2-agonists, and intravenous glucocorticoids can dramatically improve lung function in a few hours.

3. Intraoperative bronchospasm is usually manifested as wheezing, increasing peak inflation pressures (plateau pressure should remain unchanged), decreasing exhaled tidal volumes, or a slowly rising waveform on the capnograph.

4. If the bronchospasm does not resolve after deepening the anesthetic, less common causes should be considered before administering more specific drugs. Obstruction of the tracheal tube from kinking, secretions, or an overinflated balloon; bronchial intubation; active expiratory efforts (straining); pulmonary edema or embolism; and pneumothorax can all simulate bronchospasm.

5. In patients with chronic obstructive pulmonary disease (COPD), chronic hypoxemia leads to erythrocytosis, pulmonary hypertension, and eventually right ventricular failure (cor pulmonale).

6. Oxygen therapy can dangerously elevate $PaCO_2$ in patients with CO_2 retention; elevating PaO_2 above 60 mm Hg can precipitate respiratory failure.

7. Preoperative interventions in patients with COPD aimed at correcting hypoxemia, relieving bronchospasm, mobilizing and reducing secretions, and treating infections may decrease the incidence of postoperative pulmonary complications. Patients at greatest risk for complications are those with preoperative pulmonary function measurements less than 50% of predicted.

8. Patients with pulmonary bullae are at high risk of developing pneumothoraxes intraoperatively, particularly if ventilated with positive pressure.

9. Restrictive pulmonary diseases are characterized by decreased lung compliance. Lung volumes are typically reduced, with preservation of normal expiratory flow rates. Thus, both forced expiratory volume in 1 s (FEV_1) and forced vital capacity (FVC) are reduced, but the FEV_1/FVC ratio is normal.

10. Intraoperative pulmonary embolism usually presents as unexplained sudden hypotension, hypoxemia, or bronchospasm. A decrease in end-tidal CO_2 concentration is also suggestive of pulmonary embolism but not specific.

The impact of preexisting pulmonary disease on respiratory function during anesthesia and in the postoperative period is predictable: Greater degrees of preoperative pulmonary impairment are associated with more marked intraoperative alterations in respiratory function (see Chapter 22) and higher rates of postoperative pulmonary complications. Failure to recognize patients who are at increased risk is a frequent contributory factor leading to complications, as patients may not receive appropriate preoperative and intraoperative care. This chapter examines pulmonary risk in general and then reviews the anesthetic approach to patients with the most common types of respiratory disease.

PULMONARY RISK FACTORS

Six risk factors (Table 23–1) predispose patients to postoperative pulmonary dysfunction, the most common postoperative complication. The incidence of atelectasis, pneumonia, pulmonary embolism, and respiratory failure following surgery is quite high but varies widely (from 6% to 60%) depending on the patient population studied and the surgical procedures performed. With the exception of the operative site and the duration of the procedure, most are related to preoperative pulmonary dysfunction. The two strongest predictors of complications appear to be operative site and a history of dyspnea, which correlates with the degree of preexisting pulmonary disease. The least consistent factor is the duration of anesthesia.

The association between smoking and respiratory disease is well established; abnormalities in maximal midexpiratory flow (MMEF) rates are often demonstrable well before symptoms of chronic obstructive pulmonary disease (COPD) appear. Although abnormalities can be demonstrated on pulmonary function tests (PFTs), because most patients who smoke do not have PFTs performed preoperatively, it is best to assume that such patients have some degree of pulmonary compromise. Even in normal individuals, advancing age is associated with an increasing prevalence of pulmonary disease and an increase in closing capacity. Obesity decreases functional residual capacity (FRC), increases the work of breathing, and predisposes patients to deep venous thrombosis.

Table 23–1. Risk factors for postoperative pulmonary complications.

Preexisting pulmonary disease
Thoracic or upper abdominal surgery
Smoking
Obesity
Age (> 60 years)
Prolonged general anesthesia (> 3 h)

Thoracic and upper abdominal surgical procedures can have marked effects on pulmonary function. Operations near the diaphragm often result in diaphragmatic dysfunction and a restrictive ventilatory defect (see below). Upper abdominal procedures consistently decrease FRC (60–70%); the effect is maximal on the first postoperative day and usually lasts 7–10 days. Rapid shallow breathing with an ineffective cough caused by pain (splinting), a decrease in the number of sighs, and impaired mucociliary clearance lead to microatelectasis and loss of lung volume. Intrapulmonary shunting promotes hypoxemia (see Chapter 22). Residual anesthetic effects, the recumbent position, sedation from opioids, abdominal distention, and restrictive dressings may also be contributory. Complete relief of pain with regional anesthesia can decrease but does not completely reverse these abnormalities. Persistent microatelectasis and retention of secretions favor the development of postoperative pneumonia.

Although many adverse effects of general anesthesia on pulmonary function have been described (see Chapter 22), the superiority of regional over general anesthesia for patients with pulmonary impairment is not firmly established.

In summary, because of the prevalence of smoking and obesity, many patients are at increased risk of developing postoperative pulmonary dysfunction. The risk of complications increases if the patient is having a thoracotomy or laparotomy, even if the patient has no risk factors. Patients with known disease should have their pulmonary function optimized preoperatively, with careful consideration given to the choice of general versus regional anesthesia.

■ OBSTRUCTIVE PULMONARY DISEASE

Obstructive and restrictive breathing are the two most common abnormal patterns, as determined by PFTs. Obstructive lung diseases are the most common form of pulmonary dysfunction. They include asthma, emphysema, chronic bronchitis, cystic fibrosis, bronchiectasis, and bronchiolitis. The primary characteristic of these disorders is resistance to airflow. An MMEF of < 70% (forced expiratory flow [$FEF_{25-75\%}$]; see Chapter 22) is often the only abnormality early in the course of these disorders. Values for $FEF_{25-75\%}$ in adult males and females are normally > 2.0 and > 1.6 L/s, respectively. As the disease progresses, both forced expiratory volume in 1 s (FEV_1) and the FEV_1/FVC (forced vital capacity) ratio are less than 70% of the predicted values.

Elevated airway resistance and air trapping increase the work of breathing; respiratory gas exchange is impaired because of ventilation/perfusion (V/Q) imbalance. The predominance of expiratory airflow resistance results in air trapping; residual volume and total lung capacity (TLC) increase. Wheezing is a common finding and represents turbulent airflow. It is often absent with mild obstruction that may be manifested initially only by prolonged exhalation. Progressive obstruction typically results first in expiratory wheezing only, and then in both inspiratory and expiratory wheezing. With marked obstruction, wheezing may be absent when airflow has nearly ceased.

ASTHMA

Preoperative Considerations

Asthma is a common disorder affecting 5–7% of the population. Its primary characteristic is airway (bronchiolar) inflammation and hyperreactivity in response to a variety of stimuli. Clinically, asthma is manifested by episodic attacks of dyspnea, cough, and wheezing. Airway obstruction, which is generally reversible, is the result of bronchial smooth muscle constriction, edema, and increased secretions. Classically, the obstruction is precipitated by a variety of airborne substances, including pollens, animal danders, dusts, pollutants, and various chemicals. Some patients also develop bronchospasm following ingestion of aspirin, nonsteroidal antiinflammatory agents, sulfiting agents, or tartrazine and other dyes. Exercise, emotional excitement, and viral infections also precipitate bronchospasm in many patients. Asthma is classified as acute or chronic. Chronic asthma is further classified as intermittent (mild) and mild, moderate, and severe persistent disease.

The terms extrinsic (allergic) asthma (attacks related to environmental exposures) and intrinsic (idiosyncratic) asthma (attacks usually occur without provocation) were used in the past but these classifications were imperfect; many patients show features of both forms. Moreover, overlap with chronic bronchitis (see below) is common.

A. PATHOPHYSIOLOGY

The pathophysiology of asthma involves the local release of various chemical mediators in the airway and, possibly, overactivity of the parasympathetic nervous system. Inhaled substances can initiate bronchospasm through both specific and nonspecific immune mechanisms by degranulating bronchial mast cells. In classic allergic asthma, antigen binding to immunoglobulin E (IgE) on the surface of mast cells causes degranulation. Bronchoconstriction is the result of the subsequent release of histamine; bradykinin; leukotrienes C, D, and E; platelet-activating factor; prostaglandins (PG) PGE_2, $PGF_2\alpha$, and PGD_2; and neutrophil and eosinophil chemotactic factors. The role of serotonin, a potent bronchoconstrictor, is uncertain in humans. The parasympathetic nervous system plays a major role in maintaining normal bronchial tone; a normal diurnal variation in tone is recognized in most individuals with peak airway resistance early in the morning at about 6:00 AM. **Vagal afferents in the bronchi are sensitive to histamine and multiple noxious stimuli, including cold air, inhaled irritants, and instrumentation (eg, tracheal intubation).** Reflex vagal activation results in bronchoconstriction, which is mediated by an increase in intracellular cyclic guanosine monophosphate (cGMP).

During an asthma attack, bronchoconstriction, mucosal edema, and secretions increase resistance to gas flow at all levels of the lower airways. Most cells phagocytose the inciting allergen during exposure. If they are unable to digest or degrade the allergen, the allergen may subsequently, long after the original incident, be released by the mast cells, thus creating a recrudescence of the disease process. As an attack resolves, airway resistance normalizes first in the larger airways (mainstem, lobar, segmental, and subsegmental bronchi), and then in more peripheral airways. Consequently, expiratory flow rates are initially decreased throughout an FVC procedure, but during resolution of the attack the expiratory flow rate is reduced only at low lung volumes. TLC, residual volume (RV), and FRC are all increased. In acutely ill patients, RV and FRC are often increased by more than 400% and 100%, respectively. Prolonged or severe attacks markedly increase the work of breathing and can fatigue respiratory muscles. The number of alveolar units with low $\dot{V}/\dot{Q}$ ratios increases, resulting in hypoxemia. Tachypnea is likely due to stimulation of bronchial receptors and typically produces hypocapnia (see Chapter 22). A normal or high $PaCO_2$ indicates that the patient can no longer maintain the work of breathing and is often a sign of impending respiratory failure. A pulsus paradoxus and electrocardiographic signs of right ventricular strain (ST-segment changes, right-axis deviation, and right bundle branch block) are also indicative of severe airway obstruction.

B. TREATMENT

Drugs used to treat asthma include β-adrenergic agonists, methylxanthines, glucocorticoids, anticholinergics, leukotriene blockers, and mast cell-stabilizing agents; with the exception of the last, these drugs may be used for either acute or chronic treatment of asthma. Cromolyn sodium and nedocromil are effective for preventing bronchospasm only in patients with extrinsic asthma and in some with intrinsic asthma. Although devoid of any bronchodilating properties, both agents block the degranulation of mast cells.

Sympathomimetic agents (Table 23–2) are the most useful and the most commonly used. They produce bronchodilation via β₂-agonist activity. Activation of

Table 23–2. A comparison of commonly used bronchodilators.[1]

	Adrenergic Activity	
Agent	β_1	β_2
Albuterol (Ventolin)	+	+++
Bitolterol (Tornalate)	+	++++
Epinephrine (various)	++++	++
Fenoterol (Berotec)	+	+++
Formaterol (Foradil)	+	++++
Isoetharine (Bronkosol)	++	+++
Isoproterenol (Isuprel)	++++	—
Metaproterenol (Alupent)	+	+
Pirbuterol (Maxair)	+	++++
Salmeterol (Serevent)	+	++++
Terbutaline (Brethaire)	+	+++

[1] + Indicates level of activity.

β_2-adrenergic receptors on bronchiolar smooth muscle in turn activates adenylate cyclase, which results in the formation of intracellular cyclic adenosine monophosphate (cAMP). These agents are usually administered via a metered-dose inhaler or by aerosol. Use of more selective β_2-agonists, such as terbutaline or albuterol, may decrease the incidence of undesirable β_1 cardiac effects but are often not that selective in high doses.

Methylxanthines traditionally are thought to produce bronchodilation by inhibiting phosphodiesterase, the enzyme responsible for the breakdown of cAMP. Their pulmonary effects appear much more complex and include catecholamine release, blockade of histamine release, and diaphragmatic stimulation. Oral long-acting theophylline preparations are used for patients with nocturnal symptoms. Unfortunately, theophylline has a narrow therapeutic range; therapeutic blood levels are considered to be 10–20 µg/mL. Lower levels, however, may be effective. Aminophylline is the only available intravenous theophylline preparation.

Glucocorticoids are used for both acute treatment and maintenance therapy of patients with asthma because of their antiinflammatory and membrane-stabilizing effects. Beclomethasone, triamcinolone, fluticasone, and budesonide are synthetic steroids commonly used in metered-dose inhalers for maintenance therapy. Although they are associated with a low incidence of undesirable systemic effects, their use does not necessar-

ily prevent adrenal suppression. Intravenous hydrocortisone or methylprednisolone is used acutely for severe attacks, followed by tapering doses of oral prednisone. Glucocorticoids usually require several hours to become effective.

Anticholinergic agents produce bronchodilation through their antimuscarinic action and may block reflex bronchoconstriction. Ipratropium, a congener of atropine that can be given by a metered-dose inhaler or aerosol, is a moderately effective bronchodilator without appreciable systemic anticholinergic effects.

Anesthetic Considerations

A. PREOPERATIVE MANAGEMENT

The emphasis in evaluating patients with asthma should be on determining the recent course of the disease (review peak flow diary if available) and whether the patient has ever been hospitalized for an acute asthma attack, as well as on ascertaining that the patient is in optimal condition. The difference between anesthetizing an asthmatic patient who has recently been hospitalized or who has clearly audible preoperative wheezing and one without such a history or finding on examination may be a potentially life-threatening anesthetic experience versus a totally uneventful one.

The clinical history is of critical importance. No or minimal dyspnea, wheezing, or cough is optimal. Complete resolution of recent exacerbations should be confirmed by chest auscultation. Patients with frequent or chronic bronchospasm should be placed on an optimal bronchodilating regimen, including β_2-adrenergic agonists; glucocorticoids should also be considered. A chest radiograph may be useful in assessing air trapping; hyperinflation results in a flattened diaphragm, a small-appearing heart, and hyperlucent lung fields. PFTs—particularly expiratory airflow measurements such as FEV_1, FEV_1/FVC, and peak expiratory flow rate (PEFR)—should be used to confirm clinical impressions. Comparisons with previous measurements are invaluable. FEV_1 values are normally more than 3 L for men and 2 L for women. FEV_1/FVC should normally be > 70%. Normal PEFR values exceed 200 L/min (often > 500 L/min in young adult males). An FEV_1, FEV_1/FVC, or PEFR less than 50% of normal is indicative of moderate to severe asthma.

Asthmatic patients with active bronchospasm presenting for emergency surgery should be treated aggressively whenever possible. Supplemental oxygen, aerosolized β_2-agonists, and intravenous glucocorticoids can dramatically improve lung function in a few hours. Arterial blood gases may be useful in managing severe cases. Hypoxemia and hypocapnia are typical of moderate and severe disease; even slight hypercapnia is indicative of severe air trapping and may be a sign of impending respiratory failure (see above). An FEV_1 below 40% of normal may also be predictive of respiratory failure.

Some degree of preoperative sedation is desirable in asthmatic patients presenting for elective surgery—particularly in patients whose disease has an emotional component. In general, benzodiazepines are the most satisfactory agents for premedication. Anticholinergic agents are not customarily given unless very copious secretions are present or if ketamine is to be used for induction of anesthesia. In typical intramuscular doses, anticholinergics are not effective in preventing reflex bronchospasm following intubation. The use of an H_2-blocking agent (such as cimetidine, ranitidine, or famotidine) is theoretically detrimental, since H_2-receptor activation normally produces bronchodilation; in the event of histamine release, unopposed H_1 activation with H_2 blockade may accentuate bronchoconstriction.

Bronchodilators should be continued up to the time of surgery; in order of effectiveness, they are β-agonists, inhaled glucocorticoids, leukotriene blockers, mast-cell stabilizers, theophyllines, and anticholinergics. Patients who have been receiving long-term glucocorticoid therapy should be given supplemental doses to compensate for adrenal suppression. Hydrocortisone (50–100 mg preoperatively and 100 mg every 8 h for 1–3 postoperative days, depending on the degree of surgical stress) is most commonly used.

B. INTRAOPERATIVE MANAGEMENT

The most critical time for asthmatic patients undergoing anesthesia is during instrumentation of the airway. General anesthesia by mask or regional anesthesia will circumvent this problem, but neither necessarily eliminates the possibility of bronchospasm. In fact, some clinicians believe that high spinal or epidural anesthesia may aggravate bronchoconstriction by blocking sympathetic tone to the lower airways (T1–T4) and allowing unopposed parasympathetic activity. Pain, emotional stress, or stimulation during light general anesthesia can precipitate bronchospasm. Drugs often associated with histamine release (eg, curare, atracurium, mivacurium, morphine, and meperidine) should be avoided or given very slowly when used. The goal of any general anesthetic is a smooth induction and emergence, with anesthetic depth adjusted to stimulation.

Which induction agent is chosen is not as important as achieving deep anesthesia before intubation and surgical stimulation. Thiopental is most commonly used for adults but occasionally can induce bronchospasm as a result of exaggerated histamine release. Propofol and etomidate are suitable alternatives and, in fact, are preferred by some clinicians. Ketamine, the only intravenous agent with bronchodilating properties, is a good choice for patients who are also hemodynamically

unstable. Ketamine should probably not be used in patients with high theophylline levels, as the combined actions of the two drugs can precipitate seizure activity. Halothane and sevoflurane usually provide the smoothest inhalation induction with bronchodilation in asthmatic children. Isoflurane and desflurane can provide equal bronchodilation but are not normally used for inhalation induction. When used to maintain anesthesia, their concentration should be increased slowly because they exert a mild irritant effect on the airways.

Reflex bronchospasm can be blunted before intubation by an additional dose of thiopental (1–2 mg/kg), ventilating the patient with a 2–3 minimum alveolar concentration (MAC) of a volatile agent for 5 min, or administering intravenous or intratracheal lidocaine (1–2 mg/kg). Note that intratracheal lidocaine itself can initiate bronchospasm if an inadequate induction dose of thiopental is used. A large dose of an anticholinergic (atropine, 2 mg, or glycopyrrolate, 1 mg) can also block reflex bronchospasm but causes excessive tachycardia. Although succinylcholine may on occasion induce marked histamine release, it can generally be safely used in most asthmatic patients. In the absence of capnography, confirmation of correct tracheal placement by chest auscultation can be difficult in the presence of marked bronchospasm.

Volatile anesthetics are most often used for maintenance of anesthesia to take advantage of their potent bronchodilating properties. Halothane can sensitize the heart to aminophylline and β-adrenergic agonists administered during anesthesia; for that reason—together with concern over hepatotoxicity—halothane is generally avoided in adults. Ventilation should be controlled with warmed humidified gases whenever possible. Airflow obstruction during expiration is apparent on capnography as a delayed rise of the end-tidal CO_2 value (Figure 23–1); the severity of obstruction is generally inversely

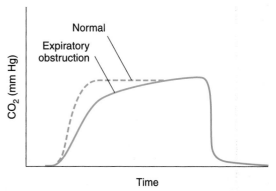

Figure 23–1. Capnograph of a patient with expiratory airway obstruction.

related to the rate of rise in end-tidal CO_2. Severe bronchospasm is manifested by rising peak inspiratory pressures and incomplete exhalation. In the past, tidal volumes of 10–12 mL/kg with ventilatory rates of 8–10 breaths/min were considered desirable. Currently, minimizing the tidal volume ($\leq$ 10 mL/kg) with prolongation of the expiratory time may allow more uniform distribution of gas flow to both lungs and may help avoid air trapping. The $PaCO_2$ may increase, which is acceptable if there is no contraindication from a cardiovascular or neurologic perspective.

    ③   Intraoperative bronchospasm is usually manifested as wheezing, increasing peak inflation pressures (plateau pressure should remain unchanged), decreasing exhaled tidal volumes, or a slowly rising waveform on the capnograph. It should be treated by increasing the concentration of the volatile **④** agent. If the bronchospasm does not resolve after deepening the anesthetic, less common causes should be considered before administering more specific drugs. Obstruction of the tracheal tube from kinking, secretions, or an overinflated balloon; bronchial intubation; active expiratory efforts (straining); pulmonary edema or embolism; and pneumothorax can all simulate bronchospasm.

Bronchospasm should be treated with a β-adrenergic agonist delivered either by aerosol or a metered-dose inhaler into the inspiratory limb of the breathing circuit. Intravenous hydrocortisone (1.5–2 mg/kg) can be given, particularly in patients with a history of glucocorticoid therapy.

At the completion of surgery, the patient should ideally be free of wheezing. Reversal of nondepolarizing neuromuscular blocking agents with anticholinesterase agents does not precipitate bronchoconstriction if preceded by the appropriate dose of an anticholinergic (see Chapter 10). Deep extubation (before airway reflexes return) prevents bronchospasm on emergence. Lidocaine as a bolus (1.5–2 mg/kg) or a continuous infusion (1–2 mg/min) may help obtund airway reflexes during emergence.

CHRONIC OBSTRUCTIVE PULMONARY DISEASE

Preoperative Considerations

COPD is the most common pulmonary disorder encountered in anesthetic practice. Its prevalence increases with age, it is strongly associated with cigarette smoking, and it has a male predominance (affecting up to 20% of men). The overwhelming majority of patients are asymptomatic or only mildly symptomatic but show expiratory airflow obstruction upon PFTs. In many patients, the obstruction has an element of reversibility, presumably from bronchospasm (as shown by improvement in response to

administration of a bronchodilator). With advancing disease, maldistribution of both ventilation and pulmonary blood flow results in areas of low $\dot{V}/\dot{Q}$ ratios (intrapulmonary shunt) as well as areas of high $\dot{V}/\dot{Q}$ ratios (dead space). Traditionally, patients have been classified as having chronic bronchitis or emphysema (Table 23–3); most patients, however, have features of both.

A. CHRONIC BRONCHITIS

The clinical diagnosis of chronic bronchitis is defined by the presence of a productive cough on most days of 3 consecutive months for at least 2 consecutive years. In addition to cigarette smoking, air pollutants, occupational exposure to dusts, recurrent pulmonary infections, and familial factors may be responsible. Secretions from hypertrophied bronchial mucous glands and mucosal edema from inflammation of the airways produce airflow obstruction. The term chronic asthmatic bronchitis may be used when bronchospasm is a major feature. Recurrent pulmonary infections (viral and bacterial) are common and often associated with bronchospasm. RV is increased but TLC is often normal. Intrapulmonary shunting is prominent, and hypoxemia is common.

    ⑤   In patients with COPD, chronic hypoxemia leads to erythrocytosis, pulmonary hypertension, and eventually right ventricular failure (cor pulmonale); this combination of findings is often referred to as the blue bloater syndrome, but < 5% of patients with COPD fit this description. In the course of disease progression, patients gradually develop chronic CO_2 retention; the normal ventilatory drive becomes less sensitive to arterial CO_2 tension and may be depressed by oxygen administration (below).

Table 23–3. Signs and symptoms of chronic obstructive pulmonary disease.

Feature	Chronic Bronchitis	Emphysema
Cough	Frequent	With exertion
Sputum	Copious	Scant
Hematocrit	Elevated	Normal
$PaCO_2$ (mm Hg)	Often elevated (> 40)	Usually normal or < 40
Chest radiograph	Increased lung markings	Hyperinflation
Elastic recoil	Normal	Decreased
Airway resistance	Increased	Normal to slightly increased
Cor pulmonale	Early	Late

B. EMPHYSEMA

Emphysema is a pathological disorder characterized by irreversible enlargement of the airways distal to terminal bronchioles and destruction of alveolar septa. The diagnosis can be reliably made with computed tomography (CT) of the chest. Mild apical emphysematous changes are a normal but clinically insignificant consequence of aging. Significant emphysema is nearly always related to cigarette smoking. Less commonly, emphysema occurs at an early age and is associated with a homozygous deficiency of α_1-antitrypsin. This is a protease inhibitor that prevents excessive activity of proteolytic enzymes (mainly elastase) in the lungs; these enzymes are produced by pulmonary neutrophils and macrophages in response to infection and pollutants. Emphysema associated with smoking may similarly be due to a relative imbalance between protease and antiprotease activities in susceptible individuals. Loss of the elastic recoil that normally supports small airways by radial traction allows premature collapse during exhalation (dynamic airway collapse). Patients characteristically have increases in RV, FRC, TLC, and the RV/TLC ratio.

Destruction of pulmonary capillaries in the alveolar septa decreases carbon monoxide diffusion capacity (see Chapter 22) and inevitably leads to pulmonary hypertension in the terminal stages of the disease. Large cystic areas, or bullae, develop in some patients. Increased dead space is a prominent feature of emphysema. **Arterial oxygen tensions are usually normal or only slightly reduced; CO_2 tension is also typically normal.** When dyspneic, patients with emphysema often purse their lips to delay closure of the small airways—which accounts for the term *pink puffers* that is often used. The majority of patients, though, have a combination of bronchitis and emphysema and carry the diagnosis of COPD.

C. TREATMENT

Treatment for COPD is primarily supportive. The most important intervention is cessation of smoking. Patients demonstrating a reversible element in airway obstruction (> 15% improvement in FEV_1 following administration of a bronchodilator) should be started on long-term bronchodilator therapy. Inhaled β_2-adrenergic agonists, glucocorticoids, and ipratropium are very useful; ipratropium has more of a role in the management of these patients than in patients with asthma. Even patients who do not show improvement in their PFTs from the use of bronchodilators may improve clinically with bronchodilator therapy. Exacerbations are often related to bouts of bronchitis, heralded by a change in sputum; frequent treatment with broad-spectrum antibiotics (eg, ampicillin, tetracycline, sulfamethoxazole-trimethoprim) may be necessary. Hypoxemia should be treated carefully with supplemental oxygen. Patients with chronic hypoxemia (PaO_2 < 55 mm Hg) and pulmonary hypertension require low-flow oxygen therapy (1–2 L/min).

Oxygen therapy can dangerously elevate $PaCO_2$ in patients with CO_2 retention; elevating PaO_2 above 60 mm Hg can precipitate respiratory failure. Abolition of a hypoxic respiratory drive or, more likely, a release of hypoxic vasoconstriction that results in greater blood flow to areas of low $\dot{V}/\dot{Q}$ may well be responsible (see Chapter 22). When cor pulmonale is present, diuretics are used to control peripheral edema; beneficial effects from digoxin and vasodilators are inconsistent. Physical conditioning has no effect on PFTs but has been shown to improve symptoms. Some studies even suggest the ability to increase oxygen consumption during exercise is inversely related to postoperative complications.

Anesthetic Considerations

A. PREOPERATIVE MANAGEMENT

Patients with COPD should be optimally prepared prior to elective surgical procedures in the same way as patients with asthma (above). They should be questioned about recent changes in dyspnea, sputum, and wheezing. Patients with an FEV_1 less than 50% of predicted (1.2–1.5 L) usually have dyspnea on exertion, whereas those with an FEV_1 less than 25% (< 1 L for men) typically have dyspnea with minimal activity. The latter finding, in patients with predominantly chronic bronchitis, is also often associated with CO_2 retention and pulmonary hypertension. PFTs, chest radiographs, and arterial blood gas measurements should be reviewed carefully. The presence of bullous changes on the radiograph should be noted. Many patients have concomitant cardiac disease and should also receive a careful cardiovascular evaluation (see Chapter 20).

In contrast to asthma, only limited improvement in respiratory function may be seen after a short period of intensive preoperative preparation. Nonetheless, preoperative interventions in patients with COPD aimed at correcting hypoxemia, relieving bronchospasm, mobilizing and reducing secretions, and treating infections may decrease the incidence of postoperative pulmonary complications. Patients at greatest risk for complications are those with preoperative pulmonary function measurements less than 50% of predicted. The possibility that postoperative ventilation may be necessary in high-risk patients should be discussed with both the patient and the surgeon.

Smoking should be discontinued for at least 6–8 weeks before the operation to decrease secretions and to reduce pulmonary complications. Cigarette smoking increases mucus production and decreases clearance.

Both gaseous and particulate phases of cigarette smoke can deplete glutathione and vitamin C and may promote oxidative injury to tissues. Unfortunately, many patients will not quit smoking for even 6–8 weeks. However, cessation of smoking for as little as 24 h has theoretical beneficial effects on the oxygen-carrying capacity of hemoglobin; acute inhalation of cigarette smoke releases carbon monoxide, which increases carboxyhemoglobin levels, and nitric oxide and nitrogen dioxide, which can lead to formation of methemoglobin.

Preoperative chest physiotherapy (chest percussion and postural drainage) and antibiotics for patients with a change in sputum are beneficial in reducing secretions. Bronchospasm should be treated with bronchodilators. Patients with moderate to severe disease may benefit from a perioperative course of glucocorticoids. Those with malnutrition should receive nutritional supplementation before major surgery. Pulmonary hypertension should be treated by optimizing oxygenation. Perioperative digitalization may be useful in patients with cor pulmonale, particularly if right ventricular failure is also present.

B. Intraoperative Management

Although regional anesthesia is often considered preferable to general anesthesia, high spinal or epidural anesthesia can decrease lung volumes, restrict the use of accessory respiratory muscles, and produce an ineffective cough, leading to dyspnea and retention of secretions. Loss of proprioception from the chest and unusual positioning, such as lithotomy or the lateral decubitus position, often accentuate dyspnea in awake patients.

Preoxygenation prior to induction of general anesthesia prevents the rapid oxygen desaturation often seen in these patients. The selection of anesthetic agents and general intraoperative management are similar to those for asthmatic patients (see above). Unfortunately, the use of bronchodilating anesthetics improves only the reversible component of airflow obstruction; significant expiratory obstruction is still often present even under deep anesthesia. Enhanced respiratory depression from anesthetics is often seen with moderate to severe disease. As with asthmatic patients, ventilation should be controlled with small to moderate tidal volumes and slow rates to avoid air trapping. Humidified gases should be used if significant bronchospasm is present and for long procedures (> 2 h). Nitrous oxide should be avoided in patients with bullae and in those who have pulmonary hypertension. Pneumothorax from expansion of bullae can occur with the former, whereas further elevations in pulmonary artery pressures may be seen with the latter. Inhibition of hypoxic pulmonary vasoconstriction by inhalation anesthetics is usually not clinically significant at the usual doses (see Chapter 22).

Measurement of arterial blood gases is desirable for, extensive intraabdominal, and all thoracic procedures.

Although pulse oximetry accurately detects significant arterial desaturation, direct measurement of arterial oxygen tensions may be necessary to detect more subtle changes in intrapulmonary shunting. Moreover, arterial CO_2 measurements should be used to guide ventilation because increased dead space widens the normal arterial-to-end-tidal CO_2 gradient. Ventilation should be adjusted to maintain a normal arterial pH. Normalization of $PaCO_2$ in patients with preoperative CO_2 retention results in alkalosis (see Chapter 30). Hemodynamic monitoring should be dictated by any underlying cardiac dysfunction as well as the extent of the surgery. In patients with pulmonary hypertension, measurements of central venous pressure reflect right ventricular function rather than intravascular volume.

Patients with pulmonary bullae are at high risk of developing pneumothoraxes intraoperatively, particularly if ventilated with positive pressure. A pneumothorax, particularly in a patient with a central line, may go undetected. In the presence of positive-pressure ventilation, however, these patients may develop a tension pneumothorax manifested by hypotension, hypoxemia, increasing peak airway pressures, and decreasing tidal volumes. In this circumstance, on examination, the patient may have a deviated trachea and absent chest movement and breath sounds (particularly if on the side of a central venous cannulation). If clinical suspicion is high, an intercatheter placed in the second intercostal space in the midclavicular line can be life saving.

At the end of surgery, the timing of extubation should balance the risk of bronchospasm with that of pulmonary insufficiency, but evidence suggests that early extubation (in the operating room) is beneficial. An awake extubation allows a more accurate assessment of immediate postoperative pulmonary function but risks bronchospasm; deep extubation decreases the risk of reflex bronchospasm but assumes that the patient will be able to maintain adequate ventilation. Patients with an FEV_1 below 50% are most likely to require a period of postoperative ventilation, particularly following upper abdominal and thoracic operations. General criteria for extubation are discussed in Chapter 49.

RESTRICTIVE PULMONARY DISEASE

Restrictive pulmonary diseases are characterized by decreased lung compliance. Lung volumes are typically reduced, with preservation of normal expiratory flow rates. Thus, both FEV_1 and FVC are reduced, but the FEV_1/FVC ratio is normal.

Restrictive pulmonary diseases include many acute and chronic intrinsic pulmonary disorders as well as extrinsic (extrapulmonary) disorders involving the pleura, chest wall, diaphragm, or neuromuscular function. Reduced lung compliance increases the work of breathing, resulting in a characteristic rapid but shallow breathing pattern. Respiratory gas exchange is usually maintained until the disease process is advanced.

ACUTE INTRINSIC PULMONARY DISORDERS

Acute intrinsic pulmonary disorders include pulmonary edema (including the acute respiratory distress syndrome [ARDS]), infectious pneumonia, and aspiration pneumonitis.

Preoperative Considerations

Reduced lung compliance in these disorders is primarily due to an increase in extravascular lung water, from either an increase in pulmonary capillary pressure or an increase in pulmonary capillary permeability (see Chapter 49). Increased pressure occurs with left ventricular failure, whereas fluid overload and increased permeability are present with ARDS. Localized or generalized increases in permeability also occur following aspiration or infectious pneumonitis.

Anesthetic Considerations

A. PREOPERATIVE MANAGEMENT

Patients with acute pulmonary disease should be spared elective surgery. In preparation for emergency procedures, oxygenation and ventilation should be optimized preoperatively to the greatest extent possible. Fluid overload should be treated with diuretics; heart failure may also require vasodilators and inotropes. Drainage of large pleural effusions should be considered. Similarly, massive abdominal distention should be relieved by nasogastric compression or drainage of ascites. Persistent hypoxemia may require positive-pressure ventilation and positive end-expiratory pressure (PEEP). Associated systemic disturbances such as hypotension or infection should be aggressively treated.

B. INTRAOPERATIVE MANAGEMENT

Selection of anesthetic agents should be tailored to each patient. Surgical patients with acute pulmonary disorders, such as ARDS, cardiogenic pulmonary edema, or pneumonia, are critically ill; anesthetic management should be a continuation of their preoperative intensive care. Anesthesia is most often provided with a combination of intravenous and inhalation agents together with a neuromuscular blocking agent. High inspired oxygen concentrations and PEEP may be required. The decreased lung compliance results in high peak inspiratory pressures during positive-pressure ventilation and increases the risk of barotrauma and volutrauma. Tidal volumes for these patients should be reduced to 4–8 mL/kg, with a compensatory increase in the ventilatory rate (14–18 breaths/min), even if the result is an increase in end-tidal CO_2. Airway pressure should generally not exceed 30 cm H_2O. The ventilator on the anesthesia machine may prove inadequate for patients with severe ARDS because of its limited gas flow capabilities, low pressure-limiting settings, and the absence of certain ventilatory modes (see Chapter 49); a more sophisticated intensive care unit ventilator should be used in such instances. Aggressive hemodynamic monitoring is recommended.

CHRONIC INTRINSIC PULMONARY DISORDERS

Chronic intrinsic pulmonary disorders are also often referred to as interstitial lung diseases. Regardless of etiology, the disease process is generally characterized by an insidious onset, chronic inflammation of alveolar walls and perialveolar tissue, and progressive pulmonary fibrosis. The latter can eventually interfere with gas exchange and ventilatory function. The inflammatory process may be primarily confined to the lungs or may be part of a generalized multiorgan process. Causes include hypersensitivity pneumonitis from occupational and environmental pollutants, drug toxicity (bleomycin and nitrofurantoin), radiation pneumonitis, idiopathic pulmonary fibrosis, autoimmune diseases, and sarcoidosis. Chronic pulmonary aspiration, oxygen toxicity, and severe ARDS can also produce chronic fibrosis.

Preoperative Considerations

Patients typically present with dyspnea on exertion and sometimes a nonproductive cough. Symptoms of cor pulmonale are present only with advanced disease. Physical examination may reveal fine (dry) crackles over the lung bases and, in late stages, evidence of right ventricular failure. The chest radiograph progresses from a "ground-glass" appearance to prominent reticulonodular markings and, finally, to a "honeycomb" appearance. Arterial blood gases usually show mild hypoxemia with normocarbia. PFTs are typical of a restrictive ventilatory defect (see above), and carbon monoxide diffusing capacity is reduced 30–50%.

Treatment is directed at abating the disease process and preventing further exposure to the causative agent (if known). Glucocorticoid and immunosuppressive therapy may be used for idiopathic pulmonary fibrosis, autoimmune disorders, and sarcoidosis. If the patient has chronic hypoxemia, oxygen therapy may be started to prevent, or attenuate, right ventricular failure.

Anesthetic Considerations

A. PREOPERATIVE MANAGEMENT

Preoperative evaluation should focus on determining the degree of pulmonary impairment as well as the underlying disease process. The latter is important in determining the potential involvement of other organs. A history of dyspnea on exertion (or at rest) should be evaluated further with PFTs and arterial blood gas analysis. A vital capacity less than 15 mL/kg is indicative of severe dysfunction (normal is > 70 mL/kg). A chest radiograph is helpful in assessing disease severity.

B. INTRAOPERATIVE MANAGEMENT

The management of these patients is complicated by a predisposition to hypoxemia and the need to control ventilation to ensure optimum gas exchange; anesthetic drug selection is generally not critical. The reduction in FRC (and oxygen stores) predisposes these patients to rapid hypoxemia following induction of anesthesia (see Chapter 22); their uptake of inhalation anesthetics may also be accelerated. Because these patients may be more susceptible to oxygen-induced toxicity, particularly patients who have received bleomycin, the inspired fractional concentration of oxygen should be kept to the minimum concentration compatible with acceptable oxygenation (SpO_2 of > 88–92%). High peak inspiratory pressures during mechanical ventilation increase the risk of pneumothorax and should prompt smaller than normal tidal volumes with a faster rate.

EXTRINSIC RESTRICTIVE PULMONARY DISORDERS

Extrinsic restrictive pulmonary disorders alter gas exchange by interfering with normal lung expansion. They include pleural effusions, pneumothorax, mediastinal masses, kyphoscoliosis, pectus excavatum, neuromuscular disorders, and increased intraabdominal pressure from ascites, pregnancy, or bleeding. Marked obesity also produces a restrictive ventilatory defect (see Chapter 36). Anesthetic considerations are similar to those discussed for intrinsic restrictive disorders.

■ PULMONARY EMBOLISM

Preoperative Considerations

Pulmonary embolism results from the entry of blood clots, fat, tumor cells, air, amniotic fluid, or foreign material into the venous system. Clots from the lower extremities (nearly always above the knee), pelvic veins, or, less commonly, the right side of the heart are usually responsible. Venous stasis or hypercoagulability is often contributory in such cases (Table 23–4). Pulmonary embolism can also occur intraoperatively in normal individuals undergoing certain procedures. Fat embolism is discussed in Chapter 40; air embolism is discussed in Chapter 26.

A. PATHOPHYSIOLOGY

Embolic occlusions in the pulmonary circulation increase dead space, and, if minute ventilation does not change, this increase in dead space should theoretically increase $PaCO_2$. However, in practice, hypoxemia is more often seen. Pulmonary emboli acutely increase pulmonary vascular resistance by reducing the cross-sectional area of the pulmonary vasculature causing reflex and humoral vasoconstriction. Localized or generalized reflex bronchoconstriction further increases areas with low $\dot{V}/\dot{Q}$ ratios. The net effect is an increase in pulmonary shunt and hypoxemia. The affected area loses its surfactant within hours and may become atelectatic within 24–48 h. Pulmonary infarction occurs if the embolus involves a large vessel and collateral blood flow from the bronchial circulation is insufficient for that part of the lung (incidence < 10%). In previously healthy persons, occlusion of more than 50% of the pulmonary circulation (massive pulmonary embolism) is necessary before sustained pulmonary hypertension is seen. Patients with preexisting cardiac or pulmonary disease can develop acute pulmonary hypertension with occlusions of lesser magnitude. A sustained increase in right ventricular afterload can precipitate acute right ventricular failure. If the patient survives acute pulmonary thromboembolism, the thrombus usually begins to resolve within 1–2 weeks.

B. DIAGNOSIS

Clinical manifestations of pulmonary embolism include sudden tachypnea, dyspnea, chest pain, or hemoptysis.

Table 23–4. Factors associated with deep venous thrombosis and pulmonary embolism.

Prolonged bed rest
Postpartum state
Fracture of the lower extremities
Surgery on the lower extremities
Carcinoma
Heart failure
Obesity
Surgery lasting more than 30 min
Hypercoagulability
Antithrombin III deficiency
Protein C deficiency
Protein S deficiency
Plasminogen-activator deficiency

The latter generally implies infarction. Symptoms are often absent or mild and nonspecific unless massive embolism has occurred. Wheezing may be present on auscultation. Arterial blood gas analysis typically shows mild hypoxemia with respiratory alkalosis (the latter due to an increase in ventilation). The chest radiograph is commonly normal but may show an area of oligemia (radiolucency), a wedge-shaped density with an infarct, atelectasis with an elevated diaphragm, or an asymmetrically enlarged proximal pulmonary artery with acute pulmonary hypertension. Cardiac signs include tachycardia and wide fixed splitting of the S_2 heart sound; hypotension with elevated central venous pressure is usually indicative of right ventricular failure. The electrocardiogram frequently shows tachycardia and may show signs of acute cor pulmonale, such as new right axis deviation, right bundle branch block, and tall peaked T waves. Impedance plethysmography is also helpful in demonstrating deep venous thrombosis above the knee. The diagnosis of embolism is more difficult to make intraoperatively (see below).

Pulmonary angiography is the most accurate means of diagnosing a pulmonary embolism, but noninvasive pulmonary perfusion and ventilation scans using γ-emitting radionucleotides may be helpful and are widely used. A normal perfusion scan usually excludes significant embolism. An abnormal perfusion scan is diagnostic only if perfusion defects are present in areas with normal ventilation. Helical CT scanning is increasingly used in large medical centers to diagnose pulmonary embolism.

C. Treatment

The best treatment for pulmonary embolism is prevention. Heparin (unfractionated heparin 5000 U subcutaneously every 12 h begun preoperatively or immediately postoperatively in high-risk patients), oral anticoagulation (warfarin), aspirin, or dextran therapy together with early ambulation can decrease the incidence of postoperative emboli. The use of high elastic stockings and pneumatic compression of the legs may also decrease the incidence of venous thrombosis in the legs but not in the pelvis or the heart.

Systemic anticoagulation prevents the formation of new blood clots or the extension of existing clots. Heparin therapy is begun with the goal of achieving an activated partial thromboplastin time of 1.5–2.4 times normal. Low-molecular-weight heparin (LMWH) is as effective and is given subcutaneously at a fixed dose (based on body weight) without laboratory monitoring. LMWH is more expensive than unfractionated heparin but is more cost-effective. In high-risk patients, LMWH is started either 12 h before surgery, 12–24 h after surgery, or at 50% the usual dose 4–6 h after surgery. All patients should start warfarin therapy concur-

rent with starting heparin therapy, and the two should overlap for 4–5 days. The international normalized ratio should be within the therapeutic range on two consecutive measurements at least 24 h apart before the heparin is stopped. Warfarin should be continued for 3–12 months. Thrombolytic therapy with tissue plasminogen activator or streptokinase is indicated for patients with massive pulmonary embolism or circulatory collapse. Recent surgery and active bleeding are contraindications to anticoagulation and thrombolytic therapy. In these cases, an inferior vena cava umbrella filter may be placed to prevent recurrent pulmonary emboli. Pulmonary embolectomy may be indicated for patients with massive embolism in whom thrombolytic therapy is contraindicated.

Anesthetic Considerations

A. Preoperative Management

Patients with acute pulmonary embolism may present in the operating room for placement of a caval filter or, rarely, for pulmonary embolectomy. In most instances, the patient will have a history of pulmonary embolism and presents for unrelated surgery; in this group of patients, the risk of interrupting anticoagulant therapy perioperatively is unknown. If the acute episode is more than 1 year old, the risk of temporarily stopping anticoagulant therapy is probably small. Moreover, except in the case of chronic recurrent pulmonary emboli, pulmonary function has usually returned to normal. The emphasis in the perioperative management of these patients should be in preventing new episodes of embolism (see above).

B. Intraoperative Management

Vena cava filters are usually placed percutaneously under local anesthesia with sedation. Patients may display enhanced sensitivity to the circulatory effects of most anesthetic agents. Decreased venous return during placement of the device can precipitate hypotension.

Although no definite recommendations can be made regarding the choice of anesthesia for patients with a history of pulmonary embolism, studies suggest that regional anesthesia for some procedures (eg, hip surgery) decreases the incidence of postoperative deep venous thrombosis and pulmonary embolism. The use of regional anesthesia is contraindicated in patients with residual anticoagulation or a prolonged bleeding time. When general anesthesia is selected, the use of short-acting agents may allow early postoperative ambulation.

Patients presenting for pulmonary embolectomy are critically ill. They are usually already intubated but tolerate positive-pressure ventilation poorly. Inotropic support is necessary until the clot is removed. They also tolerate all anesthetic agents very poorly. Small doses of an opioid, etomidate, or ketamine may be used, but the latter can theoretically increase pulmonary artery pressures. Cardiopulmonary bypass is required.

C. Intraoperative Pulmonary Embolism

Significant pulmonary embolism is a rare occurrence during anesthesia. Diagnosis requires a high index of suspicion. Air emboli are common but are often overlooked unless large amounts are entrained. Fat embolism can occur during orthopedic procedures (see Chapter 40); amniotic fluid embolism is a rare, unpredictable, and often fatal, complication of obstetrical delivery (see Chapter 43). Thromboembolism may occur intraoperatively during prolonged procedures. The clot may have been present prior to surgery or may form intraoperatively; surgical manipulations or a change in the patient's position may then dislodge the venous thrombus. Manipulation of tumors with intravascular extension can similarly produce pulmonary embolism.

 Intraoperative pulmonary embolism usually presents as unexplained sudden hypotension, hypoxemia, or bronchospasm. A decrease in end-tidal CO_2 concentration is also suggestive of pulmonary embolism but not specific. Invasive monitoring may reveal elevated central venous and pulmonary arterial pressures. Depending on the type and location of an embolism, a transesophageal echocardiogram may be helpful. **If air is identified in the right atrium, or if it is suspected, emergent central vein cannulation and aspiration of the air may be lifesaving.** For all other emboli, treatment is supportive, with intravenous fluids and inotropes. Placement of a vena cava filter should be considered postoperatively.

CASE DISCUSSION: LAPAROSCOPIC SURGERY

A 45-year-old woman is scheduled for a laparoscopic cholecystectomy. Known medical problems include obesity and a history of smoking.

What are the advantages of laparoscopic cholecystectomy compared with open cholecystectomy?

Laparoscopic techniques have rapidly increased in popularity because of the multiple benefits associated with much smaller incisions than with traditional open techniques. These benefits include decreased postoperative pain, less postoperative pulmonary impairment, a reduction in postoperative ileus, shorter hospital stays, earlier ambulation, and smaller surgical scars. Thus, laparoscopic surgery can provide substantial medical and economic advantages.

How does laparoscopic surgery affect intraoperative pulmonary function?

The hallmark of laparoscopy is the creation of a pneumoperitoneum with pressurized CO_2. The resulting increase in intraabdominal pressure displaces the diaphragm cephalad, causing a decrease in lung compliance and an increase in peak inspiratory pressure. **Atelectasis, diminished FRC, ventilation/perfusion mismatch, and pulmonary shunting contribute to a decrease in arterial oxygenation.** *These changes should be exaggerated in this obese patient with a long history of tobacco use.*

The high solubility of CO_2 increases systemic absorption by the vasculature of the peritoneum. This, combined with smaller tidal volumes because of poor lung compliance, leads to increased arterial CO_2 levels and decreased pH.

Why does patient position affect oxygenation?

A head-down (Trendelenburg) position is commonly requested during insertion of the Veress needle and cannula. This position causes a cephalad shift in abdominal viscera and the diaphragm. FRC, total lung volume, and pulmonary compliance will be decreased. Although these changes are usually well tolerated by healthy patients, this patient's obesity and presumed preexisting lung disease increase the likelihood for hypoxemia. A head-down position also tends to shift the trachea upward, so that a tracheal tube anchored at the mouth may migrate into the right mainstem bronchus. This tracheobronchial shift may be exacerbated during insufflation of the abdomen.

After insufflation, the patient's position is usually changed to a steep head-up position (reverse Trendelenburg) to facilitate surgical dissection. The respiratory effects of the head-up position are the opposite of the head-down position: FRC increases and the work of breathing decreases.

Does laparoscopic surgery affect cardiac function?

Moderate insufflation pressures usually leave heart rate, central venous pressure, and cardiac output unchanged or slightly elevated. This appears to result from increased effective cardiac filling because blood tends to be forced out of the abdomen and into the chest. **Higher insufflation pressures (> 25 cm H_2O or 18 mm Hg), however, tend to collapse the major abdominal veins (particularly the inferior vena cava), which decreases** *venous return and leads to a drop in preload and cardiac output in some patients.*

Hypercarbia, if allowed to develop, will stimulate the sympathetic nervous system and thus increase blood pressure, heart rate, and the risk of arrhythmias. Attempting to compensate by increasing the tidal volume or respiratory rate will increase the mean intrathoracic pressure, further hindering venous return and increasing mean pulmonary artery pressures. These effects can prove particularly challenging in patients with restrictive lung disease, impaired cardiac function, or intravascular volume depletion.

Although the Trendelenburg position increases preload, mean arterial pressure and cardiac output usually either remain unchanged or decrease. These seemingly paradoxical responses may be explained by carotid and aortic baroreceptor-mediated reflexes. The reverse Trendelenburg position decreases preload, cardiac output, and mean arterial pressure.

Describe the advantages and disadvantages of alternative anesthetic techniques for this patient.

Anesthetic approaches to laparoscopic surgery include infiltration of local anesthetic with an intravenous sedative, epidural or spinal anesthesia, or general anesthesia. Experience with local anesthesia has been largely limited to brief gynecologic procedures (laparoscopic tubal sterilization, intrafallopian transfers) in young, healthy, and motivated patients. Although postoperative recovery is rapid, patient discomfort and suboptimal visualization of intraabdominal organs preclude the use of this local anesthesia technique for laparoscopic cholecystectomy.

Epidural or spinal anesthesia represents another alternative for laparoscopic surgery. A high level is required for complete muscle relaxation and to prevent diaphragmatic irritation caused by gas insufflation and surgical manipulations, however. An obese patient with lung disease may not be able to increase spontaneous ventilation to maintain normocarbia in the face of a high (T2 level) regional block during insufflation and a 20° Trendelenburg position. Another disadvantage of a regional technique is the occasional occurrence of referred shoulder pain from diaphragmatic irritation. General anesthesia would therefore be the preferred technique for this patient.

Does a general anesthetic technique require tracheal intubation?

Tracheal intubation with positive-pressure ventilation is usually favored for many reasons: the risk of regurgitation from increased intraabdominal pressure during insufflation; the necessity for controlled ventilation to prevent hypercapnia; the relatively high peak inspiratory pressures required because of the pneumoperitoneum; the need for neuromuscular blockade during surgery to allow lower insufflation pressures, provide better visualization, and prevent unexpected patient movement; and the placement of a nasogastric tube and gastric decompression to minimize the risk of visceral perforation during trocar introduction and optimize visualization. The obese patient presented here would benefit from intubation to decrease the likelihood of hypoxemia, hypercarbia, and aspiration.

What special monitoring should be considered for this patient?

Monitoring end-tidal CO_2 normally provides an adequate guide for determining the minute ventilation required to maintain normocarbia. This assumes a constant gradient between arterial CO_2 and end-tidal CO_2, which is generally valid in healthy patients undergoing laparoscopy. This assumption would not apply if alveolar dead space changes during surgery. For example, any significant reduction in lung perfusion increases alveolar dead space, dilutes expired CO_2, and thereby decreases end-tidal CO_2 measurements. This may occur during laparoscopy if cardiac output drops because of high inflation pressures, the reverse Trendelenburg position, or gas embolism. Furthermore, abdominal distention lowers pulmonary compliance. Large tidal volumes are usually avoided because they are associated with high peak inspiratory pressures and can cause considerable movement of the surgical field. The resulting choice of lower tidal volumes and higher respiratory rates may lead to poor alveolar gas sampling and erroneous end-tidal CO_2 measurements. In fact, end-tidal CO_2 values have been found to be particularly unreliable in patients with significant cardiac or pulmonary disease undergoing laparoscopy. Thus, placement of an arterial catheter should be considered in patients with cardiopulmonary disease.

What are some possible complications of laparoscopic surgery?

Surgical complications include hemorrhage if a major abdominal vessel is lacerated or peritonitis if a viscus is perforated during trocar introduction. Significant intraoperative hemorrhage may go unrecognized because of the limitations of laparoscopic visualization. Fulguration has been associated with bowel burns and bowel gas explosions. The use of *pressurized gas introduces the possibility of extravasation of CO_2 along tissue planes, resulting in subcutaneous emphysema, pneumomediastinum, or pneumothorax. Nitrous oxide should be discontinued and insufflating pressures decreased as much as possible. Patients with this complication may benefit from the continuation of mechanical ventilation into the immediate postoperative period.*

Venous CO_2 embolism resulting from unintentional insufflation of gas into an open vein may lead to hypoxemia, pulmonary hypertension, pulmonary edema, and cardiovascular collapse. Unlike air embolism, end-tidal CO_2 may transiently increase during CO_2 gas embolism. Treatment includes immediate release of the pneumoperitoneum, discontinuation of nitrous oxide, insertion of a central venous catheter for gas aspiration, and placement of the patient in a head-down left lateral decubitus position.

Vagal stimulation during trocar insertion, peritoneal insufflation, or manipulation of viscera can result in bradycardia and even sinus arrest. Although this usually resolves spontaneously, elimination of the stimulus (eg, deflation of the peritoneum) and administration of a vagolytic drug (eg, atropine sulfate) should be considered. Intraoperative hypotension may be more common during laparoscopic cholecystectomy than during cholecystectomy by laparotomy. Preoperative fluid loading has been recommended to avoid this complication.

Even though laparoscopic procedures are associated with less muscle trauma and incisional pain than is open surgery, pulmonary dysfunction can persist for at least 24 h postoperatively. For example, forced expiratory volume, forced vital capacity, and forced expiratory flow are reduced by approximately 25% following laparoscopic cholecystectomy as opposed to a 50% reduction following open cholecystectomy. The cause of this dysfunction may be related to diaphragmatic tension during the pneumoperitoneum.

Nausea and vomiting are common following laparoscopic procedures, despite routine emptying of the stomach with a nasogastric tube. Pharmacological prophylaxis is recommended.

SUGGESTED READING

Benumof J: *Anesthesia and Uncommon Diseases,* 4th ed. W.B. Saunders, 1998.

Evers AS, Maze M: *Anesthetic Pharmacology. Physiologic Principles and Clinical Practice.* Churchill Livingstone, 2004. Chapters 20 and 40 are excellent chapters that provide good reviews of pulmonary function and bronchodilator therapy.

Hurford WE: The bronchospastic patient. Int Anesthesiol Clin 2000;38:77.

Lumb A, Nunn JF: *Nunn's Applied Respiratory Physiology,* 5th ed. Butterworth-Heinemann, 2000.

Reilly JJ Jr: Evidence-based preoperative evaluation candidates for thoracotomy. Chest 1999;116:474.

Anesthesia for Thoracic Surgery

KEY CONCEPTS

  During one-lung ventilation, the mixing of unoxygenated blood from the collapsed upper lung with oxygenated blood from the still-ventilated dependent lung widens the P_{A-a} (alveolar-to-arterial) O_2 gradient and often results in hypoxemia.

 Malpositioning of a double-lumen tube is usually indicated by poor lung compliance and low exhaled tidal volume.

 If epidural opioids are to be used postoperatively, their intravenous use should be limited during surgery to prevent excessive postoperative respiratory depression.

 Postoperative hemorrhage complicates about 3% of thoracotomies and may be associated with up to 20% mortality. Signs of hemorrhage include increased chest tube drainage (> 200 mL/h), hypotension, tachycardia, and a falling hematocrit.

 Bronchopleural fistula presents as a sudden large air leak from the chest tube that may be associated with an increasing pneumothorax and partial lung collapse.

 Acute herniation of the heart into the operative hemithorax can occur through the pericardial defect that is left following a radical pneumonectomy.

 Nitrous oxide is contraindicated in patients with cysts or bullae because it can expand the air space and cause rupture. The latter may be signaled by sudden hypotension, bronchospasm, or an abrupt rise in peak inflation pressure and requires immediate placement of a chest tube.

 Following transplantation, peak inspiratory pressures should be maintained at the minimum pressure compatible with good lung expansion, and the inspired oxygen concentration should be maintained at < 60%.

 Regardless of the procedure, the major anesthetic consideration for patients with esophageal disease is the risk of pulmonary aspiration.

 During the transhiatal approach to esophagectomy, substernal and diaphragmatic retractors can interfere with cardiac function.

Indications and techniques for thoracic surgery have continually evolved since its origins. Common indications are no longer restricted to complications of tuberculosis and suppurative pneumonitis but now include thoracic malignancies (mainly of the lungs and esophagus), chest trauma, esophageal disease, and mediastinal tumors. Diagnostic procedures such as bronchoscopy, mediastinoscopy, and open-lung biopsies are also common. Anesthetic techniques for separating the ventilation to each lung have allowed

the refinement of surgical techniques to the point that many procedures are increasingly performed thoracoscopically. High-frequency jet ventilation and cardiopulmonary bypass (CPB) now allow complex procedures such as tracheal resection and lung transplantation, respectively, to be performed. Anesthetic management of cardiac surgery and anesthesia for thoracic aortic aneurysms are discussed in Chapter 21; anesthesia for thoracic trauma is reviewed in Chapter 41.

■ PHYSIOLOGICAL CONSIDERATIONS DURING THORACIC ANESTHESIA

Thoracic surgery presents a unique set of physiological problems for the anesthesiologist that requires special consideration. These include physiological derangements caused by placing the patient with one side down (lateral decubitus position), opening the chest (**open pneumothorax**), and the frequent need for one-lung ventilation.

THE LATERAL DECUBITUS POSITION

The lateral decubitus position provides optimal access for most operations on the lungs, pleura, esophagus, the great vessels, other mediastinal structures, and vertebrae. Unfortunately, this position may significantly alter the normal pulmonary ventilation/perfusion relationships (see Chapter 22).

These derangements are further accentuated by induction of anesthesia, initiation of mechanical ventilation, neuromuscular blockade, opening the chest, and surgical retraction. Although perfusion continues to favor the dependent (lower) lung, ventilation progressively favors the less perfused upper lung. The resulting mismatch markedly increases the risk of hypoxemia.

The Awake State

When a supine patient assumes the lateral decubitus position, ventilation/perfusion matching is preserved during spontaneous ventilation. The lower lung receives more perfusion and more ventilation than the upper lung. The former is the result of gravity; the latter occurs because (1) contraction of the dependent hemidiaphragm is more efficient as it assumes a higher position in the chest (compared with the upper hemidiaphragm) due to its disproportionate share in supporting the weight of abdominal contents and (2) the dependent lung is on a more favorable part of the compliance curve (Figure 24–1).

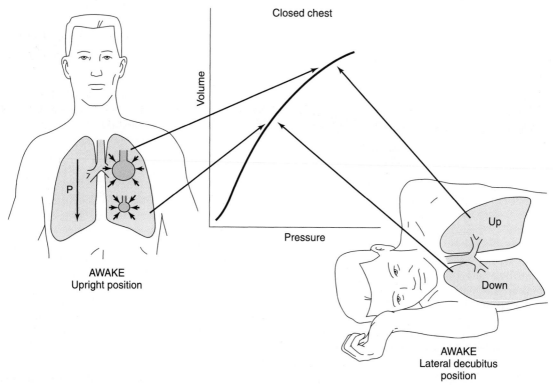

Figure 24–1. The effect of the lateral decubitus position on lung compliance.

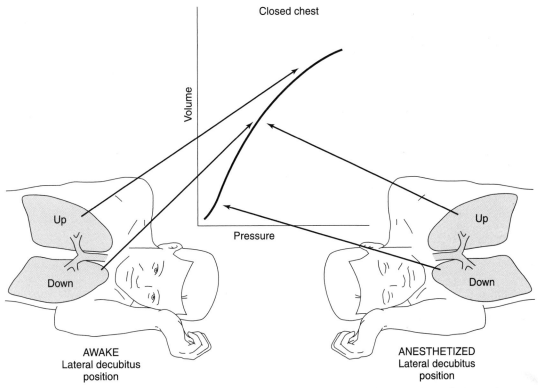

Figure 24–2. The effect of anesthesia on lung compliance in the lateral decubitus position. The upper lung assumes a more favorable position and the lower lung becomes less compliant.

Induction of Anesthesia

The decrease in functional residual capacity (FRC) with induction of general anesthesia (see Chapter 22) moves the upper lung to a more favorable part of the compliance curve but moves the lower lung to a less compliant position (Figure 24–2). As a result, the upper lung is ventilated more than the dependent lower lung; ventilation/perfusion mismatching occurs because the dependent lung continues to have greater perfusion.

Positive-Pressure Ventilation

Controlled positive-pressure ventilation favors the upper lung in the lateral position because it is more compliant than the lower one. Neuromuscular blockade enhances this effect by allowing the abdominal contents to rise up further against the dependent hemidiaphragm and impede ventilation of the lower lung. Using a rigid "bean bag" to maintain the patient in the lateral decubitus position further restricts movement of the dependent hemithorax. Finally, opening the nondependent side of the chest further accentuates differences in compliance between the two sides because the upper lung is now less restricted in movement. All these effects worsen ventilation/perfusion mismatching and predispose to hypoxemia.

THE OPEN PNEUMOTHORAX

The lungs are normally kept expanded by a negative pleural pressure—the net result of the tendency of the lung to collapse and the chest wall to expand (see Chapter 22). When one side of the chest is opened, the negative pleural pressure is lost and the elastic recoil of the lung on that side tends to collapse it. Spontaneous ventilation with an open pneumothorax in the lateral position results in paradoxical respirations and mediastinal shift. These two phenomena can cause progressive hypoxemia and hypercapnia, but, fortunately, their effects are overcome by the use of positive-pressure ventilation during general anesthesia and thoracotomy.

Mediastinal Shift

During spontaneous ventilation in the lateral position, inspiration causes pleural pressure to become more neg-

INSPIRATION

Pneumothorax

EXPIRATION

Pneumothorax

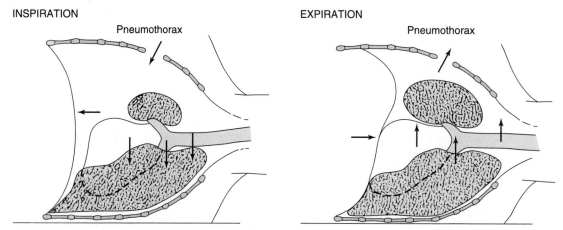

Figure 24–3. Mediastinal shift in a spontaneously breathing patient in the lateral decubitus position. (Reproduced, with permission, from Tarhan S, Moffitt EA: Principles of thoracic anesthesia. Surg Clin North Am 1973;53:813.)

ative on the dependent side but not on the side of the open pneumothorax. This results in a downward shift of the mediastinum during inspiration and an upward shift during expiration (Figure 24–3). The major effect of the mediastinal shift is to decrease the contribution of the dependent lung to the tidal volume.

Spontaneous ventilation in a patient with an open pneumothorax also results in to-and-fro gas flow between the dependent and nondependent lung (paradoxical respiration [pendeluft]). During inspiration, the pneumothorax increases, and gas flows from the upper lung across the carina to the dependent lung. During expiration, the gas flow reverses and moves from the dependent to the upper lung (Figure 24–4).

ONE-LUNG VENTILATION

Intentional collapse of the lung on the operative side facilitates most thoracic procedures but greatly complicates anesthetic management. Because the collapsed lung continues to be perfused and is deliberately no longer ventilated, the patient develops a large right-to-left intrapulmonary shunt (20–30%). During one-lung ventilation, the mixing of unoxygenated blood from the collapsed upper lung with oxygenated blood from the still-ventilated dependent lung widens the PA–a (alveolar-to-arterial) O_2 gradient and often results in hypoxemia. Fortunately, blood flow to the nonventilated lung is decreased by hypoxic pul-

INSPIRATION

Pneumothorax

EXPIRATION

Pneumothorax

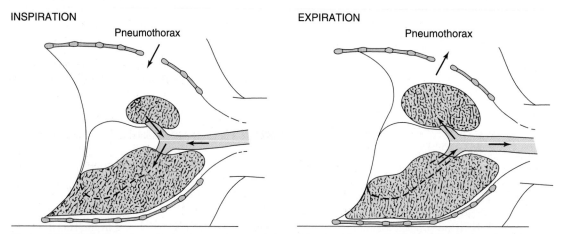

Figure 24–4. Paradoxical respiration in spontaneously breathing patients on their side. (Reproduced, with permission, from Tarhan S, Moffitt EA: Principles of thoracic anesthesia. Surg Clin North Am 1973;53:813.)

monary vasoconstriction (HPV—see Chapter 22) and possibly surgical compression of the upper lung.

Factors known to inhibit HPV and thus worsen the right-to-left shunting include (1) very high or very low pulmonary artery pressures; (2) hypocapnia; (3) high or very low mixed venous PO_2; (4) vasodilators such as nitroglycerin, nitroprusside, β-adrenergic agonists (including dobutamine and salbutamol), and calcium channel blockers; (5) pulmonary infection; and (6) inhalation anesthetics (see Chapter 22).

Factors that decrease blood flow to the ventilated lung can be equally detrimental; they counteract the effect of HPV by indirectly increasing blood flow to the collapsed lung. Such factors include (1) high mean airway pressures in the ventilated lung due to high positive end-expiratory pressure (PEEP), hyperventilation, or high peak inspiratory pressures; (2) a low FIO_2, which produces hypoxic pulmonary vasoconstriction in the ventilated lung; (3) vasoconstrictors that may have a greater effect on normoxic vessels than hypoxic ones; and (4) intrinsic PEEP that develops due to inadequate expiratory times.

Elimination of CO_2 is usually not affected by one-lung ventilation provided minute ventilation is unchanged and preexisting CO_2 retention was not present while ventilating both lungs; arterial CO_2 tension is usually not appreciably altered.

■ TECHNIQUES FOR ONE-LUNG VENTILATION

One-lung ventilation can also be utilized to isolate a lung or to facilitate ventilatory management under certain conditions (Table 24–1). Three techniques can be employed: (1) placement of a double-lumen bronchial tube, (2) use of a single-lumen tracheal tube in conjunction with a bronchial blocker, or (3) use of a single-lumen bronchial tube. Double-lumen tubes are most often used.

DOUBLE-LUMEN BRONCHIAL TUBES

The principal advantages of double-lumen tubes are relative ease of placement, the ability to ventilate either or both lungs, and the ability to suction either lung.

All double-lumen tubes (Table 24–2) share the following characteristics:

- A longer bronchial lumen that enters either the right or left main bronchus and another shorter tracheal lumen that remains in the lower trachea
- A preformed curve that allows preferential entry into either bronchus

Table 24–1. Indications for one-lung ventilation.

Patient-related
  Confine infection to one lung
  Confine bleeding to one lung
  Separate ventilation to each lung
    Bronchopleural fistula
    Tracheobronchial disruption
    Large lung cyst or bulla
  Severe hypoxemia due to unilateral lung disease
Procedure-related
  Repair of thoracic aortic aneurysm
  Lung resection
    Pneumonectomy
    Lobectomy
    Segmental resection
  Thoracoscopy
  Esophageal surgery
  Single-lung transplantation
  Anterior approach to the thoracic spine
  Bronchoalveolar lavage

- A bronchial cuff
- A tracheal cuff

Ventilation can be delivered to only one lung by clamping either the bronchial or tracheal lumen with both cuffs inflated; opening the port on the appropriate connector allows the ipsilateral lung to collapse. Because of differences in bronchial anatomy between the two sides, tubes are designed specifically for either the right or left bronchus.

The most commonly used double-lumen tubes are of the Robert-Shaw type. They are available in sizes 35, 37, 39, and 41F (internal diameters of about 5.0, 5.5, 6.0, and 6.5 mm, respectively). A 39F tube is used for most men, whereas a 37F tube is selected for most women.

Anatomic Considerations

The adult trachea is 11–13 cm long. It begins at the level of the cricoid cartilage (C6) and bifurcates behind the

Table 24–2. Types of double-lumen tubes.

Name	Bronchus Intubated	Carinal Hook	Shape of Lumen
Carlens	Left	Yes	Oval
White	Right	Yes	Oval
Robert-Shaw	Right or left	No	D-shaped

sternomanubrial joint (T5). Major differences between the right and left main bronchi are as follows: (1) the wider right bronchus diverges away from the trachea at a 25° angle, whereas the left bronchus diverges at a 45° angle (Figure 24–5); (2) the right bronchus has upper, middle, and lower lobe branches, whereas the left bronchus divides into only upper and lower lobe branches; and (3) the orifice of the right upper lobe bronchus is about 1–2.5 cm from the carina, whereas that of the left upper lobe is about 5 cm distal to the carina.

Right-sided bronchial tubes must have a slit in the bronchial cuff for ventilating the right upper lobe (Figure 24–6). Anatomic variations between individuals in the distance between the right carina and the upper lobe orifice often result in difficulties in ventilating that lobe with right-sided tubes. Right-sided tubes were designed for left thoracotomies, whereas left-sided tubes were designed for right thoracotomies. Most anesthesiologists, however, use a left-sided tube regardless of the operative side; for left-sided surgery, the tube can be withdrawn into the trachea prior to clamping of the left bronchus, if necessary.

Some tubes have carinal hooks (eg, Carlens and White), but the difficulties often encountered in placing them through the larynx have caused many clinicians to abandon them. The most widely used double-lumen tubes are disposable versions of the Robert-Shaw tube.

Placement of Double-Lumen Tubes

Laryngoscopy with a curved (MacIntosh) blade usually provides better visualization than a straight blade; the latter may be more useful if the larynx is anterior. The double-lumen tube is passed with the distal curvature concave anteriorly and is rotated 90° (toward the side of the bronchus to be intubated) after the tip enters the larynx (Figure 24–7). It is advanced until resistance is felt; the average depth of insertion is about 29 cm (at the teeth). Correct tube placement should be established using a preset protocol (Figure 24–8 and Table 24–3) and confirmed by flexible fiberoptic bronchoscopy. When problems are encountered in intubating the patient with the double-lumen tube, placement of a smaller (6.0–7.0 i.d.) regular tube should be attempted;

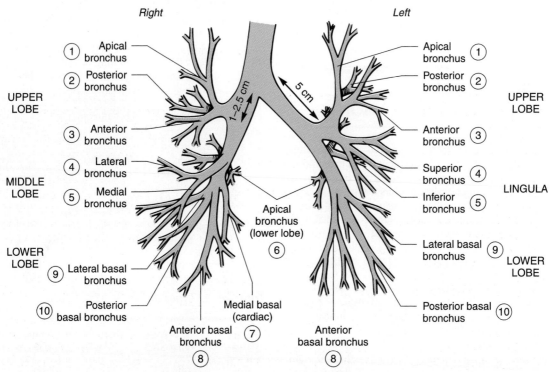

Figure 24–5. Anatomy of the tracheobronchial tree. Note bronchopulmonary segments (1–10) as numbered. (Adapted and reproduced, with permission, from Gothard JWW, Branthwaite MA: *Anesthesia for Thoracic Surgery.* Blackwell, 1982.)

Figure 24–6. Correct position of a left- and right-sided double-lumen tube.

once positioned in the trachea, the latter can be exchanged for the double-lumen tube by utilizing a specially designed catheter guide ("tube exchanger").

Most double-lumen tubes easily accommodate bronchoscopes with a 3.6- to 4.2-mm outer diameter. When the bronchoscope is introduced into the tracheal lumen and advanced to the tracheal orifice, the carina should be visible (Figure 24–9) and the bronchial tip of the tube should be seen entering the left bronchus; additionally, the top of the bronchial cuff (usually colored blue) should be visible but should not extend above the carina. If the bronchial cuff of a left-sided double-lumen tube is not visible, it may be low enough to obstruct the orifice of the left lower lobe (below); the tube should be withdrawn until the cuff becomes visible. The bronchial cuff should ideally be inflated only to a point at which the audible leak from the open tracheal lumen disappears while ventilating only through the bronchial lumen. Tube position should be reconfirmed after the patient is positioned for surgery because the tube may move relative to the carina as the patient is turned into the lateral decubitus position.

Malpositioning of a double-lumen tube is usually indicated by poor lung compliance and low exhaled tidal volume. Problems with left-sided double-lumen tubes are usually related to one of three possibilities: (1) the tube is too deep, (2) it is not deep enough, or (3) it entered the right bronchus (the wrong side). If the tube is too deep (as can readily occur in a short person), the bronchial cuff can obstruct the left upper or the left lower lobe orifice with the opening of the bronchial lumen in the left lower or left upper lobe bronchus, respectively. When the tube is not advanced far enough, the bronchial cuff can occlude the right bronchus. In both instances, deflation of the bronchial cuff improves ventilation to the affected lung and helps identify the problem. In some patients the bronchial lumen may be within the left upper or left lower lobe bronchus but with the tracheal opening remaining above the carina; this situation is suggested by collapse of only one of the left lobes when the bronchial lumen is clamped. Worse, if the surgical procedure is in the right thorax, when the tracheal lumen is clamped, only the left upper or left lower lobe will be ventilated; hypoxia usually develops rapidly.

A   B   C

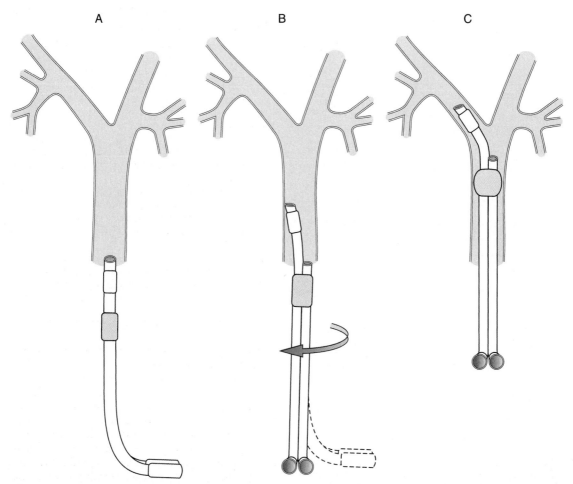

Figure 24–7. Placement of a left-sided double-lumen tube. Note that the tube is turned 90° as soon as it enters the larynx. ***A:*** Initial position. ***B:*** Rotated 90°. ***C:*** Final position.

Problems with right-sided double-lumen tubes arise because the orifice of the right upper lobe is close (1.0–2.5 cm) to the carina. It is very easy to occlude the right upper lobe orifice with the bronchial tube cuff and, hence, the preference for using left-sided double-lumen tubes.

If the tube inadvertently enters the wrong bronchus, the fiberoptic bronchoscope can be used to reposition it into the correct side: (1) the bronchoscope is passed through the bronchial lumen to the tip of the tube; (2) under direct vision, the tube and the bronchoscope are withdrawn together into the trachea just above the carina; (3) the bronchoscope alone is then advanced into the correct bronchus; and (4) the double-lumen tube is gently advanced over the bronchoscope, which functions as a stylet to guide the bronchial lumen into the correct bronchus.

Complications of Double-Lumen Tubes

Major complications of double-lumen tubes include (1) hypoxemia due to tube malplacement or occlusion, (2) traumatic laryngitis (particularly with tubes that have a carinal hook), (3) tracheobronchial rupture resulting from overinflation of the bronchial cuff, and (4) inadvertent suturing of the tube to a bronchus during surgery (detected as the inability to withdraw the tube during attempted extubation).

SINGLE-LUMEN TRACHEAL TUBES WITH A BRONCHIAL BLOCKER

Bronchial blockers are inflatable devices that are passed alongside or through a single-lumen tracheal tube to selectively occlude a bronchial orifice. A single-lumen

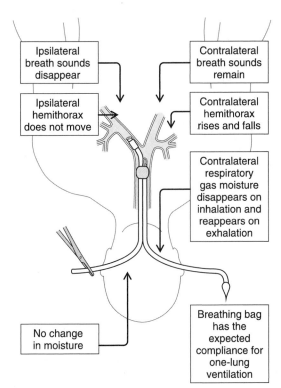

Figure 24–8. Results of unilateral clamping of the tracheal tube when the double-lumen tube is in the correct position.

Table 24–3. Protocol for checking placement of a left-sided double-lumen tube.

1. Inflate the tracheal cuff (5–10 mL of air).
2. Check for bilateral breath sounds. Unilateral breath sounds indicate that the tube is too far down (tracheal opening is bronchial).
3. Inflate the bronchial cuff (1–2 mL).
4. Clamp the tracheal lumen.
5. Check for unilateral left-sided breath sounds.
   a. Persistence of right-sided breath sounds indicates that the bronchial opening is still in the trachea (tube should be advanced).
   b. Unilateral right-sided breath sounds indicate incorrect entry of the tube in the right bronchus.
   c. Absence of breath sounds over the entire right lung and the left upper lobe indicates the tube is too far down the left bronchus.
6. Unclamp the tracheal lumen and clamp the bronchial lumen.
7. Check for unilateral right-sided breath sounds. Absence or diminution of breath sounds indicates that the tube is not far enough down and the bronchial cuff is occluding the distal trachea.

tracheal tube with a built-in side channel for a retractable bronchial blocker is commercially available (Univent tube; Vitaid, Lewiston, NY). The tube is placed with the blocker fully retracted; its natural curve is such that turning the tube with the curve concave toward the right preferentially directs the bronchial blocker toward the right bronchus. Turning the tube with the curve concave toward the left usually directs the blocker toward the left bronchus. The bronchial blocker must be advanced, positioned, and inflated under direct visualization via a flexible bronchoscope. The latter is passed through an adapter with a self-sealing diaphragm that allows uninterrupted ventilation. The cuff of the blocker is a high-pressure–low-volume cuff (see Chapter 5), so the minimum volume that prevents a leak should be used. A channel within the blocker allows the lung to deflate (though slowly) and can be used for suctioning or insufflating oxygen (below). The major advantage of this tube is that unlike a double-lumen tube, it does not need to be replaced with a regular tracheal tube if the patient is to be left intubated postoperatively (below). Its major disadvantage is that the "blocked" lung collapses slowly (and

sometimes incompletely) because of the small size of the channel within the blocker.

An inflatable (Fogarty) catheter (3 mL) can be used as a bronchial blocker in conjunction with a regular tracheal tube (inside or alongside); a guidewire in the catheter can be used to facilitate placement. This technique is occasionally used to collapse one lung when other techniques do not work. It also does not allow suctioning or ventilation of the isolated lung, and the catheter is easily dislodged. Nonetheless, bronchial blockers may be useful for one-lung anesthesia in pediatric patients

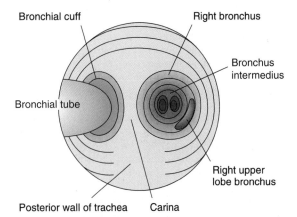

Figure 24–9. The view of the carina looking down the tracheal lumen of a properly positioned left double-lumen bronchial tube.

and for tamponading bronchial bleeding in adult patients (see below).

SINGLE-LUMEN BRONCHIAL TUBES

Single-lumen bronchial tubes are rarely used now. The Gordon–Green tube is a right-sided single-lumen tube that can be used for left thoracotomies; it has both tracheal and bronchial cuffs as well as a carinal hook. Inflating the bronchial cuff isolates and allows ventilation of only the right lung. When the bronchial cuff is deflated and the tracheal cuff is inflated, both lungs can be ventilated. A much larger slit in the bronchial cuff (compared with right-sided double-lumen tubes) results in a high success rate for ventilating the right upper lobe. The principal disadvantages of the Gordon–Green tube are the hazards of a carinal hook and the inability to suction the left lung. An ordinary, uncut single-lumen tracheal tube may be used as a bronchial tube in an emergency situation (unilateral pulmonary hemorrhage). The tube can usually be advanced blindly into the right bronchus if the source of the hemorrhage is the left lung; unfortunately, the right upper lobe may not be ventilated (see above). Positioning the tube blindly into the left bronchus is more difficult (advancing the tube with its convexity posteriorly while turning the head to the right) and should be guided by bronchoscopy, whenever possible.

■ ANESTHESIA FOR LUNG RESECTION

PREOPERATIVE CONSIDERATIONS

Lung resections are usually carried out for the diagnosis and treatment of pulmonary tumors and, less commonly, for complications of necrotizing pulmonary infections and bronchiectasis.

1. Tumors

Pulmonary tumors may be either benign or malignant, or can have an intermediate nature. This distinction often cannot be made until the time of surgery. Hamartomas account for 90% of benign pulmonary tumors; they are usually peripheral pulmonary lesions, and represent disorganized normal pulmonary tissue. Bronchial adenomas are usually central pulmonary lesions that are typically benign but occasionally may be locally invasive and rarely can metastasize. These tumors include pulmonary carcinoids, cylindromas, and mucoepidermoid adenomas. They often obstruct the bronchial lumen and cause recurrent pneumonia distal to the obstruction in the same area. Pulmonary carcinoids are derived from APUD cells and may secrete multiple hormones, including adrenocorticotropic hormone (ACTH) and arginine vasopressin; manifestations of the carcinoid syndrome are uncommon and are more likely with hepatic metastases (see Chapter 36).

Malignant pulmonary tumors are divided into small ("oat") cell (20% of tumors with a 5–10% 5-year survival) and non–small cell carcinomas (80% of tumors with a 15–20% 5-year survival). The latter includes squamous cell (epidermoid) tumors, adenocarcinomas, and large cell (anaplastic) carcinomas. All types are most commonly encountered in smokers, but adenocarcinoma also occurs in nonsmokers. Epidermoid and small cell carcinomas usually present as central masses with bronchial lesion; adenocarcinoma and large cell carcinomas are more typically peripheral lesions that often involve the pleura.

Clinical Manifestations

Symptoms may include cough, hemoptysis, dyspnea, wheezing, weight loss, fever, or productive sputum. The latter two suggest a postobstructive pneumonia. Pleuritic chest pain or pleural effusion suggests pleural extension. Involvement of mediastinal structures is suggested by hoarseness that results from compression of the recurrent laryngeal nerve, a Horner's syndrome (see Chapter 18) caused by involvement of the sympathetic chain, an elevated hemidiaphragm caused by compression of the phrenic nerve, dysphagia caused by compression of the esophagus, or the superior vena cava syndrome. Pericardial effusion or cardiomegaly suggests cardiac involvement. Extension of apical (superior sulcus) tumors can result in either shoulder or arm pain or both because of involvement of the C7–T2 roots of the brachial plexus (Pancoast syndrome). Distant metastases most commonly involve the brain, bone, liver, and adrenal glands.

Lung carcinomas—particularly small cell—can produce remote effects that are not related to malignant spread (paraneoplastic syndromes). Mechanisms include ectopic hormone production and immunologic crossreactivity between the tumor and normal tissues. Cushing's syndrome, hyponatremia, and hypercalcemia may be encountered, resulting from secretion of ACTH, arginine vasopressin, and parathyroid hormone, respectively (see Chapter 36). Lambert–Eaton (myasthenic) syndrome is characterized by a proximal myopathy in which muscle strength increases with repeated effort (in contrast to myasthenia gravis—see Chapter 37). Other paraneoplastic syndromes include hypertrophic osteoarthropathy, cerebellar degeneration, peripheral neuropathy, polymyositis, migratory thrombophlebitis, and nonbacterial carditis.

Treatment

Surgery is the treatment of choice for the curative treatment of lung cancer. Surgical resection is attempted for non–small cell carcinomas in the absence of advanced lymph node involvement, direct extension into mediastinal structures, or distant metastases. In contrast, small cell carcinomas are infrequently treated surgically because they nearly always have metastasized by the time the diagnosis is made; these cancers are treated with chemotherapy or chemotherapy and radiation.

Resectability & Operability

Resectability is determined by the anatomic stage of the tumor, whereas operability is dependent on the extent of the procedure and the physiological status of the patient. Anatomic staging includes chest radiography, computed tomography (CT), bronchoscopy, and mediastinoscopy (below). Patients with ipsilateral peribronchial or ipsilateral hilar lymph node metastases can be resected. Resection of lesions with ipsilateral mediastinal or subcarinal lymph node metastases, however, is controversial. Lesions associated with scalene, supraclavicular, contralateral mediastinal, or contralateral hilar lymph node metastases are usually considered unresectable. In the absence of mediastinal metastases, some centers also perform en bloc resections of tumors involving the chest wall; similarly, in the absence of mediastinal metastases, superior sulcus tumors may be resected after preoperative radiotherapy.

The extent of the surgery should maximize the chances for a cure but still allow for adequate residual pulmonary function postoperatively. Lobectomy via a posterior thoracotomy, through the fifth or sixth intercostal space, is the procedure of choice for most lesions. Segmental or wedge resections may be performed in patients with small peripheral lesions and poor pulmonary reserve. Pneumonectomy is necessary for curative treatment of lesions involving the left or right main bronchus or when the tumor extends to the hilum. Operative criteria for pneumonectomy are discussed below. A sleeve resection may be employed for patients with proximal lesions and limited pulmonary reserve as an alternative to pneumonectomy; in such instances, the involved lobar bronchus together with part of the right or left main bronchus is resected, and the distal bronchus is reanastomosed to the proximal bronchus or the trachea. Sleeve pneumonectomy may be considered for tumors involving the trachea. The mortality rate for pneumonectomy is generally 5–7%, compared with 2–3% for a lobectomy. Mortality is higher for right-sided pneumonectomy than for left-sided pneumonectomy, possibly because of greater loss of lung tissue. Most postoperative deaths result from cardiac causes.

Operative Criteria for Pneumonectomy

Operability is ultimately a clinical decision, but pulmonary function tests offer useful preliminary guidelines. The degree of preoperative impairment—as measured by routine pulmonary function tests—is directly related to operative risk. Standard preliminary criteria for operability are set forth in Table 24–4. Failure to meet any one of these criteria necessitates split lung function tests if pneumonectomy is still contemplated. The most commonly used criterion for operability is a predicted postoperative forced expiratory volume at 1 second (FEV_1) greater than 800 mL. The percentage contribution of each lung to total FEV_1 is assumed to be proportionate to the percentage of the total pulmonary blood flow it receives, as determined by radioisotopic scanning (^{133}Xe or ^{99}Tc).

$$\text{Postoperative } FEV_1 = \% \text{ blood flow to remaining lung} \times \text{total } FEV_1$$

Removal of extensively diseased lung (nonventilated but perfused) may not adversely affect pulmonary function and may actually improve oxygenation. If the predicted postoperative FEV_1 is less than 800 mL but resection is still considered, the ability of the remaining pulmonary vasculature to tolerate total blood flow can be tested but is rarely done. The main pulmonary artery on the diseased side is occluded with a balloon catheter; if the mean pulmonary artery pressure exceeds 40 mm Hg or the PaO_2 decreases to < 45 mm Hg, the patient is not a candidate for pneumonectomy.

The two greatest risks to lung resection involve the pulmonary and cardiac systems. It therefore makes sense to test both systems. Patients capable of climbing two to three flights of stairs without becoming too winded often tolerate surgery relatively well without

Table 24–4. Preoperative laboratory criteria for pneumonectomy.

Test	High-Risk Patients
Arterial blood gas	$PaCO_2$ > 45 mm Hg (on room air) PaO_2 < 50 mm Hg
FEV_1[1] (Predicted postoperative FEV_1)	< 2 L < 0.8 L or < 40% of predicted
FEV_1/FVC[1]	< 50% of predicted
Maximum breathing capacity	< 50% of predicted
Maximum VO_2	< 10 mL/kg/min

[1]FEV_1, forced expiratory volume in 1 s; FVC, forced vital capacity; VO_2, oxygen consumption.

further testing. Maximum oxygen consumption ($\dot{V}O_2$) during exercise also appears to be a useful predictor of postoperative morbidity and mortality. Patients with $\dot{V}O_2 > 20$ mL/kg have low complication rates, whereas those with $\dot{V}O_2 < 10$ mL/kg have unacceptably high morbidity and mortality.

2. Infection

Pulmonary infections may present as a solitary nodule or cavitary lesion (necrotizing pneumonitis). An exploratory thoracotomy may be carried out to exclude malignancy and diagnose the infectious agent. Lung resection is also indicated for cavitary lesions that are refractory to antibiotic treatment, are associated with refractory empyema, or result in massive hemoptysis. Responsible organisms include both bacteria (anaerobes, *Mycoplasma, Mycobacterium tuberculosis, Nocardia,* and a variety of enteric and nonenteric pyogenic species) and fungi (*Histoplasma, Coccidioides, Cryptococcus, Blastomyces, Mucor,* and *Aspergillus*).

3. Bronchiectasis

Bronchiectasis is a permanent dilation of bronchi. It is usually the end result of severe or recurrent inflammation and obstruction of bronchi. Causes include a variety of viral, bacterial, and fungal pathogens, as well as inhalation of toxic gases, aspiration of gastric acid, and defective mucociliary clearance (cystic fibrosis and disorders of ciliary dysfunction). Bronchial muscle and elastic tissue is typically replaced by very vascular fibrous tissue. The latter predisposes to bouts of hemoptysis. Pulmonary resection is usually indicated for massive hemoptysis when conservative measures have failed and the disease is localized. Patients with diffuse disease have a significant chronic obstructive ventilatory defect (see Chapter 23).

ANESTHETIC CONSIDERATIONS

1. Preoperative Management

The majority of patients undergoing pulmonary resections have underlying lung disease. Preoperative assessment of such patients is discussed in detail in Chapter 23. It should be emphasized that smoking is a risk factor for both chronic obstructive pulmonary disease and coronary artery disease; both disorders commonly coexist in patients presenting for thoracotomy. Echocardiography is very useful for assessing baseline cardiac function and may suggest evidence of cor pulmonale (right ventricular enlargement or hypertrophy). Dobutamine stress echocardiography may be useful in detecting occult coronary artery disease.

Patients with tumors should be evaluated for complications related to local extension of the tumor and paraneoplastic syndromes (above). Preoperative chest radiographs and CT and magnetic resonance imaging (MRI) scans should be reviewed carefully. Tracheal or bronchial deviation can complicate tracheal intubation or proper positioning of bronchial tubes. Moreover, airway compression can lead to difficulty in ventilating the patient following induction of anesthesia. Pulmonary consolidation, atelectasis, and large pleural effusions predispose to hypoxemia. The location of any bullous cysts or abscesses should be noted.

Patients undergoing thoracic procedures are at increased risk for postoperative pulmonary and cardiac complications (see Chapter 23). Good preoperative preparation may reduce pulmonary complications in high-risk patients. Perioperative arrhythmias, particularly supraventricular tachycardias, are thought to result from surgical manipulations or distention of the right atrium following reduction of the pulmonary vascular bed. The incidence of arrhythmias increases with age and with the amount of pulmonary resection.

Premedication

Patients with moderate to severe respiratory compromise should receive little or no sedative premedication. Although anticholinergics (atropine, 0.5 mg intramuscularly or intravenously, or glycopyrrolate, 0.1–0.2 mg intramuscularly or intravenously) can theoretically inspissate secretions and increase dead space; clinically they are very useful in reducing copious secretions. The latter improves visualization during repeated laryngoscopies and facilitates the use of a fiberoptic bronchoscope.

2. Intraoperative Management

Preparation

As with anesthesia for cardiac surgery, optimal preparation may help prevent potentially catastrophic problems. The frequent presence of poor pulmonary reserve, anatomic abnormalities, or compromise of the airways, and the need for one-lung ventilation predispose these patients to the rapid onset of hypoxemia. A clear and well-thought-out plan to deal with potential difficulties is necessary. Moreover, in addition to items for basic airway management (see Chapter 5), specialized and properly functioning equipment—such as multiple sizes of single- and double-lumen tubes, a flexible (pediatric) fiberoptic bronchoscope, a small-diameter "tube exchanger," a continuous positive airway pressure (CPAP) delivery system, and an anesthesia circuit adapter for administering bronchodilators—should be immediately available.

When epidural opioids or local anesthetics are to be used for postoperative analgesia (below), consideration should be given to placing the catheter prior to induction of anesthesia while the patient is still awake. This practice can facilitate placement and may be safer than placing the epidural catheter in an anesthetized patient (see Chapter 16).

Venous Access

At least one large-bore (14- or 16-gauge) intravenous line is mandatory for all thoracic surgical procedures. Central venous access (preferably on the side of the thoracotomy), a blood warmer, and a rapid infusion device are also desirable if extensive blood loss is anticipated.

Monitoring

Direct monitoring of arterial pressure is indicated for one-lung ventilation (below), for resections of large tumors (particularly those with mediastinal or chest wall extension), and for any procedure performed in patients who have limited pulmonary reserve or significant cardiovascular disease. Central venous access with monitoring of central venous pressure (CVP) is highly desirable for pneumonectomies and resections of large tumors. CVP reflects the net effect of venous capacitance, blood volume, and right ventricular function; consequently, it is only a rough guide to fluid management. Pulmonary artery catheterization is indicated in patients with pulmonary hypertension, cor pulmonale, or left ventricular dysfunction; radiographic confirmation of the position of the catheter is useful in ascertaining that the pulmonary artery catheter (PAC) is not in a lung segment that is to be resected. When the tip of the PAC is in the nondependent (upper) lung and that lung is collapsed, cardiac output and mixed venous oxygen tension may be falsely depressed during one-lung ventilation. The balloon of a PAC should be inflated carefully following pneumonectomy because the remaining pulmonary vasculature has a significantly reduced cross-sectional area; balloon inflation can acutely increase right ventricular afterload and can lower left ventricular preload.

Induction of Anesthesia

After adequate preoxygenation, an intravenous anesthetic is used for induction of most patients. The selection of an induction agent should be based on the patient's preoperative status. Direct laryngoscopy should generally be performed only after deep anesthesia to prevent reflex bronchospasm and to obtund the cardiovascular pressor response. This may be accomplished by incremental doses of the induction agent, an opioid, or both (see Chapter 20). Deepening anesthesia with a volatile inhalation agent may be preferable in patients with reactive airways.

Tracheal intubation is facilitated with succinylcholine or a nondepolarizing agent; the former may be more appropriate if difficult laryngoscopy is anticipated. Most thoracotomies can be performed with an ordinary tracheal tube, but techniques for one-lung ventilation (above) greatly facilitate most thoracic operations. Use of a single-lumen tracheal tube may be necessary, however, if the surgeon performs diagnostic bronchoscopy (below) prior to surgery; once the bronchoscopy is completed, the single-lumen tube can be replaced with a double-lumen bronchial tube (above). Controlled positive-pressure ventilation helps prevent atelectasis, paradoxical breathing, and mediastinal shift; it also allows control of the operative field to facilitate the surgery.

Positioning

Following induction, intubation, and confirmation of correct tracheal or bronchial tube position, additional venous access and monitoring may be obtained before the patient is positioned for surgery. Most lung resections are performed via posterior thoracotomy with the patient in the lateral decubitus position. Proper positioning is critical to avoid injuries and to facilitate surgical exposure. The lower arm is flexed and the upper arm is extended in front of the head, pulling the scapula away from the operative field (Figure 24–10). Pillows are placed between the arms and legs, and an axillary roll is positioned just beneath the dependent axilla to avoid injury to the brachial plexus; care is taken to avoid pressure on the eyes and the dependent ear.

Maintenance of Anesthesia

All current anesthetic techniques have been successfully used for thoracic surgery, but the combination of a potent halogenated agent (halothane, isoflurane, sevoflurane, or desflurane) and an opioid is preferred by most clinicians. Advantages of the halogenated agents include (1) potent dose-related bronchodilation, (2) depression of airway reflexes, (3) the ability to use a high inspired oxygen concentration (FIO_2), (4) the ability to make relatively rapid adjustments in anesthetic depth, and (5) minimal effects on hypoxic pulmonary vasoconstriction (see below). Halogenated agents generally have minimal effects on HPV in doses < 1 minimum alveolar concentration (MAC) (see Chapter 22). Advantages of an opioid include (1) generally minimal hemodynamic effects, (2) depression of airway reflexes, and (3) residual postoperative analgesia. If epidural opioids are to be used postoperatively, their intravenous use should be limited during surgery to prevent excessive postoperative respiratory depression. Nitrous oxide (N_2O) is generally not used because of the obligatory decrease in

Figure 24–10. Proper positioning for a lateral thoracotomy. (Reproduced, with permission, from Gothard JWW, Branthwaite MA: *Anesthesia for Thoracic Surgery.* Blackwell, 1982.)

FIO_2. Like volatile agents, nitrous oxide can also inhibit hypoxic pulmonary vasoconstriction and, in addition, can exacerbate pulmonary hypertension in some patients.

Maintenance of neuromuscular blockade with a nondepolarizing neuromuscular blocking agent (NMBA) during surgery facilitates rib spreading as well as anesthetic management. Maximal anesthetic depth is required when the ribs are spread apart. Sustained vagally mediated bradycardia due to surgical manipulations should be treated with intravenous atropine. Venous return decreases when the chest is opened because negative pleural (intrathoracic) pressure is lost on the operative side. This effect may be reversed with an intravenous fluid bolus.

Intravenous fluids should generally be restricted in patients undergoing pulmonary resections. Fluid management consists of basic maintenance requirements and replacement of blood loss (see Chapter 29); colloid or blood is usually used for the latter. Excessive fluid administration in the lateral decubitus position may promote a "lower lung syndrome," ie, gravity-dependent transudation of fluid into the dependent lung. The latter increases intrapulmonary shunting and promotes hypoxemia, particularly during one-lung ventilation. Moreover, the collapsed lung is also prone to edema following reexpansion as a result of surgical retraction.

During lung resections, the bronchus (or remaining lung tissue) is usually divided with an automated stapling device. The bronchial stump is then tested for an air leak under water by transiently sustaining 30 cm of positive pressure to the airway. During rib approximation, hand ventilation is helpful in avoiding injury to lung parenchyma from suture needles following lobectomy or wedge resection if a single-lumen tube is being used. Prior to completion of chest closure, all remaining lung segments should be fully expanded manually under direct vision. Controlled mechanical ventilation is then resumed and continued until chest tubes are connected to suction. Chest tubes are not needed following pneumonectomy.

Management of One-Lung Ventilation

The greatest risk of one-lung ventilation is hypoxemia. To reduce this risk, the period of time of one-lung ventilation should be kept to a minimum and 100% oxygen should be used. Major adjustments in ventilation are usually not necessary. If peak airway pressures rise excessively (> 30 cm H_2O), tidal volume may be reduced to 6–8 mL/kg and the ventilatory rate may be increased to maintain the same minute ventilation. Close monitoring of the pulse oximeter is mandatory. Periodic arterial blood gas analysis is helpful to ensure adequate ventilation. End-tidal CO_2 measurement may not be reliable (see Chapter 6).

Hypoxemia during one-lung anesthesia requires one or more of the following interventions:
Consistently effective measures:

(1) Periodic inflation of the collapsed lung with oxygen.
(2) Early ligation or clamping of the ipsilateral pulmonary artery (during pneumonectomy).
(3) CPAP (5–10 cm H_2O) to the collapsed lung; this is most effective when there is partial reexpansion of the lung, which unfortunately can interfere with surgery.

Marginally effective measures:

(1) PEEP (5–10 cm H_2O) to the ventilated lung.
(2) Continuous insufflation of oxygen into the collapsed lung.
(3) Changing the tidal volume and ventilatory rate.

When a patient undergoing one-lung ventilation develops hypoxia, as measured by the pulse oximeter, the anesthesiologist should first apply CPAP to the collapsed lung, and then, if the patient is still hypoxic, PEEP to the ventilated lung. Persistent hypoxemia requires immediate reexpansion of the collapsed lung. The position of the bronchial tube (or bronchial blocker) relative to the carina can change as a result of surgical manipulations or traction; repeat fiberoptic bronchoscopy through the tracheal lumen can quickly eliminate this problem. Both lumens of the tube should also be suctioned to exclude excessive secretions or obstruction as a factor. If blood is present in the airway, instillation of streptokinase into the tube may help facilitate the removal of clots. Pneumothorax on the dependent ventilated side should also be considered; the latter may be more likely to occur following extensive mediastinal dissection or with high peak inspiratory pressures.

Alternatives to One-Lung Ventilation

Ventilation can be stopped for short periods if 100% oxygen is insufflated at a rate greater than oxygen consumption (**apneic oxygenation**). Adequate oxygenation can often be maintained for prolonged periods, but progressive respiratory acidosis limits the use of this technique to 10–20 min in most patients. Arterial P_{CO_2} rises 6 mm Hg in the first minute, followed by a rise of 3–4 mm Hg during each subsequent minute.

High-frequency positive-pressure ventilation and high-frequency jet ventilation (see Chapter 49) have been used during thoracic procedures as alternatives to one-lung ventilation. A standard tracheal tube may be used with either technique. Small tidal volumes (< 2 mL/kg) allow decreased lung excursion, which may facilitate the surgery but still allow ventilation of both lungs. Unfortunately, mediastinal "bounce"—a to-and-fro movement—often interferes with the surgery.

3. Postoperative Management

General Care

Most patients are extubated early to decrease the risk of pulmonary barotrauma (particularly "blowout" [rupture] of the bronchial suture line) and pulmonary infection. Patients with marginal pulmonary reserve should be left intubated until standard extubation criteria are met; if a double-lumen tube was used for one-lung ventilation, it should be replaced with a regular single-lumen tube at the end of surgery. A catheter guide ("tube exchanger") should be used if the original laryngoscopy was difficult (above).

Patients are observed carefully in the postanesthesia care unit (PACU) and, in most instances, at least overnight or longer in an intensive care unit (ICU) or intermediate care unit. Postoperative hypoxemia and respiratory acidosis are common. These effects are largely caused by atelectasis from surgical compression of the lungs and "shallow breathing ('splinting')" due to

incisional pain. Gravity-dependent transudation of fluid into the dependent lung (above) may also be contributory. Reexpansion edema of the collapsed nondependent lung can also occur, particularly with rapid reinflation of the lung.

Postoperative hemorrhage complicates about 3% of thoracotomies and may be associated with up to 20% mortality. Signs of hemorrhage include increased chest tube drainage (> 200 mL/h), hypotension, tachycardia, and a falling hematocrit. Postoperative supraventricular tachyarrhythmias are common and should be treated aggressively (see Chapters 19 and 47). Acute right ventricular failure is suggested by a low cardiac output, elevated CVP, oliguria, and a normal pulmonary capillary occlusion pressure.

Routine postoperative care should include maintenance of a semiupright (> 30°) position, supplemental oxygen (40–50%), incentive spirometry, close electrocardiographic and hemodynamic monitoring, a postoperative radiograph, and aggressive pain relief.

Postoperative Analgesia

The balance between comfort and respiratory depression in patients with marginal lung function is difficult to achieve with parenteral opioids alone. Patients who have undergone thoracotomy clearly benefit from the use of other techniques described below that may obviate the need for any parenteral opioids. If parenteral opioids are used alone, small intravenous doses are superior to large intramuscular doses and probably are best administered via a patient-controlled analgesia (PCA) device (see Chapter 18).

A long-acting agent such as 0.5% ropivacaine (4–5 mL), injected two levels above and below the thoracotomy incision, typically provides excellent pain relief. These blocks may be done under direct vision intraoperatively or via the standard technique (see Chapter 17) postoperatively. Intercostal or paravertebral nerve blocks improve postoperative arterial blood gases and pulmonary function tests and shorten hospital stay. Alternatively, a cryoanalgesia probe may be used intraoperatively to freeze the intercostal nerves (cryoneurolysis) and produce long-lasting anesthesia; unfortunately, maximum analgesia may not be achieved until 24–48 h after the cryoanalgesia procedure. Nerve regeneration is reported to occur approximately 1 month after the cryoneurolysis.

Epidural opioids with or without a local anesthetic can also provide excellent analgesia (see Chapter 18). Equally satisfactory analgesia may be obtained with either a lumbar or thoracic epidural catheter when morphine is used. Injection of morphine 5–7 mg in 10–15 mL of saline usually provides 6–24 h of analgesia without autonomic, sensory, or motor blockade. The lumbar route may be safer because it is less likely to traumatize the spinal cord or puncture the dura, but the latter is more of a theoretical concern because it may occur (although infrequently) during cautious and correct placement of a thoracic epidural. Epidural injections of a lipophilic opioid, such as fentanyl, are more effective via a thoracic catheter than a lumbar catheter (see Chapter 18). Some clinicians prefer fentanyl given epidurally because it is less likely to cause delayed respiratory depression. In either case, patients should be closely monitored for this complication.

Some studies suggest that interpleural analgesia, also called intrapleural analgesia, can provide good analgesia following thoracotomy. Unfortunately, clinical experience has provided inconsistent results, possibly because of the necessary use of thoracostomy tubes and the presence of blood within the pleura.

Postoperative Complications

Postoperative complications following thoracotomy are relatively common, but fortunately most are minor and resolve uneventfully. Blood clots and thick secretions readily obstruct the airways and result in atelectasis; aggressive but gentle suctioning may be necessary. Significant atelectasis is suggested by tracheal deviation and shifting of the mediastinum to the operative side following segmental or lobar resections. Therapeutic bronchoscopy should be considered for persistent atelectasis, particularly when associated with thick secretions. Air leaks from the operative hemithorax are common following segmental and lobar resections because fissures are usually incomplete; resection therefore often leaves the small channels responsible for collateral ventilation open. Most air leaks stop after a few days. Bronchopleural fistula presents as a sudden large air leak from the chest tube that may be associated with an increasing pneumothorax and partial lung collapse. When it occurs within the first 24–72 h, it is usually the result of inadequate surgical closure of the bronchial stump. Delayed presentation is usually due to necrosis of the suture line associated with inadequate blood flow or infection.

Some complications are rare but deserve special consideration because they can be life-threatening, require a high index of suspicion, and may require immediate exploratory thoracotomy. Postoperative bleeding was discussed above. Torsion of a lobe or segment can occur as the remaining lung on the operative side expands to occupy the hemithorax. The torsion usually occludes the pulmonary vein to that part of the lung, causing venous outflow obstruction. Hemoptysis and infarction can rapidly follow. The diagnosis is suggested by an enlarging homogeneous density on the chest radiograph and a closed lobar orifice on bronchoscopy. Acute herniation of the heart into the operative hemithorax can occur through the pericardial defect that may be left following a radical pneumonectomy. A large pressure differential between the two hemithoraxes is thought to trigger this catastrophic event. Herniation into the right hemithorax results in sudden severe hypotension with an elevated CVP because of torsion of the central veins. Herniation into the left hemithorax following left pneumonectomy results in sudden compression of the heart at the atrioventricular groove, resulting in hypotension, ischemia, and infarction. A chest radiograph shows a shift of the cardiac shadow into the operative hemithorax.

Extensive mediastinal dissections can injure the phrenic, vagus, and left recurrent laryngeal nerves. Postoperative phrenic nerve palsy presents as elevation of the ipsilateral hemidiaphragm together with difficulty in weaning the patient from the ventilator. Large en bloc chest wall resections may also involve part of the diaphragm, causing a similar problem, in addition to a flail chest. Paraplegia can rarely follow thoracotomy for lung resection. Sacrificing the left lower intercostal arteries can produce spinal cord ischemia. Alternately, an epidural hematoma may form if the surgical dissection enters the epidural space through the chest cavity.

SPECIAL CONSIDERATIONS FOR PATIENTS UNDERGOING LUNG RESECTION

Massive Pulmonary Hemorrhage

Massive hemoptysis is usually defined as > 500–600 mL of blood loss from the tracheobronchial tree within 24 h. It complicates only 1–2% of all cases of hemoptysis and is usually the result of tuberculosis, bronchiectasis, or a neoplasm or follows transbronchial biopsies. Emergency surgical management with lung resection is reserved for "potentially lethal" massive hemoptysis. In most cases, surgery is usually carried out on a semielective rather than on a true emergent basis whenever possible; even then, operative mortality may exceed 20% (compared with > 50% for medical management). Embolization of the involved bronchial arteries may be attempted. The most common cause of death is asphyxia secondary to blood in the airway. Patients may be brought to the operating room for rigid bronchoscopy when localization is not possible with fiberoptic flexible bronchoscopy. A bronchial blocker or Fogarty catheter (above) may be placed to tamponade the bleeding or laser coagulation may be attempted.

The patient should be maintained in the lateral position as long as possible with the affected lung in a dependent position to tamponade the bleeding. Multiple large-bore intravenous catheters should be placed. Premedication should not be given to awake patients because they are usually already hypoxic; 100% oxygen should be given continuously. If the patient is already intubated and has bronchial blockers in place, sedation is helpful to prevent coughing. Moreover, the bronchial blocker should be left in position until the lung is resected. When the patient is not intubated, an awake intubation is preferable, but rapid sequence induction (ketamine or etomidate with succinylcholine) is often necessary. Patients usually swallow a large amount of blood and should be considered to have a full stomach; a semiupright position and cricoid pressure should therefore be maintained during induction of anesthesia. A large double-lumen bronchial tube is ideal for protecting the normal lung from blood and for suctioning each lung separately. If any difficulty is encountered in placing the double-lumen tube or its relatively small lumens occlude easily, a large (> 8.0-mm i.d.) single-lumen tube may be safer; a single-lumen tracheal tube with a built-in side channel for a retractable bronchial blocker (Univent) should be considered. Streptokinase can be used to facilitate the suctioning of large clots from the airways; if bleeding is active, iced saline helps slow it down.

Pulmonary Cyst & Bulla

Pulmonary cysts or bullae may be congenital or acquired as a result of emphysema. Large bullae can impair ventilation by compressing the surrounding lung. These air cavities often behave as if they have a one-way valve, predisposing them to progressively enlarge. Lung resection may be undertaken for progressive dyspnea or recurrent pneumothorax. The greatest risk of anesthesia is rupture of the air cavity during positive-pressure ventilation, resulting in tension pneumothorax; the latter may occur on either side prior to thoracotomy or on the nonoperative side during the lung resection. Induction of anesthesia with maintenance of spontaneous ventilation is desirable until the side with the cyst or bullae is isolated with a double-lumen tube or until a chest tube is placed; most patients have a large increase in dead space, so assisted ventilation is necessary to avoid excessive hypercarbia. The use of N_2O is contraindicated in patients with cysts or bullae because it can expand the air space and cause rupture. The latter may be signaled by sudden hypotension, bronchospasm, or an abrupt rise in peak inflation pressure and requires immediate placement of a chest tube.

Lung Abscess

Lung abscesses result from primary pulmonary infections, obstructing pulmonary neoplasms (above), or, rarely, hematogenous spread of systemic infections. Anesthetic management emphasizes isolating the two lungs early to prevent soiling the healthy one with pus. A rapid-sequence intravenous induction with tracheal intubation with a double-lumen tube is generally rec-

ommended while the patient is in a semiupright position with the affected lung in a dependent position; the latter helps prevent soiling of the healthy lung. As soon as the double-lumen tube is placed, both bronchial and tracheal cuffs are inflated. The bronchial cuff should make a tight seal before the patient is turned into the lateral decubitus position, with the diseased lung in a nondependent position. The diseased lung should be frequently suctioned during the procedure to decrease the likelihood of contaminating the healthy lung.

Bronchopleural Fistula

Bronchopleural fistulas occur following lung resection (usually pneumonectomy), rupture of a pulmonary abscess into a pleural cavity, pulmonary barotrauma, or spontaneous rupture of bullae. The majority of patients are treated (and cured) conservatively; patients come to surgery when chest tube drainage and antibiotics have failed. **Anesthetic management may be complicated by the inability to effectively ventilate the patient with positive pressure because of a large air leak, the potential for a tension pneumothorax, and the risk of contaminating the other lung if an empyema is present.** The empyema is usually drained as much as possible preoperatively, prior to closure of the fistula.

Some clinicians recommend an awake intubation with a double-lumen tube in the presence of a large air leak. Alternatively, a rapid sequence intravenous induction with bronchial intubation may also be utilized. The double-lumen tube greatly simplifies anesthetic management by isolating the fistula and allowing one-lung ventilation to the healthy side. The patient should be extubated after the repair whenever possible.

ANESTHESIA FOR TRACHEAL RESECTION

Preoperative Considerations

Tracheal resection is most commonly performed for tracheal stenosis, tumors, or, less commonly, congenital abnormalities. Tracheal stenosis can follow penetrating or blunt trauma as well as tracheal intubation and tracheostomy. Squamous cell and adenoid cystic carcinomas account for the majority of tumors. Compromise of the tracheal lumen results in progressive dyspnea. Wheezing or stridor may be evident only with exertion. The dyspnea may be worse when the patient is lying down, with progressive airway obstruction. Hemoptysis can also complicate tracheal tumors. CT is valuable in localizing the lesion. **Measurement of flow-volume loops confirms**

Peter Slinger, MD, FRCPC

ACUTE LUNG INJURY FOLLOWING THORACIC ANESTHESIA

Acute lung injury (ALI) following pulmonary resection has been described over the past 50 years. The most widely known report is a multicenter compilation of 10 cases following pneumonectomy published in 1984 by Zeldin et al.[1] After retrospective comparison with controls, three risk factors were identified: right pneumonectomy, increased perioperative intravenous fluids, and increased postoperative urine output. Zeldin et al[1] further demonstrated their thesis that this was an anesthetic complication caused by overhydration by producing postpneumonectomy pulmonary edema in a dog model with fluid overload. In their recommendations, they wrote that "the most important thing that we can do in terms of recognizing this problem is to watch our anesthetists as they start loading the patient up with fluid."

A recent study by Licker et al[2] found a bimodal distribution of ALI following pulmonary resection. Late onset (3–10 days postoperatively) cases (an incidence of 10 per 879, 1%) were secondary to other obvious causes such as bronchopneumonia and aspiration.

Primary ALI (an incidence of 27 per 879, 3%) presented on days 0–3, and this includes the subgroup of postpneumonectomy pulmonary edema, which had been the focus of Zeldin et al[1] and previous investigators. Licker et al[2] found four factors that were independent significant predictors of primary ALI: excessive intravascular volume, pneumonectomy, high intraoperative ventilation pressures, and preoperative alcohol abuse.

The most useful information in the search for the underlying causes of postpneumonectomy pulmonary edema in the past decade comes from a study by Waller et al.[3] They studied the postoperative permeability, assessed by scintigraphy with technetium-99m–labeled albumin, of the nonoperated lung in pulmonary resection patients. In the early postoperative period, the permeability of the nonoperated lung increased in pneumonectomy but not lobectomy patients. Although the exact reasons may not be clear, knowing that a pneumonectomy patient has a "leaky lung" is enormously important for the anesthesiologist. Knowing that the pulmonary resection patient, particularly the pneumonectomy patient, has a degree of endothelial injury in the nonoperated lung leads to obvious management principles based on what we have learned from the outcomes of therapy for patients with acute respiratory distress syndrome (ARDS).[4]

First, we should try to avoid overinflation of the nonoperated lung. Traditionally, anesthesiologists have been taught to use large tidal volumes (10–12 mL/kg) during one-lung anesthesia to prevent atelectasis in the dependent lung; this practice is still followed in many centers. However, most patients during one-lung ventilation develop auto–peak end-expiratory pressure (PEEP) and have an elevated functional residual capacity. The use of a large tidal volume in a lung that is starting at an elevated volume can lead to end-inspiratory lung volumes that approach the theoretical limits associated with ventilator-induced lung injury. Because

the location of the obstruction and aids the clinician in evaluating the severity of the lesion (Figure 24–11).

Anesthetic Considerations

Little or no premedication is given, as most patients presenting for tracheal resection have moderate to

severe airway obstruction. Use of an anticholinergic agent to dry secretions is controversial because of the theoretical risk of inspissation. Monitoring should include direct arterial pressure measurements. The left radial artery is preferred for lower tracheal resections because of the potential for compression of the innominate artery. ⓇBrachiocephalic artery ↗

of this concern, some anesthesiologists no longer use the traditional large tidal volumes for one-lung anesthesia and are using more physiological volumes (eg, 5 mL/kg), adding PEEP to those patients without auto-PEEP and limiting plateau inspiratory pressures to < 25 cm H_2O.

Not all hyperinflation of the residual lung occurs in the operating room. Overexpansion of the remaining lung after a pneumonectomy may occur postoperatively either with or without a chest drain in place. Alvarez et al[5] described their use of a balanced chest drainage system to keep the mediastinum in a neutral position and avoid hyperinflation of the residual lung following a pneumonectomy. There has been a marked decline in this complication in their practice since the introduction of this system of chest drainage.

Second, we should try to minimize pulmonary intravascular pressures. This has been commonly attempted by fluid restriction, as suggested originally by Zeldin et al.[1] Those managing thoracic cases are well aware that fluid management is a contentious issue between the anesthesiologist and surgeon. Anesthesiologists tend to focus on the undesirable consequences of regional hypoperfusion of potentially compromised organs (brain, heart, kidneys) whereas surgeons worry about the complications due to volume overload on the respiratory system. The most thorough study of this controversy was an investigation by Turnage and Lunn.[6] In a retrospective survey of 806 pneumonectomies from the Mayo Clinic, only 21 cases (2.5%) of postpneumonectomy pulmonary edema were found, one of the lowest reported incidences of this complication. There were no differences in any measure of perioperative fluid balance among cases of postpneumonectomy pulmonary edema (positive fluid balance at 24 h, 10 mL/kg) versus age- and sex-matched pneumonectomy controls (positive balance 13 mL/kg). However, the routine practice was rigorous fluid restriction. This suggests that by limiting fluids the incidence of ALI can be decreased but not eliminated. Avoidance of fluid overload in pneumonectomy patients is logical but must be appreciated in the context that severe fluid re-

striction can precipitate renal dysfunction, which also has a high postoperative mortality in the thoracic surgical population. Not all increases in pulmonary pressures postoperatively are related to intravascular volume. Other factors under the influence of the anesthesiologist, such as hypercarbia, hypoxemia, and pain, can all increase pulmonary pressures and must be treated.

One reason that ALI after lung resection has been the focus of more attention in recent years is that the other major causes of respiratory morbidity and mortality (atelectasis, pneumonia, etc) following lung resection have declined. Much of this reduction is coincident with better postoperative analgesic techniques, such as the introduction of thoracic epidural infusions. However, the incidence of ALI has not noticeably decreased, and in some centers ALI has now become the major cause of mortality following lung resection. Although aggressive nonspecific treatment, similar to that used for other types of ARDS, including the use of nitric oxide, has decreased the case-fatality rate, it still remains exceedingly high. At this time our efforts seem better directed to prevention than cure.

1. Zeldin RA, Normadin D, Landtwing BS, Peters RM: Postpneumonectomy pulmonary edema. J Thorac Cardiovasc Surg 1984;87:359.

2. Licker M, De Perrot M, Spiliopoulos A, et al: Risk factors for acute lung injury after thoracic surgery for lung cancer. Anesth Analg 2003;97:1558.

3. Waller DA, Keavey P, Woodfine L, Dark JH: Pulmonary endothelial permeability changes after major resection. Ann Thorac Surg 1996;61:1435.

4. The Acute Respiratory Distress Syndrome Network: Ventilation with lower tidal volumes as compared with traditional tidal volumes for acute lung injury and the acute respiratory distress syndrome. N Engl J Med 2000;342:1301.

5. Alvarez JM, Panda RK, Newman MAJ, et al: Postpneumonectomy pulmonary edema. J Cardiothorac Vasc Anesth 2003;17:388.

6. Turnage WS, Lunn JL: Postpneumonectomy pulmonary edema. A retrospective analysis of associated variables. Chest 1993;103:1646.

A slow inhalation induction (in 100% oxygen) is carried out for patients with severe obstruction. Halothane or sevoflurane is the preferred agent because they are least irritating to the airway. Spontaneous ventilation is maintained throughout induction. NMBAs are generally avoided because of the potential for complete airway obstruction following neuro-

muscular blockade. Laryngoscopy is performed only when the patient is judged to be under deep anesthesia. Intravenous lidocaine (1–2 mg/kg) can deepen the anesthesia without depressing respirations. The surgeon may then perform rigid bronchoscopy to evaluate and possibly dilate the lesion. Following bronchoscopy, the patient is intubated with a tra-

A NORMAL

B VARIABLE EXTRATHORACIC OBSTRUCTION

C VARIABLE INTRATHORACIC OBSTRUCTION

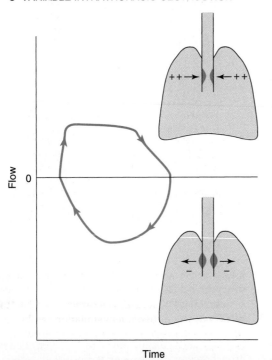

D FIXED LARGE AIRWAY OBSTRUCTION

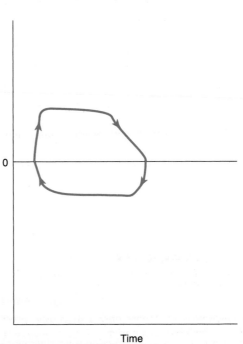

Figure 24–11. A–D: Flow–volume loops.

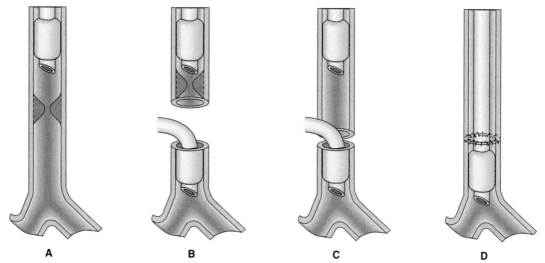

Figure 24–12. **A–D:** Airway management of a high tracheal lesion.

cheal tube small enough to be passed distal to the obstruction whenever possible.

A collar incision is utilized for high tracheal lesions. The surgeon divides the trachea in the neck and advances a sterile armored tube into the distal trachea passing off a sterile connecting hose to the anesthesiologist for ventilation during the resection. Following the resection and completion of the posterior part of the reanastomosis, the armored tube is removed and the original tracheal tube is advanced distally past the anastomosis (Figure 24–12). Alternatively, high-frequency jet ventilation may be employed during the anastomosis by passing the jet cannula past the obstruction and into the distal trachea (Figure 24–13). Return of spontaneous ventilation and early extubation at the end of the procedure are desirable. Patients should be positioned with the neck flexed immediately postoperatively after the operation to minimize tension on the suture line (Figure 24–14).

Surgical management of low tracheal lesions requires a median sternotomy or right posterior thoracotomy. Anesthetic management is similar but more regularly requires more complicated techniques such as high-frequency ventilation or even CPB (the latter for complex congenital cases).

■ ANESTHESIA FOR THORACOSCOPIC SURGERY

Thoracoscopy is no longer only a diagnostic procedure; it is now used for up to one-third to one-half of

Figure 24–13. Tracheal resection using high-frequency jet ventilation. **A:** The catheter is advanced past the obstruction and the cuff is deflated when jet ventilation is initiated. **B:** The catheter is advanced distally by the surgeon. Jet ventilation can be continued without interruption during resection and reanastomosis.

Figure 24–14. Position of the patient before (**A**) and after (**B**) tracheal resection and reanastomosis with the patient's neck flexed for the first 24–48 h.

many thoracic surgical procedures that previously required open thoracotomy. The list of procedures includes lung biopsy, segmental and lobar resections, pleurodesis, esophageal procedures (such as myomectomy), and even pericardectomy (see Chapter 21). Most procedures are performed through three or more small incisions in the chest with the patient in the lateral decubitus position.

Anesthetic management is similar to that for open procedures (above) except that one-lung ventilation is mandatory for all but the most minor procedures. Some centers may use only local anesthesia with spontaneous ventilation for minor procedures, but patient discomfort can be considerable. Opening one of the portals to the atmosphere allows the lung on the operative side to collapse; unlike lap-

aroscopy, insufflation of gas is not only unnecessary but hazardous.

■ ANESTHESIA FOR DIAGNOSTIC THORACIC PROCEDURES

Bronchoscopy

Topical and local anesthesia for flexible bronchoscopy is discussed in Chapter 5. Rigid bronchoscopy for removal of foreign bodies or for tracheal dilatation is usually performed under general anesthesia. These procedures are complicated by the need to share the airway with the surgeon or pulmonologist; fortunately, they are often of short duration (5–10 min). After a standard intravenous induction, anesthesia is usually maintained with a potent inhalation agent in 100% oxygen and a short- or intermediate-acting NMBA. Total intravenous anesthesia (such as with propofol) can also be used.

One of three techniques can then be used during rigid bronchoscopy: (1) apneic oxygenation using a small catheter positioned alongside the bronchoscope to insufflate with oxygen (above), (2) conventional ventilation through the side arm of a ventilating bronchoscope (when the proximal window of this instrument is opened for suctioning or biopsies, ventilation must be interrupted), or (3) high-frequency ventilation through an injector-type bronchoscope. In the latter instance, a narrow (16- to 18-gauge) cannula in the proximal end of the bronchoscope is used to inject oxygen at high pressures; the Venturi effect created proximally entrains an air–oxygen mixture down the trachea.

Mediastinoscopy

Mediastinoscopy provides access to the mediastinal lymph nodes and is used to establish either the diagnosis or the resectability of intrathoracic malignancies (above). Preoperative CT is essential for evaluating tracheal distortion or compression.

Mediastinoscopy is performed under general tracheal anesthesia with an NMBA. Venous access with a large-bore (14- to 16-gauge) intravenous catheter is mandatory because of the risk of excessive bleeding and the difficulty in controlling bleeding when it occurs. Because the innominate artery may be compressed during the procedure, blood pressure should be measured in the left arm.

Complications associated with mediastinoscopy include (1) vagally mediated reflex bradycardia from compression of the trachea or the great vessels, (2) excessive hemorrhage (see above), (3) cerebral ischemia from compression of the innominate artery (detected with a plethysmograph or pulse oximeter on the right hand), (4) pneumothorax (usually presents postoperatively), (5) air embolism (because of a 30° head elevation, the risk is greatest during spontaneous ventilation), (6) recurrent laryngeal nerve damage, and (7) phrenic nerve injury.

Bronchoalveolar Lavage

Bronchoalveolar lavage may be employed for patients with pulmonary alveolar proteinosis. These patients produce excessive quantities of surfactant and fail to clear it. They present with dyspnea and bilateral consolidation on the chest radiograph. Bronchoalveolar lavage may be indicated for severe hypoxemia or worsening

dyspnea. Often, one lung is lavaged, allowing the patient to recover for a few days before the other lung is lavaged; the worse lung is therefore done first. Increasingly, both lungs are lavaged during the same procedure, creating unique challenges to ensure adequate oxygenation during lavage of the second lung.

Unilateral bronchoalveolar lavage is performed under general anesthesia with a double-lumen bronchial tube. The cuffs on the tube should be properly positioned and should make a watertight seal to prevent spillage of fluid into the other side. The procedure is normally done in the supine position; although lavage with the lung in a dependent position helps minimize soiling of the other lung, this position can cause severe ventilation/perfusion mismatch. Warm normal saline is infused into the lung to be treated and is drained by gravity; treatment continues until the fluid returning is clear (about 10–20 L). At the end of the procedure, both lungs are well suctioned, and the double-lumen tracheal tube is replaced with a single-lumen tracheal tube.

■ ANESTHESIA FOR LUNG TRANSPLANTATION

PREOPERATIVE CONSIDERATIONS

Lung transplantation is indicated for end-stage pulmonary parenchymal disease or pulmonary hypertension. Candidates are functionally incapacitated by dyspnea and have a poor prognosis. Criteria vary according to the primary disease process. Common etiologies are listed in Table 24–5. The number of transplants is limited by the availability of suitable organs. Patients typically have dyspnea at rest or with minimal activity and resting hypoxemia ($PaO_2 < 50$ mm Hg) with increasing oxygen requirements. Progressive CO_2 retention is also very common. Patients may be venti-

Table 24–5. Indications for lung transplantation.

Cystic fibrosis
Bronchiectasis
Obstructive
    Chronic obstructive pulmonary disease
    α_1-Antitrypsin deficiency
    Pulmonary lymphangiomatosis
Restrictive
    Idiopathic pulmonary fibrosis
Vascular
    Primary pulmonary hypertension
    Eisenmenger syndrome (congenital heart disease)

lator dependent. Cor pulmonale does not necessarily require combined heart–lung transplantation because right ventricular function may recover when pulmonary artery pressures normalize. Patients should have normal left ventricular function and be free of coronary artery disease as well as other serious health problems.

Single-lung transplantation may be performed for selected patients with chronic obstructive pulmonary disease, whereas double-lung transplantation is typically performed for patients with cystic fibrosis, bullous emphysema, or vascular diseases. Younger patients are more likely to receive bilateral lung transplants. Patients with Eisenmenger syndrome require combined heart–lung transplantation (see Chapter 21).

Organ selection is based on size and ABO compatibility. Cytomegalovirus serology matching may also be attempted.

ANESTHETIC CONSIDERATIONS

1. Preoperative Management

Effective coordination between the organ-retrieval team and the transplant team minimizes graft ischemia time and avoids unnecessary prolongation of pretransplant anesthesia time. These procedures are performed on an emergency basis so patients may have little time to fast for surgery. Oral cyclosporine also may be given preoperatively. Administration of a clear antacid, an H_2 blocker, or metoclopramide should be considered. Patients are very sensitive to sedatives, so premedication is usually administered only in the operating room when the patient is directly attended. Intravenous azathioprine may also be administered just prior to induction.

2. Intraoperative Management

Monitoring

Strict asepsis should be observed for invasive monitoring procedures, which are similar to cardiac surgery (see Chapter 21). Because of tricuspid regurgitation, difficulty may be encountered in floating a PAC. Central venous access might be accomplished only after induction of anesthesia because patients may not be able to lie flat while awake. The PAC must, however, be withdrawn into its sterile protective sheath just prior to lung resection (if it floats to the operative side); it may be refloated back into the pulmonary artery after transplantation. Care must be taken to avoid air bubbles or clots in the intravenous fluids; patients with a patent foramen ovale are at risk for paradoxical embolism because of high right atrial pressures.

Induction & Maintenance of Anesthesia

A modified rapid-sequence induction with moderate head-up position is utilized. A slow induction with

ketamine, etomidate, an opioid, or a combination of these agents is employed to avoid precipitous drops in blood pressure. Succinylcholine or a nondepolarizing NMBA is used to facilitate laryngoscopy. Cricoid pressure is maintained throughout induction until the airway is secured with a tracheal or bronchial tube (below). Hypoxemia and hypercarbia must be avoided to prevent further increases in pulmonary artery pressure. Hypotension should be treated with vasopressors (dobutamine) instead of large fluid boluses (see below).

Anesthesia is usually maintained with an opioid infusion with or without a low dose of a volatile agent. Intraoperative difficulties in ventilation are not uncommon. Progressive retention of CO_2 can also be a problem intraoperatively. Ventilation should be adjusted to maintain a normal arterial pH to limit metabolic alkalosis (see Chapter 30). Patients with cystic fibrosis have copious secretions and require frequent suctioning.

Single-Lung Transplantation

Single-lung transplantation is often attempted without CPB. The procedure is performed through a posterior thoracotomy. A left-sided double-lumen or single-lumen tube with a built-in bronchial blocker must be used for one-lung ventilation in such instances. Whether to employ CPB during transplantation of one lung is based on the patient's response to collapsing the lung to be replaced and clamping its pulmonary artery. Persistent arterial hypoxemia ($SpO_2 < 88\%$) or a sudden increase in pulmonary artery pressures necessitates CPB. Prostaglandin E_1, amrinone (or milrinone), nitroglycerin, and dobutamine may be utilized to control pulmonary hypertension and prevent right ventricular failure. Inotropic support with dopamine may be necessary. When CPB is necessary, femoral-vein-to-femoral-artery bypass is employed during left thoracotomy, whereas right-atrium-to-aorta bypass is used during right thoracotomy.

After the recipient lung is resected, the pulmonary artery, left atrial cuff (with the pulmonary veins), and bronchus of the donor lung are anastomosed. An omental flap may be mobilized to wrap around the bronchial anastomosis (omentopexy) to promote revascularization and help prevent ischemic breakdown. Flexible bronchoscopy is used to examine the bronchial suture line after its completion.

Double-Lung Transplantation

A "clamshell" transverse sternotomy can be used for double-lung transplantation. The procedure is occasionally performed with normothermic CPB; sequential thoracotomies for double-lung transplantation without CPB is more common. Severe metabolic alkalosis can develop in patients with marked chronic CO_2 retention if the CO_2 is normalized; administration of intravenous hydrochloric acid may be necessary (see Chapter 30).

Posttransplantation Management

After anastomosis of the donor organ or organs, ventilation to both lungs is resumed. Following transplantation, peak inspiratory pressures should be maintained at the minimum pressure compatible with good lung expansion, and the inspired oxygen concentration should be maintained at < 60%. Methylprednisolone is usually given prior to release of vascular clamps. Hyperkalemia may occur as the preservative fluid (Euro-Collins) is washed out of the donor organ. The patient is separated from CPB if the latter is employed, and the PAC is refloated into the main pulmonary artery. Pulmonary vasodilators and inotropes (above) may be necessary. Transesophageal echocardiography is very helpful in differentiating right and left ventricular dysfunction as well as in evaluating blood flow in the pulmonary vessels before and after transplantation.

Transplantation disrupts the neural innervation, lymphatic drainage, and bronchial circulation of the transplanted lung. Respiratory pattern is unaffected but the cough reflex is abolished below the carina. Bronchial hyperreactivity is described in some patients. Hypoxic pulmonary vasoconstriction remains normal. Loss of lymphatic drainage increases extravascular lung water and predisposes the transplanted lung to pulmonary edema. Intraoperative fluid replacement must therefore be kept to a minimum. Loss of the bronchial circulation predisposes to ischemic breakdown of the bronchial suture line.

3. Postoperative Management

Patients are extubated after surgery as soon as feasible. A thoracic epidural catheter may be employed for postoperative analgesia when coagulation studies are normal. The postoperative course is often complicated by acute rejection, infections, and renal and hepatic dysfunction. Deteriorating lung function may result from rejection or reperfusion injury. Occasionally, temporary extracorporeal membrane oxygenation may be necessary. Frequent bronchoscopy with transbronchial biopsies and lavage are necessary to differentiate between rejection and infection. Nosocomial gram-negative bacteria, cytomegalovirus, *Candida*, *Aspergillus*, and *Pneumocystis carinii* are common pathogens. Other postoperative surgical complications include damage to the phrenic, vagus, and left recurrent laryngeal nerves.

ANESTHESIA FOR ESOPHAGEAL SURGERY

PREOPERATIVE CONSIDERATIONS

Common indications for esophageal surgery include tumors, gastroesophageal reflux, and motility disorders (achalasia). Surgical procedures include simple endoscopy, esophageal dilatation, cervical esophagomyotomy, open or thoracoscopic distal esophagomyotomy, and blunt esophagectomy, as well as en bloc esophageal resections.

Squamous cell carcinomas account for the majority of esophageal tumors; adenocarcinomas are less common, whereas benign tumors (leiomyomas) are rare. Most tumors occur in the distal esophagus. Operative treatment may be palliative or curative. Although the prognosis is generally poor, surgical therapy offers the only hope of a cure. After esophageal resection, the stomach is pulled up into the neck or the esophagus is functionally replaced with part of the colon (interposition).

Gastroesophageal reflux is treated surgically when the esophagitis is refractory to medical management or results in complications such as stricture, recurrent pulmonary aspiration, or Barrett's esophagus (columnar epithelium). A variety of antireflux operations may be performed (Nissen, Belsey, Hill, or Collis–Nissen) via thoracic or abdominal approaches, often laparoscopically. They all involve wrapping part of the stomach around the esophagus.

Achalasia and systemic sclerosis (scleroderma) account for the majority of surgical procedures performed for motility disorders. The former usually occurs as an isolated finding, whereas the latter is part of a generalized collagen–vascular disorder. Cricopharyngeal muscle dysfunction can be associated with a variety of neurogenic or myogenic disorders and often results in a Zenker's diverticulum.

ANESTHETIC CONSIDERATIONS

Regardless of the procedure, the major anesthetic consideration for patients with esophageal disease is the risk of pulmonary aspiration. This may result from obstruction, altered motility, or abnormal sphincter function. In fact, most patients typically complain of dysphagia, heartburn, regurgitation, coughing, and/or wheezing when lying flat. Dyspnea on exertion may also be prominent when chronic aspiration results in pulmonary fibrosis. Patients with malignancies may additionally present with anemia and weight loss. A history of heavy smoking is common, so patients should be evaluated for coexisting chronic obstructive pulmonary disease and coronary artery disease. Patients with systemic sclerosis (scleroderma) should be evaluated for involvement of other organs, particularly the kidneys, heart, and lungs; Raynaud's phenomena is also common.

Consideration should be given to administering metoclopramide, an H_2 blocker, or a proton-pump inhibitor preoperatively; awake nasogastric suctioning may also be helpful in decreasing the risk of aspiration. With the patient in a semiupright position, a rapid-sequence induction with cricoid pressure is used. Awake fiberoptic intubation should be considered in patients with systemic sclerosis when a difficult laryngoscopy appears likely. A double-lumen tube is used for procedures involving thoracoscopy or thoracotomy. The anesthesiologist may be asked to pass a large-diameter bougie into the esophagus as part of the surgical procedure; great caution must be exercised to help avoid pharyngeal or esophageal injury.

Transhiatal (blunt) and en bloc thoracic esophagectomies deserve special consideration. These procedures often involve considerable blood loss. The former requires an upper abdominal incision and a left cervical incision, whereas the latter requires posterior thoracotomy, a large abdominal incision, and, finally, a left cervical incision. Monitoring of arterial and central venous pressure is indicated. A PAC should also be used for patients with significant cardiac disease. Multiple large-bore intravenous access, fluid warmers, and a forced-air body warmer are advisable. During the transhiatal approach to esophagectomy, substernal and diaphragmatic retractors can interfere with cardiac function. Moreover, as the esophagus is freed up blindly from the posterior mediastinum by blunt dissection, the surgeon's hand transiently interferes with cardiac filling and produces profound hypotension. The dissection can also induce marked vagal stimulation.

Colonic interposition involves forming a pedicle graft of the colon and passing it through the posterior mediastinum up to the neck to take the place of the esophagus. This procedure is lengthy and involves considerable shifts of fluid. Maintenance of an adequate blood pressure, cardiac output, and hemoglobin concentration is necessary to ensure graft viability. Graft ischemia may be heralded by a progressive metabolic acidosis. For relatively minor procedures, the patient should be extubated on the operating room table or in the PACU. Although in most cases the risk of aspiration likely diminishes following surgery, patients should generally be extubated only when fully awake. Postoperative ventilation should be considered for patients undergoing esophagectomy. Postoperative surgical complications include

damage to the phrenic, vagus, and left recurrent laryngeal nerves.

ANESTHESIA FOR LUNG VOLUME REDUCTION SURGERY

Many patients with severe chronic obstructive pulmonary disease are being treated with lung volume reduction surgery (LVRS). The National Emphysema Treatment Trial (NETT) was a multicenter randomized clinical trial of usual medical therapy versus usual medical therapy plus LVRS. The NETT was discontinued because of a lack of efficacy of LVRS, but many surgeons and medical centers continue to offer the procedure.

PREANESTHETIC EVALUATION

It is imperative that patients be seen by the anesthesiologist prior to surgery, at which time a careful history and physical examination must be done. During the evaluation, information that must be obtained includes a history of previous anesthetics, whether the patient has a difficult airway, and possible abnormal emergence. The baseline breathing and respiratory capacity should be reviewed.

It is important for the patient and any family members to understand that the procedure is lengthy and includes the placement of intravascular lines, induction of anesthesia, placement of a tracheal tube, initiation of mechanical ventilation, positioning of the patient, and emergence (and possible extubation) with recovery initially in the PACU or in an ICU. The risks associated with general anesthesia, tracheal intubation, mechanical ventilation, and one-lung ventilation need to be addressed.

The anesthesiologist should use this opportunity to describe the use and importance of epidural analgesia to the patient, preferably allowing the patient an opportunity to become familiar with the PCA device that could be used with either the epidural or intravenous route of opioid administration. At this time, the anesthesiologist should also discuss the needs and techniques for placement of arterial lines and central venous lines, including a PAC.

Patients should continue all medications up to and including the morning of surgery, including cardiac (β-blockers, calcium channel blockers) and pulmonary (bronchodilators) medications.

The importance of incentive spirometry, coughing, and deep breathing postoperatively should be stressed.

The correct use of inhalers at appropriate intervals should be reviewed.

ANESTHETIC CONSIDERATIONS

The assessment of the airway, degree of respiratory failure with particular reference to the bullous disease component, degree of hyperinflation, oxygen requirement, and degree of resting hypercapnia are of particular importance to the anesthesiologist. Any cardiac disease, with particular reference to ischemic coronary disease, left and right ventricular function, and pulmonary vascular disease, should also be reviewed. Anyone caring for such a patient should be well trained in one-lung ventilation, fiberoptic bronchoscopy, hemodynamic monitoring, CPB, and postoperative analgesia.

Prior to induction, the anesthesiologist should also ensure that the ventilator on the anesthetic machine is capable of several different ventilator modes, all capable of achieving long expiratory times, high gas flows, and pressure-controlled ventilation. A fiberoptic bronchoscope must be available.

All preoperative medications are continued as already discussed, and sedative drugs are avoided or given in minimal dose and appropriately monitored. Although it is necessary to guard against overly aggressive fluid resuscitation, many of these patients may benefit from a fluid bolus before induction of general anesthesia, particularly if an epidural catheter with local anesthetic has been placed. Prophylactic antibiotics, deep venous thrombosis prophylaxis, and corticosteroids for those patients receiving steroids preoperatively also should be administered.

Peripheral arterial catheterization and central venous catheterization—with or without a PAC—should be performed prior to induction or immediately afterward. Transesophageal echocardiography should be considered if the transthoracic echocardiogram was not adequate and in all hemodynamically unstable patients.

There are no specific induction agents that have demonstrated superiority for LVRS. The choice of agents should be guided by the patient's medical condition. Doses should be reduced in patients who are hypovolemic or who have significant cardiac disease. Following intubation, the ventilator should be adjusted to limit the degree of positive-pressure ventilation (< 30 cm H_2O peak inspiratory pressure) and to prolong expiratory time. During induction, if there is sudden hemodynamic collapse, a tension pneumothorax must be ruled out, although the diagnosis may be very difficult because of the masking of physical signs by the preexisting pulmonary disease. Double-lumen tubes are strongly recommended to improve surgical exposure and allow selective lung ventilation. The position of the tube should be confirmed by fiberoptic bronchoscopy.

MAINTENANCE OF ANESTHESIA

Maintenance of anesthesia is often achieved either with inhalation or intravenous agents. Total intravenous anesthesia is particularly useful, particularly if propofol or other short-acting agents are used to allow for a rapid postoperative extubation. NMBAs that are easily and reliably reversed are recommended. NMBAs that cause histamine release should be avoided. Minimal intravenous opioid use is recommended, again to allow early postoperative extubation. Particular attention must be paid to maintaining core temperature; postoperative hypothermia leads to shivering, increased oxygen consumption, and perioperative adverse events.

Patients should be extubated at the conclusion of LVRS or as soon as possible. For those who require continued mechanical ventilation, the double-lumen tracheal tube should be replaced with a single-lumen tracheal tube. The FIO_2 needs to be decreased to maintain SpO_2 at around 88%–90% or greater. Corticosteroids, along with bronchodilators, should be administered to reduce airway inflammation and edema and to promote bronchodilation.

POSTOPERATIVE MANAGEMENT

Patients having LVRS should be cared for in a location with appropriate monitoring and personnel immediately available, ie, either a PACU or ICU. Noninvasive ventilation with bilevel positive airway pressure should be considered for patients who have been extubated and who have a $PaCO_2$ > 70 mm Hg. Inotropes should be considered for treatment of hypotension that may develop in patients secondary to their epidural anesthetic. Thoracic epidural analgesia is strongly recommended for patients having LVRS. Alternatives to the use of epidural analgesia include intercostal or paravertebral nerve blocks and the use of intravenous opioids, either by PCA or through an intermittent bolus, with conversion to oral opioids within the first 24–72 h postoperatively.

CASE DISCUSSION: MEDIASTINAL ADENOPATHY

A 9-year-old boy with mediastinal lymphadenopathy seen on a chest radiograph presents for biopsy of a cervical lymph node.

What is the most important preoperative consideration?

Is there any evidence of airway compromise? Tracheal compression may produce dyspnea (proximal obstruction) or a nonproductive cough (distal obstruction). Asymptomatic compression is also common and may be evident only as tracheal deviation on physical or radiographic examinations. A CT scan of the chest provides invaluable information about the presence, location, and severity of airway compression. Flow-volume loops will also detect subtle airway obstruction and provide important information regarding the location and functional importance of the obstruction (above).

Does the absence of any preoperative dyspnea make severe intraoperative respiratory compromise less likely?

No. Severe airway obstruction can occur following induction of anesthesia in these patients even in the absence of any preoperative symptoms. This mandates that the chest radiograph and CT scan be reviewed for evidence of asymptomatic airway obstruction. The point of obstruction is typically distal to the tip of the tracheal tube. Moreover, loss of spontaneous ventilation can precipitate complete airway obstruction.

What is the superior vena cava syndrome?

Superior vena cava syndrome is the result of progressive enlargement of a mediastinal mass and compression of mediastinal structures, particularly the vena cava. Lymphomas are most commonly responsible, but primary pulmonary or mediastinal neoplasms can also produce the syndrome. Superior vena cava syndrome is often associated with severe airway obstruction and cardiovascular collapse on induction of general anesthesia. The caval compression produces venous engorgement and edema of the head, neck, and arms. Direct mechanical compression as well as mucosal edema severely compromise airflow in the trachea. Most patients favor an upright posture, as recumbency worsens the airway obstruction. Cardiac output may be severely depressed due to impeded venous return from the upper body, direct mechanical compression of the heart, and (with malignancies) pericardial invasion. An echocardiogram is useful in evaluating cardiac function and detecting pericardial fluid.

What is the anesthetic of choice for a patient with superior vena cava syndrome?

The absence of signs or symptoms of airway compression or superior vena cava syndrome does not preclude potentially life-threatening complications following induction of general anesthesia. Therefore, biopsy of a peripheral node (usually cervical or scalene) under local anesthesia is safest whenever possible. Although establishing a diagnosis is of prime importance, the presence of significant airway compromise or the superior vena cava syndrome may dictate empiric treatment with corticosteroids prior to tissue diagnosis at surgery (cancer is the most common cause); preoperative radiation therapy or chemotherapy may also be considered. The patient can usually safely undergo surgery with general anesthesia once airway compromise and other manifestations of the superior vena cava syndrome are alleviated.

General anesthesia may be indicated for establishing a diagnosis in young or uncooperative patients who have no evidence of airway compromise or the superior vena cava syndrome and, rarely, for patients unresponsive to steroids, radiation, and chemotherapy.

How does the presence of airway obstruction and the superior vena cava syndrome influence management of general anesthesia?

1. Premedication: Only an anticholinergic should be given. The patient should be transported to the operating room in a semiupright position with supplemental oxygen.

2. Monitoring: In addition to standard monitors, an arterial line is mandatory, but it should be placed after induction in young patients. At least one large-bore intravenous catheter should be placed in a lower extremity, as venous drainage from the upper body may be unreliable.

3. Airway management: Difficulties with ventilation and intubation should be anticipated. Following preoxygenation, awake intubation with an armored tracheal tube may be safest in a cooperative patient. Use of a flexible bronchoscope is advantageous in the presence of airway distortion and will define the site and degree of obstruction. Coughing or straining, however, may precipitate complete airway obstruction because the resultant positive pleural pressure increases intrathoracic tracheal compression. Passing the armored tube beyond the area of compression may obviate this problem. Uncooperative patients require a careful slow inhalation induction.

4. Induction: The goal should be a smooth induction maintaining spontaneous ventilation

and hemodynamic stability. The ability to ventilate the patient with a good airway should be established prior to use of an NMBA. Using 100% oxygen, one of three induction techniques can be used: (1) intravenous ketamine (because it results in greater hemodynamic stability in patients with reduced cardiac output); (2) inhalational induction with a volatile agent (usually halothane or sevoflurane); or (3) incremental small doses of thiopental, propofol, or etomidate.

Positive-pressure ventilation can precipitate severe hypotension, and volume loading prior to induction may partly offset impaired ventricular filling secondary to caval obstruction.

5. Maintenance of anesthesia: The technique selected should be tailored to the patient's hemodynamic status. Following intubation, neuromuscular blockade prevents coughing or straining.

6. Extubation: At the end of the procedure, patients should be left intubated until the airway obstruction has resolved, as determined by flexible bronchoscopy or the presence of an air leak around the tracheal tube when the tracheal cuff is deflated.

SUGGESTED READING

Benumof JL: *Anesthesia for Thoracic Surgery,* 2nd ed. W.B. Saunders, 1995.

Cohen E: *The Practice of Thoracic Anesthesia.* Lippincott, 1995.

Ghosh S, Latimer RD: *Thoracic Anaesthesia: Principles and Practice.* Butterworth Heinemann, 1999.

Kaplan JA, Slinger PD: *Thoracic Anesthesia,* 3rd ed. Churchill Livingstone, 2003.

Reilly JJ Jr: Evidence-based preoperative evaluation of candidates for thoracotomy. Chest 1999;116:474S.

Youngberg JA: *Cardiac, Vascular, and Thoracic Anesthesia.* Churchill Livingstone, 2000.

Neurophysiology & Anesthesia

25

KEY CONCEPTS

 Cerebral perfusion pressure is the difference between mean arterial pressure and intracranial pressure (ICP) (or central venous pressure, whichever is greater).

 The cerebral autoregulation curve is shifted to the right in patients with chronic arterial hypertension.

 The most important extrinsic influences on cerebral blood flow (CBF) are respiratory gas tensions—particularly Pa_{CO_2}. CBF is directly proportionate to Pa_{CO_2} between tensions of 20 and 80 mg Hg. Blood flow changes approximately 1–2 mL/100 g/min per mm Hg change in Pa_{CO_2}.

 CBF changes 5–7% per 1°C change in temperature. Hypothermia decreases both cerebral metabolic rate and CBF, whereas pyrexia has the reverse effect.

 The movement of a given substance across the blood–brain barrier is governed simultaneously by its size, charge, lipid solubility, and degree of protein binding in blood.

 The blood–brain barrier may be disrupted by severe hypertension, tumors, trauma, strokes, infection, marked hypercapnia, hypoxia, and sustained seizure activity.

 The cranial vault is a rigid structure with a fixed total volume, consisting of brain (80%), blood (12%), and cerebrospinal fluid (8%). Any increase in one component must be offset by an equivalent decrease in another to prevent a rise in intracranial pressure.

 With the exception of ketamine, all intravenous agents either have little effect on or reduce cerebral metabolic rate and CBF.

 With normal autoregulation and an intact blood–brain barrier, vasopressors increase CBF only when mean arterial blood pressure is below 50–60 mm Hg or above 150–160 mm Hg.

 The brain is very vulnerable to ischemic injury because of its relatively high oxygen consumption and near-total dependence on aerobic glucose metabolism.

 Hypothermia is the most effective method for protecting the brain during focal and global ischemia.

 Both animal and human data suggest that barbiturates are effective for brain protection in the setting of focal ischemia.

The anesthetic care of patients who undergo neurosurgery requires a basic understanding of the physiology of the central nervous system (CNS). The effects of anesthetic agents on cerebral metabolism, blood flow, cerebrospinal fluid (CSF) dynamics, and intracranial volume and pressure are often profound. In some instances, these alterations are deleterious, whereas in others they may actually be beneficial. This chapter reviews important physiological concepts in anesthetic practice and then discusses the effects of commonly used anesthetics on cerebral physiology. Although most of the discussion focuses on the brain, the same concepts also apply, at least qualitatively, to the spinal cord.

■ CEREBRAL PHYSIOLOGY

CEREBRAL METABOLISM

The brain is normally responsible for consumption of 20% of total body oxygen. Most of cerebral oxygen consumption (60%) is used in generating adenosine triphosphate (ATP) to support neuronal electrical activity (Figure 25–1). The cerebral metabolic rate (CMR) is usually expressed in terms of oxygen consumption ($CMRO_2$), which averages 3–3.8 mL/100 g/min (50 mL/min) in adults. $CMRO_2$ is greatest in the gray matter of the cerebral cortex and generally parallels cortical electrical activity. Because of the relatively high oxygen consumption and the absence of significant oxygen reserves, interruption of cerebral perfusion usually results in unconsciousness within 10 s as oxygen tension rapidly drops below 30 mm Hg. If blood flow is not reestablished within minutes (3–8 min under most conditions), ATP stores are depleted and irreversible cellular injury begins to occur. The hippocampus and cerebellum appear to be most sensitive to hypoxic injury.

Neuronal cells normally utilize glucose as their primary energy source. Brain glucose consumption is approximately 5 mg/100 g/min, of which over 90% is metabolized aerobically. $CMRO_2$ therefore normally parallels glucose consumption. This relationship does not hold during starvation, when ketone bodies (acetoacetate and β-hydroxybutyrate) also become major energy substrates. Although the brain can also take up and metabolize some lactate, cerebral function is normally dependent on a continuous supply of glucose.

Acute sustained hypoglycemia is equally as devastating as hypoxia. Paradoxically, hyperglycemia can exacerbate global and focal hypoxic brain injury by accelerating cerebral acidosis and cellular injury.

CEREBRAL BLOOD FLOW

Cerebral blood flow (CBF) varies with metabolic activity. It is most commonly measured with a γ-emitting isotope such as xenon (^{133}Xe). Following systemic injection, detectors placed around the brain measure the rate of radioactive decay, which is directly proportionate to CBF. Newer techniques employing positron emission tomography (PET) in conjunction with short-lived isotopes such as ^{11}C and ^{15}O also allow measurement of CMR (for glucose and oxygen, respectively). Such studies confirm that regional CBF parallels metabolic activity and can vary from 10–300 mL/100 g/min. For example, motor activity of a limb is associated with a rapid increase in regional CBF of the corresponding motor cortex. Similarly, visual activity is associated with an increase in regional CBF of the corresponding occipital visual cortex.

Although total CBF averages 50 mL/100 g/min, flow in gray matter is about 80 mL/100 g/min, whereas that in white matter is estimated to be 20 mL/100 g/min. Total CBF in adults averages 750 mL/min (15–20% of cardiac output). Flow rates below 20–25 mL/100 g/min are usually associated with cerebral impairment, as evidenced by slowing on the electroencephalogram (EEG). CBF rates between 15 and 20 mL/100 g/min typically produce a flat (isoelectric) EEG, whereas values below 10 mL/100 g/min are usually associated with irreversible brain damage.

REGULATION OF CEREBRAL BLOOD FLOW

1. Cerebral Perfusion Pressure

Cerebral perfusion pressure (CPP) is the difference between mean arterial pressure (MAP) and intracranial pressure (ICP) (or central venous pressure [CVP], whichever is greater). MAP – ICP (or CVP) = CPP. When CVP is significantly greater than ICP, perfusion pressure becomes the difference between MAP and CVP. CPP is normally 80–100 mm Hg. Moreover, because ICP is normally less than 10 mm Hg, CPP is primarily dependent on MAP.

Moderate to severe increases in ICP (> 30 mm Hg) can significantly compromise CPP and CBF even in the presence of a normal MAP. Patients with CPP values less than 50 mm Hg often show slowing on the EEG, whereas those with a CPP between 25 and 40 mm Hg

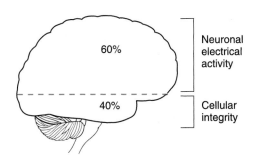

Figure 25–1. Normal brain oxygen requirements.

60% Neuronal electrical activity

40% Cellular integrity

Figure 25–2. Normal cerebral autoregulation curve.

typically have a flat EEG. Sustained perfusion pressures less than 25 mm Hg result in irreversible brain damage.

2. Autoregulation

Similar to the heart and kidneys, the brain normally tolerates wide swings in blood pressure with little change in blood flow. The cerebral vasculature rapidly (10–60 s) adapts to changes in CPP, but abrupt changes in MAP will lead to transient changes in CBF even when autoregulation is intact. Decreases in CPP result in cerebral vasodilation, whereas elevations induce vasoconstriction. In normal individuals, CBF remains nearly constant between MAPs of about 60 and 160 mm Hg (Figure 25–2). Beyond these limits, blood flow becomes pressure dependent. Pressures above 150–160 mm Hg can disrupt the blood–brain barrier (see below) and may result in cerebral edema and hemorrhage.

The cerebral autoregulation curve (Figure 25–2) is shifted to the right in patients with chronic arterial hypertension. Both upper and lower limits are shifted. Flow becomes more pressure dependent at low "normal" arterial pressures in return for cerebral protection at higher arterial pressures. Studies suggest that long-term antihypertensive therapy can restore cerebral autoregulation limits toward normal.

Both myogenic and metabolic mechanisms may explain cerebral autoregulation. Myogenic mechanisms involve an intrinsic response of smooth muscle cells in cerebral arterioles to changes in MAP. Metabolic mechanisms indicate that cerebral metabolic demands determine arteriolar tone. Thus, when tissue demand exceeds blood flow, the release of tissue metabolites causes vasodilation and increases flow. Whereas hydrogen ions were previously thought to mediate this response, other metabolites are probably involved, including nitric oxide, adenosine, prostaglandins, and perhaps ionic (electrolyte) concentration gradients.

3. Extrinsic Mechanisms

Respiratory Gas Tensions

The most important extrinsic influences on CBF are respiratory gas tensions—particularly $PaCO_2$. CBF is directly proportionate to $PaCO_2$ between tensions of 20 and 80 mm Hg (Figure 25–3). Blood flow changes approximately 1–2 mL/100 g/min per mm Hg change in $PaCO_2$. This effect is almost immediate and is thought to be secondary to changes in the pH of CSF and cerebral tissue. Because ions do not readily cross the blood–brain barrier (see below) but CO_2 does, acute changes in $PaCO_2$ but not HCO_3^- affect CBF. Thus, acute metabolic acidosis has little effect on CBF because hydrogen ions (H^+) cannot readily cross the blood–brain barrier. After 24–48 h, CSF HCO_3^- concentration adjusts to compensate for the change in $PaCO_2$, so that the effects of hypocapnia and hypercapnia are diminished. Marked hyperventilation ($PaCO_2 < 20$ mm Hg) shifts the oxygen–hemoglobin dissociation curve to the left and, with changes in CBF, may result in EEG changes suggestive of cerebral impairment even in normal individuals.

Only marked changes in PaO_2 alter CBF. Whereas hyperoxia may be associated with only minimal decreases (−10%) in CBF, severe hypoxemia ($PaO_2 < 50$ mm Hg) profoundly increases CBF (Figure 25–3).

Temperature

CBF changes 5–7% per 1°C change in temperature. Hypothermia decreases both CMR and CBF, whereas pyrexia has the reverse effect.

Figure 25–3. The relationship between cerebral blood flow and arterial respiratory gas tensions.

Between 17°C and 37°C, the Q10 for humans is approximately 2—that is, for every 10° increase in temperature, the CMR doubles. Conversely, the CMR decreases by 50% if the temperature of the brain falls by 10°C, eg, from 37°C to 27°C, and another 50% if the temperature decreases from 27°C to 17°C. At 20°C, the EEG is isoelectric, but further decreases in temperature continue to reduce CMR throughout the brain. Above 42°C, oxygen activity begins to decrease and may reflect cell damage.

Viscosity

Normally, changes in blood viscosity do not appreciably alter CBF. The most important determinant of blood viscosity is hematocrit. A decrease in hematocrit decreases viscosity and can improve CBF; unfortunately, a reduction in hematocrit also decreases the oxygen-carrying capacity and thus can potentially impair oxygen delivery. Elevated hematocrits, as may be seen with marked polycythemia, increase blood viscosity and can reduce CBF. Some studies suggest that optimal cerebral oxygen delivery may occur at hematocrits of approximately 30%.

Autonomic Influences

Intracranial vessels are innervated by sympathetic (vasoconstrictive), parasympathetic (vasodilatory), and noncholinergic nonadrenergic fibers; serotonin and vasoactive intestinal peptide appear to be the neurotransmitters for the latter. The normal physiological function of this innervation is uncertain, but it may play an important role in some pathological states. This is particularly true for the innervation of large cerebral vessels by sympathetic fibers originating in the superior cervical sympathetic ganglia. Intense sympathetic stimulation induces marked vasoconstriction in these vessels, which can limit CBF. Autonomic innervation may also play an important role in cerebral vasospasm following brain injury and stroke.

BLOOD–BRAIN BARRIER

Cerebral blood vessels are unique in that the junctions between vascular endothelial cells are nearly fused. The paucity of pores is responsible for what is termed the blood–brain barrier. This lipid barrier allows the passage of lipid-soluble substances but restricts the movement of those that are ionized or have large molecular weights. Thus, the movement of a given substance across the blood–brain barrier is governed simultaneously by its size, charge, lipid solubility, and degree of protein binding in blood. Carbon dioxide, oxygen, and lipid-soluble substances (such as most anesthetics) freely enter the brain, whereas most ions, proteins, and large substances such as mannitol penetrate poorly.

Water moves freely across the blood–brain barrier as a consequence of bulk flow, whereas movement of even small ions is impeded to some extent (the equilibration half-life for sodium is 2–4 h). As a result, rapid changes in plasma electrolyte concentrations (and, secondarily, osmolality) produce a transient osmotic gradient between plasma and the brain. Acute hypertonicity of plasma results in net movement of water out of the brain, whereas acute hypotonicity causes a net movement of water into the brain. These effects are short-lived, as equilibration eventually occurs, but, when marked, they can cause rapid fluid shifts in the brain. Thus, marked abnormalities in serum sodium or glucose concentrations should generally be corrected slowly (see Chapters 28 and 36). Mannitol, an osmotically active substance that does not normally cross the blood–brain barrier, causes a sustained decrease in brain water content and is often used to decrease brain volume.

The blood–brain barrier may be disrupted by severe hypertension, tumors, trauma, strokes, infection, marked hypercapnia, hypoxia, and sustained seizure activity. Under these conditions, fluid movement across the blood–brain barrier becomes dependent on hydrostatic pressure rather than osmotic gradients.

CEREBROSPINAL FLUID

CSF is found in the cerebral ventricles and cisterns and in the subarachnoid space surrounding the brain and spinal cord. Its major function is to protect the CNS against trauma.

Most of the CSF is formed by the choroid plexuses of the cerebral (mainly lateral) ventricles. Smaller amounts are formed directly by the ventricles' ependymal cell linings and yet smaller quantities from fluid leaking into the perivascular spaces surrounding cerebral vessels (blood–brain barrier leakage). In adults, normal total CSF production is about 21 mL/h (500 mL/d), yet total CSF volume is only about 150 mL. CSF flows from the lateral ventricles through the intraventricular foramina (of Monro) into the third ventricle, through the cerebral aqueduct (of Sylvius) into the fourth ventricle, and through the median aperture of the fourth ventricle (foramen of Magendie) and the lateral aperture of the fourth ventricle (foramina of Luschka) into the cerebellomedullary cistern (cisterna magna) (Figure 25–4). From the cerebellomedullary cistern, CSF enters the subarachnoid space, circulating around the brain and spinal cord before being absorbed in arachnoid granulations over the cerebral hemispheres.

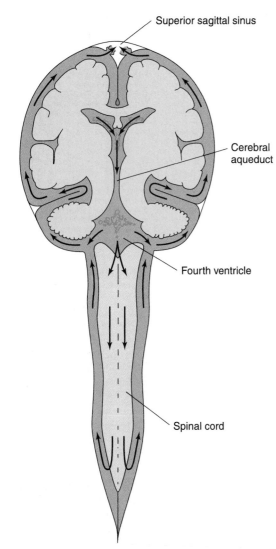

Figure 25–4. The flow of cerebrospinal fluid in the central nervous system. Reproduced, with permission, from Waxman SG: *Correlative Neuroanatomy,* 24th ed. McGraw-Hill, 2000.)

CSF formation involves active secretion of sodium in the choroid plexuses. The resulting fluid is isotonic with plasma despite lower potassium, bicarbonate, and glucose concentrations. Its protein content is limited to the very small amounts that leak into perivascular fluid. Carbonic anhydrase inhibitors (acetazolamide), corticosteroids, spironolactone, furosemide, isoflurane, and vasoconstrictors decrease CSF production.

Absorption of CSF involves the translocation of fluid from the arachnoid granulations into the cerebral

venous sinuses. Smaller amounts are absorbed at nerve root sleeves and by meningeal lymphatics. Although the mechanism remains unclear, absorption appears to be directly proportionate to ICP and inversely proportionate to cerebral venous pressure. Because the brain and spinal cord lack lymphatics, absorption of CSF is also the principal means by which perivascular and interstitial protein is returned to blood.

INTRACRANIAL PRESSURE

The cranial vault is a rigid structure with a fixed total volume, consisting of brain (80%), blood (12%), and CSF (8%). Any increase in one component must be offset by an equivalent decrease in another to prevent a rise in ICP. ICP by convention means supratentorial CSF pressure measured in the lateral ventricles or over the cerebral cortex and is normally 10 mm Hg or less. Minor variations may occur depending on the site measured, but, in the lateral recumbent position, lumbar CSF pressure normally approximates supratentorial pressure.

Intracranial compliance is determined by measuring the change in ICP in response to a change in intracranial volume. Normally, increases in volume are initially well compensated (Figure 25–5). A point is eventually reached, however, at which further increases produce precipitous rises in ICP. Major compensatory mechanisms include (1) an initial displacement of CSF from the cranial to the spinal compartment, (2) an increase in CSF absorption, (3) a decrease in CSF production, and (4) a decrease in total cerebral blood volume (primarily venous).

The concept of total intracranial compliance is useful clinically even though compliance probably varies in the

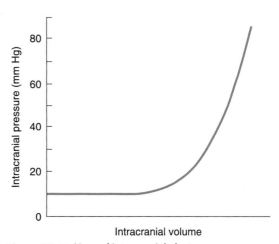

Figure 25–5. Normal intracranial elastance.

Figure 25–6. Potential sites of brain herniation. (Reproduced, with permission, from Fishman RA: Brain edema. N Engl J Med 1975;293:706.)

different compartments of the brain and is affected by arterial blood pressure and $PaCO_2$. Increases in blood pressure can reduce cerebral blood volume because autoregulation induces vasoconstriction in order to maintain CBF. In contrast, hypotension can increase cerebral blood volume as cerebral vessels dilate to maintain blood flow. Cerebral blood volume is estimated to increase 0.05 mL/100 g of brain per 1 mm Hg increase in $PaCO_2$.

Compliance can be determined in patients with intraventricular catheters by injecting sterile saline. An increase in ICP greater than 4 mm Hg following injection of 1 mL of saline indicates poor compliance. At that point, compensatory mechanisms have been exhausted and CBF is progressively compromised as ICP rises further. Sustained elevations in ICP can lead to catastrophic herniation of the brain. Herniation may occur at one of four sites (Figure 25–6): (1) the cingulate gyrus under the falx cerebri, (2) the uncinate gyrus through the tentorium cerebelli, (3) the cerebellar tonsils through the foramen magnum, or (4) any area beneath a defect in the skull (transcalvarial).

■ EFFECT OF ANESTHETIC AGENTS ON CEREBRAL PHYSIOLOGY

Overall, most general anesthetics have a favorable effect on the CNS by reducing electrical activity. Carbohy-drate metabolism decreases, whereas energy stores in the form of ATP, adenosine diphosphate, and phosphocreatine increase. Determination of the effects of the specific agents is complicated by the concomitant administration of other drugs, surgical stimulation, intracranial compliance, blood pressure, and CO_2 tension. For example, hypocapnia or prior administration of thiopental blunts the increases in CBF and ICP that usually occur with ketamine and volatile agents.

This section describes the changes generally associated with each drug when given alone. Table 25–1 summarizes and compares the effects of the various anesthetics. The effects of vasoactive agents and neuromuscular blocking agents are also discussed.

EFFECT OF INHALATION AGENTS

1. Volatile Anesthetics

Cerebral Metabolic Rate

Halothane, desflurane, sevoflurane, and isoflurane produce dose-dependent decreases in CMR. Isoflurane produces the greatest depression (up to 50% reduction), whereas halothane has the least effect (< 25% reduction). The effects of desflurane and sevoflurane appear to be similar to isoflurane. Unlike hypothermia, no further reduction in CMR is observed once the EEG is isoelectric. Moreover, the reduction is not uniform throughout the brain; isoflurane reduces metabolic rate mainly in the neocortex.

Cerebral Blood Flow & Volume

Volatile anesthetics dilate cerebral vessels and impair autoregulation in a dose-dependent manner (Figure 25–7). Halothane has the greatest effect on CBF; at concentrations greater than 1%, it nearly abolishes cerebral autoregulation. Moreover, the increase in blood flow is generalized throughout all parts of the brain. At an equivalent minimum alveolar concentration (MAC) and blood pressure, halothane increases CBF up to 200%, compared with 20% for isoflurane. Unlike halothane, isoflurane increases blood flow primarily in subcortical areas and the hindbrain. Qualitatively and quantitatively, desflurane and sevoflurane may be closest to isoflurane. The effect of volatile agents on CBF also appears to be time dependent because, with continued administration (2–5 h), blood flow begins to return to normal.

The response of the cerebral vasculature to CO_2 is generally retained with all volatile agents. Hyperventilation (hypocapnia) can therefore abolish or blunt the initial effects of these agents on CBF. The timing of the hyperventilation is important because this effect is observed only if hyperventilation is initiated prior to

Table 25–1. Comparative effects of anesthetic agents on cerebral physiology.[1]

Agent	CMR	CBF	CSF Production	CSF Absorption	CBV	ICP
Halothane	↓↓	↑↑↑	↓	↓	↑↑	↑↑
Isoflurane	↓↓↓	↑	±	↑	↑↑	↑
Desflurane	↓↓↓	↑	↑	↓	↑	↑↑
Sevoflurane	↓↓↓	↑	?	?	↑	↑↑
Nitrous oxide	↓	↑	±	±	±	↑
Barbiturates	↓↓↓↓	↓↓↓	±	↑	↓↓	↓↓↓
Etomidate	↓↓↓	↓↓	±	↑	↓↓	↓↓
Proprofol	↓↓↓	↓↓↓↓	?	?	↓↓	↓↓
Benzodiazepines	↓↓	↓	±	↑	↓	↓
Ketamine	±	↑↑	±	↓	↑↑	↑↑
Opioids	±	±	±	↑	±	±
Lidocaine	↓↓	↓↓	?	?	↓↓	↓↓

[1]↑, increase; ↓, decrease; ±, little or no change; ?, unknown; CMR, cerebral metabolic rate; CBF, cerebral blood flow; CSF, cerebrospinal fluid; CBV, cerebral blood volume; ICP, intracranial pressure.

the administration of halothane. In contrast, simultaneous hyperventilation with administration of either isoflurane or sevoflurane can prevent increases in ICP. Hypocapnia may be less effective in decreasing ICP with desflurane compared with other volatile agents.

Increases in cerebral blood volume (10–12%) generally parallel increases in CBF, but the relationship is not necessarily linear. Expansion of cerebral blood volume can markedly elevate ICP in patients with reduced intracranial compliance. Studies indicate that cerebral blood volume increases to the same extent with all volatile agents, suggesting that each affects cerebral venous capacitance to a variable degree. Moreover, these studies demonstrate that hypocapnia most effectively blunts the increase in cerebral blood volume during isoflurane anesthesia.

Altered Coupling of Cerebral Metabolic Rate & Blood Flow

As is apparent from the discussion above, volatile agents alter but do not uncouple the normal relationship of CBF and CMR. The combination of a decrease in neuronal metabolic demand with an increase in CBF (metabolic supply) has been termed luxury perfusion. This state may be desirable during induced hypotension and supports the use of a volatile agent, particularly isoflurane, during this technique. In contrast to this potentially beneficial effect during global ischemia, a detrimental

circulatory steal phenomenon is possible with volatile anesthetics in the setting of focal ischemia. Volatile agents can increase blood flow in normal areas of the brain but not in ischemic areas, where arterioles are already maximally vasodilated. The end result may be a

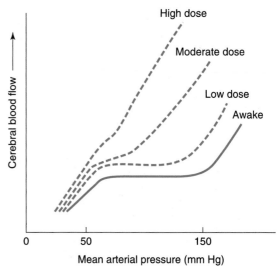

Figure 25–7. Dose-dependent depression of cerebral autoregulation by the volatile anesthetics.

redistribution of blood flow away from ischemic to normal areas.

Cerebrospinal Fluid Dynamics

Volatile anesthetics affect both formation and absorption of CSF. Halothane impedes absorption of CSF but only minimally retards formation. Isoflurane, on the other hand, facilitates absorption and is therefore the only volatile agent with favorable effects on CSF dynamics.

Intracranial Pressure

The net effect of volatile anesthetics on ICP is the result of immediate changes in cerebral blood volume, delayed alterations on CSF dynamics, and arterial CO_2 tension. Based on these factors, isoflurane appears to be the volatile agent of choice in patients with decreased intracranial compliance. Animal studies suggest that desflurane may increase ICP more than other volatile agents.

2. Nitrous Oxide

The effects of nitrous oxide are generally mild and easily overcome by other agents or changes in CO_2 tension. Thus when combined with intravenous agents, nitrous oxide has minimal effects on CBF, CMR, and ICP. Adding this agent to a volatile anesthetic, however, can further increase CBF. When given alone, nitrous oxide causes mild cerebral vasodilation and can potentially increase ICP.

EFFECT OF INTRAVENOUS AGENTS

1. Induction Agents

 With the exception of ketamine, all intravenous agents either have little effect on or reduce CMR and CBF. Moreover, with some exceptions, changes in blood flow generally parallel those in metabolic rate. Cerebral autoregulation and CO_2 responsiveness are preserved with all agents.

Barbiturates

Barbiturates have four major actions on the CNS: (1) hypnosis, (2) depression of CMR, (3) reduction of CBF due to increased cerebral vascular resistance, and (4) anticonvulsant activity. These properties make barbiturates, particularly thiopental, the most commonly used induction agents in neuroanesthesia.

Barbiturates produce dose-dependent decreases in CMR and CBF until the EEG becomes isoelectric. At that point, maximum reductions of nearly 50% are observed; additional barbiturate does not further reduce metabolic rate. Unlike isoflurane, however, barbiturates reduce metabolic rate uniformly throughout the brain. CMR is

depressed slightly more than CBF, such that metabolic supply exceeds metabolic demand (as long as CPP is maintained). Because barbiturate-induced cerebral vasoconstriction occurs only in normal areas, these agents tend to redistribute blood flow from normal to ischemic areas in the brain (Robin Hood, or reverse steal phenomenon). The cerebral vasculature in ischemic areas remains maximally dilated and is unaffected by the barbiturate because of ischemic vasomotor paralysis.

Barbiturates also appear to facilitate absorption of CSF. The resultant reduction in CSF volume, combined with decreases in CBF and cerebral blood volume, makes barbiturates highly effective in lowering ICP. Their anticonvulsant properties are also advantageous in neurosurgical patients who are at increased risk for seizures. The metabolic demand imposed by seizure activity promotes secondary injury in ischemic areas. Small doses of methohexital can activate seizure foci in patients with epilepsy, but higher doses are anticonvulsant like other barbiturates.

Other possible actions of barbiturates include blockade of sodium channels, reduction of intracellular calcium influx, scavenging or suppression of free radical formation, and retardation of cerebral edema following ischemic brain injury. All these actions represent the theoretic justification for the controversial use of barbiturates for cerebral protection. Studies suggest that barbiturate prophylaxis is effective in preventing brain injury during focal but not global ischemia.

Opioids

All opioids generally have minimal effects on CBF, CMR, and ICP, unless $PaCO_2$ rises secondary to respiratory depression. Increases in ICP have been reported in some patients with intracranial tumors following administration of sufentanil and, to a lesser degree, alfentanil. The mechanism appears to be a precipitous drop in blood pressure; reflex cerebral vasodilation likely increases intracranial blood volume and potentially ICP. Although hypotension may be more likely with sufentanil and alfentanil than with fentanyl, significant decreases in blood pressure can adversely affect CPP regardless of the opioid selected. In addition, small doses of alfentanil (< 50 mg/kg) can activate seizure foci in patients with epilepsy. Morphine is generally not considered optimal in neuroanesthesia due to poor lipid solubility. The latter results in slow CNS penetration and prolonged sedative effects. Normeperidine, a metabolite of meperidine, can induce seizures, particularly in patients with renal failure. The accumulation of normeperidine and the associated cardiac depression limit the use of meperidine during the perioperative period.

Etomidate

Etomidate decreases the CMR, CBF, and ICP in somewhat the same way as thiopental. Its effect on CMR is nonuniform, affecting the cortex more than the brain stem. Its limited effect on the brain stem may be responsible for greater hemodynamic stability in unstable patients when compared with the effect of barbiturates. Etomidate also decreases production and enhances absorption of CSF. Concern over adrenal suppression limits its long-term use (see Chapter 8).

Induction with etomidate is associated with a relatively high incidence of myoclonic movements, but these movements are not associated with seizure activity on the EEG in normal individuals. The drug has been used to treat seizures, but reports of seizure activity following etomidate suggest that the drug is best avoided in patients with a history of epilepsy. In fact, small doses of etomidate can activate seizure foci in patients with epilepsy.

Propofol

Propofol reduces CBF and CMR similar to barbiturates and etomidate; however, the decrease in CBF may exceed that in metabolic rate. The drug also appears to be useful in the CMR. Although it has been associated with dystonic and choreiform movements, propofol appears to have significant anticonvulsant activity. Moreover, its short elimination half-life (see Chapter 8) makes it a useful agent for neuroanesthesia. Unfortunately, excessive hypotension and cardiac depression in elderly or unstable patients can compromise CPP.

Benzodiazepines

Benzodiazepines lower CBF and CMR but to a lesser extent than barbiturates, etomidate, and propofol. Benzodiazepines also have useful anticonvulsant properties. Midazolam is the benzodiazepine of choice because of its short half-life. Midazolam induction frequently causes significant decreases in CPP in elderly and unstable patients and may prolong emergence in some instances, particularly in patients with renal failure or if used as a continuous infusion throughout the case.

Ketamine

Ketamine is the only intravenous anesthetic that dilates the cerebral vasculature and increases CBF (50–60%). Selective activation of certain areas (limbic and reticular) is partially offset by depression of other areas (somatosensory and auditory) such that total CMR does not change. Seizure activity in thalamic and limbic areas is also described. Ketamine may also impede absorption of CSF without affecting formation. Increases in CBF, cerebral blood volume, and CSF volume can potentially increase ICP markedly in patients with decreased intracranial compliance.

2. Anesthetic Adjuncts

Intravenous lidocaine decreases CMR, CBF, and ICP but to a lesser degree than other agents. Its principal advantage is that it decreases CBF (by increasing cerebral vascular resistance) without causing other significant hemodynamic effects. The risks of systemic toxicity and seizures, however, limit the usefulness of repeated dosing.

Droperidol has little or no effect on CMR and minimally reduces CBF. When used with an opioid as part of a neuroleptic technique, droperidol may cause undesirable prolonged sedation. Reversal of opioids or benzodiazepines with naloxone or flumazenil, respectively, can reverse any beneficial reductions in CBF and CMR. Severe hypertension may also follow the use of naloxone but not flumazenil.

3. Vasopressors

With normal autoregulation and an intact blood–brain barrier, vasopressors increase CBF only when mean arterial blood pressure is below 50–60 mm Hg or above 150–160 mm Hg. In the absence of autoregulation, vasopressors increase CBF by their effect on CPP. Changes in CMR generally parallel those in blood flow. β-Adrenergic agents seem to have a greater effect on the brain when the blood–brain barrier is disrupted; central β_1-receptor stimulation increases CMR and blood flow. β-Adrenergic blockers generally have no direct effect on CMR or CBF, whereas α_2-adrenergic agonists produce cerebral vasoconstriction. Excessive elevations in blood pressure with any agent can disrupt the blood–brain barrier.

4. Vasodilators

In the absence of hypotension, most vasodilators induce cerebral vasodilation and increase CBF in a dose-related fashion. When these agents decrease blood pressure, CBF is usually maintained and may even increase. The resultant increase in cerebral blood volume can significantly elevate ICP in patients with decreased intracranial compliance. Of this group of drugs, only trimethaphan has little or no effect on CBF and cerebral blood volume; because it constricts pupils, trimethaphan may complicate the neurological examination. Trimethaphan is no longer available in the United States, but it is available in Europe.

5. Neuromuscular Blocking Agents

Neuromuscular blocking agents (NMBAs) lack direct action on the brain but can have important secondary effects. Hypertension and histamine-mediated cerebral vasodilation increase ICP, while systemic hypotension (from histamine release or ganglionic blockade) lowers CPP. Succinylcholine can increase ICP, possibly as a result of cerebral activation associated with enhanced muscle spindle activity, but the increase is generally minimal if an adequate dose of thiopental or propofol is given and hyperventilation is initiated at induction. Moreover, a small (defasciculating) dose of a non-depolarizing NMBA appears to blunt the increase, at least partially. Agents that are likely to release histamine include tubocurarine, atracurium, metocurine, and mivacurium. Tachycardia and hypertension may follow large doses of pancuronium, whereas ganglionic blockade may be seen following the use of tubocurarine.

In the majority of instances, increases in ICP following administration of an NMBA are the result of a hypertensive response due to light anesthesia during laryngoscopy and tracheal intubation. Acute elevations in ICP will also be seen if hypercapnia or hypoxemia results from prolonged apnea.

■ PHYSIOLOGY OF BRAIN PROTECTION

PATHOPHYSIOLOGY OF CEREBRAL ISCHEMIA

The brain is very vulnerable to ischemic injury because of its relatively high oxygen consumption and near-total dependence on aerobic glucose metabolism (above). Interruption of cerebral perfusion, metabolic substrate (glucose), or severe hypoxemia rapidly results in functional impairment; reduced perfusion also impairs clearance of potentially toxic metabolites. If normal oxygen tension, blood flow, and glucose supply are not reestablished within 3–8 min under most conditions, ATP stores are depleted and irreversible neuronal injury begins. During ischemia, intracellular K^+ decreases and intracellular Na^+ increases. More important, intracellular Ca^{2+} increases because of failure of ATP-dependent pumps to either extrude the ion extracellularly or into intracellular cisterns, increased intracellular Na^+ concentration, and release of the excitatory neurotransmitter glutamate.

Sustained increases in intracellular Ca^{2+} activate lipases and proteases, which initiate and propagate structural damage to neurons. Increases in free fatty acid concentration and cyclooxygenase and lipoxygenase activities result in the formation of prostaglandins and leukotrienes, some of which are potent mediators of cellular injury. Accumulation of toxic metabolites such as lactic acid also impairs cellular function and interferes with repair mechanisms. Lastly, reperfusion of ischemic tissues can cause additional tissue damage due to the formation of oxygen-derived free radicals.

STRATEGIES FOR BRAIN PROTECTION

Ischemic brain injury is usually classified as focal (incomplete) or global (complete). On the one hand, this convention may be somewhat artificial in that differences may involve severity more than mechanism. On the other hand, this classification is useful in defining clinical settings. Global ischemia includes total circulatory arrest as well as global hypoxia. Cessation of perfusion may be caused by cardiac arrest or deliberate circulatory arrest, whereas global hypoxia may be caused by severe respiratory failure, drowning, and asphyxia (including anesthetic mishaps). Focal ischemia includes embolic, hemorrhagic, and atherosclerotic strokes as well as blunt, penetrating, and surgical trauma.

In some instances, interventions aimed at restoring perfusion and oxygenation are possible; these include reestablishing effective circulation, normalizing arterial oxygenation and oxygen-carrying capacity, or reopening an occluded vessel. With focal ischemia, the brain tissue surrounding a severely damaged area may suffer marked functional impairment but still remain viable. Such areas are thought to have very marginal perfusion (< 15 mL/100 g/min), but, if further injury can be limited and normal flow is rapidly restored, these areas (the "ischemic penumbra") may recover completely. When the above interventions are not applicable or available, the emphasis must be on limiting the extent of brain injury.

From a practical point of view, efforts aimed at preventing or limiting neuronal tissue damage are often the same whether the ischemia is focal or global. Clinical goals are usually to optimize CPP, decrease metabolic requirements (basal and electrical), and possibly block mediators of cellular injury. Clearly, the most effective strategy is prevention because once injury has occurred, measures aimed at cerebral protection become less effective.

Hypothermia

Hypothermia is the most effective method for protecting the brain during focal and global ischemia. Indeed, profound hypothermia is often used for up to 1 h of total circulatory arrest with little evidence of neurological impairment. Unlike anesthetic agents, hypothermia decreases both basal and electrical metabolic requirements throughout the brain; metabolic requirements continue to decrease even after complete electrical silence.

Even mild degrees of hypothermia (33°–35°C) have some protective effects. Moreover, mild hypothermia has fewer adverse effects than more profound reductions in temperature (see Chapter 6).

Anesthetic Agents

Barbiturates, etomidate, propofol, and isoflurane can produce complete electrical silence of the brain and eliminate the metabolic cost of electrical activity; unfortunately, these agents have no effect on basal energy requirements. Furthermore, with the exception of barbiturates, their effects are nonuniform, affecting different parts of the brain to variable extents. Lastly, barbiturates can also produce inverse steal, reduce cerebral edema and calcium influx, and inhibit free radical formation and blockade of sodium channels (above).

Both animal and human data suggest that barbiturates are effective for brain protection in the setting of focal ischemia. Although some animal data suggest that etomidate, propofol, and possibly isoflurane may be protective, the results are conflicting, and clinical experience with these agents is limited. Ketamine may also have a protective effect because of its ability to block the actions of glutamate at the *N*-methyl-D-aspartate (NMDA) receptor (see Chapter 8), but animal studies for this agent are also conflicting.

No anesthetic agent has consistently been shown to be protective against global ischemia. Only hypothermia is truly protective.

Specific Adjuncts

The calcium channel blockers, nimodipine and nicardipine, have not been shown to reduce neurological injury following hemorrhagic and ischemic strokes. Both agents have cerebral vasodilating properties; unfortunately, though they may improve CBF, they do not improve neurological outcome. However, nimodipine has a role in the management of patients with subarachnoid hemorrhage. Methylprednisolone has been shown to reduce neurological deficits following spinal cord injury if given within 8 h. Although preliminary studies were encouraging, neither the nonglucocorticoid steroid tirilazad nor acadesine, an adenosine-modulating agent, has been shown to improve outcome either with subarachnoid hemorrhage or in the incidence of stroke following coronary artery surgery. Other agents that may prove to be beneficial include magnesium, dexmedetomidine (an α_2-adrenergic agonist that also interacts with NMDA receptors), dextromethorphan (a noncompetitive NMDA blocker), 2,3-dihydroxy-6-nitro-7-sulfamoyl-benzo[*F*]quinoxaline (NBQX, an α-amino-3-hydroxy-5-methyl-4-isoxazole-propionic acid [AMPA]-receptor blocker), and vitamin E (an antioxidant).

General Measures

Maintenance of an optimal CPP is critical. Thus arterial blood pressure should be normal or slightly elevated, and increases in venous and ICP should be avoided. Oxygen-carrying capacity should ideally be maintained with a hematocrit of 30% and normal arterial oxygen tension. Hyperglycemia aggravates neurological injuries following either focal or global ischemia. Excessive hyperglycemia (> 150–180 mg/dL) should be avoided. Normocarbia should be maintained, as both hypercarbia and hypocarbia have no beneficial effect in the setting of ischemia and could prove detrimental; hypocarbia-induced cerebral vasoconstriction may aggravate the ischemia, whereas hypercarbia may induce a steal phenomena (with focal ischemia) or worsen intracellular acidosis.

EFFECT OF ANESTHESIA ON ELECTROPHYSIOLOGICAL MONITORING

Electrophysiological monitoring attempts to assess the functional integrity of the CNS. The most commonly used monitors for neurosurgical procedures are the EEG and evoked potentials. Proper application of these monitoring modalities is critically dependent on monitoring the specific area at risk and recognizing anesthetic-induced changes. Both monitoring modalities are described in Chapter 6.

The effects of anesthetic agents on the EEG and evoked potentials are summarized in Tables 25–2 and 25–3. Correct interpretation of changes requires correlation with anesthetic depth- and dose-related changes and with physiological variables such as blood pressure, body temperature, and respiratory gas tensions. EEG slowing associated with relative hypotension is of greater concern during light anesthesia and intense surgical retraction than during deep anesthesia without stimulation. Regardless of the technique employed, recordings should be bilateral (for comparison) and correlated with the intraoperative course of events.

ELECTROENCEPHALOGRAPHY

EEG monitoring is most useful for assessing the adequacy of cerebral perfusion during carotid endarterectomy (CEA) and controlled hypotension, as well as for assessing anesthetic depth. EEG changes can be simplistically described as either activation or depression. EEG activation (a shift to predominantly high-frequency and low-voltage activity) is seen with light anesthesia and surgical stimulation, whereas EEG depression (a shift to predominantly low-frequency and high-voltage activity) occurs with deep anesthesia or cerebral compromise. **Most anesthetics produce a biphasic pattern on the**

Table 25–2. Electroencephalographic changes during anesthesia.

Activation	Depression
Inhalational agents (subanesthetic)	Inhalation agents (1–2 MAC)
Barbiturates (small doses)	Barbiturates
Benzodiazepines (small doses)	Opioids
Etomidate (small doses)	Propofol
Nitrous oxide	Etomidate
Ketamine	Hypocapnia
Mild hypercapnia	Marked hypercapnia
Sensory stimulation	Hypothermia
Hypoxia (early)	Hypoxia (late)
	Ischemia

EEG consisting of an initial activation (at subanesthetic doses) followed by dose-dependent depression.

Inhalation Anesthetics

Clinically, halothane produces a typical biphasic pattern. Isoflurane is the only volatile anesthetic that can produce an isoelectric EEG at high clinical doses (1–2 MAC). **Desflurane and sevoflurane produce a burst suppression pattern at high doses (> 1.2 and > 1.5 MAC, respectively) but not electrical silence.** Nitrous oxide is also unusual in that it increases both frequency and amplitude (high-amplitude activation).

Intravenous Agents

Benzodiazepines produce a typical biphasic pattern on the EEG. Barbiturates, etomidate, and propofol produce a typical biphasic pattern and are the only intravenous agents capable of producing burst suppression and electrical silence at high doses. In contrast, opioids characteristically produce only a monophasic, dose-

Table 25–3. Effect of anesthetic agents on evoked potentials.[1]

Agent	SSEP		VER		BAER	
	Amp	*Lat*	*Amp*	*Lat*	*Amp*	*Lat*
Nitrous oxide	↓	±	↓	↑	±	±
Halothane	↓	↑	±	↑	±	↑
Isoflurane	↓	↑	↓	↑	±	↑
Barbiturates	±	±	↓	↑	±	±
Opioids[2]	±	±	±	±	±	±
Etomidate	↑	↑				
Propofol	↓	↑			↓	↑
Benzodiazepines	↓	±				
Ketamine	±	↑				

[1]↑, increase; ↓, decrease; ±, little or no change; SSEP, somatosensory evoked potentials; VER, visual evoked response; BAER, brainstem auditory evoked response; Amp, amplitude; Lat, latency.
[2]At very high doses, can decrease the latency and decrease the amplitude of SSEP.

dependent depression of the EEG. Lastly, ketamine produces an unusual activation consisting of rhythmic high-amplitude theta activity followed by very high-amplitude gamma and low-amplitude beta activities.

EVOKED POTENTIALS

Somatosensory evoked potentials (SSEPs) test the integrity of the dorsal spinal columns and the sensory cortex and may be useful during resection of spinal tumors, instrumentation of the spine, CEA, and aortic surgery. The adequacy of perfusion of the spinal cord during aortic surgery is probably better assessed with motor evoked potentials. Brain stem auditory evoked potentials test the integrity of the eighth cranial nerve and the auditory pathways above the pons and are used for surgery in the posterior fossa. Visual evoked potentials may be used to monitor the optic nerve and upper brain stem during resections of large pituitary tumors.

Interpretation of evoked potentials is more complicated than that of the EEG. Evoked potentials have poststimulus latencies that are described as short, intermediate, and long. Short-latency evoked potentials arise from the nerve stimulated or from the brain stem. Intermediate- and long-latency evoked potentials are primarily of cortical origin. In general, short-latency potentials are least affected by anesthetic agents, while long-latency potentials are affected by even subanesthetic levels of most agents. Consequently, only short and intermediate potentials are monitored intraoperatively. Visual evoked potentials are most affected by anesthetics, while brain stem auditory evoked potentials are least affected.

Inhalation Anesthetics

Of all anesthetics, volatile ones have the greatest effect on evoked potentials, causing dose-dependent decreases in wave amplitude and increases in latencies. To minimize anesthetic-induced changes, limiting isoflurane concentration to 0.5 MAC and halothane to 1 MAC has been recommended. Nitrous oxide decreases wave amplitude but has no effect on latencies.

Intravenous Anesthetics

Intravenous agents in clinical doses generally have fewer effects on evoked potentials compared with volatile agents but, in high doses can also decrease amplitude and increase latencies. It should be noted that evoked potentials are often preserved with barbiturates even when they produce an isoelectric EEG. Etomidate increases latencies of SSEPs but can increase wave amplitude. Although most opioids produce dose-dependent increases in latencies of SSEPs and more variable decreases in wave amplitude, meperidine may

increase amplitude. Ketamine has also been reported to increase SSEP wave amplitude.

CASE DISCUSSION: POSTOPERATIVE HEMIPLEGIA

A 62-year-old man has undergone a right CEA. Immediately following surgery, in the recovery room, he is noted to be weak on the contralateral side.

How is a patient undergoing CEA evaluated preoperatively?

Patients with cerebrovascular disease and, in particular, carotid stenosis are at very high risk for coronary artery and peripheral arterial disease. It would be unusual for a patient to have carotid stenosis who did not have evidence of atherosclerosis elsewhere. Patients undergoing CEA, therefore, require a preoperative cardiac evaluation. The American Heart Association and the American College of Cardiology, with input from anesthesiologists, recently revised their guidelines on how these patients should be evaluated. Evaluations are based on a patient's risk factors and the risk of the surgery. Whereas a CEA would appear to be a very high-risk procedure from a cardiac standpoint, in reality, it is a moderate-risk procedure; a femoral popliteal bypass is considered a high-risk procedure. The increase in afterload that develops when the iliac or femoral artery is clamped is much greater than when the carotid artery is crossclamped and, therefore, places a greater afterload on the left ventricle. Based on body surface area and the affected arterial distribution, the crossclamping of the carotid artery produces less than a 3–5% increase in afterload (particularly if there has not been much flow through the carotid artery) compared to an 18% increase in afterload when the iliac artery is crossclamped.

With respect to patient risk factors, the guidelines have algorithms for how patients should be evaluated and managed intraoperatively. In the patient under discussion, coronary artery disease or peripheral artery disease other than the carotid stenosis would be an unlikely cause of the patient's postoperative findings. However, all such patients require thorough evaluation for cardiac disease and appropriate management, depending on the findings. As part of this patient's preoperative evaluation, a thorough neurological examination should have been performed with special attention paid to motor function. This patient may well have been weak on the left side prior to surgery, in which case the hemiparesis might be due to a preexisting condition. If this is a new finding, it requires aggressive management.

Is general or regional anesthesia the optimal anesthetic technique for managing patients undergoing CEA?

For the past several decades, the majority of patients undergoing CEAs in the United States have had general anesthesia. General anesthesia was chosen because many surgeons operating in the neck area felt more comfortable if the airway was controlled, and the patient was completely anesthetized should evidence of cerebral ischemia develop. Unfortunately, because the patient was anesthetized, monitors of ischemia had to be developed, and so most patients were monitored with measures of CBF (xenon versus more recently transcranial Doppler [TCD]), of pressure within the cerebral vascular tree (stump pressure), or of electrophysiological activity (12-lead EEG).

More recently, regional anesthesia has been advocated as providing an adequate surgical field, a comfortable and relaxed patient (if done with monitored anesthesia care), stable hemodynamics, and ideal monitoring of cerebral function during crossclamping because an awake patient provides the best evidence of adequate cerebral perfusion. The patient can indicate or can be observed for evidence of aphasia, facial droop, or hemiparesis. Regional anesthesia is usually performed with deep and superficial cervical nerve blocks (see Chapter 17).

No studies demonstrate a superiority of general over regional anesthesia or vice versa; however, in the United States, anesthesiologists are increasingly choosing regional anesthesia as they believe it is superior to general anesthesia for monitoring of cerebral function following carotid clamping.

How should cerebral function be monitored intraoperatively in this patient?

When the carotid is crossclamped, the ability to identify inadequate cerebral circulation in the ipsilateral hemisphere is critical, as there is a window of opportunity for immediate intervention and correction of any deficit.

Global and focal neurological status can continuously be assessed in awake patients if the patient is mildly sedated when undergoing regional anesthesia. In such a situation, practical assessment consists of frequent (every 2–5 min) examination of strength using the contralateral handgrip and maintenance of constant verbal contact with the patient to assess level of consciousness.

In patients undergoing general anesthesia, indirect cerebral monitoring techniques have been used to assess the adequacy of the cerebral circulation. These techniques include stump bleeding, stump pressure, jugular venous oxygen saturation, EEG, a processed EEG (such as the bispectral index or evoked potentials), TCD, arteriography, and measurement of blood flow using xenon. Back bleeding of the distal carotid artery following crossclamp and incision of the artery suggests reasonable collateral circulation above the clamp. It is very subjective and nonquantitative.

To better qualify and quantify the adequacy of collateral perfusion (Figure 25–8), stump pressure measurements can be used. Some surgeons believe that a shunt should be used in all patients with a previous cerebrovascular accident, independent of stump pressure, and for any patient whose stump pressure is less than 25 mm Hg. However, this is controversial, as many neurosurgeons and vascular surgeons use 50 mm Hg as a cutoff.

The EEG is the gold standard for monitoring patients undergoing CEA under general anesthesia. In such a circumstance, inhalation or intravenous anesthesia can influence the EEG. However, analyzing the EEG is labor and technology intensive and requires interpretation of the data.

For this reason, techniques that employ a processed EEG, eg, the bispectral index monitor, are being explored as a monitor for cerebral ischemia. Evoked potentials, such as auditory and visual evoked potentials, have also been examined, but do not appear to have significant clinical application.

Jugular venous oxygen saturation has been studied in an attempt to identify the acute onset of cerebral ischemia. Because it is a global measure, it does not reflect regional or, in particular, focal cerebral ischemia and, therefore, is not used for routine clinical practice. TCD ultrasonography provides noninvasive assessment of blood flow in the middle cerebral artery. Though the Doppler is very useful for detection of intraoperative cerebral emboli, it is not particularly helpful or reliable in predicting the requirement of a shunt.

Because of drawbacks with all these techniques, in terms of cerebral monitoring, no measure is better than continuous assessment of global and focal neurological status in awake patients.

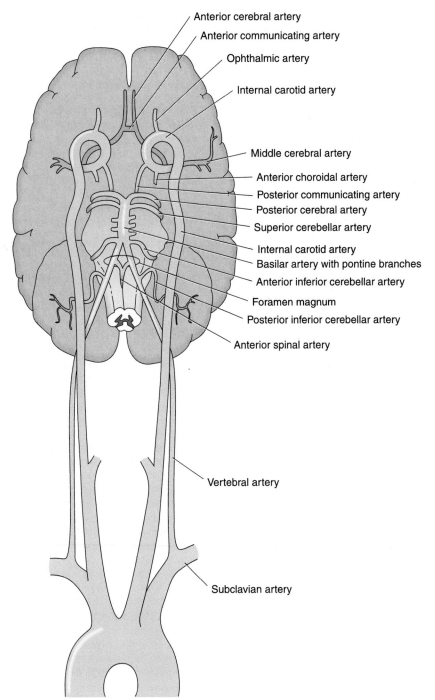

Figure 25–8. The cerebral circulation.

How should hemodynamics be controlled intraoperatively?

During carotid clamping and immediately afterward in the recovery room, patients are often hemodynamically labile. **Bradycardia can develop during surgical manipulation of the carotid sinus because of the direct stimulation of the vagus nerve.** Tachycardia may develop as a result of stress or pain or as a direct result of manipulation of the carotid sinus with release of catecholamines into the circulation.

Hypotension is also observed because of the direct vasodilating and negative ionotropic effects of anesthetic agents. Hypotension following carotid unclamping is common, particularly in patients with more severe carotid stenosis. This could be due to a cerebral protective process. Cerebral autoregulation protects the brain from reperfusion by reducing cerebral production of renin, vasopressin, and norepinephrine, which results in hypotension. Hypertension is also a frequent finding in patients undergoing CEA. Many patients have hypertension as a comorbid condition, which is often further exacerbated by the surgical stress and manipulation of the carotid body, which causes release of catecholamines and sympathetic stimulation.

Because of the nature of the problem and the wide swings in blood pressure and heart rate, many anesthesiologists place a "crow's foot" (Figure 25–9) in the intravenous line at the site of entry of the indwelling venous cannula so that a vasoconstrictor and vasodilator, along with the maintenance fluid, can be manipulated immediately should any hemodynamic changes require treatment.

What is the most likely etiology of this patient's findings?

This patient most likely has had a cerebrovascular accident due to an arterio-to-arterial embolus; more than 95% of patients will fit into this category. Weakness can also develop as a result of a hyperperfusion syndrome, which occurs in patients with severe carotid stenosis who have now reestablished flow to the affected cerebral hemisphere. Such patients usually have a greater than 95% carotid stenosis with a less than 1-mm channel in the affected carotid artery. Typically, the syndrome does not develop in the postoperative anesthesia care unit (PACU), but several hours afterward when the patient begins complaining of a headache and, in severe cases, develops hemiparesis.

Because a cerebrovascular accident is most likely, when the anesthesiologist is called to see such a patient in the PACU, a thorough neurological examination quantifying any cranial nerve involvement and the degree of weakness on the contralateral side should be performed. Any hemodynamic changes need to be treated immediately with assurance of adequate hemoglobin and oxygenation levels. The surgeon needs to be notified at once as it may be necessary to return to the operating room to explore the carotid artery. If a neurological consultation is obtained, a computerized tomographic (CT) scan, occasionally with angiography, is often performed. A magnetic resonance imaging (MRI) scan can better quantify the area of ischemia sooner than CT scanning, but MRI scanners are not as widely distributed as are CT scanners.

In the current circumstances, the patient's hemodynamics need to be treated, the neurosurgeon should be consulted, and, if a decision is made to not take the patient back to the operating room, a neurologist should be consulted. Obviously, these patients are not candidates for thrombolytic therapy because of the CEA. The use of thrombolytics could lead to oozing at the surgical site, the most feared consequence of which would be obstruction of the airway in the neck.

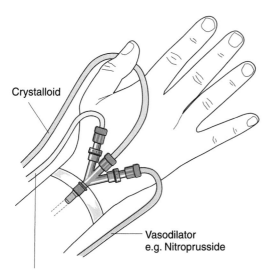

Crystalloid

Vasodilator
e.g. Nitroprusside

Vasoconstrictor
e.g. neosynephrine

Figure 25–9. A triconnector ("crow's foot") in an indwelling intravenous catheter.

SUGGESTED READING

Albin MS: *Textbook of Neuroanesthesia with Neurosurgical and Neuroscience Perspectives.* McGraw-Hill, 1997.

Cottrell JE, Smith DS: *Anesthesia and Neurosurgery,* 4th ed. Mosby Year Book, 2001.

Cucchiara RF, Black S, Michenfelder JD: *Clinical Neuroanesthesia,* 2nd ed. Churchill Livingstone, 1998.

Newfield P, Cottrell JE: *Handbook of Neuroanesthesia,* 3rd ed. Lippincott, Williams & Wilkins, 1999.

Schubert A: *Clinical Neuroanesthesia.* Butterworth-Heinemann, 1997.

Stone DJ, Sperry RJ: *The Neuroanesthesia Handbook.* Mosby, 1996.

Walters FJM, Ingram GS, Jenkinson JL: *Anaesthesia and Intensive Care for the Neurosurgical Patient.* Blackwell, 1994.

Anesthesia for Neurosurgery

26

KEY CONCEPTS

 Regardless of the cause, intracranial masses present according to growth rate, location, and intracranial pressure. Slowly growing masses are frequently asymptomatic for long periods, whereas rapidly growing ones usually present acutely.

 Computed tomographic and magnetic resonance imaging scans should be reviewed for evidence of brain edema, a midline shift greater than 0.5 cm, and ventricular size.

 Operations in the posterior fossa can injure vital circulatory and respiratory brain stem centers as well as cranial nerves or their nuclei.

 Venous air embolism can occur when the pressure within an open vein is subatmospheric. These conditions may exist in any position (and during any procedure) whenever the wound is above the level of the heart.

 Optimal recovery of air following venous air embolism is provided by a multiorificed catheter positioned high in the atrium at its junction with the superior vena cava. Confirmation of correct catheter positioning is important and is accomplished by intravascular electrocardiography or by transesophageal echocardiography.

 In a patient with head trauma, correction of hypotension and control of any bleeding take precedence over radiographic studies and definitive neurosurgical treatment because systolic arterial blood pressures of less than 80 mm Hg correlate with a poor outcome.

 Massive blood loss from aortic or vena caval injury can occur intraoperatively or postoperatively with thoracic or lumbar procedures and is often initially occult.

Harvey Cushing, one of the founders of neurosurgery, is largely responsible for the development of the anesthesia record. Out of concern for the safety of his patients, he emphasized the need to record the surgical patient's pulse, respiratory rate, temperature, and blood pressure intraoperatively. A better understanding of the effects of anesthesia on the central nervous system (CNS) (see Chapter 25) and improvements in anesthetic techniques have similarly contributed to the improved outcomes seen in modern neurosurgery. Sophisticated monitoring techniques and improved operating conditions under anesthesia have allowed increasingly difficult procedures to be performed on patients previously deemed inoperable.

Anesthetic techniques must be modified in the presence of intracranial hypertension and marginal cerebral perfusion. In addition, many neurosurgical procedures require unusual patient positions—eg, sitting, prone—further complicating management. This chapter applies the principles developed in Chapter 25 to the anesthetic care of neurosurgical patients.

INTRACRANIAL HYPERTENSION

Intracranial hypertension is defined as a sustained increase in intracranial pressure (ICP) above 15 mm Hg. Uncompensated increases in the tissue or fluid within the rigid cranial vault produce sustained ICP elevations (see Chapter 25). Intracranial hypertension may result from an expanding tissue or fluid mass, depressed skull fracture, interference with normal absorption of cerebrospinal fluid (CSF), excessive cerebral blood flow (CBF), or systemic disturbances promoting brain edema (see below). Multiple factors are often simultaneously present. For example, tumors in the posterior fossa are not only usually associated with some degree of brain edema, but they also readily obstruct CSF flow by compressing the fourth ventricle (obstructive hydrocephalus).

Although many patients with increased ICP are initially asymptomatic, all eventually develop characteristic symptoms and signs, including headache, nausea, vomiting, papilledema, focal neurological deficits, and altered consciousness. When ICP exceeds 30 mm Hg, CBF progressively decreases, and a vicious circle is established: ischemia causes brain edema, which in turn increases ICP, resulting in more ischemia. If left unchecked, this cycle continues until the patient dies of progressive neurological damage or catastrophic herniation (see Chapter 25). **Periodic increases in arterial blood pressure with reflex slowing of the heart rate (Cushing response) are often observed and can be correlated with abrupt increases in ICP (plateau or A waves) lasting 1–15 min.** This phenomena is the result of autoregulatory mechanisms periodically decreasing cerebral vascular resistance in response to cerebral ischemia; unfortunately, the latter further increases ICP as cerebral blood volume increases. Eventually, severe ischemia and acidosis completely abolish autoregulation (vasomotor paralysis), and both ICP and CBF become passive to arterial blood pressure.

CEREBRAL EDEMA

An increase in brain water content can be produced by several mechanisms. Disruption of the blood–brain barrier (vasogenic edema) is most common and allows the entry of plasma-like fluid into the brain. Increases in blood pressure enhance the formation of this type of edema. Common causes of vasogenic edema include mechanical trauma, inflammatory lesions, brain tumors, hypertension, and infarction. Cerebral edema following metabolic insults (cytotoxic edema), such as hypoxemia or ischemia, results from failure of brain cells to actively extrude sodium and progressive cellular swelling. Interstitial cerebral edema is the result of obstructive hydrocephalus and entry of CSF into brain interstitium. Cerebral edema can also be the result of intracellular movement of water secondary to acute decreases in serum osmolality (water intoxication).

TREATMENT

Treatment of intracranial hypertension and cerebral edema is ideally directed at the underlying cause. Metabolic disturbances are corrected and operative intervention is undertaken whenever possible. Vasogenic edema—particularly that associated with tumors—often responds to corticosteroids (dexamethasone), which appear to promote repair of the blood–brain barrier. Regardless of the cause, fluid restriction, osmotic agents, and loop diuretics are usually effective in temporarily decreasing brain edema and lowering ICP until more definitive measures can be undertaken. Diuresis lowers ICP chiefly by removing intracellular water from normal brain tissue. Moderate hyperventilation ($PaCO_2$ 30–33 mm Hg) is often very helpful in reducing CBF (see Chapter 25) and normalizing ICP but may aggravate ischemia in patients with focal ischemia.

Mannitol, in doses of 0.25–0.5 g/kg, is particularly effective in rapidly decreasing ICP. Its efficacy is primarily related to its effect on serum osmolality (see Chapter 26); a serum osmolality of 300–315 mOsm/L is generally considered desirable. Mannitol can transiently decrease blood pressure by virtue of its weak vasodilating properties, but its principal disadvantage is a transient increase in intravascular volume, which can precipitate pulmonary edema in patients with borderline cardiac or renal function. Mannitol should generally not be used in patients with intracranial aneurysms, arteriovenous malformations (AVMs), or intracranial hemorrhage until the cranium is opened. Osmotic diuresis in such instances can expand a hematoma as the volume of the normal brain tissue around it decreases. Rapid osmotic diuresis in elderly patients can also occasionally cause a subdural hematoma due to rupture of fragile bridging veins entering the sagittal sinus. Rebound edema may follow the use of mannitol; thus, its use is limited to procedures (such as a craniotomy for tumor resection) in which intracranial volume will be reduced.

Use of a loop diuretic (furosemide), although less effective and requiring up to 30 min, may have the additional advantage of directly decreasing formation of CSF. The combined use of mannitol and furosemide may be synergistic but requires close monitoring of the serum potassium concentration (see Chapter 28).

■ ANESTHESIA & CRANIOTOMY FOR PATIENTS WITH MASS LESIONS

Intracranial masses may be congenital, neoplastic (benign or malignant), infectious (abscess or cyst), or vascular (hematoma or arteriovenous malformation). Craniotomy is commonly undertaken for primary and metastatic neoplasms of the brain. Primary tumors usually arise from glial cells (astrocytoma, oligodendroglioma, or glioblastoma), ependymal cells (ependymoma), or supporting tissues (meningioma, schwannoma, or choroidal papilloma). Childhood tumors include medulloblastoma, neuroblastoma, and chordoma.

Regardless of the cause, intracranial masses present according to growth rate, location, and ICP. Slowly growing masses are frequently asymptomatic for long periods, whereas rapidly growing ones usually present acutely. Common presentations include headache, seizures, a general decline in cognitive or specific neurological functions, and focal neurological deficits. Supratentorial masses typically present as seizures, hemiplegia, or aphasia, whereas infratentorial masses more commonly present as cerebellar dysfunction (ataxia, nystagmus, and dysarthria) or brain stem compression (cranial nerve palsies, altered consciousness, or abnormal respiration). As ICP increases, signs of intracranial hypertension also develop (above).

PREOPERATIVE MANAGEMENT

The preanesthetic evaluation should attempt to establish the presence or absence of intracranial hypertension. Computed tomographic (CT) and magnetic resonance imaging (MRI) scans should be reviewed for evidence of brain edema, a midline shift greater than 0.5 cm, and ventricular size. Examination should include a neurological assessment documenting mental status and any existing sensory or motor deficits. Medications should be reviewed with special reference to corticosteroid, diuretic, and anticonvulsant therapy. Laboratory evaluation should rule out corticosteroid-induced hyperglycemia and electrolyte disturbances due to diuretics or abnormalities in secretion of antidiuretic hormone (see Chapter 28). Anticonvulsant levels should be measured, particularly when seizures are not well controlled.

Premedication

Premedication is best avoided when intracranial hypertension is suspected. Hypercapnia secondary to respiratory depression increases ICP and may be lethal. Patients with normal ICP are usually given a benzodiazepine (diazepam orally or midazolam intravenously or intramuscularly). Corticosteroids and anticonvulsant therapy should be continued until the time of surgery.

INTRAOPERATIVE MANAGEMENT

Monitoring

In addition to standard monitors, direct intraarterial pressure monitoring and bladder catheterization are mandatory for most patients undergoing craniotomy. Rapid changes in blood pressure during induction, hyperventilation, intubation, positioning, surgical manipulation, and emergence necessitate continuous monitoring of blood pressure to ensure optimal cerebral perfusion. Moreover, measurements of arterial blood gas are necessary to closely regulate $PaCO_2$. Many neuroanesthesiologists zero the arterial pressure transducer at the level of the head (external auditory meatus)—instead of the right atrium—to facilitate calculation of cerebral perfusion pressure (CPP). End-tidal CO_2 measurements alone cannot be relied upon for precise regulation of ventilation; the arterial to end-tidal CO_2 gradient must be determined. Central venous access and pressure monitoring should be considered for patients requiring vasoactive drugs. Use of the internal jugular vein for access is somewhat controversial because of the risk of carotid puncture and concern that the catheter might interfere with venous drainage from the brain. Many clinicians avoid this issue by passing a long catheter centrally through the median basilic vein. The external jugular and subclavian veins may be suitable alternatives. A urinary catheter is necessary because of the frequent use of diuretics, the long duration of most neurosurgical procedures, and its utility in guiding fluid therapy. Neuromuscular function should be monitored on the unaffected side in patients with hemiparesis because the twitch response is often abnormally resistant on the affected side. Monitoring visual evoked potentials may be useful in preventing optic nerve damage during resections of large pituitary tumors. Additional monitors for surgery in the posterior fossa are described below.

Management of patients with intracranial hypertension is greatly facilitated by monitoring ICP perioperatively. A ventriculostomy or subdural bolt is most commonly employed and is usually placed by the neurosurgeon preoperatively under local anesthesia. Electronic monitoring of ICP is possible utilizing saline-filled tubing with a pressure transducer. The transducer should be zeroed to the same reference level as the arterial pressure transducer (usually the external auditory meatus; see above). A ventriculostomy has the added advantage of allowing removal of CSF to decrease ICP.

Robert F. Bedford, MD

LIGHTWAND MAGIC

One of my favorite clinical techniques is lightwand-facilitated tracheal intubation, used in situations in which a traditional laryngoscopy might be disadvantageous and an awake, fiberoptic intubation seems excessive. I was first introduced to this device during the early 1970s, when colleagues at the Brooke Army Hospital Burn Center described using it to intubate the tracheas of patients with orofacial burns without need for rigid laryngoscopy (E. D. Miller, Jr., personal communication). This was more than a decade before the introduction of flexible intubating bronchoscopes, and the only other option at the time was "blind" intubation, guided primarily by listening for breath sounds through the tracheal tube.

In my neuroanesthesia practice, I am frequently confronted with problems of cervical spine pathology,

in which forcible neck motion caused by rigid laryngoscopy could aggravate a patient's neurological status. By contrast, if no symptoms result from having patients gently extend their head enough to expose the anterior surface of the thyroid cartilage and it appears that the airway can be transilluminated, then a lightwand-guided intubation usually can be performed safely after induction of general anesthesia and neuromuscular blockade. Other indications for this technique include the presence of dental prostheses that could be "dinged" with a rigid laryngoscope or, conversely, the presence of extensive periodontal disease, where teeth may fall out when even a small amount of pressure is applied. Finally, I like to use it as an intubating stylet in situations in which glottic visualization is impossible with a rigid laryngoscope. It is extremely comforting to actually see the light go into the trachea instead of blindly passing the tube over a bougie and hoping to see signs of a successful intubation.

One disadvantage of the lightwand is the need to dim the lights in the operating room so the hypopharynx and trachea transilluminate when the device is inserted. (I usually shine a low-level surgical spotlight in the direction of the scrub nurse so progress can continue in setting up for the planned operation.) If the patient's neck is very short, muscular, or deeply pigmented, transillumination is not likely to be successful, and, if the patient has a large tongue, it is often difficult to maneuver the tracheal tube to the glottic opening. Thus, I do not use the lightwand for airway situations that are anticipated to be difficult unless I am using it for an awake intubation, where I am sure patients can control their own airway. It should also be noted that use of the lightwand does not minimize hemodynamic responses to tracheal intubation.[1]

Induction

Induction of anesthesia and tracheal intubation are critical periods for patients with compromised intracranial elastance or an already elevated ICP. Intracranial elastance can be improved by osmotic diuresis, steroids, or removal of CSF via a ventriculostomy drain immediately prior to induction. The goal of any technique should be to induce anesthesia and intubate the trachea in a slow, controlled

fashion without increasing ICP or compromising CBF. Arterial hypertension during induction increases cerebral blood volume and promotes cerebral edema. Marked or sustained hypertension can lead to marked increases in ICP that can decrease CPP and risk herniation (see Chapter 25). Excessive decreases in arterial blood pressure can be equally detrimental by compromising CPP.

The most common induction technique employs thiopental or propofol together with hyperventilation

A number of approaches for using the lightwand have been published.[2,3] My favorite is to place the light at the bevel of the tracheal tube and bend the lightwand and tube at approximately a 60° angle to create a "hockey-stick" shape (Figure 1). With the

Figure 1. Lightwand intubation. Note the light at the end of the tracheal tube bevel, the approximately 60° angle of curvature of the tube/lightwand apparatus, and the gentle jaw lift before insertion of the tracheal tube into the right pyriform sinus and subsequent manipulation into the trachea.

patient's head extended (not necessarily "sniffing"), I gently lift the lower jaw and direct the tube down the right side of the mouth and tongue until the right pyriform sinus transilluminates lateral to the thyroid cartilage. Then I slightly withdraw the light cephalad to the superior aspect of the thyroid cartilage and rotate the tube toward the midline, anticipating that the dull, round glow will become a brighter, longitudinal "flash" as the light shines down the trachea. I then advance the entire apparatus until the light is transilluminating the suprasternal notch before withdrawing the lightwand. At this point, the tube tip usually measures about 20 cm from the incisors, and its depth can be adjusted further, as appropriate.

During traditional laryngoscopy and tracheal intubation, most of the movement of the cervical spine is induced when the laryngoscope is lifted to force the tongue anteriorly.[4] The beauty of the lightwand is the ability to intubate the trachea with negligible movement of the cervical vertebrae, particularly when there is nearby neuropathology to be considered.

1. Takahashi S, Mizutani T, Miyabe M, Toyooka H: Hemodynamic responses to tracheal intubation with laryngoscope versus lightwand intubating device (Trachlight) in adults with normal airway. Anesth Analg 2002;95:480.
2. Agro F, Hung OR, Cataldo R, et al: Lightwand intubation using the Trachlight: A brief review of current knowledge. Can J Anesth 2001;48:592.
3. Graham DH, Agro F: Lightwand intubation using the Trachlight: A brief review of current knowledge (letter). Can J Anesth 2001;48:1169.
4. Sawin PD, Todd MM, Traynelis VC, et al: Cervical spine motion with direct laryngoscopy and orotracheal intubation: An *in vivo* cinefluoroscopic study of subjects without cervical abnormality. Anesthesiology 1996;85:26.

to lower ICP and blunt the noxious effects of laryngoscopy and intubation. Cooperative patients can be asked to hyperventilate during preoxygenation. All patients are hyperventilated with controlled ventilation once the thiopental or propofol is injected. A neuromuscular blocking agent (NMBA) is given to facilitate ventilation and prevent straining or coughing, both of which can abruptly increase ICP. An intravenous opioid—eg, fentanyl, 5–10 mg/kg—just prior to thiopental blunts the sympathetic response, particularly in young patients. Esmolol, 0.5–1.0 μg/kg, is effective in preventing tachycardia in hypertensive patients.

The actual induction technique can be varied according to individual patient responses and coexisting diseases. Use of propofol has the added benefit of a very short recovery time, whereas substitution of etomidate for thiopental may provide greater protection against circulatory depression. The combination of a small dose of fentanyl, 5 µg/kg, with etomidate, 6–8 mg, is also useful in unstable patients. Conversely, for patients with reactive airways (bronchospastic disease), the combination of incremental doses of thiopental and low-dose isoflurane with hyperventilation may be preferable.

A nondepolarizing NMBA is generally given at induction to facilitate controlled ventilation and tracheal intubation. Rocuronium, vecuronium, pipecuronium, and doxacurium provide the greatest hemodynamic stability (see Chapter 9). Succinylcholine may increase ICP, particularly if intubation is attempted prior to the establishment of deep thiopental anesthesia and hyperventilation (see Chapter 25). Succinylcholine, however, may be the agent of choice in patients at increased risk for aspiration or with a potentially difficult airway because hypoxemia and hypercarbia are even more detrimental. Significant muscle wasting is a relative contraindication to succinylcholine because of the risk of hyperkalemia.

Hypertension during induction should be treated with esmolol or by deepening the anesthetic with additional thiopental or propofol, or by hyperventilation with low doses (< 1 minimum alveolar concentration [MAC]) of isoflurane. Because of their potentially deleterious effect on cerebral blood volume and ICP (see Chapter 25), vasodilators (such as nitroprusside, nitroglycerin, calcium channel blockers, and hydralazine) should generally be avoided until the dura is opened. Transient hypotension should generally be treated with incremental doses of vasopressors (ephedrine or phenylephrine) rather than intravenous fluids.

Positioning

Frontal, temporal, and parietooccipital craniotomies are performed in the supine position. The head is elevated 15°–30° to facilitate venous drainage and drainage of CSF. The head may also be turned to the side to facilitate exposure. Excessive flexion or rotation of the neck impedes jugular venous drainage and can increase ICP. During positioning, the tracheal tube should be well secured and all breathing circuit connections checked. The risk of unrecognized disconnections may be increased because the patient's airway is not easily assessible; the operating table is usually turned 90° or 180° away from the anesthesiologist, and both the patient and the breathing circuit are almost completely covered by surgical drapes.

Maintenance of Anesthesia

Anesthesia is usually maintained with a nitrous oxide–opioid–NMBA technique. Any opioid may be used (see Chapter 25). Persistent hypertension requires the use of low-dose (< 1 MAC) isoflurane, sevoflurane, or desflurane. Alternatively, a combination of an opioid and low-dose inhalation agent or a total intravenous technique may be used. Even though periods of stimulation are fairly limited, neuromuscular blockade is recommended—unless electromyography is used—to prevent straining, bucking, or movement. Increased anesthetic requirements can be expected during the most stimulating periods: laryngoscopy–intubation, skin incision, dural opening, periosteal manipulations, and closure.

Hyperventilation should be continued intraoperatively to maintain $PaCO_2$ between 30 mm Hg and 35 mm Hg. Lower $PaCO_2$ tensions provide little additional benefit and may be associated with cerebral ischemia and impaired oxygen dissociation from hemoglobin. Positive end-expiratory pressure (PEEP) and ventilatory patterns resulting in high mean airway pressures (a low rate with large tidal volumes) should be avoided because of a potentially adverse effect on ICP by increasing central venous pressure. Hypoxic patients may require PEEP and higher mean airway pressures; in such patients, the effect of PEEP on ICP is variable.

Intravenous fluid replacement should be limited to glucose-free isotonic crystalloid (normal saline) or colloid solutions. Hyperglycemia is common in neurosurgical patients (corticosteroid effect) and has been implicated in increasing ischemic brain injury (see Chapter 25). Although controversy still surrounds the choice between crystalloid and colloid solutions, large amounts of hypotonic crystalloid solutions clearly can worsen brain edema. Colloid solutions should generally be used to restore intravascular volume deficits, whereas isotonic crystalloid solutions are used for maintenance fluid requirements. Intraoperative fluid replacement should be below calculated maintenance requirements (see Chapter 29) for patients with severe brain edema or increased ICP. Neurosurgical procedures result in minimal redistributive fluid losses but are often associated with "occult" blood loss (underneath surgical drapes or on the floor). Medical judgment should be used for making decisions on blood transfusions (see Chapter 29).

Emergence

Most patients undergoing craniotomy can be extubated at the end of the procedure as long as neurological function is intact. Patients who remain intubated should be sedated if agitation is a problem. Extubation in the operating room requires special handling during emergence. Straining or bucking on the tracheal tube may precipitate intracranial hemorrhage or worsen cerebral edema. Like induction, emergence must be slow and controlled. As the skin is being closed, attempts should be made to have the patient breathe spontaneously. After the head dressing is applied and full access to the patient is regained (the table is turned back to its original position as at induction), anesthetic gases are completely discontinued, and the NMBA is reversed.

Many anesthesiologists give intravenous lidocaine, 1.5 mg/kg, or a small dose of propofol (20–30 mg) or thiopental (25–50 mg), just before suctioning to try to suppress coughing prior to extubation. Rapid awakening facilitates immediate neurological assessment and can generally be expected following a careful anesthetic. Delayed awakening may be seen following opioid overdose or prolonged administration of the volatile agent. Opioid overdosing is manifested by small pupils and slow respirations (< 12/min). In this circumstance, naloxone can be given in 0.04-mg increments, but it must be titrated carefully because if too much is given, the results can be dangerous. Most patients are taken to the intensive care unit postoperatively for close monitoring of neurological function. Patients generally have minimal pain.

■ ANESTHESIA FOR SURGERY IN THE POSTERIOR FOSSA

Craniotomy for a mass in the posterior fossa presents a unique set of potential problems: obstructive hydrocephalus, possible injury to vital brain stem centers, unusual positioning, pneumocephalus, postural hypotension, and **venous air embolism**.

Obstructive Hydrocephalus

Infratentorially located masses can obstruct flow of CSF at the level of the fourth ventricle or the cerebral aqueduct. Even small but critically located lesions can markedly increase ICP. In such cases, a ventriculostomy is often performed under local anesthesia to decrease ICP prior to induction of general anesthesia.

Brain Stem Injury

Operations in the posterior fossa can injure vital circulatory and respiratory brain stem centers as well as cranial nerves or their nuclei. Such injuries occur as a result of direct surgical trauma, retraction, or ischemia. Damage to respiratory centers is said to be nearly always associated with circulatory changes, so that abrupt changes in blood pressure, heart rate, or cardiac rhythm should alert the anesthesiologist to the possibility of such an injury. Communication of such changes to the surgeon is critical. Rarely, isolated damage to respiratory centers without premonitory circulatory signs has occurred during operations in the floor of the fourth ventricle; historically, spontaneous ventilation has been used during these procedures to offer an additional monitor of function. At completion of the surgery, brain stem injuries often present as

an abnormal respiratory pattern or as an inability to maintain a patent airway following extubation. Monitoring brain stem auditory evoked potentials may be useful in preventing eighth nerve damage during resections of acoustic neuromas. Electromyography is also used to avoid injury to the facial nerve, but the latter requires incomplete neuromuscular blockade intraoperatively.

Positioning

Although most explorations of the posterior fossa can be performed with the patient in either a modified lateral or prone position, the sitting position may be preferred by some surgeons. Regardless of position, the head is always elevated above the heart. The lateral position is discussed in Chapter 24, and the prone position is discussed below under spinal surgery.

The patient is actually semirecumbent in the standard sitting position (Figure 26–1); the back is elevated to 60°, and the legs are elevated with the knees flexed. The head is fixed in a three-point holder with the neck flexed; the arms remain at the sides with the hands resting on the lap.

Careful positioning helps avoid injuries. Pressure points such as the elbows, ischial spines, heels, and forehead must be protected. Excessive neck flexion has been associated with swelling of the upper airway (due to venous obstruction) and, rarely, quadriplegia (due to compression of the cervical spinal cord). Preexisting cervical spinal stenosis probably predisposes patients to the latter injury.

Pneumocephalus

The sitting position increases the likelihood of significant pneumocephalus. In this position, air readily

Figure 26–1. The sitting position for craniotomy.

enters the subarachnoid space as CSF is lost during surgery. In patients with cerebral atrophy, drainage of CSF is marked; air can replace CSF on the surface of the brain and in the lateral ventricles. Expansion of a pneumocephalus following dural closure can compress the brain. Postoperative pneumocephalus can cause delayed awakening and continued impairment of neurological function. Because of these concerns, some neuroanesthesiologists advocate not using nitrous oxide for sitting craniotomies (see also below).

Venous Air Embolism

Venous air embolism can occur when the pressure within an open vein is subatmospheric. These conditions may exist in any position (and during any procedure) whenever the wound is above the level of the heart. The incidence of venous air embolism is highest during sitting craniotomies (20–40%). Low pressure in veins and large cerebral venous sinuses increase the risk.

The physiological consequences of venous air embolism depend on the volume as well as the rate of air entry and whether the patient has a probe-patent foramen ovale (10–25% incidence). The latter is important because it can facilitate passage of air into the arterial circulation (paradoxical air embolism). Air bubbles entering the venous system ordinarily lodge in the pulmonary circulation, where their gases eventually diffuse into the alveoli and are exhaled. Small bubbles are well tolerated by most patients. When the amount entrained exceeds the rate of pulmonary clearance, pulmonary artery pressure progressively rises. Eventually, cardiac output decreases in response to increases in right ventricular afterload. Preexisting cardiac or pulmonary disease enhances the effects of venous air embolism; relatively small amounts of air may produce marked hemodynamic changes. Nitrous oxide, by increasing the volume of the entrained air, can markedly accentuate the effects of even small amounts of air. The dose for lethal venous air embolism in animals receiving nitrous oxide anesthesia is one-third to one-half that of control animals. Many clinicians are convinced that nitrous oxide should not be used for surgery on patients in the sitting position. Others continue to use it but in a concentration of 50% instead of 70% and discontinue it if venous air embolism is detected.

Clinically, signs of venous air embolism are often not apparent until large amounts of air have been entrained. A decrease in end-tidal CO_2 or arterial oxygen saturation might be noticed prior to hemodynamic changes. Arterial blood gas values may show only slight increases in $PaCO_2$ as a result of increased pulmonary dead space (areas with normal ventilation but decreased perfusion). Major hemodynamic manifestations such as sudden hypotension can occur well before hypoxemia is noted. Moreover, rapid entrainment of large amounts of air can produce sudden circulatory arrest by obstructing right ventricular outflow when intracardiac air impairs tricuspid and pulmonic valve function or blocks pulmonary arterioles.

Paradoxic air embolism can result in a stroke or coronary occlusion, which may be apparent only postoperatively. Paradoxic air emboli are more likely to occur in patients with probe-patent foramen ovale, particularly when the normal transatrial (left > right) pressure gradient is reversed. Reversal of this gradient is favored by hypovolemia and perhaps by PEEP. Some studies suggest that a right > left pressure gradient can develop at some time during the cardiac cycle even when the overall mean gradient remains left > right. Transpulmonary passage of venous air into the arterial system has also been demonstrated and suggests that even small bubbles in intravenous infusions should be avoided in all patients.

A. Central Venous Catheterization

Central venous access frequently allows aspiration of entrained air. Many clinicians consider right atrial catheterization mandatory for sitting craniotomies. Optimal recovery of air following venous air embolism is provided by a multiorificed catheter positioned high in the atrium at its junction with the superior vena cava. Confirmation of correct catheter positioning is important and is accomplished by intravascular electrocardiography or by transesophageal echocardiography (TEE). During intravascular electrocardiography, a high atrial position is indicated by the appearance of a biphasic P wave. If the catheter is advanced too far, the P wave changes from a negative to a positive deflection, and a right ventricular waveform may also be observed when the pressure is transduced (see Chapter 6).

B. Monitoring for Venous Air Embolism

The most sensitive monitors available should be used. Detecting even small amounts of venous air embolism is important because it allows surgical control of the entry site before additional air is entrained. Currently, the most sensitive intraoperative monitors are TEE and precordial Doppler sonography. These monitors can detect air bubbles as small as 0.25 mL. TEE has the added benefit of detecting the amount of the bubbles and any transatrial passage, as well as evaluating cardiac function. Doppler methods employ a probe over the right atrium (usually to the right of the sternum and between the third and sixth ribs). Interruption of the regular swishing of the Doppler signal by sporadic roaring sounds indicates venous air embolism. Changes in end-tidal respiratory gas concentrations and in pulmonary artery pressure are less sensitive but are important monitors that can also detect venous air embolism before overt clinical signs are present. Venous air embolism causes a sudden decrease in end-tidal CO_2 tension in proportion to the increase in pulmonary dead space; unfortunately, such decreases can also be seen with hemodynamic changes unrelated to venous air embolism. A reappearance (or increase) of nitrogen in expired gases may also be seen with venous air embolism. Mean pulmonary artery pressure increases in direct proportion to the amount of air entrained. Changes in blood pressure and heart sounds (mill wheel murmur) are late manifestations of venous air embolism.

C. TREATMENT OF VENOUS AIR EMBOLISM

1. The surgeon should be notified so that the surgical field can be flooded with saline or packed and bone wax applied to the skull edges until the entry site is identified.
2. Nitrous oxide (if used) should be discontinued and the inhalation anesthetic delivered in 100% oxygen.
3. The central venous catheter should be aspirated in an attempt to retrieve the entrained air.
4. Intravascular volume infusion should be given to increase central venous pressure.
5. Vasopressors should be given to treat hypotension.
6. Bilateral jugular vein compression, by increasing cranial venous pressure, may slow air entrainment and cause back bleeding, which might help the surgeon identify the source of the embolus.
7. Some clinicians advocate PEEP in an effort to increase cerebral venous pressure; however, reversal of the normal transatrial pressure gradient may promote paradoxic embolism.
8. If the above measures fail, the patient should be placed in a head-down position and the wound closed quickly.
9. Persistent circulatory arrest necessitates the supine position and institution of resuscitation efforts using advanced cardiac life support algorithms (see Chapter 47).

■ ANESTHESIA FOR STEREOTACTIC SURGERY

Stereotaxis can be employed in treating involuntary movement disorders, intractable pain, and epilepsy and can also be used when diagnosing and treating tumors that are located deep within the brain.

These procedures are often performed under local anesthesia to allow periodic evaluation of the patient. Propofol infusion may be used for sedation and amnesia. Sedation

should be omitted, however, if the patient already has increased ICP. The ability to rapidly provide controlled ventilation and general anesthesia for emergency craniotomy is mandatory but is complicated by the platform and localizing frame that is attached to the patient's head for the procedure. **Although mask ventilation or ventilation through a laryngeal mask airway (LMA) or orotracheal intubation might be readily accomplished in an emergency, awake intubation with a fiberoptic bronchoscope prior to positioning and surgery may be the safest approach when intubation is necessary for a patient whose head is in a stereotactic head frame.**

■ ANESTHESIA FOR HEAD TRAUMA

Head injuries are a contributory factor in up to 50% of deaths due to trauma. Most patients with head trauma are young, and many (10–40%) have associated intraabdominal injuries, long bone fractures, or both. A general discussion of the trauma patient is found in Chapter 41. The significance of a head injury is dependent not only on the extent of the irreversible neuronal damage at the time of injury, but also on the occurrence of any secondary insults. These additional insults include (1) systemic factors such as hypoxemia, hypercapnia, or hypotension; (2) formation and expansion of an epidural, subdural, or intracerebral hematoma; and (3) sustained intracranial hypertension. Surgical and anesthetic management of these patients is directed at preventing these secondary insults. The **Glasgow Coma Scale (GCS) score** (Table 26–1) generally correlates well with the severity of injury and outcome. A GCS score of 8 or less is associated with approximately 35% mortality. Evidence of more than a 5-mm midline shift, a lesion larger than 25 mL, and ventricular compression on the CT scan are associated with substantially increased morbidity.

Specific lesions include skull fractures, subdural and epidural hematomas, brain concussions and contusions (including intracerebral hemorrhages), penetrating head injuries, and traumatic vascular occlusions and dissections. The presence of a skull fracture greatly increases the likelihood of a significant intracranial lesion. Linear skull fractures are commonly associated with subdural or epidural hematomas. Basilar skull fractures may be associated with CSF rhinorrhea, pneumocephalus, cranial nerve palsies, or even a cavernous sinus–carotid artery fistula. Depressed skull fractures often present with an underlying brain contusion. Contusions may be limited to the surface of the brain or may involve hemorrhage in deeper hemispheric structures or the

Table 26–1. Glasgow Coma Scale.

Category	Score
Eye opening	
Spontaneous	4
To speech	3
To pain	2
Nil	1
Best motor response	
To verbal command	
Obeys	6
To pain	
Localizes	5
Withdraws	4
Decorticate flexion	3
Extensor response	2
Nil	1
Best verbal response	
Oriented	5
Confused conversation	4
Inappropriate words	3
Incomprehensible sounds	2
Nil	1

brain stem. Deceleration injuries often produce both coup and contrecoup lesions. Subdural and epidural hematomas can occur as isolated lesions as well as in association with cerebral contusions.

Operative treatment is usually elected for depressed skull fractures; evacuation of epidural, subdural, and some intracerebral hematomas; and debridement of penetrating injuries.

ICP monitoring is usually indicated for patients with significant contusions, intracerebral hemorrhage, or tissue shifts. Intracranial hypertension should be treated with moderate hyperventilation, mannitol, barbiturates, or propofol (see Chapter 25). Studies suggest that sustained increases in ICP greater than 60 mm Hg result in irreversible brain edema. Unlike treatment following spinal cord trauma, the early use of large doses of glucocorticoids does not clearly improve outcome in patients with head trauma. ICP monitoring should also be considered for patients with signs of intracranial hypertension who are undergoing nonneurological procedures.

PREOPERATIVE MANAGEMENT

Anesthetic care of patients with severe head trauma ideally begins in the emergency department. Measures to ensure the patency of the airway, the adequacy of ventilation and oxygenation, and correction of systemic hypotension should go forward simultaneously with neu-

rological evaluation. Airway obstruction and hypoventilation are common. Up to 70% of such patients have hypoxemia, which may be complicated by pulmonary contusion, fat emboli, or neurogenic pulmonary edema. The latter is the result of marked systemic and pulmonary hypertension secondary to intense sympathetic nervous system activity. Supplemental oxygen should be given to all patients while the airway and ventilation are evaluated. All patients must be assumed to have a cervical spine injury (up to 10% incidence) until the contrary is proven radiographically. In-line stabilization should be used during airway manipulation to maintain the head in a neutral position (see Chapter 41). Patients with obvious hypoventilation, an absent gag reflex, or a persistent total score below 8 on the GCS (Table 26–1) require tracheal intubation and hyperventilation. All other patients should be carefully observed for deterioration.

Intubation

All patients should be regarded as having a full stomach and should have cricoid pressure applied during ventilation and tracheal intubation. Following adequate preoxygenation and hyperventilation by mask, the adverse effects of intubation on ICP are blunted by prior administration of thiopental, 2–4 mg/kg, or propofol, 1.5–3.0 mg/kg, and a rapid-onset NMBA. If the patient is hypotensive (systolic blood pressure < 100 mm Hg), either a smaller dose of thiopental or propofol should be used or etomidate should be substituted. The use of succinylcholine in closed head injury is controversial because of its potential for increasing ICP and the rare occurrence of hyperkalemia in these patients; rocuronium or mivacurium is a suitable alternative. If a difficult intubation is anticipated, awake intubation, fiberoptic techniques, or tracheostomy may be necessary. Blind nasal intubation is contraindicated in the presence of a basilar skull fracture, which is suggested by CSF rhinorrhea or otorrhea, hemotympanum, or ecchymosis into periorbital tissues (raccoon sign) or behind the ear (Battle's sign).

Hypotension

Hypotension in the setting of head trauma is nearly always related to other associated injuries (usually intraabdominal). Bleeding from scalp lacerations may be responsible in children. Hypotension may be seen with spinal cord injuries because of the sympathectomy associated with spinal shock. In a patient with head trauma, correction of hypotension and control of any bleeding take precedence over radiographic studies and definitive neurosurgical treatment because systolic arterial blood pressures of less than 80 mm Hg correlate with a poor outcome. Many anesthesiologists believe that fluid resuscitation with primarily colloid solutions and blood may be more advantageous than crystalloid solutions in preventing brain edema; temporary infusion of a vasopressor is often necessary for severe hypotension. Glucose-containing or hypotonic solutions should not be used (see above). The hematocrit should be maintained above 30%. Invasive monitoring of intraarterial pressure, central venous or pulmonary artery pressure, and ICP is extremely valuable but should not delay diagnosis and treatment. Arrhythmias and electrocardiographic abnormalities in the T wave, U wave, ST segment, and QT interval are common following head injuries but are not necessarily associated with cardiac injury; they likely represent altered autonomic function.

Diagnostic Studies

The choice between operative and medical management of head trauma is based on radiographic as well as clinical findings. Patients should be stabilized prior to any CT or angiographic studies. Critically ill patients should be closely monitored during such studies. Restless or uncooperative patients may additionally require general anesthesia. Sedation without control of the airway should generally be avoided because of the risk of further increases in ICP from hypercapnia or hypoxemia. In the event of neurological deterioration prior to completion of these studies, intravenous mannitol should be considered.

INTRAOPERATIVE MANAGEMENT

Anesthetic management is generally similar to that for other mass lesions associated with intracranial hypertension. Management of the airway is discussed above. Intraarterial and central venous (or pulmonary artery) pressure monitoring should be established if not already present but should not delay surgical decompression in a rapidly deteriorating patient.

A barbiturate–opioid–nitrous oxide–NMBA technique is commonly used. Nitrous oxide should be avoided when air is entrapped within the cranium and during periods of hypotension. Hypotension may occur after induction of anesthesia as a result of the combined effects of vasodilation and hypovolemia and should be treated with an α-adrenergic agonist and volume infusion if necessary. Subsequent hypertension is common with surgical stimulation but may also occur with acute elevations in ICP. The latter is often associated with bradycardia (Cushing phenomenon).

Hypertension can be treated with additional doses of the induction agent, with increased concentrations of the inhalation anesthetic, or with antihypertensives. Hyperventilation to a $PaCO_2$ < 30 should be avoided in trauma patients to avoid excessive decreases in CBF. β-Adrenergic blockade is usually effective in controlling hypertension associated with tachycardia. CPP should be maintained between 70 and 110 mm Hg. Vasodilators should be avoided until the dura is opened. Excessive vagal tone should be treated with atropine or glycopyrrolate.

Disseminated intravascular coagulation (DIC) may be seen with severe head injuries. Such injuries cause release of large amounts of brain thromboplastin and may also be associated with the acute respiratory distress syndrome (ARDS) (see Chapter 49). DIC should be diagnosed by coagulation testing and treated with platelets, fresh-frozen plasma, and cryoprecipitate, whereas ARDS may require mechanical ventilation. Pulmonary aspiration and neurogenic pulmonary edema may also be responsible for deteriorating lung function. PEEP should be applied on the ventilator only if ICP is monitored or when the dura is opened. Diabetes insipidus, characterized by copious dilute urine, is frequently seen following injuries to the pituitary stalk. Other likely causes of polyuria should be excluded and the diagnosis confirmed by measurement of urine and serum osmolality prior to treatment with fluid restriction and vasopressin (see Chapter 28). Gastrointestinal hemorrhage may complicate management after several days; it is usually due to stress ulceration.

The decision whether to extubate the trachea at the conclusion of the surgical procedure depends on the severity of the injury, the presence of concomitant abdominal or thoracic injuries, preexisting illnesses, and the preoperative level of consciousness. Young patients who were conscious preoperatively may be extubated following the removal of a localized lesion, whereas patients with diffuse brain injury should remain intubated. Moreover, persistent intracranial hypertension requires continued paralysis, sedation, hyperventilation, and perhaps a pentobarbital infusion postoperatively.

■ ANESTHESIA & CRANIOTOMY FOR INTRACRANIAL ANEURYSMS & ARTERIOVENOUS MALFORMATIONS

Saccular aneurysms and AVMs are common causes of nontraumatic intracranial hemorrhages. Surgical treatment may be undertaken either electively to prevent hemorrhage or emergently to prevent further complications once hemorrhage has taken place. Other causes of nontraumatic hemorrhage, including hypertensive and spontaneous lobar hemorrhages, are usually treated medically.

CEREBRAL ANEURYSMS

Preoperative Considerations

Cerebral aneurysms typically occur at the bifurcation of the large arteries at the base of the brain; the vast majority are located in the anterior circle of Willis. Approximately 10–30% of patients have more than one aneurysm. The general incidence of saccular aneurysms in some estimates is reported to be 5%, but only a minority of individuals have complications. Rupture of a saccular aneurysm is the most common cause of subarachnoid hemorrhage. The acute mortality following rupture is approximately 10%. Of those that survive the initial hemorrhage, about 25% subsequently die within 3 months from delayed complications. Moreover, up to 50% of survivors are left with significant neurological deficits. As a result, the emphasis in management is on prevention of rupture. Although anatomic correlates for the probability of rupture are not established, those larger than 7 mm are usually considered for surgical obliteration. Unfortunately, most patients present only after rupture has already occurred.

Unruptured Aneurysms

Patients often present with prodromal symptoms and signs suggesting progressive enlargement. The most common symptom is headache, and the most common sign is a third-nerve palsy. Other manifestations might include brain stem dysfunction, visual field defects, trigeminal neuralgia, cavernous sinus syndrome, seizures, and hypothalamic–pituitary dysfunction. The most commonly used techniques to diagnose an aneurysm are angiography, MRI angiography, and helical CT angiography. Following diagnosis, patients are brought to the operating room for elective clipping or obliteration of the aneurysm. Most patients are in the 40- to 60-year age group and in otherwise good health.

Ruptured Aneurysms

Ruptured aneurysms usually present acutely as subarachnoid hemorrhage, and less commonly they hemorrhage into the epidural space or the brain. Patients typically complain of a sudden severe headache without focal neurological deficits but often associated with nausea and vomiting. Transient loss of consciousness may occur and may result from a sudden rise in ICP and precipitous drop in CPP. If ICP does not decrease rapidly after the initial sudden increase, death usually follows. Large blood clots can cause focal neurological signs in some patients. Minor bleeding may cause only a mild headache, vomiting, and nuchal rigidity. Unfortunately, even minor bleeding in the subarachnoid space appears to predispose to delayed complications.

Delayed complications include cerebral vasospasm, rerupture, and hydrocephalus. Cerebral vasospasm occurs in 30% of patients (usually after 4–14 days) and is the major cause of morbidity and mortality. The mechanism is unknown but is related to the presence of a blood clot around the cerebral vessels. Manifestations, which are principally due to cerebral ischemia and infarction, may vary and depend on the severity and distribution of the involved vessels. The calcium channel antagonist nimodipine is useful in preventing vasospasm, but is usually ineffective once it is established. **In patients with symptomatic vasospasm, intravascular volume expansion and induced hypertension (triple H therapy: hypervolemia, hemodilution, and hypertension) are added as part of the therapeutic regimen.** Dopamine is usually used to induce mild hypertension because marked hypertension can increase the risk of rebleeding. Glucocorticoids do not reduce cerebral edema following rupture. Cerebral edema should be managed as it is in patients with head trauma; ICP monitoring is often indicated.

Neurosurgical management of patients surviving a ruptured aneurysm is complicated by the risk of rebleeding and vasospasm. The incidence of rerupture is 10–30%. Early surgical obliteration of the aneurysm (within 24–72 h) is usually recommended for stable patients because rerupture carries a 60% mortality rate. Emergency surgical intervention is also indicated for neurological deterioration associated with a subdural or intracerebral hematoma. Acute hydrocephalus requires emergency ventricular drainage, whereas chronic hydrocephalus requires delayed ventricular shunting.

PREOPERATIVE MANAGEMENT

Preanesthetic evaluation should determine whether rupture has occurred; signs of intracranial hypertension (above) should be sought. Generally, most patients have normal ICP by the time they come for surgery. A small group of patients, however, may have persistent elevation in ICP. Hydrocephalus develops in these patients as a result of interference with absorption of CSF and is usually evidenced by ventricular enlargement on the CT scan. In addition to neurological findings, evaluation should include a search for coexisting diseases that may modify the use of elective hypotension intraoperatively. Preexisting hypertension and renal, cardiac, or ischemic cerebrovascular disease are relative contraindications to controlled hypotension. Electrocardiographic abnormalities are commonly seen in patients with subarachnoid hemorrhage but do not necessarily reflect underlying heart disease. Most conscious patients with normal ICP are sedated following rupture to prevent rebleeding; such sedation should be continued until induction of anesthesia. Patients with persistent elevation in ICP should receive little or no premedication to avoid hypercapnia.

INTRAOPERATIVE MANAGEMENT

Aneurysm surgery can result in exsanguinating hemorrhage as a consequence of rupture or rebleeding. Blood should be available prior to the start of these operations.

Regardless of the anesthetic technique employed, anesthetic management should focus on preventing rupture (or rebleeding) and avoiding factors that promote cerebral ischemia or vasospasm. Intraarterial and central venous (or pulmonary artery) pressure monitoring are mandatory. Sudden increases in blood pressure with tracheal intubation or surgical stimulation should be avoided. Judicious intravascular volume loading, guided by the central venous pressure, allows surgical levels of anesthesia without excessive decreases in blood pressure. Because calcium channel blockers cause systemic vasodilation and reduce systemic vascular resistance, patients receiving these agents preoperatively may be particularly prone to hypotension. Hyperventilation is unlikely to overcome ischemia-induced vasodilation. Once the dura is opened, mannitol is often given to facilitate surgical exposure and reduce tissue trauma from surgical retraction. Rapid decreases in ICP prior to dural opening may promote rebleeding by removing a tamponading effect on the aneurysm.

Elective (controlled) hypotension is useful in aneurysm surgery. Decreasing mean arterial blood pressure reduces the transmural tension across the aneurysm, making rupture (or rebleeding) less likely and facilitating surgical clipping. Controlled hypotension can also decrease blood loss and improve surgical visualization in the event of bleeding. The combination of a slightly head-up position with a volatile anesthetic (isoflurane) enhances the effects of any of the commonly used hypotensive agents (see Chapter 13). Technical improvements in temporary vascular clips have enabled surgeons to use them more often to interrupt blood flow during aneurysm surgery; use of these clips has obviated the need for controlled hypotension and has made normotension or even mild hypertension at least theoretically possible for protecting cerebral perfusion during aneurysm clipping. Administration of thiopental and mild hypothermia may protect the brain during periods of prolonged or excessive hypotension or vascular occlusion. Rarely, hypothermic circulatory arrest is used for large basilar artery aneurysms.

Depending on neurological condition, most patients should be extubated at the end of surgery. Extubation should be handled similarly to other craniotomies (see above). A rapid awakening allows neurological evaluation in the operating room prior to transfer to the intensive care unit.

ARTERIOVENOUS MALFORMATION

AVMs cause intracerebral hemorrhage more often than does subarachnoid hemorrhage. These lesions are developmental abnormalities that result in arteriovenous fistulas; they typically grow in size with time. AVMs may present at any age but bleeding is most common between 10 and 30 years of age. Other common presentations include headache and seizures. The combination of high blood flow with low vascular resistance can rarely result in high-output cardiac failure. Acutely, neuroradiologists try to embolize AVMs; subacute or chronic problems due to AVMs will respond to irradiation. When embolization and irradiation are not successful or available, surgical excision may be undertaken.

Anesthetic management of patients with AVMs is often complicated by extensive blood loss. Venous access with multiple large-bore cannulas and direct arterial pressure monitoring is necessary. Embolization may be carried out prior to surgery in an attempt to reduce operative blood loss. Hyperventilation and mannitol may be used to facilitate surgical access. Pharmacological brain protection should be considered for large lesions. Hyperemia and swelling can develop following resection, possibly because of altered autoregulation in the remaining normal brain. Blood pressure must therefore be controlled carefully (usually with β-blockers) so as not to aggravate this problem.

■ ANESTHESIA FOR SURGERY ON THE SPINE

Spinal surgery is most often performed for symptomatic nerve root or cord compression secondary to degenerative disorders. Compression may occur from protrusion of an intervertebral disk or osteophytic bone (spondylosis) into the spinal canal (or an intervertebral foramen). Herniation of an intervertebral disk usually occurs at either the fourth or fifth lumbar or the fifth or sixth cervical levels in patients 30–50 years old. Spondylosis tends to affect the lower cervical spine more than the lumbar spine and typically afflicts older patients. Operations on the spinal column can help correct deformities such as scoliosis, decompress the cord, and fuse the spine if disrupted by blunt trauma. Spinal surgery may also be performed to resect a tumor or vascular malformation or to drain an abscess or hematoma.

PREOPERATIVE MANAGEMENT

Preoperative evaluation should focus on any existing ventilatory impairment and the airway. Anatomic abnormalities and limited neck movements due to disease, traction, or braces complicate airway management and necessitate special techniques (see Chapter 5). Neurological deficits should be documented. Most patients with degenerative disease have considerable pain preoperatively and should be given an opioid with premedication. Conversely, premedication should be used sparingly in patients with difficult airways or ventilatory impairment.

INTRAOPERATIVE MANAGEMENT

Anesthetic management is complicated primarily by the prone position. Spinal operations involving multiple levels, fusion, and instrumentation are also complicated by the potential for large intraoperative blood losses; a red-cell salvage device is often used. Excessive distraction during spinal instrumentation (Harrington rod or pedicle screw fixation) can additionally injure the spinal cord. A transthoracic approach to the spine requires one-lung ventilation (see Chapter 24).

Positioning

Most surgical procedures are carried out in the prone position. Use of the supine position (with head traction) for an anterior approach to the cervical spine facilitates anesthetic management but may be associated with injuries to the trachea, esophagus, recurrent laryngeal nerve, sympathetic chain, carotid artery, or jugular vein. A sitting or lateral decubitus position may occasionally be used.

Following induction of anesthesia and tracheal intubation in the supine position, the patient is turned prone. Care must be taken to maintain the neck in a neutral position. Once in the prone position, the head may be turned to the side (not exceeding the patient's normal range of motion) or can remain face down on a cushioned holder. Extreme caution is necessary to avoid corneal abrasions or retinal ischemia from pressure on either globe or pressure necrosis of the nose, ears, forehead, chin, breasts (females), or genitalia (males). The chest should rest on parallel rolls (foam) or special supports—if a frame is used—to facilitate ventilation. The arms may be at the sides in a comfortable position or extended with the elbows flexed (avoiding excessive abduction at the shoulder).

Turning the patient prone is a critical maneuver, often complicated by hypotension resulting from blunted postural sympathetic reflexes. Abdominal compression, particularly in obese patients, may impede venous return and contributes to excessive intraoperative blood loss from engorgement of epidural veins. The use of specially designed frames that allow the abdomen to hang free may alleviate these problems.

Monitoring

When significant blood loss is anticipated or the patient has preexisting cardiac disease, intraarterial and possibly central venous pressure monitoring should be undertaken prior to "positioning" or "turning." In suitable candidates, elective hypotension or infiltration of the wound with a weak epinephrine solution may decrease intraoperative blood loss. Massive blood loss from aortic or vena caval injury can occur intraoperatively or postoperatively with thoracic or lumbar spine procedures and is often initially occult.

Instrumentation of the spine requires the ability to intraoperatively detect spinal cord injury from excessive distraction. Intraoperative wake-up techniques, employing balanced or total intravenous anesthesia, allow testing of motor function following distraction. Once preservation of motor function is established, the patient's anesthetic is deepened. Monitoring somatosensory evoked potentials and motor evoked potentials (see Chapter 6) is an alternative that avoids the problems associated with intraoperative awakening.

> ### CASE DISCUSSION: RESECTION OF A PITUITARY TUMOR

A 41-year-old woman presents to the operating room for resection of a 10-mm pituitary tumor. She had complained of amenorrhea and had started noticing some decrease in visual acuity.

What hormones does the pituitary gland normally secrete?

Functionally and anatomically, the pituitary is divided into two parts: anterior and posterior. The latter is part of the neurohypophysis, which also includes the pituitary stalk and the median eminence.

The anterior pituitary is composed of several cell types, each secreting a specific hormone. Anterior pituitary hormones include adrenocorticotropic hormone (ACTH), thyroid-stimulating hormone (TSH), growth hormone (GH), the gonadotropins (follicle-stimulating hormone [FSH] and luteinizing hormone [LH]), and prolactin (PRL). Secretion of each of these hormones is regulated by hypothalamic peptides (releasing hormones) that are transported to the adenohypophysis by a capillary portal system. The secretion of FSH, LH, ACTH, TSH, and their respective releasing hormones is also under negative feedback control by the products of their target organs. For example, an increase in circulating thyroid hormone inhibits the secretion of TSH-releasing factor and TSH.

The posterior pituitary secretes antidiuretic hormone (ADH, also called vasopressin) and oxytocin. These hormones are actually formed in supraoptic and paraventricular neurons, respectively, and are transported down axons that terminate in the posterior pituitary. Hypothalamic osmoreceptors and, to a lesser extent, peripheral vascular stretch receptors regulate secretion of ADH (see Chapter 28).

What is the function of these hormones?

ACTH stimulates the adrenal cortex to secrete glucocorticoids. Unlike production of mineralocorticoids, production of glucocorticoids is dependent on ACTH secretion. TSH accelerates the synthesis and release of thyroid hormone (thyroxine). Normal thyroid function is dependent on production of TSH. The gonadotropins FSH and LH are necessary for normal production of testosterone and spermatogenesis in males and cyclic ovarian function in females. GH promotes tissue growth and increases protein synthesis as well as fatty acid mobilization. Its effects on carbohydrate metabolism are to decrease cellular glucose uptake and utilization and increase insulin secretion. PRL functions to support breast development during pregnancy. Dopamine receptor antagonists are known to increase secretion of PRL.

Through its effect on water permeability in renal collecting ducts, ADH regulates extracellular osmolarity and blood volume (see Chapter 28). Oxytocin acts on areolar myoepithelial cells as part of the milk letdown reflex during suckling and enhances uterine activity during labor.

What factors determine the surgical approach in this patient?

The pituitary gland is attached to the brain by a stalk and extends downward to lie in the sella turcica of the sphenoid bone. Anteriorly, posteriorly, and inferiorly, it is bordered by bone. Laterally it is bordered by the cavernous sinus, which contains cranial nerves III, IV, V_1, and VI, as well as the cavernous portion of the carotid artery. Superiorly, the diaphragma sella, a thick dural reflection, usually tightly encircles the stalk and forms the roof of the sella turcica. In close proximity to the stalk lie the optic nerves and chiasm. Contiguous and superior to the stalk lies the hypothalamus.

Tumors under 10 mm in diameter are usually approached via the transsphenoidal route, whereas tumors larger than 20 mm in diameter and with significant suprasellar extension are approached via a bifrontal craniotomy. With use of prophylactic antibiotics, morbidity and mortality rates are significantly less with the transsphenoidal approach; the operation is carried out with the aid of a microscope through an incision in the gingival mucosa beneath the upper lip. The surgeon enters the nasal cavity, dissects through the nasal septum, and finally penetrates the roof of the sphenoid sinus to enter the floor of the sella turcica.

What are the major problems associated with the transsphenoidal approach?

Problems include (1) the need for mucosal injections of epinephrine-containing solution to reduce bleeding, (2) the accumulation of blood and tissue debris in the pharynx and stomach, (3) the risks of hemorrhage from inadvertent entry into the cavernous sinus or the internal carotid artery, (4) cranial nerve damage, and (5) pituitary hypofunction. Prophylactic administration of glucocorticoids is routinely used in most centers. Diabetes insipidus (see Chapter 29) develops postoperatively in up to 40% of patients but is usually transient. Less commonly, the diabetes insipidus presents intraoperatively. The supine and slightly head-up position used for this procedure may also predispose to venous air embolism.

What type of tumor does this patient have?

Tumors in or around the sella turcica account for 10–15% of intracranial neoplasms. Pituitary adenomas are most common, followed by craniopharyngiomas and then parasellar meningiomas. Primary malignant pituitary and metastatic tumors are rare. Pituitary tumors that secrete hormones (functional tumors) usually present early when they are still relatively small (< 10 mm). Other tumors present late, with signs of increased ICP (headache, nausea and vomiting) or compression of contiguous structures (visual disturbances or pituitary hypofunction). Compression of the optic chiasm classically results in bitemporal hemianopia. Compression of normal pituitary tissue produces progressive endocrine dysfunction. Failure of hormonal secretion usually progresses in the order of gonadotropins, GH, ACTH, and TSH. Diabetes insipidus can also be seen preoperatively. Rarely, hemorrhage into the pituitary results in acute panhypopituitarism (pituitary apoplexy) with signs of a rapidly expanding mass, hemodynamic instability, and hypoglycemia.

This patient has the most common type of secretory adenoma—that producing hyperprolactinemia. Women with this tumor typically have amenorrhea, galactorrhea, or both. Men with prolactin-secreting adenomas may have galactorrhea or infertility but more commonly present with symptoms of an expanding mass.

What other types of secretory hormones are seen?

Adenomas secreting ACTH (Cushing's disease) produce classic manifestations of Cushing's syndrome: truncal obesity, moon facies, abdominal striae, proximal muscle weakness, hypertension, and osteoporosis. Glucose tolerance is typically impaired, but frank diabetes is less common (< 20%). Hirsutism, acne, and amenorrhea are also commonly seen in women.

Adenomas that secrete GH are often large and result in either gigantism (prepubertal patients) or acromegaly (adults). Excessive growth prior to epiphyseal fusion results in massive growth of the entire skeleton. After epiphyseal closure, the abnormal growth is limited to soft tissues and acral parts: hands, feet, nose, and mandible. Patients develop osteoarthritis, which often affects the temporomandibular joint and spine. Diabetes, myopathies, and neuropathies are common. Cardiovascular complications include hypertension, premature coronary disease, and cardiomyopathy in some patients. The most serious anesthetic problem encountered in these patients is difficulty in intubating the trachea.

Are any special monitors required for transsphenoidal surgery?

Monitoring should be carried out in somewhat the same way as for craniotomies. Visual evoked potentials may be employed with large tumors that involve the optic nerves. Precordial Doppler sonography may be used for detecting venous air embolism. Venous access with large-bore catheters is desirable in the event of massive hemorrhage.

What modifications, if any, are necessary in the anesthetic technique?

The same principles discussed for craniotomies apply, particularly if the patient has evidence of increased ICP. Intravenous antibiotic prophylaxis and glucocorticoid coverage (hydrocortisone, 100 mg) are usually given prior to induction. Many clinicians avoid nitrous oxide to prevent problems with a postoperative pneumocephalus (see above). Intense neuromuscular blockade is important to prevent movement while the surgeon is using the microscope. In some circumstances, the surgeon may request placement of a lumbar intrathecal catheter to drain CSF, thereby facilitating surgical exposure. The management of diabetes insipidus is discussed in Chapter 28.

SUGGESTED READING

Albin M: *Textbook of Neuroanesthesia with Neurosurgical and Neuroscience Perspectives.* McGraw-Hill, 1997.

Cottrell JE, Smith DS: *Anesthesia and Neurosurgery,* 3rd ed. Mosby Year Book, 1994.

Cucchiara RF, Black S, Michenfelder JD: *Clinical Neuroanesthesia,* 2nd ed. Churchill Livingstone, 1998.

Newfield P, Cottrell JE: *Handbook of Neuroanesthesia,* 3rd ed. Lippincott, Williams & Wilkins, 1999.

Schubert A: *Clinical Neuroanesthesia.* Butterworth-Heinemann, 1997.

Stone DJ, Sperry RJ: *The Neuroanesthesia Handbook.* Mosby, 1996.

Anesthesia for Patients with Neurologic & Psychiatric Diseases

27

KEY CONCEPTS

 An asymptomatic cervical bruit does not appear to increase the risk of stroke following surgery but increases the likelihood of coexisting coronary artery disease.

 Resistance to neuromuscular blockade—as assessed by train-of-four monitoring—may be observed in paretic extremities; neuromuscular blockade should therefore be monitored on the nonparetic side. Succinylcholine should be avoided in patients with a history of recent stroke as well as in those with extensive muscle wasting because of the risks of hyperkalemia.

 If a seizure occurs, maintaining an open airway and adequate oxygenation are the first priorities. Intravenous thiopental (50–100 mg), phenytoin (500–1000 mg slowly), or a benzodiazepine such as diazepam (5–10 mg) or midazolam (1–5 mg) can be used to terminate the seizure.

 Induction of anesthesia in patients receiving long-term levodopa therapy may result in either marked hypotension or hypertension.

 Increases in body temperature cause exacerbation of symptoms, presumably by decreasing nerve conduction.

 The major risk of anesthesia in patients with autonomic dysfunction is severe hypotension, compromising cerebral and coronary blood flow.

 Patients with high transections often have impaired airway reflexes and are further predisposed to hypoxemia by a decrease in functional residual capacity. Hypotension and bradycardia are often present prior to induction.

 Autonomic hyperreflexia should be expected in patients with lesions above T6 and can be precipitated by surgical manipulations.

 The most important interaction between anesthetic agents and tricyclic antidepressants is an exaggerated response to both indirect-acting vasopressors and sympathetic stimulation.

 Opioids should generally be used with caution in patients receiving monoamine oxidase inhibitors because rare but serious reactions to opioids have been reported. Most serious reactions are associated with meperidine, resulting in hyperthermia, seizures, and coma.

Cerebrovascular disease is a major cause of morbidity and death. Patients with a history of stroke, transient ischemic attacks (TIAs), or asymptomatic extracranial vascular obstructions frequently present to the operating room for unrelated procedures. This chapter discusses a general approach to these patients as well as patients with

other common neurologic disorders. Chapter 21 discusses anesthetic management of patients undergoing carotid artery surgery.

Nonvascular neurologic diseases and psychiatric disorders are less frequently encountered in surgical patients and are often overlooked. Fortunately, unless increased intracranial pressure (ICP) is present, special anesthetic techniques are not usually required. Nonetheless, the anesthesiologist must have a basic understanding of the major neurologic and psychiatric disorders and their drug therapy; failure to recognize potentially adverse anesthetic interactions may result in avoidable perioperative morbidity.

■ CEREBROVASCULAR DISEASE

Preoperative Considerations

The incidence of significant cerebrovascular disease in surgical patients is unknown but increases with age. Patients with known cerebrovascular disease typically have a history of TIAs or stroke. Asymptomatic cervical bruits occur in up to 4% of patients over age 40 but do not necessarily indicate significant carotid artery obstruction. Fewer than 10% of patients with completely asymptomatic bruits have hemodynamically significant carotid artery lesions. Moreover, the absence of a bruit does not exclude significant carotid obstruction.

The risk of postoperative stroke increases with patient age and varies with the type of surgery. The overall risk of stroke following nonneurologic surgery is low, but it is higher in patients undergoing cardiovascular surgery. Rates of stroke after general anesthesia and surgery range from 0.08 to 0.4%. Even in patients with known cerebrovascular disease, the risk is only 0.4–3.3%. An asymptomatic cervical bruit does not appear to increase the risk of stroke following surgery but increases the likelihood of coexisting coronary artery disease (see Chapter 20). Patients undergoing open heart procedures for valvular disease are at highest risk for postoperative stroke (incidence of about 4%), as are patients undergoing operations on the thoracic aorta. The mortality rate following postoperative stroke may be as high as 26%. Strokes following open heart surgery are usually due to emboli of air, fibrin, or calcium debris. Strokes following thoracic aortic surgery are most likely due to emboli or ischemia secondary to prolonged cross-clamping from a clamp close to the take off of the carotid artery. The pathophysiology of postoperative strokes following noncardiovascular surgery is less clear but may involve severe sustained hypotension or hypertension. Hypotension with severe hypoperfusion can result in intracerebral thrombosis and infarction, whereas hypertension can result in hemorrhage into a carotid plaque or intracerebral hemorrhage (hemorrhagic stroke); sustained hypertension can also disrupt the blood–brain barrier and promote cerebral edema (see Chapter 25). The period of time after which a patient may be safely anesthetized following a stroke has not been determined. Abnormalities in regional blood flow and metabolic rate usually resolve after 2 weeks, whereas alterations in CO_2 responsiveness and in the blood–brain barrier may require more than 4 weeks. Most clinicians postpone elective procedures a minimum of 6–26 weeks following a completed stroke.

Patients with TIAs have a history of transient (< 24 h) impairment and, by definition, have no residual neurologic impairment. These attacks are thought to result from emboli of fibrin-platelet aggregates or atheromatous debris from plaques in extracranial vessels. Unilateral visual impairment, numbness or weakness of an extremity, or aphasia is suggestive of carotid disease, whereas bilateral visual impairment, dizziness, ataxia, dysarthria, bilateral weakness, or amnesia is suggestive of vertebral-basilar disease. Patients with TIAs have a 30–40% chance of developing a thrombotic stroke within 5 years; most (50%) occur within the first year. Patients with TIAs should not undergo any elective surgical procedure without an adequate medical evaluation that generally includes at least noninvasive (Doppler) flow and imaging studies. The presence of an ulcerative plaque of greater than 60% occlusion is generally an indication for carotid endarterectomy provided the patient does not have significant comorbid conditions. If the patient is symptomatic, then surgical intervention is favored over medical therapy if the stenosis is > 50%.

PREOPERATIVE MANAGEMENT

Preoperative assessment requires careful neurologic and cardiovascular evaluations. The type of stroke, the presence of neurologic deficits, and the extent of residual impairment should be determined. Thrombotic strokes are most common and usually occur in patients with generalized atherosclerosis. Most patients are elderly and have comorbid conditions such as hypertension, hyperlipidemia, and diabetes. Coexisting coronary artery disease and renal impairment are common. Embolic strokes are most often associated with mitral valve disease or endocarditis or follow valve replacement. Hemorrhagic strokes are typically due to accelerated hypertension, rupture of a cerebral aneurysm, or an arteriovenous malformation. Many patients, following nonhemorrhagic strokes or TIAs, are placed on long-term warfarin or antiplatelet therapy. The risk of stopping such therapy perioperatively for a few days appears small. Clotting studies and a bleeding time should be used to confirm reversal of their effect prior to operation. Once surgical hemostasis has been achieved (12–48 h), anticoagulants or aspirin may be resumed postoperatively.

Regardless of the procedure or the type of anesthetic to be administered, hypertension, angina, congestive heart failure, and hyperglycemia should be under good control preoperatively. With the exception of diuretics and insulin, all patients should receive their usual medications up to the time of surgery. The management of diabetes and hyperglycemia is discussed in Chapter 36.

INTRAOPERATIVE MANAGEMENT

Although some clinicians believe that regional anesthesia may be safer than general anesthesia for these patients, supporting studies are lacking. No one anesthetic technique is clearly superior to another. Blood pressure should be maintained at or slightly higher than normal levels because of a rightward shift in cerebral autoregulation (Figure 27–1) (see Chapter 25). Vasopressors should not be relied upon to maintain blood pressure, as their overuse can precipitate myocardial ischemia. Vasodilators or adrenergic blockade may be necessary during periods of intense stimulation and during emergence. Use of a neuromuscular blocking agent (NMBA) facilitates anesthetic management by providing optimal surgical conditions yet allowing appropriate adjustments in anesthetic depth. Wide swings in blood pressure are undesirable and may contribute to postoperative cardiac and cerebral complications.

The use of a paretic or paralyzed extremity for monitoring neuromuscular blockade can result in overdosage. Resistance to neuromuscular blockade—as assessed by train-of-four monitoring—may be observed in paretic extremities; neuromuscular blockade should therefore be monitored on the nonparetic side. Succinylcholine should be avoided in patients with a history of recent stroke as well as in those with extensive muscle wasting because of the risks of hyperkalemia.

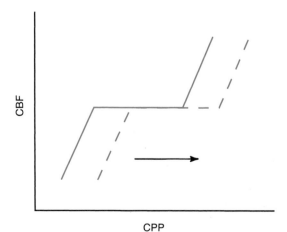

Figure 27–1. Rightward shift in cerebral blood flow (CBF) seen in patients with chronic hypertension. CPP, cerebral perfusion pressure.

SEIZURE DISORDERS

Preoperative Considerations

Seizures represent abnormal synchronized electrical activity in the brain. They may be a manifestation of an underlying central nervous system disease, a systemic disorder, or may be idiopathic. Mechanisms are thought to include (1) loss of inhibitory γ-aminobutyric acid (GABA) activity, (2) enhanced release of excitatory amino acids (glutamate), and (3) enhanced neuronal firing due to abnormal voltage-mediated calcium currents. Up to 2% of the population may experience a seizure in their lifetime. Epilepsy is a disorder characterized by recurrent paroxysmal seizure activity. Healthy individuals who experience an isolated nonrecurrent seizure are not considered to have epilepsy.

Seizure activity may be localized to a specific area in the brain or may be generalized. Moreover, initially localized (focal) seizures can subsequently spread, becoming generalized. A simple classification scheme is presented in Table 27–1. Partial seizures (also called focal) are clinically manifested by motor, sensory, autonomic, or psychiatric symptoms, depending on the cortical area affected. Focal seizures associated with impairment in consciousness are termed "complex partial" (psychomotor or temporal lobe) seizures. Generalized seizures characteristically produce bilaterally symmetric electrical activity without local onset. They result in abnormal motor activity, loss of consciousness, or both. Generalized activity resulting in isolated and transient lapses in consciousness are called absence (petit mal) seizures. Other generalized seizures are usually classified according to the type of motor activity. Tonic–clonic (grand mal) seizures are most common and are characterized by a loss of consciousness followed by clonic and then tonic motor activity.

PREOPERATIVE MANAGEMENT

Preoperative evaluation of patients with a seizure disorder should focus on determining the cause and type of seizure activity and on the drugs with which the patient is being treated. Seizures in adults are most commonly due to structural brain lesions (head trauma, tumor, degeneration, or stroke) or metabolic abnormalities (uremia, hepatic failure, hypoglycemia, hypocalcemia, or drug toxicity or withdrawal). Idiopathic seizures occur most often in children but may persist into adulthood. Anesthetic evaluation should focus primarily on the underlying disorder and secondarily on the seizures. Management of patients with a mass lesion or increased ICP is discussed in Chapter 26.

Table 27–1. Classification of seizures.

Partial (focal)
Simple
Complex
Secondarily generalized tonic–clonic
Generalized
Absence (petit mal)
Myoclonic
Clonic
Tonic
Tonic–clonic (grand mal)
Atonic
Unclassified

Characterization of the type of seizure is important in detecting such activity perioperatively. Seizures—particularly grand mal seizures—are serious complicating factors in surgical patients and should be treated aggressively to prevent musculoskeletal injury, hypoventilation, hypoxemia, and aspiration of gastrointestinal content. Even partial seizures can progress to grand mal seizures. If a seizure occurs, maintaining an open airway and adequate oxygenation are the first priorities. Intravenous thiopental (50–100 mg), phenytoin (500–1000 mg slowly), or a benzodiazepine such as diazepam (5–10 mg) or midazolam (1–5 mg) can be used to terminate the seizure.

Most patients with seizure disorders receive antiepileptic drugs ([AEDs] anticonvulsants) preoperatively (Table 27–2). Drug therapy should be reviewed for effi-

cacy and toxicity. Phenytoin, carbamazepine, and valproate are used for generalized tonic–clonic seizures. Phenytoin and valproate are often used for partial seizures. Adverse side effects and signs of toxicity should be excluded clinically and by laboratory investigations. Carbamazepine, ethosuximide, felbamate, and valproate may cause bone marrow depression and hepatotoxicity. At toxic levels, most agents cause ataxia, dizziness, confusion, and sedation. Blood levels of AEDs are usually readily available from the hospital laboratory and should be checked in patients with signs of toxicity and those who give a history of recent seizures. AEDs should ideally be continued throughout the perioperative period to maintain therapeutic levels. Fortunately, most agents have a relatively long half-life, so that a delayed or even a missed dose is often not critical.

INTRAOPERATIVE MANAGEMENT

In selecting anesthetic agents, drugs with possible epileptogenic potential should be avoided. Ketamine and methohexital (in small doses) theoretically can precipitate seizure activity and should be avoided. Theoretically, large doses of atracurium or cisatracurium or meperidine may be contraindicated because of the reported epileptogenic potential of their metabolites, laudanosine and normeperidine. Hepatic microsomal enzyme induction should be expected from chronic AED therapy. Enzyme induction may increase dose requirement and frequency for intravenous anesthetics and nondepolarizing NMBAs and may increase the potential for hepatotoxicity from halothane.

Table 27–2. Commonly used anticonvulsants and their dose.[1]

Drug	Daily Dose[2] (mg)
Carbamazepine	800–1600
Felbamate	2400–3600
Gabapentin	900–3600
Lamotrigine	300–500
Phenytoin	300–400
Tiagabine	32–56
Topiramate	200–400
Valproate	1000–3000

[1]Reprinted, with permission, from Samuels MA: Update in neurology. Ann Intern Med 1998;129:878.
[2]Usual total daily dose for adults.

■ DEGENERATIVE & DEMYELINATING DISEASES

PARKINSON DISEASE

Preoperative Considerations

Parkinson disease (PD) is a common movement disorder that typically afflicts individuals aged 50–70 years; it has a prevalence of 3% in the United States and Canada. This neurodegenerative disease is characterized by bradykinesia, rigidity, postural instability, and resting (pill-rolling) tremor. Additional frequently occurring findings include facial masking, hypophonia, dysphagia, and festination. Increasing problems with freezing, rigidity, and tremor eventually result in physical incapacitation. Early in the course of the disease, intellectual function is usually preserved, but declines in intellectual function can occur and may be severe over the course of the disease. PD is caused by a progressive loss of dopamine in the nigrostriatum, with severity of loss of dopamine correlating with bradykinesia. As the loss of dopamine occurs, the activity of the GABA nuclei in the basal ganglia increases, leading to an inhibition of thalamic and brain stem nuclei. Thalamic inhibition, in turn, suppresses the motor system in the cortex, resulting in the dyskinesia, rigidity, postural instability, and tremor that are characteristic of the disease.

Treatment is directed at controlling the symptoms. A variety of drugs may be used for mild disease, including the anticholinergic agents trihexyphenidyl, benztropine, and ethopropazine; the irreversible monoamine oxidase (MAO) inhibitors, selegiline and rasagiline; and the antiviral drug, amantadine. Moderate to severe disease is typically treated pharmacologically with dopaminergic agents, either levodopa (a precursor of dopamine) or a dopamine-receptor agonist. Levodopa, which is given with a decarboxylase inhibitor to retard the peripheral breakdown of the drug (thereby increasing its central delivery and decreasing the dose of levodopa that is required to control symptoms), is the most effective therapy and is used to treat moderate to severe symptoms. Catechol methyltransferase (COMT) inhibitors are also used to prevent the decarboxylation of levodopa and include Stalevo, and Tolcapone. Levodopa is available in either an immediate- or sustained-release formulation, with a duration of action of 2–4 h and 3–6 h, respectively, and can be crushed and mixed with liquid. Side effects include nausea, vomiting, dyskinesias, sudden onset of sleepiness, motor fluctuations, cardiac irritability, and orthostatic hypotension. The latter may be due to catecholamine depletion (chronic negative feedback inhibition) and volume depletion, perhaps secondary to a natriuretic effect.

Dopamine-receptor agonists include both ergot (bromocriptine, cabergoline, lisuride, and apomorphine) and nonergot derivatives (pramipexole and ropinirole). Apomorphine may be administered as an intravenous or subcutaneous injection for rapid rescue therapy during off periods, the severe motor fluctuations for PD. The nonergot derivatives have been shown to be beneficial when used as monotherapy in early PD; all dopamine-receptor agonists are effective when given as combination therapy with levodopa in the treatment of moderate to severe PD. Side effects are similar to those found with the use of levodopa and, in addition, include headache, confusion, and hallucinations. Pulmonary and retroperitoneal fibrosis, pleural effusion and thickening, Raynaud syndrome, and erythromyalgia are more common side effects with the use of ergot derivatives than with nonergot derivitives.

The surgical treatment of PD includes both ablative procedures (thalamotomy and pallidotomy), as well as electrical stimulation of the ventral intermediate nucleus of the thalamus, the globus pallidus internus, or the sub-

thalamic nucleus. Pallidotomy is effective for treating the dyskinesia and wearing-off symptoms of PD (70–90%) as well as the tremor, rigidity, bradykinesia, and gait symptoms (30–50%) of the disorder. Thalamotomy is most effective in treating the contralateral tremor, but not the other symptoms of the disease, and has been largely replaced by the use of thalamic stimulation. The efficacy of deep brain stimulation of the thalamus is related to the effect on tremor; it has little to no effect on the other symptoms of PD. Subthalamic stimulation has been shown to improve all the primary symptoms of PD and to decrease the amount of off time and the amount of medication necessary for symptom relief, with bilateral, as compared with unilateral, simulation having better efficacy. Some decrease in cognitive function may occur with this treatment and, therefore, it should be used with caution in patients with cognitive impairment. The effects of globus pallidus internus stimulation are similar to those of pallidotomy, with improvements in dyskinesia and, to a lesser extent, off times.

Anesthetic Considerations

Medication for PD should be continued perioperatively, including the morning of surgery, because the half-life of levodopa is short. Abrupt withdrawal of levodopa can cause worsening of muscle rigidity and may interfere with ventilation. Phenothiazines, butyrophenones (droperidol), and metoclopramide can exacerbate symptoms as a consequence of their antidopaminergic activity and should be avoided. Anticholinergics (atropine) or antihistamines (diphenhydramine) may be used for acute exacerbation of symptoms. Diphenhydramine is particularly valuable for premedication and intraoperative sedation in patients with tremor. Induction of anesthesia in patients receiving long-term levodopa therapy may result in either marked hypotension or hypertension. Relative hypovolemia, catecholamine depletion, autonomic instability, and sensitization to catecholamines are probably contributory. Arterial blood pressure should be monitored carefully. Significant hypotension should be treated with small doses of a direct-acting vasopressor such as phenylephrine. Cardiac irritability readily produces arrhythmias, so halothane, ketamine, and local anesthetic solutions containing epinephrine should be used cautiously if at all. Although the response to NMBAs is generally normal, a rare occurrence of hyperkalemia following succinylcholine has been reported. Adequacy of ventilation and airway reflexes should be carefully assessed prior to extubation of patients with moderate to severe disease.

As mentioned previously, patients who fail medical treatment are candidates for surgical intervention, eg, an ablative therapy such as a thalamotomy or pallidotomy or implantation of a deep brain stimulator of the subthalamic nucleus, the ventral intermediate nucleus, or the globus pallidus internus. Because general anesthesia alters the threshold for stimulation, correct placement of the electrodes can be affected. An awake craniotomy has been the norm for epilepsy surgery for some time, and, increasingly, it is being used for deep brain stimulation procedures as well. Two techniques are advocated—a true awake craniotomy with heavy sedation and an approach in which the patient receives a general anesthetic, usually a total intravenous anesthetic with propofol and remifentanil, and a laryngeal mask airway for control of the airway. Following appropriate surgical exposure, the intravenous infusions are discontinued, and the laryngeal mask airway is removed. The patient can be reanesthetized once the implantation of leads is complete. The same goals could be achieved with a short-acting inhalation anesthetic such as sevoflurane or desflurane.

ALZHEIMER DISEASE

Preoperative Considerations

Neurodegenerative diseases, increasingly common in patients 70 years of age or older, often lead to dementia. Along with a loss of gray matter, elderly patients have altered pharmacokinetic and pharmacodynamic responses to many drugs that present a challenge when attempting to induce and maintain anesthesia or sedation. Alzheimer disease (AD) is the most common neurodegenerative disease, causing approximately 40–80% of all cases of dementia, with a prevalence of approximately 20% in patients aged over 80 years. The disease is characterized by a slow decline in intellectual function (dementia). Progressive impairment of memory, judgment, and decision making and emotional lability are hallmarks of the disease. Late in the course of the disease, severe extrapyramidal signs, apraxias, and aphasia are often present. Although some degree of brain atrophy is normal with advancing age, patients with AD usually show marked cortical atrophy with ventricular enlargement; the pathological hallmarks of AD include neurofibrillary tangles that contain the phosphorylated microtubular protein tau and neuritic plaques composed of the peptide β-amyloid.

In the absence of an effective cure, treatment is aimed at preventing further deterioration and, if not possible, slowing the rate of deterioration and treating symptoms. The cholinesterase inhibitors, which include tacrine, donepezil, galantamine, and rivastigmine, are often prescribed to slow deterioration of mental status.

Anesthetic Considerations

Anesthetic management of patients with moderate to severe disease is often complicated by disorientation and uncooperativeness. Significant cognitive impairment is a frequent observation in elderly patients and often persists for 1–3 days following surgery. Such patients require repeated reassurance and explanation. Consent must be obtained from the next of kin or a legal guardian if the patient is legally incompetent, but patients may still be asked to sign the consent form if able, as they are "assenting" to the operation. Because the use of centrally acting drugs must be minimized, premedication is usually not given, and if it is, at smaller doses than usual. Regional anesthesia should be attempted only if the patient is cooperative. Inhalation agents may be preferable for general anesthesia because of their rapid elimination. Centrally acting anticholinergics, such as atropine and scopolamine, could theoretically contribute to postoperative confusion. Glycopyrrolate, which does not cross the blood–brain barrier, may be the preferred agent when an anticholinergic is required.

MULTIPLE SCLEROSIS

Preoperative Considerations

Multiple sclerosis is characterized by reversible demyelination at random and multiple sites in the brain and spinal cord; chronic inflammation, however, eventually produces scarring (gliosis). The disease may be an autoimmune disorder that is initiated by a viral infection. It primarily affects patients between 20 and 40 years of age, with a 2:1 female predominance, and typically follows an unpredictable course of frequent attacks and remissions. With time, remissions become less complete, and the disease is progressive and incapacitating; almost 50% of patients will require help with walking within 15 years of diagnosis. Clinical manifestations depend on the sites affected but frequently include sensory disturbances (paresthesias), visual problems (optic neuritis and diplopia), and motor weakness. Symptoms develop over the course of days and remit over weeks to months. Early diagnosis of exacerbations can often be confirmed by analysis of cerebrospinal fluid and magnetic resonance imaging. Remyelination is limited and often fails to occur. Moreover, axonal loss can develop. Changes in neurological function appear to be related to changes in axonal conduction. Conduction can occur across demyelinated axons but appears to be affected by multiple factors, particularly temperature. Increases in body temperature cause exacerbation of symptoms, presumably by decreasing nerve conduction.

Treatment of multiple sclerosis may be primarily symptomatic or may be used in an attempt to arrest the disease process. Diazepam, dantrolene, or baclofen and, in refractory cases, an intrathecal delivery system for baclofen are used to control spasticity;

bethanechol and other anticholinergics are useful for urinary retention. Painful dysesthesia may respond to carbamazepine, phenytoin, or antidepressants (see Chapter 18). Glucocorticoids may decrease the severity and duration of acute attacks. Corticosteroid-resistant relapses may respond to five to seven courses of plasma exchange offered on alternate days. Interferon β_{1b}, interferon β_{1a}, and glatiramer acetate reduce the frequency of relapse by up to 30%. Immunosuppression with azathioprine or cyclophosphamide may also be attempted to halt disease progression, but there is limited "evidence-based" support for these approaches. The Food and Drug Administration (FDA) has recently approved mitoxantrone for aggressive relapsing and progressive multiple sclerosis.

Anesthetic Considerations

The effect of stress, anesthesia, and surgery on the course of the disease is controversial. A detrimental effect has been suggested but not substantiated. Overall, the effect of anesthesia is unpredictable. Elective surgery should be avoided during relapse regardless of the anesthetic technique employed. The preoperative consent record should document counseling of the patient to the effect that the stress of surgery and anesthesia might worsen the symptoms. Spinal anesthesia has been reported to cause exacerbation of the disease. Epidural and other regional techniques appear to have no adverse effect, particularly in obstetrics. No specific interactions with general anesthetics are usually recognized. Patients with advanced disease may have a labile cardiovascular system due to autonomic dysfunction. In the setting of paresis or paralysis, succinylcholine should be avoided because of hyperkalemia. Regardless of the anesthetic technique employed, increases in body temperatures should be avoided. Demyelinated fibers are extremely sensitive to increases in temperature; an increase of as little as 0.5°C may completely block conduction.

AMYOTROPHIC LATERAL SCLEROSIS

Motor neuron disease is another common neurodegenerative disease, with amyotrophic lateral sclerosis (ALS) the most prevalent. The cause of ALS is unknown, although small numbers of patients with the familial form of the disease have a defect in the superoxide dismutase-1 (SOD_1) gene. ALS is a rapidly progressive disorder of both upper and lower motor neurons. Clinically, patients present in the fifth or sixth decade of life with muscular weakness, atrophy, fasciculation, and spasticity. The disease may initially be asymmetric but over the course of 2–3 years becomes generalized, involving all skeletal and bulbar muscles. Progressive respiratory muscle weakness makes the patient susceptible to aspiration and eventually leads to death from ventilatory failure. Although the heart is unaffected, autonomic dysfunction can be seen. There is no specific treatment for ALS.

The primary emphasis in management is judicious respiratory care. As with other patients with lower motor neuron disease, succinylcholine is contraindicated because of the risk of hyperkalemia. Nondepolarizing NMBAs should be used sparingly, if at all, because patients often display enhanced sensitivity. Adequacy of ventilation should be carefully assessed both intraoperatively and postoperatively; an awake extubation is desirable. Difficulty in weaning patients off mechanical ventilation postoperatively is not uncommon in patients with moderate to advanced disease.

GUILLAIN–BARRÉ SYNDROME

Guillain–Barré syndrome (GBS), a relatively common disorder affecting one to four individuals per 100,000 population, is characterized by a sudden onset of ascending motor paralysis, areflexia, and variable paresthesias. Subtypes of GBS include acute inflammatory demyelinating polyneuropathy (about 75% of cases), acute motor axonal neuropathy (with antibodies against gangliosides), and acute motor sensory axonal neuropathy. Bulbar involvement, including respiratory muscle paralysis, is a frequent complication. Pathologically, the disease appears to be an immunologic reaction against the myelin sheath of peripheral nerves, particularly lower motor neurons. In most instances, the syndrome appears to follow viral respiratory or gastrointestinal infections; the disorder can also present as a paraneoplastic syndrome associated with Hodgkin's disease or as a complication of human immunodeficiency virus (HIV) infection. Some patients respond to plasmapheresis. The prognosis is relatively good, with most patients recovering completely, but unfortunately approximately 10% will die of complications and another 10% are left with long-term neurologic sequelae.

In addition to the respiratory complications, anesthetic management is complicated by lability of the autonomic nervous system. Exaggerated hypotensive and hypertensive responses during anesthesia may be seen. As with other lower motor neuron disorders, succinylcholine should not be used because of the risk of hyperkalemia. The use of regional anesthesia in these patients remains controversial, as there are several case reports of patients who, after its use, developed GBS or whose GBS became worse.

AUTONOMIC DYSFUNCTION
Preoperative Considerations

Autonomic dysfunction, or dysautonomia, may be due to generalized or segmental disorders of the central or peripheral nervous system. Symptoms can be generalized, segmental, or focal. These disorders may be congenital, familial, or acquired. Common manifestations include impotence; bladder and gastrointestinal dysfunction; abnormal regulation of body fluids; decreased sweating, lacrimation, and salivation; and orthostatic hypotension. The latter is often the most serious manifestation of the dysfunction.

Acquired autonomic dysfunction can be isolated (pure autonomic failure), part of a more generalized degenerative process (Shy–Drager syndrome, PD, olivopontocerebellar atrophy), part of a segmental neurological process (multiple sclerosis, syringomyelia, reflex sympathetic dystrophy, or spinal cord injury), or a manifestation of disorders affecting peripheral nerves (GBS, diabetes, chronic alcoholism, amyloidosis, or porphyria). Treatment includes increasing salt intake, sleeping in a reverse Trendelenburg position (to minimize nocturnal diuresis), and various drug therapies. The latter may include a mineralocorticoid (fludrocortisone—Florinef), prostaglandin inhibitor (ibuprofen), β-adrenergic blocker, sympathomimetic, or dopamine antagonist (metoclopramide). The vasopressin analogue desmopressin (DDAVP) or the somatostatin analogue octreotide (Sandostatin) may also be tried.

Congenital or familial dysautonomia occurs most frequently in Ashkenazi Jewish children and is usually referred to as Riley–Day syndrome. Autonomic dysfunction is prominent and is associated with generalized diminished sensation and emotional lability. Moreover, patients are predisposed to dysautonomic crises triggered by stress and characterized by marked hypertension, tachycardia, abdominal pain, diaphoresis, and vomiting. Intravenous diazepam is effective in resolving such episodes. Hereditary dysautonomia associated with a deficiency of dopamine β-hydroxylase is described. Administration of α-dihydroxyphenylserine (α-DOPS) improves symptoms in these patients.

Anesthetic Considerations

The major risk of anesthesia in patients with autonomic dysfunction is severe hypotension, compromising cerebral and coronary blood flow. Marked hypertension can be equally deleterious. Most patients are chronically hypovolemic. The vasodilatory effects of spinal and epidural anesthesia are poorly tolerated. Similarly, the vasodilatory and cardiac depressant effects of most general anesthetic agents combined with positive airway pressure can be equally deleterious. Continuous intraarterial blood pressure monitoring is desirable. Hypotension should be treated with fluids and direct-acting vasopressors. The latter are preferable to indirect-acting agents. Enhanced sensitivity to vasopressors due to denervation sensitivity may be observed. Blood loss also is usually poorly tolerated; monitoring of central venous or pulmonary artery pressure is invaluable

when significant fluid shifts are expected. Body temperature should be monitored closely. Patients with anhidrosis are particularly susceptible to hyperpyrexia.

SYRINGOMYELIA

Syringomyelia results in progressive cavitation of the spinal cord. In many cases, obstruction of cerebrospinal fluid outflow from the fourth ventricle appears to be contributory. Many patients have craniovertebral abnormalities, particularly the Arnold–Chiari malformation. Increased pressure in the central canal of the spinal cord produces enlargement or diverticulation to the point of cavitation. Syringomyelia typically affects the cervical spine, producing sensory and motor deficits in the upper extremities and, frequently, thoracic scoliosis. Extension upward into the medulla (syringobulbia) leads to cranial nerve deficits. Ventricular-peritoneal shunting and other decompressive procedures have variable success in arresting the disease.

Anesthetic evaluation should focus on defining existing neurologic deficits as well as any pulmonary impairment due to scoliosis. Pulmonary function testing and arterial blood gas analysis may be useful. Autonomic instability should be expected in patients with extensive lesions. Succinylcholine should be avoided when muscle wasting is present because of the risk of hyperkalemia. Adequacy of ventilation and reversal of nondepolarizing NMBAs should be achieved prior to extubation.

■ SPINAL CORD INJURY

Preoperative Considerations

Most spinal cord injuries are traumatic and often result in partial or complete transection. The majority of injuries are due to fracture and dislocation of the vertebral column. The mechanism is usually either compression and flexion at the thoracic spine or extension at the cervical spine. Clinical manifestations depend on the level of the transection. Injuries above C3–5 (diaphragmatic innervation) require patients to receive ventilatory support to stay alive. Transections above T1 result in quadriplegia, whereas those above L4 result in paraplegia. The most common sites of transection are C5–6 and T12–L1. Acute spinal cord transection produces loss of sensation, flaccid paralysis, and loss of spinal reflexes below the level of injury. These findings characterize a period of spinal shock that typically lasts 1–3 weeks.

Over the course of the next few weeks, spinal reflexes gradually return, together with muscle spasms and signs of sympathetic overactivity. Compression in the low thoracic or lumbar spine results in cauda equina (conus medullaris) syndrome. The latter usually consists of incomplete injury to nerve roots rather than the spinal cord.

Overactivity of the sympathetic nervous system is common with transections at T5 or above but is unusual with injuries below T10. Interruption of normal descending inhibitory impulses in the cord results in autonomic hyperreflexia. Cutaneous or visceral stimulation below the level of injury can induce intense autonomic reflexes: sympathetic discharge produces hypertension and vasoconstricltion below the transection and a baroreceptor-mediated reflex bradycardia and vasodilation above the transection. Cardiac arrhythmias are not unusual.

Emergent surgical management is undertaken whenever there is potentially reversible compression of the spinal cord due to dislocation of a vertebral body or bony fragment. Operative treatment is also indicated for spinal instability to prevent further injury. Patients can also present to the operating room as a result of delayed complications or unrelated disorders.

Anesthetic Considerations

A. ACUTE TRANSECTION

Anesthetic management depends on the age of the injury. In the early care of acute injuries, the emphasis should be on preventing further spinal cord damage during patient movement, airway manipulation, and positioning. High-dose corticosteroid therapy (methylprednisolone: 30 mg/kg over the first hour followed by 5.4 mg/kg/h for 23 h) is used for the first 24 h following injury to improve neurologic outcome. The head should be maintained in a neutral position using in-line stabilization with the help of an assistant or should remain in traction during intubation. Awake fiberoptic intubation after topical anesthesia may

 be safest. Patients with high transections often have impaired airway reflexes and are further predisposed to hypoxemia by a decrease in functional residual capacity. Hypotension and bradycardia are often present prior to induction. Direct arterial pressure monitoring is indicated. Monitoring of central venous and pulmonary artery pressure also facilitates management. An intravenous fluid bolus and the use of ketamine for anesthesia may help prevent further decreases in blood pressure; vasopressors may also be required. Succinylcholine can be used safely in the first 24 h but should not be used thereafter because of the risk of hyperkalemia. The latter can occur within the first week following injury and is due to excessive release of potassium secondary to the proliferation of acetylcholine receptors outside the neuromuscular synaptic cleft.

B. CHRONIC TRANSECTION

Anesthetic management of patients with nonacute transections is complicated by the possibility of autonomic hyper-

reflexia in addition to the risk of hyperkalemia. Autonomic hyperreflexia should be expected in patients with lesions above T6 and can be precipitated by surgical manipulations. **Regional anesthesia and deep general anesthesia are effective in preventing hyperreflexia.** Many clinicians, however, are reluctant to administer spinal and epidural anesthesia in these patients because of the difficulties encountered in determining anesthetic level, exaggerated hypotension, and technical problems resulting from deformities. Severe hypertension can result in pulmonary edema, myocardial ischemia, or cerebral hemorrhage and should be treated aggressively. Direct arterial vasodilators and α-adrenergic blocking agents should be readily available. Although the risk of succinylcholine-induced hyperkalemia is reported to decrease 6 months after the injury, the use of nondepolarizing NMBAs are preferred. Administration of a small dose of a nondepolarizing NMBA does not reliably prevent hyperkalemia. Body temperature should be monitored carefully, particularly in patients with transections above T1, because chronic vasodilation and loss of normal reflex cutaneous vasoconstriction predispose to hypothermia.

Many patients eventually develop progressive renal insufficiency due to recurrent calculi and amyloid deposition. Drugs that are primarily excreted renally should be avoided in these patients (see Chapter 31).

■ PSYCHIATRIC DISORDERS

DEPRESSION

Depression is a mood disorder characterized by sadness and pessimism. Its cause is multifactorial, but pharmacological treatment is based on the presumption that its manifestations are due to a brain deficiency of dopamine, norepinephrine, and serotonin or altered receptor activities. Up to 50% of patients with major depression hypersecrete cortisol and have abnormal circadian secretion. Current pharmacological therapy utilizes three classes of drugs that increase brain levels of these neurotransmitters: tricyclic antidepressants, monoamine oxidase (MAO) inhibitors, and atypical antidepressants. The mechanisms of action of these drugs result in some potentially serious anesthetic interactions. Electroconvulsive therapy (ECT) is increasingly used for refractory and severe cases and prophylactically once the patient returns to baseline. The use of general anesthesia for ECT is largely responsible for its safety and widespread acceptance.

Tricyclic Antidepressants

Tricyclic antidepressants may be used for the treatment of depression and chronic pain syndromes (see Chapter 18)

Table 27–3. Classification of antidepressants.[1,2]

Class	Mechanism of Action	Generic Name (US Trade Name)
Selected newer antidepressants Selective serotonin reuptake inhibitors	Inhibit reuptake of 5-HT at the presynaptic nerve membrane	Fluoxetine (Prozac) Fluvoxamine (Luvox) Paroxetine (Paxil) Sertraline (Zoloft) Citalopram (Celexa)
Serotonin and noradrenaline reuptake inhibitors	Potent inhibitors of 5-HT and NEPI uptake	Venlafaxine (Effexor) Mirtazapine (Remeron)
NEPI reuptake inhibitors	Selectively inhibit NEPI reuptake	Viloxazine[3] Reboxetine[4]
Reversible inhibitors of monoamine oxidase A	Selective, reversible inhibitors of monoamine oxidase A, increases NEPI, 5-HT, and dopamine	Moclobemide[4] Brofaromine[4]
5-HT$_2$ receptor antagonists	Mixed serotonin effects	Nefazodone (Serzone) Ritanserin[4]
5-HT$_{1\alpha}$ receptor agonists	Partial agonist of serotonin 5-HT$_{1\alpha}$	Gepirone[4] ipaspirone,[4] tandospirone,[4] felsinoxan[4]
GABAmimetics	GABA$_A$ and GABA$_B$ receptor agonists	Fengamine[4]
Dopamine reuptake inhibitor	Increases activity of NEPI and dopamine only; no affect on serotonin	Buproprion (Wellbutrin, Zyban)
Herbal remedies	Unclear	Hypericum (also known as St. John's wort)

Selected older antidepressants
  Mixed serotonin and NEPI reuptake inhibitors
    First-generation tricyclic antidepressants
 	
    Second-generation tricyclic antidepressants
    Tetracyclic antidepressant
	Potentiate serotonin and NEPI activity; potency and selectivity differ by agent	
		
		Amitriptyline (Elavil, Endep)[5]
		Clomipramine (Anafranil)
		Doxepin (Adapin, Sinequan)[5]
		Imipramine (Tofranil)[5]
		Trimipramine (Surmontil)
		Desipramine (Norpramin)[5]
		Nortriptyline (Pamelor)[5]
		Maprotiline (Ludiomil)[5]

Triazolopyridine	Mixed serotonin effects	Trazodone (Desyrel)
Monoamine oxidase inhibitors	Nonselective inhibitor of monoamine oxidase A and B	Phenelzine (Nardil) Tranylcypromine (Parnate)

[1]Modified with permission from Williams JW et al: Ann Intern Med 2000;132:743.
[2]HT, hydroxytryptophan; NEPI, norepinephrine; GABA, γ-aminobutyric acid.
[3]Brand name drugs are produced by the following manufacturers: Adapin, Fisons Pharmaceuticals, Rochester, NY; Anafranil and Tofranil, Novartis, East Hanover, NJ; Celexa, Forest Pharmaceuticals, Inc., St. Louis, MO; Desyrel and Serzone, Bristol-Myers Squibb, Princeton, NJ; Effexor and Surmontil, Wyeth-Ayerst, Philadelphia, PA; Elavil, Zeneca Pharmaceuticals, Wilmington, DE; Endep, Hoffmann-LaRoche, Nutley, NJ; Luvox, Solvay Pharmaceuticals, Inc., Marietta, GA; Nardil, Parke-Davis, Morris Plains, NJ; Norpramine, Aventis Pharmaceuticals, Parsippany, NJ; Pamelor and Ludiomil, Novartis, East Hanover, NJ; Paxil and Parnate, SmithKline Beecham Pharmaceuticals, Philadelphia, PA; Prozac, Eli Lilly and Co., Indianapolis, IN; Remeron, Organon, Inc., West Orange, NJ; Wellbutrin and Zyban, Glaxo Wellcome, Research Triangle Park, NC; Zoloft and Sinequan, Pfizer, New York, NY.
[4]Not available in the United States.
[5]Generic form available.

(Table 27–3). All tricyclic antidepressants work at nerve synapses by blocking neuronal reuptake of catecholamines, serotonin, or both (see Table 18–8). Desipramine (Norpramin and Pertofrane) and nortriptyline (Pamelor and Aventyl) are commonly used because they are less sedating and tend to have fewer side effects. Other agents are generally more sedating and include amitriptyline (Elavil [withdrawn from the U.S. market]), imipramine (Tofranil and Janamine), protriptyline (Vivactil), amoxapine (Asendin), doxepin (Sinequan and Adapin), and trimipramine (Surmontil). Clomipramine (Anafranil) is used in the treatment of obsessive–compulsive disorders. Most tricyclic antidepressants also have significant anticholinergic (antimuscarinic) actions: dry mouth, blurred vision, prolonged gastric emptying, and urinary retention. Quinidine-like cardiac effects include tachycardia, T-wave flattening or inversion, and prolongation of the PR, QRS, and QT intervals. Amitriptyline has the most marked anticholinergic effects, whereas doxepin has the fewest cardiac effects.

St. John's wort is being used with increased frequency as an over-the-counter therapy for depression. Because it induces hepatic enzymes, blood levels of other drugs may decrease, sometimes with serious complications. During the preoperative evaluation, the use of all over-the-counter medications should be reviewed.

Anti-depressant drugs are generally continued perioperatively. Increased anesthetic requirements, presumably from enhanced brain catecholamine activity, have been reported with these agents. Potentiation of centrally acting anticholinergic agents (atropine and scopolamine) may increase the likelihood of postoperative confusion and delirium. The most important interaction between anesthetic agents and tricyclic antidepressants is an exaggerated response to both indirect-acting vasopressors and sympathetic stimulation. Pancuronium, ketamine, meperidine, and epinephrine-containing local anesthetic solutions should be avoided (particularly during halothane anesthesia). Chronic therapy with tricyclic antidepressants is reported to deplete cardiac catecholamines, theoretically potentiating the cardiac depressant effects of anesthetics. If hypotension occurs, small doses of a direct-acting vasopressor should be used instead of an indirect-acting agent. Amitriptyline's anticholinergic action may occasionally contribute to postoperative delirium.

Monoamine Oxidase Inhibitors

MAO inhibitors may be more effective for patients with depression accompanied by panic attacks and prominent anxiety. They block the oxidative deamination of naturally occurring amines. At least two MAO isoenzymes (types A and B) with differential substrate selectivities have been identified. MAO A is selective for serotonin, dopamine, and norepinephrine, whereas MAO B is selective for tyramine and phenylethylamine. Currently available agents that are effective in treating depression are nonselective MAO inhibitors. They include phenelzine (Nardil), isocarboxazid (Marplan), and tranylcypromine (Parnate). Selective MAO-B inhibitors (see above) are not effective in the treatment of depression. Nonselective agents also appear to interfere with many enzymes other than MAO. Side effects include orthostatic hypotension, agitation, tremor, seizures, muscle spasms, urinary retention, paresthesias, and jaundice. Their hypotensive effect may be related to the accumulation of false neurotransmitters (octopamine). The most serious sequela is a hypertensive crisis that occurs following ingestion of tyramine-containing foods (cheeses and red wines).

The practice of discontinuing MAO inhibitors at least 2 weeks prior to elective surgery is no longer recommended. With the exception of tranylcypromine, these agents produce irreversible enzyme inhibition; the 2-week delay allows sufficient regeneration of new enzyme. Studies suggest that patients may be safely anesthetized, at least for ECT, without this waiting period. Phenelzine can decrease plasma cholinesterase activity and prolong the duration of succinylcholine. Opioids should generally be used with caution in patients receiving MAO inhibitors, as rare but serious reactions to opioids have been reported. Most serious reactions are associated with meperidine, resulting in hyperthermia, seizures, and coma. As with tricyclic antidepressants, exaggerated responses to vasopressors and sympathetic stimulation should be expected. If a vasopressor is necessary, a direct-acting agent in small doses should be employed. Drugs that enhance sympathetic activity such as ketamine, pancuronium, and epinephrine (in local anesthetic solutions) should be avoided.

Atypical Antidepressants

Most atypical antidepressants are primarily selective serotonin reuptake inhibitors (SSRIs). These include fluoxetine (Prozac), which is available in a once-weekly preparation, sertraline (Zoloft), and paroxetine (Paxil), which some clinicians consider first-line agents of choice for depression. These agents have little or no anticholinergic activity and do not affect cardiac conduction. Their principal side effects are headache, agitation, and insomnia. Other atypical agents include bupropion (Welbutrin), venlafaxine (Effexor), also available in an extended-release formulation, trazodone (Desyrel), nefazodone (Serzone), fluvoxamine (Luvox), maprotiline (Ludiomil), and mirtazapine (Remeron), which is available in an oral-disintegrating tablet (Remeron SolTab). Maprotiline is not commonly used because of a relatively high incidence of seizures. Bupropion may primarily inhibit dopamine reuptake. Anesthetic interactions with atypical antidepressants are not well documented.

MANIA

Mania is a mood disorder characterized by elation, hyperactivity, and flight of ideas. Manic episodes may alternate with depression in patients with a bipolar disorder. Mania is thought to be related to excessive norepinephrine activity in the brain. Lithium (Eskalith, Lithobid) and lamotrigine (Lamictal) are the drugs of choice for treating acute manic episodes and preventing their recurrence, as well as suppressing episodes of depression. Concomitant administration of an antipsychotic (haloperidol) or a benzodiazepine (lorazepam) is usually necessary during acute mania. Alternative treatments include valproic acid, carbamazepine, and aripiprazole (Abilify), as well as ECT.

The mechanism of action of lithium is poorly understood. It has a narrow therapeutic range, with a desirable blood concentration between 0.8 and 1.0 mEq/L. Side effects include reversible T-wave changes, mild leukocytosis, and, on rare occasions, hypothyroidism or a vasopressin-resistant diabetes insipidus-like syndrome. Toxic blood concentrations produce confusion, sedation, muscle weakness, tremor, and slurred speech. Still higher concentrations result in widening of the QRS complex, atrioventricular block, hypotension, and seizures.

Although lithium is reported to decrease minimum alveolar concentration and prolong the duration of some NMBAs, clinically these effects appear to be minor. Nonetheless, neuromuscular function should be closely monitored when NMBAs are used. The greatest concern is the possibility of perioperative toxicity. Blood levels should be checked perioperatively. Sodium depletion decreases renal excretion of lithium and can lead to lithium toxicity. Fluid restriction and overdiuresis should be avoided.

SCHIZOPHRENIA

Patients with schizophrenia display disordered thinking, withdrawal, paranoid delusions, and auditory hallucinations. This disorder is thought to be related to an excess of dopaminergic activity in the brain. Antipsychotic drugs remain the only effective treatment for controlling this disease.

The most commonly used antipsychotics include phenothiazines, thioxanthenes, phenylbutylpiperadines, dihydroindolones, dibenzapines, benzisoxazoles, and a quinolone derivative. Commonly used agents include haloperidol (Haldol), chlorpromazine (Thorazine), risperidone (Risperdal), molindone (Moban), clozapine (Clozaril), fluphenazine (Prolixin), trifluoperazine (Stelazine), thiothixene (Navane), perphenazine (Trilafon), aripiprazole (Abilify), and thioridazine (Mellaril). All these agents have similar properties with minor variations. Clozapine may be effective in patients refractory to other drugs. The antipsychotic effect of these agents appears to be due to dopamine antagonist activity. Most are sedating and mildly anxiolytic. With the exception of thioridazine, all

are potent antiemetics (see Chapter 8). Mild α-adrenergic blockade and anticholinergic activity are also observed. Side effects include orthostatic hypotension, acute dystonic reactions, and parkinsonism-like manifestations. Risperidone and clozapine have little extrapyramidal activity, but the latter is associated with a significant incidence of granulocytopenia. T-wave flattening, ST segment depression, and prolongation of the PR and QT intervals may be seen, particularly in patients taking thioridazine.

Generally, patients whose disease is controlled by antipsychotics present few problems. Continuing antipsychotic medication perioperatively is desirable. Reduced anesthetic requirements may be observed in some patients. α-Adrenergic blockade is usually well compensated. Ketamine should probably be avoided, as antipsychotics decrease the seizure threshold.

NEUROLEPTIC MALIGNANT SYNDROME

Neuroleptic malignant syndrome is a rare complication of antipsychotic therapy that may occur hours or weeks after drug administration. Meperidine and metoclopramide can also precipitate the disorder. The mechanism is related to dopamine blockade in the basal ganglia and hypothalamus and impairment of thermoregulation. In its most severe form, the presentation is similar to that of malignant hyperthermia. Muscle rigidity, hyperthermia, rhabdomyolysis, autonomic instability, and altered consciousness are seen. Creatine kinase levels are often high. The mortality rate approaches 20–30%, with deaths occurring primarily as a result of renal failure or arrhythmias. Treatment with dantrolene appears to be effective; bromocriptine, a dopamine agonist, may also be effective. Although muscle biopsy is often normal, patients with a history of **neuroleptic malignant syndrome** should be treated in the same way as patients susceptible to malignant hyperthermia (see Chapter 44).

SUBSTANCE ABUSE

Behavioral disorders from abuse of psychotropic (mind-altering) substances may involve a socially acceptable drug (alcohol), a medically prescribed drug (eg, diazepam), or an illegal substance (eg, cocaine). Environmental, social, and perhaps genetic factors lead to this type of behavior. A "need" for the substance develops, ranging in intensity from a simple desire to a compulsion that consumes the patient's life. Characteristically, with chronic abuse, patients develop tolerance to the drug and varying degrees of psychological and physical dependence. Physical dependence is most often seen with opioids, barbiturates, alcohol, and benzodiazepines. Life-threatening complications primarily due to sympathetic overactivity can develop during abstention. Barbiturate withdrawal is potentially the most lethal and dangerous of the withdrawal syndromes.

Table 27–4. Effect of acute and chronic substance abuse on anesthetic requirements.[1]

Substance	Acute	Chronic
Opioids	↓	↑
Barbiturates	↓	↑
Alcohol	↓	↑
Marijuana	↓	0
Benzodiazepines	↓	↑
Amphetamines	↑[2]	↓
Cocaine	↑[2]	0
Phencyclidine	↓	?

[1]↓, decreases; ↑, increases; 0, no effect; ?, unknown.
[2]Associated with marked sympathetic stimulation.

Knowledge of a patient's substance abuse preoperatively may prevent adverse drug interactions, predict tolerance to anesthetic agents, and facilitate the recognition of drug withdrawal. The history of substance abuse may be volunteered by the patient (usually only on direct questioning) or deliberately hidden. A high index of suspicion is often required. Sociopathic tendencies are difficult to detect during a short interview. The presence of numerous punctate scars with difficult venous access strongly suggests intravenous drug abuse. Such injecting drug users have a relatively high incidence of skin infections, thrombophlebitis, malnutrition, endocarditis, hepatitis B and C, and HIV infection.

Anesthetic requirements for substance abusers vary depending on whether the drug exposure is acute or chronic (see Table 27–4). Elective procedures should be postponed for acutely intoxicated patients and those with signs of withdrawal. When surgery is deemed necessary in patients with physical dependence, perioperative doses of the abused substance should be provided or specific agents should be given to prevent withdrawal. In the case of opioid dependence, any opioid can be used, whereas for alcohol, a benzodiazepine is usually substituted. Tolerance to most anesthetic agents is often seen but is not always predictable. Regional anesthetics should be considered whenever possible. For general anesthesia, a technique primarily relying on a volatile inhalation agent may be preferable so that anesthetic depth can be readily adjusted according to individual need. Opioids with mixed agonist–antagonist activity should be avoided in opioid-dependent patients because such agents can precipitate acute withdrawal. Clonidine is a useful adjuvant in the treatment of postoperative withdrawal syndromes.

CASE DISCUSSION:
ANESTHESIA FOR
ELECTROCONVULSIVE THERAPY

A 64-year-old man with depression refractory to drug therapy is scheduled for electroconvulsive therapy (ECT).

How is ECT administered?

The electroconvulsive shock is applied to one or both cerebral hemispheres to induce a seizure. Variables include stimulus pattern, amplitude, and duration. The goal is to produce a therapeutic generalized seizure 30–60 s in duration. Electrical stimuli are usually administered until a therapeutic seizure is induced. A good therapeutic effect is generally not achieved until a total of 400–700 seizure seconds have been induced. Because only one treatment is given per day, patients are usually scheduled for a series of treatments, generally two or three a week. Progressive memory loss often occurs with an increasing number of treatments, particularly when electrodes are applied bilaterally.

Why is anesthesia necessary?

When the efficacy of ECT was discovered, enthusiasm was tempered in the medical community because drugs were not used to control the violent seizures caused by the procedure, thus engendering a relatively high incidence of musculoskeletal injuries. Moreover, when an NMBA was used alone, patients sometimes recalled being paralyzed and awake just prior to the shock. The routine use of general anesthesia to ensure amnesia and neuromuscular blockade to prevent injuries has renewed interest in ECT. The current mortality rate for ECT is estimated to be one death per 10,000 treatments. Although some psychiatrists administer the anesthetic, the presence of an anesthesiologist is optimal for airway management and cardiovascular monitoring.

What are the physiological effects of ECT-induced seizures?

Seizure activity is characteristically associated with an initial parasympathetic discharge followed by a more sustained sympathetic discharge. The initial phase is characterized by bradycardia and increased secretions. Marked bradycardia (< 30 beats/min) and even transient asystole (up to 6 s) are occasionally seen. The hypertension and tachycardia that follow are typically sustained for several min-

utes. Transient autonomic imbalance can produce arrhythmias and T-wave abnormalities on the electrocardiogram. Cerebral blood flow and ICP, intragastric pressure, and intraocular pressure all transiently increase.

Are there any contraindications to ECT?

Contraindications are a recent myocardial infarction (usually < 3 months), a recent stroke (usually < 1 month), an intracranial mass, or increased ICP from any cause. More relative contraindications include angina, poorly controlled heart failure, significant pulmonary disease, bone fractures, severe osteoporosis, pregnancy, glaucoma, and retinal detachment.

What are the important considerations in selecting anesthetic agents?

Amnesia is required only for the brief period (1–5 min) from when the NMBA is given to when a therapeutic seizure has been successfully induced. The seizure itself usually results in a brief period of anterograde amnesia, somnolence, and often confusion. Consequently, only a short-acting induction agent is necessary. Moreover, because most induction agents (barbiturates, etomidate, benzodiazepines, and propofol) have anticonvulsant properties, small doses must be used. Seizure threshold is increased and **seizure duration** is decreased by all these agents.

Following adequate preoxygenation, methohexital, 0.5–1 mg/kg, is most commonly employed. Propofol, 1–1.5 mg/kg, may be used but higher doses reduce seizure duration. Benzodiazepines raise the seizure threshold and decrease duration. Ketamine increases seizure duration but is generally not used because it also increases the incidence of delayed awakening, nausea, and ataxia and is also associated with hallucinations during emergence. Use of etomidate also prolongs recovery. Short-acting opioids such as alfentanil are not given alone because they do not consistently produce amnesia. However, alfentanil (10–25 mg/kg) can be a useful adjunct when very small doses of methohexital (10–20 mg) are required in patients with a high seizure threshold. In very small doses, methohexital may actually enhance seizure activity. Increases in seizure threshold are often observed with each subsequent ECT.

Neuromuscular blockade is required from the time of electrical stimulation until the end of the seizure. A short-acting agent such as succinylcholine (0.25–0.5 mg/kg) is most often selected. Controlled mask ventilation using a self-inflating bag device or an anesthesia circle system is required until spontaneous respirations resume.

Can seizure duration be increased without increasing the electrical stimulus?

Hyperventilation can increase seizure duration and is routinely employed in some centers. Intravenous caffeine, 125–250 mg (given slowly), has also been reported to increase seizure duration.

What monitors should be used during ECT?

Monitoring should be similar to what is appropriate with the use of any other general anesthetic. Seizure activity is sometimes monitored by an unprocessed electroencephalogram. It can also be monitored in an isolated limb: a tourniquet is inflated around one arm prior to injection of succinylcholine, preventing entry of the NMBA and allowing observation of convulsive motor activity in that arm.

How can the adverse hemodynamic effects of the seizure be controlled in patients with limited cardiovascular reserve?

Exaggerated parasympathetic effects should be treated with atropine. In fact, premedication with glycopyrrolate is desirable both to prevent the profuse secretions associated with seizures and to attenuate bradycardia. Nitroglycerin, nifedipine, and α- and β-adrenergic blockers have all been employed successfully to control sympathetic manifestations. High doses of β-adrenergic blockers (esmolol, 200 mg), however, are reported to decrease seizure duration.

What if the patient has a pacemaker?

Patients with pacemakers may safely undergo electroconvulsive treatments, but a magnet should be readily available to convert the pacemaker to a fixed mode if necessary.

SUGGESTED READING

Atlee JL: *Complications in Anesthesia*. W.B. Saunders, 1999.

Cucchiara RF, Black S, Michenfelder JD: *Clinical Neuroanesthesia*, 2nd ed. Churchill Livingstone, 1998.

Grunze H, Kasper S, Goodwin G, et al: The World Federation of Societies of Biological Psychiatry (WFSBP). Guidelines for the biological treatment of bipolar disorders, Part II: Treatment of mania. World J Biol Psychiatr 2003;4:5. Recently published guidelines for managing patients with mania.

MRC Asyptomatic Carotid Surgery Trial (ACST) Collaborative Group: Prevention of disabling and fatal strokes by successful carotid endarterectomy in patients without recent neurological symptoms: randomised controlled trial. Lancet 2004; 363:1491. Recent prospective, randomized controlled trial that has defined criteria for carotid endarterectomy.

Newfield P, Cottrell JE: *Handbook of Neuroanesthesia,* 3rd ed. Lippincott, Williams & Wilkins, 1999.

Nussbaum RL, Ellis CE: Alzheimer's disease and Parkinson's disease. N Engl J Med 2003;348:1356. Excellent recent review of the most current thinking on these two most common diseases.

Richards KJC, Cohen AT: Guillain–Barré syndrome. Br J Anaesth 2003;3:46. Recent summary of Guillain–Barré syndrome that appeared in British literature.

Sarang A, Dinsmore J: Anaesthesia for awake craniotomy—evolution of a technique that facilitates awake neurological testing. Br J Anaesth 2003;90:161. Excellent discussion of how to manage patients who need to be awake for craniotomy.

Management of Patients with Fluid & Electrolyte Disturbances

28

KEY CONCEPTS

 Osmotic pressure is generally dependent only on the number of nondiffusible solute particles. This is because the average kinetic energy of particles in solution is similar regardless of their mass.

 Potassium is the most important determinant of intracellular osmotic pressure, whereas sodium is the most important determinant of extracellular osmotic pressure.

 Fluid exchange between the intracellular and interstitial spaces is governed by the osmotic forces created by differences in nondiffusible solute concentrations.

 Serious manifestations of hyponatremia are generally associated with plasma sodium concentrations < 120 mEq/L.

 Very rapid correction of hyponatremia has been associated with demyelinating lesions in the pons (central pontine myelinolysis), resulting in serious permanent neurological sequelae.

 The major hazard of increases in extracellular volume is impaired gas exchange due to pulmonary interstitial edema, alveolar edema, or large collections of pleural or ascitic fluid.

 Intravenous replacement of potassium chloride should usually be reserved for patients with or at risk for serious cardiac manifestations or muscle weakness.

 Because of its lethal potential, hyperkalemia exceeding 6 mEq/L should always be treated.

 Symptomatic hypercalcemia requires rapid treatment. The most effective initial treatment is rehydration followed by a brisk diuresis (urinary output 200–300 mL/h) with administration of intravenous saline infusion and a loop diuretic to accelerate calcium excretion.

 Symptomatic hypocalcemia is a medical emergency and should be treated immediately with intravenous calcium chloride (3–5 mL of a 10% solution) or calcium gluconate (10–20 mL of a 10% solution).

 Some patients with severe hypophosphatemia may require mechanical ventilation postoperatively.

 Marked hypermagnesemia can lead to respiratory arrest.

 Isolated hypomagnesemia should be corrected prior to elective procedures because of its potential for causing cardiac arrhythmias.

Fluid and electrolyte disturbances are extremely common in the perioperative period. Large amounts of intravenous fluids are frequently required to correct fluid deficits and compensate for blood loss during surgery. Anesthesiologists must therefore have a clear understanding of normal water and electrolyte physiology. Major disturbances in fluid and electrolyte balance can rapidly alter cardiovascular, neurological, and neuromuscular functions. This chapter examines the body's fluid compartments and common water and electrolyte derangements, their treatment, and anesthetic implications. Acid–base disorders and intravenous fluid therapy are discussed in subsequent chapters.

NOMENCLATURE OF SOLUTIONS

The system of international units (SI) has still not gained universal acceptance in clinical practice, and many older expressions of concentration remain in common use. Thus, for example, the quantity of a solute in a solution may be expressed in grams, moles, or equivalents. To complicate matters further, the concentration of a solution may be expressed either as quantity of solute per volume of solution or quantity of solute per weight of solvent.

MOLARITY, MOLALITY, & EQUIVALENCY

One mole of a substance represents 6.02×10^{23} molecules. The weight of this quantity in grams is commonly referred to as gram-molecular weight. Molarity is the standard SI unit of concentration that expresses the number of moles of solute per *liter* of solution. Molality is an alternative term that expresses moles of solute per *kilogram* of solvent. Equivalency is also commonly used for substances that ionize: the number of equivalents of an ion in solution is the number of moles multiplied by its charge (valence). Thus, a 1 M solution of $MgCl_2$ yields 2 equivalents of magnesium per liter and 2 equivalents of chloride per liter.

OSMOLARITY, OSMOLALITY, & TONICITY

Osmosis is the net movement of water across a semipermeable membrane as a result of a difference in nondiffusible solute concentrations between the two sides. Osmotic pressure is the pressure that must be applied to the side with more solute to prevent a net movement of water across the membrane to dilute the solute.

Osmotic pressure is generally dependent only on the number of nondiffusible solute particles. This is because the average kinetic energy of particles in solution is similar regardless of their mass. One osmole equals 1 mol of nondissociable substances. For substances that ionize, however, each mole results in n Osm, where n is the number of ionic species produced. Thus, 1 mol of a highly ionized substance such as NaCl dissolved in solution should produce 2

Osm; in reality ionic interaction between the cation and anion reduces the effective activity of each such that NaCl behaves as if it is only 75% ionized. A difference of 1 mOsm/L between two solutions results in an osmotic pressure of 19.3 mm Hg. The osmolarity of a solution is equal to the number of osmoles per *liter* of solution, whereas its osmolality equals the number of osmoles per *kilogram* of solvent. Tonicity is a term that is often used interchangeably with osmolarity and osmolality. More correctly, tonicity refers to the effect a solution has on cell volume. An isotonic solution has no effect on cell volume, whereas hypotonic and hypertonic solutions increase and decrease cell volume, respectively.

FLUID COMPARTMENTS

The average adult male is approximately 60% water by weight; females are 50%. This water is distributed between two major fluid compartments separated by cell membranes: intracellular fluid (ICF) and extracellular fluid (ECF). The latter can be further subdivided into intravascular and interstitial compartments. The interstitium includes all fluid that is both outside cells and outside the vascular endothelium. The relative contributions of each compartment to total body water (TBW) and body weight are set forth in Table 28–1.

The volume of fluid (water) within a compartment is determined by its solute composition and concentrations (Table 28–2). Differences in solute concentrations are largely due to the characteristics of the physical barriers that separate compartments (see below). The osmotic forces created by "trapped" solutes govern the distribution of water between compartments and ultimately each compartment's volume.

INTRACELLULAR FLUID

The outer membrane of cells plays an important role in regulating intracellular volume and composition. A membrane-bound adenosine-triphosphate (ATP)-dependent pump exchanges Na^+ for K^+ in a 3:2 ratio. Because cell membranes are relatively impermeable to sodium and to a lesser extent potassium ions, potassium is concentrated intracellularly, whereas sodium is concentrated extracellularly. As a result, potassium is the most important determinant of intracellular osmotic pressure, whereas sodium is the most important determinant of extracellular osmotic pressure.

The impermeability of cell membranes to most proteins results in a high intracellular protein concentra-

TBW

IC (2/3)   EC (1/3)

Intra
Cellular   Inter
stitial
25%   75%

Table 28–1. Body fluid compartments (based on average 70-kg male).

Compartment	Fluid as Percent Body Weight (%)	Total Body Water (%)	Fluid Volume (L)
Intracellular	40	67	28
Extracellular			
Interstitial	15	25	10.5
Intravascular	5	8	3.5
Total	60	100	42

tion. Because proteins act as nondiffusible solutes (anions), the unequal exchange ratio of 3 Na^+ for 2 K^+ by the cell membrane pump is critical in preventing relative intracellular hyperosmolality. Interference with Na^+–K^+ ATPase activity, as occurs during ischemia or hypoxia, results in progressive swelling of cells.

EXTRACELLULAR FLUID

The principal function of extracellular fluid is to provide a medium for cell nutrients and electrolytes and for cellular waste products. Maintenance of a normal extracellular volume—particularly the circulating component (intravascular volume)—is critical. For the reasons described above, sodium is quantitatively the most important extracellular cation and the major determinant of extracellular osmotic pressure and volume. Changes in extracellular fluid volume are therefore related to changes in total body sodium content. The latter is a function of sodium intake, renal sodium excretion, and extrarenal sodium losses (see below).

Interstitial Fluid

Very little interstitial fluid is normally in the form of free fluid. Most interstitial water is in chemical association with extracellular proteoglycans, forming a gel. Interstitial fluid pressure is generally thought to be negative (about –5 mm Hg). As interstitial fluid volume increases, interstitial pressure also rises and eventually becomes positive. When the latter occurs, the free fluid in the gel increases rapidly and appears clinically as edema.

Because only small quantities of plasma proteins can normally cross capillary clefts, the protein content of interstitial fluid is relatively low (2 g/dL). Protein enter-

Table 28–2. The composition of fluid compartments.

	Gram-Molecular Weight	Intracellular (mEq/L)	Extracellular	
			Intravascular (mEq/L)	Interstitial (mEq/L)
Sodium	23.0	10	145	142
Potassium	39.1	140	4	4
Calcium	40.1	< 1	3	3
Magnesium	24.3	50	2	2
Chloride	35.5	4	105	110
Bicarbonate	61.0	10	24	28
Phosphorus	31.0[1]	75	2	2
Protein (g/dL)		16	7	2

[1] PO_4^{3-} is 95 g.

Figure 28–1. The relationship between blood volume and extracellular fluid volume. (Modified and reproduced, with permission, from Guyton AC: *Textbook of Medical Physiology,* 7th ed. W.B. Saunders, 1986.)

ing the interstitial space is returned to the vascular system via the lymphatic system.

Intravascular Fluid

Intravascular fluid, commonly referred to as plasma, is restricted to the intravascular space by the vascular endothelium. Most electrolytes (small ions) freely pass between plasma and the interstitium, resulting in nearly identical electrolyte composition. However, the tight intercellular junctions between adjacent endothelial cells impede the passage of plasma proteins outside the intravascular compartment. As a result, plasma proteins (mainly albumin) are the only osmotically active solutes in fluid not normally exchanged between plasma and interstitial fluid.

Increases in extracellular volume are normally proportionately reflected in intravascular and interstitial volume. When interstitial pressure becomes positive, continued increases in ECF result in expansion of only the interstitial fluid compartment (Figure 28–1). In this way, the interstitial compartment acts as an overflow reservoir for the intravascular compartment. This can be seen clinically in the form of tissue edema.

EXCHANGE BETWEEN FLUID COMPARTMENTS

Diffusion is the random movement of molecules due to their kinetic energy and is responsible for the majority of fluid and solute exchange between compartments. The rate of diffusion of a substance across a membrane depends on (1) the permeability of that substance through that membrane, (2) the concentration difference for that substance between the two sides, (3) the pressure difference between either side because pressure imparts greater kinetic energy, and (4) the electrical potential across the membrane for charged substances.

Diffusion Through Cell Membranes

Diffusion between interstitial fluid and intracellular fluid may take place by one of several mechanisms: (1) directly through the lipid bilayer of the cell membrane, (2) through protein channels within the membrane, or (3) by reversible binding to a carrier protein that can traverse the membrane (facilitated diffusion). Oxygen, CO_2, water, and lipid-soluble molecules penetrate the cell membrane directly. Cations such as Na^+, K^+, and Ca^{2+} penetrate the membrane poorly because of the cell transmembrane voltage potential (which is positive to the outside) created by the Na^+–K^+ pump. Therefore, these cations can diffuse only through specific protein channels. Passage through these channels is dependent on membrane voltage and the binding of ligands (such as acetylcholine) to the membrane receptors. Glucose and amino acids diffuse with the help of membrane-bound carrier proteins.

Fluid exchange between the intracellular and interstitial spaces is governed by the osmotic forces created by differences in nondiffusible solute concentrations. Relative changes in osmolality between the intracellular and interstitial compartments result in a net water movement from the hypoosmolar to the hyperosmolar compartment.

Diffusion Through Capillary Endothelium

Capillary walls are typically 0.5 μm thick, consisting of a single layer of endothelial cells with their basement membrane. Intercellular clefts, 6–7 nm wide, separate each cell from its neighbors. Oxygen, CO_2, water, and lipid-soluble substances can penetrate directly through both sides of the endothelial cell membrane. Only low-molecular-weight water-soluble substances such as sodium, chloride, potassium, and glucose readily cross intercellular clefts. High-molecular-weight substances such as plasma proteins penetrate the endothelial clefts poorly (except in the liver and the lungs, where the clefts are larger).

Fluid exchange across capillaries differs from that across cell membranes in that it is governed by significant differences in hydrostatic pressures in addition to osmotic forces (Figure 28–2). These forces are operative on both arterial and venous ends of capillaries. As a result, there is a tendency for fluid to move out of capillaries at the arterial end and back into capillaries at the venous end. Moreover, the magnitude of these forces differs between the various tissue beds. Arterial capillary pressure is determined by precapillary sphincter tone. Thus capillaries that require a high pressure such as glomeruli have low precapillary sphincter tone, whereas the normally low-pressure capillaries of muscle have high precapillary sphincter tone. Normally, all but 10% of

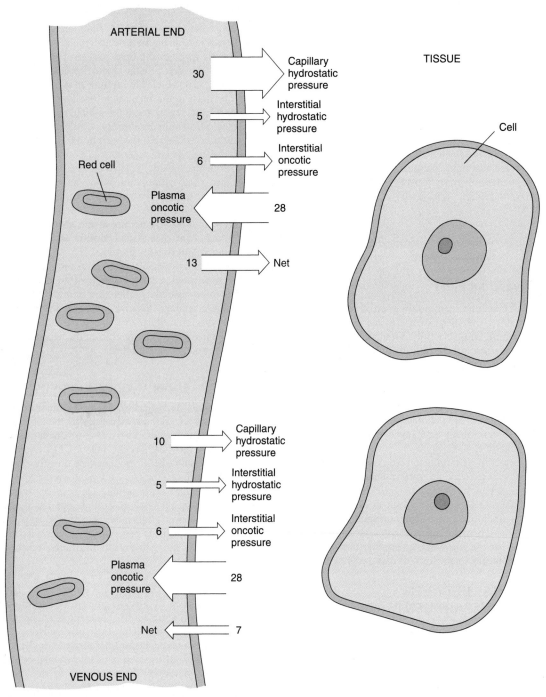

Figure 28–2. Capillary fluid exchange. The numbers in this figure are in mm Hg and indicate the pressure gradient for the respective pressures. "Net" refers to the net pressure at either end of the capillary, ie, 13 mm Hg at the arterial and 7 mm Hg at the venous end of the capillary.

the fluid filtered is reabsorbed back into capillaries. What is not reabsorbed (about 2 mL/min) enters the interstitial fluid and is then returned by lymphatic flow to the intravascular compartment.

■ DISORDERS OF WATER BALANCE

The human body at birth is approximately 75% water by weight. By 1 month this value decreases to 65%, and by adulthood to 60% for males and 50% for females. The higher fat content in females decreases water content. For the same reason, obesity and advanced age further decrease water content.

NORMAL WATER BALANCE

The normal adult daily water intake averages 2500 mL, which includes approximately 300 mL as a by-product of the metabolism of energy substrates. Daily water loss necessarily averages 2500 mL and can roughly be accounted for by 1500 mL in urine, 400 mL in respiratory tract evaporation, 400 mL in skin evaporation, 100 mL in sweat, and 100 mL in feces. The evaporative losses are very important in thermoregulation because they normally account for 20–25% of heat loss.

Both ICF and ECF osmolalities are closely regulated in such a way as to maintain a normal water content in tissues. Changes in water content and cell volume can induce serious impairment of function, particularly in the brain (see below).

RELATIONSHIP OF PLASMA SODIUM CONCENTRATION, EXTRACELLULAR OSMOLALITY, & INTRACELLULAR OSMOLALITY

The osmolality of ECF is equal to the sum of the concentrations of all dissolved solutes. Because Na^+ and its anions account for nearly 90% of these solutes, the following approximation is valid:

$$Plasma\ osmality = 2 \times Plasma\ sodium\ concentration$$

Moreover, because ICF and ECF are in osmotic equilibrium, plasma sodium concentration $[Na^+]_{plasma}$ generally reflects total body osmolality:

$$Total\ body\ osmolality = \frac{Extracellular\ solutes + intracellular\ solutes}{TBW}$$

Because sodium and potassium are the major intra- and extracellular solutes, respectively:

$$Total\ body\ osmolality = \frac{(Na^+_{extracellular} \times 2) + (K^+_{intracellular\ solutes} \times 2)}{TBW}$$

Combining the two approximations:

$$[Na^+]_{plasma} \approx \frac{Na^+_{extracellular} + K^+_{intracellular}}{TBW}$$

Using these principles, the effect of isotonic, hypotonic, and hypertonic fluid loads on compartmental water content and plasma osmolality can be calculated (Table 28–3). The potential importance of intracellular potassium concentration is readily apparent from this equation. Thus significant potassium losses may contribute to hyponatremia.

In pathological states, glucose and—to a much lesser extent—urea can contribute significantly to extracellular osmolality. A more accurate approximation of plasma osmolality is therefore given by the following equation:

$$Plasma\ osmolality\ (mOsm/kg) = [Na^+] \times 2 + \frac{BUN}{2.8} + \frac{glucose}{18}$$

where $[Na^+]$ is expressed as mEq/L and blood urea nitrogen (BUN) and glucose as mg/dL. Urea is an ineffective osmole because it readily permeates cell membranes and is therefore frequently omitted from this calculation:

$$Effective\ plasma\ osmolality = [Na^+] \times 2 + \frac{glucose}{18}$$

Plasma osmolality normally varies between 280 and 290 mOsm/L. Plasma sodium concentration decreases approximately 1 mEq/L for every 62 mg/dL increase in glucose concentration. A discrepancy between the measured and calculated osmolality is referred to as an osmolal gap. Significant osmolal gaps indicate a high concentration of an abnormal osmotically active molecule in plasma such as ethanol, mannitol, methanol, ethylene glycol, or isopropyl alcohol. Osmolal gaps may also be seen in patients with chronic renal failure (attributed to retention of small solutes), patients with ketoacidosis (as a result of a high concentration of ketone bodies), and those receiving large amounts of glycine (as during transurethral resection of the prostate). Lastly, osmolal gaps may also be present in patients with marked hyperlipidemia or hyperproteinemia. In such instances, the protein or lipid part of plasma contributes significantly to plasma volume; although plasma $[Na^+]$ is decreased, $[Na^+]$ in the water

Table 28–3. Effect of different fluid loads on extracellular and intracellular water contents.[1]

A. Normal

Total body solute	= 280 mOsm/kg × 42 kg = 11,760 mOsm
Intracellular solute	= 280 mOsm/kg × 25 kg = 7000 mOsm
Extracellular solute	= 280 mOsm/kg × 17 kg = 4760 mOsm

Extracellular sodium concentration = 280 ÷ 2 = 140 mEq/L

	Intracellular	Extracellular
Osmolality	280	280
Volume (L)	25	17
Net water gain	0	0

B. Isotonic load: 2 L of Isotonic saline (NaCl)

Total body solute	= 280 mOsm/kg × 44 kg = 12,320 mOsm
Intracellular solute	= 280 mOsm/kg × 25 kg = 7000 mOsm
Extracellular solute	= 280 mOsm/kg × 19 kg = 5320 mOsm

	Intracellular	Extracellular
Osmolality	280	280
Volume (L)	25	19
Net water gain	0	2

Net effect: Fluid remains in extracellular compartment.

C. Free water (hypotonic) load: 2 L water

New body water	= 42 + 2 = 44 kg
New body osmolality	= 11,760 mOsm ÷ 44 kg = 267 mOsm/kg
New intracellular volume	= 7000 mOsm ÷ 267 mOsm/kg = 26.2 kg

New extracellular sodium concentration = 267 ÷ 2 = 133 mEq/L

	Intracellular	Extracellular
Osmolality	267.0	267.0
Volume (L)	26.2	17.8
Net water gain	+1.2	+0.8

Net effect: Fluid distributes between both compartments.

D. Hypertonic load: 600 mEq NaCl (no water)

Total body solute	= 11,760 + 600 = 12,360 mOsm/kg
New body osmolality	= 12,360 mOsm/kg ÷ 42 kg = 294 mOsm
New extracellular solute	= 600 + 4760 = 5360 mOsm
New extracellular volume	= 5360 mOsm ÷ 294 mOsm/kg = 18.2 kg
New intracellular volume	= 42 − 18.2 = 23.8 kg

New extracellular sodium concentration = 294 ÷ 2 = 147 mEq/L

	Intracellular	Extracellular
Osmolality	294.0	294.0
Volume (L)	23.8	18.2
Net water gain	−1.2	+1.2

Net effect: An intracellular to extracellular movement of water.

---

[1]Based on a 70-kg adult male.

phase of plasma (true plasma osmolality) remains normal. The water phase of plasma is normally only 93% of its volume; the remaining 7% consists of plasma lipids and proteins.

CONTROL OF PLASMA OSMOLALITY

Plasma osmolality is closely regulated by osmoreceptors in the hypothalamus. These specialized neurons control the secretion of antidiuretic hormone (ADH) and the thirst mechanism. Plasma osmolality is therefore maintained within relatively narrow limits by varying both water intake and water excretion.

Secretion of Antidiuretic Hormone

Specialized neurons in the supraoptic and paraventricular nuclei of the hypothalamus are very sensitive to changes in extracellular osmolality. When ECF osmolality increases, these cells shrink and release ADH (arginine vasopressin) from the posterior pituitary. ADH markedly increases water reabsorption in renal-collecting tubules (see Chapter 31), which tends to reduce plasma osmolality to normal again. Conversely, a decrease in extracellular osmolality causes osmoreceptors to swell and suppresses the release of ADH. Decreased ADH secretion allows a water diuresis, which tends to increase osmolality to normal. Peak diuresis occurs once circulating ADH is metabolized (90–120 min). With complete suppression of ADH secretion, the kidneys can excrete up to 10–20 L of water per day (see below).

Nonosmotic Release of Antidiuretic Hormone

The carotid baroreceptors and possibly atrial stretch receptors can also stimulate ADH release following a 5–10% decrease in blood volume (see below). Other nonosmotic stimuli include pain, emotional stress, and hypoxia.

Thirst

Osmoreceptors in the lateral preoptic area of the hypothalamus are also very sensitive to changes in extracellular osmolality. Activation of these neurons by increases in ECF osmolality induces thirst and causes the individual to drink water. Conversely, hypoosmolality suppresses thirst.

Thirst is the major defense mechanism against hyperosmolality and hypernatremia, because it is the only mechanism that increases water intake. Unfortunately, the thirst mechanism is only operative in conscious individuals who are capable of drinking.

HYPEROSMOLALITY & HYPERNATREMIA

Hyperosmolality occurs whenever total body solute content increases relative to TBW and is usually but not always associated with hypernatremia ($[Na^+] > 145$ mEq/L). Hyperosmolality without hypernatremia may be seen during marked hyperglycemia or following the accumulation of abnormal osmotically active substances in plasma (see above). In the latter two instances, plasma sodium concentration may actually decrease as water is drawn from the intracellular to the extracellular compartment. For every 100 mg/dL increase in plasma glucose concentration, plasma sodium decreases approximately 1.6 mEq/L.

Hypernatremia is nearly always the result of either a loss of water in excess of sodium (hypotonic fluid loss) or the retention of large quantities of sodium. Even when renal concentrating ability is impaired, thirst is normally highly effective in preventing hypernatremia. Hypernatremia is therefore most commonly seen in debilitated patients who are unable to drink, the very aged, the very young, and patients with altered consciousness. Patients with hypernatremia may have a low, normal, or high total body sodium content (Table 28–4).

Hypernatremia & Low Total Body Sodium Content

These patients have lost both sodium and water, but the water loss is in excess of the sodium loss. Hypotonic losses can be renal (osmotic diuresis) or extrarenal (diarrhea or sweat). In either case, patients usually manifest signs of hypovolemia (see Chapter 29). Urinary sodium concentration is generally greater than 20 mEq/L with renal losses and less than 10 mEq/L with extrarenal losses.

Table 28–4. Major causes of hypernatremia.

Impaired thirst
Coma
Essential hypernatremia
Solute diuresis
Osmotic diuresis: diabetic ketoacidosis, nonketotic hyperosmolar coma, mannitol administration
Excessive water losses
Renal
Neurogenic diabetes insipidus
Nephrogenic diabetes insipidus
Extrarenal
Sweating
Combined disorders
Coma plus hypertonic nasogastric feeding

Hypernatremia & Normal Total Body Sodium Content

This group of patients generally manifests signs of water loss without overt hypovolemia unless the water loss is massive. Total body sodium content is generally normal. Nearly pure water losses can occur via the skin, respiratory tract, or kidneys. Occasionally transient hypernatremia is observed with movement of water into cells following exercise, seizures, or rhabdomyolysis. The most common cause of hypernatremia with a normal total body sodium content is **diabetes insipidus** (in conscious individuals). Diabetes insipidus is characterized by marked impairment in renal concentrating ability that is due either to decreased ADH secretion (central diabetes insipidus) or failure of the renal tubules to respond normally to circulating ADH (nephrogenic diabetes insipidus). Rarely, "essential hypernatremia" may be encountered in patients with central nervous system disorders. These patients appear to have reset osmoreceptors that function at a higher baseline osmolality.

A. CENTRAL DIABETES INSIPIDUS

Lesions in or around the hypothalamus and the pituitary stalk frequently produce diabetes insipidus. Diabetes insipidus frequently develops with brain death. Transient diabetes insipidus is also commonly seen following neurosurgical procedures and head trauma. The diagnosis is suggested by a history of polydipsia, polyuria (often > 6 L/d), and the absence of hyperglycemia. In the perioperative setting, the diagnosis of diabetes insipidus is suggested by marked polyuria without glycosuria and a urinary osmolality lower than plasma osmolality. The absence of thirst in unconscious individuals leads to marked water losses and can rapidly produce hypovolemia. The diagnosis of central diabetes insipidus is confirmed by an increase in urinary osmolality following the administration of exogenous ADH. Aqueous vasopressin (5 U subcutaneously every 4 h) is the treatment of choice for acute central diabetes insipidus. Vasopressin in oil (0.3 mL intramuscularly every day) is longer lasting but is more likely to cause water intoxication. Desmopressin (DDAVP), a synthetic analogue of ADH with a 12- to 24-h duration of action, is available as an intranasal preparation (5–10 mg every day or twice daily) that can be used both in the ambulatory and perioperative settings.

B. NEPHROGENIC DIABETES INSIPIDUS

Nephrogenic diabetes insipidus can be congenital but is more commonly secondary to other disorders. These include chronic renal disease, certain electrolyte disorders (hypokalemia and hypercalcemia), and a variety of other disorders (sickle cell disease, hyperproteinemias).

Nephrogenic diabetes insipidus can also be secondary to the side effects of some drugs (amphotericin B, lithium, demeclocycline, ifosfamide, mannitol). ADH secretion in all the above patients is normal, but the kidneys fail to respond to ADH. Urinary concentrating ability is therefore impaired. The mechanism may be either a decreased response to circulating ADH or interference with the renal countercurrent mechanism. The diagnosis is confirmed by failure of the kidneys to produce a hypertonic urine following the administration of exogenous ADH. Treatment is generally directed at the underlying illness and ensuring an adequate fluid intake. Volume depletion by a thiazide diuretic can paradoxically decrease urinary output by reducing water delivery to collecting tubules. Sodium and protein restriction can similarly reduce urinary output.

Hypernatremia & Increased Total Body Sodium Content

This condition most commonly results from the administration of large quantities of hypertonic saline solutions (3% NaCl or 7.5% $NaHCO_3$). Patients with primary hyperaldosteronism and Cushing's syndrome may also have small elevations in serum sodium concentration along with signs of increased sodium retention.

Clinical Manifestations of Hypernatremia

Neurological manifestations predominate in patients with hypernatremia and are generally thought to result from cellular dehydration. Restlessness, lethargy, and hyperreflexia can progress to seizures, coma, and ultimately death. Symptoms correlate more closely with the rate of movement of water out of brain cells than with the absolute level of hypernatremia. Rapid decreases in brain volume can rupture cerebral veins and result in focal intracerebral or subarachnoid hemorrhage. Seizures and serious neurological damage are common, particularly in children with acute hypernatremia when plasma [Na^+] exceeds 158 mEq/L. Chronic hypernatremia is generally better tolerated than the acute form. After 24–48 h, intracellular osmolality begins to rise as a result of increases in intracellular inositol and amino acid (glutamine and taurine) concentrations. As intracellular solute concentration increases, neuronal water content slowly returns to normal.

Treatment of Hypernatremia

The treatment of hypernatremia is aimed at restoring plasma osmolality to normal as well as correcting the underlying problem. Water deficits should generally be corrected over 48 h with a hypotonic solution such as 5% dextrose in water (see below). Abnormalities in extracellular volume must also be corrected (Figure 28–3).

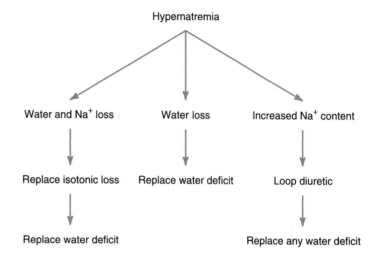

Figure 28–3. Algorithm for treatment of hypernatremia.

Hypernatremic patients with decreased total body sodium should be given isotonic fluids to restore plasma volume to normal *prior* to treatment with a hypotonic solution. Hypernatremic patients with increased total body sodium should be treated with a loop diuretic along with intravenous 5% dextrose in water. The treatment of diabetes insipidus is discussed above.

Rapid correction of hypernatremia can result in seizures, brain edema, permanent neurological damage, and even death. Serial Na^+ osmolalities should be obtained during treatment. In general, plasma sodium concentration should not be decreased faster than 0.5 mEq/L/h.

EXAMPLE

A 70-kg man is found to have a plasma $[Na^+]$ of 160 mEq/L. What is his water deficit?

If one assumes that the hypernatremia is from water loss only, then total body osmoles are unchanged. Thus, assuming he had a normal $[Na^+]$ of 140 mEq/L and a TBW content that is 60% of body weight:

Normal TBW × 140 = present TBW × $[Na^+]_{plasma}$
or (70 × 0.6) × 140 = present TBW × 160

Solving the equation:

Present TBW = 3.67 L
Water deficit = normal TBW − present TBW
or (70 × 0.6) − 36.7 = 5.3 L

To replace this deficit over 48 h, it is necessary to give 5% dextrose in water intravenously, 5300 mL over 48 h, or 110 mL/h.

Note that this method ignores any coexisting isotonic fluid deficits, which if present should be replaced with an isotonic solution.

Anesthetic Considerations

Hypernatremia increases the minimum alveolar concentration for inhalation anesthetics in animal studies, but its clinical significance is more closely related to the associated fluid deficits. Hypovolemia accentuates any vasodilation or cardiac depression from anesthetic agents and predisposes to hypotension and hypoperfusion of tissues. Decreases in the volume of distribution for drugs necessitate dose reductions for most intravenous agents, whereas decreases in cardiac output enhance the uptake of inhalation anesthetics.

Elective surgery should be postponed in patients with significant hypernatremia (> 150 mEq/L) until the cause is established and fluid deficits are corrected. Both water and isotonic fluid deficits should be completely corrected prior to surgery.

HYPOOSMOLALITY & HYPONATREMIA

Hypoosmolality is nearly always associated with hyponatremia ($[Na^+]$ < 135 mEq/L). Table 28–5 lists rare

Table 28–5. Causes of pseudohyponatremia.[1]

Hyponatremia with a normal plasma osmolality
Asymptomatic
Marked hyperlipidemia
Marked hyperproteinemia
Symptomatic
Marked glycine absorption during transurethral surgery
Hyponatremia with an elevated plasma osmolality
Hyperglycemia
Administration of mannitol

[1]Adapted from Rose RD: *Clinical Physiology of Acid-Base and Electrolyte Disorders,* 3rd ed. McGraw-Hill, 1989.

instances in which hyponatremia does not necessarily reflect hypoosmolality (pseudohyponatremia). Routine measurement of plasma osmolality in hyponatremic patients rapidly excludes pseudohyponatremia.

Hyponatremia invariably reflects water retention from either an absolute increase in TBW or a loss of sodium in excess of water. The kidneys' normal capacity to produce dilute urine with an osmolality as low as 40 mOsm/kg (specific gravity 1.001) allows them to excrete over 10 L of free water per day if necessary. Because of this tremendous reserve, hyponatremia is nearly always the result of a defect in urinary diluting capacity (urinary osmolality > 100 mOsm/kg or specific gravity > 1.003). Rare instances of hyponatremia without an abnormality in renal diluting capacity (urinary osmolality < 100 mOsm/kg) are generally attributed to primary polydipsia or "reset" osmoreceptors; the latter two conditions can be differentiated by water restriction.

Clinically, hyponatremia is best classified according to total body sodium content (Table 28–6). Hyponatremia associated with transurethral resection of the prostate is discussed in Chapter 33.

Hyponatremia & Low Total Body Sodium

Progressive losses of both sodium and water eventually lead to extracellular volume depletion. As the intravascular volume deficit reaches 5–10%, nonosmotic ADH secretion is activated (see above). With further volume

Table 28–6. Classification of hypoosmolal hyponatremia.

Decreased total sodium content
  Renal
    Diuretics
    Mineralocorticoid deficiency
    Salt-losing nephropathies
    Osmotic diuresis (glucose, mannitol)
    Renal tubular acidosis
  Extrarenal
    Vomiting
    Diarrhea
    Integumentary loss (sweating, burns)
    "Third-spacing"
Normal total sodium content
  Primary polydipsia
  Syndrome of inappropriate antidiuretic hormone
  Glucocorticoid deficiency
  Hypothyroidism
  Drug-induced
Increased total sodium content
  Congestive heart failure
  Cirrhosis
  Nephrotic syndrome

---

depletion, the stimuli for nonosmotic ADH release overcome any hyponatremia-induced suppression of ADH. Preservation of circulatory volume takes place at the expense of plasma osmolality.

Fluid losses resulting in hyponatremia may be renal or extrarenal in origin. Renal losses are most commonly related to thiazide diuretics and result in a urinary [Na⁺] greater than 20 mEq/L. Extrarenal losses are typically gastrointestinal and usually produce a urine [Na⁺] of less than 10 mEq/L. A major exception to the latter is hyponatremia due to vomiting, which can result in a urinary [Na⁺] greater than 20 mEq/L. In those instances, bicarbonaturia from the associated metabolic alkalosis obligates concomitant excretion of Na⁺ with HCO_3 to maintain electrical neutrality in the urine; urinary chloride concentration, however, is usually less than 10 mEq/L.

Hyponatremia & Increased Total Body Sodium

Edematous disorders are characterized by an increase in both total body sodium and TBW. When the increase in water exceeds that in sodium, hyponatremia occurs. Edematous disorders include congestive heart failure, cirrhosis, renal failure, and nephrotic syndrome. Hyponatremia in these settings results from progressive impairment of renal free water excretion and generally parallels underlying disease severity. Pathophysiological mechanisms include nonosmotic ADH release and decreased delivery of fluid to the distal diluting segment in nephrons (see Chapter 31). The "effective" circulating blood volume is reduced (see below).

Hyponatremia with Normal Total Body Sodium

Hyponatremia in the absence of edema or hypovolemia may be seen with glucocorticoid insufficiency, hypothyroidism, drug therapy (chlorpropamide and cyclophosphamide), and the syndrome of inappropriate antidiuretic hormone secretion (SIADH). The hyponatremia associated with adrenal hypofunction may be due to cosecretion of ADH with corticotropin-releasing factor (CRF). Patients with AIDS often exhibit hyponatremia, which may due to adrenal infection by cytomegalovirus or mycobacteria. Diagnosis of SIADH requires exclusion of other causes of hyponatremia and the absence of hypovolemia, edema, and adrenal, renal, or thyroid disease. A variety of malignant tumors, pulmonary diseases, and central nervous system disorders are commonly associated with SIADH. In most such instances, plasma ADH concentration is not elevated but is inadequately suppressed relative to the degree of hypoosmolality in plasma; urine osmolality is usually > 100 mOsm/kg and urine sodium concentration is > 40 mEq/L.

Clinical Manifestations of Hyponatremia

Symptoms of hyponatremia are primarily neurological and result from an increase in intracellular water. Their severity is generally related to the rapidity with which extracellular hypoosmolality develops. Patients with mild to moderate hyponatremia ($[Na^+] > 125$ mEq/L) are frequently asymptomatic. Early symptoms are typically nonspecific and may include anorexia, nausea, and weakness. Progressive cerebral edema, however, results in lethargy, confusion, seizures, coma, and finally death. Serious manifestations of hyponatremia are generally associated with plasma sodium concentrations < 120 mEq/L. Compared with men, premenopausal women appear to be at greater risk of neurological impairment and damage from hyponatremia.

Patients with slowly developing or chronic hyponatremia are generally less symptomatic. A gradual compensatory loss of intracellular solutes (primarily Na^+, K^+, and amino acids) appears to restore cell volume to normal. Neurological symptoms in patients with chronic hyponatremia may be related more closely to changes in cell membrane potential (due to a low extracellular $[Na^+]$) than to changes in cell volume.

Treatment of Hyponatremia

As with hypernatremia, the treatment of hyponatremia (Figure 28–4) is directed at correcting both the underlying disorder as well as the plasma $[Na^+]$. **Isotonic saline is generally the treatment of choice for hyponatremic patients with decreased total body sodium content.** Once the extracellular fluid deficit is corrected, spontaneous water diuresis returns plasma $[Na^+]$ to normal. Conversely, water restriction is the primary treatment for hyponatremic patients with normal or increased total

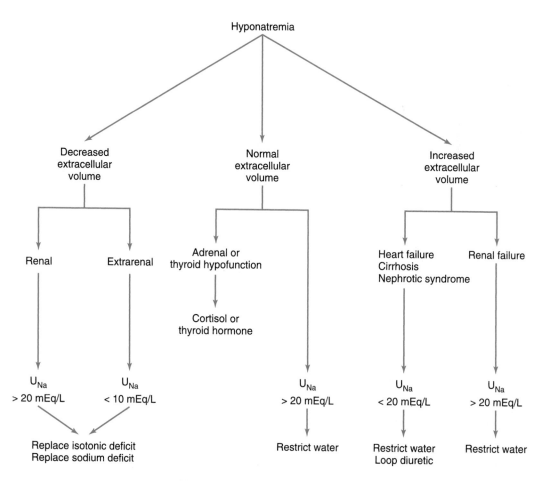

U_{Na} = Urinary sodium concentration

Figure 28–4. Algorithm for treatment of hyponatremia.

body sodium. More specific treatments such as hormone replacement in patients with adrenal or thyroid hypofunction and measures aimed at improving cardiac output in patients with heart failure may also be indicated. Demeclocycline, a drug that antagonizes ADH activity at the renal tubules, has proved to be a useful adjunct to water restriction in the treatment of patients with SIADH.

Acute symptomatic hyponatremia requires prompt treatment. In such instances, correction of plasma [Na⁺] to > 125 mEq/L is usually sufficient to alleviate symptoms. **The amount of NaCl necessary to raise plasma [Na⁺] to the desired value, the Na⁺ deficit, can be estimated by the following formula:**

$$Na^+ \text{ deficit} = TBW \times (\text{desired}[Na^+] - \text{present}[Na^+])$$

 Very rapid correction of hyponatremia has been associated with demyelinating lesions in the pons (central pontine myelinolysis), resulting in serious permanent neurological sequelae. The rapidity with which hyponatremia is corrected should be tailored to the severity of symptoms. The following correction rates have been suggested: for mild symptoms, 0.5 mEq/L/h or less; for moderate symptoms, 1 mEq/L/h or less; and for severe symptoms, 1.5 mEq/L/h or less.

EXAMPLE

An 80-kg woman is lethargic and is found to have a plasma [Na⁺] of 118 mEq/L. How much NaCl must be given to raise her plasma [Na⁺] to 130 mEq/L?

$$Na^+ \text{ deficit} = TBW \times (130 - 118)$$

TBW is approximately 50% of body weight in females:

$$Na^+ \text{ deficit} = 80 \times 0.5 \times (130 - 118) = 480 \text{ mEq}$$

Because normal (isotonic) saline contains 154 mEq/L, the patient should receive 480 mEq ÷ 154 mEq/L, or 3.12 L of normal saline. For a correction rate of 0.5 mEq/L/h, this amount of saline should be given over 24 h (130 mL/h).

Note that this calculation does not take into account any coexisting isotonic fluid deficits, which, if present, should also be replaced. More rapid correction of hyponatremia can be achieved by giving a loop diuretic to induce water diuresis while replacing urinary Na⁺ losses with isotonic saline. Even more rapid corrections can be achieved with intravenous hypertonic saline (3% NaCl). Hypertonic saline may be indicated in markedly symptomatic patients with a plasma [Na⁺] less than 110 mEq/L. Three percent NaCl should be given cautiously as it can precipitate pulmonary edema, hypokalemia, hyperchloremic metabolic acidosis, and transient hypotension;

bleeding has been associated with prolongation of the prothrombin time and activated partial thromboplastin time.

Anesthetic Considerations

Hyponatremia is often a manifestation of a serious underlying disorder and requires careful evaluation preoperatively. Plasma sodium concentrations above 130 mEq/L are generally considered safe for patients undergoing general anesthesia. Plasma [Na⁺] should be corrected above 130 mEq/L for all elective procedures, even in the absence of symptoms. Lower concentrations may result in significant cerebral edema that can be manifested intraoperatively as a decrease in minimum alveolar concentration or postoperatively as agitation, confusion, or somnolence. Patients undergoing transurethral resection of the prostate can absorb significant amounts of water from irrigation fluids (as much as 20 mL/min) and are at high risk for rapid development of profound acute water intoxication.

■ DISORDERS OF SODIUM BALANCE

Extracellular fluid volume is directly proportionate to total body sodium content. Variations in ECF volume result from changes in total body sodium content. A positive sodium balance increases ECF volume, whereas a negative sodium balance decreases ECF volume. It is important to reemphasize that *extracellular (plasma)* Na⁺ *concentration is more indicative of water balance than total body sodium content.*

NORMAL SODIUM BALANCE

Net sodium balance is equal to total sodium intake (adults average 170 mEq/d) minus both renal sodium excretion and extrarenal sodium losses. (One gram of sodium yields 43 mEq of Na⁺ ions, whereas 1 g of sodium chloride yields 17 mEq of Na⁺ ions.) The kidneys' ability to vary urinary Na⁺ excretion from less than 1 mEq/L to more than 100 mEq/L allows them to play a critical role in sodium balance (see Chapter 31).

REGULATION OF SODIUM BALANCE & EXTRACELLULAR FLUID VOLUME

Because of the relationship between ECF volume and total body sodium content, regulation of one is intimately tied to the other. This regulation is achieved via sensors (see below) that detect changes in the most important component of ECF, namely, the "effective" intravascular volume. The latter correlates more closely with the rate of perfusion in renal capillaries than with measurable intravascular fluid (plasma) volume. Indeed, with edematous disorders (heart failure, cirrhosis, and renal failure), "effective" intravascular volume can be independent of the measurable plasma volume, ECF volume, and even cardiac output.

Extracellular fluid volume and total body sodium content are ultimately controlled by appropriate adjustments in renal Na$^+$ excretion. In the absence of renal disease, diuretic therapy, and selective renal ischemia, urinary Na$^+$ concentration reflects "effective" intravascular volume. A low urine Na$^+$ concentration (< 10 mEq/L) is therefore generally indicative of a low "effective" intravascular fluid volume and reflects secondary retention of Na$^+$ by the kidneys.

Control Mechanisms

The multiple mechanisms involved in regulating ECF volume and sodium balance normally complement one another but can function completely independently of one another. In addition to altering renal Na$^+$ excretion, some mechanisms also produce more rapid compensatory hemodynamic responses when "effective" intravascular volume is reduced.

A. Sensors of Volume

The principal volume receptors in the body are really baroreceptors. Because blood pressure is the product of cardiac output and systemic vascular resistance (see Chapter 19), significant changes in intravascular volume (preload) not only affect cardiac output but also transiently affect arterial blood pressure. Thus, the baroreceptors at the carotid sinus and afferent renal arterioles (juxtaglomerular apparatus) indirectly function as sensors of intravascular volume. **Changes in blood pressure at the carotid sinus modulate sympathetic nervous system activity and nonosmotic ADH secretion, whereas changes at the afferent renal arterioles modulate the renin–angiotensin–aldosterone system.** Stretch receptors in both atria are also known to sense changes in intravascular volume; the degree of atrial distention modulates the release of atrial natriuretic hormone and ADH.

B. Effectors of Volume Change

Regardless of the mechanism, effectors of volume change ultimately alter urinary Na$^+$ excretion. Decreases in "effective" intravascular volume decrease urinary Na$^+$ excretion, whereas increases in the "effective" intravascular volume increase urinary Na$^+$ excretion. These mechanisms include the following:

1. Renin–angiotensin–aldosterone—Renin secretion increases the formation of angiotensin II. The latter increases the secretion of aldosterone and has some direct effect in enhancing Na$^+$ reabsorption in the proximal renal

tubules. Angiotensin II is also a potent direct vasoconstrictor and potentiates the actions of norepinephrine. Secretion of aldosterone enhances Na$^+$ reabsorption in the distal nephron (see Chapter 31) and is a major determinant of urinary Na$^+$ excretion.

2. Atrial natriuretic peptide (ANP)—This peptide is normally released from both right and left atrial cells following atrial distention. Atrial natriuretic peptide appears to have two major actions: arterial vasodilation and increased urinary sodium and water excretion in the renal collecting tubules. Na$^+$-mediated afferent arteriolar dilation and efferent arteriolar constriction can also increase glomerular filtration rate (GFR). Other reported effects include the inhibition of both renin and aldosterone secretion and antagonism of ADH.

3. Brain natriuretic peptide (BNP)—ANP, BNP, and C-type natriuretic peptide are structurally related peptides. BNP is released by the ventricles in response to increased ventricular volume and pressure, and ventricular overdistention. BNP levels are usually ~20% of ANP levels, but during an episode of acute congestive heart failure BNP levels may exceed those of ANP. BNP levels can be measured clinically, and a recombinant form of BNP, nesiritide (Natrecor), is available to treat acute decompensated congestive heart failure.

4. Pressure natriuresis—Even small elevations of blood pressure can result in a relatively large increase in urinary Na$^+$ excretion. Pressure diuresis appears to be independent of any known humorally or neurally mediated mechanism.

5. Sympathetic nervous system activity—Enhanced sympathetic activity increases Na$^+$ reabsorption in the proximal renal tubules, resulting in Na$^+$ retention, and mediates renal vasoconstriction, which reduces renal blood flow (see Chapter 31). Conversely, stimulation of left atrial stretch receptors results in decreases in renal sympathetic tone and increases renal blood flow (cardiorenal reflex) and, potentially, glomerular filtration.

6. Glomerular filtration rate and plasma sodium concentration—The amount of Na$^+$ filtered in the kidneys is directly proportionate to the product of the GFR and plasma Na$^+$ concentration. Because GFR is generally directly proportionate to intravascular volume, intravascular volume expansion can increase Na$^+$ excretion. Conversely, intravascular volume depletion decreases Na$^+$ excretion.

7. Tubuloglomerular balance—Despite wide variations in the amount of Na$^+$ filtered in nephrons, Na$^+$ reabsorption in the proximal renal tubules is normally controlled within narrow limits. Factors considered to be responsible for tubuloglomerular balance include the rate of renal tubular flow and changes in peritubular capillary hydrostatic and oncotic pressures. Altered Na$^+$ reabsorption in the proximal tubules can have a marked effect on renal Na$^+$ excretion.

Table 28–7. Osmoregulation versus volume regulation.[1]

	Volume Regulation	Osmoregulation
Purpose	Control extracellular volume	Control extracellular osmolality
Mechanism	Vary renal Na⁺ excretion	Vary water intake Vary renal water excretion
Sensors	Afferent renal arterioles Carotid baroreceptors Atrial stretch receptors	Hypothalamic osmoreceptors
Effectors	Renin–angiotensin–aldosterone Sympathetic nervous system Tubuloglomerular balance Renal pressure natriuresis Atrial natriuretic peptide Antidiuretic hormone Brain natriuretic peptide	Thirst Antidiuretic hormone

[1]Adapted from Rose RD: *Clinical Physiology of Acid-Base and Electrolyte Disorders,* 3rd ed. McGraw-Hill, 1989.

8. Antidiuretic hormone—Although ADH secretion has little effect on Na⁺ excretion, nonosmotic secretion of this hormone (see above) can play an important part in maintaining extracellular volume with moderate to severe decreases in the "effective" intravascular volume.

Extracellular Osmoregulation versus Volume Regulation

Osmoregulation protects the normal ratio of solutes to water, whereas extracellular volume regulation preserves absolute solute and water content. Differences between the two mechanisms are highlighted in Table 28–7. As noted previously, volume regulation generally takes precedence over osmoregulation.

Anesthetic Implications

Problems related to altered sodium balance result from its manifestations as well as the underlying disorder. Disorders of sodium balance present either as hypovolemia (sodium deficit) or hypervolemia (sodium excess). Both disturbances require correction prior to elective surgical procedures. Cardiac, liver, and renal function should also be carefully evaluated in the presence of sodium excess (generally manifested as tissue edema).

Hypovolemic patients are sensitive to the vasodilating and negative inotropic effects of the volatile anesthetics, barbiturates, and agents associated with histamine release (morphine, meperidine, curare, atracurium). Dosage requirements for other drugs must also be reduced to compensate for decreases in their volume of distribution. Hypovolemic patients are particularly sensitive to sympathetic blockade from spinal or epidural anesthesia. If an anesthetic must be administered prior to complete correction of the hypovolemia, ketamine may be the induction agent of choice for general anesthesia; etomidate may be a suitable alternative.

Hypervolemia should generally be corrected preoperatively with diuretics. Abnormalities in cardiac, renal, and hepatic function should also be corrected whenever possible. The major hazard of increases in extracellular volume is impaired gas exchange due to pulmonary interstitial edema, alveolar edema, or large collections of pleural or ascitic fluid.

■ DISORDERS OF POTASSIUM BALANCE

Potassium plays a major role in the electrophysiology of cell membranes as well as carbohydrate and protein synthesis (see below). The resting cell membrane potential is normally dependent on the ratio of intracellular to extracellular potassium concentrations. Intracellular potassium concentration is estimated to be 140 mEq/L, whereas extracellular potassium concentration is normally about 4 mEq/L. Although the regulation of intracellular [K⁺] is poorly understood, extracellular [K⁺] generally reflects the balance between potassium intake and excretion.

Under some conditions (see below), a redistribution of K⁺ between the ECF and ICF compartments can result in marked changes in extracellular [K⁺] without a change in total body potassium content.

NORMAL POTASSIUM BALANCE

Dietary potassium intake averages 80 mEq/d in adults (range, 40–140 mEq/d). About 70 mEq of that amount is normally excreted in urine, whereas the remaining 10 mEq is lost through the gastrointestinal tract.

Renal excretion of potassium can vary from as little as 5 mEq/L to over 100 mEq/L. Nearly all the potassium filtered in glomeruli is normally reabsorbed in the proximal tubule and the loop of Henle. The potassium excreted in urine is the result of distal tubular secretion. Potassium secretion in the distal tubules is coupled to aldosterone-mediated reabsorption of sodium (see Chapter 31).

REGULATION OF EXTRACELLULAR POTASSIUM CONCENTRATION

Extracellular potassium concentration is closely regulated by cell membrane Na^+–K^+ ATPase activity as well as plasma $[K^+]$. The former regulates the distribution of potassium between cells and ECF, whereas the latter is the major determinant of urinary potassium excretion.

INTERCOMPARTMENTAL SHIFTS OF POTASSIUM

Intercompartmental shifts of potassium are known to occur following changes in extracellular pH (see Chapter 30), circulating insulin levels, circulating catecholamine activity, plasma osmolality, and possibly hypothermia. Insulin and catecholamines are known to directly affect Na^+–K^+ ATPase activity and decrease plasma $[K^+]$. Exercise can also transiently increase plasma $[K^+]$ as a result of the release of K^+ by muscle cells; the increase in plasma $[K^+]$ (0.3–2 mEq/L) is proportionate to the intensity and duration of muscle activity. Intercompartmental potassium shifts are also thought to be responsible for changes in plasma $[K^+]$ in syndromes of periodic paralysis (see Chapter 37).

Changes in extracellular hydrogen ion concentration (pH) directly affect extracellular $[K^+]$ because the ICF may buffer up to 60% of an acid load (see Chapter 30). During acidosis, extracellular hydrogen ions enter cells, displacing intracellular potassium ions; the movement of potassium ions out of cells maintains electrical balance but increases extracellular and plasma $[K^+]$. Conversely, during alkalosis, extracellular potassium ions move into cells to balance the movement of hydrogen ions out of cells; as a result, plasma $[K^+]$ decreases. Although the relationship can be quite variable, a useful rule of thumb is that plasma potassium concentration changes approximately 0.6 mEq/L per 0.1 U change in arterial pH (range 0.2–1.2 mEq/L per 0.1 U).

Changes in circulating insulin levels can directly alter plasma $[K^+]$ independent of glucose transport. Insulin enhances the activity of membrane-bound Na^+–K^+ ATPase, increasing cellular uptake of potassium in the liver and in skeletal muscle. In fact, insulin secretion may play an important role in the basal control of plasma potassium concentration and facilitates the handling of increased potassium loads.

Sympathetic stimulation also increases intracellular uptake of potassium by enhancing Na^+–K^+ ATPase activity. This effect is mediated through activation of β_2-adrenergic receptors. In contrast, α-adrenergic activity may impair the intracellular movement of K^+. Plasma $[K^+]$ often decreases following the administration of β_2-adrenergic agonists as a result of uptake of potassium by muscle and the liver. Moreover, β-adrenergic blockade can impair the handling of a potassium load in some patients.

Acute increases in plasma osmolality (hypernatremia, hyperglycemia, or mannitol administration) are reported to increase plasma $[K^+]$ (about 0.6 mEq/L per 10 mOsm/L). In such instances, the movement of water out of cells (down its osmotic gradient) is accompanied by movement of K^+ out of cells. The latter may be the result of "solvent drag" or the increase in intracellular $[K^+]$ that follows cellular dehydration.

Hypothermia has been reported to lower plasma $[K^+]$ as a result of cellular uptake. Rewarming reverses this shift and may result in transient hyperkalemia if potassium was given during the hypothermia.

Urinary Excretion of Potassium

Urinary potassium excretion generally parallels its extracellular concentration. Potassium is secreted by tubular cells in the distal nephron. Extracellular $[K^+]$ is a major determinant of aldosterone secretion from the adrenal gland. Hyperkalemia stimulates aldosterone secretion, whereas hypokalemia suppresses aldosterone secretion. Renal tubular flow in the distal nephron may also be an important determinant of potassium secretion because high tubular flow rates (as during osmotic diuresis) increase potassium secretion by keeping the capillary to renal tubular gradient for potassium secretion high. Conversely, slow tubular flow rates increase $[K^+]$ in tubular fluid and decrease the gradient for K^+ secretion.

HYPOKALEMIA

Hypokalemia is defined as plasma $[K^+]$ less than 3.5 mEq/L and can occur as a result of (1) an intercompartmental shift of K^+ (see above), (2) increased potassium loss, or (3) an inadequate potassium intake (Table 28–8). Plasma potassium concentration typically correlates poorly with the total potassium deficit. A decrease in plasma $[K^+]$ from 4 mEq/L to 3 mEq/L usually represents a 100- to 200-mEq deficit, whereas a plasma $[K^+]$ below 3 mEq/L can represent a deficit anywhere between 200 mEq and 400 mEq.

Table 28–8. Major causes of hypokalemia.

Excess renal loss
  Mineralocorticoid excess
    Primary hyperaldosteronism (Conn's syndrome)
    Glucocorticoid-remediable hyperaldosteronism
  Renin excess
    Renovascular hypertension
  Bartter's syndrome
  Liddle's syndrome
  Diuresis
  Chronic metabolic alkalosis
  Antibiotics
    Carbenicillin
    Gentamicin
    Amphotericin B
  Renal tubular acidosis
    Distal, gradient-limited
    Proximal
    Ureterosigmoidostomy
Gastrointestinal losses
  Vomiting
  Diarrhea, particularly secretory diarrheas
ECF → ICF shifts
  Acute alkalosis
  Hypokalemic periodic paralysis
  Barium ingestion
  Insulin therapy
  Vitamin B_{12} therapy
  Thyrotoxicosis (rarely)
Inadequate intake

Hypokalemia due to the Intracellular Movement of Potassium

Hypokalemia due to the intracellular movement of potassium occurs with alkalosis, insulin therapy, β_2-adrenergic agonists, and hypothermia and during attacks of hypokalemic periodic paralysis (see above). Hypokalemia may also be seen following transfusion of frozen red cells; these cells lose potassium in the preservation process and take up potassium following reinfusion. Cellular K^+ uptake by red blood cells (and platelets) also accounts for the hypokalemia seen in patients recently treated with folate or vitamin B_{12} for megaloblastic anemia.

Hypokalemia due to Increased Potassium Losses

Increased potassium losses are nearly always either renal or gastrointestinal. Renal wasting of potassium is most commonly the result of a diuresis or enhanced mineralocorticoid activity. Other renal causes include hypomagnesemia (see below), renal tubular acidosis (see Chapter 30), ketoacidosis, salt-wasting nephropathies, and some drug therapies (carbenicillin and amphotericin

B). Increased gastrointestinal loss of potassium is most commonly due to vomiting, nasogastric suctioning, or diarrhea. Other gastrointestinal causes include losses from fistulae, laxative abuse, villous adenomas, and pancreatic tumors secreting vasoactive intestinal peptide.

Chronic increased sweat formation occasionally causes hypokalemia, particularly when potassium intake is limited. Dialysis with a low-potassium-containing dialysate solution can also cause hypokalemia. Uremic patients may actually have a total body potassium deficit (primarily intracellular) despite a normal or even high plasma concentration; the absence of hypokalemia in these instances is probably due to an intercompartmental shift from the acidosis. Dialysis in these patients unmasks the total body potassium deficit and often results in hypokalemia.

A urinary $[K^+]$ less than 20 mEq/L is generally indicative of increased extrarenal losses, whereas concentrations greater than 20 mEq/L suggest renal wasting of K^+.

Hypokalemia due to Decreased Potassium Intake

Because of the kidney's ability to decrease urinary potassium excretion to as low as 5–20 mEq/L, marked reductions in potassium intake are required to produce hypokalemia. Low potassium intakes, however, often accentuate the effects of increased potassium losses.

Clinical Manifestations of Hypokalemia

Hypokalemia can produce widespread organ dysfunction (Table 28–9). Most patients are asymptomatic

Table 28–9. Effects of hypokalemia.[1]

Cardiovascular
  Electrocardiographic changes/arrhythmias
  Myocardial dysfunction
Neuromuscular
  Skeletal muscle weakness
  Tetany
  Rhabdomyolysis
  Ileus
Renal
  Polyuria (nephrogenic diabetes insipidus)
  Increased ammonia production
  Increased bicarbonate reabsorption
Hormonal
  Decreased insulin secretion
  Decreased aldosterone secretion
Metabolic
  Negative nitrogen balance
  Encephalopathy in patients with liver disease

---

[1]Adapted from Schrier RW, ed: *Renal and Electrolyte Disorders*, 3rd ed. Little, Brown and Company, 1986.

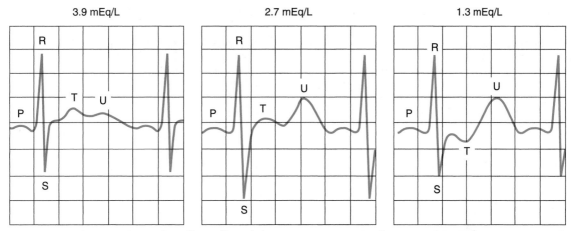

Figure 28–5. Electrocardiographic effects of hypokalemia. Note progressive flattening of the T wave, an increasingly prominent U wave, increased amplitude of the P wave, prolongation of the P–R interval, and ST-segment depression.

until plasma $[K^+]$ falls below 3 mEq/L. Cardiovascular effects are most prominent and include an abnormal electrocardiogram (ECG), arrhythmias, decreased cardiac contractility, and a labile arterial blood pressure due to autonomic dysfunction. Chronic hypokalemia has also been reported to cause myocardial fibrosis. **ECG manifestations are primarily due to delayed ventricular repolarization and include T-wave flattening and inversion, an increasingly prominent U wave, ST-segment depression, increased P-wave amplitude, and prolongation of the P–R interval** (Figure 28–5). Increased myocardial cell automaticity and delayed repolarization promote both atrial and ventricular arrhythmias.

Neuromuscular effects of hypokalemia include skeletal muscle weakness (particularly the quadriceps), ileus, muscle cramping, tetany, and, rarely, rhabdomyolysis. Hypokalemia induced by diuretics is often associated with metabolic alkalosis; as the kidneys absorb sodium to compensate for intravascular volume depletion and in the presence of diuretic-induced hypochloremia, bicarbonate is absorbed. The end result is hypokalemia and hypochloremic metabolic alkalosis. Renal dysfunction is seen due to impaired concentrating ability (resistance to ADH, resulting in polyuria) and increased production of ammonia resulting in impairment of urinary acidification. Increased ammonia production represents intracellular acidosis; hydrogen ions move intracellularly to compensate for intracellular potassium losses. The resulting metabolic alkalosis, together with increased ammonia production, can precipitate encephalopathy in patients with advanced liver disease. Chronic hypokalemia has been associated with renal fibrosis (tubulointerstitial nephropathy).

Treatment of Hypokalemia

The treatment of hypokalemia depends on the presence and severity of any associated organ dysfunction. Significant ECG changes such as ST-segment changes or arrhythmias mandate continuous ECG monitoring, particularly during intravenous K^+ replacement. Digoxin therapy—as well as the hypokalemia itself—sensitizes the heart to changes in potassium ion concentration. Muscle strength should also be periodically assessed in patients with weakness.

Oral replacement with potassium chloride solutions is generally safest (60–80 mEq/d). Replacement of the potassium deficit usually requires several days. Intravenous replacement of potassium chloride should usually be reserved for patients with or at risk for serious cardiac manifestations or muscle weakness. The goal of intravenous therapy is to remove the patient from immediate danger and not necessarily to correct the entire potassium deficit. Peripheral intravenous replacement should not exceed 8 mEq/h because of the irritative effect of potassium on peripheral veins. Dextrose-containing solutions should generally be avoided because the resulting hyperglycemia and secondary insulin secretion may actually lower plasma $[K^+]$ even further. Faster intravenous replacement (10–20 mEq/h) requires a central venous catheter and close monitoring of the ECG. Higher replacement rates may be safest through a femoral catheter, because very high localized K^+ concentrations may occur within the heart with standard central venous catheters. Intravenous replacement should generally not exceed 240 mEq/d.

Potassium chloride is the preferred potassium salt when a metabolic alkalosis is also present because it also corrects the chloride deficit discussed above. Potassium bicarbonate or equivalent (K^+ acetate or K^+ citrate) is preferable for patients with metabolic acidosis. Potassium phosphate is a suitable alternative with concomitant hypophosphatemia (diabetic ketoacidosis).

Anesthetic Considerations

Hypokalemia is a common preoperative finding. The decision to proceed with elective surgery is often arbitrarily based on lower limits somewhere between 3 and 3.5 mEq/L. The decision, however, should also be based on the rate at which the hypokalemia developed as well as the presence or absence of secondary organ dysfunction. In general, chronic mild hypokalemia (3–3.5 mEq/L) without ECG changes does not appear to substantially increase anesthetic risk. The latter may not apply to patients receiving digoxin, who may be at increased risk of developing digoxin toxicity from the hypokalemia; plasma [K^+] values above 4 mEq/L are desirable in such patients.

The intraoperative management of hypokalemia requires vigilant ECG monitoring. Intravenous potassium should be given if atrial or ventricular arrhythmias develop. Glucose-free intravenous solutions should be used and hyperventilation avoided to prevent further decreases in plasma [K^+]. Increased sensitivity to neuromuscular blocking agents (NMBAs) may be seen in some patients. Dosages of NMBAs should therefore be reduced 25–50%, and a nerve stimulator should be used to follow the degree of paralysis and the adequacy of reversal.

HYPERKALEMIA

Hyperkalemia exists when plasma [K^+] exceeds 5.5 mEq/L. Hyperkalemia rarely occurs in normal individuals because of the kidney's tremendous capacity to excrete potassium. When potassium intake is increased slowly, the kidneys can excrete as much as 500 mEq of K^+ per day. The sympathetic system and insulin secretion also appear to play important roles in preventing acute increases in plasma [K^+] following potassium loads.

Hyperkalemia can result from (1) an intercompartmental shift of potassium ions, (2) decreased urinary excretion of potassium, or, rarely, (3) an increased potassium intake (Table 28–10). Measurements of plasma potassium concentration can be spuriously elevated if red cells hemolyze in a blood specimen (most commonly due to prolonged application of a tourniquet while obtaining a venous sample). *In vitro* release of potassium from white cells in a blood specimen can also falsely indicate increased levels in the measured plasma [K^+] when the leukocyte count exceeds 70,000 $\times 10^9$/L. A similar release of potassium from platelets

Table 28–10. Causes of hyperkalemia.

Pseudohyperkalemia
Red cell hemolysis
Marked leukocytosis/thrombocytosis
Intercompartmental shifts
Acidosis
Hypertonicity
Rhabdomyolysis
Excessive exercise
Periodic paralysis
Succinylcholine
Decreased renal potassium excretion
Renal failure
Decreased mineralocorticoid activity and impaired Na^+ reabsorption
Acquired immunodeficiency syndrome
Competitive potassium-sparing diuretics
Spironolactone
ACE[1] inhibitors
Nonsteroidal antiinflammatory drugs
Pentamidine
Trimethoprim
Enhanced Cl^- reabsorption
Gordon's syndrome
Cyclosporine
Increased potassium intake
Salt substitutes

[1]ACE, angiotensin-converting enzyme.

occurs when the platelet count exceeds 1,000,000 $\times 10^9$/L.

Hyperkalemia due to Extracellular Movement of Potassium

Movement of K^+ out of cells can be seen with administration of succinylcholine, acidosis, cell lysis following chemotherapy, hemolysis, rhabdomyolysis, massive tissue trauma, hyperosmolality, digitalis overdoses, administration of arginine hydrochloride, and β_2-adrenergic blockade, and during episodes of hyperkalemic periodic paralysis. The average increase in plasma [K^+] of 0.5 mEq/L following succinylcholine can be exaggerated following large burns or severe muscle trauma and in patients with muscle denervation.

β_2-Adrenergic blockade accentuates the increase in plasma [K^+] that occurs following exercise. Digitalis inhibits Na^+–K^+ ATPase in cell membranes; digitalis overdose has been reported to cause hyperkalemia in some patients. Arginine hydrochloride, which is used to treat metabolic alkalosis, can cause hyperkalemia as the cationic arginine ions enter cells and potassium ions move out to maintain electroneutrality.

Hyperkalemia due to Decreased Renal Excretion of Potassium

Decreased renal excretion of potassium can result from (1) marked reductions in glomerular filtration, (2) decreased aldosterone activity, or (3) a defect in potassium secretion in the distal nephron.

Glomerular filtration rates less than 5 mL/min are nearly always associated with hyperkalemia. Patients with decreased degrees of renal impairment can also readily develop hyperkalemia when faced with increased potassium loads (dietary, catabolic, or iatrogenic). Uremia may also impair Na^+–K^+ ATPase activity.

Hypokalemia due to decreased aldosterone activity can result from a primary defect in adrenal hormone synthesis or a defect in the renin-aldosterone system. Patients with primary adrenal insufficiency (Addison's disease) and those with isolated 21-hydroxylase adrenal enzyme deficiency have marked impairment of aldosterone synthesis. Patients with the syndrome of isolated hypoaldosteronism (also called hyporeninemic hypoaldosteronism, or type IV renal tubular acidosis) are usually diabetics with some degree of renal impairment; they appear to have an impaired ability to increase aldosterone secretion in response to hyperkalemia. Although usually asymptomatic, these patients develop hyperkalemia when they increase their potassium intake or when given potassium-sparing diuretics. They also often have varying degrees of Na^+ wasting and a hyperchloremic metabolic acidosis. Similar findings have been reported in some patients with AIDS who may have relative adrenal insufficiency (due to cytomegalovirus infection).

Drugs interfering with the renin–aldosterone system have the potential to cause hyperkalemia, particularly in the presence of any degree of renal impairment. Nonsteroidal antiinflammatory drugs (NSAIDs) inhibit prostaglandin-mediated renin release. Angiotensin-converting enzyme (ACE) inhibitors interfere with angiotensin II-mediated release of aldosterone. Large doses of heparin can interfere with aldosterone secretion. The potassium-sparing diuretic spironolactone directly antagonizes aldosterone activity at the kidneys.

Decreased renal excretion of potassium can also occur as a result of an intrinsic or acquired defect in the distal nephron's ability to secrete potassium. Such defects may occur even in the presence of normal renal function and are characteristically unresponsive to mineralocorticoid therapy. The kidneys of patients with pseudohypoaldosteronism display an intrinsic resistance to aldosterone. Acquired defects have been associated with systemic lupus erythematosus, sickle cell anemia, obstructive uropathies, and cyclosporine nephropathy in transplanted kidneys.

Hyperkalemia due to Increased Potassium Intake

Increased potassium loads rarely cause hyperkalemia in normal individuals unless large amounts are given rapidly and intravenously. Hyperkalemia, however, may be seen when potassium intake is increased in patients receiving β-blockers or those with renal impairment or insulin deficiency. Unrecognized sources of potassium include potassium penicillin, sodium substitutes (primarily potassium salts), and transfusion of stored whole blood. The plasma $[K^+]$ in a unit of whole blood can increase to 30 mEq/L after 21 days of storage. The risk of hyperkalemia from multiple transfusions is reduced (but not eliminated) by minimizing the volume of plasma given through the use of packed red blood cell transfusions (see Chapter 29).

Clinical Manifestations of Hyperkalemia

The most important effects of hyperkalemia are on skeletal and cardiac muscle. Skeletal muscle weakness is generally not seen until plasma $[K^+]$ is greater than 8 mEq/L. The weakness is due to sustained spontaneous depolarization and inactivation of Na^+ channels of muscle membrane (similar to succinylcholine), eventually resulting in ascending paralysis. Cardiac manifestations (Figure 28–6) are primarily due to delayed depolarization and consistently present when plasma $[K^+]$ is greater than 7 mEq/L. ECG changes characteristically progress (in order) from symmetrically peaked T waves (often with a shortened QT interval) → widening of the QRS complex → prolongation of the P–R interval → loss of the P wave → loss of R-wave amplitude → ST-segment depression (occasionally elevation) → an ECG that resembles a sine wave—before progression to ventricular fibrillation and asystole. Contractility appears to be relatively well preserved. Hypocalcemia, hyponatremia, and acidosis accentuate the cardiac effects of hyperkalemia.

Treatment of Hyperkalemia

Because of its lethal potential, hyperkalemia exceeding 6 mEq/L should always be treated. Treatment is directed at reversing cardiac manifestations, and skeletal muscle weakness, and restoring of plasma [K+] to normal. The number of treatment modalities employed (see below) depends on the severity of manifestations as well as the cause of hyperkalemia. Hyperkalemia associated with hypoaldosteronism can be treated with mineralocorticoid replacement. Drugs contributing to hyperkalemia should be discontinued and sources of increased potassium intake reduced or stopped.

Calcium (5–10 mL of 10% calcium gluconate or 3–5 mL of 10% calcium chloride) partially antagonizes the cardiac effects of hyperkalemia and is useful in

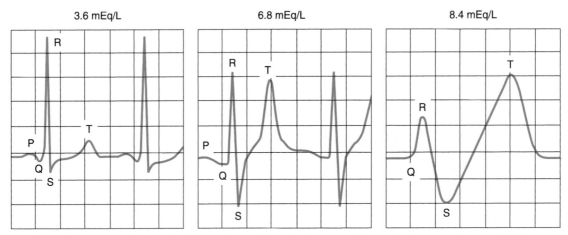

Figure 28–6. Electrocardiographic effects of hyperkalemia. Electrocardiographic changes characteristically progress from symmetrically peaked T waves, often with a shortened QT interval, to widening of the QRS complex, prolongation of the P–R interval, loss of the P wave, loss of R-wave amplitude, and ST-segment depression (occasionally elevation)—to an ECG that resembles a sine wave—before final progression into ventricular fibrillation or asystole.

patients with marked hyperkalemia. Its effects are rapid but unfortunately short lived. Care must be exercised in patients taking digoxin, as calcium potentiates digoxin toxicity.

When metabolic acidosis is present, intravenous sodium bicarbonate (usually 45 mEq) will promote cellular uptake of potassium and can decrease plasma [K$^+$] within 15 min. β-Agonists promote cellular uptake of potassium and may be useful in acute hyperkalemia associated with massive transfusions; low doses of epinephrine (0.5–2 mg/min) often rapidly decrease plasma [K$^+$] and provide inotropic support in this setting. An intravenous infusion of glucose and insulin (30–50 g of glucose with 10 units of insulin) is also effective in promoting cellular uptake of potassium and lowering plasma [K$^+$], but often takes up to 1 h for peak effect.

For patients with some renal function, furosemide is a useful adjunct in increasing urinary excretion of potassium. In the absence of renal function, elimination of excess potassium can be accomplished only with nonabsorbable cation-exchange resins such as oral or rectal sodium polystyrene sulfonate (Kayexalate). Each gram of resin binds up to 1 mEq of K$^+$ and releases 1.5 mEq of Na$^+$; the oral dose is 20 g in 100 mL of 20% sorbitol.

Dialysis is indicated in symptomatic patients with severe or refractory hyperkalemia. Hemodialysis is faster and more effective than peritoneal dialysis in decreasing plasma [K$^+$]. Maximal potassium removal with hemodialysis approaches 50 mEq/h, compared with 10–15 mEq/h for peritoneal dialysis.

Anesthetic Considerations

Elective surgery should not be undertaken in patients with hyperkalemia. Anesthetic management of hyperkalemic surgical patients is directed at both lowering the plasma potassium concentration and preventing any further increases. The ECG should be carefully monitored. Succinylcholine is contraindicated, as is the use of any potassium-containing intravenous solutions such as lactated Ringer's injection. The avoidance of metabolic or respiratory acidosis is critical to prevent further increases in plasma [K$^+$]. Ventilation should be controlled under general anesthesia; mild hyperventilation may even be desirable. Lastly, neuromuscular function should be monitored closely, as hyperkalemia can accentuate the effects of NMBAs.

■ DISORDERS OF CALCIUM BALANCE

Although 98% of total body calcium is in bone, maintenance of a normal extracellular calcium concentration is critical to homeostasis. Calcium ions are involved in nearly all essential biological functions, including muscle contraction, the release of neurotransmitters and hormones, blood coagulation, and bone metabolism. It is not surprising that abnormalities in calcium balance can result in profound physiological derangements.

NORMAL CALCIUM BALANCE

Calcium intake in adults averages 600–800 mg/d. Intestinal absorption of calcium occurs primarily in the proximal small bowel but is quite variable. Calcium is also secreted into the intestinal tract; moreover, this secretion appears to be constant and independent of absorption. Up to 80% of the daily calcium intake is normally lost in feces.

The kidneys are responsible for calcium excretion. Renal calcium excretion averages 100 mg/d but can be varied from as low as 50 mg/d to more than 300 mg/d. Normally, 98% of the filterable calcium is reabsorbed. Calcium reabsorption parallels that of sodium in the proximal renal tubules and the ascending loop of Henle. In the distal tubules, however, calcium reabsorption is dependent on parathyroid hormone secretion, whereas sodium reabsorption is dependent on aldosterone secretion. Increased parathyroid hormone levels enhance distal calcium reabsorption and decrease urinary calcium excretion.

Plasma Calcium Concentration

The normal plasma calcium concentration is 8.5–10.5 mg/dL (2.1–2.6 mmol/L). Approximately 50% is in the free ionized form, 40% is protein bound (mainly to albumin), and 10% is complexed with anions such as citrate and amino acids. It is the free ionized calcium concentration ($[Ca^{2+}]$) that is physiologically most important. Plasma $[Ca^{2+}]$ is normally 4.75–5.3 mg/dL (2.38–2.66 mEq/L or 1.19–1.33 mmol/L). Changes in plasma albumin concentration affect total but not ionized calcium concentrations: for each increase or decrease of 1 g/dL in albumin, the total plasma calcium concentration increases or decreases approximately 0.8–1.0 mg/dL, respectively.

Changes in plasma pH directly affect the degree of protein binding and thus ionized calcium concentration. Ionized calcium increases approximately 0.16 mg/dL for each decrease of 0.1 unit in plasma pH and decreases by the same amount for each 0.1 unit increase in pH.

Regulation of Extracellular Ionized Calcium Concentration

Calcium normally enters extracellular fluid by either absorption from the intestinal tract or resorption of bone; only 0.5–1% of calcium in bone is exchangeable with extracellular fluid. In contrast, calcium normally leaves the extracellular compartment by (1) deposition into bone, (2) urinary excretion, (3) secretion into the intestinal tract, and (4) sweat formation. Extracellular $[Ca^{2+}]$ is closely regulated by three hormones: parathyroid hormone (PTH), vitamin D, and calcitonin. These hormones act primarily on bone, the distal renal tubules, and the small bowel.

PTH is the most important regulator of plasma $[Ca^{2+}]$. Decreases in plasma $[Ca^{2+}]$ stimulate PTH secretion, while increases in plasma $[Ca^{2+}]$ inhibit PTH secretion. The calcemic effect of PTH is due to (1) mobilization of calcium from bone, (2) enhancement of calcium reabsorption in the distal renal tubules, and (3) an indirect increase in intestinal absorption of calcium via acceleration of 1,25-dihydroxycholecalciferol synthesis in the kidneys (see below).

Vitamin D exists in several forms in the body, but 1,25-dihydroxycholecalciferol has the most important biological activity. It is the product of the metabolic conversion of (primarily endogenous) cholecalciferol, first by the liver to 25-cholecalciferol and then by the kidneys to 1,25-dihydroxycholecalciferol. The latter transformation is enhanced by secretion of PTH as well as hypophosphatemia. Vitamin D augments intestinal absorption of calcium, facilitates the action of PTH on bone, and appears to augment renal reabsorption of calcium in the distal tubules.

Calcitonin is a polypeptide hormone that is secreted by parafollicular cells in the thyroid gland. Its secretion is stimulated by hypercalcemia and inhibited by hypocalcemia. Calcitonin inhibits bone reabsorption and increases urinary calcium excretion.

HYPERCALCEMIA

Hypercalcemia can occur as a result of a variety of disorders (Table 28–11). In primary hyperparathyroidism, secretion of PTH is increased and is independent of $[Ca^{2+}]$. In contrast, in secondary hyperparathyroidism (chronic renal failure or malabsorption), the elevated PTH levels are in response to chronic hypocalcemia. Prolonged secondary hyperparathyroidism, however, can occasionally result in autonomous secretion of PTH, resulting in a normal or elevated $[Ca^{2+}]$ (tertiary hyperparathyroidism).

Table 28–11. Causes of hypercalcemia.

Hyperparathyroidism
Malignancy
Excessive vitamin D intake
Paget's disease of bone
Granulomatous disorders (sarcoidosis, tuberculosis)
Chronic immobilization
Milk-alkali syndrome
Adrenal insufficiency
Drug-induced
Thiazide diuretics
Lithium

Patients with cancer can present with hypercalcemia whether or not bone metastases are present. Direct bony destruction or secretion of humoral mediators of hypercalcemia (PTH-like substances, cytokines, or prostaglandins) is probably responsible in most patients. Hypercalcemia due to increased turnover of calcium from bone can also be encountered in patients with benign conditions such as Paget's disease and chronic immobilization. Increased gastrointestinal absorption of calcium can lead to hypercalcemia in patients with the milk-alkali syndrome (marked increase in calcium intake), hypervitaminosis D, or granulomatous diseases (enhanced sensitivity to vitamin D). The mechanisms responsible for other causes of hypercalcemia are poorly understood.

Clinical Manifestations of Hypercalcemia

Hypercalcemia often produces anorexia, nausea, vomiting, weakness, and polyuria. Ataxia, irritability, lethargy, or confusion can rapidly progress to coma. Hypertension is often present initially before hypovolemia supervenes. ECG signs include a shortened ST segment and a shortened QT interval. Hypercalcemia increases cardiac sensitivity to digitalis. Pancreatitis, peptic ulcer disease, and renal failure can also complicate hypercalcemia.

Treatment of Hypercalcemia

Symptomatic hypercalcemia requires rapid treatment. The most effective initial treatment is rehydration followed by a brisk diuresis (urinary output 200–300 mL/h) with administration of intravenous saline infusion and a loop diuretic to accelerate calcium excretion. Premature diuretic therapy prior to rehydration may aggravate the hypercalcemia by additional volume depletion. Renal loss of potassium and magnesium usually occurs during diuresis, and laboratory monitoring and intravenous replacement should be performed as necessary. Although hydration and diuresis may remove the potential risk of cardiovascular and neurological complications of hypercalcemia, the serum calcium usually remains elevated above normal. Additional therapy with a bisphosphonate or calcitonin may be required to further lower the serum calcium. Severe hypercalcemia (> 15 mg/dL) usually requires additional therapy after saline hydration and lasix calciuresis. Bisphosphonates (pamidronate 60–90 mg intravenously) or calcitonin (2–8 U/kg subcutaneously) are preferred agents. Pamidronate has become the agent of choice in this setting because of its prolonged duration of action (but may be replaced by zoledronate, a bisphosphonate with an even longer duration of action), but it likely should be avoided in the setting of renal insufficiency (serum creatinine > 2.5 mg/dL). Dialysis may be necessary in the presence of renal or cardiac failure. Additional treatment depends on the underlying cause of the hypercalcemia and may include glucocorticoids in the setting of vita-

min D–induced hypercalcemia such as granulomatous disease states. Older agents such as plicamycin (mithramycin) or phosphates are seldom used today because of their potential adverse effects.

It is necessary to look for the underlying etiology and direct appropriate treatment toward the cause of the hypercalcemia once the initial threat of hypercalcemia has been removed. Approximately 90% of all hypercalcemia is due to either malignancy or hyperparathyroidism. The best laboratory test for discriminating between these two main categories of hypercalcemia is the double-antibody PTH assay. The serum PTH concentration will usually be suppressed in malignancy states and elevated in hyperparathyroidism.

Anesthetic Considerations

Hypercalcemia is a medical emergency and should be corrected, if possible, prior to administration of any anesthetic. Ionized calcium levels should be monitored closely. If surgery must be performed, saline diuresis should be continued intraoperatively with great care to avoid hypovolemia; central venous or pulmonary artery pressure monitoring may be advisable for patients with decreased cardiac reserve. Serial measurements of $[K^+]$ and $[Mg^{2+}]$ are helpful in detecting iatrogenic hypokalemia and hypomagnesemia. Responses to anesthetic agents are not predictable. Ventilation should be controlled under general anesthesia. Acidosis should be avoided so as not to raise plasma $[Ca^{2+}]$ any further.

HYPOCALCEMIA

Hypocalcemia should be diagnosed only on the basis of the plasma ionized calcium concentration. When direct measurements of plasma $[Ca^{2+}]$ are not available, the total calcium concentration must be corrected for decreases in plasma albumin concentration (see above). The causes of hypocalcemia are listed in Table 28–12.

Hypocalcemia due to hypoparathyroidism is a relatively common cause of symptomatic hypocalcemia. Hypoparathyroidism may be surgical, idiopathic, or part of multiple endocrine defects (most often with adrenal insufficiency), or may be associated with hypomagnesemia. Magnesium deficiency is postulated to impair the secretion of PTH and antagonize its effects on bone. Hypocalcemia during sepsis is also thought to be due to suppression of PTH release. Hyperphosphatemia (see below) is also a relatively common cause of hypocalcemia, particularly in patients with chronic renal failure. Hypocalcemia due to vitamin D deficiency may be the result of a markedly reduced intake (nutritional), vitamin D malabsorption, or abnormal vitamin D metabolism.

Chelation of calcium ions with the citrate ions in blood preservatives is an important cause of perioperative hypocalcemia; similar transient decreases in $[Ca^{2+}]$ are

Table 28–12. Causes of hypocalcemia.

Hypoparathyroidism
Pseudohypoparathyroidism
Vitamin D deficiency
  Nutritional
  Malabsorption
    Postsurgical (gastrectomy, short bowel)
    Inflammatory bowel disease
  Altered vitamin D metabolism
Hyperphosphatemia
Precipitation of calcium
  Pancreatitis
  Rhabdomyolysis
  Fat embolism
Chelation of calcium
  Multiple rapid red blood transfusions or rapid infusion of
    large amounts of albumin

also theoretically possible following rapid infusions of large volumes of albumin. Hypocalcemia following acute pancreatitis is thought to be due to precipitation of calcium with fats (soaps) following the release of lipolytic enzymes and fat necrosis; hypocalcemia following fat embolism may have a similar basis. Precipitation of calcium (in injured muscle) may also be seen following rhabdomyolysis.

Less common causes of hypocalcemia include calcitonin-secreting medullary carcinomas of the thyroid, osteoblastic metastatic disease (breast and prostate cancer), and pseudohypoparathyroidism (familial unresponsiveness to parathyroid hormone). Transient hypocalcemia may also be seen following heparin, protamine, or glucagon administration and massive blood transfusion (from citrate).

Clinical Manifestations of Hypocalcemia

Manifestations include paresthesias, confusion, laryngeal stridor (laryngospasm), carpopedal spasm (Trousseau's sign), masseter spasm (Chvostek's sign), and seizures. Biliary colic and bronchospasm have also been described. Cardiac irritability can lead to arrhythmias. Decreased cardiac contractility may result in heart failure, hypotension, or both. Decreased responsiveness to digoxin and β-adrenergic agonists has also been reported. ECG signs include prolongation of the QT interval. The severity of ECG manifestations is not necessarily correlated with the degree of hypocalcemia.

Treatment of Hypocalcemia

 Symptomatic hypocalcemia is a medical emergency and should be treated immediately with intravenous calcium chloride (3–5 mL of a

10% solution) or calcium gluconate (10–20 mL of a 10% solution). (Ten milliliters of 10% $CaCl_2$ contains 272 mg of Ca^{2+}, whereas 10 mL of 10% calcium gluconate contains only 93 mg of Ca^{2+}.) To avoid precipitation, intravenous calcium should not be given with bicarbonate- or phosphate-containing solutions. Serial ionized calcium measurements are mandatory. Repeat boluses or a continuous infusion (Ca^{2+} 1–2 mg/kg/h) may be necessary. Plasma magnesium concentration should be checked to exclude hypomagnesemia. In chronic hypocalcemia, oral calcium ($CaCO_3$) and vitamin D replacement are usually necessary. Treatment for hyperphosphatemia is discussed below.

Anesthetic Considerations

Hypocalcemia should be corrected preoperatively. Serial ionized calcium levels should be monitored intraoperatively in patients with a history of hypocalcemia. Alkalosis should be avoided to prevent further decreases in $[Ca^{2+}]$. Intravenous calcium may be necessary following rapid transfusions of citrated blood products or large volumes of albumin solutions. Potentiation of the negative inotropic effects of barbiturates and volatile anesthetics should be expected. Responses to NMBAs are inconsistent and require close monitoring with a nerve stimulator.

■ DISORDERS OF PHOSPHORUS BALANCE

Phosphorus is an important intracellular constituent. Its presence is required for the synthesis of (1) the phospholipids and phosphoproteins in cell membranes and intracellular organelles, (2) the phosphonucleotides involved in protein synthesis and reproduction, and (3) ATP used for the storage of energy. Only 0.1% of total body phosphorus is in extracellular fluid; 85% is in bone and 15% is intracellular.

NORMAL PHOSPHORUS BALANCE

Phosphorus intake averages 800–1500 mg/d in adults. About 80% of that amount is normally absorbed in the proximal small bowel. Vitamin D increases intestinal absorption of phosphorus. The kidneys are the major route for phosphorus excretion and are responsible for regulating total body phosphorus content. Urinary excretion of phosphorus depends on both intake and plasma concentration. Secretion of PTH can augment urinary phosphorus excretion by inhibiting its proximal tubular reabsorption. The latter effect may be offset by PTH-induced release of phosphate from bone.

Plasma Phosphorus Concentration

Plasma phosphorus exists in both organic and inorganic forms. Organic phosphorus is mainly in the form of phospholipids. Of the inorganic phosphorus fraction, 80% is filterable in the kidneys and 20% is protein bound. The majority of inorganic phosphorus is in the form of $H_2PO_4^-$ and HPO_4^{2-} in a 1:4 ratio. By convention, plasma phosphorus is measured as milligrams of elemental phosphorus. Normal plasma phosphorus concentration is 2.5–4.5 mg/dL (0.8–1.45 mmol/L) in adults and up to 6 mg/dL in children. Plasma phosphorus concentration is usually measured during fasting, because a recent carbohydrate intake transiently decreases the plasma phosphorus concentration. Hypophosphatemia increases vitamin D production, whereas hyperphosphatemia depresses it. The latter plays an important role in the genesis of secondary hyperparathyroidism in patients with chronic renal failure (see Chapter 32).

HYPERPHOSPHATEMIA

Hyperphosphatemia may be seen with increased phosphorus intakes (abuse of phosphate laxatives or excessive potassium phosphate administration), decreased phosphorus excretion (renal insufficiency), or massive cell lysis (following chemotherapy for lymphoma or leukemia).

Clinical Manifestations of Hyperphosphatemia

Although hyperphosphatemia itself does not appear to be directly responsible for any functional disturbances, its secondary effect on plasma [Ca^{2+}] can be important. Marked hyperphosphatemia is thought to lower plasma [Ca^{2+}] by precipitation and deposition of calcium phosphate in bone and soft tissues.

Treatment of Hyperphosphatemia

Hyperphosphatemia is generally treated with phosphate-binding antacids such as aluminum hydroxide or aluminum carbonate.

Anesthetic Considerations

Although specific interactions between hyperphosphatemia and anesthesia are generally not described, renal function should be carefully evaluated. Secondary hypocalcemia should also be excluded.

HYPOPHOSPHATEMIA

Hypophosphatemia is usually the result of either a negative phosphorus balance or cellular uptake of extracellular phosphorus (an intercompartmental shift). Intercompartmental shifts of phosphorus can occur during alkalosis and following carbohydrate ingestion or insulin administration. Large doses of aluminum- or magnesium-containing antacids, severe burns, inadequate phosphorus supplementation during hyperalimentation, diabetic ketoacidosis, alcohol withdrawal, and prolonged respiratory alkalosis can all produce a negative phosphorus balance and lead to severe hypophosphatemia (< 0.3 mmol/dL or < 1.0 mg/dL). In contrast to respiratory alkalosis, metabolic alkalosis rarely leads to severe hypophosphatemia.

Clinical Manifestations of Hypophosphatemia

Mild to moderate hypophosphatemia (1.5–2.5 mg/dL) is generally asymptomatic. In contrast, severe hypophosphatemia (< 1.0 mg/dL) is often associated with widespread organ dysfunction. Cardiomyopathy, impaired oxygen delivery (decreased 2,3-diphosphoglycerate levels), hemolysis, impaired leukocyte function, platelet dysfunction, encephalopathy, skeletal myopathy, respiratory failure, rhabdomyolysis, skeletal demineralization, metabolic acidosis, and hepatic dysfunction have all been associated with severe hypophosphatemia.

Treatment of Hypophosphatemia

Oral phosphorus replacement is generally preferable to parenteral replacement because of the risk of hypocalcemia and metastatic calcification. Potassium or sodium phosphate (2–5 mg of elemental phosphorus per kilogram, or 10–45 mmol slowly over 6–12 h) is generally used for intravenous correction of severe symptomatic hypophosphatemia.

Anesthetic Considerations

Anesthetic management of patients with hypophosphatemia requires familiarity with its complications (see above). Hyperglycemia and respiratory alkalosis should be avoided to prevent further decreases in plasma phosphorus concentration. Neuromuscular function must be monitored carefully when NMBAs are given. Some patients with severe hypophosphatemia may require mechanical ventilation postoperatively.

◼ DISORDERS OF MAGNESIUM BALANCE

Magnesium is an important intracellular cation that functions as a cofactor in many enzyme pathways. Only 1–2% of total body magnesium stores is in the ECF compartment; 67% is contained in bone whereas the remaining 31% is intracellular.

NORMAL MAGNESIUM BALANCE

Magnesium intake averages 20–30 mEq/d (240–370 mg/d) in adults. Of that amount, only 30–40% is absorbed, mainly in the distal small bowel. Renal excretion is the primary route for elimination, averaging 6–12 mEq/d. Magnesium reabsorption by the kidneys is very efficient. Twenty-five percent of filtered magnesium is reabsorbed in the proximal tubule, whereas 50–60% is reabsorbed in the thick ascending limb of the loop of Henle. Factors known to increase magnesium reabsorption in the kidneys include hypomagnesemia, parathyroid hormone, hypocalcemia, ECF depletion, and metabolic alkalosis. Factors known to increase renal excretion include hypermagnesemia, acute volume expansion, hyperaldosteronism, hypercalcemia, ketoacidosis, diuretics, phosphate depletion, and alcohol ingestion.

Plasma Magnesium Concentration

Plasma $[Mg^{2+}]$ is closely regulated between 1.7 and 2.1 mEq/L (0.7–1 mmol/L or 1.7–2.4 mg/dL). Although the exact mechanisms involved remain unclear, they involve interaction of the gastrointestinal tract (absorption), bone (storage), and the kidneys (excretion). Approximately 50–60% of plasma magnesium is unbound and diffusible.

HYPERMAGNESEMIA

Increases in plasma $[Mg^{2+}]$ are nearly always due to excessive intake (magnesium-containing antacids or laxatives), renal impairment (GFR < 30 mL/min), or both. Iatrogenic hypermagnesemia can also occur during magnesium sulfate therapy for gestational hypertension in the mother as well as the fetus. Less common causes include adrenal insufficiency, hypothyroidism, rhabdomyolysis, and lithium administration.

Clinical Manifestations of Hypermagnesemia

Symptomatic hypermagnesemia typically presents with neurological, neuromuscular, or cardiac manifestations. Hyporeflexia, sedation, and skeletal muscle weakness are characteristic features. Hypermagnesemia appears to impair the release of acetylcholine and decreases motor end-plate sensitivity to acetylcholine in muscle. Vasodilation, bradycardia, and myocardial depression can lead to hypotension at levels > 10 mmol/dL (> 24 mg/dL). ECG signs are inconsistent but often include prolongation of the P–R interval and widening of the QRS complex. Marked hypermagnesemia can lead to respiratory arrest.

Treatment of Hypermagnesemia

All sources of magnesium intake (most often antacids) should be stopped. Intravenous calcium (1 g calcium gluconate) can temporarily antagonize most of the effects of hypermagnesemia. A loop diuretic along with an infusion of $^{1}/_{2}$-normal saline in 5% dextrose enhances urinary magnesium excretion. Diuresis with normal saline is generally not recommended to decrease the likelihood of iatrogenic hypocalcemia, because the latter potentiates the effects of hypermagnesemia. Dialysis may be necessary in patients with marked renal impairment.

Anesthetic Considerations

Hypermagnesemia requires close monitoring of the ECG, blood pressure, and neuromuscular function. Potentiation of the vasodilating and negative inotropic properties of anesthetics should be expected. Dosages of NMBAs should be reduced by 25–50%. A urinary catheter is required when diuretic and saline infusions are used to enhance magnesium excretion (see above). Serial measurements of $[Ca^{2+}]$ and $[Mg^{2+}]$ may be useful.

HYPOMAGNESEMIA

Hypomagnesemia is a common and frequently overlooked problem, particularly in critically ill patients. Associated deficiencies of other intracellular components such as potassium and phosphorus are common. Deficiencies of magnesium are generally the result of inadequate intake, reduced gastrointestinal absorption, or increased renal excretion (Table 28–13). β-Adrenergic agonists may cause transient hypomagnesemia as the ion is taken up by adipose tissues. Drugs that cause renal wasting of magnesium include ethanol, theophylline, diuretics, cisplatin, aminoglycosides, cyclosporine, amphotericin B, pentamidine, and granulocyte colony-stimulating factor.

Clinical Manifestations of Hypomagnesemia

Most patients with hypomagnesemia are asymptomatic, but anorexia, weakness, fasciculation, paresthesias, confusion, ataxia, and seizures may be encountered. Hypomagnesemia is frequently associated with both hypocalcemia (impaired parathyroid hormone secretion) and hypokalemia (due to renal K^+ wasting). Cardiac manifestations include electrical irritability and potentiation of digoxin toxicity; both factors are aggravated by hypokalemia. Hypomagnesemia is associated with an increased incidence of atrial fibrillation. Prolongation of the P–R and QT intervals may also be present and usually reflects concomitant hypocalcemia.

Table 28–13. Causes of hypomagnesemia.

Inadequate intake
  Nutritional
Reduced gastrointestinal absorption
  Malabsorption syndromes
  Small bowel or biliary fistulas
  Prolonged nasogastric suctioning
  Severe diarrhea
Increased renal losses
  Diuresis
  Diabetic ketoacidosis
  Hyperparathyroidism
  Hyperaldosteronism
  Hypophosphatemia
  Drugs
  Postobstructive diuresis
Multifactorial
  Chronic alcoholism
  Protein–calorie malnutrition
  Hyperthyroidism
  Pancreatitis
  Burns

Treatment of Hypomagnesemia

Asymptomatic hypomagnesemia can be treated orally (magnesium sulfate heptahydrate or magnesium oxide) or intramuscularly (magnesium sulfate). Serious manifestations such as seizures should be treated with intravenous magnesium sulfate, 1–2 g (8–16 mEq or 4–8 mmol) given slowly over 15–60 min.

Anesthetic Considerations

Although no specific anesthetic interactions are described, coexistent electrolyte disturbances such as hypokalemia, hypophosphatemia, and hypocalcemia are often present and should be corrected prior to surgery (see above). Isolated hypomagnesemia should be corrected prior to elective procedures because of its potential for causing cardiac arrhythmias. Moreover, magnesium appears to have intrinsic antiarrhythmic properties and possibly cerebral protective effects (see Chapter 25), such that it is increasingly being administered prior to coming off cardiopulmonary bypass.

CASE DISCUSSION:
ELECTROLYTE ABNORMALITIES
FOLLOWING URINARY
DIVERSION

A 70-year-old man with carcinoma of the bladder presents for radical cystectomy and ileal loop urinary diversion. He weighs 70 kg and has a 20-year history of hypertension. Preoperative laboratory measurements revealed normal plasma electrolyte concentrations and a blood urea nitrogen (BUN) of 20 mg/dL with a serum creatinine of 1.5 mg/dL. The operation lasts 4 h and is performed under uncomplicated general anesthesia. The estimated blood loss is 900 mL. Fluid replacement consists of 3500 mL of lactated Ringer's injection and 750 mL of 5% albumin.

One hour after admission to the recovery room, the patient is awake, his blood pressure is 130/70 mm Hg, and he appears to be breathing well (18 breaths/min, $F_{IO_2} = 0.4$). Urinary output has been only 20 mL in the last hour. Laboratory measurements are as follows: Hb, 10.4 g/dL; plasma Na^+, 133 mEq/L; K^+, 3.8 mEq/L; Cl^-, 104 mEq/L; total CO_2, 20 mmol/L; Pa_{O_2}, 156 mm Hg; arterial blood pH, 7.29; Pa_{CO_2}, 38 mm Hg; and calculated HCO_3^-, 18 mEq/L.

What is the most likely explanation for the hyponatremia?

Multiple factors tend to promote hyponatremia postoperatively, including nonosmotic ADH secretion (surgical stress, hypovolemia, and pain), large evaporative and functional fluid losses (tissue sequestration), and the administration of hypotonic intravenous fluids. Hyponatremia is particularly common postoperatively in patients who have received relatively large amounts of lactated Ringer's injection ([Na^+] 130 mEq/L); the postoperative plasma [Na^+] generally approaches 130 mEq/L in such patients. (Fluid replacement in this patient was appropriate considering basic maintenance requirements, blood loss, and the additional fluid losses usually associated with this type of surgery.)

Why is the patient hyperchloremic and acidotic (normal arterial blood pH is 7.35–7.45)?

Operations for supravesical urinary diversion utilize a segment of bowel (ileum, ileocecal segment, jejunum, or sigmoid colon) that is made to function as a conduit or reservoir. The simplest and most common procedure utilizes an isolated loop of ileum as a conduit: the proximal end is anastomosed to the ureters, and the distal end is brought through the skin, forming a stoma.

Whenever urine comes in contact with bowel mucosa, the potential for significant fluid and electrolyte exchange exists. The ileum actively absorbs chloride in exchange for bicarbonate and sodium in exchange for potassium or hydrogen ions. When chloride absorption exceeds sodium absorption, plasma chloride concentration increases, whereas plasma bicarbonate concentration decreases—a hyperchloremic metabolic acidosis is established. In addition, the colon absorbs NH_4^+ directly from urine; the latter may also be produced by urea-splitting bacteria. Hypokalemia results if significant amounts of Na^+ are exchanged for K^+. Potassium losses through the conduit are increased by high urinary sodium concentrations. Moreover, a potassium deficit may be present—even in the absence of hypokalemia—because movement of K^+ out of cells (secondary to the acidosis) can prevent an appreciable decrease in extracellular plasma $[K^+]$.

Are there any factors that tend to increase the likelihood of hyperchloremic metabolic acidosis following urinary diversion?

The longer the urine is in contact with bowel, the greater the chance that hyperchloremia and acidosis will occur. Mechanical problems such as poor emptying or redundancy of a conduit—along with hypovolemia—thus predispose to hyperchloremic metabolic acidosis. Preexisting renal impairment also appears to be a major risk factor and probably represents an inability to compensate for the excessive bicarbonate losses.

What treatment, if any, is required for this patient?

The ileal loop should be irrigated with saline—through the indwelling catheter or stent—to exclude partial obstruction and ensure free drainage of urine. Hypovolemia should be considered and treated based on central venous pressure measurements or the response to a fluid challenge (see Chapter 29). A mild to moderate systemic acidosis (arterial pH > 7.25) is generally well tolerated by most patients. Moreover, hyperchloremic metabolic acidosis following ileal conduits is often transient and usually due to urinary stasis. Persistent or more severe acidosis requires treatment with sodium bicarbonate. Potassium replacement may also be required if hypokalemia is present.

Are electrolyte abnormalities seen with other types of urinary diversion?

Procedures employing bowel as a conduit (ileal or colonic) are less likely to result in a hyperchloremic metabolic acidosis than those where bowel functions as a reservoir. The incidence of hyperchloremic metabolic acidosis approaches 80% following ureterosigmoidostomies. In contrast, newer techniques for continent reservoirs such as the Kock pouch and Indiana pouch appear to be associated with a very low incidence of electrolyte abnormalities postoperatively.

SUGGESTED READING

Boldt J: Volume replacement in the surgical patient—does the type of fluid make a difference? Br J Anaesth 2000;84:783.

Paradis OC: *Fluids and Electrolytes,* 2nd ed. Lippincott, 1999.

Vincent JL: Strategies in body fluid replacement. Minerva Anesthesiol 2000;66:278.

Palmer BF: Managing hyperkalemia caused by inhibitors of the rennin-angiotensin-aldosterone system. N Engl J Med 2004;351:585. ACE inhibitors are being used with increased frequency. This article is a good review of one of their side effects.

Fluid Management & Transfusion

29

KEY CONCEPTS

 Although the intravascular half-life of a crystalloid solution is 20–30 min, most colloid solutions have intravascular half-lives between 3 and 6 h.

 Patients with a normal hematocrit should generally be transfused only after losses greater than 10–20% of their blood volume. The exact point is based on the patient's medical condition and the surgical procedure.

 The most severe transfusion reactions are due to ABO incompatibility; naturally acquired antibodies can react against the transfused (foreign) antigens, activate complement, and result in intravascular hemolysis.

 In anesthetized patients, an acute hemolytic reaction is manifested by a rise in temperature, unexplained tachycardia, hypotension, hemoglobinuria, and diffuse oozing in the surgical field.

 Transfusion of leukocyte-containing blood products appears to be immunosuppressive.

 Immunocompromised and immunosuppressed patients (eg, premature infants and organ transplant recipients) are particularly susceptible to severe cytomegalovirus (CMV) infections through transfusions. Such patients should receive only CMV-negative units.

 The most common cause of bleeding following massive blood transfusion is dilutional thrombocytopenia.

 Clinically significant hypocalcemia, causing cardiac depression, does not occur in most normal patients unless the transfusion rate exceeds 1 U every 5 min.

 The most consistent acid–base abnormality after massive blood transfusion is postoperative metabolic alkalosis.

All patients except those undergoing the most minor surgical procedures require venous access and intravenous fluid therapy. Some patients may require transfusion of blood or blood components. Maintenance of a normal intravascular volume is highly desirable in the perioperative period. The anesthesiologist should be able to assess intravascular volume accurately and to replace any fluid or electrolyte deficits and ongoing losses. Errors in fluid replacement or transfusion may result in considerable morbidity or even death.

■ EVALUATION OF INTRAVASCULAR VOLUME

Clinical evaluation and assessment of intravascular volume must generally be relied upon, because measurements of fluid compartment volumes are not readily available. Intravascular volume can be assessed using physical or laboratory examinations or with the aid of sophisticated hemodynamic monitoring techniques. Regardless of the method employed, serial evaluations are necessary to confirm initial impressions and guide fluid therapy. Moreover, modalities should complement one another, because all parameters are indirect, nonspecific measures of volume; reliance on any one parameter may be erroneous and, therefore, hazardous.

PHYSICAL EXAMINATION

Physical examination is most reliable preoperatively. Invaluable clues to hypovolemia (Table 29–1) include skin turgor, the hydration of mucous membranes, fullness of a peripheral pulse, the resting heart rate and blood pressure and the (orthostatic) changes from the supine to sitting or standing positions, and urinary flow rate. Unfortunately, many drugs used during anesthesia, as well as the physiological effects of surgical stress, alter these signs and render them unreliable in the immediate postoperative period. Intraoperatively, the fullness of a peripheral pulse (radial or dorsalis pedis), urinary flow rate, and indirect signs, such as the response of blood pressure to positive-pressure ventilation and the vasodilating or negative inotropic effects of anesthetics, are most often used.

Pitting edema—presacral in the bedridden patient or pretibial in the ambulatory patient—and increased urinary flow are signs of hypervolemia in patients with normal cardiac, hepatic, and renal function. Late signs of hypervolemia include tachycardia, pulmonary crackles, wheezing, cyanosis, and pink, frothy pulmonary secretions.

LABORATORY EVALUATION

Several laboratory measurements may be used as surrogates of intravascular volume and adequacy of tissue perfusion. These measurements include serial hematocrits, arterial blood pH, urinary specific gravity or osmolality, urinary sodium or chloride concentration, serum sodium, and the serum creatinine to blood urea nitrogen (BUN) ratio. These measurements are only indirect indices of intravascular volume and often cannot be relied upon intraoperatively because they are affected by many other variables and results are often delayed. Laboratory signs of dehydration include a rising hematocrit, a progressive metabolic acidosis, a urinary specific gravity greater than 1.010, a urinary sodium less than 10 mEq/L, a urinary osmolality greater than 450 mOsm/kg, hypernatremia, and a BUN-to-creatinine ratio greater than 10:1. Only radiographic signs of increased pulmonary vascular and interstitial markings (Kerly "B" lines) or diffuse alveolar infiltrates are reliable measures of volume overload.

HEMODYNAMIC MEASUREMENTS

Hemodynamic monitoring is discussed in Chapter 6. Central venous pressure monitoring is indicated in patients with normal cardiac and pulmonary function when volume status is difficult to assess by other means or when rapid or major alterations are expected. Central venous pressure readings must be interpreted in view of the clinical setting. Low values (< 5 mm Hg) may be normal unless associated with other signs of hypovolemia. Moreover, the response to a fluid bolus (250 mL)

Table 29–1. Signs of fluid loss (hypovolemia).

| Sign | Fluid Loss (Expressed as Percentage of Body Weight) | | |
	5%	*10%*	*15%*
Mucous membranes	Dry	Very dry	Parched
Sensorium	Normal	Lethargic	Obtunded
Orthostatic changes	None	Present	Marked
In heart rate			>15 bpm↑[1]
In blood pressure			>10 mm Hg↓
Urinary flow rate	Mildly decreased	Decreased	Markedly decreased
Pulse rate	Normal or increased	Increased > 100 bpm	Markedly increased >120 bpm
Blood pressure	Normal	Mildly decreased with respiratory variation	Decreased

[1]bpm, beats per minute.

is equally as important: a small elevation (1–2 mm Hg) may indicate the need for more fluid, whereas a large increase (> 5 mm Hg) suggests the need for a slower rate of administration and a reevaluation of volume status. Central venous pressure readings greater than 12 mm Hg are considered elevated and imply hypervolemia in the absence of right ventricular dysfunction, increased intrathoracic pressure, or restrictive pericardial disease.

Pulmonary artery pressure monitoring is necessary if central venous pressures do not correlate with the clinical assessment or if the patient has primary or secondary right ventricular dysfunction; the latter is usually due to pulmonary or left ventricular disease, respectively. Pulmonary artery occlusion pressure (PAOP) readings of less than 8 mm Hg indicate hypovolemia in the presence of confirmatory clinical signs; however, values less than 15 mm Hg may be associated with relative hypovolemia in patients with poor ventricular compliance. PAOP measurements greater than 18 mm Hg are elevated and generally imply left ventricular volume overload. The presence of mitral valve disease (particularly stenosis), severe aortic stenosis, or a left atrial myxoma or thrombus alters the normal relationship between PAOP and left ventricular end-diastolic volume (see Chapters 6, 19, 20, and 21). Increased thoracic and pulmonary airway pressures also introduce errors; consequently, all pressure measurements should always be obtained at end expiration and interpreted in the context of the clinical setting.

Newer techniques of measuring ventricular volumes with transesophageal echocardiography or by radioisotopes are more accurate but are not as widely available.

■ INTRAVENOUS FLUIDS

Intravenous fluid therapy may consist of infusions of crystalloids, colloids, or a combination of both. Crystalloid solutions are aqueous solutions of low-molecular-weight ions (salts) with or without glucose, whereas colloid solutions also contain high-molecular-weight substances such as proteins or large glucose polymers. Colloid solutions maintain plasma colloid oncotic pressure (see Chapter 28) and for the most part remain intravascular, whereas crystalloid solutions rapidly equilibrate with and distribute throughout the entire extracellular fluid space.

Controversy exists regarding the use of colloid versus crystalloid fluids for surgical patients. Proponents of colloids justifiably argue that by maintaining plasma oncotic pressure, colloids are more effective in restoring normal intravascular volume and cardiac output. Crys-

talloid proponents, on the other hand, maintain that the crystalloid solutions are equally as effective when given in sufficient amounts. Concerns that colloids may enhance the formation of pulmonary edema fluid in patients with increased pulmonary capillary permeability appear to be unfounded, because pulmonary interstitial oncotic pressure parallels that of plasma (see Chapter 22). Several generalizations can be made:

(1) Crystalloids, when given in sufficient amounts, are just as effective as colloids in restoring intravascular volume.

(2) Replacing an intravascular volume deficit with crystalloids generally requires three to four times the volume needed when using colloids.

(3) Most surgical patients have an extracellular fluid deficit that exceeds the intravascular deficit.

(4) Severe intravascular fluid deficits can be more rapidly corrected using colloid solutions.

(5) The rapid administration of large amounts of crystalloids (> 4–5 L) is more frequently associated with significant tissue edema.

Some evidence suggests—but does not prove—that marked tissue edema can impair oxygen transport, tissue healing, and return of bowel function following major surgery.

CRYSTALLOID SOLUTIONS

Crystalloids should be considered as the initial resuscitation fluid in patients with hemorrhagic and septic shock, in burn patients, in patients with head injury to maintain cerebral perfusion pressure, and in patients undergoing plasmapheresis and hepatic resection. If 3–4 L of crystalloid has been given, and the hemodynamic response is inadequate, colloids may be added.

A wide variety of solutions is available (Table 29–2). Solutions are chosen according to the type of fluid loss being replaced. For losses primarily involving water, replacement is with hypotonic solutions, also called maintenance-type solutions. If losses involve both water and electrolytes, replacement is with isotonic electrolyte solutions, also called replacement-type solutions. Glucose is provided in some solutions to maintain tonicity or to prevent ketosis and hypoglycemia due to fasting. Children are prone to developing hypoglycemia (< 50 mg/dL) following 4- to 8-h fasts. Women may be more likely to develop hypoglycemia following extended fasts (> 24 h) than men.

Because most intraoperative fluid losses are isotonic, replacement-type solutions are generally used. The most commonly used fluid is lactated Ringer's solution. Although it is slightly hypotonic, providing approximately 100 mL of free water per liter and tending to lower serum sodium to 130 mEq/L, lactated Ringer's

Table 29–2. Composition of crystalloid solutions.

Solution	Toxicity (mOsm/L)	Na⁺ (mEq/L)	Cl⁻ (mEq/L)	K⁺ (mEq/L)	Ca²⁺ (mEq/L)	Mg²⁺ (mEq/L)	Glucose (g/L)	Lactate (mEq/L)	HCO₃⁻ (mEq/L)	Acetate (mEq/L)	Gluconate (mEq/L)
5% dextrose in water (D$_5$W)	Hypo (253)						50				
Normal saline (NS)	Iso (308)	154	154								
D$_5$¹/₄NS	Iso (355)	38.5	38.5				50				
D$_5$¹/₂NS	Hyper (432)	77	77				50				
D$_5$NS	Hyper (586)	154	154				50				
Lactated Ringer's injection (LR)	Iso (273)	130	109	4	3			28			
D$_5$LR	Hyper (525)	130	109	4	3		50	28			
¹/₂NS	Hypo (154)	77	77								
3% S	Hyper (1026)	513	513								
5% S	Hyper (1710)	855	855								
7.5% NaHCO₃	Hyper (1786)	893							893		
Plasmalyte	Iso (294)	140	98	5		3				27	23

generally has the least effect on extracellular fluid composition and appears to be the most physiological solution when large volumes are necessary. The lactate in this solution is converted by the liver into bicarbonate. **When given in large volumes, normal saline produces a dilutional hyperchloremic acidosis because of its high sodium and chloride content (154 mEq/L): plasma bicarbonate concentration decreases as chloride concentration increases.** Normal saline is the preferred solution for hypochloremic metabolic alkalosis and for diluting packed red blood cells prior to transfusion. Five percent dextrose in water (D_5W) is used for replacement of pure water deficits and as a maintenance fluid for patients on sodium restriction. Hypertonic 3% saline is employed in therapy of severe symptomatic hyponatremia (see Chapter 28). Three to 7.5% saline solutions have been advocated for the resuscitation of patients in hypovolemic shock. These solutions must be administered slowly (preferably through a central venous catheter) because they readily cause hemolysis.

COLLOID SOLUTIONS

The osmotic activity of the high-molecular-weight substances in colloids tends to maintain these solutions intravascularly. Although the intravascular half-life of a crystalloid solution is 20–30 min, most colloid solutions have intravascular half-lives between 3 and 6 h. The substantial cost and occasional complications associated with colloids tend to limit their use. Generally accepted indications for colloids include (1) fluid resuscitation in patients with severe intravascular fluid deficits (eg, hemorrhagic shock) prior to the arrival of blood for transfusion, and (2) fluid resuscitation in the presence of severe hypoalbuminemia or conditions associated with large protein losses such as burns. In burn patients colloids should also be considered if the injury involves more than 30% of the body surface area or if more than 3–4 L of crystalloid has been given over 18–24 h postinjury.

Many clinicians also use colloid solutions in conjunction with crystalloids when fluid replacement needs exceed 3–4 L prior to transfusion. It should be noted that these solutions are prepared in normal saline (Cl–145–154 mEq/L) and can also cause hyperchloremic metabolic acidosis (above).

Several colloid solutions are generally available. All are derived from either plasma proteins or synthetic glucose polymers and are supplied in isotonic electrolyte solutions.

Blood-derived colloids include albumin (5% and 25% solutions) and plasma protein fraction (5%). Both are heated to 60°C for at least 10 h to minimize the risk of transmitting hepatitis and other virally transmitted diseases. Plasma protein fraction contains α- and β-globulins in addition to albumin and has occasionally resulted in hypotensive reactions. These reactions are allergic in nature and may involve activators of prekallikrein.

Synthetic colloids include dextrose starches and gelatins. Gelatins are associated with histamine-mediated allergic reactions and are not available in the United States. **Dextran** is available as dextran 70 (Macrodex) and dextran 40 (Rheomacrodex), which have average molecular weights of 70,000 and 40,000, respectively. Although dextran 70 is a better volume expander than dextran 40, the latter also improves blood flow through the microcirculation, presumably by decreasing blood viscosity. Antiplatelet effects are also described for dextrans. Infusions exceeding 20 mL/kg per day can interfere with blood typing, may prolong bleeding time (dextran 40), and have been associated with renal failure. Dextrans can also be antigenic, and both mild and severe anaphylactoid and anaphylactic reactions are described. Dextran 1 (Promit) may be administered prior to dextran 40 or dextran 70 to prevent severe anaphylactic reactions; it acts as a hapten and binds any circulating dextran antibodies.

Hetastarch (hydroxyethyl starch) is available as a 6% solution with an average molecular weight of 450,000. Small molecules are eliminated by the kidneys, whereas large molecules must be first broken down by amylase. Hetastarch is highly effective as a plasma expander and is less expensive than albumin. Moreover, hetastarch is nonantigenic, and anaphylactoid reactions are rare. Coagulation studies and bleeding times are generally not significantly affected following infusions of up to 0.5–1.0 L. Whether kidney transplant patients do worse following hetastarch infusions is controversial. Similarly, controversy exists as to an association between hetastarch use in patients undergoing cardiopulmonary bypass. Pentastarch, a lower molecular weight starch solution, is less likely to cause adverse effects and may replace hetastarch.

■ PERIOPERATIVE FLUID THERAPY

Perioperative fluid therapy includes replacement of preexisting fluid deficits, of normal losses (maintenance requirements), and of surgical wound losses including blood loss.

NORMAL MAINTENANCE REQUIREMENTS

In the absence of oral intake, fluid and electrolyte deficits can rapidly develop as a result of continued urine forma-

Table 29–3. Estimating maintenance fluid requirements.[1]

Weight	Rate
For the first 10 kg	4 mL/kg/h
For the next 10–20 kg	Add 2 mL/kg/h
For each kg above 20 kg	Add 1 mL/kg/h

[1]Example: What are the maintenance fluid requirements for a 25-kg child? Answer: 40 + 20 + 5 = 65 mL/h.

tion, gastrointestinal secretions, sweating, and insensible losses from the skin and lungs. Normal maintenance requirements can be estimated from Table 29–3.

PREEXISTING DEFICITS

Patients presenting for surgery after an overnight fast without any fluid intake will have a preexisting deficit proportionate to the duration of the fast. The deficit can be estimated by multiplying the normal maintenance rate by the length of the fast. For the average 70-kg person fasting for 8 h, this amounts to (40 + 20 + 50) mL/h × 8 h, or 880 mL. (In reality, this deficit will be somewhat less as a result of renal conservation.)

Abnormal fluid losses frequently contribute to preoperative deficits. Preoperative bleeding, vomiting, diuresis, and diarrhea are often contributory. Occult losses (really redistribution; see below) due to fluid sequestration by traumatized or infected tissues or ascites can also be substantial. Increased insensible losses due to hyperventilation, fever, and sweating are often overlooked.

Ideally, all deficits should be replaced preoperatively in all patients. The fluids used should be similar in composition to the fluids lost (Table 29–4).

SURGICAL FLUID LOSSES

Blood Loss

One of the most important and difficult tasks of the anesthesiologist is to continually monitor and estimate blood loss. Although estimates are complicated by occult bleeding into the wound or under the surgical drapes, accuracy is important to guide fluid therapy and transfusions.

The most commonly used method for estimating blood loss is measurement of blood in the surgical suction container and visually estimating the blood on surgical sponges and laparotomy pads ("laps"). A fully soaked sponge (4 × 4) is said to hold 10 mL of blood, whereas a soaked "lap" holds 100–150 mL. More accurate estimates are obtained if sponges and "laps" are weighed before and after use (particularly during pediatric procedures). Use of irrigating solutions complicates estimates, but their use should be noted and some attempt made to compensate for them. Serial hematocrits or hemoglobin concentrations reflect the ratio of blood cells to plasma, not necessarily blood loss; moreover, rapid fluid shifts and intravenous replacement affect measurements. Hematocrits may be useful during long procedures or when estimates are difficult.

Other Fluid Losses

Many surgical procedures are associated with obligatory losses of fluids other than blood. Such losses are due mainly to evaporation and internal redistribution of body fluids. Evaporative losses are most apparent with

Table 29–4. Electrolyte content of body fluids.

Fluid	Na$^+$ (mEq/L)	K$^+$ (mEq/L)	Cl$^-$ (mEq/L)	HCO$_3^-$ (mEq/L)
Sweat	30–50	5	45–55	
Saliva	2–40	10–30	6–30	30
Gastric juice				
High acidity	10–30	5–40	80–150	
Low acidity	70–140	5–40	55–95	5–25
Pancreatic secretions	115–180	5	55–95	60–110
Biliary secretions	130–160	5	90–120	30–40
Ileal fluid	40–135	5–30	20–90	20–30
Diarrheal stool	20–160	10–40	30–120	30–50

large wounds and directly proportionate to the surface area exposed and the duration of the surgical procedure.

Internal redistribution of fluids—often called "third spacing"—can cause massive fluid shifts and severe intravascular depletion. Traumatized, inflamed, or infected tissue (as occurs with burns, extensive injuries, surgical dissections, or peritonitis) can sequester large amounts of fluid in its interstitial space and can translocate fluid across serosal surfaces (ascites) or into bowel lumen. The result is an obligatory increase in a nonfunctional component of the extracellular compartment, as this fluid does not readily equilibrate with the rest of the compartments. This fluid shift cannot be prevented by fluid restriction and is at the expense of both the functional extracellular and intracellular fluid compartments. Cellular dysfunction as a result of hypoxia can produce an increase of the intracellular fluid volume, also at the expense of the functional extracellular compartment. Lastly, significant losses of lymphatic fluid may occur during extensive retroperitoneal dissections.

INTRAOPERATIVE FLUID REPLACEMENT

Intraoperative fluid therapy should include supplying basic fluid requirements and replacing residual preoperative deficits as well as intraoperative losses (blood, fluid redistribution, and evaporation). Selection of the type of intravenous solution depends upon the surgical procedure and the expected blood loss. For procedures involving minimal blood loss and fluid shifts, maintenance solutions can be used. For all other procedures, lactated Ringer's solution or fluid is generally used even for maintenance requirements.

Replacing Blood Loss

Ideally, blood loss should be replaced with crystalloid or colloid solutions to maintain intravascular volume (normovolemia) until the danger of anemia outweighs the risks of transfusion. At that point, further blood loss is replaced with transfusions of red blood cells to maintain hemoglobin concentration (or hematocrit) at that level. For most patients, that point corresponds to a hemoglobin between 7 and 8 g/dL (or a hematocrit of 21–24%).

Below a hemoglobin concentration of 7 g/dL, the resting cardiac output increases to maintain a normal oxygen delivery. A level of 10 g/dL is generally used for elderly patients and those with significant cardiac or pulmonary disease. Higher limits may be used if continuing rapid blood loss is expected.

In practice, most clinicians give lactated Ringer's solution in approximately three to four times the volume of the blood lost, or colloid in a 1:1 ratio, until the

Table 29–5. Average blood volumes.

Age	Blood Volume
Neonates	
Premature	95 mL/kg
Full-term	85 mL/kg
Infants	80 mL/kg
Adults	
Men	75 mL/kg
Women	65 mL/kg

transfusion point is reached. At that time, blood is replaced unit for unit as it is lost, with reconstituted packed red blood cells.

The transfusion point can be determined preoperatively from the hematocrit and by estimating blood volume (Table 29–5). Patients with a normal hematocrit should generally be transfused only after losses greater than 10–20% of their blood volume. The exact point is based on the patient's medical condition and the surgical procedure. The amount of blood loss necessary for the hematocrit to fall to 30% can be calculated as follows:

(1) Estimate blood volume from Table 29–5.

(2) Estimate the red blood cell volume (RBCV) at the preoperative hematocrit ($RBCV_{preop}$).

(3) Estimate RBCV at a hematocrit of 30% ($RBCV_{30\%}$), assuming normal blood volume is maintained.

(4) Calculate the red cell volume lost when the hematocrit is 30%; $RBCV_{lost} = RBCV_{preop} - RBCV_{30\%}$.

(5) Allowable blood loss = $RBCV_{lost} \times 3$.

EXAMPLE

An 85-kg woman has a preoperative hematocrit of 35%. How much blood loss will decrease her hematocrit to 30%?

Estimated blood volume = 65 mL/kg × 85 kg = 5525 mL.
$RBCV_{35\%}$ = 5525 × 35% = 1934 mL.
$RBCV_{30\%}$ = 5525 × 30% = 1658 mL.
Red cell loss at 30% = 1934 – 1658 = 276 mL.
Allowable blood loss = 3 × 276 mL = 828 mL.

Therefore, transfusion should be considered only when this patient's blood loss exceeds 800 mL. Increasingly, transfusions are not recommended until the hematocrit decreases to 24% (hemoglobin < 8.0 g/dL), but it is necessary to take into account the rate of blood loss and comorbid conditions, ie, cardiac disease in which case transfusion might be indicated if only 800 mL of blood is lost.

Table 29–6. Redistribution and evaporative surgical fluid losses.

Degree of Tissue Trauma	Additional Fluid Requirement
Minimal (eg, herniorrhaphy)	0–2 mL/kg
Moderate (eg, cholecystectomy)	2–4 mL/kg
Severe (eg, bowel resection)	4–8 mL/kg

Other useful guidelines commonly used are as follows: (1) one unit of red blood cells will increase hemoglobin 1 g/dL and the hematocrit 2–3% (in adults); and (2) a 10-mL/kg transfusion of red blood cells will increase hemoglobin concentration by 3 g/dL and the hematocrit by 10%.

Replacing Redistributive & Evaporative Losses

Because these losses are primarily related to wound size and the extent of surgical dissections and manipulations, procedures can be classified according to the degree of tissue trauma. These additional fluid losses can be replaced according to Table 29–6, based on whether tissue trauma is minimal, moderate, or severe. These values are only guidelines, and actual needs vary considerably from patient to patient.

■ TRANSFUSION

BLOOD GROUPS

Human red cell membranes are estimated to contain at least 300 different antigenic determinants. At least 20 separate blood group antigen systems are known; the expression of each is under genetic control from separate chromosomal loci. Fortunately, only the ABO and the Rh systems are important in the majority of blood transfusions. Individuals often produce antibodies (alloantibodies) to the alleles they lack within each system. Such antibodies are responsible for the most serious reactions to transfusions. Antibodies may occur "naturally" or in response to sensitization from a previous transfusion or pregnancy.

The ABO System

Simplistically, the chromosomal locus for this system produces two alleles: A and B. Each represents an enzyme that modifies a cell surface glycoprotein, producing a different antigen. (Actually, there are multiple variants of A and B.) Almost all individuals not having A or B "naturally" produce antibodies (mainly immunoglobulin M (IgM) against those antigens (Table 29–7) within the first year of life. The H antigen is the structural precursor of the ABO system but is produced by a different chromosomal locus. Absence of the H antigen (hh genotype, also called the Bombay phenotype) prevents expression of the A or B genes; individuals with this very rare condition will have anti-A, anti-B, and anti-H antibodies.

The Rh System

The Rh system is encoded by two genes located on chromosome 1. There are about 46 Rh-related antigens, but in most clinical settings, the five principal antigens (D, C, c, E, and e) and their corresponding antibodies account for most issues involving the Rh system. For simplicity, only the presence or absence of the most common and most immunogenic allele, the D antigen, is considered. Approximately 80–85% of the white population has the D antigen. Individuals lacking this allele are called Rh-negative and usually develop antibodies against the D antigen only after exposure to a previous (Rh-positive) transfusion or pregnancy (an Rh-negative mother delivering an Rh-positive baby).

Other Systems

Other systems include the Lewis, P, Ii, MNS, Kidd, Kell, Duffy, Lutheran, Xg, Sid, Cartright, YK, and Chido Rodgers antigens. Fortunately, with some exceptions (Kell, Kidd, Duffy, and S), alloantibodies against these systems rarely cause serious hemolytic reactions.

COMPATIBILITY TESTING

The purpose of compatibility testing is to predict and to prevent antigen–antibody reactions as a result of red

Table 29–7. ABO blood grouping.

Type	Naturally Occurring Antibodies in Serum	Incidence[1]
A	Anti-B	45%
B	Anti-A	8%
AB	—	4%
O	Anti-A, anti-B	43%

[1]Rates are based on persons of western European ancestry.

blood cell transfusions. Donor and recipient blood are typed and checked for the presence of adverse antibodies.

ABO-Rh Testing

The most severe transfusion reactions are due to ABO incompatibility; naturally acquired antibodies can react against the transfused (foreign) antigens, activate complement, and result in intravascular hemolysis. The patient's red cells are tested with serum known to have antibodies against A and against B to determine blood type. Because of the almost universal prevalence of natural ABO antibodies, confirmation of blood type is then made by testing the patient's serum against red cells with a known antigen type.

The patient's red cells are also tested with anti-D antibodies to determine Rh. If the subject is Rh-negative, the presence of anti-D antibody is checked by mixing the patient's serum against Rh-positive red cells. The probability of developing anti-D antibodies after a single exposure to the Rh antigen is 50–70%.

Crossmatching

A crossmatch mimics the transfusion: donor cells are mixed with recipient serum. Crossmatching serves three functions: (1) it confirms ABO and Rh typing (in less than 5 min), (2) it detects antibodies to the other blood group systems, and (3) it detects antibodies in low titers or those that do not agglutinate easily. The latter two require at least 45 min.

Antibody Screen

The purpose of this test is to detect in the serum the presence of the antibodies that are most commonly associated with non-ABO hemolytic reactions. The test (also known as the indirect Coombs test) requires 45 min and involves mixing the subject's serum with red cells of known antigenic composition; if specific antibodies are present, they will coat the red cell membrane, and addition of an antiglobulin antibody results in red cell agglutination. Screens are routinely done on all donor blood and may be done for a potential recipient instead of a crossmatch (below).

Type & Crossmatch versus Type & Screen

The incidence of a serious hemolytic reaction after transfusion of an ABO- and Rh-compatible transfusion with a negative screen but without a crossmatch is less than 1%. Crossmatching, however, assures optimal safety and detects the presence of less common antibodies not usually tested for in a screen. Crossmatches are now performed only for elective surgical procedures in which the probability of transfusion is high. Because of the time involved, (45 min) if two previous type and screen procedures have been documented, some centers have

begun computer crossmatching—no actual crossmatch is performed.

Maximum Surgical Blood Ordering Schedule

Most hospitals compile a list of their most commonly performed operations and the maximum number of units that can be crossmatched preoperatively. Such practices prevent needless, excessive crossmatching of blood. Lists are usually based on each institution's own experience. A crossmatch-to-transfusion ratio less than 2.5:1 is considered acceptable. Only a type and screen is performed if the incidence of transfusion for a procedure is less than 10%. If transfusion is required, a crossmatch is performed. Allowances are typically made for anemic patients and those with coagulation disorders.

EMERGENCY TRANSFUSIONS

When a patient is exsanguinating, the need to transfuse arises prior to completion of a crossmatch, screen, or even blood typing. If the patient's blood type is known, an abbreviated crossmatch, requiring less than 5 min, will confirm ABO compatibility. **If the recipient's blood type is not known with certainty and transfusion must be started before determination, type O Rh-negative (universal donor) blood may be used.**

BLOOD BANK PRACTICES

Blood donors are screened to exclude medical conditions that might adversely affect the donor or the recipient. The hematocrit is determined, and if it is greater than 37% for allogeneic or 32% for autologous donors, the blood is collected, typed, screened for antibodies, and tested for hepatitis B, hepatitis C, syphilis, human T cell leukemia virus (HTLV)-1 and HTLV-2, and human immunodeficiency virus (HIV)-1 and HIV-2. Most centers are doing nucleic acid testing for viral RNA to detect hepatitis B and C, and HIV viruses, and work is on-going to detect West Nile virus. There are extremely sensitive tests, and they should narrow even further the window of positive virus but negative test.

Once blood is collected, a preservative–anticoagulant solution is added. The most commonly used solution is **CPDA-1,** which contains citrate as an anticoagulant (by binding calcium), phosphate as a buffer, dextrose as a red cell energy source, and adenosine as a precursor for adenosine triphosphate (ATP) synthesis. CPDA-1-preserved blood can be stored for 35 days, after which the viability of the red cells rapidly decreases. Alternatively, use of either AS-1 (Adsol) or AS-3 (Nutrice) extends the shelf-life to 6 weeks.

All units collected are separated into their component parts, namely, red blood cells, platelets, and plasma.

When centrifuged, one unit of whole blood yields about 250 mL of packed red blood cells (hematocrit 70%); following the addition of more saline preservative, the volume of a unit of packed red cells often reaches 350 mL. Red cells are normally stored at 1–6°C. Red cells may be frozen in a hypertonic glycerol solution for up to 10 years. The latter technique is usually reserved for storage of blood with rare phenotypes.

The supernatant is centrifuged to yield platelets and plasma. The unit of platelets obtained generally contains 50–70 mL of plasma and can be stored at 20–24°C for 5 days. The remaining plasma supernatant is further processed and frozen to yield fresh frozen plasma; rapid freezing helps prevent inactivation of labile coagulation factors (V and VIII). Slow thawing of fresh frozen plasma yields a gelatinous precipitate (cryoprecipitate) that contains high concentrations of Factor VIII and fibrinogen. Once separated, this cryoprecipitate can be refrozen for storage. One unit of blood yields about 200 mL of plasma, which is frozen for storage; once thawed, it must be transfused within 24 h. Platelets may alternatively be obtained by automated plateletpheresis, which yields the equivalent of up to six regular units from a single patient.

INTRAOPERATIVE TRANSFUSION PRACTICES

Packed Red Blood Cells

Blood transfusions should be given as packed red blood cells, which allows optimal utilization of blood bank resources. Packed red blood cells are ideal for patients requiring red cells but not volume replacement (eg, anemic patients in compensated congestive heart failure). Surgical patients require volume as well as red blood cells; crystalloid can be infused simultaneously through a second intravenous line for volume replacement.

Prior to transfusion, each unit should be carefully checked against the blood bank slip and the recipient's identity bracelet. The transfusion tubing should contain a 170-μm filter to trap any clots or debris. A similar sized but charged filter is used to reduce leukocyte content to prevent febrile transfusion reactions in sensitized patients (see below). Blood for intraoperative transfusion should be warmed to 37°C during infusion, particularly if more than 2–3 units is going to be transfused; failure to do so can result in profound hypothermia. The additive effects of hypothermia and the typically low levels of 2,3-diphosphoglycerate (2,3-DPG) in stored blood can cause a marked leftward shift of the hemoglobin–oxygen dissociation curve (see Chapter 22) and, at least theoretically, promote tissue hypoxia. Blood warmers should be able to maintain blood temperature > 30°C even at flow rates up to 150 mL/min.

Fresh Frozen Plasma

Fresh frozen plasma (FFP) contains all plasma proteins, including all clotting factors. Transfusions of FFP are indicated in the treatment of isolated factor deficiencies, the reversal of warfarin therapy, and the correction of coagulopathy associated with liver disease. Each unit of FFP generally increases the level of each clotting factor by 2–3% in adults. The initial therapeutic dose is usually 10–15 mL/kg. The goal is to achieve 30% of the normal coagulation factor concentration.

FFP may also be used in patients who have received massive blood transfusions (see below) and continue to bleed following platelet transfusions. Patients with antithrombin III deficiency or thrombotic thrombocytopenic purpura also benefit from FFP transfusions.

Each unit of FFP carries the same infectious risk as a unit of whole blood. In addition, occasional patients may become sensitized to plasma proteins. ABO-compatible units should generally be given but are not mandatory. As with red cells, FFP should generally be warmed to 37°C prior to transfusion.

Platelets

Platelet transfusions should be given to patients with thrombocytopenia or dysfunctional platelets in the presence of bleeding. Prophylactic platelet transfusions are also indicated in patients with platelet counts below 10,000–20,000 × 10⁹/L because of an increased risk of spontaneous hemorrhage.

Platelet counts less than 50,000 × 10⁹/L are associated with increased blood loss during surgery. Thrombocytopenic patients about to undergo surgery or invasive procedures should receive prophylactic platelet transfusions preoperatively: the platelet count should be increased to approximately 100,000 × 10⁹/L. Vaginal delivery and minor surgical procedures may be performed in patients with lower platelet counts but with normal platelet function and counts greater than 50,000 × 10⁹/L.

Each single unit of platelets may be expected to increase the count by 10,000–20,000 × 10⁹/L. Plateletpheresis units contain the equivalent of six regular, single donor units (above). Lesser increases can be expected in patients with a history of prior platelet transfusions. Platelet dysfunction can also increase surgical bleeding even when the platelet count is normal and can be diagnosed preoperatively with a bleeding time. Platelet transfusions may also be indicated in patients with dysfunctional platelets and increased surgical bleeding.

ABO-compatible platelet transfusions are desirable but not necessary. Transfused platelets generally survive only 1–7 days following transfusion. ABO compatibility may increase platelet survival. Rh sensitization can occur in Rh-negative recipients due to the presence of a few red cells in Rh-positive platelet units. Moreover, anti-A or anti-B antibodies in the 70 mL of plasma in each platelet unit can cause a hemolytic reaction against the recipient's red cells when a large number of ABO-incompatible platelet units is given. Administration of Rh immunoglobulin to Rh-negative individuals can protect against Rh sensitization following Rh-positive platelet transfusions. Patients who develop antibodies against HLA antigens (present on lymphocytes in platelet concentrates) or specific platelet antigens require HLA-compatible or single-donor units. Use of plateletpheresis transfusions may decrease the likelihood of sensitization.

Granulocyte Transfusions

Granulocyte transfusions, prepared by leukapheresis, may be indicated in neutropenic patients with bacterial infections not responding to antibiotics. Transfused granulocytes have a very short circulatory life span, so that daily transfusions of 10^{10} granulocytes are usually required. Irradiation of these units decreases the incidence of graft-versus-host reactions, pulmonary endothelial damage, and other problems associated with transfusion of leukocytes (see below), but may adversely affect granulocyte function. The availability of filgrastim (granulocyte colony-stimulating factor, or G-CSF) and sargramostim (granulocyte-macrophage colony-stimulating factor, or GM-CSF) has greatly reduced the use of granulocyte transfusions.

■ COMPLICATIONS OF BLOOD TRANSFUSION

IMMUNE COMPLICATIONS

Immune complications following blood transfusions are primarily due to sensitization of the recipient to donor red cells, white cells, platelets, or plasma proteins. Less commonly, the transfused cells or serum may mount an immune response against the recipient.

1. Hemolytic Reactions

Hemolytic reactions usually involve specific destruction of the transfused red blood cells by the recipient's antibodies. Less commonly, hemolysis of a recipient's red blood cells occurs as a result of the transfusion of red cell antibodies. Incompatible units of platelet concentrates, FFP, clotting factor concentrates, or cryoprecipitate may contain small amounts of plasma with anti-A or anti-B (or both) alloantibodies. Transfusions of large volumes of such units can lead to intravascular

hemolysis. Hemolytic reactions are commonly classified as either acute (intravascular) or delayed (extravascular).

Acute Hemolytic Reactions

Acute intravascular hemolysis is usually due to ABO blood incompatibility and the reported frequency is approximately 1:38,000 transfusions. The most common cause is misidentification of a patient, blood specimen, or transfusion unit. These reaction are often severe. The risk of a fatal hemolytic reaction is about 1 in 100,000 transfusions. In awake patients, symptoms include chills, fever, nausea, and chest and flank pain. In anesthetized patients, an acute hemolytic reaction is manifested by a rise in temperature, unexplained tachycardia, hypotension, hemoglobinuria, and diffuse oozing in the surgical field. Disseminated intravascular coagulation, shock, and renal shutdown can develop rapidly. The severity of a reaction often depends on how much incompatible blood has been given. Severe symptoms can occur after infusion of as little as 10–15 mL of ABO-incompatible blood.

Management of hemolytic reactions can be summarized as follows:

(1) Once a hemolytic reaction is suspected, the transfusion should be stopped immediately.

(2) The unit should be rechecked against the blood slip and the patient's identity bracelet.

(3) Blood should be drawn to identify hemoglobin in plasma, to repeat compatibility testing, and to obtain coagulation studies and a platelet count.

(4) A urinary catheter should be inserted, and the urine should be checked for hemoglobin.

(5) Osmotic diuresis should be initiated with mannitol and intravenous fluids.

(6) In the presence of rapid blood loss, platelets and FFP are indicated.

Delayed Hemolytic Reactions

A delayed hemolytic reaction—also called extravascular hemolysis—is generally mild and is caused by antibodies to non-D antigens of the Rh system or to foreign alleles in other systems such as the Kell, Duffy, or Kidd antigens. Following an ABO and Rh D-compatible transfusion, patients have a 1–1.6% chance of forming antibodies directed against foreign antigens in these other systems. By the time significant amounts of these antibodies have formed (weeks to months), the transfused red cells have been cleared from the circulation. Moreover, the titer of these antibodies subsequently decreases and may become undetectable. Reexposure to the same foreign antigen during a subsequent red cell transfusion, however, triggers an anamnestic antibody response against the foreign antigen. This phenomenon is seen more with the Kidd antigen system. The hemolytic reaction is therefore typically delayed 2–21 days after transfusion, and symptoms are generally mild, consisting of malaise, jaundice, and fever. The patient's hematocrit typically fails to rise in spite of the transfusion and the absence of bleeding. The serum unconjugated bilirubin increases as a result of hemoglobin breakdown.

Diagnosis of delayed antibody-mediated hemolytic reactions may be facilitated by the antiglobulin (Coombs) test. The direct Coombs test detects the presence of antibodies on the membrane of red cells. In this setting, however, this test cannot distinguish between recipient antibodies coated on donor red cells and donor antibodies coated on recipient red cells. The latter requires a more detailed reexamination of pretransfusion specimens from both the patient and the donor.

The treatment of delayed hemolytic reactions is primarily supportive. The frequency of delayed hemolytic transfusion reactions is estimated to be approximately 1:12,000 transfusions. Pregnancy (exposure to fetal red cells) can also be responsible for the formation of alloantibodies to red cells.

2. Nonhemolytic Immune Reactions

Nonhemolytic immune reactions are due to sensitization of the recipient to the donor's white cells, platelets, or plasma proteins.

Febrile Reactions

White cell or platelet sensitization is typically manifested as a febrile reaction. Such reactions are relatively common (1–3% of transfusion episodes) and are characterized by an increase in temperature without evidence of hemolysis. Patients with a history of repeated febrile reactions should receive white cell-poor red cell transfusions only. Red cell transfusions can be made leukocyte-poor by centrifugation, filtration, or freeze–thaw techniques.

Urticarial Reactions

Urticarial reactions are usually characterized by erythema, hives, and itching without fever. They are relatively common (1% of transfusions) and are thought to be due to sensitization of the patient to transfused plasma proteins. Urticarial reactions can be treated with antihistaminic drugs (H_1 and perhaps H_2 blockers) and steroids.

Anaphylactic Reactions

Anaphylactic reactions are rare (approximately 1 in 150,000 transfusions). These severe reactions may occur after only a few milliliters of blood has been given, typically in IgA-deficient patients with anti-IgA antibodies who receive IgA-containing blood transfusions. The prevalence of IgA deficiency is estimated to be 1:600–800 in the general population. Such reactions call for treatment with epinephrine, fluids, corticosteroids, and H_1 and H_2 blockers. Patients with IgA deficiency should receive thoroughly washed packed red cells, deglycerolized frozen red cells, or IgA-free blood units.

Noncardiogenic Pulmonary Edema

An acute lung injury syndrome (*Transfusion-Related Acute Lung Injury* [TRALI]) is a rare complication of blood transfusion (< 1:10,000). It is thought to be due to transfusion of antileukocytic or anti-HLA antibodies that interact with and cause the patient's white cells to aggregate in the pulmonary circulation. Damage to the alveolar/capillary membrane triggers the syndrome. Alternatively, transfused white cells can interact with leukoagglutinins in the patient. Initial treatment of TRALI is similar to that for acute respiratory distress syndrome (ARDS) (see Chapter 49), but it typically resolves within 12–48 h with supportive therapy.

Graft-Versus-Host Disease

This type of reaction may be seen in immune-compromised patients. Cellular blood products contain lymphocytes capable of mounting an immune response against the compromised (recipient) host. Use of special leukocyte filters alone does not reliably prevent graft-versus-host disease; irradiation (1500–3000 cGy) of red cell, granulocyte, and platelet transfusions effectively inactivates lymphocytes without altering the efficacy of such transfusions.

Posttransfusion Purpura

Profound thrombocytopenia can rarely occur following blood transfusions and is due to the development of platelet alloantibodies. For unknown reasons, these antibodies also destroy the patient's own platelets. The platelet count typically drops precipitously 1 week after transfusion. Plasmapheresis is generally recommended.

Immune Suppression

Transfusion of leukocyte-containing blood products appears to be immunosuppressive. This is most clearly evident in renal transplant recipients, in whom preoperative blood transfusions appear to improve graft survival. Some studies suggest that recurrence of malignant growths may be more likely in patients who receive a blood transfusion during surgery. Available evidence also suggests that transfusion of allogenic leukocytes can activate latent viruses in the recipient. Lastly, blood transfusion may increase the incidence of serious infections following surgery or trauma.

INFECTIOUS COMPLICATIONS

Viral Infections

A. HEPATITIS

Until routine testing for hepatitis viruses was implemented, the incidence of hepatitis following blood transfusion was 7–10%. At least 90% of these cases were due to the hepatitis C virus. The incidence of posttransfusion hepatitis is presently between 1:63,000 and 1:1,600,000; 75% of these cases are anicteric, and at least 50% develop chronic liver disease. Moreover, of this latter group, at least 10–20% develop cirrhosis.

B. ACQUIRED IMMUNODEFICIENCY SYNDROME (AIDS)

The virus responsible for this disease, HIV-1, is transmissible by blood transfusion. All blood is tested for the presence of anti-HIV-1 and -2 antibodies. The requirement of nucleic acid testing by the Food and Drug Administration (FDA) greatly narrows the window to less than a week and decreases the risk of transfusion-transmitted HIV to 1:1,900,000 transfusions.

C. OTHER VIRAL INFECTIONS

Cytomegalovirus (CMV) and Epstein–Barr virus usually cause asymptomatic or mild systemic illness. Unfortunately, some individuals become asymptomatic infectious carriers; the white cells in blood units from such donors are capable of transmitting either virus. Immunocompromised and immunosuppressed patients (eg, premature infants and organ transplant recipients) are particularly susceptible to severe CMV infections through transfusions. Ideally, such patients should receive only CMV-negative units. However, recent studies indicate that the risk of CMV transmission from transfusion of leukocyte-reduced blood products is equivalent to CMV test-negative units. Therefore, issuing leukocyte-reduced units is clinically appropriate for such patients. Human T cell lymphotropic viruses I and II (HTLV-1 and HTLV-2) are leukemia and lymphoma viruses, respectively, that have been reported to be transmitted by blood transfusion; the former has also been associated with myelopathy. Parvovirus transmission has been reported following transfusion of coagulation factor concentrates and can result in transient aplastic crises in immunocompromised hosts. The use of special leukocyte filters appears to reduce but not eliminate the incidence of these complications.

Parasitic Infections

Parasitic diseases that can be transmitted by transfusion include malaria, toxoplasmosis, and Chagas' disease. Fortunately, such cases are very rare.

Bacterial Infections

Bacterial contamination of blood products is the second leading cause of transfusion-associated death. The prevalence of positive culture from the blood bag ranges from 1/2000 for platelet products to 1/7000 for pRBC. The prevalence of sepsis due to blood transfusion ranges from 1/25,000 for platelets to 1/250,000 for pRBC. These numbers are relatively large when compared to risks of HIV or hepatitis, which are in the range of 1/1–2 million. Both gram-positive (*Staphylococcus*) and gram-negative (*Yersinia* and *Citrobacter*) bacteria can rarely contaminate blood transfusions and transmit disease. To avoid the possibility of significant bacterial contamination, blood products should be administered over a period shorter than 4 h. Specific bacterial diseases transmitted by blood transfusions from donors include syphilis, brucellosis, salmonellosis, yersiniosis, and various rickettsioses.

MASSIVE BLOOD TRANSFUSION

Massive transfusion is generally defined as the need to transfuse one to two times the patient's blood volume. For most adult patients, that is the equivalent of 10–20 units.

Coagulopathy

The most common cause of bleeding following massive blood transfusion is dilutional thrombocytopenia. Clinically significant dilution of the coagulation factors is unusual in previously normal patients. Coagulation studies and platelet counts, if readily available, ideally should guide platelet and FFP transfusion. Viscoelastic analysis of whole blood clotting (thromboelastography and Sonoclot analysis) may also be useful.

Citrate Toxicity

Calcium binding by the citrate preservative can theoretically become significant following transfusion of large volumes of blood or blood products. Clinically significant hypocalcemia, causing cardiac depression, does not occur in most normal patients unless the transfusion rate exceeds 1 U every 5 min. Because citrate metabolism is primarily hepatic, patients with hepatic disease or dysfunction (and possibly hypothermic patients) may require calcium infusion during massive transfusion.

Hypothermia

Massive blood transfusion is an absolute indication for warming all blood products and intravenous fluids to normal body temperature. Ventricular arrhythmias progressing to fibrillation often occur at temperatures close to 30°C. Hypothermia can hamper cardiac resuscitation. The use of rapid infusion devices with very efficient heat transfer has remarkably decreased the incidence of transfusion-related hypothermia.

Acid–Base Balance

Although stored blood is acidic due to the citric acid anticoagulant and accumulation of red cell metabolites (carbon dioxide and lactic acid), significant metabolic acidosis due to transfusion is not common. The most consistent acid–base abnormality after massive blood transfusion is postoperative metabolic alkalosis. Once normal perfusion is restored, any metabolic acidosis typically resolves, and a progressive metabolic alkalosis supervenes as citrate and lactate contained in transfusions and resuscitation fluids are converted to bicarbonate by the liver.

Serum Potassium Concentration

The extracellular concentration of potassium in stored blood steadily increases with time. The amount of extracellular potassium transfused with each unit is typically less than 4 mEq per unit. Hyperkalemia can develop regardless of the age of the blood when transfusion rates exceed 100 mL/min. The treatment of hyperkalemia is discussed in Chapter 28. Hypokalemia is commonly encountered postoperatively, particularly in association with metabolic alkalosis (see Chapters 28 and 30).

■ ALTERNATIVE STRATEGIES FOR MANAGEMENT OF BLOOD LOSS DURING SURGERY

AUTOLOGOUS TRANSFUSIONS

Patients undergoing elective surgical procedures with a high probability for transfusion can donate their own blood for use during that surgery. Collection is usually started 4–5 weeks prior to the procedure. The patient is allowed to donate a unit as long as the hematocrit is at least 34% or hemoglobin at least 11 g/dL. A minimum of 72 h is required between donations to make certain that plasma volume returns to normal. With iron sup-

plementation and recombinant erythropoietin therapy (400 U weekly), at least three or four units can usually be collected prior to the operation. Some studies suggest that autologous blood transfusions do not adversely affect survival in patients undergoing operations for cancer. Although autologous transfusions likely reduce the risk of infection and transfusion reactions, they are not completely free of hazard. Risks include those of immunological reactions due to clerical errors in collection and labeling, contamination, and improper storage. Allergic reactions can occur due to allergens (eg, ethylene oxide) that dissolve into the blood from collection and storage equipment. Preoperative autologous blood collection is being used with decreasing frequency.

BLOOD SALVAGE & REINFUSION

This technique is used widely during cardiac and major reconstructive vascular and orthopedic surgery (see Chapter 21). The shed blood is aspirated intraoperatively together with an anticoagulant (heparin) into a reservoir. After a sufficient amount of blood is collected, the red blood cells are concentrated and washed to remove debris and anticoagulant and then reinfused into the patient. The concentrates obtained usually have hematocrits of 50–60%. To be used effectively, this technique requires blood losses greater than 1000–1500 mL. Contraindications include septic contamination of the wound and perhaps a malignant tumor, though concerns about the possibility of reinfusing malignant cells via this technique may not be justified. Newer, simpler systems allow reinfusion of shed blood without centrifugation.

NORMOVOLEMIC HEMODILUTION

Acute normovolemic hemodilution relies on the premise that if the concentration of red blood cells is decreased, total red cell loss is reduced when large amounts of blood are shed; moreover, cardiac output remains normal because intravascular volume is maintained. Blood is typically removed just prior to surgery from a large bore intravenous catheter and is replaced with crystalloid and colloids such that the patient remains normovolemic but has a hematocrit of 21–25%. The blood that is removed is stored in a CPD bag at room temperature (up to 6 h) to preserve platelet function; the blood is given back to the patient after the blood loss or sooner if necessary.

DONOR-DIRECTED TRANSFUSIONS

Patients can request donated blood from family members or friends known to be ABO compatible. Most blood banks discourage this practice and generally require donation at least 7 days prior to surgery to process the donated blood and confirm compatibility.

Studies comparing the safety of donor-directed units to that of random donor units have found either no difference, or that blood bank units are safer.

CASE DISCUSSION: A PATIENT WITH SICKLE CELL DISEASE

A 24-year-old black woman with a history of a hereditary sickle cell anemia presents with abdominal pain and is scheduled for cholecystectomy. The patient thinks she may have sickle cell anemia.

What is sickle cell anemia?

Sickle cell anemia is a hereditary hemolytic anemia resulting from the formation of an abnormal hemoglobin (HbS). HbS differs structurally from the normal adult hemoglobin (HbA) only in the substitution of valine for glutamic acid at the sixth position of the β chain. Functionally, sickle hemoglobin has less affinity for oxygen (P_{50} = 31 mm Hg) as well as decreased solubility. Upon deoxygenation, HbS readily polymerizes and precipitates inside red blood cells, causing them to sickle. Patients produce variable amounts (2–20%) of fetal hemoglobin (HbF). It is likely that cells with large amounts of HbF are somewhat protected from sickling. The continuous formation and destruction of irreversibly sickled cells lead to anemia. Hematocrits are typically 18–30% due to extravascular hemolysis. Red cell survival is reduced to 10–15 days, compared with up to 120 days in normal individuals.

What is the difference between sickle cell anemia and sickle cell trait?

When the genetic defect for adult hemoglobin is on both the maternally and paternally derived chromosomes (No. 11), the patient is homozygous for HbS and has sickle cell anemia (HbSS). When only one chromosome has the sickle gene, the patient is heterozygous and has the sickle cell trait (HbAS). Patients with the sickle trait produce variable amounts of HbA (55–60%) and HbS (35–40%). Unlike those with HbSS, they are generally not anemic, are asymptomatic, and have a normal life span. Sickling occurs only under extreme hypoxemia or in low-flow states. Sickling is particularly apt to occur in the renal medulla; indeed, many patients with the sickle trait have impaired renal concentrating ability. Some patients with HbAS have been reported to have renal medullary, splenic, and pulmonary infarcts.

What is the prevalence of the sickle cell gene in black Americans?

Sickle cell anemia is primarily a disease of blacks of Central African ancestry. Approximately 0.2–0.5% of black Americans are homozygous for the sickle gene and approximately 8–10% are heterozygous. Sickle cell anemia is found less commonly in patients of Mediterranean ancestry.

What is the pathophysiology?

Conditions favoring the formation of deoxyhemoglobin—eg, hypoxemia, acidosis, intracellular hypertonicity or dehydration, increased 2,3-DPG levels, or increased temperature—can precipitate sickling in patients with HbSS. Hypothermia may also be detrimental because of the associated vasoconstriction (see below). Intracellular polymerization of HbS distorts red cells, makes them less pliable and "more sticky," and increases blood viscosity. Sickling may initially be reversible but eventually becomes irreversible in some cells. Formation of red cell aggregates in capillaries can obstruct the microcirculation in tissues. A vicious cycle is established in which circulatory stasis leads to localized hypoxia, which, in turn, causes more sickling.

With what symptoms do patients with sickle cell anemia usually present?

Patients with HbSS generally first develop symptoms in infancy, when levels of fetal hemoglobin (HbF) decline appreciably. The disease is characterized by both acute episodic crises and chronic and progressive features (Table 29–8). Children display retarded growth and have recurrent infections. Recurrent splenic infarction leads to splenic atrophy and functional asplenism by adolescence. Patients usually die from recurrent infections or renal failure. Crises are often precipitated by infection, cold weather, dehydration, or other forms of stress. Crises may be divided into three types:

1. *Vasoocclusive crises: Depending on the vessels involved, these acute episodes can result in micro- or macroinfarctions. Most painful crises are thought to be due to microinfarcts in the various tissues. Clinically, they present as acute abdominal, chest, back, or joint pain. Differentiation between surgical and nonsurgical causes of abdominal pain is difficult. Most patients form pigmented gallstones by adulthood, and many present with acute cholecystitis. Vasooc-*

Table 29–8. Manifestations of sickle cell anemia.

Neurological
  Stroke
  Subarachnoid hemorrhage
  Coma
  Seizures
Ocular
  Vitreous hemorrhage
  Retinal infarcts
  Proliferative retinopathy
  Retinal detachment
Pulmonary
  Increased intrapulmonary shunting
  Pleuritis
  Recurrent pulmonary infections
  Pulmonary infarcts
Cardiovascular
  Congestive heart failure
  Cor pulmonale
  Pericarditis
  Myocardial infarction
Gastrointestinal
  Cholelithiasis (pigmented stones)
  Cholecystitis
  Hepatic infarcts
  Hepatic abscesses
  Hepatic fibrosis
Hematological
  Anemia
  Aplastic anemia
  Recurrent infections
  Splenic infarcts
  Splenic sequestration
  Functional asplenia
Genitourinary
  Hematuria
  Renal papillary necrosis
  Impaired renal concentrating ability (isosthenuria)
  Nephrotic syndrome
  Renal insufficiency
  Renal failure
  Priapism
Skeletal
  Synovitis
  Arthritis
  Aseptic necrosis of femoral head
  Small bone infarcts in hand and feet (dactylitis)
  Biconcave ("fishmouth") vertebrae
  Osteomyelitis
Skin
  Chronic ulcers

clusive phenomena in larger vessels can produce thromboses resulting in splenic, cerebral, pulmonary, hepatic, renal, and, less commonly, myocardial infarctions.

2. Aplastic crisis: *Profound anemia (Hb 2–3 g/dL) can rapidly occur when red cell production in the bone marrow is exhausted or suppressed. Infections and folate deficiency may play a major role. Some patients also develop leukopenia.*

3. Splenic sequestration crisis: *Sudden pooling of blood in the spleen can occur in infants and young children and can cause life-threatening hypotension. The mechanism is thought to be partial or complete occlusion of venous drainage from the spleen.*

How is sickle cell anemia diagnosed?

Red blood cells from patients with sickle cell anemia readily sickle following addition of an oxygen-consuming reagent (metabisulfite) or a hypertonic ionic solution (solubility test). Confirmation requires hemoglobin electrophoresis.

What would be the best way to prepare patients with sickle cell anemia for surgery?

Optimal preoperative preparation is desirable for all patients undergoing surgery. Patients should be well hydrated, infections should be controlled, and the hemoglobin concentration should be at an acceptable level. Preoperative transfusion therapy must be individualized to the patient and to the surgical procedure. Partial exchange transfusions before major surgical procedures are usually advocated. Unlike simple transfusions, exchange transfusions decrease blood viscosity. They also increase oxygen-carrying capacity and decrease the likelihood of sickling. The goal of such transfusions is generally to achieve a hematocrit of 35–40% with 40–50% normal hemoglobin (HbA$_1$). Although the benefits of exchange transfusions for patients undergoing anesthesia have yet to be demonstrated, they clearly help patients experiencing a crisis.

Are there any special intraoperative considerations?

Conditions that might promote hemoglobin desaturation or low-flow states should be avoided. Every effort must be made to avoid hypothermia and hyperthermia, acidosis, and even mild degrees of hypoxemia, hypotension, or hypovolemia. Gen-

erous hydration and a relatively high (> 50%) inspired oxygen tension are desirable. The major compensatory mechanism in these patients is an increased cardiac output, which should be maintained intraoperatively. Monitoring central venous pressure or pulmonary artery pressure with mixed venous oxygen saturation may be useful in some patients. Mild alkalosis may help avoid sickling, but even moderate degrees of respiratory alkalosis may have an adverse effect on cerebral blood flow. Many clinicians will also avoid the use of tourniquets. Studies are not available to support or reject the use of any one regional or general anesthetic technique.

Are there any special postoperative considerations?

The same principles applied intraoperatively hold for the postoperative period. Most perioperative deaths occur in the postoperative period. Hypoxemia and pulmonary complications appear to be major risk factors. Supplemental oxygen, optimal pain control, pulmonary physiotherapy, and early ambulation are desirable to avoid such complications.

What is the significance of sickle cell anemia and thalassemia in the same patient?

The combination of HbS and thalassemia, most commonly sickle β-thalassemia, has a variable and unpredictable effect on disease severity. In general, the combination tends to be milder in black patients than in those of Mediterranean ancestry.

What is the pathophysiology of thalassemia?

Thalassemia is a hereditary defect in the production of one or more of the normal subunits of hemoglobin. Patients with thalassemia may be able to produce normal HbA but have reduced amounts of α- or β-chain production. The severity of this defect depends on the subunit affected and the degree with which hemoglobin production is affected. Symptoms may be absent or severe. Patients with α-thalassemia produce reduced amounts of α-subunit, whereas patients with β-thalassemia produce reduced amounts of the β-subunit. The formation of hemoglobins with abnormal subunit composition can alter the red cell membrane and lead to variable degrees of hemolysis as well as ineffective hematopoiesis. The latter can result in hypertrophy

of the bone marrow and often an abnormal skeleton. Maxillary hypertrophy may make tracheal intubation difficult. Thalassemias are most common in patients of Southeast Asian, African, Mediterranean, and Indian ancestry.

What is hemoglobin C disease?

Substitution of lysine for glutamic acid at position 6 on the β-subunit results in hemoglobin C (HbC). Approximately 0.05% of black Americans carry the gene for HbC. Patients homozygous for HbC generally have only a mild hemolytic anemia and splenomegaly. They rarely develop significant complications. The tendency for HbC to crystallize in hypertonic environments is probably responsible for the hemolysis and characteristically produces target cells on the peripheral blood smear.

What is the significance of the genotype HbSC?

Nearly 0.1% of black Americans are simultaneously heterozygous for both HbS and HbC (HbSC). These patients generally have a mild to moderate hemolytic anemia. Some patients occasionally have painful crises, splenic infarcts, and hepatic dysfunction. Eye manifestations similar to those associated with HbSS disease are particularly prominent. Females with HbSC have a high rate of complications during the third trimester of pregnancy and delivery.

What is hemoglobin E?

Hemoglobin E is the result of a single substitution on the β-chain and is the second most common hemoglobin variant worldwide. It is most often encountered in patients from Southeast Asia. Although oxygen-binding affinity is normal, the substitution impairs production of β-chains (similar to β-thalassemia). Homozygous patients have marked microcytosis and prominent target cells, but are not usually anemic and lack any other manifestations.

What is the hematologic significance of glucose-6-phosphate dehydrogenase deficiency?

Red blood cells are normally well protected against oxidizing agents. The sulfhydryl groups on hemoglobin are protected by reduced glutathione. The latter is regenerated by NADPH (reduced nicotinamide adenine dinucleotide phosphate), which

Table 29–9. Drugs to avoid in patients with G6PD[1] deficiency.

Drugs that may cause hemolysis
Sulfonamides
Antimalarial drugs
Nitrofurantoin
Nalidixic acid
Probenecid
Aminosalicylic acid
Phenacetin
Acetanilid
Ascorbic acid (in large doses)
Vitamin K
Methylene blue
Quinine[2]
Quinidine[3]
Chloramphenicol
Penicillamine
Dimercaprol
Other drugs
Prilocaine
Nitroprusside

[1]G6PD, glucose-6-phosphate dehydrogenase.
[2]May be safe in patients with A⁻ variant.
[3]Should be avoided because of their potential to cause methemoglobinemia.

itself is regenerated by glucose metabolism in the hexose monophosphate shunt. Glucose-6-phosphate dehydrogenase (G6PD) is a critical enzyme in this pathway. A defect in this pathway results in an inadequate amount of reduced glutathione, which can potentially result in the oxidation and precipitation of hemoglobin in red cells (seen as Heinz bodies) and hemolysis.

Abnormalities in G6PD are relatively common. Over 400 variants are described. Depending on the functional significance of the enzyme abnormality, clinical manifestations can be quite variable. Up to 15% of black American males have the common clinically significant A⁻ variant. A second variant is common in individuals of eastern Mediterranean ancestry, and a third in individuals of Chinese ancestry. Because the locus for the enzyme is on the X chromosome, abnormalities are X-linked traits, with males being primarily affected. As red blood cells age, G6PD activity normally decreases. Consequently, aging red cells are most susceptible to oxidation. This decay is markedly accelerated in patients with the Mediterranean variant but only moderately so in patients with the A⁻ variant. Most patients are typically not anemic but can develop hemolysis following oxidant stresses such as viral and bacterial infections or ingestions of some drugs (Table 29–9). Hemolysis can also be precipitated by metabolic acidosis. Hemolytic episodes can present with hemoglobinuria and hypotension. They are generally self-limited because only the older population of cells is destroyed. Mediterranean variants may be associated with some degree of chronic hemolytic anemia, and some patients are exquisitely sensitive to fava beans.

Treatment is primarily preventive. Measures aimed at preserving renal function (see above) are indicated in patients who develop hemoglobinuria.

SUGGESTED READING

Boldt J: New light on intravascular volume replacement regimens: what did we learn from the past three years? Anesth Analg 2003;97:1595. Metaanalysis of 40 studies of intraoperative intravascular volume resuscitation.

Mollison PL, Engelfriet CP, Contreras M: *Blood Transfusion in Clinical Medicine,* 10th ed. Blackwell Science, 1997.

Pestana C: *Fluids and Electrolytes in the Surgical Patient,* 5th ed. Lippincott, Williams & Wilkins, 2000.

Practice Guidelines for blood component therapy: a report by the American Society of Anesthesiologists Task Force on Blood Component Therapy. Park Ridge, IL: American Society of Anesthesiologists. Anesthesiology 1996;84:732.

University Hospital Consortium Clinical Practice Advancement Center: Technology assessment: albumin, nonprotein colloid, and crystalloid solutions. Oak Brook, IL, May 2000. Excellent evidence-based guidelines useful for guiding intravenous fluid therapy during the perioperative period.

van Hilten JA, van de Watering LMG, van Bockel JH, et al: Effects of transfusion with red cells filtered to remove leucocytes: randomised controlled trial in patients undergoing major surgery. BMJ 2004;328:1281. Good review of the effects of transfusing leukocyte-poor RBCs.

Acid–Base Balance

30

Nearly all biochemical reactions in the body are dependent on maintenance of a physiological hydrogen ion concentration. The latter is closely regulated because changes in hydrogen ion concentration produce widespread organ dysfunction.

This regulation—often referred to as acid–base balance—is of prime importance to anesthesiologists. Changes in ventilation and perfusion and the infusion of electrolyte-containing solutions are common during anesthesia and can rapidly alter acid–base balance. A thorough understanding of acid–base disturbances, their physiological effects, and treatment is thus essential for proper anesthetic management.

Our understanding of acid–base balance is evolving. In the past, we focused on the concentration of hydrogen ions [H^+], CO_2 balance, and the base excess/deficit. We now understand that the strong ion difference (SID), P_{CO_2}, and total weak acid concentration (A_{TOT}) best explain acid–base balance in physiological systems.

This chapter examines acid–base physiology, common disturbances, and their anesthetic implications. Clinical measurements of blood gases and their interpretation are also discussed.

■ DEFINITIONS

ACID–BASE CHEMISTRY

Hydrogen Ion Concentration & pH

In any aqueous solution, water molecules reversibly dissociate into hydrogen and hydroxide ions:

$$H_2O \leftrightarrow H^+ + OH^-$$

This process is described by the dissociation constant, K_W:

$$K_W = [H^+] + [OH^-] = 10^{-14}$$

The concentration of water is omitted from the denominator of this expression because it does not vary appreciably and is already included in the constant. Therefore, given $[H^+]$ or $[OH^-]$, the concentration of the other ion can be readily calculated.

Example: If $[H^+] = 10^{-8}$ nEq/L, then $[OH^-] = 10^{-14} \div 10^{-8} = 10^{-6}$ nEq/L.

Arterial $[H^+]$ is normally 40 nEq/L, or 40×10^{-9} mol/L. Hydrogen ion concentration is more commonly expressed as pH, because dealing with numbers of this order of magnitude is awkward. The pH of a solution is defined as the negative logarithm (base 10) of $[H^+]$ (Figure 30–1). Normal arterial pH is therefore $-\log (40 \times 10^{-9}) = 7.40$. Hydrogen ion concentrations between 16 and 160 nEq/L (pH 6.8–7.8) are compatible with life.

Like most dissociation constants, K_W is affected by changes in temperature. Thus the electroneutrality point for water occurs at a pH of 7.0 at 25°C but at about a pH of 6.8 at 37°C; temperature-related changes may be important during hypothermia (see Chapter 21).

Because physiological fluids are complex aqueous solutions, other factors that affect the dissociation of water into H^+ and OH^- are the SID, the P_{CO_2}, and A_{TOT}.

Acids & Bases

An acid is usually defined as a chemical species that can act as a proton (H^+) donor, whereas a base is a species that can act as a proton acceptor (Brönsted–Lowry definitions). In physiological solutions, it is probably better to use Arrhenius' definitions: An acid is a compound that contains hydrogen and reacts with water to form hydrogen ions. A

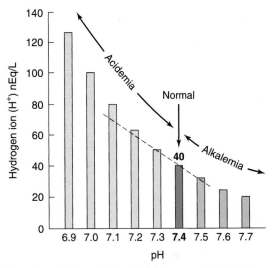

Figure 30–1. The relationship between pH and $[H^+]$. Note that between a pH of 7.10 and 7.50, the relationship between pH and $[H^+]$ is nearly linear. (Reproduced, with permission, from Narins RG, Emmett M: Simple and mixed acid–base disorders: a practical approach. *Medicine* 1980;49:161.)

base is a compound that produces hydroxide ions in water. Using these definitions, the SID becomes important as other ions in solutions (cations and anions) will affect the dissociation constant for water and, therefore, the hydrogen ion concentration. A strong acid is a substance that readily and almost irreversibly gives up an H^+ and increases $[H^+]$, whereas a strong base avidly binds H^+ and decreases $[H^+]$. In contrast, weak acids reversibly donate H^+, whereas weak bases reversibly bind H^+; both tend to have less of an effect on $[H^+]$. Biological compounds are either weak acids or weak bases.

For a solution containing the weak acid HA, where

$$HA \leftrightarrow H^+ + A^-$$

a dissociation constant, K, can be defined as follows:

$$K = \frac{[H^+][A^-]}{[HA]} \quad \text{or} \quad [H^+] = \frac{K[HA]}{[A^-]}$$

The negative logarithmic form of the latter equation is called the Henderson–Hasselbalch equation:

$$pH = pK + \log\left(\frac{[A^-]}{[HA]}\right)$$

From this equation, it is apparent that the pH of this solution is related to the ratio of the dissociated anion to the undissociated acid.

Figure 30–2. The strong ion difference (SID). SIDa, apparent strong ion difference. SIDe, effective strong ion difference. The strong ion gap (SIG) is the difference between SIDa and SIDe and represents the anion gap. (Reproduced, with permission, from Kellum JA: Metabolic acidosis in the critically ill: lessons from physical chemistry [clinical management of acute renal failure in the ICU]. Kidney Int 1998;53:S-81.)

The problem with this approach is that it is phenomenological—measure the pH and bicarbonate, and then other variables can be manipulated mathematically. This approach works well with pure water—the concentration of $[H^+]$ must equal $[OH^-]$. But physiological solutions, although aqueous, are far more complex. Even in such a complex solution, the $[H^+]$ can be predicted using three variables: the SID, the P_{CO_2}, and the total weak acid concentration $[A_{TOT}]$.

Strong Ion Difference

The SID is the sum of all the strong, completely or almost completely dissociated, cations (Na^+, K^+, Ca^{2+}, Mg^{2+}) minus the strong anions (Cl^-, lactate$^-$, etc) (Figure 30–2). Although we can calculate an SID, because the laws of electroneutrality must be observed, if there is an SID, other unmeasured ions must be present. P_{CO_2} is an independent variable assuming ventilation is ongoing. The conjugate base of HA is A^- and is composed mostly of phosphates and proteins that do not change independent of the other two variables. A^- plus AH is an independent variable because its value is not determined by any other variable. Note that $[H^+]$ is not a strong ion (water does not completely dissociate), but it can, does, and must change in response to any change in SID, P_{CO_2}, or A_{TOT} to comply with the laws of electroneutrality and conservation of mass. Strong ions cannot be made to achieve electroneutrality but

hydrogen ions, H^+, are created or consumed based on changes in the dissociation of water.

Conjugate Pairs & Buffers

As discussed above, when the weak acid HA is in solution, HA can act as an acid by donating an H^+ and A^- can act as a base by taking up H^+. A^- is therefore often referred to as the conjugate base of HA. A similar concept can be applied for weak bases. Consider the weak base B, where

$$B + H^+ \leftrightarrow BH^+$$

BH^+ is therefore the conjugate acid of B.

A buffer is a solution that contains a weak acid and its conjugate base or a weak base and its conjugate acid (conjugate pairs). Buffers minimize any change in $[H^+]$ by readily accepting or giving up hydrogen ions. It is readily apparent that buffers are most efficient in minimizing changes in the $[H^+]$ of a solution (ie, $[A^-] = [HA]$) when pH = pK. Moreover, the conjugate pair must be present in significant quantities in solution to act as an effective buffer.

CLINICAL DISORDERS

A clear understanding of acid–base disorders and compensatory physiological responses requires precise terminology (Table 30–1). The suffix "-osis" is used here to denote any pathological process that alters arterial pH. Thus, any disorder that tends to lower pH is an acidosis, whereas one tending to increase pH is termed an alkalosis. If the disorder primarily affects $[HCO_3^-]$, it is termed metabolic. If the disorder primarily affects P_{aCO_2}, it is termed respiratory. Secondary compensatory responses (see below) should be referred to as just that and not as an "-osis." One might therefore refer to a metabolic acidosis with respiratory compensation.

When only one pathological process occurs by itself, the acid–base disorder is considered to be simple. The presence of two or more primary processes indicates a mixed acid–base disorder.

Table 30–1. Defining acid-based disorders.

Disorder	Primary Change	Compensatory Response
Respiratory		
Acidosis	↑P_{aCO_2}	↑HCO_3^-
Alkalosis	↓P_{aCO_2}	↓HCO_3^-
Metabolic		
Acidosis	↓HCO_3^-	↓P_{aCO_2}
Alkalosis	↑HCO_3^-	↑P_{aCO_2}

The suffix "-emia" is used to denote the net effect of all primary processes and compensatory physiological responses (see below) on arterial blood pH. Because arterial blood pH is normally 7.35–7.45 in adults, the term "acidemia" signifies a pH < 7.35 while alkalemia signifies a pH > 7.45.

■ COMPENSATORY MECHANISMS

Physiological responses to changes in [H⁺] are characterized by three phases: (1) immediate chemical buffering, (2) respiratory compensation (whenever possible), and (3) a slower but more effective renal compensatory response that may nearly normalize arterial pH even if the pathological process is still present.

BODY BUFFERS

Physiologically important buffers in humans include bicarbonate (H_2CO_3/HCO_3^-), hemoglobin (HbH/Hb^-), other intracellular proteins (PrH/Pr^-), phosphates ($H_2PO_4^-$/ HPO_4^{2-}), and ammonia (NH_3/NH_4^+). The effectiveness of these buffers in the various fluid compartments is related to their concentration. Bicarbonate is the most important buffer in the extracellular fluid compartment. Hemoglobin, though restricted inside red blood cells, also functions as an important buffer in blood. Other proteins probably play a major role in buffering the intracellular fluid compartment. Phosphate and ammonium ions are important urinary buffers.

Buffering of the extracellular compartment can also be accomplished by the exchange of extracellular H⁺ for Na⁺ and Ca^{2+} ions from bone and by the exchange of extracellular H⁺ for intracellular K⁺. Acid loads can also demineralize bone and release alkaline compounds ($CaCO_3$ and $CaHPO_4$). Alkaline loads ($NaHCO_3$) increase the deposition of carbonate in bone.

Buffering by plasma bicarbonate is almost immediate whereas that due to interstitial bicarbonate requires 15–20 min. In contrast, buffering by intracellular proteins and bone is slower (2–4 h). Up to 50–60% of acid loads may ultimately be buffered by bone and intracellular buffers.

The Bicarbonate Buffer

Although in the strictest sense, the bicarbonate buffer consists of H_2CO_3 and HCO_3^-, CO_2 tension (PCO_2) may be substituted for H_2CO_3, because:

$$H_2O + CO_2 \leftrightarrow H_2CO_3 \leftrightarrow H^+ + HCO_3^-$$

This hydration of CO_2 is catalyzed by carbonic anhydrase. If adjustments are made in the dissociation

constant for the bicarbonate buffer and if the solubility coefficient for CO_2 (0.03 mEq/L) is taken into consideration, the Henderson–Hasselbalch equation for bicarbonate can be written as follows:

$$pH = pK' + \left(\frac{[HCO_3^-]}{0.03\ Paco_2} \right)$$

where $pK' = 6.1$.

Note that its pK' is not close to the normal arterial pH of 7.40, which means that bicarbonate would not be expected to be an efficient extracellular buffer (see above). The bicarbonate system is, however, important for two reasons: (1) bicarbonate (HCO_3^-) is present in relatively high concentrations in extracellular fluid, and (2) more importantly—$Paco_2$ and plasma [HCO_3^-] are closely regulated by the lungs and the kidneys, respectively. The ability of these two organs to alter the [HCO_3^-]/$Paco_2$ ratio allows them to exert important influences on arterial pH.

A simplified and more practical derivation of the Henderson–Hasselbalch equation for the bicarbonate buffer is as follows:

$$[H^+] = 24 \times \frac{Paco_2}{[HCO_3^-]}$$

This equation is very useful clinically because pH can be readily converted to [H⁺] (Table 30–2). Note that below 7.40, [H⁺] increases 1.25 nEq/L for each 0.01 decrease in pH; above 7.40, [H⁺] decreases 0.8 nEq/L for each 0.01 increase in pH.

Table 30–2. The relationship between pH and [H⁺].

pH	[H⁺] nEq/L
6.80	158
6.90	126
7.00	100
7.10	79
7.20	63
7.30	50
7.40	40
7.50	32
7.60	25
7.70	20

Example: If arterial pH = 7.28 and $PaCO_2$ = 24 mm Hg, what should the plasma $[HCO_3^-]$ be?

$$[H^+] = 40 + [(40 - 28) \times 1.25] = 55 \, nEq/L$$

Therefore,

$$55 = 24 \times \frac{24}{[HCO_3^-]} \text{ and } [HCO_3^-] =$$

$$\frac{(24 \times 24)}{55} = 10.5 \, mEq/L$$

It should be emphasized that the bicarbonate buffer is effective against metabolic but *not* respiratory acid–base disturbances. If 3 mEq/L of a strong nonvolatile acid such as HCl is added to extracellular fluid, the following reaction takes place:

$$3 \, mEq/L \text{ of } H^+ + 24 \, mEq/L \text{ of } HCO_3^- \rightarrow H_2CO_3 + H_2O +$$

$$3 \, mEq/L \text{ of } CO_2 + 21 \, mEq/L \text{ of } HCO_3^-$$

Note that HCO_3^- reacts with H^+ to produce CO_2. Moreover, the CO_2 generated is normally eliminated by the lungs such that $PaCO_2$ does not change. Consequently, $[H^+] = 24 \times 40 \div 21 = 45.7 \, nEq/L$ and pH = 7.34. Furthermore, the decrease in $[HCO_3^-]$ reflects the amount of nonvolatile acid added.

In contrast, an increase in CO_2 tension (volatile acid) has a minimal effect on $[HCO_3^-]$. If, for example, $PaCO_2$ increases from 40 to 80 mm Hg, the dissolved CO_2 increases only from 1.2 mEq/L to 2.2 mEq/L. Moreover, the equilibrium constant for the hydration of CO_2 is such that an increase of this magnitude minimally drives the reaction to the left:

$$H_2O + CO_2 \leftrightarrow H_2CO_3 \leftrightarrow H^+ + HCO_3^-$$

If the valid assumption is made that $[HCO_3^-]$ does not appreciably change, then

$$[H^+] = \frac{(24 \times 80)}{24} = 80 \, nEq/L \text{ and pH} = 7.10$$

$[H^+]$ therefore increases by 40 nEq/L, and since HCO_3^- is produced in a 1:1 ratio with H^+, $[HCO_3^-]$ also increases by 40 nEq/L. Thus, extracellular $[HCO_3^-]$ increases negligibly, from 24 mEq/L to 24.000040 mEq/L. Therefore, the bicarbonate buffer is not effective against increases in $PaCO_2$, and changes in $[HCO_3^-]$ do not reflect the severity of a respiratory acidosis.

Hemoglobin as a Buffer

Hemoglobin is rich in histidine, which is an effective buffer from pH 5.7 to 7.7 (pK_a 6.8). Hemoglobin is the most important noncarbonic buffer in extracellular fluid. Simplistically, hemoglobin may be thought of as existing in red blood cells in equilibrium as a weak acid (HHb) and a potassium salt (KHb). In contrast to the bicarbonate buffer, hemoglobin is capable of buffering both carbonic (CO_2) and noncarbonic (nonvolatile) acids:

$$H^+ + KHb \leftrightarrow HHb + K^+ \text{ and}$$

$$H_2CO_3 + KHb \leftrightarrow HHb + HCO_3^-$$

PULMONARY COMPENSATION

Changes in alveolar ventilation responsible for pulmonary compensation of $PaCO_2$ are mediated by chemoreceptors within the brain stem (see Chapter 22). These receptors respond to changes in cerebrospinal spinal fluid pH. Minute ventilation increases 1–4 L/min for every 1 mm Hg increase in $PaCO_2$. In fact, the lungs are responsible for eliminating the approximately 15 mEq of carbon dioxide produced every day as a byproduct of carbohydrate and fat metabolism. Pulmonary compensatory responses are also important in defending against marked changes in pH during metabolic disturbances.

Pulmonary Compensation during Metabolic Acidosis

Decreases in arterial blood pH stimulate medullary respiratory centers. The resulting increase in alveolar ventilation lowers $PaCO_2$ and tends to restore arterial pH toward normal. The pulmonary response to lower $PaCO_2$ occurs rapidly but may not reach a predictably steady state until 12–24 h; pH is never completely restored to normal. $PaCO_2$ normally decreases 1–1.5 mm Hg below 40 mm Hg for every 1 mEq/L decrease in plasma $[HCO_3^-]$.

Pulmonary Compensation during Metabolic Alkalosis

Increases in arterial blood pH depress respiratory centers. The resulting alveolar hypoventilation tends to elevate $PaCO_2$ and restore arterial pH toward normal. The pulmonary response to metabolic alkalosis is generally less predictable than the response to metabolic acidosis. Hypoxemia, as a result of progressive hypoventilation, eventually activates oxygen-sensitive chemoreceptors; the latter stimulates ventilation and limits the compensatory pulmonary response. Consequently, $PaCO_2$ usually does not rise above 55 mm Hg in response to metabolic alkalosis. As a general rule, $PaCO_2$ can be expected to increase 0.25–1 mm Hg for each 1 mEq/L increase in $[HCO_3^-]$.

RENAL COMPENSATION

The ability of the kidneys to control the amount of HCO_3^- reabsorbed from filtered tubular fluid, form new HCO_3^-, and eliminate H^+ in the form of titratable acids and ammonium ions (see Chapter 31) allows them to exert a major influence on pH during both metabolic and respiratory acid–base disturbances. In fact, the kidneys are responsible for eliminating the approximately 1 mEq/kg per day of sulfuric acid, phosphoric acid, and incompletely oxidized organic acids that are normally produced by the metabolism of dietary and endogenous proteins, nucleoproteins, and organic phosphates (from phosphoproteins and phospholipids). Metabolism of nucleoproteins also produces uric acid. Incomplete combustion of fatty acids and glucose produces keto acids and lactic acid. Endogenous alkali are produced during the metabolism of some anionic amino acids (glutamate and aspartate) and other organic compounds (citrate, acetate, and lactate), but the quantity is insufficient to offset the endogenous acid production.

Renal Compensation during Acidosis

The renal response to acidemia is 3-fold: (1) increased reabsorption of the filtered HCO_3^-, (2) increased excretion of titratable acids, and (3) increased production of ammonia.

Although these mechanisms are probably activated immediately, their effects are generally not appreciable for 12–24 h and may not be maximal for up to 5 days.

A. INCREASED REABSORPTION OF HCO_3^-

Bicarbonate reabsorption is shown in Figure 30–3. CO_2 within renal tubular cells combines with water in the presence of carbonic anhydrase. The carbonic acid (H_2CO_3) formed rapidly dissociates into H^+ and HCO_3^-. Bicarbonate ion then enters the bloodstream while the H^+ is secreted into the renal tubule, where it reacts with filtered HCO_3^- to form H_2CO_3. Carbonic anhydrase associated with the luminal brush border catalyzes the dissociation of H_2CO_3 into CO_2 and H_2O. The CO_2 thus formed can diffuse back into the renal tubular cell to replace the CO_2 originally consumed. The proximal tubules normally reabsorb 80–90% of the filtered bicarbonate load along with sodium, whereas the distal tubules are responsible for the remaining 10–20%. Unlike the proximal H^+ pump, the H^+ pump in the distal tubule is not necessarily linked to sodium reabsorption, and is capable of generating steep H^+ gradients between tubular fluid and tubular cells. Urinary pH can decrease to as low as 4.4 (compared with a pH of 7.40 in plasma).

B. INCREASED EXCRETION OF TITRATABLE ACIDS

After all the HCO_3^- in tubular fluid is reclaimed, the H^+ secreted into the tubular lumen can combine with HPO_4^{2-} to form $H_2PO_4^-$ (Figure 30–4); the latter is

Figure 30–3. Reclamation of filtered HCO_3^- by the proximal renal tubules.

not readily reabsorbed because of its charge and is eliminated in urine. The net result is that H^+ is excreted from the body as $H_2PO_4^-$, and the HCO_3^- that is generated in the process can enter the bloodstream. With a pK of 6.8, the $H_2PO_4^-/HPO_4^{2-}$ pair is normally an ideal urinary buffer. When urinary pH approaches 4.4, however, all the phosphate reaching the distal tubule is in the $H_2PO_4^-$ form; HPO_4^{2-} ions are no longer available for eliminating H^+.

C. INCREASED FORMATION OF AMMONIA

After complete reabsorption of HCO_3^- and consumption of the phosphate buffer, the NH_3/NH_4^+ pair becomes the most important urinary buffer (Figure 30–5). Deamination of glutamine within the mitochondria of proximal tubular cells is the principal source of NH_3 production in the kidneys. Acidemia markedly increases renal NH_3 production. The ammonia formed is then able to passively cross the cell's luminal membrane, enter the tubular fluid, and react with H^+ to form NH_4^+. Unlike NH_3, NH_4^+ does not readily penetrate the luminal membrane and is therefore trapped within the tubules. Thus, excretion of NH_4^+ in urine effectively eliminates H^+.

Figure 30–4. Formation of a titratable acid in urine.

Renal Compensation during Alkalosis

The tremendous amount of HCO_3^- normally filtered and subsequently reabsorbed allows the kidneys to rapidly excrete large amounts of bicarbonate if necessary (see Chapter 28). As a result, the kidneys are highly effective in protecting against metabolic alkalosis, which therefore generally occurs only in association with concomitant sodium deficiency or mineralocorticoid excess. Sodium depletion decreases extracellular fluid volume and enhances Na^+ reabsorption in the proximal tubule. To maintain neutrality, the Na^+ ion is brought across with a Cl^- ion. As Cl^- ions decrease in number (< 10 mEq/L of urine), HCO_3^- must be reabsorbed. In addition, increased H^+ secretion in exchange for augmented Na^+ reabsorption favors continued HCO_3^- formation with metabolic alkalosis. Similarly, increased mineralocorticoid activity augments aldosterone-mediated Na^+ reabsorption in exchange for H^+ secretion in the distal tubules. The resulting increase in HCO_3^- formation can initiate or propagate metabolic alkalosis. Metabolic alkalosis is commonly associated with increased mineralocorticoid activity even in the absence of sodium and chloride depletion.

Base Excess

Base excess is the amount of acid or base that must be added for blood pH to return to 7.40 and $PaCO_2$ to return to 40 mm Hg at full O_2 saturation and 37°C. Moreover, it adjusts for noncarbonic buffering in the blood. Simplistically, base excess represents the metabolic component of an acid–base disturbance. A positive value indicates metabolic alkalosis, whereas a negative value reveals metabolic acidosis. Base excess is usually derived graphically or electronically from a nomogram originally developed by Siggaard-Andersen and requires measurement of hemoglobin concentration (Figure 30–6).

■ ACIDOSIS

PHYSIOLOGICAL EFFECTS OF ACIDEMIA

[H^+] is strictly regulated in the nanomole/liter (36–43 nmol/L) range as H^+ ions have high charge densities and "large" electric fields that can affect the strength of hydro-

Figure 30–5. Formation of ammonia in urine.

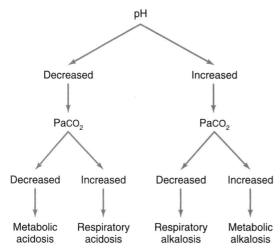

Figure 30–6. Diagnosis of simple acid–base disorders.

gen bonds that are present on most physiological biochemicals. Biochemical reactions are very sensitive to changes in [H⁺]. The overall effects of acidemia seen in patients represent the balance between its direct effects and sympathoadrenal activation. With worsening acidosis (pH < 7.20), direct depressant effects predominate. Direct myocardial and smooth muscle depression reduces cardiac contractility and peripheral vascular resistance, resulting in progressive hypotension. Severe acidosis can lead to tissue hypoxia despite a rightward shift in hemoglobin affinity for oxygen. Both cardiac and vascular smooth muscle become less responsive to endogenous and exogenous catecholamines, and the threshold for ventricular fibrillation is decreased. Progressive hyperkalemia as a result of the movement of K^+ out of cells in exchange for extracellular H^+ is also potentially lethal. Plasma [K⁺] increases approximately 0.6 mEq/L for each 0.10 decrease in pH.

Central nervous system depression is more prominent with respiratory acidosis than with metabolic acidosis. This effect, often termed **CO₂ narcosis,** may be the result of intracranial hypertension secondary to increased cerebral blood flow and of severe intracellular acidosis. Unlike CO_2, H^+ ions do not readily penetrate the blood–brain barrier.

RESPIRATORY ACIDOSIS

Respiratory acidosis is defined as a primary increase in $PaCO_2$. This increase drives the reaction

$$H_2O + CO_2 \leftrightarrow H_2CO_3 \leftrightarrow H^+ + HCO_3^-$$

to the right, leading to an increase in [H⁺] and a decrease in arterial pH. For the reasons described above, [HCO₃⁻] is minimally affected.

$PaCO_2$ represents the balance between CO_2 production and CO_2 elimination:

$$PaCO_2 = \frac{CO_2 \text{ production}}{\text{Alveolar ventilation}}$$

Carbon dioxide production is a byproduct of fat and carbohydrate metabolism. Muscle activity, body temperature, and thyroid hormone activity can all have major influences on CO_2 production. Because CO_2 production does not appreciably vary under most circumstances, respiratory acidosis is usually the result of alveolar hypoventilation (Table 30–3). In patients with a limited capacity to increase alveolar ventilation, however, increased CO_2 production can precipitate respiratory acidosis.

Acute Respiratory Acidosis

The compensatory response to acute (6–12 h) elevations in $PaCO_2$ is limited. Buffering is primarily provided by hemoglobin and the exchange of extracellular H^+ for Na^+ and K^+ from bone and the intracellular fluid compartment (see above). The renal response to retain more bicarbonate is very limited acutely. As a result, plasma [HCO₃⁻] increases only about 1 mEq/L for each 10 mm Hg increase in $PaCO_2$ above 40 mm Hg.

Chronic Respiratory Acidosis

"Full" renal compensation characterizes chronic respiratory acidosis. Renal compensation is appreciable only after 12–24 h and may not peak until 3–5 days. During that time, the sustained increase in $PaCO_2$ has been present long enough to permit maximal renal compensation. During chronic respiratory acidosis, plasma [HCO₃⁻] increases approximately 4 mEq/L for each 10 mm Hg increase in $PaCO_2$ above 40 mm Hg.

Treatment of Respiratory Acidosis

Respiratory acidosis is treated by reversing the imbalance between CO_2 production and alveolar ventilation. In most instances, this is accomplished by increasing alveolar ventilation. Measures aimed at reducing CO_2 production are useful only in specific instances (eg, dantrolene for malignant hyperthermia, muscle paralysis for tetanus, antithyroid medication for thyroid storm, and reduced caloric intake). Temporizing measures aimed at improving alveolar ventilation include bronchodilation, reversal of narcosis, administration of a respiratory stimulant (doxapram), or improving lung compliance (diuresis). Moderate to severe acidosis (pH < 7.20), CO_2 narcosis, and impending respiratory muscle fatigue are indications for mechanical ventilation. An increased inspired oxygen concentration is also usually necessary, as coexistent hypoxemia is common.

Table 30–3. Causes of respiratory acidosis.

Alveolar hypoventilation
  Central nervous system depression
    Drug-induced
    Sleep disorders
    Obesity hypoventilation (Pickwickian) syndrome
    Cerebral ischemia
    Cerebral trauma
  Neuromuscular disorders
    Myopathies
    Neuropathies
  Chest wall abnormalities
    Flail chest
    Kyphoscoliosis
  Pleural abnormalities
    Pneumothorax
    Pleural effusion
  Airway obstruction
    Upper airway
      Foreign body
      Tumor
      Laryngospasm
      Sleep disorders
    Lower airway
      Severe asthma
      Chronic obstructive pulmonary disease
      Tumor
  Parenchymal lung disease
    Pulmonary edema
      Cardiogenic
      Noncardiogenic
    Pulmonary emboli
    Pneumonia
    Aspiration
    Interstitial lung disease
  Ventilator malfunction
Increased CO_2 production
  Large caloric loads
  Malignant hyperthermia
  Intensive shivering
  Prolonged seizure activity
  Thyroid storm
  Extensive thermal injury (burns)

Intravenous $NaHCO_3$ is rarely necessary unless pH is < 7.10 and HCO_3^- is < 15 mEq/L. Sodium bicarbonate therapy will transiently increase $PaCO_2$:

$$H^+ + HCO_3^- \leftrightarrow CO_2 + H_2O$$

Buffers that do not produce CO_2, such as carbicarb or tromethamine (THAM), have been proposed as alternatives but are not of proven benefit (below). Carbicarb is a mixture of 0.3 M sodium bicarbonate and 0.3 M sodium carbonate; buffering by this mix-

ture mainly produces sodium bicarbonate instead of CO_2. Tromethamine has the added advantage of lacking sodium and may be a more effective intracellular buffer.

Patients with a baseline chronic respiratory acidosis require special consideration. When such patients develop acute ventilatory failure, the goal of therapy should be to return $PaCO_2$ to the patient's "normal" baseline. Normalizing the patient's $PaCO_2$ to 40 mm Hg will result in respiratory alkalosis (see below). Oxygen therapy must also be carefully controlled, because the respiratory drive in these patients may be dependent on hypoxemia, not $PaCO_2$; or may increase physiological dead space. "Normalization" of $PaCO_2$ or relative hyperoxia can precipitate severe hypoventilation.

METABOLIC ACIDOSIS

Metabolic acidosis is defined as a primary decrease in $[HCO_3^-]$. Pathological processes can initiate metabolic acidosis by one of three mechanisms: (1) consumption of HCO_3^- by a strong nonvolatile acid, (2) renal or gastrointestinal wasting of bicarbonate, or (3) rapid dilution of the extracellular fluid compartment with a bicarbonate-free fluid.

A fall in plasma $[HCO_3^-]$ without a proportionate reduction in $PaCO_2$ decreases arterial pH. The pulmonary compensatory response in a simple metabolic acidosis (see above) characteristically does not reduce $PaCO_2$ to a level that completely normalizes pH but can produce marked hyperventilation (Kussmaul's respiration).

Table 30–4 lists disorders that can cause metabolic acidosis. Note that differential diagnosis of metabolic acidosis may be facilitated by calculation of the anion gap.

The Anion Gap

The anion gap in plasma is most commonly defined as the difference between the major measured cations and the major measured anions:

Anion Gap =
    Major plasma cations – Major plasma anions

or

$$\text{Anion Gap} = [Na^+] - ([Cl^-] + [HCO_3^-])$$

Some physicians include plasma K^+ in the calculation. Using normal values,

$$\text{Anion Gap} = 140 - (104 + 24) = 12 \text{ mEq/L}$$
$$(\text{normal range} = 7 - 14 \text{ mEq/L})$$

Table 30–4. Causes of metabolic acidosis.

Increased anion gap
  Increased production of endogenous nonvolatile acids
    Renal failure
    Ketoacidosis
      Diabetic
      Starvation
    Lactic acidosis
    Mixed
      Nonketotic hyperosmolar coma
      Alcoholic
    Inborn errors of metabolism
  Ingestion of toxin
    Salicylate
    Methanol
    Ethylene glycol
    Paraldehyde
    Toluene
    Sulfur
  Rhabdomyolysis
Normal anion gap (hyperchloremic)
  Increased gastrointestinal losses of HCO_3^-
    Diarrhea
    Anion exchange resins (cholestyramine)
    Ingestion of $CaCl_2$, $MgCl_2$
    Fistulas (pancreatic, biliary, or small bowel)
    Ureterosigmoidostomy or obstructed ileal loop
  Increased renal losses of HCO_3^-
    Renal tubular acidosis
    Carbonic anhydrase inhibitors
    Hypoaldosteronism
  Dilutional
    Large amount of bicarbonate-free fluids
  Total parenteral nutrition (Cl^- salts of amino acids)
  Increased intake of chloride-containing acids
    Ammonium chloride
    Lysine hydrochloride
    Arginine hydrochloride

In reality, an anion gap cannot exist because electroneutrality must be maintained in the body; the sum of all anions must equal the sum of all cations. Therefore,

$$\text{Anion Gap} = \text{Unmeasured anions} - \text{Unmeasured cations}$$

"Unmeasured cations" include K^+, Ca^{2+}, and Mg^{2+}, whereas "unmeasured anions" include all organic anions (including plasma proteins), phosphates, and sulfates. Plasma albumin normally accounts for the largest fraction of the anion gap (about 11 mEq/L). The anion gap decreases by 2.5 mEq/L for every 1 g/dL reduction in plasma albumin concentration. Any process that increases "unmeasured anions" or decreases "unmeasured cations" will increase the anion gap. Conversely, any pro-

cess that decreases "unmeasured anions" or increases "unmeasured cations" will decrease the anion gap.

Mild elevations of plasma anion gap up to 20 mEq/L may not be helpful diagnostically during acidosis, but values > 30 mEq/L usually indicate the presence of a high anion gap acidosis (below). Metabolic alkalosis can also produce a high anion gap because of extracellular volume depletion, an increased charge on albumin, and a compensatory increase in lactate production. A low plasma anion gap may be encountered with hypoalbuminemia, bromide or lithium intoxication, and multiple myeloma.

High Anion Gap Metabolic Acidosis

Metabolic acidosis with a high anion gap is characterized by an increase in relatively strong nonvolatile acids. These acids dissociate into H^+ and their respective anions; the H^+ consumes HCO_3^- to produce CO_2, whereas their anions (conjugate bases) accumulate and take the place of HCO_3^- in extracellular fluid (hence the anion gap increases). Nonvolatile acids can be endogenously produced or ingested.

A. FAILURE TO EXCRETE ENDOGENOUS NONVOLATILE ACIDS

Endogenously produced organic acids are normally eliminated by the kidneys in urine (above). Glomerular filtration rates below 20 mL/min (renal failure) typically result in progressive metabolic acidosis from the accumulation of these acids.

B. INCREASED ENDOGENOUS NONVOLATILE ACID PRODUCTION

Severe tissue hypoxia following hypoxemia, hypoperfusion (ischemia), or inability to utilize oxygen (cyanide poisoning) can result in lactic acidosis. Lactic acid is the end product of the anaerobic metabolism of glucose (glycolysis) and can rapidly accumulate under these conditions. Decreased utilization of lactate by the liver, and to a lesser extent by the kidneys, is less commonly responsible for lactic acidosis; causes include hypoperfusion, alcoholism, and liver disease. Lactate levels can be readily measured and are normally 0.3–1.3 mEq/L. Acidosis resulting from D-lactic acid, which is not recognized by α-lactate dehydrogenase (and not measured by routine assays), may be encountered in patients with short bowel syndromes; D-lactic acid is formed by colonic bacteria from dietary glucose and starch and is absorbed systemically.

An absolute or relative lack of insulin can result in hyperglycemia and progressive ketoacidosis from accumulation of β-hydroxybutyric and acetoacetic acids. Ketoacidosis may also be seen following starvation and alcoholic binges. The pathophysiology of the acidosis often associated with severe alcoholic intoxication and nonketotic hyperosmolar coma is complex and may represent a build-up of lactic, keto, or other unknown acids.

Some inborn errors of metabolism, such as maple syrup urine disease, methylmalonic aciduria, propionic acidemia, and isovaleric acidemia, produce a high anion gap metabolic acidosis as a result of accumulation of abnormal amino acids.

C. Ingestion of Exogenous Nonvolatile Acids

Ingestion of large amounts of salicylates frequently results in metabolic acidosis. Salicylic acid as well as other acid intermediates rapidly accumulate and produce a high anion gap acidosis. Because salicylates also produce direct respiratory stimulation, most adults develop mixed metabolic acidosis with superimposed respiratory alkalosis. Ingestion of methanol (methyl alcohol) frequently produces acidosis and visual disturbances (retinitis). Symptoms are typically delayed until the slow oxidation of methanol by alcohol dehydrogenase produces formic acid, which is highly toxic to the retina. The high anion gap represents the accumulation of many organic acids, including acetic acid. The toxicity of ethylene glycol is also the result of the action of alcohol dehydrogenase to produce glycolic acid. Glycolic acid, the principal cause of the acidosis, is further metabolized to form oxalic acid, which can be deposited in the renal tubules and result in renal failure.

Normal Anion Gap Metabolic Acidosis

Metabolic acidosis associated with a normal anion gap is typically characterized by hyperchloremia. Plasma $[Cl^-]$ increases to take the place of the HCO_3^- ions that are lost. Hyperchloremic metabolic acidosis most commonly results from abnormal gastrointestinal or renal losses of HCO_3^-.

Calculation of the anion gap in urine can be helpful in diagnosing a normal anion gap acidosis.

$$\text{Urine anion Gap} = ([Na^+] + [K^+]) - [Cl^-]$$

The urine anion gap is normally positive or close to zero. The principal unmeasured urinary cation is normally NH_4^+, which should increase (along with Cl^-) during a metabolic acidosis; the latter results in a negative urinary anion gap. Impairment of H^+ or NH_4^+ secretion, as occurs in renal failure or renal tubular acidosis (below), results in a positive urine anion gap in spite of systemic acidosis.

A. Increased Gastrointestinal Loss of HCO_3^-

 Diarrhea is the most common cause of hyperchloremic metabolic acidosis. Diarrheal fluid contains 20–50 mEq/L of HCO_3^-. Small bowel, biliary, and pancreatic fluids are all rich in HCO_3^-. Loss of large volumes of these fluids can lead to hyperchloremic metabolic acidosis. Patients with ureterosigmoidostomies and those with ileal loops that are too long or that become partially obstructed frequently develop hyperchloremic metabolic acidosis. The ingestion of chloride-containing anion-exchange resins (cholestyramine) or large amounts of calcium or magnesium chloride can result in increased absorption of chloride and loss of bicarbonate ions. These nonabsorbable resins bind bicarbonate ions, whereas calcium and magnesium combine with bicarbonate to form insoluble salts within the intestines.

B. Increased Renal Loss of HCO_3^-

Renal wasting of HCO_3^- can occur as a result of failure to reabsorb filtered HCO_3^- or to secrete adequate amounts of H^+ in the form of titratable acid or ammonium ion. These defects are encountered in patients taking carbonic anhydrase inhibitors such as acetazolamide and in those with renal tubular acidosis.

Renal tubular acidosis comprises a group of nonazotemic defects of H^+ secretion by the renal tubules, resulting in a urinary pH that is too high for the systemic acidemia. These defects may be a result of a primary renal defect or may be secondary to a systemic disorder. The site of the H^+-secreting defect may be in the distal (type 1) or proximal (type 2) renal tubule. Hyporeninemic hypoaldosteronism is commonly referred to as type 4 renal tubular acidosis. With distal renal tubular acidosis, the defect occurs at a site after most of the filtered HCO_3^- has been reclaimed. As a result, there is a failure to acidify the urine, so that net acid excretion is less than daily net acid production. This disorder is frequently associated with hypokalemia, demineralization of bone, nephrolithiasis, and nephrocalcinosis. Alkali ($NaHCO_3$) therapy (1–3 mEq/kg/d) is usually sufficient to reverse those side effects. With the less common proximal renal tubular acidosis, defective H^+ secretion in the proximal tubule results in massive wasting of HCO_3^-. Concomitant defects in tubular reabsorption of other substances such as glucose, amino acids, or phosphates are common. The hyperchloremic acidosis results in volume depletion and hypokalemia. Treatment involves giving alkali (as much as 10–25 mEq/kg per day) and potassium supplements.

C. Other Causes of Hyperchloremic Acidosis

A dilutional hyperchloremic acidosis can occur when extracellular volume is rapidly expanded with a bicarbonate-free fluid such as normal saline. The plasma HCO_3^- decreases in proportion to the amount of fluid infused as extracellular HCO_3^- is diluted. Amino acid infusions (parenteral hyperalimentation) contain organic cations in excess of organic anions and can produce hyperchloremic metabolic acidosis because chloride is commonly used as the anion for the cationic amino acids. Lastly, the administration of excessive quantities of chloride-containing acids such as ammonium chloride or arginine hydrochloride (usually given to treat a metabolic alkalosis) can cause hyperchloremic metabolic acidosis.

Treatment of Metabolic Acidosis

Several general measures can be undertaken to control the severity of acidemia until the underlying processes are corrected. Any respiratory component of the acidemia should be corrected. Respiration should be controlled if necessary; a $PaCO_2$ in the low 30s may be desirable to partially return pH to normal. If arterial blood pH remains below 7.20, alkali therapy, usually in the form of $NaHCO_3$ (usually a 7.5% solution), may be necessary. $PaCO_2$ may transiently rise as HCO_3^- is consumed by acids (emphasizing the need to control ventilation in severe acidemia). The amount of $NaHCO_3$ given is decided empirically as a fixed dose (1 mEq/kg) or is derived from the base excess and the calculated bicarbonate space (see below). In either case, serial blood gas measurements are mandatory to avoid complications (eg, overshoot alkalosis and sodium overload) and to guide further therapy. Raising arterial pH to > 7.25 is usually sufficient to overcome the adverse physiological effects of the acidemia. Profound or refractory acidemia may require acute hemodialysis with a bicarbonate dialysate.

The routine use of large amounts of $NaHCO_3$ in treating cardiac arrest and low flow states is no longer recommended. Paradoxical intracellular acidosis may occur, particularly when CO_2 elimination is impaired, because the CO_2 formed readily enters cells but bicarbonate ion does not. Alternate buffers that do not produce CO_2 may be theoretically preferable, but are unproven clinically.

Specific therapy for diabetic ketoacidosis includes replacement of the existing fluid deficit (as a result of a hyperglycemic osmotic diuresis) first as well as insulin, potassium, phosphate, and magnesium. The treatment of lactic acidosis should be directed first at restoring adequate oxygenation and tissue perfusion. Alkalinization of the urine with $NaHCO_3$ to a pH greater than 7.0 increases elimination of salicylate following salicylate poisoning. Ethanol infusions (an intravenous loading dose of 8–10 mL/kg of a 10% ethanol in D_5 solution over 30 min with the concomitant administration of a continuous infusion at 0.15 mL/kg/h to achieve a blood ethanol level of 100–130 mg/dL) are indicated following methanol or ethylene glycol intoxication. Ethanol competes for alcohol dehydrogenase and slows down the formation of formic acid from methanol and glycolic and oxalic acids from ethylene glycol, respectively.

BICARBONATE SPACE

The bicarbonate space is defined as the volume to which HCO_3^- will distribute when it is given intravenously. Although this theoretically should equal the extracellular fluid space (approximately 25% of body weight), in reality it ranges anywhere between 25% and 60% of body weight depending on the severity and duration of the acidosis. This variation is at least partly related to the amount of intracellular and bone buffering that has taken place.

Example: Calculate the amount of $NaHCO_3$ necessary to correct a base deficit (BD) of –10 mEq/L for a 70-kg man with an estimated HCO_3^- space of 30%:

$$NaHCO_3 = BD \times 30\% \times \text{body weight in L}$$

$$NaHCO_3 = -10 \text{ mEq/L} \times 30\% \times 70 \text{ L} = 210 \text{ mEq}$$

In practice, only 50% of the calculated dose (105 mEq) is usually given, after which another blood gas is measured.

ANESTHETIC CONSIDERATIONS IN PATIENTS WITH ACIDOSIS

Acidemia can potentiate the depressant effects of most sedatives and anesthetic agents on the central nervous and circulatory systems. Because most opioids are weak bases, acidosis can increase the fraction of the drug in the nonionized form and facilitate penetration of the opioid into the brain. Increased sedation and depression of airway reflexes may predispose to pulmonary aspiration. The circulatory depressant effects of both volatile and intravenous anesthetics can also be exaggerated. Moreover, any agent that rapidly decreases sympathetic tone can potentially allow unopposed circulatory depression in the setting of acidosis. Halothane is more arrhythmogenic in the presence of acidosis. Succinylcholine should generally be avoided in acidotic patients with hyperkalemia to prevent further increases in plasma [K$^+$]. Lastly, respiratory—but not metabolic—acidosis augments nondepolarizing neuromuscular blockade and may prevent its antagonism by reversal agents.

◼ ALKALOSIS

PHYSIOLOGICAL EFFECTS OF ALKALOSIS

Alkalosis increases the affinity of hemoglobin for oxygen and shifts the oxygen dissociation curve to the left, making it more difficult for hemoglobin to give up oxygen to tissues. Movement of H$^+$ out of cells in exchange for

Table 30–5. Causes of respiratory alkalosis.

Central stimulation
Pain
Anxiety
Ischemia
Stroke
Tumor
Infection
Fever
Drug-induced
Salicylates
Progesterone (pregnancy)
Analeptics (doxapram)
Peripheral stimulation
Hypoxemia
High altitude
Pulmonary disease
Congestive heart failure
Noncardiogenic pulmonary edema
Asthma
Pulmonary embolism
Severe anemia
Unknown mechanism
Sepsis
Metabolic encephalopathies
Iatrogenic
Ventilator-induced

the movement of extracellular K^+ into cells can produce hypokalemia. Alkalosis increases the number of anionic binding sites for Ca^{2+} on plasma proteins and can therefore decrease ionized plasma $[Ca^{2+}]$, leading to circulatory depression and neuromuscular irritability. Respiratory alkalosis reduces cerebral blood flow, increases systemic vascular resistance, and may precipitate coronary vasospasm. In the lungs, respiratory alkalosis increases bronchial smooth muscle tone (bronchoconstriction) but decreases pulmonary vascular resistance.

RESPIRATORY ALKALOSIS

Respiratory alkalosis is defined as a primary decrease in $PaCO_2$. The mechanism is usually an inappropriate increase in alveolar ventilation relative to CO_2 production. Table 30–5 lists the most common causes of respiratory alkalosis. *Plasma* $[HCO_3^-]$ usually decreases 2 mEq/L for each 10 mm Hg acute decrease in $PaCO_2$ below 40 mm Hg. The distinction between acute and chronic respiratory alkalosis is not always made, because the compensatory response to chronic respiratory alkalosis is quite variable: plasma $[HCO_3^-]$ decreases 2–5 mEq/L for each 10 mm Hg decrease in $PaCO_2$ below 40 mm Hg.

Treatment of Respiratory Alkalosis

Correction of the underlying process is the only treatment for respiratory alkalosis. For severe alkalemia (arterial pH > 7.60), intravenous hydrochloric acid, arginine chloride, or ammonium chloride may be indicated (see below).

METABOLIC ALKALOSIS

Metabolic alkalosis is defined as a primary increase in plasma $[HCO_3^-]$. Most cases of metabolic alkalosis can be divided into (1) those associated with NaCl deficiency and extracellular fluid depletion, often described as chloride sensitive, and (2) those associated with enhanced mineralocorticoid activity, commonly referred to as chloride resistant (Table 30–6).

Chloride-Sensitive Metabolic Alkalosis

Depletion of extracellular fluid causes the renal tubules to avidly reabsorb Na^+. Because not enough Cl^- is avail-

Table 30–6. Causes of metabolic alkalosis.

Chloride-sensitive
Gastrointestinal
Vomiting
Gastric drainage
Chloride diarrhea
Villous adenoma
Renal
Diuretics
Posthypercapnic
Low chloride intake
Sweat
Cystic fibrosis
Chloride-resistant
Increased mineralocorticoid activity
Primary hyperaldosteronism
Edematous disorders (secondary hyperaldosteronism)
Cushing's syndrome
Licorice ingestion
Bartter's syndrome
Severe hypokalemia
Miscellaneous
Massive blood transfusion
Acetate-containing colloid solutions
Alkaline administration with renal insufficiency
Alkali therapy
Combined antacid and cation-exchange resin therapy
Hypercalcemia
Milk-alkali syndrome
Bone metastases
Sodium penicillins
Glucose feeding after starvation

able to accompany all the Na^+ ions reabsorbed, increased H^+ secretion must take place to maintain electroneutrality. In effect, HCO_3^- ions that might otherwise have been excreted are reabsorbed, resulting in metabolic alkalosis. Physiologically, maintenance of extracellular fluid volume is therefore given priority over acid–base balance. Because secretion of K^+ ion can also maintain electroneutrality, potassium secretion is also enhanced. Moreover, hypokalemia augments H^+ secretion (and HCO_3^- reabsorption) and will also propagate metabolic alkalosis. Indeed, severe hypokalemia alone can cause alkalosis. Urinary chloride concentrations during a chloride-sensitive metabolic alkalosis are characteristically low (< 10 mEq/L).

Diuretic therapy is the most common cause of chloride-sensitive metabolic alkalosis. Diuretics such as furosemide, ethacrynic acid, and thiazides increase Na^+, Cl^-, and K^+ excretion, resulting in NaCl depletion, hypokalemia, and usually mild metabolic alkalosis. Loss of gastric fluid is also a common cause of chloride-sensitive metabolic alkalosis. Gastric secretions contain 25–100 mEq/L of H^+, 40–160 mEq/L of Na^+, about 15 mEq/L of K^+, and approximately 200 mEq/L of Cl^-. Vomiting or continuous loss of gastric fluid by gastric drainage (nasogastric suctioning) can result in marked metabolic alkalosis, extracellular volume depletion, and hypokalemia. Rapid normalization of $PaCO_2$ after plasma [HCO_3^-] has risen in chronic respiratory acidosis results in metabolic alkalosis (posthypercapnic alkalosis; see above). Infants being fed formulas containing Na^+ without chloride readily develop metabolic alkalosis because of the increased H^+ (or K^+) secretion that must accompany sodium absorption.

Chloride-Resistant Metabolic Alkalosis

Increased mineralocorticoid activity commonly results in metabolic alkalosis even when it is not associated with extracellular volume depletion. Inappropriate (unregulated) increases in mineralocorticoid activity cause sodium retention and expansion of extracellular fluid volume. Increased H^+ and K^+ secretion takes place to balance enhanced mineralocorticoid-mediated sodium reabsorption, resulting in metabolic alkalosis and hypokalemia. Urinary chloride concentrations are typically greater than 20 mEq/L in such cases.

Other Causes of Metabolic Alkalosis

Metabolic alkalosis is rarely encountered in patients given even large doses of $NaHCO_3$ unless renal excretion of HCO_3^- is impaired. The administration of large amounts of blood products and some plasma protein-containing colloid solution frequently results in metabolic alkalosis. The citrate, lactate, and acetate contained in these fluids are converted by the liver into HCO_3^-. Patients receiving high doses of sodium penicillin (particularly carbenicillin) can develop metabolic alkalosis. Because penicillins act as nonabsorbable anions in the renal tubules, increased H^+ (or K^+) secretion must accompany sodium absorption. For reasons that are not clear, hypercalcemia that results from nonparathyroid causes (milk-alkali syndrome and bone metastases) is also often associated with metabolic alkalosis. The pathophysiology of alkalosis following refeeding is also unknown.

Treatment of Metabolic Alkalosis

As with other acid–base disorders, correction of metabolic alkalosis is never complete until the underlying disorder is treated. When ventilation is controlled, any respiratory component contributing to alkalemia should be corrected by decreasing minute ventilation to normalize $PaCO_2$. The treatment of choice for chloride-sensitive metabolic alkalosis is administration of intravenous saline (NaCl) and potassium (KCl). H_2-blocker therapy is useful when excessive loss of gastric fluid is a factor. Acetazolamide may also be useful in edematous patients. Alkalosis associated with primary increases in mineralocorticoid activity readily responds to aldosterone antagonists (spironolactone). When arterial blood pH is greater than 7.60, treatment with intravenous hydrochloric acid (0.1 mol/L), ammonium chloride (0.1 mol/L), arginine hydrochloride, or hemodialysis should be considered.

ANESTHETIC CONSIDERATIONS IN PATIENTS WITH ALKALEMIA

Respiratory alkalosis appears to prolong the duration of opioid-induced respiratory depression; this effect may result from increased protein binding of opioids. Cerebral ischemia can occur from marked reduction in cerebral blood flow during respiratory alkalosis, particularly during hypotension. The combination of alkalemia and hypokalemia can precipitate severe atrial and ventricular arrhythmias. Potentiation of nondepolarizing neuromuscular blockade is reported with alkalemia but may be more directly related to concomitant hypokalemia.

◼ DIAGNOSIS OF ACID–BASE DISORDERS

Interpretation of acid–base status from analysis of blood gases requires a systematic approach. A recommended approach follows (Figure 30–6):

(1) Examine arterial pH: Is acidemia or alkalemia present?

(2) Examine $PaCO_2$: Is the change in $PaCO_2$ consistent with a respiratory component?

(3) If the change in $PaCO_2$ does not explain the change in arterial pH, does the change in $[HCO_3^-]$ indicate a metabolic component?

(4) Make a tentative diagnosis (see Table 30–1).

(5) Compare the change in $[HCO_3^-]$ with the change in $PaCO_2$. Does a compensatory response exist (Table 30–7)? Because arterial pH is related to the ratio of $PaCO_2$ to $[HCO_3^-]$, both pulmonary and renal compensatory mechanisms are always such that $PaCO_2$ and $[HCO_3^-]$ change in the same direction. A change in opposite directions implies a mixed acid–base disorder.

(6) If the compensatory response is more or less than expected, by definition a mixed acid–base disorder exists.

(7) Calculate the plasma anion gap in the case of metabolic acidosis.

(8) Measure urinary chloride concentration in the case of metabolic alkalosis.

An alternative approach that is rapid but perhaps less precise is to correlate changes in pH with changes in CO_2 or HCO_3. For a respiratory disturbance, every 10 mm Hg change in CO_2 should change arterial pH

Table 30–7. Normal compensatory responses in acid–base disturbances.

Disturbance	Response	Expected Change
Respiratory acidosis		
Acute	↑ $[HCO_3^-]$	1 mEq/L/10 mm Hg increase in $PaCO_2$
Chronic	↑ $[HCO_3^-]$	4 mEq/L/10 mm Hg increase in $PaCO_2$
Respiratory alkalosis		
Acute	↓ $[HCO_3^-]$	2 mEq/L/10 mm Hg decrease in $PaCO_2^-$
Chronic	↓ $[HCO_3^-]$	4 mEq/L/10 mm Hg decrease in $PaCO_2$
Metabolic acidosis	↓ $PaCO_2$	1.2× the decrease in $[HCO_3^-]$
Metabolic alkalosis	↑ $PaCO_2$	0.7× the increase in $[HCO_3^-]$

by approximately 0.08 U in the opposite direction. During metabolic disturbances, every 6 mEq change in HCO_3 also changes arterial pH by 0.1 in the same direction. If the change in pH exceeds or is less than predicated, a mixed acid–base disorder is likely to be present.

MEASUREMENT OF BLOOD GAS TENSIONS & PH

Values obtained by routine blood gas measurement include oxygen and carbon dioxide tensions (PO_2 and PCO_2), pH, $[HCO_3^-]$, base excess, hemoglobin, and the percentage oxygen saturation of hemoglobin. As a rule, only PO_2, PCO_2, and pH are measured. Hemoglobin and percentage oxygen saturation are measured with a cooximeter. $[HCO_3^-]$ is derived using the Henderson–Hasselbalch equation and base excess from the Siggaard-Andersen nomogram.

Sample Source & Collection

Arterial blood samples are most commonly utilized clinically, though capillary or venous blood can be used if the limitations of such samples are recognized. Oxygen tension in venous blood (normally 40 mm Hg) reflects tissue extraction, not pulmonary function. Venous PCO_2 is usually 4–6 mm Hg higher than $PaCO_2$. Consequently, venous blood pH is usually 0.05 U lower than arterial blood pH. Despite these limitations, venous blood is often useful in determining acid–base status. Capillary blood represents a mixture of arterial and venous blood, and the values obtained reflect this fact. Samples are usually collected in heparin-coated syringes and should be analyzed as soon as possible. Air bubbles should be eliminated, and the sample should be capped and placed on ice to prevent significant uptake of gas from blood cells or loss of gases to the atmosphere. Although heparin is highly acidic, excessive amounts of heparin in the sample syringe usually lower pH only minimally but decrease PCO_2 in direct proportion to percentage dilution, and have a variable effect on PO_2.

Temperature Correction

 Changes in temperature affect measurements of PCO_2 and PO_2 directly and measurements of pH indirectly. Decreases in temperature lower the partial pressure of a gas in solution—even though the total gas content does not change—because gas solubility is inversely proportionate to temperature. Both PCO_2 and PO_2 therefore decrease during hypothermia, but pH increases because temperature does not appreciably alter $[HCO_3^-]$: $PaCO_2$ decreases, but $[HCO_3^-]$ is unchanged. Because blood gas tensions and pH are always measured at 37°C, controversy exists over whether to correct the measured values to the patient's actual temperature. "Normal" values at temperatures other than 37°C are not known. Many clinicians use the measurements at 37°C directly, regardless of the patient's actual temperature (see Chapter 21).

PH MEASUREMENT

When a metal is placed in solution with its salt, the tendency of the metal to ionize into the solution leaves the metal with a negative charge. If two different metals (electrodes) and their salts are separated by a porous partition (allowing transfer of charge), the tendency for one metal to go into solution more than the other results in an electromotive force between the two electrodes. For pH measurements, a silver/silver chloride electrode and a mercury/mercurous chloride (calomel) electrode are most commonly used. The silver electrode is in contact with the test solution through pH-sensitive glass. The calomel electrode interfaces with the test solution through a potassium chloride solution and a porous plug. The electromotive force developed between the two electrodes is proportionate to $[H^+]$.

CARBON DIOXIDE MEASUREMENT

Modification of the pH electrode system allows measurement of P_{CO_2}. In this system (the Severinghaus electrode), the two electrodes are separated by a sodium bicarbonate and potassium chloride solution. The test sample is in contact with the bicarbonate solution through a thin Teflon membrane that allows CO_2 to equilibrate between the two. As a result, the pH of the bicarbonate solution reflects the P_{CO_2} of the test solution.

OXYGEN MEASUREMENT

P_{O_2} is most commonly measured polarographically using the Clark electrode. In this system, platinum communicates with a silver/silver chloride electrode through an electrolyte solution (NaCl and KCl). The test sample is separated from the electrolyte solution by a membrane allowing oxygen to diffuse freely. When a negative voltage is applied to the platinum electrode, the electrical current that flows between the two electrodes is directly related to P_{O_2}. In the process, molecules of oxygen take up electrons from the cathode and react with water to form hydroxide ions.

CASE DISCUSSION:
A COMPLEX ACID–BASE
DISTURBANCE

A 1-month-old male infant with an anorectal malformation undergoes anoplasty. Postopera-

tively, he is found to be in congestive heart failure resulting from coarctation of the aorta. He is noted to have tachypnea, decreased urinary output, poor peripheral perfusion, hepatomegaly, and cardiomegaly. Following tracheal intubation, the infant is placed on a ventilator (pressure support ventilation, fraction of inspired oxygen [F_{IO_2}] = 1.0). Initial arterial blood gas, hemoglobin, and electrolyte measurements are as follows:

  Pa_{CO_2} = 11 mm Hg
  pH = 7.47
  Pa_{O_2} = 209 mm Hg
  Calculated [HCO_3^-] = 7.7 mEq/L
  Base deficit = –14.6 mEq/L
  Hb = 9.5 g/dL
  [Na^+] = 135 mEq/L
  [Cl^-] = 95 mEq/L
  [K^+] = 5.5 mEq/L
  [Total CO_2] = 8 mEq/L

Note that the [total CO_2] normally measured with electrolytes includes both plasma [HCO_3^-] and dissolved CO_2 in plasma.

What is the acid–base disturbance?

Using the approach described above, the patient clearly has an alkalosis (pH > 7.45), which is at least partly respiratory in origin (Pa_{CO_2} < 40 mm Hg). Because Pa_{CO_2} has decreased by nearly 30 mm Hg, we would expect [HCO_3^-] to be 18 mEq/L:

$$(40 - 10) \times \frac{2 \text{ mEq/L}}{10} = 6 \text{ mEq/L below 24 mEq/L}$$

In fact, the patient's [HCO_3^-] is nearly 10 mEq/L less than that! The patient therefore also has a mixed acid–base disturbance: primary respiratory alkalosis and primary metabolic acidosis. Note that the difference between the patient's [HCO_3^-] and the [HCO_3^-] expected for a pure respiratory alkalosis roughly corresponds to the base excess.

What are likely causes of these disturbances?

The respiratory alkalosis is probably the result of congestive heart failure, whereas the metabolic acidosis results from lactic acidosis secondary to poor perfusion. The latter is suggested by the calculated plasma anion gap:

$$\text{Anion Gap} = 135 - (95 + 8) = 32 \text{ mEq/L}$$

The lactate level was in fact measured and found to be elevated at 14.4 mEq/L. It is probable that fluid overload precipitated the congestive heart failure.

What treatment is indicated?

Treatment should be directed at the primary process, ie, the congestive heart failure. The patient was treated with digoxin and furosemide. The hemoglobin concentration is low for this infant's age (normal, 14–16 g/L), so transfusion following diuresis is also probably indicated.

Following diuresis, the patient's tachypnea has improved, but perfusion still appears to be poor. Repeat laboratory measurements are as follows ($F_{IO_2} = 0.5$):

$Pa_{CO_2} = 23$ mm Hg
pH = 7.52
$Pa_{O_2} = 136$ mm Hg
Calculated $[HCO_3^-] = 18$ mEq/L
Base deficit = –3.0 mEq/L
Hb = 10.3 g/dL
$[Na^+] = 137$ mEq/L
$[Cl^-] = 92$ mEq/L
$[K^+] = 3.9$ mEq/L
$[Total\ CO_2] = 18.5$ mEq/L

What is the acid–base disturbance?

Respiratory alkalosis is still present, whereas the base deficit appears to have improved. Note that hemoglobin concentration has increased slightly, but $[K^+]$ has decreased as a result of the diuresis. With the new Pa_{CO_2}, the expected $[HCO_3^-]$ should be 20.6 mEq/L:

$$(40 - 23) \times \frac{2\ mEq/L}{10} = 3.4\ mEq/L\ below\ 24\ mEq/L$$

Therefore, the patient still has metabolic acidosis because the $[HCO_3^-]$ is 2 mEq/L less. Note again that this difference is close to the given base deficit and the anion gap is still high:

$$Anion\ Gap = 137 - (92 + 18) = 27$$

The repeat lactate measurement is now 13.2 mEq/L.

The high anion gap and lactate level explain why the patient is still not doing well and indicate that a new process is masking the severity of the metabolic acidosis (which is essentially unchanged).

Given the clinical course, it is likely that the patient now has a triple acid–base disorder: respiratory alkalosis, metabolic acidosis, and now metabolic alkalosis. The latter probably resulted from hypovolemia secondary to excessive diuresis (chloride-sensitive metabolic alkalosis). Note also that the metabolic alkalosis is nearly equal in magnitude to the metabolic acidosis.

The patient was subsequently given packed red blood cells in saline, and within 24 h all three disorders began to improve:

$Pa_{CO_2} = 35$ mm Hg
pH = 7.51
$Pa_{O_2} = 124$ mm Hg
Calculated $[HCO_3^-] = 26.8$ mEq/L
Base excess = +5.0 mEq/L
Hb = 15 g/dL
$[Na^+] = 136$ mEq/L
$[Cl^-] = 91$ mEq/L
$[K^+] = 3.2$ mEq/L
$[Total\ CO_2] = 27$ mEq/L
Lactate = 2.7 mEq/L

Outcome

The respiratory alkalosis and the metabolic acidosis have now resolved, and the metabolic alkalosis is now most prominent.

Intravenous KCl replacement and a small amount of saline were judiciously given, followed by complete resolution of metabolic alkalosis. The patient subsequently underwent surgical correction of the coarctation.

SUGGESTED READING

Kellum JA: Metabolic acidosis in the critically ill: lessons from physical chemistry [clinical management of acute renal failure in the ICU]. Kidney Int 1998;53:S-81. An outstanding review of the changes in understanding of acid–base balance using the work of Stewart and others.

Kraut JA, Madias NE: Approach to patients with acid–base disorders. Respir Care 2001;46:392.

Longenecker JC: *High-Yield Acid-Base.* Williams & Wilkins, 1998.

Pestana C: *Fluids and Electrolytes in the Surgical Patient,* 5th ed. Lippincott, Williams & Wilkins, 2000.

Renal Physiology & Anesthesia

31

KEY CONCEPTS

 The combined blood flow through both kidneys normally accounts for 20–25% of total cardiac output.

 Autoregulation of renal blood flow normally occurs between mean arterial blood pressures of 80 and 180 mm Hg.

 Renal synthesis of vasodilating prostaglandins (PGD_2, PGE_2, and PGI_2) is an important protective mechanism during periods of systemic hypotension and renal ischemia.

 Dopamine and fenoldopam dilate afferent and efferent arterioles via D_1-receptor activation. Fenoldopam and low-dose dopamine infusion can at least partially reverse norepinephrine-induced renal vasoconstriction.

 Reversible decreases in renal blood flow, glomerular filtration rate, urinary flow, and sodium excretion occur during both regional and general anesthesia. These effects can be at least partially overcome by maintenance of an adequate intravascular volume and a normal blood pressure.

 The endocrine response to surgery and anesthesia is probably at least partly responsible for the transient postoperative fluid retention that is seen in many patients.

 Methoxyflurane has been associated with a syndrome of polyuric renal failure. Its nephrotoxicity is dose related and is the result of release of fluoride ions from its metabolic degradation.

 High plasma fluoride concentrations following prolonged enflurane anesthesia may also occur in obese patients and those receiving isoniazid therapy,

 Compound A, a breakdown product of sevoflurane that is formed at low flows, can cause renal damage in laboratory animals. Clinical studies have not detected significant renal injury in humans during sevoflurane anesthesia.

 Certain surgical procedures can significantly alter renal physiology. The pneumoperitoneum produced during laparoscopy produces an abdominal compartment syndrome–like state. The increase in intraabdominal pressure typically produces oliguria (or anuria). Other surgical procedures that can significantly compromise renal function include cardiopulmonary bypass, cross-clamping of the aorta, and dissection near the renal arteries.

The kidneys play a vital role in regulating the volume and composition of body fluids, eliminating toxins, and elaborating hormones such as renin, erythropoietin, and the active form of vitamin D. Surgery and anesthesia can have important effects on renal function. Failure to take these effects into consideration could result in serious errors in patient management. Fluid overload, hypovolemia, and postoperative renal failure are major causes of postoperative morbidity and mortality.

Figure 31–1. Major anatomic divisions of the nephron. (Modified and reproduced, with permission, from Ganong WF: *Review of Medical Physiology,* 20th ed. McGraw-Hill, 2001.)

Diuretics are an important class of drugs that is frequently employed in the perioperative period. Preoperative diuretic therapy is common in patients with hypertension and with cardiac, hepatic, and renal disease. Diuretics are also used intraoperatively, particularly during neurosurgical, cardiac, major vascular, ophthalmic, and urological procedures. Familiarity with the various types of diuretics, their mechanisms of action, side effects, and potential anesthetic interactions is therefore essential.

THE NEPHRON

Each kidney is made up of approximately 1 million functional units called nephrons. Anatomically, a nephron consists of a tortuous tubule with at least six specialized segments. At its proximal end (Bowman's capsule), an ultrafiltrate of blood is formed, and as this fluid passes through the nephron, its volume and composition are modified by both the reabsorption and the secretion of solutes. The final product is eliminated as urine.

The six major anatomic and functional divisions of the nephron include the glomerular capillaries, the proximal convoluted tubule, the loop of Henle, the distal renal tubule, the collecting tubule, and the juxtaglomerular apparatus (Figure 31–1 and Table 31–1).

The Glomerular Capillaries

The glomerulus is composed of tufts of capillaries that jut into Bowman's capsule, providing a large surface area for the filtration of blood. Blood flow is provided by a single afferent arteriole and is drained by a single efferent arteriole (see below). Endothelial cells in glomeruli are separated from the epithelial cells of Bowman's capsule only by their fused basement membranes. The endothelial cells are perforated with relatively large fenestrae (70–100 nm), but the epithelial cells interdigitate tightly with one another, leaving relatively small filtration slits (about 25 nm). The two cell types with their basement membranes provide an effective filtration barrier for cells and large-molecular-weight substances. This barrier appears to have multiple anionic sites that give it a net negative charge, which favors the filtration of cations but somewhat hinders filtration of anions. A third cell type, mesangial cells, are located between the basement membrane and epithelial cells near adjacent capillaries. Mesangial cells are thought to play a significant role in the regulation of glomerular filtration. They contain contractile proteins that respond to vasoactive substance, secrete various substances, and take up immune complexes. Mesangial cells contract, reducing glomerular filtration, in response to angiotensin II, vasopressin, norepinephrine, histamine, endothelins, thromboxane A_2, leukotrienes (C_4 and D_4), prostaglandin F_2, and platelet-activating factor. They relax, increasing filtration, in response to atrial natriuretic peptide (ANP), prostaglandin E_2, and dopamine.

Glomerular filtration pressure (about 60 mm Hg) is normally about 60% of mean arterial pressure and is opposed by both plasma oncotic pressure (about 25 mm Hg) and renal interstitial pressure (about 10 mm Hg). Both afferent and efferent arteriolar tones are important determinants of filtration pressure: Filtration pressure is directly proportional to efferent arteriolar tone, but inversely proportional to afferent arteriolar tone. Approximately 20% of plasma is normally filtered as blood passes through the glomerulus.

The Proximal Tubule

Of the ultrafiltrate formed in Bowman's capsule 65–75% is normally reabsorbed isotonically (proportional amounts of water and sodium) in the proximal renal tubules (Figure 31–2). To be reabsorbed, most substances must first

Table 31–1. Functional divisions of a nephron.[1]

Segment	Function
Glomerulus	Ultrafiltration of blood

Proximal tubule	Reabsorption
	    Sodium[2] chloride
	    Water
	    Bicarbonate
	    Glucose, protein, amino acids
	    Potassium, magnesium, calcium
	    Phosphates,[3] uric acid, urea
	Secretion
	    Organic anions
	    Organic cations
	Ammonia production

Loop of Henle	Reabsorption
	    Sodium, chloride
	    Water
	    Potassium, calcium, magnesium
	Countercurrent multiplier

Distal tubule	Reabsorption
	    Sodium[4] chloride
	    Water
	    Potassium
	    Calcium[5]
	    Bicarbonate
	Secretion
	    Hydrogen ion[4]
	    Potassium[4]
	    Calcium

Collecting tubule	Reabsorption
	    Sodium[4,6] chloride
	    Water[6,7]
	    Potassium
	    Bicarbonate
	Secretion
	    Potassium[4]
	    Hydrogen ion[4]
	Ammonia production

Juxtaglomerular apparatus	Secretion of renin

[1]Adapted from Rose BD: *Clinical Physiology of Acid-Base and Electrolyte Disorders,* 3rd ed. McGraw-Hill, 1989.
[2]Partially augmented by angiotensin II.
[3]Inhibited by parathyroid hormone.
[4]At least partly aldosterone mediated.
[5]Augmented by parathyroid hormone.
[6]Inhibited by atrial natriuretic peptide.
[7]Antidiuretic hormone mediated.

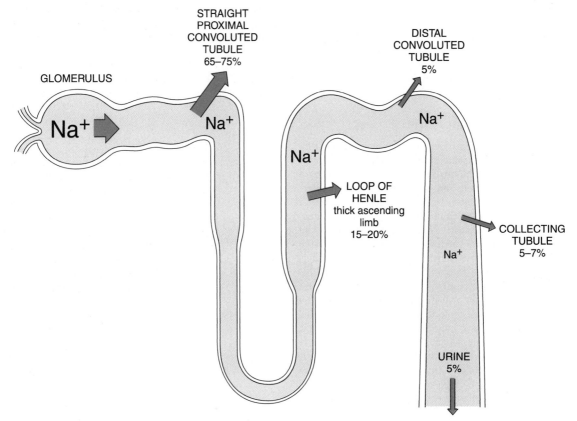

Figure 31–2. Sodium reabsorption in the nephron. Numbers represent the percentage of the filtered sodium reabsorbed at each site. (Modified and reproduced, with permission, from Cogan MG: *Fluid and Electrolytes: Physiology and Pathophysiology.* Appleton & Lange, 1991.)

traverse the tubular (apical) side of the cell membrane, and then cross the basolateral cell membrane into the renal interstitium before entering peritubular capillaries. The major function of the proximal tubule is Na^+ reabsorption. Sodium is actively transported out of proximal tubular cells at their capillary side by membrane-bound Na^+–K^+-adenosine triphosphatase (ATPase) (Figure 31–3). The resulting low intracellular concentration of Na^+ allows passive movement of Na^+ down its gradient from tubular fluid into epithelial cells. Angiotensin II and norepinephrine enhance Na^+ reabsorption in the early proximal tubule. In contrast, dopamine and fenoldopam decrease the proximal reabsorption of sodium via D_1-receptor activation.

Sodium reabsorption is coupled with the reabsorption of other solutes and the secretion of H^+ (Figure 31–3). Specific carrier proteins use the low concentration of Na^+ inside cells to transport phosphate, glucose, and amino acids. The net loss of intracellular positive charges, the result of Na^+–K^+-ATPase activity

(exchanging $3Na^+$ for $2K^+$), favors the absorption of other cations (K^+, Ca^{2+}, and Mg^{2+}). Thus, the Na^+–K^+-ATPase at the basolateral side of the renal cells provides the energy for the reabsorption of most solutes. Sodium reabsorption at the luminal membrane is also coupled with countertransport (secretion) of H^+. The latter mechanism is responsible for reabsorption of 90% of the filtered bicarbonate ions (see Figure 30–3). Unlike other solutes, chloride can traverse the tight junctions between adjacent tubular epithelial cells. As a result, chloride reabsorption is generally passive and follows its concentration gradient. Active chloride reabsorption may also take place as a result of a K^+–Cl^- cotransporter that extrudes both ions at the capillary side of the cell membrane (Figure 31–3). Water moves passively out the proximal tubule along osmotic gradients. Specialized water channels, composed of a membrane protein called aquaporin-1, in the apical membranes of epithelial cells facilitate water movement.

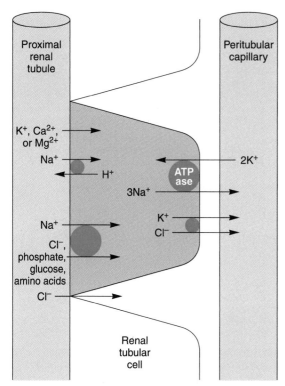

Figure 31–3. Reabsorption of solutes in proximal tubules. Note that Na+–K+-ATPase supplies the energy for reabsorption of most solutes by maintaining a low intracellular concentration of sodium.

The proximal tubules are capable of secreting organic cations and anions. Organic cations such as creatinine, cimetidine, and quinidine may share the same pump mechanism and thus can interfere with the excretion of one another. Organic anions such as urate, keto acids, penicillins, cephalosporins, diuretics, salicylates, and most x-ray dyes also appear to share common secretory mechanisms. Both pumps probably play a major role in the elimination of many circulating toxins. Low-molecular-weight proteins, which are filtered by glomeruli, are normally reabsorbed by proximal tubular cells but are metabolized intracellularly.

The Loop of Henle

The loop of Henle consists of descending and ascending portions. The thin descending segment is a continuation of the proximal tubule and descends from the renal cortex into the renal medulla. In the medulla, the descending portion acutely turns back upon itself and rises back up toward the cortex as the ascending portion. The ascending portion consists of a functionally distinct, thin ascending limb, a medullary thick ascending limb, and a cortical thick ascending limb (Figure 31–1). Cortical nephrons (30–40%) have relatively short loops of Henle, whereas those near the medulla (juxtamedullary nephrons, 10%) loop deeply into the medulla. Cortical nephrons with short loops lack a thin ascending limb. Cortical nephrons outnumber juxtamedullary nephrons by approximately 7:1. The loop of Henle is responsible for maintaining a hypertonic medullary interstitium and indirectly provides the collecting tubules with the ability to concentrate urine.

Only 25–35% of the ultrafiltrate formed in Bowman's capsule normally reaches the loop of Henle. This part of the nephron usually reabsorbs 15–20% of the filtered sodium load. With the notable exception of the ascending thick segments, solute and water reabsorption in the loop of Henle is passive and follows concentration and osmotic gradients, respectively. In the ascending thick segment, however, Na+ and Cl− are reabsorbed in excess of water; moreover, Na+ reabsorption in this part of the nephron is directly coupled to both K+ and Cl− reabsorption (Figure 31–4), and [Cl−] in tubular fluid

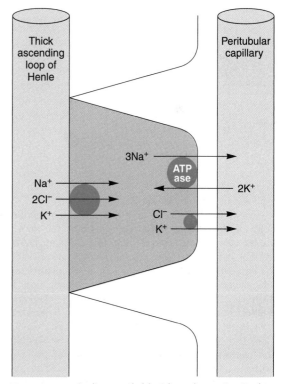

Figure 31–4. Sodium and chloride reabsorption in the thick ascending loop of Henle. All four sites on the luminal carrier protein must be occupied for transport to occur. The rate-limiting factor appears to be chloride concentration in tubular fluid.

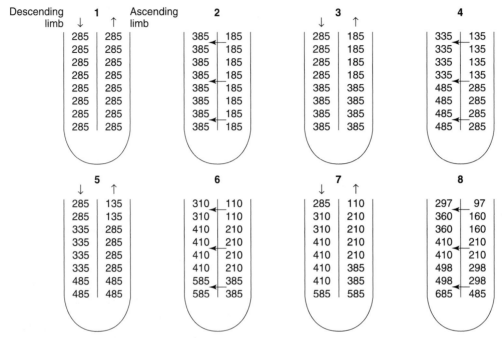

Figure 31–5. The countercurrent multiplier mechanism. This mechanism is dependent on differential permeability and transport characteristics between the descending and ascending limbs. The descending limb and the thin ascending limb are permeable to water, Na^+, Cl^-, and urea. The thick ascending limb is impermeable to water and urea, actively reabsorbs Na^+ and Cl^-, and therefore can generate an osmotic gradient. This figure depicts from "time zero" a progressive 200 mOsm/kg gradient between the descending and ascending limbs. Note that as urine flows, the gradient remains unchanged but the osmolality progressively increases at the bottom of the loop. (Adapted from Pitts RF: *Physiology of the Kidney and Body Fluids,* 3rd ed. Year Book, 1974.)

appears to be the rate-limiting factor. Active Na^+ reabsorption still results from Na^+–K^+-ATPase activity on the capillary side of epithelial cells.

Unlike the descending limb and the thin ascending limb, the thick parts of the ascending limb are impermeable to water. As a result, tubular fluid flowing out of the loop of Henle is hypotonic (100–200 mOsm/L) and the interstitium surrounding the loop of Henle is therefore hypertonic. A countercurrent multiplier mechanism is established such that both the tubular fluid and medullary interstitium become increasingly hypertonic with increasing depth into the medulla (Figure 31–5). Urea also reaches high concentrations in the medulla and contributes substantially to its hypertonicity. The countercurrent mechanism includes the loop of Henle, the cortical and medullary collecting tubules, and their respective capillaries (vasa recta).

The thick ascending loop of Henle is also an important site for calcium and magnesium reabsorption. Parathyroid hormone may augment calcium reabsorption at this site.

The Distal Tubule

The distal tubule receives hypotonic fluid from the loop of Henle and is normally responsible for only minor modifications of tubular fluid. In contrast to more proximal portions, the distal nephron has very tight junctions between tubular cells and is relatively impermeable to water and sodium. It can therefore maintain the gradients generated by the loop of Henle. Sodium reabsorption in the distal tubule normally accounts for only about 5% of the filtered sodium load. As in other parts of the nephron, the energy is derived from Na^+–K^+-ATPase activity on the capillary side, but on the luminal side Na^+ is reabsorbed by an Na^+–Cl^- carrier. Sodium reabsorption in this segment is directly proportional to Na^+ delivery. The distal tubule is the major site of parathyroid hormone– and vitamin D–mediated calcium reabsorption.

The late distal tubule is referred to as the connecting segment. Although it is also involved in hormone-mediated calcium reabsorption, unlike more proximal portions, it participates in aldosterone-mediated Na^+ reabsorption.

Figure 31–6. Secretion of hydrogen ions and reabsorption of bicarbonate and potassium in the cortical collecting tubule.

The Collecting Tubule

This tubule can be divided into cortical and medullary portions. Together, they normally account for the reabsorption of 5–7% of the filtered sodium load.

A. CORTICAL COLLECTING TUBULE

This part of the nephron consists of two cell types: (1) principal cells (P cells), which primarily secrete potassium and participate in aldosterone-mediated Na^+ reabsorption, and (2) intercalated cells (I cells), which are responsible for acid–base regulation. Because P cells reabsorb Na^+ via an electrogenic pump, either Cl^- must also be reabsorbed or K^+ must be secreted to maintain electroneutrality. Increases in intracellular $[K^+]$ favor K^+ secretion. Aldosterone enhances Na^+–K^+-ATPase activity in this part of the nephron by increasing the number of open K^+ and Na^+ channels in the luminal membrane. Aldosterone also enhances the H^+-secreting ATPase on the luminal border of I cells (Figure 31–6). I cells additionally have a luminal K^+–H^+-ATPase pump, which reabsorbs K^+ and secretes H^+. Some I cells are capable of secreting bicarbonate ion in response to large alkaline loads.

B. MEDULLARY COLLECTING TUBULE

The medullary collecting tubule courses down from the cortex through the hypertonic medulla before joining collecting tubules from other nephrons to form a single ureter in each kidney. This part of the collecting tubule is the principal site of action for antidiuretic hormone (ADH), also called arginine vasopressin (AVP); this hormone activates adenylate cyclase via V_2 receptors. (V_1 receptors increase vascular resistance.) ADH stimulates the expression of a water channel protein, aquaporin-2, in the cell membrane. The permeability of the luminal membrane to water is entirely dependent of the presence of ADH (see Chapter 28). Dehydration increases ADH secretion, rendering the luminal membrane permeable to water. As a result, water is osmotically drawn out of the tubular fluid passing through the medulla, and a concentrated urine (up to 1400 mOsm/L) is produced. Conversely, adequate hydration suppresses ADH secretion; the fluid in the collecting tubules therefore passes through the medulla unchanged and remains hypotonic (100–200 mOsm/L). The medullary collecting tubule also possesses P and I cells, but the latter predominate. Moreover, this part of the nephron is responsible for acidifying urine; the hydrogen ions secreted are excreted in the form of titratable acids (phosphates) and ammonium ions (see Chapter 30).

C. ROLE OF THE COLLECTING TUBULE IN MAINTAINING A HYPERTONIC MEDULLA

Differential permeability for urea between the cortical and medullary collecting tubules accounts for up to half the hypertonicity of the renal medulla. Cortical collecting tubules are freely permeable to urea, whereas medullary collecting tubules are normally impermeable. In the presence of ADH, the innermost part of the medullary collecting tubules becomes even more permeable to urea. Thus, when ADH is secreted, water moves out of the collecting tubules and the urea becomes highly concentrated. Urea can then diffuse out deeply into the medullary interstitium, increasing its tonicity.

The Juxtaglomerular Apparatus

This small organ within each nephron consists of a specialized segment of the afferent arteriole, containing juxtaglomerular cells within its wall, and the end of the thick, ascending cortical segment of the loop of Henle, the macula densa (Figure 31–7). Juxtaglomerular cells contain the enzyme renin and are innervated by the sympathetic nervous system. Release of renin depends on β_1-adrenergic sympathetic stimulation, changes in afferent arteriolar wall pressure (see Chapter 28), and changes in chloride flow past the macula densa. Renin released into the bloodstream acts on angiotensinogen, a protein synthesized by the liver, to form angiotensin I. This inert decapeptide is then rapidly converted, primarily in the

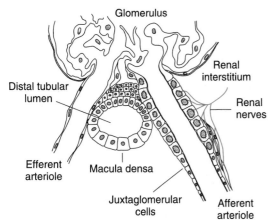

Glomerulus

Distal tubular lumen

Renal interstitium

Renal nerves

Efferent arteriole

Macula densa

Juxtaglomerular cells

Afferent arteriole

Figure 31–7. The juxtaglomerular apparatus. (Modified and reproduced, with permission, from Ganong WF: *Review of Medical Physiology,* 20th ed. McGraw-Hill, 2001.)

lungs, by angiotensin-converting enzyme (ACE) to form the octapeptide angiotensin II. Angiotensin II plays a major role in blood pressure regulation (see Chapter 19) and aldosterone secretion (see Chapter 28). Proximal renal tubular cells have converting enzyme as well as angiotensin II receptors. Moreover, intrarenal formation of angiotensin II enhances sodium reabsorption in proximal tubules. Some extrarenal production of renin and angiotensin II also takes place in the vascular endothelium, the adrenal glands, and the brain.

■ THE RENAL CIRCULATION

Renal function is intimately related to renal blood flow (RBF). In fact, the kidneys are the only organs for which oxygen consumption is determined by blood flow; the reverse is true in other organs. The combined blood flow through both kidneys normally accounts for 20–25% of total cardiac output. Approximately 80% of RBF normally goes to cortical nephrons, and only 10–15% goes to juxtamedullary nephrons. The renal cortex extracts relatively little oxygen, having an oxygen tension of about 50 mm Hg, because of the relatively high blood flow with a mostly filtration function. In contrast, the renal medulla maintains high metabolic activity because of solute reabsorption and requires low blood flow to maintain high osmotic gradients. The medulla has an oxygen tension of only about 15 mm Hg and is readily vulnerable to ischemia.

Redistribution of RBF away from cortical nephrons with short loops of Henle to larger juxtamedullary neph-

rons with long loops is known to occur under certain conditions. Sympathetic stimulation, increased levels of catecholamines and angiotensin II, and heart failure can cause redistribution of RBF to the medulla. Although the significance of this redistribution remains controversial, it appears to be clinically associated with sodium retention.

In most persons, each kidney is supplied by a single renal artery arising from the aorta. The renal artery then divides at the renal pelvis into interlobar arteries, which in turn give rise to arcuate arteries at the junction between the renal cortex and medulla (Figure 31–8). Arcuate arteries further divide into interlobular branches that eventually supply each nephron via a single afferent arteriole. Blood from each glomerulus is drained via a single efferent arteriole and then travels alongside adjacent renal tubules in a second (peritubular) system of capillaries. In contrast to the glomerular capillaries, which favor filtration, peritubular capillaries are primarily "reabsorptive." Venules draining the second capillary plexus finally return blood to the inferior vena cava via a single renal vein on each side.

RENAL BLOOD FLOW & GLOMERULAR FILTRATION

Clearance

The concept of clearance is frequently used in measurements of renal blood flow and the glomerular filtration rate (GFR). The renal clearance of a substance is defined as the volume of blood that is completely cleared of that substance per unit of time (usually, per minute).

Renal Blood Flow

Renal plasma flow (RPF) is most commonly measured by *p*-aminohippurate (PAH) clearance. PAH at low plasma concentrations can be assumed to be completely cleared from plasma by filtration and secretion in one passage through the kidneys. Consequently

$$\text{RPF} = \text{Clearance of PAH} = \left(\frac{[\text{PAH}]_U}{[\text{PAH}]_P}\right) \times \text{Urine flow}$$

where $[\text{PAH}]_U$ = urinary concentration of PAH and $[\text{PAH}]_P$ = plasma PAH concentration.

If the hematocrit is known, then

$$\text{RBF} = \frac{\text{RPF}}{(1 - \text{Hematocrit})}$$

RPF and RBF are normally about 660 and 1200 mL/min, respectively.

Glomerular Filtration Rate

The GFR is normally about 20% of RPF. Clearance of inulin, a fructose polysaccharide that is completely fil-

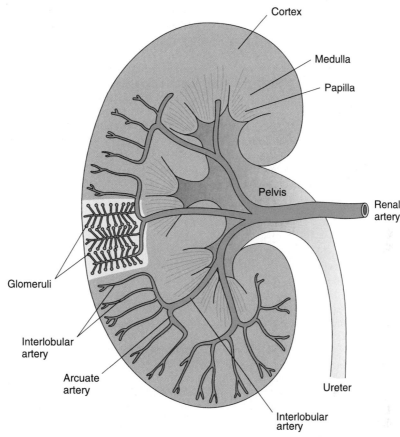

Figure 31–8. The renal circulation. (Modified and reproduced, with permission, from Leaf A, Cotran RS: *Renal Pathophysiology.* Oxford University Press, 1976.)

tered but is neither secreted nor reabsorbed, is a good measure of GFR. Normal values for GFR are about 120 ± 25 mL/min in men and 95 ± 20 mL/min in women. Although less accurate than measuring inulin clearance, creatinine clearance is a much more practical measurement of GFR (see Chapter 32). Creatinine clearance tends to overestimate GFR because some creatinine is normally secreted by renal tubules. Creatinine is a product of phosphocreatine breakdown in muscle. Creatinine clearance is calculated as follows:

$$\text{Creatinine clearance} = \frac{([\text{Creatinine}]_U \times \text{Urinary flow rate})}{[\text{Creatinine}]_P}$$

where $[\text{creatinine}]_U$ = creatinine concentration in urine and $[\text{creatinine}]_P$ = creatinine concentration in plasma.

The ratio of GFR to RPF is called the filtration fraction (FF) and is normally 20%. GFR is dependent on the relative tones of both the afferent and efferent arterioles (see above). Afferent arteriolar dilatation or efferent arteriolar vasoconstriction can increase the FF and maintain GFR, even when RPF decreases. Afferent arteriolar tone appears to be responsible for maintaining GFR nearly constant over a wide range of blood pressures.

Control Mechanisms

Regulation of renal blood flow represents a complex interplay between intrinsic autoregulation, tubuloglomerular balance, and hormonal and neuronal influences.

A. INTRINSIC REGULATION

Autoregulation of RBF normally occurs between mean arterial blood pressures of 80 and 180 mm Hg. Blood flow is generally decreased at mean arterial pressures less than 70 mm Hg. Although the exact mechanism is not known, it is thought to be an intrinsic myogenic response of the afferent arterioles to changes in blood pressure. Within these limits, RBF (and GFR) can be kept relatively constant by afferent arteriolar vasoconstriction or vasodilation. Outside the autoregulation limits, RBF becomes pressure dependent. Glomerular filtration generally ceases when mean systemic arterial pressure is less than 40–50 mm Hg.

B. TUBULOGLOMERULAR BALANCE AND FEEDBACK

Changes in renal tubular flow rates affect GFR: Increases in tubular flow tend to reduce GFR, whereas decreases in flow tend to favor increases in GFR. Tubuloglomerular feedback probably plays an important role in maintaining GFR constant over a wide range of perfusion pressures. Although the mechanism is poorly understood, the macula densa appears to be responsible for tubuloglomerular feedback by inducing reflex changes in afferent arteriolar tone and possibly glomerular capillary permeability. Angiotensin II probably plays a permissive role in this mechanism. Local release of adenosine (which occurs in response to volume expansion) may inhibit renin release and dilate the afferent arteriole. The phenomenon of pressure natriuresis, or decreased sodium reabsorption in response to increases in blood pressure, likely reflects tubuloglomerular feedback.

C. HORMONAL REGULATION

Increases in afferent arteriolar pressure stimulate renin release and formation of angiotensin II. Angiotensin II causes generalized arterial vasoconstriction and secondarily reduces RBF. Both afferent and efferent arterioles are constricted but because the efferent arteriole is smaller, its resistance becomes greater than that of the afferent arteriole; GFR therefore tends to be relatively preserved. Very high levels of angiotensin II constrict both arterioles and can markedly decrease GFR. Adrenal catecholamines (epinephrine and norepinephrine) directly and preferentially increase afferent arteriolar tone, but marked decreases in GFR are minimized indirectly through activation of renin release and angiotensin II formation. Relative preservation of GFR during increased aldosterone or catecholamine secretion appears to be at least partly mediated by angiotensin-induced prostaglandin synthesis and is blocked by inhibitors of prostaglandin synthesis (nonsteroidal antiinflammatory drugs). Renal synthesis of vasodilating prostaglandins (PGD_2, PGE_2, and PGI_2) is an important protective mechanism during periods of systemic hypotension and renal ischemia.

ANP is released from atrial myocytes in response to distention. ANP is a direct smooth muscle dilator and antagonizes the vasoconstrictive action of norepinephrine and angiotensin II. It appears to preferentially dilate the afferent arteriole, may constrict the efferent arteriole, and relaxes mesangial cells, effectively increasing GFR (see Chapter 28). ANP also inhibits both the release of renin and angiotensin-induced secretion of aldosterone, and antagonizes the action of aldosterone in the distal and collecting tubules.

D. NEURONAL REGULATION

Sympathetic outflow from the spinal cord at T4–L1 reaches the kidneys via the celiac and renal plexuses. Sympathetic nerves innervate the juxtaglomerular apparatus (β_1) as well as the renal vasculature (α_1). This innervation is probably responsible for stress-induced reductions in RBF (below). α_1-Adrenergic receptors enhance sodium reabsorption in proximal tubules, whereas α_2-receptors decrease such reabsorption and promote water excretion.

Dopamine and fenoldopam dilate afferent and efferent arterioles via D_1-receptor activation. Unlike dopamine, fenoldopam is selective for the D_1-receptor. Fenoldopam and low-dose dopamine infusion can at least partially reverse norepinephrine-induced renal vasoconstriction. Activation of D_2-receptors on presynaptic postganglionic sympathetic neurons can also vasodilate arterioles through inhibition of norepinephrine secretion (negative feedback). Dopamine, which is formed in the proximal tubules as well as released from nerve endings, reduces proximal reabsorption of Na^+. Some cholinergic vagal fibers are also present, but their role is poorly understood.

■ EFFECTS OF ANESTHESIA & SURGERY ON RENAL FUNCTION

Clinical studies attempting to define the effects of anesthetic agents on renal function are complicated by difficulties in differentiating between direct and indirect effects and often fail to control many important variables. These variables include the type of surgical procedure, fluid administration, and preexisting cardiac and renal function. Several conclusions, however, can be stated:

(1) Reversible decreases in RBF, GFR, urinary flow, and sodium excretion occur during both regional and general anesthesia.

(2) Changes are generally less marked during regional anesthesia.

(3) Most of these changes are indirect and are mediated by autonomic and hormonal influences.

(4) These effects can be at least partially overcome by maintenance of an adequate intravascular volume and a normal blood pressure.

(5) Only a few anesthetics (methoxyflurane and, theoretically, enflurane and sevoflurane) in high doses can cause specific renal toxicity.

INDIRECT EFFECTS

Cardiovascular Effects

Most inhalation and intravenous anesthetics cause some degree of cardiac depression or vasodilation and therefore are capable of decreasing arterial blood pressure. The sympathetic blockade associated with regional anesthesia (spinal or epidural) can similarly cause hypotension as a result of increased venous capacitance and arterial vasodilation. Decreases in blood pressure below the limits of autoregulation can therefore be expected to reduce RBF, GFR, urinary flow, and sodium excretion. Intravenous fluid administration often at least partially reverses the hypotension and ameliorates its effects on renal function.

Neural Effects

Sympathetic activation commonly occurs in the perioperative period as a result of light anesthesia, intense surgical stimulation, tissue trauma, or anesthetic-induced circulatory depression. Sympathetic overactivity increases renal vascular resistance and activates various hormonal systems. Both effects tend to reduce RBF, GFR, and urinary output.

Endocrine Effects

Endocrine changes during anesthesia generally reflect a stress response that may be induced by surgical stimulation, circulatory depression, hypoxia, or acidosis. Increases in catecholamines (epinephrine and norepinephrine), renin, angiotensin II, aldosterone, ADH, adrenocorticotropic hormone, and cortisol are common. Catecholamines, ADH, and angiotensin II all reduce RBF by inducing renal arterial constriction. Aldosterone enhances sodium reabsorption in the distal tubule and collecting tubule, resulting in sodium retention and expansion of the extracellular fluid compartment (see Chapter 28). Nonosmotic release of ADH also favors water retention and, if marked, may result in hyponatremia (see Chapter 28). The endocrine response to surgery and anesthesia is probably at least partly responsible for the transient postoperative fluid retention that is seen in many patients.

DIRECT ANESTHETIC EFFECTS

The direct effects of anesthetics on renal function are minor compared with the secondary effects described above.

Volatile Agents

Halothane, enflurane, and isoflurane have been reported to decrease renal vascular resistance. Studies of their effect on autoregulation have had conflicting results. In some animal studies, halothane appears to depress sodium reabsorption.

Methoxyflurane has been associated with a syndrome of polyuric renal failure. Its nephrotoxicity is dose related and is the result of release of fluoride ions from its metabolic degradation. Plasma fluoride concentrations greater than 50 μmol/L have been associated with renal toxicity that is characterized by a defect in urinary concentrating ability. Methoxyflurane doses greater than 1 minimum alveolar concentration for 2 h are associated with a high incidence of renal impairment. Fluoride production is negligible during halothane, desflurane, and isoflurane anesthesia but can become significant following the prolonged administration of enflurane and possibly sevoflurane. Because fluoride excretion is dependent on GFR, patients with preexisting renal impairment may be more susceptible to this syndrome. High plasma fluoride concentrations following prolonged enflurane anesthesia may also occur in obese patients and those receiving isoniazid therapy, but an increased incidence of renal dysfunction has not been reported.

Compound A, a breakdown product of sevoflurane that is formed at low flows, can cause renal damage in laboratory animals. Clinical studies have not detected significant renal injury in humans during sevoflurane anesthesia. Nonetheless, most authorities recommend fresh gas flow of at least 2 L/min with sevoflurane to prevent significant production of compound A.

Intravenous Agents

Studies on opioids and barbiturates generally show minor effects when they are used alone. In the presence of nitrous oxide, these agents can produce effects similar to those observed with volatile agents. Ketamine is reported to minimally affect renal function and to preserve renal function during hemorrhagic hypovolemia. Agents with α-adrenergic blocking activity, such as droperidol, may prevent catecholamine-induced redistribution of RBF. Drugs with antidopaminergic activity—such as metoclopramide, phenothiazines, and droperidol—may impair the renal response to dopamine. Inhibition of prostaglandin synthesis by analgesics such as ketorolac prevents the renal production of vasodilatory prostaglandins in patients with high levels of angiotensin II and norepinephrine; attenuation of this protective response can decrease GFR and produce renal dysfunction in some patients. ACE inhibitors can similarly potentiate the detrimental effects of anesthetic agents on renal perfusion; these drugs block the protective effects of angiotensin II and may result in additional reductions in GFR during anesthesia.

Other Drugs

Many drugs and dyes that are used in the perioperative period can adversely affect renal function, particularly in the setting of preexisting renal dysfunction. These include antibiotics (eg, aminoglycosides and amphotericin B), immunosuppressive agents (eg, cyclosporin and tacrolimus), and radiocontrast dyes. Liposomal amphotericin B has less renal toxicity than amphotericin B. Mechanisms of injury include renal arterial vasospasm, direct cytotoxic properties, and renal microvascular or tubular obstruction.

Pretreatment with acetylcysteine (1200 mg orally in divided doses on the day before and on the day of the administration of the radiocontrast) has been shown to protect against radiocontrast dye–induced renal failure in patients with preexisting renal dysfunction. Acetylcysteine's protective action may be due to its free radical scavenging or sulfhydryl donor (reducing) properties. Calcium channel agents (diltiazem) may protect against cyclosporine-induced nephrotoxicity. Fenoldopam does not appear to be protective. Although anecdotal experience suggests otherwise, clinical studies have not clearly demonstrated that mannitol has renal protective effects against nephrotoxins.

DIRECT SURGICAL EFFECTS

In addition to the physiological changes associated with the neuroendocrine stress response to surgery, certain surgical procedures can significantly alter renal physiology. The pneumoperitoneum produced during laparoscopy produces an abdominal compartment syndrome–like state. The increase in intra-abdominal pressure typically produces oliguria (or anuria) that is generally proportional to the insufflation pressures. Mechanisms include central venous compression (renal vein and vena cava); renal parenchymal compression; decreased cardiac output; and increases in plasma levels of renin, aldosterone, and ADH. Other surgical procedures that can significantly compromise renal function include cardiopulmonary bypass (see Chapter 21), cross-clamping of the aorta (see Chapter 21), and dissection near the renal arteries (see Chapter 33). The potential effects of neurosurgical procedures on ADH physiology are discussed in Chapters 26 and 28.

■ DIURETICS

Diuretics increase urinary output by decreasing the reabsorption of Na$^+$ and water. They are most commonly classified according to their mechanism of action. Unfortunately, many diuretics have more than one such mechanism, so the classification system is imperfect; only major mechanisms will be reviewed here.

The majority of diuretics exert their action on the luminal cell membrane from within the renal tubules. Because nearly all diuretics are highly protein bound, relatively little of the free drug enters the tubules by filtration. Most diuretics must therefore be secreted by the proximal tubule (usually via the organic anion pump) to exert their action. Impaired delivery into the renal tubules accounts for resistance to diuretics in patients with impaired renal function.

OSMOTIC DIURETICS (MANNITOL)

Osmotically active diuretics are filtered at the glomerulus and undergo limited or no reabsorption in the proximal tubule. Their presence in the proximal tubule limits the passive water reabsorption that normally follows active sodium reabsorption. Although their major effect is to increase water excretion, in large doses, osmotically active diuretics also increase electrolyte (sodium and potassium) excretion. The same mechanism also impairs water and solute reabsorption in the loop of Henle.

Mannitol is the most commonly used osmotic diuretic. It is a six-carbon sugar that normally undergoes little or no reabsorption. In addition to its diuretic effect, mannitol appears to increase RBF. The latter can wash out some of the medullary hypertonicity and interfere with renal concentrating ability. Mannitol appears to activate the intrarenal synthesis of vasodilating prostaglandins. It also appears to be a free radical scavenger.

Uses

A. PROPHYLAXIS AGAINST ACUTE RENAL FAILURE IN HIGH-RISK PATIENTS

High-risk patients include those with massive trauma, major hemolytic reactions, rhabdomyolysis, and severe jaundice as well as those undergoing cardiac or aortic operations. The efficacy of prophylaxis in these instances may be related to dilution of nephrotoxic substances within the renal tubules, prevention of sludging and obstruction within the tubules, maintenance of RBF, and perhaps reduction of cellular swelling and preservation of the cellular architecture.

B. EVALUATION OF ACUTE OLIGURIA

Mannitol in the presence of hypovolemia will augment urinary output. In contrast, it will have little effect in the presence of severe glomerular or tubular injury.

C. CONVERSION OF OLIGURIC RENAL FAILURE TO NONOLIGURIC RENAL FAILURE

Although this indication is controversial, the lower mortality rate associated with nonoliguric renal failure still prompts many clinicians to use mannitol in that setting.

D. Acute Reduction of Intracranial Pressure and Cerebral Edema

See Chapter 26.

E. Acute Reduction of Intraocular Pressure in the Perioperative Period

See Chapter 38.

Intravenous Dosage

For mannitol, the intravenous dose is 0.25–1 g/kg.

Side Effects

Mannitol solutions are hypertonic and acutely raise plasma and extracellular osmolality. A rapid intracellular to extracellular shift of water can transiently increase intravascular volume and precipitate cardiac decompensation and pulmonary edema in patients with limited cardiac reserve. Transient hyponatremia and reductions in hemoglobin concentration are also common and represent acute hemodilution resulting from rapid movement of water out of cells; a modest, transient increase in plasma potassium concentration may also be observed (see Chapter 28). It is also important to note that the initial hyponatremia does not represent hypoosmolality but reflects the presence of mannitol (see Chapter 28). If fluid and electrolyte losses are not replaced following diuresis, mannitol can result in hypovolemia, hypokalemia, and hypernatremia. The hypernatremia occurs because water is lost in excess of sodium.

LOOP DIURETICS

The loop diuretics include furosemide (Lasix), bumetanide (Bumex), ethacrynic acid (Edecrin), and torsemide (Demadex). All loop diuretics inhibit Na$^+$ and Cl$^-$ reabsorption in the thick ascending limb. Sodium reabsorption at that site requires that all four sites on the Na$^+$–K$^+$–2Cl$^-$ luminal carrier protein be occupied. Loop diuretics compete with Cl$^-$ for its binding site on the carrier protein (see Figure 31–4). With a maximal effect, they can lead to excretion of 15–20% of the filtered sodium load. Both urinary concentrating and urinary diluting capacities are impaired. The large amounts of Na$^+$ and Cl$^-$ presented to the distal nephron overwhelm its limited reabsorptive capability. The resulting urine remains hypotonic. The reason for the latter is not clear but may relate to rapid urinary flow rates that prevent equilibration with the hypertonic renal medulla or interference with the action of ADH on the collecting tubules. A marked increase in diuresis may occur when loop diuretics are combined with thiazides, particularly metolazone.

Some studies suggest that furosemide increases RBF and can reverse the redistribution of blood flow from the cortex to the medulla.

Loop diuretics increase urinary calcium and magnesium excretion. Ethacrynic acid is the only diuretic (other than mannitol and filtration diuretics) that is not a sulfonamide derivative, and it may for that reason be the diuretic of choice in patients allergic to sulfonamide drugs. Torsemide may have an antihypertensive action independent of its diuretic effect.

Uses

A. Edematous States (Sodium Overload)

These disorders include heart failure, cirrhosis, the nephrotic syndrome, and renal insufficiency. When given intravenously, these agents can rapidly reverse cardiac and pulmonary manifestations.

B. Hypertension

Loop diuretics may be used as adjuncts to other hypotensive agents, particularly when thiazides (below) are ineffective.

C. Evaluation of Acute Oliguria

The response to a small dose (10–20 mg) of furosemide may be useful in differentiating between oliguria resulting from hypovolemia and oliguria that results from redistribution of RBF to juxtamedullary nephrons. Little or no response is seen with hypovolemia, whereas resumption of normal urinary output occurs with the latter.

D. Conversion of Oliguric Renal Failure to Nonoliguric Renal Failure

Use of these drugs in this setting is as controversial as with mannitol. Moreover, mannitol may be more effective.

E. Treatment of Hypercalcemia

See Chapter 28.

F. Rapid Correction of Hyponatremia

See Chapter 28.

Intravenous Dosages

The intravenous doses are furosemide, 20–100 mg; bumetanide, 0.5–1 mg; ethacrynic acid, 50–100 mg; and torsemide 10–100 mg.

Side Effects

Increased delivery of Na$^+$ to the distal and collecting tubules increases K$^+$ and H$^+$ secretion at those sites and can result in hypokalemia and metabolic alkalosis. Marked Na$^+$ losses will also lead to hypovolemia and prerenal azotemia (see Chapter 47); secondary hyperaldosteronism often accentuates the hypokalemia and metabolic alkalosis. Hypercalciuria can result in stone formation and occasionally hypocalcemia. Hypomagnesemia may be seen in patients receiving long-term therapy. Hyperuricemia is thought to result from increased urate reabsorption and competitive inhibition of urate secretion in the proximal tubule. Reversible hearing loss has been reported with both furosemide and ethacrynic acid but may be more common with ethacrynic acid.

THIAZIDE-TYPE DIURETICS

This group of agents includes thiazides, chlorthalidone (Thalitone), quinethazone (Hydromox), metolazone (Zaroxolyn), and indapamide (Lozol). These diuretics act at the distal tubule, including the connecting segment. Inhibition of sodium reabsorption at this site impairs the diluting but not the concentrating ability of urine. The thiazide diuretics compete for the Cl^- site on the luminal Na^+–Cl^- carrier protein. When given alone, thiazide-type diuretics increase Na^+ excretion to only 3–5% of the filtered load because of enhanced compensatory Na^+ reabsorption in the collecting tubules. They also have some carbonic anhydrase inhibiting activity in the proximal tubule. The latter is normally masked by sodium reabsorption in the loop of Henle but is probably responsible for the often marked ("high ceiling") diuresis seen when thiazides are combined with loop diuretics. In contrast to their effects on sodium excretion, thiazide-type diuretics augment Ca^{2+} reabsorption in the distal tubule. Indapamide has some vasodilating properties and is the only thiazide-type diuretic with significant hepatic excretion.

Uses

A. HYPERTENSION

Thiazides are often selected as first-line agents in the treatment of hypertension (see Chapter 20).

B. EDEMATOUS DISORDERS (SODIUM OVERLOAD)

These agents are exclusively used as oral agents for mild to moderate sodium overload.

C. HYPERCALCIURIA

Thiazide diuretics are often used to decrease calcium excretion in patients with hypercalciuria who form renal stones.

D. NEPHROGENIC DIABETES INSIPIDUS

The efficacy of these agents in this disorder reflects their ability to impair diluting capacity and increase urine osmolality (see Chapter 28).

Intravenous Dosages

These agents are only given orally.

Side Effects

Although thiazide-type diuretics deliver less sodium to the collecting tubules than loop diuretics, the increase in sodium excretion is enough to enhance K^+ secretion and frequently results in hypokalemia. Enhanced H^+ secretion can also occur, enough to result in metabolic alkalosis. Impairment of renal diluting capacity may produce hyponatremia in some patients. Hyperuricemia, hyperglycemia, hypercalcemia, and hyperlipidemia may also be seen.

POTASSIUM-SPARING DIURETICS

These weak agents characteristically do not increase potassium excretion. Potassium-sparing diuretics inhibit Na^+ reabsorption in the collecting tubules and therefore can maximally excrete only 1–2% of the filtered Na^+ load. They are usually used in conjunction with more potent diuretics for their potassium-sparing effect.

1. Aldosterone Antagonists (Spironolactone)

Spironolactone (Aldactone) is a direct aldosterone receptor antagonist in collecting tubules. It acts to inhibit aldosterone-mediated Na^+ reabsorption and K^+ secretion. As a result, spironolactone is effective only in patients with hyperaldosteronism. This agent also has some antiandrogenic properties.

Uses

A. PRIMARY AND SECONDARY HYPERALDOSTERONISM

Spironolactone is usually used as an adjuvant in the treatment of refractory edematous states associated with secondary hyperaldosteronism (see Chapter 28). It is particularly effective in patients with advanced liver disease.

B. HIRSUTISM

This less common indication relies on spironolactone's antiandrogenic properties.

Intravenous Dosage

Spironolactone is only given orally.

Side Effects

Spironolactone can result in hyperkalemia in patients with high potassium intake or renal insufficiency and in those receiving β-blockers or ACE inhibitors. Metabolic acidosis may also be seen. Other side effects include diarrhea, lethargy, ataxia, gynecomastia, and sexual dysfunction.

2. Noncompetitive Potassium-Sparing Diuretics

Triamterene (Dyrenium) and amiloride (Midamor) are not dependent on aldosterone activity in the collecting tubule. They inhibit Na^+ reabsorption and K^+ secretion by decreasing the number of open sodium channels in the luminal membrane of collecting tubules. Amiloride may also inhibit Na^+–K^+-ATPase activity in the collecting tubule.

Uses

A. HYPERTENSION

These agents are often combined with thiazides to prevent hypokalemia.

B. CONGESTIVE HEART FAILURE

They are often added to more potent (loop) diuretics in patients with marked potassium wasting.

Intravenous Dosages

These agents are only given orally.

Side Effects

Amiloride and triamterene can cause hyperkalemia and metabolic acidosis similar to spironolactone (see above). Both can also cause nausea, vomiting, and diarrhea. Amiloride is generally associated with fewer side effects, but paresthesias, depression, muscle weakness, and cramping may occasionally be seen. Triamterene on rare occasions has resulted in renal stones and is potentially nephrotoxic, particularly when combined with nonsteroidal antiinflammatory agents.

CARBONIC ANHYDRASE INHIBITORS

Carbonic anhydrase inhibitors such as acetazolamide (Diamox) interfere with Na^+ reabsorption and H^+ secretion in proximal tubules. They are weak diuretics because the former effect is limited by the reabsorptive capacities of more distal segments of nephrons. Nonetheless, these agents significantly interfere with H^+ secretion in the proximal tubule and impair HCO_3^- reabsorption (see Chapter 30).

Uses

A. CORRECTION OF METABOLIC ALKALOSIS IN EDEMATOUS PATIENTS

Carbonic anhydrase inhibitors often potentiate the effects of other diuretics.

B. ALKALINIZATION OF URINE

Alkalinization enhances urinary excretion of weakly acidic compounds such as uric acid.

C. REDUCTION OF INTRAOCULAR PRESSURE

Inhibition of carbonic anhydrase in the ciliary processes reduces the formation of aqueous humor and, secondarily, intraocular pressure. This is a common indication during ophthalmic surgery.

Intravenous Dosage

For acetazolamide, the intravenous dose is 250–500 mg.

Side Effects

Carbonic anhydrase inhibitors generally produce only a mild hyperchloremic metabolic acidosis because of an apparently limited effect on the distal nephron. Large doses of acetazolamide have been reported to cause drowsiness, paresthesias, and confusion. Alkalinization of the urine can interfere with the excretion of amine drugs, such as quinidine.

OTHER "DIURETICS"

These agents may increase GFR by elevating cardiac output or arterial blood pressure. Drugs in this category are not primarily classified as diuretics because of their other major actions. These agents include methylxanthines (theophylline), cardiac glycosides (digitalis), fenoldopam, inotropes (dopamine), and saline infusions. Methylxanthines also appear to decrease sodium reabsorption in both the proximal and distal renal tubules. The renal effects of dopamine are discussed above.

CASE DISCUSSION: INTRAOPERATIVE OLIGURIA

A 58-year-old woman is undergoing radical hysterectomy under general anesthesia. She was in good health prior to the diagnosis of uterine carcinoma. An indwelling urinary catheter is placed following induction of general anesthesia. Total urinary output was 60 mL for the first 2 h of surgery. After the third hour of surgery, only 5 mL of urine is noted in the drainage reservoir.

Should the anesthesiologist be concerned?

Decreases in urinary output during anesthesia are very common. Although decreases may be expected owing to the physiological effects of surgery and anesthesia (above), a urinary output of less than 20 mL/h in adults generally requires evaluation.

What issues should be addressed?

The following questions should be answered:

(1) Is there a problem with the urinary catheter and drainage system?

(2) Are hemodynamic parameters compatible with adequate renal function?

(3) Could the decrease in urinary output be directly related to surgical manipulations?

How can the urinary catheter and drainage system be evaluated intraoperatively?

Incorrect catheter placement is not uncommon and should be suspected if there has been a total absence of urine flow since the time of catheter insertion. The catheter may be inadvertently placed and inflated in the urethra in men or the vagina in women. Catheter displacement, kinking, obstruction, or disconnection from the reservoir tubing can all present with features similar to this case, with complete or near-complete cessation of urinary flow. The diagnosis of such mechanical problems requires retracing and inspecting the path of urine (often under the surgical drapes) from the catheter to the collection reservoir. Obstruction of the catheter can be confirmed by an inability to irrigate the bladder with saline through the catheter.

What hemodynamic parameters should be evaluated?

Decreased urinary output during surgery is most commonly the result of hemodynamic changes. In most instances, a decrease in intravascular volume (hypovolemia), cardiac output, or mean arterial blood pressure is responsible. Redistribution of renal blood flow from the renal cortex to the medulla may also play a role.

Intravascular volume depletion can rapidly develop when intravenous fluid replacements do not match intraoperative blood loss, insensible fluid losses, and sequestration of fluid by traumatized tissues (third-spacing). Oliguria requires careful assessment of intravascular volume to exclude hypovolemia (see Chapter 29). An increase in urinary output following an intravenous fluid bolus is highly suggestive of hypovolemia. In contrast, oliguria in patients with a history of congestive heart failure may require inotropes, vasodilators, or diuretics. Central venous or pulmonary artery pressure monitoring is useful in patients with underlying cardiac, renal, or advanced hepatic disease, as well as in patients experiencing extensive blood loss (see Chapter 6).

When mean arterial blood pressure drops below the lower limit of renal autoregulation (80 mm Hg), urinary flow may become blood pressure dependent. The latter may be particularly true in patients with chronic systemic hypertension, in whom renal autoregulation occurs at higher mean arterial blood pressures. Reductions in anesthetic depth, intravenous fluid boluses, or the administration of a vasopressor may increase blood pressure and urinary output in such instances.

Occasionally, otherwise normal patients may exhibit decreased urinary output in spite of normal intravascular volume, cardiac output, and mean arterial blood pressure. A small dose of a loop diuretic (furosemide, 5–10 mg) usually restores normal urinary flow in such instances.

How can surgical manipulations influence urinary output?

In addition to the neuroendocrine response to surgery, mechanical factors related to the surgery itself can alter urinary output. This is particularly true during pelvic surgery, when compression of the bladder by retractors, unintentional cystotomy, and ligation or severing of one or both ureters can dramatically affect urinary output. Retractor compression combined with a head-down (Trendelenburg) position commonly impedes emptying of the bladder. Excessive pressure on the bladder will often produce hematuria. When mechanical problems with the urinary catheter drainage system and hemodynamic factors are excluded (see above), a surgical explanation should be sought. The surgeon should be notified so that the position of the retractors can be checked, the ureters identified, and their path retraced in the operative area. Intravenous methylene blue or indigo carmine—both dyes that are excreted in urine—are useful in identifying the site of an unintentional cystotomy or the end of a severed ureter. Note that the appearance of the dye in the urinary drainage reservoir does not exclude unilateral ligation of one ureter. Methylene blue and, to a much lesser extent, indigo carmine can transiently give falsely low pulse oximeter readings (see Chapter 6).

What was the outcome?

After the integrity of the urinary catheter and drainage system was checked, 2 L of lactated Ringer's injection along with 250 mL of 5% albumin and 10 mg of furosemide were administered intravenously but failed to increase urinary output. Indigo carmine was given intravenously, and the proximal end of a severed left ureter was subsequently identified. A urologist was called and the ureter was reanastomosed.

SUGGESTED READING

Asif A, Epstein M: Prevention of radiocontrast-induced nephropathy. Am J Kidney Dis 2004;44:12.

Colson P, Ryckwaert F, Coriat P: Renin-angiotensin system antagonists and anesthesia. Anesth Analg 1999;89:1143.

Evers SA, Maze M: *Anesthetic Pharmacology: Physiologic Principles and Clinical Practice.* Churchill Livingstone, 2004.

Ganong WF: *Review of Medical Physiology,* 21st ed. McGraw-Hill, 2003.

Murphy MB, Murray C, Shorten GD. Fenoldopam—a selective peripheral dopamine-receptor agonist for the treatment of severe hypertension. N Engl J Med 2001;345:1548.

Anesthesia for Patients with Renal Disease

32

KEY CONCEPTS

 1 Creatinine clearance measurements are the most accurate method available for clinically assessing overall renal function.

 2 The accumulation of morphine and meperidine metabolites has been reported to prolong respiratory depression in some patients with renal failure.

 3 Succinylcholine can be used safely in the presence of renal failure if the serum potassium concentration is less than 5 mEq/L at the time of induction.

 4 The extracellular fluid overload from sodium retention—together with the increased demand imposed by anemia and hypertension—makes patients with chronic renal failure particularly prone to congestive heart failure and pulmonary edema.

 5 Delayed gastric emptying secondary to autonomic neuropathy in some patients can predispose patients with chronic renal failure to aspiration perioperatively.

 6 Controlled ventilation should be considered for patients with renal failure. Inadequate spontaneous or assisted ventilation with progressive

hypercarbia under anesthesia can result in respiratory acidosis that may exacerbate preexisting acidemia, lead to potentially severe circulatory depression, and dangerously increase serum potassium concentration.

 7 Procedures associated with a relatively high incidence of postoperative renal failure include cardiac and aortic reconstructive surgery.

 8 Intravascular volume depletion, sepsis, obstructive jaundice, crush injuries, recent contrast dye injections, and aminoglycoside, angiotensin-converting enzyme inhibitor, or nonsteroidal antiinflammatory drug therapy are additional major risk factors for an acute deterioration in renal function. Prophylaxis against renal failure with generous hydration together with solute diuresis appears to be effective and indicated in high-risk patients undergoing cardiac, major aortic reconstructive, and possibly other surgical procedures.

 9 The consequences of excessive fluid overload—namely, pulmonary congestion or edema—are easier to treat than those of acute renal failure.

Diseases affecting the kidneys are often grouped into syndromes based on common clinical and laboratory findings: nephrotic syndrome, acute renal failure, chronic renal failure, nephritis, nephrolithiasis, and urinary tract obstruction and infection. The anesthetic care of patients with these syndromes is facilitated by grouping patients according to the status of their preoperative renal function rather than by syndrome. This chapter examines the basis for this approach and the anesthetic considerations applicable within each group. Renal physiology and the effects of anesthesia on renal function are discussed in Chapter 31.

■ EVALUATING RENAL FUNCTION

Accurate assessment of renal function relies heavily on laboratory determinations (Table 32–1). Renal impairment can be due to glomerular dysfunction, tubular dysfunction, or obstruction of the urinary tract. Because abnormalities of glomerular function cause the greatest derangements and are most readily detectable, the most useful laboratory tests are those related to the glomerular filtration rate (GFR; see Chapter 31).

BLOOD UREA NITROGEN

The primary source of urea in the body is the liver. During protein catabolism, ammonia is produced from the deamination of amino acids. Hepatic conversion of ammonia to urea prevents the build-up of toxic ammonia levels:

$$2NH_3 + CO_2 \rightarrow H_2N - CO - NH_2 + H_2O$$

Blood urea nitrogen (BUN) is therefore directly related to protein catabolism and inversely related to glomerular filtration. As a result, BUN is not a reliable indicator of the GFR unless protein catabolism is normal and constant. Moreover, 40–50% of the filtrate is normally reabsorbed passively by the renal tubules; hypovolemia increases this fraction (below). Renal handling of urea is discussed in Chapter 31.

The normal BUN concentration is 10–20 mg/dL. Lower values can be seen with starvation or liver disease; elevations usually result from decreases in GFR or increases in protein catabolism. The latter may be due to a high catabolic state (trauma or sepsis), degradation of blood either in the gastrointestinal tract or in a large hematoma, or a high-protein diet. BUN concentrations greater than 50 mg/dL are generally associated with renal impairment.

Figure 32–1. The relationship between the serum creatinine concentration and the glomerular filtration rate.

SERUM CREATININE

Creatine is a product of muscle metabolism that is nonenzymatically converted to creatinine. Creatinine production in most persons is relatively constant and related to muscle mass, averaging 20–25 mg/kg in men and 15–20 mg/kg in women. Creatinine is then filtered (and to a minor extent secreted) but not reabsorbed in the kidneys (see Chapter 31). Serum creatinine concentration is therefore directly related to body muscle mass but inversely related to glomerular filtration (Figure 32–1). Because body muscle mass is usually fairly constant, serum creatinine measurements are generally reliable indices of GFR. The normal serum creatinine concentration is 0.8–1.3 mg/dL in men and 0.6–1 mg/dL in women. Note from Figure 32–1 that each doubling of the serum creatinine represents a 50% reduction in GFR. Large meat meals, cimetidine therapy, and increases in acetoacetate (as during ketoacidosis) can increase serum creatinine measurements without a change in GFR. Meat meals increase the creatinine load, and high acetoacetate concentrations interfere with the most common laboratory method for measuring creatinine. Cimetidine appears to inhibit creatinine secretion by the renal tubules.

GFR declines with increasing age in most persons (5% per decade after age 20), but because muscle mass also declines, the serum creatinine remains relatively normal; creatinine production may decrease to 10 mg/kg. Thus, in elderly patients, small increases in serum creatinine may represent large changes in GFR. Using age and lean body weight (in kilograms), GFR can be estimated by the following formula for men:

Creatinine clearance =
$$\frac{[(140 - age) \times lean\ body\ weight]}{(72 \times plasma\ creatinine)}$$

Table 32–1. Grouping of patients according to glomerular function.

	Creatinine Clearance (mL/min)
Normal	100–120
Decreased renal reserve	60–100
Mild renal impairment	40–60
Moderate renal insufficiency	25–40
Renal failure	< 25
End-stage renal disease[1]	< 10

[1]This term applies to patients with chronic renal failure.

For women, this equation must be multiplied by 0.85 to compensate for a smaller muscle mass.

The serum creatinine concentration requires 48–72 h to equilibrate at a new level following acute changes in GFR.

BLOOD UREA NITROGEN: CREATININE RATIO

Low renal tubular flow rates enhance urea reabsorption but do not affect creatinine handling. As a result, the BUN to serum creatinine ratio increases above 10:1. Decreases in tubular flow can be caused by decreased renal perfusion or obstruction of the urinary tract. **BUN:creatinine ratios greater than 15:1 are therefore seen in volume depletion and in edematous disorders associated with decreased tubular flow (eg, heart failure, cirrhosis, nephrotic syndrome) as well as in obstructive uropathies.** Increases in protein catabolism can also increase this ratio (see above).

CREATININE CLEARANCE

As discussed in Chapter 31, creatinine clearance measurements are the most accurate method available for clinically assessing overall renal function (really GFR). Although measurements are usually performed over 24 h, 2-h creatinine clearance determinations are reasonably accurate and easier to perform. Mild renal impairment generally results in creatinine clearances of 40–60 mL/min. Clearances between 25 and 40 mL/min produce moderate renal dysfunction and nearly always cause symptoms. Creatinine clearances less than 25 mL/min are indicative of overt renal failure.

Progressive renal disease enhances creatinine secretion in the proximal tubule. As a result, with declining renal function the creatinine clearance progressively overestimates the true GFR. Moreover, relative preservation of GFR may occur early in the course of progressive renal disease due to compensatory hyperfiltration in the remaining nephrons and increases in glomerular filtration pressure. It is therefore important to look for other signs of deteriorating renal function such as hypertension, proteinuria, or other abnormalities in urine sediment.

URINALYSIS

Urinalysis continues to be the most common test routinely performed for evaluating renal function. Although its utility for that purpose is justifiably questionable, urinalysis can be helpful in identifying some disorders of renal tubular dysfunction as well as some nonrenal disturbances. A routine urinalysis typically includes pH, specific gravity, detection and quantification of glucose, protein, and bilirubin content, and microscopic examination of the urinary sediment. Urinary pH is helpful only when arterial pH is also known. A urinary pH greater than 7.0 in the presence of systemic acidosis is suggestive of renal tubular acidosis (see Chapter 30). Specific gravity is related to urinary osmolality; 1.010 usually corresponds to 290 mOsm/kg. A specific gravity greater than 1.018 after an overnight fast is indicative of adequate renal concentrating ability. A lower specific gravity in the presence of hyperosmolality in plasma is consistent with diabetes insipidus.

Glycosuria is the result of either a low tubular threshold for glucose (normally 180 mg/dL) or hyperglycemia. Proteinuria detected by routine urinalysis should be evaluated by means of 24-h urine collection. Urinary protein excretions greater than 150 mg/d are significant. Elevated levels of bilirubin in the urine are seen with biliary obstruction.

Microscopic analysis of the urinary sediment detects the presence of red or white blood cells, bacteria, casts, and crystals. Red cells may be indicative of bleeding due to tumor, stones, infection, coagulopathy, or trauma. White cells and bacteria are generally associated with infection. Disease processes at the level of the nephron produce tubular casts. Crystals may be indicative of abnormalities in oxalic acid, uric acid, or cystine metabolism.

◼ ALTERED RENAL FUNCTION & THE EFFECTS OF ANESTHETIC AGENTS

Most drugs commonly employed during anesthesia are at least partly dependent on renal excretion for elimination. In the presence of renal impairment, dosage modifications may be required to prevent accumulation of the drug or active metabolites. Moreover, the systemic effects of azotemia can potentiate the pharmacological actions of many of these agents. This latter observation may be the result of decreased protein binding of the drug, greater brain penetration due to some breach of the blood–brain barrier, or a synergistic effect with the toxins retained in renal failure.

INTRAVENOUS AGENTS

Propofol & Etomidate

The pharmacokinetics of both propofol and etomidate are not significantly affected by impaired renal function. Decreased protein binding of etomidate in patients with hypoalbuminemia may enhance its pharmacological effects.

Barbiturates

Patients with renal disease often exhibit increased sensitivity to barbiturates during induction, even though pharmacokinetic profiles appear to be unchanged. The mechanism appears to be an increase in free circulating barbiturate as a result of decreased protein binding. Acidosis may also favor a more rapid entry of these agents into the brain by increasing the nonionized fraction of the drug (see Chapter 25).

Ketamine

Ketamine pharmacokinetics are minimally altered by renal disease. Some active hepatic metabolites are dependent on renal excretion and can potentially accumulate in renal failure. Ketamine's secondary hypertensive effect may be undesirable in hypertensive renal patients.

Benzodiazepines

Benzodiazepines undergo hepatic metabolism and conjugation prior to elimination in urine. Because most are highly protein bound, increased sensitivity may be seen in patients with hypoalbuminemia. Diazepam should be used cautiously in the presence of renal impairment because of a potential for the accumulation of active metabolites.

Opioids

Most opioids currently in use in anesthetic management (morphine, meperidine, fentanyl, sufentanil, and alfentanil) are inactivated by the liver; some of these metabolites are then excreted in urine. Remifentanil pharmacokinetics are unaffected by renal function due to rapid ester hydrolysis in blood. With the exception of morphine and meperidine, significant accumulation of active metabolites generally does not occur with these agents. The accumulation of morphine (morphine-6-glucuronide) and meperidine metabolites has been reported to prolong respiratory depression in some patients with renal failure. Increased levels of normeperidine, a meperidine metabolite, have been associated with seizures. The pharmacokinetics of the most commonly used opioid agonist–antagonists (butorphanol, nalbuphine, and buprenorphine) are unaffected by renal failure.

Anticholinergic Agents

In doses used for premedication, atropine and glycopyrrolate can generally be used safely in patients with renal impairment. Because up to 50% of these drugs and their active metabolites are normally excreted in urine, however, the potential for accumulation exists following repeated doses. Scopolamine is less dependent on renal excretion, but its central nervous system effects can be enhanced by azotemia.

Phenothiazines, H₂ Blockers, & Related Agents

Most phenothiazines, such as promethazine, are metabolized to inactive compounds by the liver. Although pharmacokinetic profiles are not appreciably altered by renal impairment, potentiation of their central depressant effects by azotemia can also occur. Their antiemetic actions are particularly useful in the setting of preoperative nausea. Droperidol may be partly dependent on the kidneys for excretion. Although accumulation may be seen following large doses in patients with renal impairment, relatively small doses of droperidol (< 2.5 mg) are usually used clinically.

All H_2-receptor blockers are very dependent on renal excretion. Metoclopramide is partly excreted unchanged in urine and will also accumulate in renal failure. Although up to 50% of dolasetron is excreted in urine, no dosage adjustments are recommended for any of the 5-HT$_3$ blockers in patients with renal insufficiency.

INHALATION AGENTS

Volatile Agents

Volatile anesthetic agents are nearly ideal for patients with renal dysfunction because of their lack of dependence on the kidneys for elimination, their ability to control blood pressure, and generally minimal direct effects on renal blood flow (see Chapter 31). Although patients with mild to moderate renal impairment do not exhibit altered uptake or distribution, accelerated induction and emergence may be seen in severely anemic patients (hemoglobin < 5 g/dL) with chronic renal failure; this observation may be explained by a decrease in the blood:gas partition coefficient or a decrease in minimum alveolar concentration. Enflurane and sevoflurane (with < 2 L/min gas flows) are considered undesirable for patients with renal disease undergoing long procedures because of the potential for fluoride accumulation (see Chapter 7).

Nitrous Oxide

Many clinicians omit or limit the use of nitrous oxide to 50% in patients with renal failure in an attempt to increase arterial oxygen content in the presence of anemia. This rationale may be justified only in severely anemic patients (hemoglobin < 7 g/dL), in whom even a small increase in the dissolved oxygen content may represent a significant percentage of the arterial to venous oxygen difference (see Chapter 22).

MUSCLE RELAXANTS

Succinylcholine

 Succinylcholine can be safely used in the presence of renal failure, provided the serum potassium concentration is known to be less than 5 mEq/L at the time of induction. When the serum potassium is higher or is in doubt, a nondepolarizing muscle relaxant should be used instead. Although decreased pseudocholinesterase levels have been reported in a few uremic patients following dialysis, significant prolongation of neuromuscular blockade is rarely seen.

Cisatracurium, Atracurium, & Mivacurium

Mivacurium is minimally dependent on the kidneys for elimination. Minor prolongation of effect may be observed due to reduced plasma pseudocholinesterase. Cisatracurium and atracurium are degraded in plasma by enzymatic ester hydrolysis and nonenzymatic Hofmann elimination. These agents may be the drugs of choice for muscle relaxation in patients with renal failure.

Vecuronium & Rocuronium

The elimination of vecuronium is primarily hepatic, but up to 20% of the drug is eliminated in urine. The effects of large doses of vecuronium (> 0.1 mg/kg) are only modestly prolonged in patients with renal insufficiency. Rocuronium primarily undergoes hepatic elimination, but prolongation by severe renal disease has been reported.

Curare

Elimination of curare is dependent on both renal and biliary excretion; 40–60% of a dose of curare is normally excreted in urine. Increasingly prolonged effects are observed following repeated doses in patients with significant renal impairment. Smaller doses and longer dosing intervals are therefore required for maintenance of optimal muscle relaxation.

Pancuronium, Pipecuronium, Alcuronium, & Doxacurium

These agents are all primarily dependent on renal excretion (60–90%). Although pancuronium is metabolized by the liver into less active intermediates, its elimination half-life is still primarily dependent on renal excretion (60–80%). Neuromuscular function should be closely monitored if these agents are used in patients with abnormal renal function.

Metocurine, Gallamine, & Decamethonium

All three agents are almost entirely dependent on renal excretion for elimination and should generally be avoided in patients with impaired renal function.

Reversal Agents

Renal excretion is the principal route of elimination for edrophonium, neostigmine, and pyridostigmine. The half-lives of these agents in patients with renal impairment are therefore prolonged at least as much as any of the above relaxants. Problems with inadequate reversal of neuromuscular blockade are usually related to other factors (see Chapter 9).

■ ANESTHESIA FOR PATIENTS WITH RENAL FAILURE

PREOPERATIVE CONSIDERATIONS

Acute Renal Failure

This syndrome is a rapid deterioration in renal function that results in retention of nitrogenous waste products (azotemia). These substances, many of which behave as toxins, are by-products of protein and amino acid metabolism. They include urea, guanidine compounds (including creatine and creatinine), urates, aliphatic amines, and various peptides and metabolites of aromatic amino acids. Impaired renal metabolism of circulating proteins and peptides may also contribute to widespread organ dysfunction.

Azotemia can be divided into prerenal, renal, and postrenal types depending on its causes (see Chapter 49). Prerenal azotemia results from an acute decrease in renal perfusion. Renal azotemia is usually due to intrinsic renal disease, renal ischemia, or nephrotoxins. Postrenal azotemia is the result of urinary tract obstruction or disruption. Both prerenal and postrenal azotemia are readily reversible in their initial stages but with time progress to renal azotemia. Most adult patients with renal failure develop oliguria. Nonoliguric patients (those with urinary outputs > 400 mL/d) continue to form urine that is qualitatively poor; these patients tend to have greater preservation of GFR. Although glomerular filtration and tubular function are impaired in both cases, abnormalities tend to be less severe in nonoliguric renal failure.

The course of acute renal failure varies widely, but the oliguria typically lasts for 2 weeks and is followed by a diuretic phase marked by a progressive increase in urinary output. This diuretic phase often results in very large urinary outputs and is usually absent in nonoliguric renal failure. Urinary function improves over the course of several weeks but may not return to normal for up to 1 year. A more complete discussion of acute renal failure is found in Chapter 49.

Table 32–2. Manifestations of uremia.

Neurological
Peripheral neuropathy
Autonomic neuropathy
Muscle twitching
Encephalopathy
  Asterixis
  Myoclonus
  Lethargy
  Confusion
  Seizures
  Coma
Cardiovascular
Fluid overload
Congestive heart failure
Hypertension
Pericarditis
Arrhythmia
Conduction blocks
Vascular calcification
Accelerated atherosclerosis
Pulmonary
Hyperventilation
Interstitial edema
Alveolar edema
Pleural effusion
Gastrointestinal
Anorexia
Nausea and vomiting
Delayed gastric emptying
Hyperacidity
Mucosal ulcerations
Hemorrhage
Adynamic ileus
Metabolic
Metabolic acidosis
Hyperkalemia
Hyponatremia
Hypermagnesemia
Hyperphosphatemia
Hypocalcemia
Hyperuricemia
Hypoalbuminemia
Hematological
Anemia
Platelet dysfunction
Leukocyte dysfunction
Endocrine
Glucose intolerance
Secondary hyperparathyroidism
Hypertriglyceridemia
Skeletal
Osteodystrophy
Periarticular calcification
Skin
Hyperpigmentation
Ecchymosis
Pruritus

Chronic Renal Failure

This syndrome is characterized by a progressive and irreversible decline in renal function over the course of at least 3–6 months. The most common causes are hypertensive nephrosclerosis, diabetic nephropathy, chronic glomerulonephritis, and polycystic renal disease.

The full manifestations of this syndrome (Table 32–2)—often referred to as uremia—are seen only after the GFR decreases below 25 mL/min. Patients with clearances below 10 mL/min (often said to have end-stage renal disease) are dependent on dialysis for survival until they receive a successful transplant. Dialysis may take the form of intermittent hemodialysis employing an arteriovenous fistula or continuous peritoneal dialysis via an implanted catheter.

The generalized effects of uremia can usually be controlled by dialysis. Indeed many patients on daily dialysis generally feel entirely normal and many do not develop the discoloration associated with end-stage renal disease and dialysis. The majority of patients, however, are dialyzed three times a week. With time some uremic complications may become refractory. Moreover, some complications are directly related to the dialysis itself (Table 32–3). Hypotension, neutropenia, hypoxemia, and the disequilibrium syndrome are

Table 32–3. Complications of dialysis.

Neurological
Disequilibrium syndrome
Dementia
Cardiovascular
Intravascular volume depletion
Hypotension
Arrhythmia
Pulmonary
Hypoxemia
Gastrointestinal
Ascites
Hematological
Anemia
Transient neutropenia
Residual anticoagulation
Hypocomplementemia
Metabolic
Hypokalemia
Large protein losses
Skeletal
Osteomalacia
Arthropathy
Myopathy
Infectious
Peritonitis
Transfusion-related hepatitis

generally transient and resolve within hours after dialysis. Factors contributing to hypotension during dialysis include the vasodilating effects of acetate dialysate solutions, autonomic neuropathy, and rapid removal of fluid. The interaction of white cells with cellophane-derived dialysis membranes can result in neutropenia and leukocyte-mediated pulmonary dysfunction leading to hypoxemia. Disequilibrium syndrome is characterized by transient neurological symptoms that appear to be related to a more rapid lowering of extracellular osmolality than intracellular osmolality.

Manifestations of Renal Failure

A. METABOLIC

Multiple metabolic abnormalities, including hyperkalemia, hyperphosphatemia, hypocalcemia, hypermagnesemia, hyperuricemia, and hypoalbuminemia typically develop in patients with overt renal failure. Water and sodium retention can result in worsening hyponatremia and extracellular fluid overload, respectively. Failure to excrete nonvolatile acids produces a high anion gap metabolic acidosis (see Chapter 30). Hypernatremia and hypokalemia are uncommon complications.

Hyperkalemia is the most lethal of these abnormalities because of its effect on the heart (see Chapter 28). It is usually present in patients with creatinine clearances of less than 5 mL/min, but it can develop rapidly in patients with higher clearances when challenged with large potassium loads (trauma, hemolysis, infections, or potassium administration).

The hypermagnesemia is generally mild unless magnesium intake is increased (most commonly from magnesium-containing antacids). Hypocalcemia develops for unclear reasons. Proposed mechanisms include deposition of calcium into bone secondary to the hyperphosphatemia, resistance to parathyroid hormone, and decreased intestinal absorption secondary to decreased renal synthesis of 1,25-dihydroxycholecalciferol (see Chapter 28). Symptoms of hypocalcemia rarely develop unless patients are also made alkalotic.

Patients with renal failure also rapidly lose tissue proteins and readily develop hypoalbuminemia. Anorexia, protein restriction, and dialysis (particularly peritoneal dialysis) are contributory.

B. HEMATOLOGICAL

Anemia is nearly always present when the creatinine clearance is below 30 mL/min. Hemoglobin concentrations are generally 6–8 g/dL. Decreased erythropoietin production, decreased red cell production, and decreased cell survival are thought to be responsible. Additional factors include gastrointestinal blood loss, hemodilution, and bone marrow suppression from recurrent infections. Even with transfusions, hemoglobin concentrations greater than 9 g/dL are often difficult to maintain. Erythropoietin administration appears to at least partially correct the anemia. Increased levels of 2,3-diphosphoglycerate (2,3-DPG) develop in response to the decrease in oxygen-carrying capacity. 2,3-DPG facilitates the unloading of oxygen from hemoglobin (see Chapter 22). The metabolic acidosis (see above) also favors a rightward shift in the hemoglobin–oxygen dissociation curve. In the absence of symptomatic heart disease, most patients tolerate the anemia remarkably well.

Both platelet and white cell function are impaired in patients with renal failure. Clinically, this is manifested as a prolonged bleeding time and increased susceptibility to infections, respectively. Most patients have decreased platelet factor III activity as well as decreased platelet adhesiveness and aggregation. Patients who have recently undergone hemodialysis may also have residual anticoagulant effects from heparin.

C. CARDIOVASCULAR

Cardiac output has to increase in renal failure to maintain oxygen delivery in the face of a decrease in oxygen-carrying capacity. Sodium retention and abnormalities in the renin–angiotensin system result in systemic arterial hypertension. Left ventricular hypertrophy is a common finding in chronic renal failure. The extracellular fluid overload from sodium retention—together with the increased demand imposed by anemia and hypertension—makes these patients particularly prone to congestive heart failure and pulmonary edema. Increased permeability of the alveolar–capillary membrane may also be a predisposing factor (below). Conduction blocks are not uncommon and may be due to deposition of calcium in the conduction system. Arrhythmias are common and may in part be related to the metabolic abnormalities. Uremic pericarditis may develop in some patients; patients may be asymptomatic, may present with chest pain, or may develop cardiac tamponade. Patients with chronic renal failure also characteristically develop accelerated peripheral vascular and coronary artery disease.

Intravascular volume depletion may occur during the diuretic phase of acute renal failure if fluid replacement is inadequate. Hypovolemia also develops if too much fluid is removed during dialysis.

D. PULMONARY

Without dialysis or bicarbonate therapy, patients may be dependent on an increase in minute ventilation to compensate for the metabolic acidosis (see Chapter 30). Pulmonary extravascular water is often increased in the form of interstitial edema, resulting in a widening of the alveolar to arterial oxygen gradient and predisposing to hypoxemia. Increased permeability of the alveolar–capillary membrane in some patients can result in pulmonary edema even with normal pulmonary capillary pressures; a characteristic picture resembling "butterfly wings" may be seen on the chest film.

E. ENDOCRINE

Abnormal glucose tolerance is characteristic of renal failure and is thought to result from peripheral resistance to insulin; patients therefore often handle large glucose loads poorly. Secondary hyperparathyroidism in patients with chronic renal failure can produce metabolic bone disease, which may predispose to fractures. Abnormalities in lipid metabolism frequently lead to hypertriglyceridemia and probably contribute to accelerated atherosclerosis. Increases in the circulating levels of proteins and polypeptides normally degraded in the kidneys are often seen; these include parathyroid hormone, insulin, glucagon, growth hormone, luteinizing hormone, and prolactin.

F. GASTROINTESTINAL

Anorexia, nausea, vomiting, and adynamic ileus are commonly associated with azotemia. Hypersecretion of gastric acid increases the incidence of peptic ulceration and gastrointestinal hemorrhage, which occurs in 10–30% of patients. Delayed gastric emptying secondary to autonomic neuropathy in some patients can predispose to aspiration perioperatively. Patients with chronic renal failure also have a high incidence of viral hepatitis (types B and C), often followed by residual hepatic dysfunction.

G. NEUROLOGICAL

Asterixis, lethargy, confusion, seizures, and coma are manifestations of uremic encephalopathy. Symptoms generally correlate with the degree of azotemia. Autonomic and peripheral neuropathies are common in patients with chronic renal failure. Peripheral neuropathies are typically sensory and involve the distal lower extremities.

Preoperative Evaluation

The generalized effects of azotemia mandate a thorough evaluation of patients in renal failure. Most patients with acute renal failure requiring surgery are critically ill. Their renal failure is frequently associated with a postoperative complication or trauma. Patients with acute renal failure also tend to have accelerated protein breakdown. Optimal perioperative management is dependent on preoperative dialysis. Hemodialysis is more effective than peritoneal dialysis and can be readily accomplished via a temporary internal jugular, subclavian, or femoral dialysis catheter. The need for dialysis in nonoliguric patients should be assessed on an individual basis. Indications for dialysis are listed in Table 32–4.

Table 32–4. Indications for dialysis.

Fluid overload
Hyperkalemia
Severe acidosis
Metabolic encephalopathy
Pericarditis
Coagulopathy
Refractory gastrointestinal symptoms
Drug toxicity

Patients with chronic renal failure most commonly present to the operating room for creation or revision of an arteriovenous fistula under local or regional anesthesia. Regardless of the procedure or the anesthetic employed, complete evaluation is required to make certain that they are in optimal medical condition; all reversible manifestations (Table 32–2) of uremia should be controlled. Preoperative dialysis on the day of surgery or on the previous day is usually necessary.

Physical and laboratory evaluation should focus on both cardiac and respiratory functions. Signs of fluid overload or hypovolemia should be sought (see Chapter 29). Intravascular volume depletion often results from overzealous dialysis. A comparison of the patient's current weight with previous predialysis and postdialysis weights may be helpful. Hemodynamic data, if available, and a chest film are invaluable in confirming clinical impressions. Arterial blood gas analysis is useful in detecting hypoxemia and evaluating acid–base status in patients who complain of or appear to have dyspnea. The electrocardiogram should be examined carefully for signs of hyperkalemia or hypocalcemia (see Chapter 28) as well as ischemia, conduction blocks, and ventricular hypertrophy. Echocardiography can be invaluable for assessing cardiac function in patients undergoing major surgical procedures because it can evaluate the ventricular ejection fraction as well as detect and quantitate hypertrophy, wall motion abnormalities, and pericardial fluid. A friction rub may not be audible on auscultation in patients with a pericardial effusion.

Preoperative red blood cell transfusions should generally be given only to severely anemic patients (hemoglobin < 6–7 g/dL) or when significant intraoperative blood loss is expected. A bleeding time and coagulation studies are advisable, particularly if regional anesthesia is being considered. Serum electrolyte, BUN, and creatinine measurements can assess the adequacy of dialysis. Glucose measurements are helpful in evaluating the potential need for perioperative insulin therapy.

Preoperative drug therapy should be carefully reviewed for drugs with significant renal elimination (Table 32–5). Dosage adjustments and measurements of blood levels (when available) are necessary to prevent drug toxicity.

Table 32–5. Drugs with a potential for significant accumulation in patients with renal impairment.

Muscle relaxants
 Metocurine
 Gallamine
 Decamethonium
 Pancuronium
 Pipecurium
 Doxacurium
 Alcuronium
Anticholinergics
 Atropine
 Glycopyrrolate
Metoclopramide
H$_2$-receptor antagonists
 Cimetidine
 Ranitidine
Digitalis
Diuretics
Calcium channel antagonists
 Nifedipine
 Diltiazem
β-Adrenergic blockers
 Propranolol
 Nadolol
 Pindolol
 Atenolol
Antihypertensives
 Clonidine
 Methyldopa
 Captopril
 Enalapril
 Lisinopril
 Hydralazine
 Nitroprusside (thiocyanate)
Antiarrhythmics
 Procainamide
 Disopyramide
 Bretylium
 Tocainide
 Encainide (genetically determined)
Bronchodilators
 Terbutaline
Psychiatric
 Lithium
Antibiotics
 Penicillins
 Cephalosporins
 Aminoglycosides
 Tetracycline
 Vancomycin
Anticonvulsants
 Carbamazepine
 Ethosuximide
 Primidone

Premedication

Alert patients who are relatively stable can be given reduced doses of an opioid (see Table 8–6) or a benzodiazepine (see Table 8–3). Promethazine, 12.5–25 mg intramuscularly, is a useful adjunct for additional sedation and for its antiemetic properties. Aspiration prophylaxis with an H$_2$ blocker may be indicated in patients with nausea, vomiting, or gastrointestinal bleeding (see Chapter 15). Metoclopramide, 10 mg orally or slowly intravenously, may also be useful in accelerating gastric emptying, preventing nausea, and decreasing the risk of aspiration. Preoperative medications—particularly antihypertensive agents—should be continued until the time of surgery (see Chapter 20). The management of diabetic patients is discussed in Chapter 36.

INTRAOPERATIVE CONSIDERATIONS

Monitoring

The surgical procedure as well as the patient's general medical condition dictate monitoring requirements. Because of the danger of occlusion, blood pressure should not be measured by a cuff in an arm with an arteriovenous fistula. Intraarterial, central venous, and pulmonary artery monitoring are often indicated, particularly for patients undergoing procedures associated with major fluid shifts (see Chapter 6); intravascular volume is often difficult to assess based on clinical signs alone. Direct intraarterial blood pressure monitoring may also be indicated in poorly controlled hypertensive patients regardless of the procedure. Aggressive invasive monitoring may be indicated, particularly in diabetic patients with advanced renal disease undergoing major surgery; this group of patients may have up to 10 times the perioperative morbidity of diabetic patients without renal disease. The latter probably reflects the high incidence of advanced cardiovascular complications in the first group.

Induction

Patients with nausea, vomiting, or gastrointestinal bleeding should undergo rapid-sequence induction with cricoid pressure (see Chapter 15). The dose of the induction agent should be reduced in debilitated or critically ill patients. Thiopental, 2–3 mg/kg, or propofol, 1–2 mg/kg, is often used. Etomidate, 0.2–0.4 mg/kg, may be preferable in hemodynamically unstable patients. An opioid, β-blocker (esmolol), or lidocaine may be used to blunt the hypertensive response to intubation (see Chapter 20). Succinylcholine, 1.5 mg/kg, can be used for endotracheal intubation if the serum potassium is less than 5 mEq/L. Rocuronium (0.6 mg/kg), cisatracurium (0.15 mg/kg), atracurium (0.4 mg/

kg), or mivacurium (0.15 mg/kg) should be used for intubating patients with hyperkalemia. Atracurium in this dosage generally causes little histamine release (see Chapter 9). Vecuronium, 0.1 mg/kg, may be a suitable alternative, but some prolongation of its effects should be expected. Use of a laryngeal mask airway, when appropriate (see Chapter 5), usually avoids the excessive sympathetic (hypertensive) response sometimes associated with intubation and the need for muscle paralysis.

Maintenance

The ideal maintenance technique should be able to control hypertension with minimal effects on cardiac output, because an increase in cardiac output is the principal compensatory mechanism for anemia. Volatile anesthetics, nitrous oxide, propofol, fentanyl, sufentanil, alfentanil, remifentanil, hydromorphone, and morphine are generally regarded as satisfactory maintenance agents. Isoflurane and desflurane may be the preferred volatile agents because they have the least effect on cardiac output (see Chapter 7). Nitrous oxide should be used cautiously in patients with poor ventricular function and should probably not be used in patients with very low hemoglobin concentrations (< 7 g/dL) to allow the administration of 100% oxygen (see above). Meperidine may not be a good choice because of the accumulation of normeperidine (see above). Morphine may be used, but some prolongation of its effects should be expected.

Controlled ventilation should be considered for patients with renal failure. Inadequate spontaneous ventilation with progressive hypercarbia under anesthesia can result in respiratory acidosis that may exacerbate preexisting acidemia, lead to potentially severe circulatory depression, and dangerously increase serum potassium concentration (see Chapter 30). Respiratory alkalosis may also be detrimental because it shifts the hemoglobin dissociation curve to the left (see Chapter 22), can exacerbate preexisting hypocalcemia (see Chapter 28), and may reduce cerebral blood flow (see Chapter 25).

Fluid Therapy

Superficial operations involving minimal tissue trauma require replacement of only insensible fluid losses with 5% dextrose in water. Procedures associated with major fluid losses or shifts require isotonic crystalloids, colloids, or both (see Chapter 29). Lactated Ringer's injection is best avoided in hyperkalemic patients when large volumes of fluid may be required, because it contains potassium (4 mEq/L); normal saline may be used instead. Glucose-free solutions should generally be used because of the glucose intolerance associated with uremia. Blood that is lost should generally be replaced with

packed red blood cells. Blood transfusion either has no effect or may be beneficial for patients in renal failure who are candidates for renal transplant; transfusion may decrease the likelihood of rejection following renal transplantation in some patients.

■ ANESTHESIA FOR PATIENTS WITH MILD TO MODERATE RENAL IMPAIRMENT

PREOPERATIVE CONSIDERATIONS

The kidneys normally exhibit a large reserve in function. GFR, as determined by creatinine clearance, can decrease from 120 to 60 mL/min without any clinically perceptible change in renal function. Even patients with creatinine clearances of 40–60 mL/min usually are asymptomatic. These patients have only mild renal impairment but should still be thought of as having decreased renal reserve. The emphasis in the care of these patients is preservation of the remaining renal function, which is best accomplished by maintaining normovolemia.

When creatinine clearance reaches 25–40 mL/min, renal impairment is moderate, and patients can be said to have renal insufficiency: Significant azotemia is always present and hypertension and anemia are common. Correct anesthetic management of this group of patients is as critical as management of those with frank renal failure.

The latter is particularly true during procedures associated with a relatively high incidence of postoperative renal failure, such as cardiac and aortic reconstructive surgery. Intravascular volume depletion, sepsis, obstructive jaundice, crush injuries, recent contrast dye injections, and aminoglycoside, angiotensin-converting enzyme inhibitor, or nonsteroidal antiinflammatory drug therapy are additional major risk factors for an acute deterioration in renal function. Hypovolemia appears to be a particularly important factor in the development of acute postoperative renal failure. The emphasis in management of these patients is on prevention, because the mortality rate of postoperative renal failure is as high as 50–60%. The increased perioperative risk associated with the combination of advanced renal disease and diabetes has previously been alluded to.

Prophylaxis against renal failure *with generous hydration* together with solute diuresis appears to be effective and is indicated in high-risk patients undergoing cardiac, major aortic reconstructive, and possibly other surgical procedures. Mannitol (0.5 g/kg) is generally employed and should be started prior to or at the time

Neal H. Cohen, MD, MPH, MS

INTEGRATING NEW TECHNOLOGIES INTO CLINICAL PRACTICE: CONTINUOUS RENAL REPLACEMENT THERAPY

Introduction

As anesthetic and surgical management have improved, patients with significant underlying clinical problems now routinely and safely undergo complex surgical procedures. Associated with this increasing complexity of surgical and anesthetic management, technologies often initially used to diagnose and treat problems outside the operating room (OR) find their way to the OR.

Multiple examples of the clinical transformation of technological advances can be provided. Blood gas analysis, capnography, automated noninvasive blood pressure monitoring, as well as the intraarterial line have all become common devices used routinely to facilitate perioperative care. Probably the best representation of the importance of the application of technology to anesthetic management is the evolution of the pulse oximeter, from a very complicated and technologically immature device to the easy to apply, safe, and incredibly important monitor that has become the standard of care in the operating room and elsewhere.

Acute renal failure (ARF) has become more common in the hospitalized patient population in general and in patients requiring anesthesia and surgery. Continuous renal replacement therapy (CRRT)

represents a major therapeutic advance for the management of patients with ARF, metabolic instability, and fluid overload. Although the therapy has been used successfully in the care of patients in the intensive care unit (ICU) setting, the potential value of the therapeutic intervention in the care of patients in the OR and as part of the overall perioperative management of many patients is significant.

What Are the Options?

A number of approaches to the delivery of CRRT are available. In general, CRRT refers to any continuous mode of extracorporeal solute or fluid removal. Each of the modalities includes an extracorporeal circuit with a hemofilter that has a semipermeable membrane. The rate of fluid removal is determined by the hydrostatic pressure gradient across the filter. In most cases the connection to the patient is through a venous cannula that incorporates an extracorporeal pump to remove blood from the patient, pass it through the filter, and return the filtered blood back to the patient.

A major advantage of CRRT is that large volumes of ultrafiltrate can be removed. As it is removed, fluid is administered through the system to effectively control volume and electrolytes. The fluid infusion rate and composition of the replacement fluid can be adjusted based on the ultrafiltration rate, the volume of fluids and blood products administered through other intravenous lines to the patient, and the fluid balance goal (positive or negative). To normalize electrolytes and acid–base balance, an isotonic, buffered electrolyte solution is used as the replacement fluid. Acetate, citrate, lactate, or bicarbonate can be used as the buffering solution. Recently most clinicians use citrate because it is both a buffer and an anticoagulant and can help minimize clotting in the filter.[1]

In addition to allowing careful control over fluid balance using hemofiltration, CRRT can be used to dialyze patients with renal insufficiency. When dialysis is required, a dialysate can be run through the hemofilter in a countercurrent direction to create a concentration gradient across the hemofilter membrane to provide solute clearance.

Does It Work?

The data that document the value of CRRT in perioperative management are limited.[2–4] In other settings,

CRRT has been shown to be effective,[4] although there are few data to demonstrate reduced morbidity and mortality associated with its use. The nonsurgical situations in which CRRT has been demonstrated to be preferable to intermittent hemodialysis or other therapies include the management of severe azotemia, the ability to remove fluid with less hemodynamic instability, and fluid, electrolyte, and nutritional management in critically ill patients.

What Do We Need to Know?

Because of the demonstrated value and advantages of CRRT in the management of surgical patients, it is becoming a more commonly utilized therapy in the perioperative period. To decide when to use CRRT as part of perioperative management and how to do so effectively, it is important to understand the effects of the therapy, how it can be initiated, and its impact on overall anesthetic management.

First, the perioperative management of patients with renal failure or fluid overload is always challenging. Many of the patients who require surgery will be receiving CRRT preoperatively. It is therefore important for the anesthesiologist to understand why the therapy was initiated, to understand the goals of therapy (optimize intravascular volume, correct metabolic abnormalities, or for dialysis), and to determine whether the treatment has accomplished the desired goals. In addition, a decision must be made as to whether to continue (or initiate) CRRT during surgery. For patients undergoing relatively short or minor procedures, CRRT can be safely discontinued for a short period of time with minimal sequelae. The decision to continue CRRT intraoperatively for the patient who is already receiving the therapy and is scheduled for a major procedure requires a more thorough understanding of the underlying medical problems, the goals of CRRT, and the patient's response to the treatment. The primary indications for providing CRRT during surgery include persistent increased intravascular volume, particularly with hemodynamic instability, pulmonary edema compromising gas exchange, and severe, ongoing metabolic acidosis.

Second, if the therapy is to be continued during surgery, the transition to the OR must be managed carefully. Currently CRRT has to be temporarily discontinued and reinstituted in the OR. A new setup is re-

quired and reinstitution must be completed after safe transport to the OR. The same transition is required when the patient is returned to the ICU.

Third, when using CRRT, the anesthesiologist must be aware of the complications and potential risks associated with the therapy. For most patients, anticoagulation is provided during the therapy. Anticoagulants are administered prefilter, minimizing the risk of anticoagulation to the patient, although the effect is often unpredictable. Fluid management must also be monitored closely to ensure that the fluid replacement is appropriate for the goals of the therapy and the electrolyte content of the replacement fluid is adjusted to normalize the acid–base balance. Because the patient is connected to an extracorporeal circuit, the catheters and flows through the circuit must be monitored closely. As a result of the large extracorporeal circuit, patients receiving CRRT can become hypothermic. Patients may require a warming blanket and more careful monitoring for signs of infection, as the temperature may not be a reliable indicator.

What Else Can We Learn?

The anesthesiologist should become familiar with CRRTs and their indications and applications in the care of patients in the OR. With increasing application of the therapy to the surgical patient, the technology will be modified to more effectively address the patient's unique needs and to reduce the complexity of the procedure. This technology is one of the most significant advances in the clinical management of the critically ill patient to become available in a long time and its potential value is yet to be fully realized.

1. Monchi M, Berghmans D, Ledoux D, et al: Citrate vs. heparin for anticoagulation in continuous venovenous hemofiltration: A prospective randomized study. Intensive Care Med 2004;30:260.

2. Ronco C, Bellomo R, Kellum JA: Continuous renal replacement therapy: Opinions and evidence. Adv Renal Replace Ther 2002;9:229.

3. Cole L, Bellomo R, Hart G, et al: A phase II randomized, controlled trial of continuous hemofiltration in sepsis. Crit Care Med 2002;30:100.

4. Weksler N, Chorni I, Gurman GM, et al: Continuous venovenous hemofiltration improves intensive care unit, but not hospital survival rate, in nonoliguric septic patients. J Crit Care 2001;16:69.

of induction (see Chapter 31). Although controversial, the beneficial effect of mannitol appears to be related to the solute diuresis rather than its antioxidant properties. *Intravenous fluids should be given concomitantly to prevent intravascular volume depletion.* Intravenous infusions of fenoldopam or low-dose dopamine can increase renal blood flow and promote diuresis via activation of vasodilatory D_1-receptors in the renal vasculature. Some studies suggest that fenoldopam, unlike dopamine, may help preserve renal function during aortic surgery. A small dose of a loop diuretic is usually necessary to help establish the diuresis, maintain an adequate urinary output, and prevent fluid overload. The value of prophylaxis with acetylcysteine prior to the administration of radiocontrast dyes is discussed in Chapter 31.

INTRAOPERATIVE CONSIDERATIONS

Monitoring

Standard monitors are used for procedures involving minimal fluid losses. For operations associated with significant blood or fluid losses, monitoring hourly urinary output and intravascular volume is critical (see Chapter 29). Although an adequate urinary output does not ensure preservation of renal function, urinary outputs greater than 0.5 mL/kg/h are generally desirable. Intraarterial pressure monitoring is also desirable if rapid changes in blood pressure may be encountered, such as in poorly controlled hypertensive patients and in those undergoing procedures associated with abrupt changes in cardiac preload or afterload.

Induction

Selection of an induction agent is not as critical as ensuring an adequate intravascular volume prior to induction. Induction of anesthesia in patients with renal insufficiency frequently results in hypotension when hypovolemia is present. Unless a vasopressor is given, the hypotension typically resolves only following intubation or surgical stimulation. Renal perfusion, which may already be compromised by the hypovolemia, deteriorates further, first as a result of hypotension and then from sympathetically or pharmacologically mediated renal vasoconstriction. If sustained, the decrease in renal perfusion could contribute to postoperative renal impairment. Preoperative hydration usually prevents this sequence of events.

Maintenance

All maintenance agents are acceptable with the possible exception of sevoflurane administered with low gas flows (< 2 L/min). Although enflurane can be used safely for short procedures, it is best avoided in patients with renal insufficiency because of the availability of other satisfactory

agents. Deterioration in renal function during this period may result from any adverse hemodynamic effects of surgery (hemorrhage) or anesthesia (cardiac depression or hypotension), indirect hormonal effects (sympathoadrenal activation or antidiuretic hormone secretion), or positive-pressure ventilation (impeded venous return; see Chapter 31). These effects are almost completely reversible when sufficient intravenous fluids are given to maintain a normal or slightly expanded intravascular volume. The administration of large doses of predominantly α-adrenergic vasopressors (phenylephrine and norepinephrine) may also be detrimental. Small intermittent doses or brief infusions may be useful in maintaining renal blood flow until other measures (eg, transfusion) are undertaken to correct hypotension. Once mean arterial blood pressure, cardiac output, and intravascular volume are adequate, a low-dose dopamine infusion (2–5 μg/kg/min) can be used in patients with marginal urinary output in an attempt to preserve renal blood flow and renal function. "Renal dose dopamine" has also been shown to at least partially reverse renal arterial vasoconstriction during infusions of α-adrenergic vasopressors (norepinephrine). Fenoldopam also appears to have the same effect.

Fluid Therapy

As discussed above, judicious fluid administration is critical in managing patients with decreased renal reserve or renal insufficiency. Concern over fluid overload is justified, but problems are rarely encountered in patients with normal urinary outputs if rational guidelines and appropriate monitors are employed (see Chapter 29). Indeed, the consequences of excessive fluid overload—namely, pulmonary congestion or edema—are easier to treat than those of acute renal failure.

**CASE DISCUSSION:
A PATIENT WITH
UNCOLLED HYPERTENSION**

A 59-year-old man with a recent onset of hypertension is scheduled for reconstruction of a stenotic left renal artery. His preoperative blood pressure is 180/110 mm Hg.

What is the cause of this man's hypertension?

Renovascular hypertension is one of the few surgically correctable forms of hypertension. Others include coarctation of the aorta, pheochromocytoma, Cushing's disease, and primary hyperaldosteronism.

Most studies suggest that renovascular hypertension accounts for 2–5% of all cases of hyper-

tension. It characteristically presents either as a relatively sudden onset of hypertension in persons younger than 35 years or older than 55 years of age. Renal artery stenosis can also be responsible for the development of accelerated or malignant hypertension in previously hypertensive persons of any age.

What is the pathophysiology of the hypertension?

Unilateral or bilateral stenosis of the renal artery decreases the perfusion pressure to the kidneys distal to the obstruction. Activation of the juxtaglomerular apparatus and release of renin increase circulating levels of angiotensin II and aldosterone, resulting in peripheral vascular constriction and sodium retention, respectively (see Chapter 31). The resulting systemic arterial hypertension is often marked.

In nearly two-thirds of patients, the stenosis results from an atheromatous plaque in the proximal renal artery. These patients are typically men over the age of 55 years. In the remaining third, the stenosis is more distal and is due to malformations of the arterial wall, commonly referred to as fibromuscular hyperplasia (or dysplasia). This latter lesion most commonly presents in women below the age of 35 years. Bilateral renal artery stenosis is present in 30–50% of patients with renovascular hypertension. Less common causes of stenosis include dissecting aneurysms, emboli, polyarteritis nodosa, radiation, trauma, extrinsic compression from retroperitoneal fibrosis or tumors, and hypoplasia of the renal arteries.

What clinical manifestations other than hypertension may be present?

Signs of secondary hyperaldosteronism can be prominent. These include sodium retention in the form of edema, a metabolic alkalosis, and hypokalemia. The latter can cause muscle weakness, polyuria, and even tetany.

How is the diagnosis made?

The diagnosis is suggested by the clinical presentation previously described. A midabdominal bruit may also be present, but the diagnosis requires laboratory and radiographic confirmation. The most sensitive diagnostic screening test is a gadolinium-enhanced magnetic resonance angiography (MRA). Alternative tests include a captopril-enhanced radionucleotide renal scan or Doppler ultrasound of the renal arteries. A defini-

tive diagnosis is made only by radiocontrast (X-ray) renal arteriography. Moreover, percutaneous balloon angioplasty with stenting may be performed at the same time. Restenosis rates are estimated to be < 15% after 1 year. Patients who are not candidates for angioplasty and stenting are referred for surgery. Long-term follow-up suggests that surgical treatment may be superior to angioplasty in preserving renal function.

Which patients are most likely to benefit from surgery?

The functional significance of the lesion may be evaluated by selective catheterization of both renal veins and measurement of plasma renin activity in blood from each kidney. Plasma renin activity is typically elevated on the stenotic side. Patients with renal artery stenosis with a plasma renin activity ratio on the two sides greater than 1.5:1 have a greater than 90% cure rate following surgery. Administration of an angiotensin-converting enzyme (ACE) inhibitor greatly magnifies the difference in renal vein plasma renin activity between the two sides. If the stenosis is bilateral, the split plasma renin activity ratios may be less than 1.5:1, yet the patient may still benefit from surgery.

Should this patient undergo the procedure given his present blood pressure?

Optimal medical therapy is important in preparing these patients for surgery. When compared with well-controlled patients, those with poorly controlled hypertension have a high incidence of problems intraoperatively: marked hypertension, hypotension, myocardial ischemia, and arrhythmias. Ideally, arterial blood pressure should be well controlled—preferably in the normal range—prior to surgery. Metabolic disturbances such as hypokalemia should be corrected. Patients should be evaluated for preexisting renal dysfunction (see Chapter 31). Patients older than 50 years of age should also be evaluated for the presence and severity of coexisting atherosclerotic disease, particularly of the coronary arteries (see Chapter 20).

What antihypertensive agents are most useful for controlling blood pressure perioperatively in these patients?

The most useful agents in unilateral renovascular hypertension are those that decrease renin–angiotensin system activity, namely ACE inhibitors, angiotensin II antagonists, β-blockers, and centrally acting agents that decrease sympathetic activity. It should be noted that ACE inhibitors and angiotensin II antagonists are contraindicated in the setting of bilateral renal artery stenosis because they can precipitate renal failure. Many ACE inhibitors are available, but only enalaprilat is available as an intravenous preparation (see Chapter 20). Side effects include transient hypotension, hyperkalemia, neutropenia, angioedema, urticaria, and rashes. Their role in perioperative blood pressure management is restricted to the preoperative period.

In contrast, β-adrenergic blocking drugs can be readily used intraoperatively and postoperatively for blood pressure control. They are particularly effective because secretion of renin is partly mediated by $β_1$-adrenergic receptors. Although parenteral selective $β_1$-blocking agents such as metoprolol and esmolol would be expected to be most effective, nonselective agents such as propranolol appear equally effective. Esmolol may be the agent of choice because of its short half-life and titratability.

Direct vasodilators such as nitroprusside and nitroglycerin are also invaluable in controlling intraoperative hypertension. Fenoldopam offers the additional benefit of increasing renal blood flow and may have renal protective properties.

What intraoperative considerations are important for the anesthesiologist?

Revascularization of a kidney is a major procedure, with the potential for major blood loss, fluid shifts, and hemodynamic changes. One of several procedures may be performed, including transaortic renal endarterectomy, aortorenal bypass (using a saphenous vein, synthetic graft, or segment of the hypogastric artery), a splenic to (left) renal artery bypass, a hepatic or gastroduodenal to (right) renal artery bypass, or excision of the stenotic segment with reanastomosis of the renal artery to the aorta. Rarely, nephrectomy may be performed. Regardless of the procedure, an extensive retroperitoneal dissection usually necessitates relatively large volumes of intravenous fluid replacement. Large-bore intravenous access is mandatory because of the potential for extensive blood loss. Heparinization contributes to increased blood loss. Depending on the surgical technique, aortic cross-clamping, with its associated hemodynamic consequences, often complicates anesthetic management (see Chapter 21). Direct intraarterial and central venous pressure monitoring are mandatory. Pulmonary artery pressure monitoring is indicated for patients with poor ventricular function and may be advisable in most patients to guide fluid management (see Chapter 6). The choice of anesthetic technique is generally determined by the patient's cardiovascular function.

Urinary output should be followed carefully. Measures to protect the affected as well as the normal kidney against ischemic injury are necessary. Generous hydration together with solute diuresis with mannitol are generally recommended (see Chapter 31). Fenoldopam may be useful in maximizing renal blood flow and controlling hypertension intraoperatively. Topical cooling of the affected kidney during the anastomosis may also be employed.

What postoperative considerations are important?

Although in most patients hypertension is ultimately cured or significantly improved, arterial blood pressure is often quite labile in the early postoperative period. Close hemodynamic monitoring should be continued well into the postoperative period. Reported operative mortality rates range from 1% to 6%, and most deaths are associated with myocardial infarction. The latter probably reflects the relatively high prevalence of coronary artery disease in older patients with renovascular hypertension.

SUGGESTED READING

Asif A, Epstein M: Prevention of radiocontrast-induced nephropathy. Am J Kidney Dis 2004;44:12.

Bambaro G, Bertaglia G, Puma G, D'Angelo A: Diuretics and dopamine for the prevention and treatment of acute renal failure: A critical reappraisal. J Nephrol 2002;15:213.

Better OS, Rubinstein I, Winaver JM, Knochel JP: Mannitol therapy revisited (1940–1997). Kidney Int 1997;52:886.

Evers SA, Maze M: *Anesthetic Pharmacology: Physiologic Principles and Clinical Practice.* Churchill Livingstone, 2004.

Murphy MB, Murray C, Shorten GD: Fenoldopam—a selective peripheral dopamine-receptor agonist for the treatment of severe hypertension. N Engl J Med 2001;345:1548.

Sadovnikoff N: Perioperative acute renal failure. Int Anesthesiol Clin 2001;39:95.

Schrier RW (editor): *Renal and Electrolyte Disorders,* 6th ed. Lippincott, Williams & Wilkins, 2002.

Sladen RN: Anesthetic considerations for the patient with renal failure. Anesthesiol Clin North Am 2000;18:863.

Stoelting RK, Dierdorf SE: *Anesthesia and Co-existing Disease,* 4th ed. Churchill Livingstone, 2002.

Thapa S, Brull SJ: Succinylcholine-induced hyperkalemia in patients with renal failure: An old question revisited. Anesth Analg 2000;91:237.

Anesthesia for Genitourinary Surgery

33

KEY CONCEPTS

 The lithotomy position is the most commonly used position for patients undergoing urological and gynecological procedures. Failure to properly position patients can result in iatrogenic injuries.

 The lithotomy position is associated with major physiological alterations. Functional residual capacity decreases, predisposing patients to atelectasis and hypoxia. Elevation of the legs increases venous return acutely. Mean blood pressure often increases, but cardiac output does not change significantly. Conversely, rapid lowering of the legs acutely decreases venous return and can result in hypotension. Blood pressure measurements should always be taken immediately after the legs are lowered.

 Because of the short duration (15–20 min) and the outpatient setting of most cystoscopies, general anesthesia is usually used.

 Both epidural and spinal blocks can provide satisfactory anesthesia. A sensory level to T10 provides excellent anesthesia for nearly all cystoscopic procedures.

 Manifestations of the TURP (transurethral resection of the prostate) syndrome are primarily those of circulatory fluid overload, water intoxication, and, occasionally, toxicity from the solute in the irrigating fluid.

 Absorption of irrigation fluid appears to be dependent on the duration of the resection as well as the height (pressure) of the irrigation fluid.

 When compared with general anesthesia, regional anesthesia appears to reduce the incidence of postoperative venous thrombosis; it is also less likely to mask symptoms and signs of the TURP syndrome or bladder perforation.

 Patients with a history of cardiac arrhythmias and those with a pacemaker or internal cardiac defibrillator (ICD) may be at risk for developing arrhythmias induced by shock waves during extracorporeal shock wave lithotripsy (ESWL). Shock waves can damage the internal components of pacemaker and ICD devices.

 Patients who are undergoing retroperitoneal lymph node dissection and who are receiving bleomycin preoperatively are at increased risk for developing postoperative pulmonary insufficiency. These patients appear to be particularly sensitive to oxygen toxicity and fluid overload, and are at increased risk for developing acute respiratory distress syndrome postoperatively. Excessive intravenous fluid administration may also be contributory.

 The serum potassium concentration should be below 5.5 mEq/L and existing coagulopathies should be corrected in patients undergoing renal transplantation. Hyperkalemia has been reported after release of the vascular clamp following completion of the arterial anastomosis, particularly in small patients and pediatric patients. Release of potassium contained in the preservative solution has been implicated in those cases.

Urological procedures account for 10–20% of most anesthetic practices. Patients undergoing genitourinary procedures may be of any age, but most are elderly and many have coexisting medical illnesses, particularly renal dysfunction. Anesthetic management of patients with renal impairment is discussed in Chapter 32, and the effects of anesthesia on renal function are discussed in Chapter 31. This chapter reviews the anesthetic management of common urological procedures. Use of the lithotomy position, the transurethral approach, and extracorporeal shock waves (lithotripsy) complicates many of these procedures. Moreover, advances in surgical technique allow more patients to undergo radical procedures for urological cancer, urinary diversion with bladder reconstruction, and renal transplantation.

CYSTOSCOPY

Preoperative Considerations

Cystoscopy is the most commonly performed urological procedure. Indications for cystoscopy include hematuria, recurrent urinary infections, renal calculi, and urinary obstruction. Bladder biopsies, retrograde pyelograms, resection of bladder tumors, extraction or laser lithotripsy of renal stones, and placement or manipulation of ureteral catheters (stents) can also be performed through the cystoscope.

Anesthetic management varies with the age and gender of the patient and the purpose of the procedure. General anesthesia is necessary for children. Topical anesthesia in the form of viscous lidocaine with or without sedation is used for diagnostic studies in most women, because of a short urethra. Operative cystoscopies involving biopsies, cauterization, or manipulation of ureteral catheters require regional or general anesthesia. Most males prefer regional or general anesthesia even for diagnostic studies.

Intraoperative Considerations

A. LITHOTOMY POSITION

Next to the supine position, the lithotomy position is the most commonly used position for patients undergoing urological and gynecological procedures. Failure to properly position patients can result in iatrogenic injuries. Two persons are required to safely move the patient's legs simultaneously up or down. Straps around the ankles or special holders support the legs in position (Figure 33–1). The leg supports should be padded, and the legs should hang freely. Caution should be exercised to prevent the fingers from being caught between the mid and lower sections of the operating room table when the lower section is lowered and raised. Injury to the common peroneal nerve, resulting in loss of dorsiflexion of the foot, may result if the lateral

thigh rests on the strap support. If the legs are allowed to rest on medially placed strap supports, compression of the saphenous nerve can result in numbness along the medial calf. Excessive flexion of the thigh against the groin can injure the obturator and, less commonly, the femoral nerves. Extreme flexion at the thigh can also stretch the sciatic nerve. It should be noted that the most common nerve injury associated with the lithotomy position involves the brachial plexus (see Chapter 46). A compartment syndrome of the lower extremities with rhabdomyolysis has been reported with prolonged time in the lithotomy position.

The lithotomy position is associated with major physiological alterations. Functional residual capacity decreases, predisposing patients to atelectasis and hypoxia. This effect is accentuated by the head-down (Trendelenburg) position (> 30°). Elevation of the legs increases venous return acutely and may exacerbate congestive heart failure. Mean blood pressure often increases, but cardiac output does not change significantly. Conversely, rapid lowering of the legs acutely decreases venous return and can result in hypotension. Vasodilation from either general or regional anesthesia accentuates the hypotension. For this reason, blood pressure measurements should always be taken immediately after the legs are lowered.

The Trendelenburg position may also be used with the lithotomy position.

B. CHOICE OF ANESTHESIA

1. General anesthesia—Because of the short duration (15–20 min) and the outpatient setting of most cystoscopies, general anesthesia is usually used. Most patients are apprehensive about the procedure and prefer to be asleep. Any anesthetic technique suitable for outpatients may be used. Oxygen saturation should be closely monitored when obese or elderly patients or those with marginal pulmonary reserve are placed in the lithotomy or Trendelenburg position. A laryngeal mask airway (LMA) is often used.

2. Regional anesthesia—Both epidural and spinal blocks can provide satisfactory anesthesia. However, satisfactory sensory blockade may require 15–20 min for epidural anesthesia compared with 5 min for spinal anesthesia. Consequently, most clinicians prefer spinal anesthesia, particularly for procedures lasting more than 30 min with elderly and high-risk patients. Some clinicians believe that the sensory level following injection of a hyperbaric anesthetic solution should be well established ("fixed") before the patient is moved into the lithotomy position; however, studies fail to demonstrate that immediate elevation of the legs following intrathecal injection increases the level of anesthesia or increases the likelihood of severe hypotension. A sensory level to T10 provides excellent anesthesia for nearly all cystoscopic pro-

Figure 33–1. The lithotomy position. ***A:*** Strap stirrups. ***B:*** Bier–Hoff stirrups. ***C:*** Allen stirrups. (Modified and reproduced, with permission, from Martin JT: *Positioning in Anesthesia.* W.B. Saunders, 1988.)

cedures. Regional anesthesia, however, does not abolish the **obturator reflex** (external rotation and adduction of the thigh secondary to stimulation of the obturator nerve by electrocautery current through the lateral bladder wall). The reflex (muscle contraction) is reliably blocked only by muscle paralysis during general anesthesia.

TRANSURETHRAL SURGERY OF THE PROSTATE

Preoperative Considerations

Benign prostatic hypertrophy frequently leads to symptomatic bladder outlet obstruction in men older than 60

years. Indications of surgery include moderate to severe lower urinary tract symptoms (LUTS) in patients who do not respond to or decline medical therapy, persistent gross hematuria, recurrent urinary infections, renal insufficiency, or bladder stones. One of several operations may be selected to remove the hypertrophied and hyperplastic prostatic tissue: **transurethral resection of the prostate (TURP),** transurethral electrovaporization, transurethral incision, transurethral laser techniques, suprapubic (transvesical) prostatectomy, perineal prostatectomy, or retropubic prostatectomy. All require general or regional anesthesia. Some less invasive procedures, such as transurethral microwave treatments, may be performed with just topical anesthesia. The transurethral approach for surgery is nearly always selected for patients with prostate gland volumes less than 40–50 mL. An alternative approach is chosen if the prostate is over 80 mL. Patients with advanced prostatic carcinoma may also present for transurethral resections to relieve symptomatic urinary obstruction. Regardless of its cause, long-standing obstruction can lead to impaired renal function.

Patients undergoing prostate surgery should be carefully evaluated for coexistent cardiac and pulmonary disease as well as renal dysfunction (see Chapters 20, 23, and 32). Because of their age these patients have a relatively high (30–60%) prevalence of both cardiovascular and pulmonary disorders. TURP is reported to carry a 0.2–6% mortality rate, which correlates best with the American Society of Anesthesiologists' (ASA) physical status scale. Common causes of death include myocardial infarction, pulmonary edema, and renal failure.

Although a type and screen (see Chapter 29) are adequate for most patients, blood should be available and crossmatched for anemic patients as well as patients with large glands (> 40 mL). Prostatic bleeding can be difficult to control through the cystoscope.

Intraoperative Considerations

TURP is performed by passing a loop through a special cystoscope (resectoscope). Using continuous irrigation and direct visualization, prostatic tissue is resected by applying a cutting current to the loop. Because of the characteristics of the prostate and the large amounts of irrigation fluid often used, TURP can be associated with a number of serious complications (Table 33–1). Although experience is more limited with other transurethral prostate procedures, their complication rate (and possible efficacy) may be less.

A. TURP SYNDROME

Transurethral prostatic resection often opens the extensive network of venous sinuses in the prostate and potentially allows systemic absorption of the irrigating fluid. The absorption of large amounts of fluid (2 L or more) results in a constellation of symptoms and signs commonly referred to as the TURP syndrome (Table 33–2). This syndrome presents intraoperatively or postopera-

Table 33–1. Major complications associated with TURP.

Hemorrhage
TURP syndrome
Bladder perforation
Hypothermia
Septicemia
Disseminated intravascular coagulation

Table 33–2. Manifestations of the TURP syndrome.

Hyponatremia
Hypoosmolality
Fluid overload
Congestive heart failure
Pulmonary edema
Hypotension
Hemolysis
Solute toxicity
Hyperglycinemia (glycine)
Hyperammonemia (glycine)
Hyperglycemia (sorbitol)
Intravascular volume expansion (mannitol)

tively as headache, restlessness, confusion, cyanosis, dyspnea, arrhythmias, hypotension, or seizures. Moreover, it can be rapidly fatal. The manifestations are primarily those of circulatory fluid overload, water intoxication, and, occasionally, toxicity from the solute in the irrigating fluid.

Electrolyte solutions cannot be used for irrigation during TURP because they disperse the electrocautery current. Water provides excellent visibility because its hypotonicity lyses red blood cells, but significant absorption can readily result in acute water intoxication. Water irrigation is generally restricted to transurethral resection of bladder tumors only. For TURP, slightly hypotonic nonelectrolyte irrigating solutions such as glycine 1.5% (230 mOsm/L) or a mixture of sorbitol 2.7% and mannitol 0.54% (195 mOsm/L) are most commonly used. Less commonly used solutions include sorbitol 3.3%, mannitol 3%, dextrose 2.5–4%, and urea 1%. Because all these fluids are still hypotonic, significant absorption of water can nevertheless occur. Solute absorption can also occur because the irrigation fluid is under pressure. High irrigation pressures (bottle height) increase fluid absorption.

Absorption of irrigation fluid appears to be dependent on the duration of the resection as well as the height (pressure) of the irrigation fluid. Most resections last 45–60 min, and, on average, 20 mL/min of the irrigating fluid is absorbed. Pulmonary congestion or florid pulmonary edema can readily result from the absorption of large amounts of irrigation fluid, particularly in patients with limited cardiac reserve. The hypotonicity of these fluids also results in acute hyponatremia and hypoosmolality, which can lead to serious neurological manifestations (see Chapter 28). Symptoms of hyponatremia usually do not develop until the serum sodium concentration decreases below 120 mEq/L. Marked hypotonicity in plasma ($[Na^+]$ < 100 mEq/L) may also result in acute intravascular hemolysis (see Chapter 29).

Toxicity may also arise from absorption of the solutes in these fluids. Marked **hyperglycinemia** has been reported with glycine solutions and is thought to contribute to circulatory depression and central nervous system toxicity. Plasma glycine concentrations in excess of 1000 mg/L have been recorded (normal is 13–17 mg/L). Glycine is known to be an inhibitory neurotransmitter in the central nervous system and has also been implicated in rare instances of transient blindness following TURP. Hyperammonemia, presumably from the degradation of glycine, has also been documented in a few patients with marked central nervous system toxicity following TURP. Blood ammonia levels in some patients exceeded 500 μmol/L (normal is 5–50 μmol/L). The use of large amounts of sorbitol or dextrose irrigating solutions can lead to hyperglycemia, which can be marked in diabetic patients. Absorption of mannitol solutions causes intravascular volume expansion and exacerbates fluid overload.

Treatment of TURP syndrome depends on early recognition and should be based on the severity of the symptoms. The absorbed water must be eliminated, and hypoxemia and hypoperfusion must be avoided. Most patients can be managed with fluid restriction and a loop diuretic. Symptomatic hyponatremia resulting in seizures or coma should be treated with hypertonic saline (see Chapter 28). Seizure activity can be terminated with small doses of midazolam (2–4 mg), diazepam (3–5 mg), or thiopental (50–100 mg). Phenytoin, 10–20 mg/kg intravenously (no faster than 50 mg/min), should also be considered to provide more sustained anticonvulsant activity. Endotracheal intubation is generally advisable to prevent aspiration until the patient's mental status normalizes. The amount and rate of hypertonic saline solution (3% or 5%) needed to correct the hyponatremia to a safe level should be based on the patient's serum sodium concentration (see Chapter 28). Hypertonic saline solution should not be given at a rate faster than 100 mL/h so as not to exacerbate circulatory fluid overload.

B. HYPOTHERMIA

Large volumes of irrigating fluids at room temperature can be a major source of heat loss in patients. Irrigating solutions should be warmed to body temperature prior to use to prevent hypothermia. Postoperative shivering associated with hypothermia is particularly undesirable, as it can dislodge clots and promote postoperative bleeding.

C. BLADDER PERFORATION

The incidence of **bladder perforation** during TURP is estimated to be approximately 1%. Perforation may result from the resectoscope going through the bladder wall or from overdistention of the bladder with irrigation fluid. Most bladder perforations are extraperitoneal and are signaled by poor return of the irrigating fluid. Awake patients will typically complain of nausea, diaphoresis, and retropubic or lower abdominal pain. Large extraperitoneal and most intraperitoneal perforations are usually

even more obvious, presenting as sudden unexplained hypotension (or hypertension) with generalized abdominal pain (in awake patients). Regardless of the anesthetic technique employed, perforation should be suspected in settings of sudden hypotension or hypertension, particularly with bradycardia (vagally mediated).

D. COAGULOPATHY

Disseminated intravascular coagulation (DIC) has on rare occasions been reported following TURP and is thought to result from the release of thromboplastins from the prostate into the circulation during surgery. Up to 6% of patients may have evidence of subclinical DIC. A dilutional thrombocytopenia can also develop during surgery as part of the TURP syndrome from absorption of irrigation fluids. Rarely, patients with metastatic carcinoma of the prostate develop a coagulopathy from primary fibrinolysis; the tumor is thought to secrete a fibrinolytic enzyme in such instances. The diagnosis of coagulopathy may be suspected from diffuse uncontrollable bleeding, but must be confirmed by laboratory tests (see Case Discussion, Chapter 34). Primary fibrinolysis should be treated with ε-aminocaproic acid (Amicar) 5 g followed by 1 g/h intravenously. The treatment of DIC in this setting may require heparin in addition to replacement of clotting factors and platelets. Consultation with a hematologist is advisable.

E. SEPTICEMIA

The prostate is often colonized with bacteria and may harbor chronic infection. Extensive surgical manipulation of the gland together with the opening of venous sinuses can allow entry of organisms into the bloodstream. Bacteremia following transurethral surgery is not uncommon and can lead to septicemia or septic shock (see Chapter 49). Prophylactic antibiotic therapy (most commonly gentamicin, levofloxacin, or cephazolin) prior to TURP may decrease the likelihood of bacteremic and septic episodes.

F. CHOICE OF ANESTHESIA

Either spinal or epidural anesthesia with a T10 sensory level provides excellent anesthesia and good operating conditions for TURP. When compared with general anesthesia, regional anesthesia appears to reduce the incidence of postoperative venous thrombosis; it is also less likely to mask symptoms and signs of the TURP syndrome or bladder perforation. Clinical studies have failed to show any differences in blood loss, postoperative cognitive function, and mortality between regional and general anesthesia. The possibility of vertebral metastasis must be considered in patients with carcinoma, particularly those with back pain. Metastatic disease to the lumbar spine is a contraindication to regional anesthesia. Acute hyponatremia from the TURP syndrome may delay or prevent emergence from general anesthesia.

G. MONITORING

Evaluation of mental status in the awake patient is the best monitor for detection of early signs of the TURP syndrome and bladder perforation. A decrease in arterial oxygen saturation may be an early sign of fluid overload. Some studies have reported perioperative ischemic electrocardiographic changes in up to 18% of patients. Temperature monitoring should be used during long resections to detect hypothermia. Blood loss is particularly difficult to assess because of the use of irrigating solutions, so it is necessary to rely on clinical signs of hypovolemia (see Chapter 29). Blood loss averages about 3–5 mL/min of resection (usually 200–300 mL total) but is rarely life-threatening. Transient, postoperative decreases in hematocrit may simply reflect hemodilution from absorption of irrigation fluid. About 2.5% of patients require intraoperative transfusion; factors associated with transfusion include a procedure whose duration is longer than 90 min and resection of greater than 45 g of prostate tissue.

LITHOTRIPSY

The treatment of kidney stones has changed significantly over the past two decades from primarily open surgical procedures to less invasive or completely noninvasive techniques. Stones in the bladder and lower ureters are now usually treated with cystoscopic procedures, including flexible and rigid ureteroscopy, stone extraction, stent placement, and intracorporeal lithotripsy (laser or electrohydraulic). Laser lithotripsy typically utilizes a holmium:YAG laser. In contrast, stones in the upper two-thirds of the ureters or kidneys are treated with extracorporeal shock wave lithotripsy (ESWL) or percutaneous nephrolithotomy. The latter is reserved for large stones (> 2 cm) and involves techniques similar to ureteroscopy; however, application is via a percutaneous sheath over the kidney in the prone position. Some stones (eg, cystine, uric acid, and calcium oxalate monohydrate) are particularly hard and are more likely to require retreatment.

During ESWL, repetitive high-energy shocks (sound waves) are generated and focused on the stone, causing it to fragment as tensile and shear forces develop inside the stone and cavitation occurs outside on its surface. Water or a conducting gel couples the generator to the patient. Because tissue has the same acoustic density as water, the waves travel through the body without damaging tissue. However, the change in acoustic impedance at the tissue–stone interface creates shear and tear forces on the stone. The stone is fragmented enough to allow its passage in small pieces down the urinary tract. Ureteral stents are often placed cystoscopically prior to the procedure to facilitate the passage of large particles of stone. Tissue

destruction can occur if the waves are focused at air–tissue interfaces such as in the lung and intestine. The inability to position the patient so that lung and intestine are away from the wave focus is a contraindication to the procedure. Other contraindications include urinary obstruction below the stone, untreated infection, a bleeding diathesis, and pregnancy. The presence of a nearby aortic aneurysm or orthopedic prosthetic device is considered a relative contraindication in some centers. Ecchymosis, bruising, or blistering of the skin over the treatment site is not uncommon. Rarely, a large perinephric hematoma can develop and may be responsible for a significant decrease in hematocrit postoperatively.

Electrohydraulic, electromagnetic, or piezoelectric shock wave generators may be used for ESWL. With older electrohydraulic units (Dornier HM3), the patient is placed in a hydraulic chair, immersed in a heated water bath, and positioned with the aid of two image intensifiers such that the stone is in the second focus of an elliptical reflector, while the source of the shock waves, an underwater capacitor (spark plug), is in the first focus (Figure 33–2). One electrohydraulic lithotriptor is tubless (Dornier MFL 5000). Most modern lithotriptors generate shock waves either electromagnetically (Dornier DoLi, Compact Delta and Sigma; Siemens Lithostar; and Storz Modulith) or from piezoelectric crystals (Wolf Piezolith); the generator is enclosed in a water-filled casing and comes in contact with the patient via a conducting gel on a plastic membrane (Figure 33–3). Newer units allow both fluoroscopic and ultrasound localization. In the case of electromagnetic machines, the vibration of a metallic plate in front of an electromagnet produces the shock waves. With piezoelectric models, the

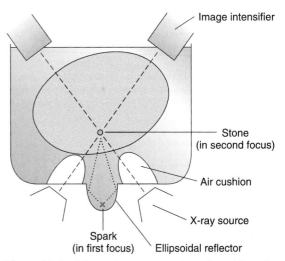

Figure 33–2. Schematic representation of an older tub lithotripsy unit (Dornier HM3).

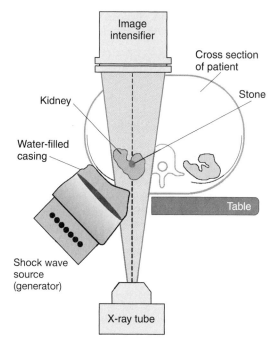

Figure 33–3. Schematic representation of a newer tubless lithotripsy unit.

waves are the result of changes in the external dimensions of ceramic crystals when electric current is applied.

Preoperative Considerations

Patients with a history of cardiac arrhythmias and those with a pacemaker or internal cardiac defibrillator (ICD) may be at risk for developing arrhythmias induced by shock waves during ESWL. Shock waves can damage the internal components of pacemaker and ICD devices. The manufacturer should be contacted as to the best method for managing the device (eg, reprogramming or applying a magnet). Synchronization of the shock waves to the R wave from the electrocardiogram (ECG) decreases the incidence of arrhythmias during ESWL. The shock waves are usually timed to be 20 ms after the R wave to correspond to the ventricular refractory period (see Chapter 19). Studies suggest that asynchronous delivery of shocks can be safe in patients without heart disease.

Intraoperative Considerations

Anesthetic considerations for ureteroscopy, stone manipulation, and laser lithotripsy are similar to those for cystoscopic procedures. ESWL requires special considerations, particularly when older lithotriptors (Dornier

HM3), which require the patient to be immersed in water, are used.

A. Effects of Immersion

Immersion into a heated water bath (36–37°C) initially results in vasodilation that can transiently lead to hypotension. Arterial blood pressure, however, subsequently rises as venous blood is redistributed centrally from the hydrostatic pressure of water on the legs and abdomen. Systemic vascular resistance (SVR) rises and cardiac output often decreases. The sudden increase in venous return and SVR can precipitate congestive heart failure in patients with marginal cardiac reserve. Moreover, the increase in intrathoracic blood volume significantly reduces functional residual capacity (30–60%) and predisposes some patients to hypoxemia.

B. Choice of Anesthesia

Pain during lithotripsy is from dissipation of a small amount of energy as shock waves enter the body through the skin. The pain is therefore localized to the skin and proportionate to the intensity of the shock waves. Older lithotripsy with units employing a water bath (Dornier HM3) requires 1000–2400 relatively high-intensity shock waves (18–22 kV) that most patients do not tolerate without either regional or general anesthesia. In contrast, newer lithotripsy units that are coupled directly to the skin utilize 2000–3000 lower-intensity shock waves (10–18 kV) that usually require only light sedation.

C. Regional Anesthesia

Continuous epidural anesthesia is commonly used for ESWL using a water bath. A T6 sensory level ensures adequate anesthesia, as renal innervation is derived from T10 to L2. Supplementation of the block with fentanyl, 50–100 mg epidurally, is often useful. As little air as possible should be used with the loss of resistance technique during insertion (see Chapter 16); large amounts of air in the epidural space can dissipate shock waves and theoretically may promote injury to neural tissue. Foam tape should not be used to secure the epidural catheter as this type of tape has been shown to dissipate the energy of the shocks when it is in their path. Light sedation is also generally desirable for most patients. Supplemental oxygen by face mask or nasal cannula is also useful in avoiding hypoxemia. Spinal anesthesia can also be used satisfactorily, but because of the potential for an increased incidence of postdural puncture headache in a seated patient and less control over the sensory level with spinal anesthesia, epidural anesthesia is usually preferred. Regional anesthesia greatly facilitates positioning and monitoring. Prior intravascular volume expansion with 1000–1500 mL of lactated Ringer's injection may help prevent severe postural hypotension following the onset of neuraxial anesthesia, positioning in the hydraulic chair, and immersion in the warm bath.

A major disadvantage of regional anesthesia is the inability to control diaphragmatic movement. Excessive diaphragmatic excursion during spontaneous ventilation can move the stone in and out of the wave focus and may prolong the procedure. This problem can be partially solved by asking the patient to breathe in a more rapid but shallow respiratory pattern. Bradycardia from high sympathetic blockade also prolongs the procedure when shock waves are coupled to the ECG.

D. GENERAL ANESTHESIA

General endotracheal anesthesia allows control of diaphragmatic excursion during tub lithotripsy (Dornier HM3) and is preferred by many patients. The procedure is complicated by the inherent risks associated with placing a supine anesthetized patient in a chair, elevating and then lowering the chair into a water bath to shoulder depth, and then reversing the sequence at the end. A light general anesthetic technique in conjunction with a muscle relaxant is preferable. The muscle relaxant ensures patient immobility and control of diaphragmatic movement. As with regional anesthesia, intravenous fluid loading with 1000 mL of lactated Ringer's injection is generally advisable prior to moving patients upright into the hydraulic chair to prevent postural hypotension.

E. MONITORED ANESTHESIA CARE

Intravenous sedation is usually adequate for low-energy lithotripsy. Low-dose propofol infusions together with midazolam and opioid supplementation may be used.

F. MONITORING

Electrocardiograph pads should be attached securely with waterproof dressing prior to immersion. **Even with R wave–riggered shocks, supraventricular arrhythmias can still occur and may require treatment.** Changes in functional residual capacity with immersion mandate close monitoring of oxygen saturation, particularly in patients at high risk for developing hypoxemia (see Chapter 22). The temperature of the bath and the patient should be monitored to prevent hypothermia or hyperthermia.

G. FLUID MANAGEMENT

Intravenous fluid therapy is typically generous. Following the initial intravenous fluid bolus (above), an additional 1000–2000 mL of lactated Ringer's injection is usually given with a small dose of furosemide (10–20 mg) to maintain brisk urinary flow and flush stone debris and blood clots. Patients with poor cardiac reserve require more conservative fluid therapy.

NONCANCER SURGERY ON THE UPPER URETER & KIDNEY

Laparoscopic techniques are increasingly utilized in urology. Advantages include shorter hospital stays, faster recovery, and less pain. Laparoscopic procedures include live donor nephrectomy, nephrectomy, partial nephrectomy, and pyeloplasty. Both transperitoneal and retroperitoneal approaches have been developed. A hand-assisted technique employs an additional larger incision that allows the surgeon to insert one hand for tactile sensation and dissection. Anesthetic management is similar to that for any laparoscopic procedures (Chapter 23). Open procedures for kidney stones in the upper ureter and renal pelvis and nephrectomies for nonmalignant disease are often carried out in the "kidney rest position," also more accurately described as the lateral flexed position. With the patient in a full lateral position, the dependent leg is flexed and the other leg is extended. An axillary roll is placed underneath the dependent upper chest to prevent injury to the brachial plexus. The operating table is then extended to achieve maximal separation between the iliac crest and the costal margin on the operative side, and the kidney rest (a bar in the groove where the table bends) is elevated to raise the nondependent iliac crest higher and increase surgical exposure.

The lateral flexed position is associated with significant adverse respiratory and circulatory effects. Functional residual capacity is reduced in the dependent lung but may increase in the nondependent lung. In the anesthetized patient receiving controlled ventilation, ventilation/perfusion mismatching occurs because the dependent lung receives greater blood flow than the nondependent lung, whereas the nondependent lung receives greater ventilation, predisposing the patient to atelectasis in the dependent lung and hypoxemia. The arterial to end-tidal gradient for carbon dioxide progressively increases during general anesthesia in this position, indicating that dead space ventilation also increases in the nondependent lung. Moreover, elevation of the kidney rest can significantly decrease venous return to the heart in some patients by compressing the inferior vena cava. Venous pooling in the legs decreases venous return and aggravates any anesthesia-induced vasodilation.

Because of the potential for large blood loss and limited access to major vascular structures in the lateral flexed position, a large-bore intravenous catheter is advisable. Inadvertent entry into the pleural space can produce a pneumothorax. Diagnosis requires a high index of suspicion. The pneumothorax may be

Figure 33–4. The hyperextended position. (Modified and reproduced, with permission, from Skinner DG, Lieskovsky G: *Diagnosis and Management of Genitourinary Cancer.* W.B. Saunders, 1988.)

subclinical intraoperatively but can be diagnosed postoperatively with a chest radiograph.

RADICAL SURGERY FOR UROLOGICAL MALIGNANCIES

Demographic changes resulting in an increasingly elderly population together with improved survival rates for patients with urological cancer following radical surgical resections have resulted in an increase in the number of procedures performed for prostatic, bladder, testicular, and renal cancer. Curative and palliative surgery plays an important role in treatment of these malignancies.

The desire for a quicker recovery with smaller, less painful incisions has prompted the successful development of laparoscopic operations for radical prostatectomy with pelvic lymph node dissection, nephrectomy, and laparoscopic retroperitoneal lymph node dissections for early malignancies. Robotic-assisted technology has also been applied to laparoscopic prostatectomy (da Vinci prostatectomy). The short-term results of these less invasive procedures appear to be comparable to standard open operations, at least for early malignancies. Whether long-term results are the same remains to be determined.

Many urological procedures are carried out in a hyperextended supine position to facilitate exposure of the pelvis during pelvic lymph node dissection, retropubic prostatectomy, or cystectomy (Figure 33–4). The patient is positioned supine with the iliac crest over the break in the operating table, and the table is extended such that distance between the iliac crest and the costal margin increases maximally. Care must be taken not to put excessive strain on the patient's back. The operating room table is also tilted head-down to make the operative field horizontal. In the frog-leg position, a variation of the hyperextended supine position, the knees are also flexed and the hips are abducted and externally rotated. For thoracoabdominal surgery, the patient is placed in a hyperextended supine position close to the edge of the table on the operative side; the leg on the nonoperative side is flexed 30° while the knee is flexed 90°, and the leg on the operative side remains straight (Figure 33–5). The shoulder on the ipsilateral side is elevated 30° with a roll to allow that arm to come across the chest into an adjustable arm rest ("airplane"), while the other arm is extended on an arm board. Although the adverse effects

of the hyperextended supine position have not been studied, the physiological consequences of this position appear to be similar to the Trendelenburg position. The potential for neurological injuries and back injury exists because of the complex nature of the position. Careful positioning and generous padding of the arms and legs are therefore warranted. Positioning the pelvis above the heart may predispose patients to venous air embolism; however, this appears to be a rare complication.

1. Prostate Cancer

Preoperative Considerations

Adenocarcinoma of the prostate is the most common cancer in men. It is the second most common cause of cancer

Figure 33–5. The thoracoabdominal incision. (Modified and reproduced, with permission, from Skinner DG, Lieskovsky G: *Diagnosis and Management of Genitourinary Cancer.* W.B. Saunders, 1988.)

deaths in men older than 55 years. The incidence of prostate cancer increases with age and is estimated to be 75% in patients over 75 years. Because of the tumor's wide spectrum of clinical behavior, management varies widely from surveillance to aggressive surgical therapy. Important variables include the grade and stage of the malignancy, the patient's age, and the presence of other medical illnesses. Transrectal ultrasound is used to evaluate tumor size and the presence or absence of extracapsular extension. Clinical staging is also based on the Gleason score of the biopsy, computed tomography (CT) scan or magnetic resonance imaging (MRI), and bone scan.

Intraoperative Considerations

Patients with prostate cancer may present to the operating room for a laparoscopic prostatectomy with pelvic lymph node dissection, radical prostatectomy, salvage prostatectomy (following failure of radiation therapy), or bilateral orchiectomy for hormonal therapy.

A. Laparoscopic Radical Prostatectomy

Laparoscopic radical prostatectomy with pelvic lymph node dissection differs from most other laparoscopic procedures in (1) the use of a steep (> 30°) Trendelenburg position for surgical exposure, and (2) the potential for greater carbon dioxide absorption from the retroperitoneum. The procedure is carried out under general endotracheal anesthesia because of the length of the procedure, steep Trendelenburg position, necessity for abdominal distention, and desirability of being able to increase the patient's minute ventilation. Most clinicians avoid nitrous oxide to prevent bowel distention and expansion of residual intraabdominal gas.

B. Radical Retropubic Prostatectomy

Radical retropubic prostatectomy is usually performed together with a pelvic lymph node dissection through a lower, midline, abdominal position. It may be curative for localized prostatic cancer or occasionally used as a salvage procedure after failure of radiation. The prostate is removed en bloc with the seminal vesicles, ejaculatory ducts, and part of the bladder neck. A "nerve-sparing" technique may be used to help preserve sexual function. Following the prostatectomy, the remaining bladder neck is anastomosed directly to the urethra over an indwelling urinary catheter. The surgeon may ask for intravenous administration of indigo carmine for visualization of the ureters. This dye can be associated with hypertension or hypotension.

Radical retropubic prostatectomy is often associated with significant operative blood loss. Direct arterial pressure monitoring is generally advisable and allows controlled hypotension (see Chapter 13). Routine use of central venous pressure monitoring has also been advocated. Blood loss appears to vary considerably from center to center; values less than 500 mL are common. Factors that may affect blood loss include positioning, pelvic anatomy, and size of the prostate; early ligation of the dorsal vein complex of the penis and temporary clamping of the hypogastric artery appear to reduce blood loss. Blood loss is similar in patients receiving general anesthesia and those receiving regional anesthesia; operative morbidity and mortality also appear to be similar. Neuraxial anesthesia requires a T6 sensory level but awake patients typically do not tolerate regional anesthesia without heavy sedation because of the hyperextended supine position. Moreover, the combination of a prolonged Trendelenburg position together with administration of large amounts of intravenous fluids can produce edema of the upper airway.

Clinical studies have found no differences in pain relief or recovery between patients receiving epidural opioids and those receiving intravenous patient-controlled analgesia. Ketorolac can be used as an analgesic adjuvant and has been reported to decrease opioid requirements, improve analgesia, and promote earlier return of bowel function without increasing transfusion requirements. Extensive surgical dissection around the pelvic veins increases the risk of thromboembolic complications. Although epidural anesthesia appears to reduce the incidence of postoperative deep venous thrombosis following prostatectomy, this beneficial effect may be negated by the routine use of warfarin or low-molecular-weight heparin prophylaxis postoperatively. Moreover, postoperative anticoagulation increases the risk of epidural hematoma. Prophylactic minidose unfractionated heparin has been reported to increase operative loss and transfusion requirements, whereas sequential pneumatic (leg) compression devices appear to delay but not reduce deep venous thrombosis. Other postoperative complications include hemorrhage; injuries to the obturator nerve, ureter, and rectum; as well as urinary incontinence and impotence.

C. Bilateral Orchiectomy

Bilateral orchiectomy is usually performed for local control of metastatic adenocarcinoma of the prostate. The procedure is relatively short (20–45 min) and is performed through a single midline scrotal incision. Although bilateral orchiectomy can be performed under local anesthesia, most patients and many clinicians prefer general anesthesia, which is usually administered with an LMA.

2. Bladder Cancer

Preoperative Considerations

Bladder cancer occurs at an average patient age of 65 years with a 3:1 male to female ratio. Transitional cell carcinoma of the bladder is the second most common malignancy of the genitourinary tract. The association of cigarette smoking with bladder carcinoma results in coexistent coronary artery and chronic obstructive pulmonary disease in many of these patients. Moreover, underlying renal impairment may be age related or secondary to urinary tract obstruction. Staging includes cystoscopy and CT or MRI scans. Intravesical chemotherapy is used for superficial tumors and transurethral resection is carried out for low-grade noninvasive bladder tumors. Some patients may receive preoperative radiation to shrink the tumor before radical cystectomy. Urinary diversion is usually performed immediately following the cystectomy.

Intraoperative Considerations

A. Radical Cystectomy

Radical cystectomy is a major operation that is often associated with significant blood loss. It is usually performed through a midline incision that extends from the pubis to the xiphoid process. All anterior pelvic organs including the bladder, prostate, and seminal vesicles are removed in males; the uterus, cervix, ovaries, and part of the anterior vaginal vault may also be removed in females. Pelvic node dissection and urinary diversion are also carried out.

These procedures typically require 4–6 h and frequently necessitate blood transfusion. General endotracheal anesthesia with a muscle relaxant provides optimal operating conditions. Controlled hypotensive anesthesia may reduce intraoperative blood loss and transfusion requirements. Many surgeons also believe controlled hypotension improves surgical visualization. Supplementation of general anesthesia with spinal or continuous epidural anesthesia can facilitate the induced hypotension, decrease general anesthetic requirements, and provide a highly effective postoperative analgesia. A major drawback of the use of neuraxial anesthesia is the hyperperistalsis that produces a very small contracted bowel, which complicates construction of a urinary reservoir.

Close monitoring of blood pressure, intravascular volume, and blood loss is essential. Direct intraarterial pressure monitoring is indicated in all patients, central venous pressure monitoring is advisable in patients with limited cardiac reserve, and pulmonary artery pressure monitoring is indicated in patients with a history of ventricular dysfunction. Urinary output should be monitored continuously and correlated with the progress of the operation, as the urinary path is interrupted at an early point during most of these procedures. An upper body forced-air warming blanket is essential in preventing hypothermia.

B. Urinary Diversion

Urinary diversion is usually performed immediately following radical cystectomy. Many procedures are currently used, but all entail implanting the ureters into a segment of bowel. The selected bowel segment is either left *in situ*, such as in ureterosigmoidostomy, or divided with its mesenteric blood supply intact and attached to a cutaneous stoma or urethra. Moreover, the isolated bowel can either function as a conduit (eg, ileal conduit) or be reconstructed to form a continent reservoir (neobladder). Conduits may be formed from ileum, jejunum, or colon. Continent urinary diversions include ureterosigmoidostomy, small bowel (Kock, Camey, T-pouch), and large bowel (Indiana).

Major anesthetic goals include keeping the patient well hydrated and maintaining a brisk urinary output once the ureters are opened. Central venous pressure monitoring is often employed to guide intravenous fluid administration. Neuraxial anesthesia often produces unopposed parasympathetic activity due to sympathetic blockade, which results in a very contracted, hyperactive bowel that makes construction of a continent ileal reservoir technically difficult. Papaverine (100–150 mg as a slow intravenous infusion over 2–3 h), a large dose of an anticholinergic (glycopyrrolate, 1 mg), or glucagon (1 mg) may alleviate this problem.

Prolonged contact of urine with bowel mucosa (slow urine flow) may produce significant metabolic disturbances. Hyponatremia, hypochloremia, hyperkalemia, and metabolic acidosis can occur following jejunal conduits. In contrast, colonic and ileal conduits may be associated with hyperchloremic metabolic acidosis. The use of temporary ureteral stents and maintenance of high urinary flow help alleviate this problem in the early postoperative period.

3. Testicular Cancer

Preoperative Considerations

Testicular tumors are classified either as seminomas or nonseminomas. The initial treatment for all tumors is radical (inguinal) orchiectomy. Subsequent management depends on tumor histology. Nonseminomas include embryonal teratoma, choriocarcinoma, and mixed tumors. Retroperitoneal lymph node dissection (RPLND) plays a major role in the treatment of patients with nonseminomatous germ cell tumors. Low-stage disease is managed with RPLND or in some instances surveillance. High-stage disease is usually treated with chemotherapy followed by RPLND.

In contrast to nonseminomas, seminomas are very radiosensitive tumors that are primarily treated with retroperitoneal radiotherapy. Chemotherapy is used for patients who relapse after radiation. Patients with large bulky seminomas or those with increased α-fetoprotein levels (usually associated with nonseminomas) are treated primarily with chemotherapy. Chemotherapeutic agents commonly include cisplatin, vincristine, vinblastine, cyclophosphamide, dactinomycin, bleomycin, and etoposide. RPLND is usually undertaken for patients with residual tumor after chemotherapy.

Patients undergoing RPLND for testicular cancer are typically young (15–35 years old) but are at increased risk for morbidity from the residual effects of preoperative chemotherapy. In addition to bone marrow suppression, specific organ toxicity may be encountered such as renal impairment following cisplatin, pulmonary fibrosis following bleomycin, and neuropathy following vincristine.

Intraoperative Considerations

A. Radical Orchiectomy

Inguinal orchiectomy can be carried out with regional or general anesthesia; most patients prefer the latter. Anesthetic management may be complicated by reflex bradycardia from traction on the spermatic cord.

B. Retroperitoneal Lymph Node Dissection

The retroperitoneum is usually accessed through a large thoracoabdominal incision that extends from the posterior axillary line over the eighth to tenth ribs to a paramedian line halfway between the xiphoid and the umbilicus (Figure 33–5). Alternatively, some surgeons use a transabdominal approach through a midline incision from the xiphoid to the pubis. A laparoscopic technique may be increasingly utilized. Regardless of the approach, all lymphatic tissue between the ureters from the renal vessels to the iliac bifurcation is removed. With the standard RPLND, all sympathetic fibers are disrupted resulting in loss of normal ejaculation and infertility; a modified technique that may help preserve fertility limits the dissection below the inferior mesenteric artery to include lymphatic tissue only on the ipsilateral side of the tumor.

Patients receiving bleomycin preoperatively appear to be particularly sensitive to oxygen toxicity and fluid overload, and are at increased risk of developing pulmonary insufficiency or acute respiratory distress syndrome postoperatively. Excessive intravenous fluid administration may also be contributory. Anesthetic management should generally include use of the lowest inspired concentration of oxygen compatible with acceptable oxygen saturation (> 90%). Positive end-expiratory pressure (5–10 cm H_2O) may be helpful in optimizing oxygenation. An air–oxygen mixture is generally used because prolonged administration of nitrous oxide can produce bone marrow suppression.

Evaporative and redistributive fluid losses ("third spacing") can be considerable as a result of the large wound and the extensive surgical dissection. Fluid replacement should be sufficient to maintain an adequate urinary output (> 0.5 mL/kg/h); the combined use of both colloid and crystalloid solutions in a ratio of 1:2 or 1:3 may be more effective in preserving urinary output than crystalloid alone. Mannitol (0.25–0.5 g/kg) is usually given prior to dissection near the renal arteries to prevent ischemic renal injury from surgically induced renal vasospasm. Retraction of the inferior vena cava during surgery often results in transient arterial hypotension.

The postoperative pain associated with thoracoabdominal incisions is severe and is typically associated with considerable splinting. Aggressive postoperative analgesia is necessary to avoid atelectasis. Continuous epidural analgesia, interpleural analgesia, and intercostal nerve blocks can facilitate management. Because ligation of intercostal arteries during left-sided dissections has resulted in paraplegia—albeit rarely—it may be prudent to document normal motor function postoperatively prior to institution of epidural anesthesia. The arteria radicularis magna (artery of Adamkiewicz), which is supplied by these vessels and is responsible for most of the arterial blood to the lower half of the spinal cord (see Chapters 16 and 21), arises on the left side in most persons. It should be noted that unilateral sympathectomy following modified RPLND usually results in the ipsilateral leg being warmer than the contralateral one.

4. Renal Cancer

Preoperative Considerations

Adenocarcinoma of the kidney (renal cell carcinoma or hypernephroma) is often termed the internist's tumor because of a frequent association with paraneoplastic syndromes, such as erythrocytosis, hypercalcemia, hypertension, and nonmetastatic hepatic dysfunction. The classic triad of hematuria, flank pain, and palpable mass occurs in only 10% of patients. Unfortunately, the tumor often causes symptoms only after it has grown considerably in size. It has a peak incidence between the fifth and sixth decades of life with 2:1 male to female ratio. Surgical treatment is undertaken for carcinomas confined to the kidneys. In approximately 5–10% of patients, the tumor extends into the renal vein and inferior vena cava as a thrombus, which does not necessarily preclude surgery. Staging includes CT or MRI scans and an arteriogram. Preoperative arterial embolization may reduce operative blood loss.

Preoperative evaluation should focus on defining the degree of renal impairment as well as searching for the presence of associated systemic diseases. Preexisting renal impairment depends on both tumor size in the affected kidney as well as underlying systemic disorders such as hypertension and diabetes. Smoking is a well-established risk factor for renal adenocarcinoma; not surprisingly, patients have a high incidence of underlying coronary artery and chronic obstructive lung disease. Although some patients present with erythrocytosis, the majority of patients are anemic. Preoperative blood transfusion may be advisable to increase hemoglobin concentration > 10 g/dL when a large tumor is to be resected.

Intraoperative Considerations

A. RADICAL NEPHRECTOMY

The operation may be carried out via an anterior subcostal, flank, midline, or thoracoabdominal incision. Smaller tumors may be resected with a hand-assisted laparoscopic technique. Many centers prefer a thoracoabdominal approach for large tumors, particularly when a tumor thrombus is present. The kidney, adrenal gland, and perinephric fat are removed en bloc with the surrounding (Gerota's) fascia. General endotracheal anesthesia is used. The operation has the potential for extensive blood loss because these tumors are very vascular and often very large at presentation. Retraction of the inferior vena cava may be associated with transient arterial hypotension. Direct arterial pressure monitoring is indicated in most patients. Central venous cannulation is used for pressure monitoring as well as for rapid transfusion when necessary; pulmonary artery catheterization may be indicated for patients with impaired left ventricular function. Only brief periods of controlled hypotension should be used to reduce blood loss because of its potential to impair renal function. Reflex renal vasoconstriction in the nonaffected kidney can result in postoperative renal dysfunction. A mannitol infusion should be initiated prior to the surgical dissection.

B. RADICAL NEPHRECTOMY WITH EXCISION OF TUMOR THROMBUS

Some medical centers routinely perform complicated resections of renal cancers with tumor thrombus extending into the inferior vena cava. A thoracoabdominal approach allows the use of cardiopulmonary bypass when necessary. The thrombus may extend only into the inferior vena cava but below the liver (level I), up to the liver but below the diaphragm (level II), or above the diaphragm into the right atrium (level III). Surgery can significantly prolong life and improve the quality of life in selected patients, and in some patients, metastases may regress after resection of the primary tumor. A preoperative ventilation to perfusion scan can detect preexisting embolization of the thrombus.

The presence of a large thrombus (level II or III) greatly complicates anesthetic management. Invasive pressure monitoring and multiple large-bore intravenous catheters are necessary because transfusion requirements are often 10–15 units of packed red blood cells and may exceed 50 units. Transfusion of platelets, fresh frozen plasma, and cryoprecipitate is usually required. Problems associated with massive blood transfusion should be

expected (see Chapter 29). Central venous or pulmonary cannulation should be performed cautiously to prevent dislodgement and embolization of the tumor thrombus. A high central venous pressure is typical and reflects the degree of venous obstruction by the thrombus. The presence of a level III thrombus contraindicates flotation of a pulmonary artery catheter. A low-lying central venous catheter may be equally detrimental, particularly on the right side. Intraoperative transesophageal echocardiography is useful in defining the extent of the thrombus and hemodynamic management.

Complete obstruction of the inferior vena cava increases blood loss because it markedly dilates venous collaterals from the lower body that traverse the abdominal wall, the retroperitoneum, and the epidural space. Patients are also at significant risk for potentially catastrophic pulmonary embolization of the tumor. Tumor embolization may be heralded by sudden supraventricular arrhythmias, arterial desaturation, and/or profound systemic hypotension. Cardiopulmonary bypass is used when the tumor occupies more than 40% of the right atrium. Hypothermic circulatory arrest has been used in some centers (see Chapter 21). Heparinization and hypothermia greatly increase surgical blood loss.

RENAL TRANSPLANTATION

The success of renal transplantation, which is largely due to advances in immunosuppressive therapy, has greatly improved the quality of life for patients with end-stage renal disease. With modern immunosuppressive regimens, cadaveric transplants have achieved almost the same 3-year graft survival rates (80–90%) as living-related donor grafts. In addition, restrictions on candidates for renal transplantation have gradually decreased. Infection and cancer are the only remaining absolute contraindications. Advanced age (> 60 years) and severe cardiovascular disease are relative contraindications.

Preoperative Considerations

Preoperative optimization of the patient's medical condition with dialysis is mandatory (see Chapter 32). Current organ preservation techniques allow ample time (24–48 h) for preoperative dialysis of cadaveric recipients. Living-related transplants are performed electively with the donor and recipient anesthetized simultaneously but in separate rooms. The recipient's serum potassium concentration should be below 5.5 mEq/L, and existing coagulopathies should be corrected.

Intraoperative Considerations

The transplant is carried out by placing the donor kidney retroperitoneally in the iliac fossa and anastomosing the renal vessels to the iliac vessels and the ureter to the bladder. Prior to temporary clamping of the iliac vessels, heparin is administered. Injection of a calcium channel blocker (verapamil) into the arterial circulation of the graft just prior to revascularization helps protect the kidney from reperfusion injury. Intravenous mannitol may also act as a radical free scavenger and helps establish an osmotic diuresis after reperfusion. Nephrectomy is performed only in the presence of intractable hypertension or chronic infection. Immunosuppression is started on the day of surgery with combinations of corticosteroids, cyclosporine (or tacrolimus), and azathioprine (or mycophenolate mofetil). Some centers avoid cyclosporine and tacrolimus in the first few days and instead use antithymocyte globulin, monoclonal antibodies directed against specific subsets of T lymphocytes (OKT3), or interleukin-2 receptor antibodies (daclizumab or basiliximab). Sirolimus may be used instead of tacrolimus or in combination with it as a steroid-sparing regimen.

A. CHOICE OF ANESTHESIA

Although both spinal and epidural anesthesia have been successfully employed, most transplants are done under general anesthesia. All general anesthetic agents, including enflurane and sevoflurane, have been employed without any apparent detrimental effect on graft function; nonetheless, these two agents are best avoided (see Chapter 32). Atracurium, cisatracurium, and rocuronium may be the muscle relaxants of choice, as they are not primarily dependent on renal excretion for elimination. Similarly, vecuronium may be used with only modest prolongation of its effects.

B. MONITORING

Central venous pressure monitoring is very useful in ensuring adequate hydration but avoiding fluid overload. Normal saline or half-normal saline solutions are commonly used. A urinary catheter is placed preoperatively. A brisk urine flow following the arterial anastomosis generally indicates good graft function. The diuresis that follows may resemble nonoliguric renal failure (see Chapter 32). If the graft ischemic time was prolonged, an oliguric phase may precede the diuretic phase, in which case fluid therapy must be adjusted appropriately. The judicious use of furosemide or additional mannitol may be indicated in such cases. Hyperkalemia has been reported after release of the vascular clamp following completion of the arterial anastomosis, particularly in small patients and pediatric patients. Release of potassium contained in the preservative solution has been implicated in those cases. Washout of the preservative solution with ice-cold lactated Ringer's solution just prior to the vascular anastomosis may help avoid this problem. Serum electrolyte concentrations should be monitored closely after completion of the anastomosis. Hyperkalemia may be suspected from peaking of

the T wave on the ECG. Most patients can generally be extubated immediately after the procedure.

CASE DISCUSSION: HYPOTENSION IN THE RECOVERY ROOM

A 69-year-old man with a history of an inferior myocardial infarction was admitted to the recovery room following TURP under general anesthesia. The procedure took 90 min and was reported to be uncomplicated. On admission, the patient is extubated but still unresponsive, and vital signs are stable. Twenty minutes later, he is noted to be awake but restless. He begins to shiver intensely, his blood pressure decreases to 80/35 mm Hg, and his respirations increase to 40 breaths/min. The bedside monitor shows a sinus tachycardia of 140 beats/min and an oxygen saturation of 92%.

What is the differential diagnosis?

The differential diagnosis of hypotension following TURP should always include (1) hemorrhage, (2) TURP syndrome, (3) bladder perforation, (4) myocardial infarction or ischemia, (5) septicemia, and (6) disseminated intravascular coagulation (DIC).

Other possibilities (see Chapter 48) are less likely in this setting but should always be considered, particularly when the patient fails to respond to appropriate measures (see below).

Based on the history, what is the most likely diagnosis?

A diagnosis cannot be made with reasonable certainty at this point, and the patient requires further evaluation. Nonetheless, the hypotension and shivering must be treated rapidly because of the history of coronary artery disease. The hypotension seriously compromises coronary perfusion, and the shivering markedly increases myocardial oxygen demand (see Chapter 20).

What diagnostic aids would be helpful?

A quick examination of the patient is extremely useful in narrowing down the possibilities. Hemorrhage from the prostate should be apparent from effluent of the continuous bladder irrigation system placed after the procedure. Relatively little blood in the urine makes it look red; brisk hemorrhage is often apparent as grossly bloody drainage. Occasionally, the drainage may be scant because of clots blocking the drainage catheter; irrigation of the catheter is indicated in such cases.

Clinical signs of peripheral perfusion are invaluable. Hypovolemic patients have decreased peripheral (radial) pulses, and their extremities are usually cool and may be cyanotic. Poor perfusion is consistent with hemorrhage, bladder perforation, DIC, and severe myocardial ischemia or infarction. A full bounding peripheral pulse with warm extremities is suggestive of, but not always present in, septicemia (see Chapter 49). Signs of fluid overload should be searched for, such as jugular venous distention, pulmonary crackles, and an S_3 gallop. Fluid overload is more consistent with TURP syndrome, but may also be seen in myocardial infarction or ischemia.

The abdomen should be examined for signs of perforation. A rigid and tender or distended abdomen is very suggestive of perforation and should prompt immediate evaluation for laparotomy. When the abdomen is soft and nontender, perforation can reasonably be excluded.

Further evaluation requires laboratory measurements, an ECG, a chest radiograph, and a transthoracic echocardiogram. Blood should be immediately obtained for arterial blood gas analysis and measurements of hematocrit, hemoglobin, electrolytes, glucose, a platelet count, and prothrombin and partial thromboplastin tests. If DIC is suggested by diffuse oozing, fibrinogen and fibrin split product measurements will confirm the diagnosis. A 12-lead ECG should be evaluated for signs of ischemia, electrolyte abnormalities (see Chapter 28), or an evolving myocardial infarction. A chest film should be obtained to search for evidence of pulmonary congestion, aspiration, pneumothorax, or cardiomegaly. An echocardiogram helps determine end-diastolic volume, systolic function (particularly the presence or absence of regional wall motion abnormalities), and can detect valvular abnormalities; comparison to prior studies would be invaluable.

While laboratory measurements are being performed, what therapeutic and diagnostic measures should be undertaken?

Immediate measures aimed at avoiding hypoxemia and hypoperfusion should be instituted. Oxygen supplementation protects against hypoxemia and may increase oxygen delivery to tissues. If hypoventilation or respiratory distress is apparent, endotracheal intubation is indicated. Frequent blood pressure measurements should be obtained. If signs of fluid overload are absent, a diagnostic fluid challenge with 500 mL of crystalloid or 250 mL of colloid is helpful. A favorable response, as indicated by an increase in blood pressure and a decrease in heart rate, is suggestive of hypovolemia and indicates the need for additional fluid boluses. Obvious bleeding in the setting of hypotension necessitates blood transfusion. The absence of a quick response should prompt further evaluation with invasive monitors. Administration of an inotrope, such as dopamine, is appropriate while the evaluation is being completed. Direct intraarterial pressure measurement is invaluable in this setting. Central venous access should be established to measure central venous pressure and for possible placement of a pulmonary artery catheter. The latter is useful in patients with a history of congestive heart failure and when clinical signs are ambiguous. Cardiac output can then be measured by thermodilution, and pulmonary capillary wedge pressure measurements can be used to guide fluid or vasodilator therapy.

If signs of fluid overload are present, intravenous furosemide in addition to an inotrope is indicated. Further treatment with vasodilator therapy should be initiated only after full hemodynamic monitoring is established.

The patient's axillary temperature is 35.5°C. Does the absence of obvious fever exclude sepsis?

No. Anesthesia is commonly associated with altered temperature regulation. Moreover, correlation between axillary and core temperatures is quite variable (see Chapter 6). A high index of suspicion is therefore required to diagnose sepsis. Leukocytosis is common following surgery and is not a reliable indicator of sepsis in this setting.

The mechanism of shivering in patients recovering from anesthesia is poorly understood. Although shivering is common in patients who become hypothermic during surgery (and presumably functions to raise body temperature back to normal), its relation to body temperature is inconsistent. Anesthetics probably alter the normal behavior of hypothalamic thermoregulatory centers in the brain. In contrast, infectious agents, circulating toxins, or immune reactions cause the release of cytokines (interleukin-1 and tumor necrosis factor) that stimulate the hypothalamus to synthesize prostaglandin (PG) E_2. The latter, in turn, activates neurons responsible for heat production, resulting in intense shivering.

How can the shivering be stopped?

Regardless of its cause, shivering has the undesirable effects of markedly increasing oxygen consumption (100–200%) and CO_2 production. Both cardiac output and minute ventilation must therefore increase. These effects are often poorly tolerated by patients with limited cardiac or pulmonary reserve. Although the ultimate therapeutic goal is to correct the underlying problem (such as hypothermia or sepsis), additional measures are indicated in this patient. Supplemental oxygen therapy (high FIO_2) helps prevent hypoxemia from the low mixed venous oxygen tension commonly associated with shivering; a low mixed venous oxygen tension tends to accentuate the effects of any intrapulmonary shunting (see Chapter 22). Unlike other opioid agonists, meperidine in small doses (20–50 mg intravenously) frequently terminates shivering regardless of the cause. Chlorpromazine, 10–25 mg, and butorphanol, 1–2 mg, may also be effective. These agents may have specific actions on temperature regulation centers in the hypothalamus. Shivering associated with sepsis and immune reactions can also be blocked by inhibitors of prostaglandin synthetase (aspirin, acetaminophen, and nonsteroidal antiinflammatory agents) as well as glucocorticoids. Acetaminophen, which can be given rectally, is generally preferred perioperatively because it does not affect platelet function. Rectal suppositories are, however, generally avoided following prostatic surgery to prevent bleeding from minor trauma to the gland during insertion.

What was the outcome?

Examination of the patient reveals warm extremities with a good pulse, even with the low blood pressure. The abdomen is soft and nontender. The irrigation fluid from the bladder is only slightly pink. A diagnosis of probable septicemia is made. Blood cultures are obtained and antibiotic therapy is initiated to cover gram-negative organisms and enterococci (the most common pathogens). The patient receives intravenous gentamicin, 80 mg, and ampicillin, 1 g, and an intravenous dopamine infusion is started. The shivering ceases following administration of meperidine, 20 mg intravenously. The blood pressure increases to 110/60 mm Hg and the pulse slows to 110 beats/min following a 1000-mL intravenous fluid bolus and 5 mg/kg/min of dopamine. The serum sodium concentration was found to be 130 mEq/L. Four hours later, the dopamine was no longer needed, and the patient recovered uneventfully.

SUGGESTED READING

Battillo JA, Hendler MA: Effects of patient positioning during anesthesia. In: *Anesthesia for Urological Surgery.* Lebowitz RW (editor). Int Anesthesiol Clin 1993;31:67.

Dobson PM, Caldicott LD, Gerrish SP, et al: Changes in hemodynamic variables during transurethral resection of the prostate: Comparison of general and spinal anaesthesia. Br J Anaesth 1994;72:267.

Eide TR: Anesthetic considerations for extracorporeal shock wave lithotripsy. In: *Anesthesia for Urological Surgery.* Lebowitz RW (editor). Int Anesthesiol Clin 1993;31:47.

Gravenstein D: Transurethral resection of the prostate (TURP) syndrome: A review of the pathophysiology and management. Anesth Analg 1997;84:438.

Malhotra V: *Anesthesia for Renal and Genito-Urological Surgery.* McGraw-Hill, 1996.

Mathes DD: Bleomycin and hyperoxia exposure in the operating room. Anesth Analg 1995;81:624.

Mebust WK, Holtgrewe HL, Cockett ATK, et al: Transurethral prostatectomy—immediate and postoperative complications: A cooperative study of 13 participating institutions evaluating 3885 patients. J Urol 1989;141:243.

Monk TG, Goodnough LT, Brechner ME, et al: A prospective randomized comparison of three blood conservation strategies for radical prostatectomy. Anesthesiology 1999;91:24.

Richardson MG, Dooley JW: The effects of general versus epidural anesthesia for outpatient extracorporeal shock wave lithotripsy. Anesth Analg 1998;86:1214.

Shir Y, Frank SM, Brendler, et al: Postoperative morbidity is similar in patients anesthetized with epidural and general anesthesia for radical prostatectomy. Urology 1994;44:232.

Shir Y, Raja SN, Frank SM: The effect of epidural versus general anesthesia on postoperative pain and analgesic requirements in patients undergoing radical prostatectomy. Anesthesiology 1994;80:49.

Sprung J, Kapural L, Bourke DL, O'Hara JF Jr: Anesthesia for kidney transplant surgery. Anesthesiol Clin North Am 2000;18:919.

Warner MA, Martin JT, Schroeder DR, et al: Lower-extremity motor neuropathy associated with surgery performed on patients in a lithotomy position. Anesthesiology 1994;81:6.

Whalley DG, Berrigan MJ: Anesthesia for radical prostatectomy, cystectomy, nephrectomy, pheochromocytoma, and laparoscopic procedures. Anesthesiol Clin North Am 2000;18:899.

WEB SITE

http://www.auanet.org/guidelines/

This site includes clinical guidelines of the American Urological Association.

Hepatic Physiology & Anesthesia

34

KEY CONCEPTS

 The hepatic artery supplies 45–50% of the liver's oxygen requirements and the portal vein supplies the remaining 50–55%.

 All coagulation factors—with the exception of factor VIII and von Willebrand factor—are produced by the liver. Vitamin K is a necessary cofactor in the synthesis of prothrombin (factor II) and factors VII, IX, and X.

 Liver tests that measure hepatic synthetic function include serum albumin, prothrombin time (PT, or international normalized ratio [INR]), cholesterol, and pseudocholinesterase.

 Albumin values less than 2.5 g/dL are generally indicative of chronic liver disease, acute stress, or severe malnutrition.

 The PT, which is normally 11–14 s (depending on the control), measures the activity of fibrinogen, prothrombin, and factors V, VII, and X.

 If an adequate intravascular volume is maintained, spinal and epidural anesthesia decrease hepatic blood flow primarily by lowering arterial blood pressure, whereas general anesthesia usu-

ally decreases it through reductions in blood pressure and cardiac output and sympathetic stimulation.

 The surgical stress response is characterized by elevated circulating levels of catecholamines, glucagon, and cortisol. Mobilization of carbohydrate stores and proteins results in hyperglycemia and a negative nitrogen balance (catabolism), respectively.

 Anesthetic interactions with bile formation and storage have not been reported. However, all opioids can potentially cause spasm of the sphincter of Oddi and increase biliary pressure (fentanyl > morphine > meperidine > butorphanol > nalbuphine).

 When the results of liver tests are elevated postoperatively, the usual cause is underlying liver disease or the surgical procedure itself.

 Epidemiological studies have identified several risk factors that are associated with halothane-associated hepatitis, including middle age, obesity, female sex, and a repeat exposure to halothane (particularly within 28 days).

The liver, which weighs approximately 1500–1600 g in adults, is the largest organ in the body. It is responsible for a seemingly endless number of complex and interrelated functions. Fortunately, because of the liver's large functional reserves, clinically significant hepatic dysfunction following anesthesia and surgery is uncommon. Such dysfunction is limited primarily to patients with preexisting hepatic impairment and to those with rare idiosyncratic reactions to halogenated volatile anesthetics. This chapter reviews normal hepatic physiol-

ogy, laboratory evaluation of hepatic function, and the effects of anesthesia on hepatic function. The anesthetic management of patients with liver disease is discussed in Chapter 35.

FUNCTIONAL ANATOMY

The liver is separated by the falciform ligament into right and left anatomic lobes; the larger right lobe has two additional smaller lobes at its posterior–inferior surface, the caudate and quadrate lobes. In contrast, surgical anatomy divides the liver based on its blood supply. Thus the right and left surgical lobes are defined by the point of bifurcation of the hepatic artery and portal vein (porta hepatis); the falciform ligament therefore divides the left surgical lobe into medial and lateral segments. Surgical anatomy defines a total of eight segments.

The liver is made up of 50,000–100,000 discrete anatomic units called lobules. Each lobule is composed of plates of hepatocytes arranged cylindrically around a centrilobular vein (Figure 34–1). Four to five portal tracts, composed of hepatic arterioles, portal venules, bile canaliculi, lymphatics, and nerves, surround each lobule.

In contrast to a lobule, an acinus, the functional unit of the liver, is defined by a portal tract in the middle and centrilobular veins at the periphery. Cells closest to the portal tract (zone 1) are well oxygenated; those closest to centrilobular veins (zone 3) receive the least oxygen and are most susceptible to injury.

Blood from hepatic arterioles and portal venules commingles in the sinusoidal channels, which lie between the cellular plates and serve as capillaries. Two types of cells line the hepatic sinusoids: endothelial cells and macrophages (Kupffer cells). The space of Disse lies between the sinusoidal capillaries and the hepatocytes. Venous drainage from the central veins of hepatic lobules coalesces to form the hepatic veins (right, middle, and left), which empty into the inferior vena cava (Figure 34–2). The caudate lobe is usually drained by its own set of veins.

Bile canaliculi originate between hepatocytes within each plate and join to form bile ducts. An extensive system of lymphatic channels also forms within the plates and is in direct communication with the space of Disse.

The liver is supplied by sympathetic nerve fibers (T6–T11), parasympathetic fibers (right and left vagus), and fibers from the right phrenic nerve. Some autonomic fibers synapse first in the celiac plexus whereas others reach the liver directly via splanchnic nerves and vagal branches before forming the hepatic plexus. The majority of sensory afferent fibers travel with sympathetic fibers.

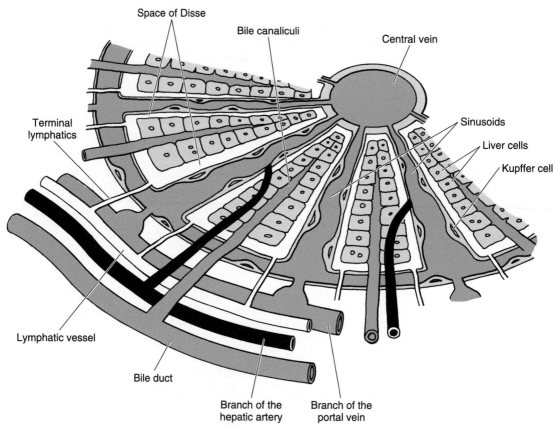

Figure 34–1. The hepatic lobule.

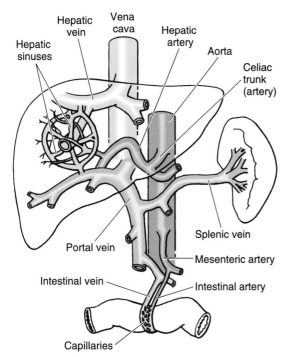

Figure 34–2. Hepatic blood flow. (Modified and reproduced, with permission, from Guyton AC: *Textbook of Medical Physiology,* 7th ed. W.B. Saunders, 1986.)

VASCULAR FUNCTIONS OF THE LIVER

Control of Hepatic Blood Flow

Normal **hepatic blood flow** is about 1500 mL/min in adults, of which 25–30% is derived from the hepatic artery and 70–75% from the portal vein (Figure 34–2). The time it takes for red blood cells to traverse from the portal vein to the central vein is approximately 8–9 s, allowing sufficient time for contact with hepatocytes and Kupffer cells. The hepatic artery supplies 45–50% of the liver's oxygen requirements and the portal vein supplies the remaining 50–55%. The pressure within the former is arterial, whereas that in the latter is normally less than 10 mm Hg. Portal vein oxygen saturation is normally 85%. The total blood flow from this dual supply represents 25–30% of the total cardiac output. Hepatic arterial flow appears dependent on metabolic demand postprandially (autoregulation), whereas flow through the portal vein is dependent on blood flow to the gastrointestinal tract and the spleen. Although autoregulation of hepatic arterial flow may not be appreciable during fasting, a reciprocal though somewhat limited mechanism exists such that a decrease in either hepatic arterial or portal venous flow results in a compensatory increase in the other.

The hepatic artery has α_1-adrenergic vasoconstricting receptors as well as β_2-adrenergic, dopaminergic (D_1), and cholinergic vasodilator receptors. The portal vein has only α_1-adrenergic and dopaminergic (D_1) receptors. Sympathetic activation results in vasoconstriction of the hepatic artery and mesenteric vessels, decreasing hepatic blood flow. β-Adrenergic stimulation vasodilates the hepatic artery; β-blockers reduce blood flow and, therefore, decrease portal pressure.

Reservoir Function

Portal vein pressure is normally only about 7–10 mm Hg, but the low resistance of the hepatic sinusoids allows relatively large blood flows through the portal vein. Small changes in hepatic venous tone (and pressure) thus can result in large changes in hepatic blood volume, allowing the liver to act as a blood reservoir.

Normal hepatic blood volume is about 450 mL (almost 10% of total blood volume). A decrease in hepatic venous pressure, as occurs during hemorrhage, shifts blood from hepatic veins and sinusoids into the central venous circulation and augments circulating blood volume as much as 300 mL. In patients with congestive heart failure, the increase in central venous pressure is transmitted to the hepatic veins and causes blood to accumulate within the liver. As much as 1 L of blood can effectively be removed from the circulation in this way at the expense of causing hepatic congestion.

Blood-Cleansing Function

The Kupffer cells lining the sinusoids are part of the monocyte–macrophage (reticuloendothelial) system. Their functions include phagocytosis, processing of antigens, as well as the release of various proteins, enzymes, cytokines, and other chemical mediators. Their phagocytic activity is responsible for removing colonic bacteria and endotoxin entering the bloodstream from the portal circulation. Cellular debris, viruses, proteins, and particulate matter in the blood are also phagocytosed.

METABOLIC FUNCTIONS

The abundance of enzymatic pathways in the liver allows it to play a key role in the metabolism of carbohydrates, fats, proteins (Figure 34–3), and other substances (Table 34–1).

Carbohydrate Metabolism

The final products of carbohydrate digestion are glucose, fructose, and galactose. With the exception of the large amount of fructose that is converted by the liver to lactate, hepatic conversion of fructose and galactose

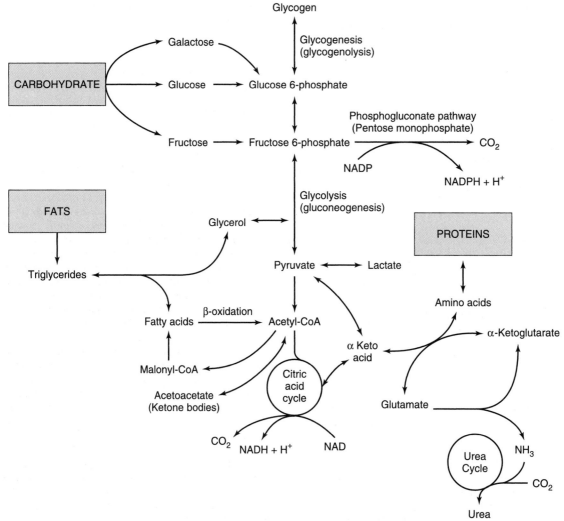

Figure 34–3. Important metabolic pathways in hepatocytes. Although small amounts of ATP are derived directly from some intermediary reactions, the overwhelming majority of ATP produced is the result of oxidative phosphorylation of the reduced forms of nicotinamide adenine dinucleotide (NADH) and nicotinamide adenine dinucleotide phosphate (NADPH).

into glucose makes glucose metabolism the final common pathway for most carbohydrates.

All cells utilize glucose to produce energy in the form of adenosine triphosphate (ATP) via glycolysis (anaerobically) or the citric acid cycle (aerobically). The liver (and adipose tissue) can also utilize the phosphogluconate pathway, and the latter not only provides energy but also produces an important cofactor in the synthesis of fatty acids. Most of the glucose absorbed following a meal is normally stored as glycogen. When glycogen storage capacity is exceeded, excess glucose is converted into fat. Glycogen is a readily available source of glucose that does

not contribute to intracellular osmolality. Only the liver and (to a lesser extent) muscle are able to store significant amounts of glycogen. Insulin enhances glycogen synthesis and epinephrine and glucagon enhance glycogenolysis. Because hepatic glycogen stores are normally only about 70 g whereas glucose consumption averages 150 g/d, glycogen stores are depleted after 24 h of fasting. After this period of fasting, *de novo* synthesis of glucose (gluconeogenesis) is necessary to provide an uninterrupted supply of glucose for other organs.

The liver and kidney are unique in their capacity to form glucose from lactate, pyruvate, amino acids (mainly

Table 34–1. Metabolic functions of the liver.

Creation and secretion of bile
Nutrient metabolism
    Amino acids
    Monosaccharides (sugars)
    Lipids (fatty acids, cholesterol, phospholipids, lipoproteins)
    Vitamins
Phase I and II biotransformation
    Toxins
    Drugs
    Hormones (steroids)
Synthesis
    Albumin, α_1-antitrypsin, proteases
    Clotting factors
    Acute phase proteins
    Plasma cholinesterase
Immune function
    Kupffer cells

---

alanine), and glycerol (derived from fat metabolism). Hepatic gluconeogenesis is vital in the maintenance of a normal blood glucose concentration. Glucocorticoids, catecholamines, glucagon, and thyroid hormone greatly enhance gluconeogenesis, whereas insulin inhibits it.

Fat Metabolism

When carbohydrate stores are saturated, the liver converts the excess ingested carbohydrates (and proteins) into fat. The fatty acids thus formed can be used immediately for fuel or stored in adipose tissue or the liver for later consumption. Nearly all cells utilize directly, as an energy source, fatty acids derived from ingested fats or those synthesized from intermediary metabolites of carbohydrates and protein. Only red blood cells and the renal medulla can utilize only glucose. Neurons normally utilize only glucose, but after a few days of starvation they can switch to break down products of fatty acids (ketone bodies) that have been made by the liver as an energy source.

To oxidize fatty acids, they are converted into acetylcoenzyme A (acetyl-CoA), which is then oxidized via the citric acid cycle to produce ATP. The liver is capable of high rates of fatty acid oxidation and can form acetoacetic acid (one of the ketone bodies) from excess acetyl-CoA. The acetoacetate released by hepatocytes serves as alternative circulating and readily available fuel (by reconversion into acetyl-CoA) for other cell types. Under some conditions (low insulin availability), glucagon increases whereas insulin inhibits ketone body production by the liver.

Acetyl-CoA is also used by the liver for production of cholesterol and phospholipids, which are necessary in the synthesis of cellular membranes throughout the body. Hepatic synthesis of lipoproteins is also important in lipid transport by blood.

Protein Metabolism

The liver performs a critical role in protein metabolism. Without this function, death usually occurs within several days. The steps involved include (1) deamination of amino acids, (2) formation of urea (to eliminate the ammonia produced from deamination), (3) interconversions between nonessential amino acids, and (4) formation of plasma proteins.

Deamination is necessary for conversion of excess amino acids into carbohydrates and fats. The enzymatic processes (most commonly transamination) convert amino acids into their respective keto acids and produce ammonia as a byproduct. The deamination of alanine plays a major role in hepatic gluconeogenesis. Although deamination also occurs to a minor extent in the kidneys (primarily glutamine; see Chapter 30), the liver is its principal site. With the exception of branched-chain amino acids (leucine, isoleucine, and valine), the liver normally deaminates most of the amino acids derived from dietary proteins. Branched-chain amino acids are primarily metabolized by skeletal muscle.

The ammonia formed from deamination (as well as that produced by colonic bacteria and absorbed through the gut) is highly toxic to tissues. Through a series of enzymatic steps, the liver combines two molecules of ammonia with CO_2 to form urea. The urea thus formed readily diffuses out of the liver and can then be excreted by the kidneys.

Hepatic transamination of the appropriate keto acid allows formation of nonessential amino acids and compensation for any dietary deficiency in these amino acids. Essential amino acids, by definition, cannot be readily synthesized through this mechanism and must be supplied exogenously.

Nearly all plasma proteins with the notable exception of immunoglobulins are formed by the liver. Quantitatively, the most important of these proteins are albumin, α_1-antitrypsin, and other proteases/elastases. Qualitatively, the coagulation factors are the most important proteins. Albumin is responsible for maintaining a normal plasma oncotic pressure and is the principal binding and transport protein for fatty acids and a large number of hormones and drugs. Consequently, changes in albumin concentration can affect the concentration of the pharmacologically active, unbound fraction of many drugs.

All coagulation factors—with the exception of factor VIII and von Willebrand factor—are produced by the liver. Vitamin K is a necessary cofactor in the synthesis of prothrombin (factor II) and factors VII, IX, and X. The liver also produces plasma cholinesterase (pseudocholinesterase), an enzyme that hydrolyzes esters, including some local anesthetics and succinylcholine. Other important proteins formed by the liver include protease inhibitors (antithrombin III, α_2-antiplasmin, and α_1-antitrypsin), transport proteins (transferrin, haptoglobin, and ceruloplasmin), complement, α_1-acid glycoprotein, C-reactive protein, and serum amyloid A.

Drug Metabolism

Many exogenous substances, including most drugs, undergo hepatic biotransformation. The end products of these reactions are generally either inactivated or more water-soluble substances that can be readily excreted in bile or urine. Hepatic biotransformations are often categorized as one of two types of reactions. Phase I reactions modify reactive chemical groups through mixed-function oxidases or the cytochrome P-450 enzyme systems, resulting in oxidation, reduction, deamination, sulfoxidation, dealkylation, or methylation. Barbiturates and benzodiazepines are inactivated by phase I reactions. Phase II reactions, which may or may not follow a phase I reaction, involve conjugation of the substance with glucuronide, sulfate, taurine, or glycine. The conjugated compound can then be readily eliminated in urine or bile.

Some enzyme systems, such as those of cytochrome P-450, can be induced by a few drugs. Ethanol, barbiturates, ketamine, and perhaps benzodiazepines (eg, diazepam) are capable of enzyme induction, increasing production of the enzymes that metabolize those drugs. This can result in increased tolerance to the drugs' effects. Moreover, enzyme induction often promotes tolerance to other drugs that are metabolized by the same enzymes (cross-tolerance). Conversely, some agents, such as cimetidine and chloramphenicol, can prolong the effects of other drugs by inhibiting these enzymes.

Products of phase I reactions may in a few instances be more active than the parent compound or may be cytotoxic. Such reactions are thought to be important in the toxicity of acetaminophen, isoniazid, and perhaps halothane (see below).

The metabolism of a few drugs—including lidocaine, morphine, verapamil, labetalol, and propranolol—is highly dependent on hepatic blood flow. These drugs have very high rates of hepatic extraction from the circulation. As a result, a decrease in their metabolic clearance usually reflects decreased hepatic blood flow rather than hepatocellular dysfunction.

Other Metabolic Functions

The liver plays a major role in hormone, vitamin, and mineral metabolism. Normal thyroid function is dependent on hepatic formation of the more active triiodo-

Table 34–2. Composition of bile.

97% water
< 1% bile salts
Pigments
Inorganic salts
Lipids
Cholesterol
Fatty acids
Lecithin
Alkaline phosphatase

thyronine (T_3) from thyroxine (T_4). Degradation of thyroid hormone is principally hepatic. The liver is also the major site of degradation for insulin, steroid hormones (estrogen, aldosterone, and cortisol), glucagon, and antidiuretic hormone. Hepatocytes are the principal storage sites for vitamins A, B_{12}, E, D, and K. Lastly, hepatic production of transferrin and haptoglobin is important because these proteins are involved in iron hemostasis, whereas ceruloplasmin is important in copper regulation.

BILE FORMATION & EXCRETION

Bile (Table 34–2) plays an important role in absorption of fat and in excretion of bilirubin, cholesterol, and many drugs. Hepatocytes continuously secrete bile salts, cholesterol, phospholipids, conjugated bilirubin, and other substances into bile canaliculi. Several mechanisms are responsible for bile formation: (1) osmotic filtration primarily due to secretion of bile salts into canaliculi (bile salt-dependent fraction), (2) Na^+–K^+-adenosine triphosphatase–mediated ion transport (bile salt-independent fraction), and (3) secretin-mediated sodium and bicarbonate transport by ductules.

Bile ducts from hepatic lobules join and eventually form the right and left hepatic ducts. These ducts, in turn, combine to form the hepatic duct, which together with the cystic duct from the gallbladder becomes the common bile duct (Figure 34–4). Biliary flow from the common bile duct into the duodenum is controlled by the sphincter of Oddi. The gallbladder serves as a reservoir for bile. Through active sodium transport and passive water reabsorption, the gallbladder concentrates biliary fluid between meals. Cholecystokinin, a hormone released by the intestinal mucosa in response to fat and protein, causes contraction of the gallbladder, relaxation of the sphincter of Oddi, and propulsion of bile into the small intestine.

Bile Acids & Fat Absorption

The bile acids formed by hepatocytes from cholesterol are essential for emulsifying the insoluble components of

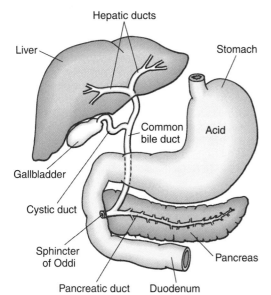

Figure 34–4. The biliary system. (Modified and reproduced, with permission, from Guyton AC: *Textbook of Medical Physiology,* 7th ed. W.B. Saunders, 1986.)

bile as well as facilitating the intestinal absorption of lipids. Bile acids also represent the major route of cholesterol elimination. Salts of the two principal acids formed, cholic acid and chenodeoxycholic acid, are usually conjugated with glycine and taurine before secretion into bile. In the colon, bacteria convert cholic acid to deoxycholic acid and chemodeoxycholic acid to lithocholic acid, secondary bile acids. Defects in the formation or secretion of bile salts interfere with the absorption of fats and fat-soluble vitamins (A, D, E, and K). Because of normally limited stores of vitamin K, a deficiency can develop in a few days. **Vitamin K deficiency is manifested as a coagulopathy due to impaired formation of prothrombin and of factors VII, IX, and X.**

Bilirubin Excretion

Bilirubin is primarily the end product of hemoglobin metabolism. It is formed from degradation of the heme ring in Kupffer cells. A much smaller amount is formed as a result of the breakdown of myoglobin and cytochrome enzymes. Heme oxygenase first breaks down hemoglobin into biliverdin, carbon monoxide, and iron; biliverdin reductase then converts the former into bilirubin. Bilirubin is then released into blood, where it readily binds to albumin. Hepatic uptake of bilirubin from the circulation is passive, but binding to intracellular proteins traps the bilirubin inside hepatocytes. Inside the hepatocyte, bilirubin is conjugated (primarily with glucuronide) and actively excreted into bile cana-

liculi. A small fraction of the conjugated bilirubin is reabsorbed into the bloodstream. Half the bilirubin secreted into the intestine is converted by colonic bacteria into urobilinogen. A small amount of this substance is normally reabsorbed by the intestine, only to be excreted into bile again (enterohepatic recirculation). Urobilinogen is also renally excreted to a minor extent.

LIVER TESTS

Unfortunately, the most commonly performed liver tests are neither very sensitive nor very specific. Many tests such as serum transaminase measurements reflect hepatocellular integrity more than hepatic function. Liver tests that measure hepatic synthetic function include serum albumin, prothrombin time (PT, or international normalized ratio [INR]), cholesterol, and pseudocholinesterase. Moreover, because of the liver's large functional reserves, cirrhosis may be present with few or no laboratory abnormalities.

No one test reflects overall hepatic function. Each test generally reflects one aspect of hepatic function and must be interpreted in conjunction with the other tests along with clinical assessment of the patient.

Liver abnormalities can often be divided into either parenchymal disorders or obstructive disorders based on laboratory tests (Table 34–3). Obstructive disorders

Table 34–3. Abnormalities in liver tests.[1,2]

	Parenchymal (Hepatocellular) Dysfunction	Biliary Obstruction or Cholestasis
AST (SGOT)	↑ to ↑↑↑[3]	↑
ALT (SGPT)	↑ to ↑↑↑	↑
Albumin	0 to ↓↓↓	0
Prothrombin time	0 to ↑↑↑	0 to ↑↑[4]
Bilirubin	0 to ↑↑↑	0 to ↑↑↑
Alkaline phosphatase	↑	↑ to ↑↑↑
5′-Nucleotidase	0 to ↑	↑ to ↑↑↑
γ-Glutamyl transpeptidase	↑ to ↑↑↑	↑↑↑

[1]Adapted from Wilson JD et al (editors): *Harrison's Principles of Internal Medicine,* 12th ed. McGraw-Hill, 1991.
[2]AST, aspartate aminotransferase; SGOT, serum glutamic-oxaloacetic transaminase; ALT, alanine aminotransferase; SGPT, serum glutamic pyruvictransferase.
[3]↑, increases; 0, no change; ↓, decreases.
[4]Usually corrects with vitamin K.

primarily affect biliary excretion of substances, whereas parenchymal disorders result in generalized hepatocellular dysfunction.

Serum Bilirubin

The normal total bilirubin concentration (conjugated [direct] and unconjugated [indirect]) is less than 1.5 mg/dL (< 25 mmol/L) and reflects the balance between production and biliary excretion. Jaundice is usually clinically obvious when total bilirubin exceeds 3 mg/dL. A predominantly conjugated hyperbilirubinemia (> 50%) is associated with increased urinary urobilinogen and may reflect hepatocellular dysfunction, intrahepatic cholestasis, or extrahepatic biliary obstruction. Hyperbilirubinemia that is primarily unconjugated may be seen with hemolysis or with congenital or acquired defects in bilirubin conjugation. In contrast to the conjugated form, unconjugated bilirubin is nontoxic to cells.

Serum Aminotransferases (Transaminases)

These enzymes are released into the circulation as a result of hepatocellular injury or death. Two aminotransferases are most commonly measured: serum aspartate aminotransferase (AST), also known as glutamic-oxaloacetic transaminase (SGOT), and serum alanine aminotransferase (ALT), also called glutamic pyruvic-transferase (SGPT). AST is present in many tissues, including the liver, heart, skeletal muscle, and kidneys. ALT is primarily located in the liver and is more specific for hepatic dysfunction. Normal AST and ALT levels are below 35–45 U/L. The circulating half-lives of these enzymes are about 18 and 36 h, respectively. Mild elevations (< 300 U/L) can be seen with cholestasis or metastatic liver disease. Absolute levels correlate poorly with degree of hepatic injury in chronic conditions but are of great value in acute liver disease (drug overdose, ischemic injury, and fulminant hepatitis, for example).

Serum Alkaline Phosphatase

Alkaline phosphatase is produced by the liver, bone, small bowel, kidneys, and placenta and is excreted into bile. Normal serum alkaline phosphatase activity is generally 25–85 IU/L in most laboratories; children and adolescents have much higher levels reflecting active growth. Most of the circulating enzyme is normally derived from bone, but with biliary obstruction more hepatic alkaline phosphatase is synthesized and released into the circulation. The circulating half-life of the enzyme is about 7 days. Although mild elevations (up to twice normal) may be seen with hepatocellular injury or hepatic metastatic disease, higher levels are indicative of intrahepatic cholestasis or biliary obstruction.

Increased serum alkaline phosphatase levels may also be encountered with pregnancy (see Chapter 40) or bone disease (Paget's disease or bone metastases). Electrophoretic separation allows differentiation of hepatobiliary from other isoenzymes. It may be more practical to measure 5'-nucleotidase (5'-NT), leucine aminopeptidase (LAP), or serum γ-glutamyl transpeptidase to help exclude an extrahepatic source of alkaline phosphatase elevations. The combination of an elevated γ-glutamyl transpeptidase level together with an elevated alkaline phosphatase level strongly suggests hepatobiliary disease. In fact, elevated serum γ-glutamyl transpeptidase activity is the most sensitive indicator of hepatobiliary disease. Measurement of 5'-NT or LAP can also be used in nonpregnant patients; unlike γ-glutamyl transpeptidase, the latter two enzymes normally increase during late pregnancy.

Serum Albumin

The normal serum albumin concentration is 3.5–5.5 g/dL. Because its half-life is about 2–3 weeks, albumin concentration may initially be normal with acute liver disease. Albumin values less than 2.5 g/dL are generally indicative of chronic liver disease, acute stress, or severe malnutrition. Increased losses of albumin in the urine (nephrotic syndrome) or the gastrointestinal tract (protein-losing enteropathy) can also produce hypoalbuminemia.

Blood Ammonia

Significant elevations of blood ammonia levels usually reflect disruption of hepatic urea synthesis. Normal whole blood ammonia levels are 47–65 mmol/L (80–110 mg/dL). Marked elevations usually reflect severe hepatocellular damage. There is only a rough correlation between arterial ammonia levels and hepatic encephalopathy.

Prothrombin Time

The PT, which is normally 11–14 s (depending on the control), measures the activity of fibrinogen, prothrombin, and factors V, VII, and X. The relatively short half-life of factor VII (4–6 h) makes the PT useful in evaluating hepatic synthetic function of patients with acute or chronic liver disease. Prolongations of the PT greater than 3–4 s from the control are considered significant. This usually corresponds to an INR greater than 1.5. Because only 20–30% of normal factor activity is required for normal coagulation, prolongation of the PT usually reflects severe liver disease unless vitamin K deficiency is present. Failure of the PT to correct following parenteral administration of vitamin K implies severe liver disease; correction normally requires 24 h.

EFFECT OF ANESTHESIA ON HEPATIC FUNCTION

Hepatic Blood Flow

Hepatic blood flow usually decreases during regional and general anesthesia. Multiple factors are probably responsible, including both direct and indirect effects of anesthetic agents, the type of ventilation employed, and the type of surgery being performed.

All volatile anesthetic agents reduce portal hepatic blood flow. This decrease is greatest with halothane and least with isoflurane. Moreover, isoflurane appears to be the only volatile agent causing significant direct arterial vasodilation that can increase hepatic arterial blood flow. Nonetheless, even with isoflurane, total hepatic blood flow decreases because the decrease in portal blood flow usually offsets any increase in hepatic artery flow. All anesthetic agents indirectly reduce hepatic blood flow in proportion to any decrease in mean arterial blood pressure or cardiac output. Decreases in cardiac output reduce hepatic blood flow via reflex sympathetic activation, which vasoconstricts both the arterial and the venous splanchnic vasculature. If an adequate intravascular volume is maintained, spinal and epidural anesthesia decrease hepatic blood flow primarily by lowering arterial blood pressure, whereas general anesthesia usually decreases it through reductions in blood pressure and cardiac output and sympathetic stimulation.

The hemodynamic effects of ventilation can also have a significant impact on hepatic blood flow. Controlled positive pressure ventilation with high mean airway pressures reduces venous return to the heart and decreases cardiac output; both mechanisms can compromise hepatic blood flow. The former increases hepatic venous pressure, whereas the latter can reduce blood pressure and increase sympathetic tone. Positive end-expiratory pressure (PEEP) further accentuates these effects. Spontaneous ventilation therefore may be more advantageous in maintaining hepatic blood flow. Hypoxemia decreases hepatic blood flow via sympathetic activation. Hypocapnia, hypercapnia, acidosis, and alkalosis have variable effects due to the complex interaction between direct effects (increased flow with hypercapnia and acidosis but decreased flow with hypocapnia and alkalosis), secondary effects on the sympathetic system (activation with hypercapnia and acidosis), the ventilatory mode (spontaneous versus controlled ventilation), and the anesthetic agent used.

Surgical procedures near the liver can reduce hepatic blood flow up to 60%. Although the mechanisms are not clear, they most likely involve sympathetic activation, local reflexes, and direct compression of vessels in the portal and hepatic circulations.

β-Adrenergic blockers, α_1-adrenergic agonists, H_2-receptor blockers, and vasopressin reduce hepatic blood flow. Low-dose dopamine infusions may increase liver blood flow.

Metabolic Functions

The effects of the various anesthetic agents on hepatic intermediary metabolism (carbohydrate, fat, and protein) are poorly defined. An endocrine stress response secondary to fasting and surgical trauma is generally observed. The surgical stress response is characterized by elevated circulating levels of catecholamines, glucagon, and cortisol. Mobilization of carbohydrate stores and proteins results in hyperglycemia and a negative nitrogen balance (catabolism), respectively. The endocrine stress response may be at least partially blunted by regional anesthesia, deep general anesthesia, or pharmacological blockade of the sympathetic system, with regional anesthesia having the most salutary effect on catabolism.

Drug Metabolism

Although halothane has been reported to directly inhibit the metabolism of several drugs (phenytoin, warfarin, and ketamine), it is probably the decreased hepatic blood flow associated with halothane and other anesthetics that is responsible for altered pharmacokinetics of other drugs (fentanyl, verapamil, and propranolol).

Biliary Function

Anesthetic interactions with bile formation and storage have not been reported. However, all opioids can potentially cause spasm of the sphincter of Oddi and increase biliary pressure (fentanyl > morphine > meperidine > butorphanol > nalbuphine). The effects of alfentanil are similar to those of fentanyl but more short-lived. Intravenous opioid administration can therefore induce biliary colic or result in false-positive cholangiograms. Sphincter spasm may be less likely when the opioid is given slowly in small increments. Halothane and to a lesser extent enflurane may further blunt the increase in biliary pressure following opioid administration. Naloxone and glucagon (1–3 mg) are also reported to relieve opioid-induced spasm.

Liver Tests

Mild postoperative liver dysfunction in healthy persons is not uncommon if sensitive tests are employed. A combination of factors is probably responsible, including decreased blood flow that results from anesthesia, sympathetic stimulation, and the surgical procedure itself. Procedures in close proximity to the liver frequently result in modest elevations in lactate dehydrogenase and transaminase concentrations regardless of the anesthetic agent or technique employed.

Table 34–4. Causes of postoperative jaundice.

Prehepatic (increased bilirubin production)
  Resorption of hematomas
  Hemolytic anemia transfusion
    Senescent red cell breakdown
    Hemolytic reactions
Hepatic (hepatocellular dysfunction)
  Preexisting liver disease
  Ischemic or hypoxemic injury
  Drug-induced
  Gilbert's syndrome
  Intrahepatic cholestasis
  Halothane
Posthepatic (biliary obstruction)
  Postoperative cholecystitis
  Postoperative pancreatitis
  Retained common bile duct stone
  Bile duct injury
Miscellaneous

When the results of liver function tests are elevated postoperatively, the usual cause is underlying liver disease or the surgical procedure itself. Persistent abnormalities in liver tests may be indicative of viral hepatitis (usually transfusion related), sepsis, idiosyncratic drug reactions, or surgical complications. **Postoperative jaundice can result from a variety of factors (Table 34–4), but the most common cause is overproduction of bilirubin because of resorption of a large hematoma or red cell breakdown following transfusion.** Nonetheless, all other causes should be considered. Correct diagnosis requires a careful review of preoperative liver function as well as intraoperative and postoperative events such as transfusions, sustained hypotension or hypoxemia, and drug exposure.

HEPATIC DYSFUNCTION ASSOCIATED WITH HALOGENATED ANESTHETICS

Halothane, the first halogenated volatile anesthetic, was introduced in 1956, and shortly afterward the first cases of "halothane hepatitis" were reported. Since then, this disorder has been widely recognized, and cases associated with methoxyflurane, enflurane, and isoflurane have been described. Desflurane- and sevoflurane-related hepatitis have not been described.

Several mechanisms have been proposed for halothane-associated hepatitis, including the formation of hepatotoxic metabolic intermediates and immune hypersensitivity. Antibodies directed against hepatocyte components have been identified in some patients. A

genetic susceptibility has been shown in rats and may also be operative in humans. Reductive metabolism under hypoxic conditions can produce hepatotoxic intermediates in some strains of laboratory animals. In contrast, oxidative metabolism, which produces trifluoroacetic acid, appears to be responsible in other models; trifluoroacetylation of tissue proteins can cause hepatotoxicity.

Halothane-associated hepatitis is a diagnosis of exclusion. Viral hepatitis—including that caused by hepatitis viruses (types A, B, and C), cytomegalovirus, Epstein–Barr virus, and herpes viruses—should be excluded. The severity of this syndrome can vary from an asymptomatic elevation in serum transaminases to fulminant hepatic necrosis. Although the incidence of a mild form of this syndrome has been reported as high as 20% in adults following a second exposure to halothane, the incidence of fatal hepatic necrosis is estimated to be approximately 1:35,000. Epidemiological studies have identified several risk factors that are associated with halothane-associated hepatitis, including middle age, obesity, female sex, and a repeat exposure to halothane (particularly within 28 days). Prepubertal children appear to be more resistant to this condition, with reported incidences of 1:80,000–1:200,000.

Hepatitis due to isoflurane or enflurane is very rare (estimated to be 1:300,000–1:500,000); indeed, the association between hepatitis and these two agents—particularly isoflurane—is still questioned by many investigators.

CASE DISCUSSION: COAGULOPATHY IN A PATIENT WITH LIVER DISEASE

A 52-year-old man with a long history of alcohol abuse presents for a splenorenal shunt after three major episodes of upper gastrointestinal hemorrhage from esophageal varices. Coagulation studies reveal a prothrombin time of 17 s (control: 12 s), INR 1.7, and a partial prothrombin time of 43 s (control: 29 s). The platelet count is 75,000/μL.

What factors can contribute to excessive bleeding during and following surgery?

Hemostasis following trauma or surgery is dependent on three major processes: (1) vascular spasm, (2) formation of a platelet plug (primary hemostasis), and (3) coagulation of blood (secondary hemostasis). The first two are nearly immediate (seconds), whereas the last is delayed (minutes). A defect in any of these processes can lead to a bleeding diathesis and increased blood loss.

Outline the mechanisms involved in primary hemostasis.

Injury to blood vessels normally causes localized spasm as a result of the release of humoral factors (from platelets) as well as local myogenic reflexes. Sympathetic-mediated vasoconstriction is also probably operative in medium-sized vessels. Exposure of circulating platelets to the damaged endothelial surface causes them to undergo a series of changes that results in the formation of a platelet plug. If the break in a vessel is small, the plug itself can often completely stop bleeding. If the break is large, however, coagulation of blood is also necessary to stop the bleeding.

Formation of the platelet plug can be broken down into three stages: (1) adhesion, (2) release of platelet granules, and (3) aggregation. Following injury, circulating platelets adhere to subendothelial collagen via specific glycoprotein (GP) receptors on their membrane. This interaction is stabilized by a circulating GP called von Willebrand factor (vWF), which forms additional bridges between subendothelial collagen and platelets via GPIb. Collagen (as well as epinephrine and thrombin) activates platelet membrane-bound phospholipases A and C, which, in turn, result in the formation of thromboxane A$_2$ (TXA$_2$) and degranulation, respectively. TXA$_2$ is a potent vasoconstrictor that also promotes platelet aggregation. Platelet granules contain a large number of substances, including adenosine diphosphate (ADP), factor V, vWF, fibrinogen, and fibronectin. These factors attract and activate additional platelets. ADP alters a platelet membrane GPIIb/IIIa, which facilitates the binding of fibrinogen to activated platelets.

Describe the mechanisms involved in normal coagulation.

Coagulation, often referred to as secondary hemostasis, involves formation of a fibrin clot, which usually binds and strengthens a platelet plug. Fibrin can be formed via one of two mechanisms (pathways) that involve activation of soluble coagulation precursor proteins in blood (Table 34–5). Regardless of which pathway is activated, the coagulation cascade ends in the conversion of fibrinogen to fibrin. The extrinsic pathway of the coagulation cascade is

Table 34–5. Coagulation factors.

	Factor	Approximate Half-Life (h)
I	Fibrinogen	100
II	Prothrombin	80
III	Tissue thromboplastin	—
IV	Calcium	—
V	Proaccelerin	18
VII	Proconvertin	6
VIII	Antihemophilic factor	10
IX	Christmas factor	24
X	Stuart factor	50
XI	Plasma thromboplastin antecedents	25
XII	Hageman factor	60
XIII	Fibrin-stabilizing factor	90

triggered by the release of a tissue lipoprotein (thromboplastin) from the membranes of injured cells and is likely the more important pathway in humans. The intrinsic pathway (Figure 34–5) can be triggered by the interaction between subendothelial collagen with circulating Hageman factor (XII), high-molecular-weight kininogen, and prekallikrein. The latter two substances are also involved in the formation of bradykinin.

Thrombin plays a central role in coagulation because it not only activates platelets (above) but also accelerates conversion of factors V, VIII, and XIII to their active forms. Conversion of prothrombin to thrombin is markedly accelerated by activated platelets. Thrombin then converts fibrinogen to soluble fibrin monomers that polymerize on the platelet plug. Cross-linking of fibrin polymers by factor XIII is necessary to form a strong, insoluble fibrin clot. Finally, retraction of the clot (which requires platelets) expresses fluid from the clot and helps pull the walls of the damaged blood vessel together.

What prevents coagulation of blood in normal tissues?

The coagulation process is limited to injured areas by localization of platelets to the injured area and maintenance of normal blood flow in uninjured areas. Normal endothelium produc-

EXTRINSIC PATHWAY

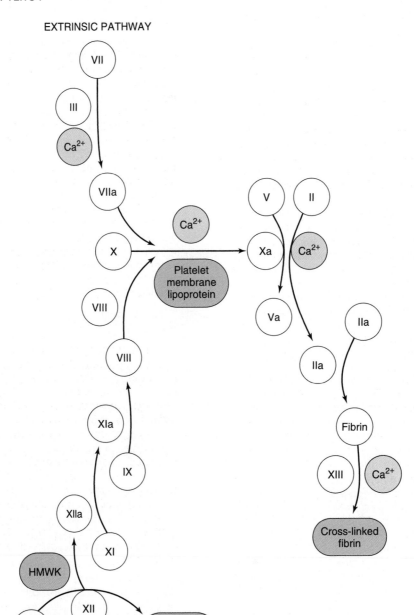

INTRINSIC PATHWAY

Figure 34–5. The intrinsic and extrinsic coagulation pathways.

es prostacyclin (prostaglandin I_2 [PGI_2]), which is a potent vasodilator that also inhibits platelet activation and helps confine the primary hemostatic process to the injured area. Normal blood flow is important in clearing activated coagulation factors, which are taken up by the monocyte–macrophage scavenger system (above). Multiple inhibitors of coagulation are normally present in plasma, including antithrombin III and proteins C and S, and tissue factor pathway inhibitor. Antithrombin III complexes with and inactivates circulating coagulation factors (with the notable exception of factor VII), whereas protein C specifically inactivates factors V and VIII. Heparin exerts its anticoagulant activity by augmenting the activity of antithrombin III. Protein S enhances the activity of protein C; deficiencies of these two proteins lead to hypercoagulability. Tissue factor pathway inhibitor antagonizes the action of activated factor VII.

What is the role of the fibrinolytic system in normal hemostasis?

The fibrinolytic system is normally activated simultaneously with the coagulation cascade and functions to maintain the fluidity of blood during coagulation. It is also responsible for clot lysis once tissue repair begins. When a clot is formed, a large amount of the protein plasminogen is incorporated. Plasminogen is then activated either by tissue plasminogen activator (tPA), which is usually released by endothelial cells in response to thrombin and fragments of Hageman factor. The resulting formation of plasmin degrades fibrin and fibrinogen as well as other coagulation factors. Urokinase (found in urine) and streptokinase (a product of bacteria) are also potent activators of plasminogen. The action of tPA is localized because (1) it is absorbed into the fibrin clot, (2) it activates plasminogen more effectively on the clot, (3) free plasmin is rapidly neutralized by a circulating α_2-antiplasmin, and (4) circulating tPA is cleared by the liver. Plasmin degrades fibrin and fibrinogen into small fragments. These fibrin degradation products possess anticoagulant activity because they compete with fibrinogen for thrombin; they are normally cleared by the monocyte–macrophage system. The drugs ε-aminocaproic acid (EACA) and tranexamic acid inhibit the conversion of plasminogen to plasmin. Endothelium also normally secretes a plasminogen activator inhibitor (PAI-1) that antagonizes tPA.

What hemostatic defects are likely to be present in this patient?

Multifactorial coagulopathy often develops in patients with advanced liver disease. Three major causes are usually responsible: (1) vitamin K deficiency (impaired storage or absorption), (2) impaired hepatic synthesis of coagulation factors, and (3) splenic sequestration of platelets resulting from hypersplenism. To complicate matters further, patients with cirrhosis typically have multiple potential bleeding sites (esophageal varices, gastritis, peptic ulcers, and hemorrhoids) and frequently require multiple blood transfusions. With severe liver disease, patients may also have decreased synthesis of coagulation inhibitors and fail to clear activated coagulation factors and fibrin split products (impaired Kupffer cell function); the coagulation defect resembles and becomes indistinguishable from disseminated intravascular coagulation (DIC).

What is DIC?

In DIC, the coagulation cascade is activated by the release of endogenous tissue thromboplastin or thromboplastin-like substances, or by direct activation of factor XII by endotoxin or foreign surfaces. Widespread deposition of fibrin in the microcirculation results in consumption of coagulation factors, secondary fibrinolysis, thrombocytopenia, and a microangiopathic hemolytic anemia. Diffuse bleeding and in some cases thromboembolic phenomena usually follow. Treatment is generally aimed at the underlying cause. Supportive measures include transfusion of coagulation factors and platelets. Heparin therapy is controversial but may benefit patients with thromboembolic phenomena.

What is primary fibrinolysis?

This bleeding disorder is due to uncontrolled fibrinolysis. Patients may have a deficiency of α_2-antiplasmin or impaired clearance of tPA. The latter may be common in patients with severe liver disease and during the anhepatic phase of liver transplantation. The disorder may occasionally be encountered in patients with carcinoma of the prostate (see Chapter 33). Diagnosis is often difficult but is suggested by a bleeding diathesis with a low fibrinogen level but relatively normal coagulation tests and platelet count (below). Treatment includes fresh *frozen plasma or cryoprecipitate and possibly either EACA or tranexamic acid.*

How are coagulation tests helpful in evaluating hemostasis?

The diagnosis of coagulation abnormalities can be facilitated by measurement of the activated partial thromboplastin time (aPTT), prothrombin time (PT), thrombin time (TT), and fibrinogen level (Table 34–6). The aPTT measures the intrinsic pathway (factors I, II, V, VIII, IX, X, XI, and XII). The whole blood clotting time and activated clotting time (ACT) also measure the intrinsic pathway. In contrast, the PT measures the extrinsic pathway (factors I, II, V, and VII). The TT specifically measures conversion of fibrinogen to fibrin (factors I and II). The normal plasma fibrinogen level is 200–400 mg/dL (5.9–11.7 µmol/L). Because heparin therapy primarily affects the intrinsic pathway, in low doses it usually prolongs the PTT only. In high doses, heparin also prolongs the PT. In contrast, warfarin primarily affects vitamin K-dependent factors (II, VII, IX, and X), so the PT is prolonged at usual doses and the PTT is prolonged only at high doses. In vivo plasmin activity can be evaluated by measuring circulating levels of peptides cleaved from fibrin and fibrinogen by plasmin, namely fibrin degradation products (FDP) and D-dimers. Patients with primary fibrinolysis usually have elevated FDPs but normal D-dimer levels.

Table 34–6. Coagulation test abnormalities.[1]

	PT	PTT	TT	Fibrinogen
Advanced liver disease	↑	↑	N or↑	N or↓
DIC	↑	↑	↑	↓
Vitamin K deficiency	↑↑	↑	N	N
Warfarin therapy	↑↑	↑	N	N
Heparin therapy	↑	↑↑	↑	N
Hemophilia				
Factor VIII deficiency	N	↑	N	N
Factor IX deficiency	N	↑	N	N
Factor VII deficiency	↑	N	N	N
Factor XIII deficiency	N	N	N	N

[1]PT, prothrombin time; PTT, partial thromboplastin time; TT, thrombin time; N, normal; DIC, disseminated intravascular coagulation.

What tests are most helpful in evaluating primary hemostasis?

The most commonly performed tests include a platelet count and a bleeding time. The bleeding time is generally not affected by the platelet count when the latter is greater than 100,000/µL. The normal platelet count is 150,000–450,000/µL. Patients with normally functioning platelets and platelet counts above 100,000/µL have normal primary hemostasis. When the platelet count is 50,000–100,000/µL, excessive bleeding generally occurs only with severe trauma or extensive surgery. In contrast, patients with platelet counts under 50,000/µL develop significant bleeding following even minor trauma. When the platelet count is under 20,000/µL, spontaneous bleeding is not unusual. Thrombocytopenia usually results from one of three mechanisms: (1) decreased platelet production, (2) splenic sequestration of platelets, or (3) increased platelet destruction. The last may fall under one of two categories of destruction: immune or nonimmune. Nonimmune destruction includes vasculitis or DIC.

A prolonged bleeding time with a normal platelet count implies a qualitative platelet defect. Although the bleeding time is somewhat dependent on the technique employed, values longer than 10 min are generally considered abnormal. Significant intraoperative and postoperative bleeding may be expected when the bleeding time exceeds 15 min. Specialized testing is required to diagnose specific platelet functional defects.

What are the most common causes of qualitative platelet defects?

The most common platelet defect is due to inhibition of TXA_2 production by aspirin and nonsteroidal antiinflammatory drugs (NSAIDs). In contrast to aspirin, which irreversibly acetylates and inactivates cyclooxygenase for the life of the platelet (up to 8 days), enzyme inhibition by NSAIDs is reversible and generally lasts only 24 h.

What is von Willebrand's disease?

The most common inherited bleeding disorder (1:800–1000 patients) is **von Willebrand's disease.** Patients with this disorder produce a defective vWF or low levels of a normal vWF (normal: 5–10 mg/L). Most patients are heterozygous and have relatively mild hemostatic defects that become apparent clinically when they are subjected to major surgery or trauma or following ingestion of aspirin or NSAIDs. In addition to helping link platelets, vWF serves as a carrier for coagulation factor VIII. As a result, patients typically have a prolonged bleeding time, decreased plasma vWF concentration, and decreased factor VIII activity. Acquired forms of von Willebrand's disease may be encountered in patients with some immune disorders and those with tumors that absorb vWF onto their surface. At least three forms of the disease are recognized, ranging in severity from mild to severe.

Treatment with desmopressin (DDAVP) can raise vWF levels in some patients with mild von Willebrand's disease (as well as normal individuals). The drug is usually administered at a dose of 0.3 μg/kg 30 min before surgery. Patients who do not respond to DDAVP should receive cryoprecipitate or factor VIII concentrates, both of which are rich in vWF; prophylactic infusions are generally recommended before and after surgery twice a day for 2–4 days to guarantee surgical hemostasis. The risk of transmitting viral diseases is decreased with the use of purified and heat-treated factor VIII concentrates (see Chapter 29).

What other hereditary hemostatic defects may be encountered in anesthetic practice?

The most common inherited defect in secondary hemostasis is **factor VIII deficiency** (hemophilia A). This X-linked abnormality is estimated to affect 1:10,000 males. Disease severity is generally inversely related to factor VIII activity. Most symptomatic patients experience hemarthrosis, bleeding into deep tissues, and hematuria. Symptomatic patients generally have less than 5% of normal factor VIII activity. Classically, patients present with a prolonged aPTT but a normal PT and bleeding time. The diagnosis is confirmed by measuring factor VIII activity in blood. Affected patients generally do not experience increased bleeding during surgery when factor VIII levels are over 30%, but most clinicians recommend increasing factor VIII levels to more than 50% prior to surgery. Normal (fresh frozen) plasma, by definition, is considered to have 1 U of factor VIII activity per milliliter. In contrast, cryoprecipitate has 5–10 U/mL, whereas factor VIII concentrates have approximately 40 U/mL. Each

unit of factor VIII transfused is estimated to raise factor VIII levels 2% per kilogram of body weight. Justifiable concern over transmission of viral disease has led to the development and increasing use of recombinant or monoclonal purified factor VIII. Twice-a-day transfusions are generally recommended following surgery because of the relatively short half-life of factor VIII (8–12 h). Administration of DDAVP can raise factor VIII levels 2- to 3-fold in some patients. EACA or tranexamic acid may also be used as adjuncts.

Hemophilia B (also known as Christmas disease) is the result of an X-linked hereditary deficiency of factor IX. The disease is very similar to hemophilia A but much less common (1:100,000 males). Measurement of factor IX levels establishes the diagnosis. Perioperative administration of fresh frozen plasma is generally recommended to maintain factor IX activity at more than 30% of normal. Recombinant or monoclonal purified factor IX should preferably be used when available.

Factor XIII deficiency is extremely rare but notable in that the aPTT, PT, TT, and bleeding times are normal. The diagnosis requires measurement of factor XIII levels. Because only 1% of normal factor XIII activity is generally required, patients are treated by a single transfusion of fresh frozen plasma.

Do normal laboratory values exclude a hemostatic defect?

A bleeding diathesis may exist even in the absence of gross abnormalities on routine laboratory tests. Some hemostatic defects are often not detected by routine testing but require additional specialized tests. A history of excessive bleeding after dental extractions, childbirth, minor surgery, minor trauma, or even during menstruation suggests a hemostatic defect. A family history of a bleeding diathesis may suggest an inherited coagulation defect but is often absent because the increased bleeding is often minor and goes unnoticed.

Hemostatic defects can often be differentiated by their clinical presentation. Bleeding in patients with primary hemostatic defects usually immediately follows minor trauma, is confined to superficial sites (skin or mucosal surfaces), and often can be controlled by local compression. Pinpoint small hemorrhages from capillaries in the dermis (petechiae) are typically present on examination. Bleeding into subcutaneous tissues (ecchymosis) from small arterioles or venules is also common in patients with platelet disorders. In contrast, bleeding that results from secondary hemostatic defects is usually delayed following injury, is typically deep (subcutaneous tissues, joints, body cavities, or muscles), and is often difficult to stop even with compression. Hemorrhages may be palpable as hematomas or may go unnoticed when located deeper (retroperitoneal). Coagulation may be impaired by systemic hypothermic or subnormal temperature of the site of bleeding even when coagulation test (PT, activated aPTT, bleeding time) results are normal and there is no history of hemostatic defects.

SUGGESTED READING

Ganong WF: *Review of Medical Physiology*, 2nd ed. McGraw-Hill, 2005.

Kaplowitz N: *Liver and Biliary Diseases*, 2nd ed. Williams & Wilkins, 1996.

Stoelting RK, Dierdorf SF: *Handbook for Anesthesia and Co-existing Disease*, 2nd ed. Churchill Livingstone, 2002.

Anesthesia for Patients with Liver Disease

35

KEY CONCEPTS

 Patients with acute hepatitis should have any elective surgery postponed until the acute hepatitis has resolved, as indicated by normalization of liver tests. Studies indicate increased perioperative morbidity (12%) and mortality (up to 10% with laparotomy) during acute viral hepatitis.

 Isoflurane is the volatile agent of choice because it has the least effect on hepatic blood flow. Factors known to reduce hepatic blood flow, such as hypotension, excessive sympathetic activation, and high mean airway pressures during controlled ventilation, should be avoided.

 In evaluating patients for chronic hepatitis, laboratory test results may show only a mild elevation in serum aminotransferase activity and often correlate poorly with disease severity.

4 Approximately 10% of patients with cirrhosis also develop at least one episode of spontaneous bacterial peritonitis, and some may eventually develop hepatocellular carcinoma.

 In patients with cirrhosis, massive bleeding from gastroesophageal varices is a major cause of morbidity and mortality.

 Cirrhosis is typically characterized by a hyperdynamic circulatory state.

 Hypoxemia is frequently present and is due to right-to-left shunting (up to 40% of cardiac output).

 The hepatorenal syndrome is a functional renal defect in patients with cirrhosis that usually follows gastrointestinal bleeding, aggressive diuresis, sepsis, or major surgery. It is characterized by progressive oliguria with avid sodium retention, azotemia, intractable ascites, and a very high mortality rate.

 Factors known to precipitate hepatic encephalopathy in patients with cirrhosis include gastrointestinal bleeding, increased dietary protein intake, hypokalemic alkalosis (from vomiting or diuresis), infections, and worsening liver function.

 Following the removal of large amounts of ascitic fluid, intravenous colloid fluid replacement is often necessary to prevent profound hypotension and renal shutdown.

The prevalence of liver disease is increasing in the United States. Cirrhosis, the terminal pathology in a majority of liver diseases, appears to have a general incidence in some autopsy series as high as 5%. It is a major cause of death of men in their fourth and fifth decades, and mortality rates are increasing. Ten percent of the patients with liver disease undergo operative procedures during the final 2 years of their lives. The liver has remarkable functional reserve, and clinical manifestations of hepatic disease are often absent until extensive damage has occurred. Consequently, when these marginal patients with little reserve come to the operating room, effects from anesthetics and surgery (see Chapter 34) can precipitate further hepatic decompensation, leading to overt hepatic failure.

This chapter discusses the anesthetic management of patients with known liver disease. With some important exceptions, the anesthetic considerations tend to be similar in both acute and chronic liver disease. Although patients with cholelithiasis often have minimal hepatic impairment, the effects of anesthesia on the biliary system also require comment.

■ HEPATITIS

ACUTE HEPATITIS

Acute hepatitis is usually the result of viral infection, a drug reaction, or exposure to a hepatotoxin. The illness represents acute hepatocellular injury with variable amounts of cell necrosis. Clinical manifestations generally depend both on the severity of the inflammatory reaction and, more importantly, on the amount of necrosis. Mild inflammatory reactions may present as asymptomatic elevations in the serum transaminases, whereas massive hepatic necrosis presents as acute fulminant hepatic failure.

Viral Hepatitis

Viral hepatitis is most commonly due to hepatitis A, hepatitis B, or hepatitis C viruses (previously called blood-borne non-A, non-B). At least two other hepatitis viruses have also been identified: hepatitis D (delta virus) and hepatitis E (enteric non-A, non-B). Hepatitis types A and E are transmitted by the oral–fecal route, whereas types B and C are transmitted primarily percutaneously and by contact with body fluids. Hepatitis D is unique in that it may be transmitted by either route and requires the presence of hepatitis B virus in the host to be infective. Other viruses, including Epstein–Barr, herpes simplex, cytomegalovirus, and coxsackieviruses, may also cause hepatitis.

Patients with viral hepatitis often have a 1- to 2-week mild prodromal illness (fatigue, malaise, low-grade fever, or nausea and vomiting) that may or may not be followed by jaundice. The jaundice typically lasts 2–12 weeks, but complete recovery, as evidenced by serum transaminase measurements, usually takes 4 months. Because clinical manifestations overlap, serological testing is necessary to determine the causative viral agent. The clinical course tends to be more complicated and prolonged with hepatitis B and C viruses. Less commonly, cholestasis (see below) is the major manifestation. Rarely, fulminant hepatic failure (massive hepatic necrosis) can develop.

The incidence of chronic active hepatitis (see below) is 3–10% following infection with hepatitis B virus and at least 50% following infection with hepatitis C virus.

A small percentage of patients (mainly immunosuppressed patients and those on long-term hemodialysis regimens) become asymptomatic infectious carriers following infection with hepatitis B virus. Depending on the patient group studied, anywhere between 0.3% and 30% of patients remain infectious with the B surface antigen (HBsAg) persisting in their blood. Approximately 0.5–1% of patients with hepatitis C infection become asymptomatic infectious carriers. Infectivity correlates with detection of hepatitis C viral RNA in peripheral blood. Most patients with chronic hepatitis C infection appear to have very low, intermittent, or absent circulating viral particles and are therefore not highly infective. However, infectious carriers pose a major health hazard to operating room personnel. In addition to "universal precautions" for avoiding direct contact with blood and secretions (gloves, mask, protective eyewear, and not recapping needles), immunization of health care personnel is highly effective against hepatitis B infection. A vaccine for hepatitis C is not available; moreover, unlike hepatitis B infection, hepatitis C infection does not appear to confer immunity to subsequent exposure. Postexposure prophylaxis with hyperimmune globulin is effective for hepatitis B but not for hepatitis C.

Drug-Induced Hepatitis

Drug-induced hepatitis (Table 35–1) can result from direct dose-dependent toxicity of a drug (or a metabolite), from an idiosyncratic drug reaction, or from a combination of the two causes. The clinical course often resembles viral hepatitis, making diagnosis difficult. Alcoholic hepatitis is probably the most commonly encountered type of drug-induced hepatitis, but the cause may not be obvious from the history. Chronic alcohol ingestion can also result in hepatomegaly from fatty infiltration of the liver, which reflects (1) impaired fatty acid oxidation, (2) increased uptake and esterification of fatty acids, and (3) diminished lipoprotein synthesis and secretion. Acetaminophen ingestion of 25 g or more usually results in fatal fulminant disease. A few drugs such as chlorpromazine and oral contraceptives characteristically cause cholestatic-type reactions (see below). Ingestion of potent hepatotoxins, such as carbon tetrachloride and certain species of mushrooms (*Amanita, Galerina*), is often associated with acute hepatic failure. Volatile anesthetics, most notably halothane, are associated with an idiosyncratic reaction hepatitis.

Preoperative Considerations

 Patients with acute hepatitis should have any elective surgery postponed until the acute hepatitis has resolved, as indicated by normaliza-

Table 35–1. Drugs and substances associated with hepatitis.

Toxic
Alcohol
Acetaminophen
Salicylates
Tetracyclines
Trichloroethylene
Vinyl chloride
Carbon tetrachloride
Yellow phosphorus
Poisonous mushrooms (*Amanita, Galerina*)
Idiosyncratic
Volatile anesthetics (halothane)
Phenytoin
Sulfonamides
Rifampin
Indomethacin
Toxic and idiosyncratic
Methyldopa
Isoniazid
Sodium valproate
Amiodarone
Primarily cholestatic
Chlorpromazine
Cyclosporine
Oral contraceptives
Anabolic steroids
Erythromycin estolate
Methimazole

tion of liver tests. Studies indicate increased perioperative morbidity (12%) and mortality (up to 10% with laparotomy) during acute viral hepatitis. Although the risk with alcoholic hepatitis may not be as great, acute alcohol toxicity greatly complicates anesthetic management. Moreover, alcohol withdrawal during surgery may be associated with a mortality rate as high as 50%. Only truly emergent surgery should be considered in such instances. Patients with hepatitis are at risk for deterioration of hepatic function and the development of complications from hepatic failure, such as encephalopathy, coagulopathy, or hepatorenal syndrome (see below).

Laboratory evaluation should include blood urea nitrogen, serum electrolytes, creatinine, glucose, transaminases, bilirubin, alkaline phosphatase, and albumin as well as a prothrombin time (PT) and platelet count. Serum should also be checked for HBsAg whenever possible. A blood alcohol level is useful if the history or mental status is compatible with intoxication. Hypokalemia and metabolic alkalosis are not uncommon and are usually due to vomiting. Concomitant hypomagnesemia may be present in chronic alcoholics and predisposes to arrhythmias. The ele-

vation in serum transaminases does not necessarily correlate with the amount of necrosis. The serum alanine aminotransferase (ALT) is generally higher than the serum aspartate aminotransferase (AST) except in alcoholic hepatitis, where the reverse occurs. Bilirubin and alkaline phosphatase are usually only moderately elevated, except with the cholestatic variant of hepatitis. The PT is the best indicator of hepatic synthetic function. Persistent prolongation greater than 3 s (international normalized ratio [INR] > 1.5) following administration of vitamin K is indicative of severe hepatic dysfunction. Hypoglycemia is not uncommon. Hypoalbuminemia is usually not present except in protracted cases, with severe malnutrition, or when chronic liver disease is present.

If a patient with acute hepatitis must undergo an emergent operation, the preanesthetic evaluation should focus on determining the cause and the degree of hepatic impairment. Information should be obtained regarding recent drug exposures, including alcohol intake, intravenous drug use, recent transfusions, and prior anesthetics. The presence of nausea or vomiting should be noted and dehydration and electrolyte abnormalities should be corrected. Changes in mental status usually indicate severe hepatic impairment. Inappropriate behavior or obtundation in alcoholic patients may be signs of acute intoxication, whereas tremulousness and irritability usually reflect withdrawal. Hypertension and tachycardia are often also prominent with the latter. Vitamin K or fresh frozen plasma (FFP) may be necessary to correct a coagulopathy. Premedication is generally not given, in an effort to minimize drug exposure and not confound hepatic encephalopathy in patients with advanced liver disease. However, benzodiazepines and thiamine are indicated for alcoholic patients with acute withdrawal.

Intraoperative Considerations

The goal of intraoperative management is to preserve existing hepatic function and avoid factors that may be detrimental to the liver. Drug selection and dosage should be individualized. Some patients with viral hepatitis may exhibit increased central nervous system sensitivity to anesthetics, whereas alcoholic patients will often display cross-tolerance to both intravenous and volatile anesthetics. Alcoholic patients also require close cardiovascular monitoring, because the cardiac depressant effects of alcohol are additive to those of anesthetics; moreover, alcoholic cardiomyopathy develops in many alcoholic patients.

By definition, all anesthetics are central nervous system depressants, and for that reason the fewest number of agents should be used. Inhalation anesthetics are generally preferable to intravenous agents because most of the latter are dependent on the liver for metabolism or elimination. Standard induction doses of intravenous induction agents can generally be used because their action is terminated by redistribution rather than metabolism or excretion. A prolonged duration of action, however, may be encountered with large or repeated doses of intravenous agents, particularly opioids. Isoflurane is the volatile agent of choice because it has the least effect on hepatic blood flow. Factors known to reduce hepatic blood flow, such as hypotension, excessive sympathetic activation, and high mean airway pressures during controlled ventilation, should be avoided. Regional anesthesia may be employed in the absence of coagulopathy, provided hypotension is avoided.

CHRONIC HEPATITIS

Chronic hepatitis is defined as persistent hepatic inflammation for longer than 6 months, as evidenced by elevated serum aminotransferases. Patients can usually be classified as having one of three distinct syndromes based on a liver biopsy: chronic persistent hepatitis, chronic lobular hepatitis, or chronic active hepatitis. Those with chronic persistent hepatitis manifest chronic inflammation of portal tracts with preservation of normal cellular architecture on the biopsy; this type usually does not progress to cirrhosis. Clinically, these patients present with acute hepatitis (usually hepatitis B or C) that has a protracted course but eventually resolves. A recently described variant called chronic lobular hepatitis is characterized by acute hepatitis that resolves but is followed by recurrent exacerbations; foci of inflammation and necrosis are present in hepatic lobules. Like chronic persistent hepatitis, however, chronic lobular hepatitis usually does not progress to cirrhosis.

Patients with chronic active hepatitis have chronic hepatic inflammation with destruction of normal cellular architecture (piecemeal necrosis) on the biopsy. Evidence of cirrhosis is often present initially (20–50% of patients) or eventually develops. Although chronic active hepatitis appears to have many causes, it occurs most commonly as a sequela of hepatitis B or hepatitis C. Other postulated causes include drugs (methyldopa, oxyphenisatin, isoniazid, and nitrofurantoin) and autoimmune disorders. Both immunological factors and a genetic predisposition appear to be responsible in most cases. Patients usually present with a history of fatigue and recurrent jaundice; extrahepatic manifestations, such as arthritis and serositis, are not uncommon. Manifestations of cirrhosis eventually predominate in patients with progressive disease. In evaluating patients for chronic hepatitis, laboratory test results may show only a mild elevation in serum aminotransferase activity and often correlate poorly with disease severity. Patients without chronic hepatitis B or C infection usually have a favorable response to immunosuppressants and are treated with long-term corticosteroid therapy with or without azathioprine.

Anesthetic Management

Patients with chronic persistent or chronic lobular hepatitis should be treated similarly to those with acute hepatitis (see above). In contrast, those with chronic active hepatitis should be assumed to already have cirrhosis and should be treated accordingly (see below). Patients with autoimmune chronic active hepatitis may also present problems related to other autoimmune manifestations (such as diabetes or thyroiditis) as well as long-term corticosteroid therapy.

■ CIRRHOSIS

Cirrhosis is a serious and progressive disease that eventually results in hepatic failure. The most common cause of cirrhosis in the United States is alcohol (Laennec's cirrhosis). Other causes include chronic active hepatitis (postnecrotic cirrhosis), chronic biliary inflammation or obstruction (primary biliary cirrhosis, sclerosing cholangitis), chronic right-sided congestive heart failure (cardiac cirrhosis), autoimmune hepatitis, hemochromatosis, Wilson's disease, α_1-antitrypsin deficiency, nonalcoholic steatohepatitis, and cryptogenic cirrhosis. Regardless of the cause, hepatocyte necrosis is followed by fibrosis and nodular regeneration. Distortion of the liver's normal cellular and vascular architecture obstructs portal venous flow and leads to portal hypertension, whereas impairment of the liver's normal synthetic and other diverse metabolic functions results in multisystem disease. Clinically, signs and symptoms often do not correlate with disease severity. Manifestations are typically absent initially, but jaundice and ascites eventually develop in most patients. Other signs include spider angiomas, palmar erythema, gynecomastia, and splenomegaly. Moreover, cirrhosis is generally associated with the development of three major complications: (1) variceal hemorrhage from portal hypertension, (2) intractable fluid retention in the form of ascites and the hepatorenal syndrome, and (3) hepatic encephalopathy or coma. Approximately 10% of patients with cirrhosis also develop at least one episode of spontaneous bacterial peritonitis, and some may eventually develop hepatocellular carcinoma.

Few diseases can produce hepatic fibrosis without hepatocellular necrosis or nodular regeneration. They result mainly in portal hypertension and its associated complications (see below); hepatocellular function is often but not always preserved. These disorders include schistosomiasis, idiopathic portal fibrosis (Banti's syndrome), and congenital hepatic fibrosis. Obstruction of the hepatic veins or inferior vena cava (Budd–Chiari syndrome) can also cause portal hypertension. The latter may be the result of venous thrombosis (hypercoagulable state), a tumor thrombus (renal carcinoma), or occlusive disease of the sublobular hepatic veins.

Preoperative Considerations

The detrimental effects of anesthesia and surgery on hepatic blood flow are discussed in Chapter 34. Patients with cirrhosis are at increased risk for deterioration of liver function because of their limited functional reserves. Successful anesthetic management of these patients is dependent on recognizing the multisystem nature of cirrhosis and controlling or preventing its complications (Table 35–2).

A. GASTROINTESTINAL MANIFESTATIONS

Portal hypertension (> 10 mm Hg) leads to the development of extensive portal-systemic venous collateral channels. Four major collateral sites are generally recognized: gastroesophageal, hemorrhoidal, periumbilical, and retroperitoneal. Portal hypertension is often apparent preoperatively as evidenced by dilated abdominal wall veins (caput medusae). In patients with cirrhosis, massive bleeding from gastroesophageal varices is a major cause of morbidity and mortality. In addition to the effects of acute blood loss, the increased nitrogen load (from the breakdown of blood in the intestinal tract) can precipitate hepatic encephalopathy. Endoscopy is a valuable diagnostic and therapeutic tool. Identification of the site of bleeding is crucial because these patients may present with bleeding from a peptic ulcer or gastritis, which require different therapy.

The treatment of variceal bleeding is generally supportive (medical). Blood loss should be replaced with intravenous fluids and blood products (see Chapter 29). Nonsurgical treatment includes vasopressin (0.1–0.9 U/min intravenously), somatostatin (250 μg followed by 250 μg/h), propranolol, balloon tamponade (with a Sengstaken–Blakemore tube), and endoscopic sclerosis of the varices. Vasopressin, somatostatin, and propranolol reduce the rate of blood loss. High doses of vasopressin can result in congestive heart failure or myocardial ischemia; concomitant infusion of intravenous nitroglycerin may decrease the likelihood of these complications as well as the bleeding. Endoscopic sclerosis or ligation of the varices is usually effective in stopping the hemorrhage in 90% of bleeding episodes. Percutaneous transjugular intrahepatic portosystemic shunts (TIPS) can reduce portal hypertension and subsequent bleeding (however, it may increase the incidence of encephalopathy). When the bleeding fails to stop or it recurs, emergency surgery may be indicated. Surgical risk has been shown to correlate with the degree of hepatic impairment, based on clinical and laboratory findings (Child's classification; see Table 35–3). Shunting procedures are generally performed on low-risk patients,

Table 35–2. Manifestations of cirrhosis.

Gastrointestinal
  Portal hypertension
    Ascites
    Esophageal varices
    Hemorrhoids
    Gastrointestinal bleeding
Circulatory
  Hyperdynamic state (high cardiac output)
  Systemic arteriovenous shunts
  Low systemic vascular resistance
  Cirrhotic cardiomyopathy
Pulmonary
  Increased intrapulmonary shunting
  Decreased functional residual capacity
  Pleural effusions
  Restrictive ventilatory defect
  Respiratory alkalosis
Renal
  Increased proximal reabsorption of sodium
  Increased distal reabsorption of sodium
  Impaired free water clearance
    Decreased renal perfusion
    Hepatorenal syndrome
Hematological
  Anemia
  Coagulopathy
    Hypersplenism
    Thrombocytopenia
    Leukopenia
Infectious
  Spontaneous bacterial peritonitis
Metabolic
  Hyponatremia
  Hypokalemia
  Hypomagnesemia
  Hypoalbuminemia
  Hypoglycemia
Neurological
  Encephalopathy

whereas ablative surgery, esophageal transection, and gastric devascularization are reserved for high-risk patients. Nonselective shunts (portacaval and proximal splenorenal) have generally been abandoned in favor of selective shunts (distal splenorenal). The latter decompress the varices but do not impair hepatic blood flow as much and are less likely to cause encephalopathy postoperatively (see below).

B. HEMATOLOGICAL MANIFESTATIONS

Anemia, thrombocytopenia, and, less commonly, leukopenia, may be present. The cause of the anemia is usually multifactorial and includes blood loss, increased red cell destruction, bone marrow suppression, and nutritional deficiencies. Congestive splenomegaly (from

Table 35–3. Child's classification for evaluating hepatic reserve.[1]

Risk Group	A	B	C
Bilirubin (mg/dL)	< 2.0	2.0–3.0	> 3.0
Serum albumin (g/dL)	> 3.5	3.0–3.5	< 3.0
Ascites	None	Controlled	Poorly controlled
Encephalopathy	Absent	Minimal	Coma
Nutrition	Excellent	Good	Poor
Mortality rate (%)	2–5	10	50

[1]Adapted from Child CG: *The Liver and Portal Hypertension.* W.B. Saunders, 1964.

portal hypertension) is largely responsible for the thrombocytopenia and leukopenia. Coagulation factor deficiencies arise as a result of decreased hepatic synthesis. Enhanced fibrinolysis secondary to decreased clearance of activators of the fibrinolytic system may also contribute to the coagulopathy.

The need for preoperative blood transfusions should be balanced against the obligatory increase in nitrogen load. Protein breakdown from excessive blood transfusions can precipitate encephalopathy. However, coagulopathy should be corrected before surgery. Clotting factors should be replaced with appropriate blood products such as FFP and cryoprecipitate. Platelet transfusions should be considered immediately prior to surgery for counts less than 100,000/μL.

C. CIRCULATORY MANIFESTATIONS

Cirrhosis is typically characterized by a hyperdynamic circulatory state. Cardiac output is often increased, and generalized peripheral vasodilation is present. Arteriovenous shunting can occur in both the systemic and pulmonary circulations. **The arteriovenous shunting together with the decrease in blood viscosity from anemia are partly responsible for the increased cardiac output, which is dependent upon above normal filling pressures and below normal systemic vascular resistance (cirrhotic cardiomyopathy).** Patients with a superimposed alcoholic cardiomyopathy readily develop congestive heart failure.

D. RESPIRATORY MANIFESTATIONS

Disturbances in pulmonary gas exchange as well as ventilatory mechanics are often present. Hyperventilation is common and results in a primary respiratory alkalosis. Hypoxemia is frequently present and is due to right-to-left shunting (up to 40% of cardiac output). Shunting is due to an increase in both pulmonary arteriovenous communications (absolute) and ventilation/perfusion mismatching (relative). Elevation of the diaphragm from ascites decreases lung volumes, particularly functional residual capacity, and predisposes to atelectasis. Moreover, large amounts of ascites produce a restrictive ventilatory defect that increases the work of breathing.

Review of the chest film and arterial blood gas measurements is very useful preoperatively because atelectasis and hypoxemia are often not evident on clinical examination. Paracentesis should be considered for patients with massive ascites and pulmonary compromise but should be done with caution because removal of too much fluid can lead to circulatory collapse.

E. RENAL MANIFESTATIONS AND FLUID BALANCE

Derangements of fluid and electrolyte balance are manifested as ascites, edema, electrolyte disturbances, or the hepatorenal syndrome. Important mechanisms thought to be responsible for ascites include (1) portal hypertension, which increases the hydrostatic pressure and favors transudation of fluid across the intestine into the peritoneal cavity; (2) hypoalbuminemia, which decreases plasma oncotic pressure and favors fluid transudation; (3) seepage of protein-rich lymphatic fluid from the serosal surface of the liver secondary to distortion and obstruction of lymphatic channels in the liver; and (4) avid renal sodium (and often water) retention (see below). Both "underfilling" and "overflow" theories have been proposed to explain the sodium retention. The "underfilling" theory states that although the measurable total extracellular fluid and plasma volumes are increased in cirrhotic patients with ascites, "effective plasma volume" is decreased: sodium retention is secondary to relative hypovolemia and secondary hyperaldosteronism. The apparent discrepancy between the measured and "effective" plasma volumes may be accounted for by an increase in splanchnic blood volume. In contrast, the "overflow" theory holds that the primary abnormality is sodium retention by the kidneys and that the ascites represents transudation secondary to an expanded plasma volume. Patients with ascites have elevated levels of circulating catecholamines, which are thought to be due to enhanced sympathetic outflow. In addition to increased renin and angiotensin II, patients demonstrate an insensitivity to circulating atrial natriuretic peptide.

Regardless of the mechanisms involved, patients with cirrhosis and ascites have decreased renal perfusion, altered intrarenal hemodynamics, enhanced proximal and distal sodium reabsorption, and often an impairment of free water clearance. Hyponatremia and hypokalemia are common. The former is dilutional, whereas the latter is due to excessive urinary potassium losses (from secondary hyperaldosteronism or diuretics). The most severe expression of these abnormalities is seen with development of the hepatorenal syndrome.

The hepatorenal syndrome is a functional renal defect in patients with cirrhosis that usually follows gastrointestinal bleeding, aggressive diuresis, sepsis, or major surgery. It is characterized by progressive oliguria with avid sodium retention, azotemia, intractable ascites, and a very high mortality rate. Treatment is supportive and often unsuccessful unless liver transplantation is undertaken.

Judicious perioperative fluid management in patients with advanced liver disease is critical. The importance of preserving renal function perioperatively cannot be overemphasized. Overzealous preoperative diuresis should be avoided, and acute intravascular fluid deficits should be corrected with colloid infusions. Diuresis of ascites and edema fluid should be accomplished over several days. Loop diuretics are administered only after measures such as bed rest, sodium restriction (< 2 g NaCl/d), and spironolactone therapy are deemed ineffective. Daily body weight measurements are useful in preventing intravascular volume depletion during diuresis. For patients with both ascites and peripheral edema, no more than 1 kg/d should be lost during diuresis; for those with ascites alone, no more than 0.5 kg/d should be lost. Hyponatremia (serum $[Na^+] < 130$ mEq/L) also requires water restriction (< 1.5 L/d) and potassium deficits should be replaced preoperatively. Prophylactic perioperative mannitol infusions may be effective in preventing renal failure, but this has not been conclusively demonstrated.

F. Central Nervous System Manifestations

Hepatic encephalopathy is characterized by alterations in mental status with fluctuating neurological signs (asterixis, hyperreflexia, or an inverted plantar reflex) and characteristic electroencephalographic changes (symmetric high-voltage, slow-wave activity). Some patients also have elevated intracranial pressure. Metabolic encephalopathy appears to be related to both the amount of hepatocellular damage present as well as the degree of shunting of portal blood away from the liver and directly into the systemic circulation. The accumulation of substances originating in the gastrointestinal tract but normally metabolized by the liver has been implicated. These proposed toxins include ammonia, methionine metabolites (mercaptans), short-chain fatty acids, and phenols. Other reported abnormalities include increased blood levels of aromatic amino acids, decreased blood levels of branched-chain amino acids, increased permeability of the blood–brain barrier, and abnormally high levels of γ-aminobutyric acid in the brain.

Factors known to precipitate hepatic encephalopathy include gastrointestinal bleeding, increased dietary protein intake, hypokalemic alkalosis

(from vomiting or diuresis), infections, and worsening liver function.

Encephalopathy should be aggressively treated preoperatively. Precipitating causes should be corrected. Oral lactulose 30–50 mL every 8 h or neomycin 500 mg every 6 h is useful in reducing intestinal ammonia absorption. Lactulose acts as an osmotic laxative and like neomycin likely inhibits ammonia production by intestinal bacteria. Avoidance of sedatives in patients with encephalopathy is recommended.

Intraoperative Considerations

Patients with postnecrotic cirrhosis due to hepatitis B or C who are carriers of the virus may be infectious. Extra caution is indicated in preventing contact with blood and body fluids from these patients.

A. Drug Responses

The response to anesthetic agents is unpredictable in patients with cirrhosis. Changes in central nervous system sensitivity, volumes of distribution, protein binding, drug metabolism, and drug elimination are common. An increase in the volume of distribution for highly ionized drugs, such as neuromuscular blocking agents (NMBAs), is due to the expanded extracellular fluid compartment; an apparent resistance may be observed, requiring larger than normal loading doses. However, smaller than normal maintenance doses of NMBAs dependent on hepatic elimination (pancuronium, rocuronium, and vecuronium) are needed. There may be a prolonged duration of action for succinylcholine as a result of reduced levels of pseudocholinesterase, but it is rarely of clinical consequence.

B. Anesthetic Technique

Because portal venous blood flow is reduced in cirrhosis, the liver becomes very dependent on hepatic arterial perfusion. Preservation of hepatic arterial blood flow and avoidance of agents with potentially adverse effects on hepatic function are critical. Regional anesthesia may be used in patients without thrombocytopenia or coagulopathy, but more care than normal must be directed to avoid hypotension. A barbiturate or propofol induction followed by isoflurane in oxygen or an oxygen–air mixture is most commonly employed for general anesthesia (see above). The use of halothane is generally avoided so as not to confuse the diagnosis if liver tests deteriorate postoperatively. Opioid supplementation reduces the dose of the volatile agent required, but the half-lives of opioids are often significantly prolonged, leading to prolonged respiratory depression. Cisatracurium may be the NMBA of choice because of its unique nonhepatic metabolism.

Preoperative nausea, vomiting, upper gastrointestinal bleeding, and abdominal distention due to massive ascites require a well-planned, methodical anesthetic induction. Preoxygenation and a rapid-sequence induction with cricoid pressure are most often performed. For unstable patients and those with active bleeding, either an awake intubation or a rapid-sequence induction with cricoid pressure using ketamine (or etomidate) and succinylcholine is best advised.

C. MONITORING

Close respiratory and cardiovascular monitoring is necessary for patients undergoing abdominal procedures. Five-lead electrocardiographic monitoring of patients receiving vasopressin infusions is necessary to detect myocardial ischemia from coronary vasoconstriction. Pulse oximetry should be supplemented with arterial blood gas measurements to evaluate acid–base status. Patients with large right-to-left intrapulmonary shunts may not tolerate the addition of nitrous oxide and may require positive end-expiratory pressure (PEEP) to treat ventilation/perfusion inequalities and subsequent hypoxemia.

Intraarterial pressure monitoring is generally indicated for most patients. Rapid changes in blood pressure occur as a result of excessive bleeding, rapid intercompartmental fluid shifts, and surgical manipulations. Intravascular volume status is often difficult to assess without central venous or pulmonary artery pressure monitoring. Such monitoring may be critical in preventing the hepatorenal syndrome. Urinary output must be followed closely; mannitol should be considered for persistently low urinary outputs in spite of adequate intravascular fluid replacement (see Chapter 31).

D. FLUID REPLACEMENT

Preoperatively, most patients are on sodium restriction, but intraoperatively preservation of intravascular volume and urinary output takes priority. The use of predominantly colloid intravenous fluids (albumin) may be preferable to avoid sodium overload and to increase oncotic pressure. Intravenous fluid replacement should take into account the excessive bleeding and fluid shifts that often occur in these patients during abdominal procedures. Venous engorgement from portal hypertension, lysis of adhesions from previous surgery, and coagulopathy lead to excessive bleeding during surgical procedures, whereas evacuation of ascites and prolonged surgical procedures result in large fluid shifts. Following the removal of large amounts of ascitic fluid, intravenous colloid fluid replacement is often necessary to prevent profound hypotension and renal shutdown.

Because most patients are anemic preoperatively and coagulopathic, red cell transfusions perioperatively are common. Significant transfusions may result in citrate toxicity. Citrate, the anticoagulant in stored red blood cell preparations, is normally readily metabolized by the liver. Toxicity occurs in patients with cirrhosis because metabolism is impaired. Citrate binds with serum calcium leading to the sequelae of hypocalcemia. Intravenous calcium is often necessary to reverse the negative inotropic effects of a decrease in the blood ionized calcium concentration.

■ HEPATOBILIARY DISEASE

Hepatobiliary disease is often characterized by cholestasis, the suppression or stoppage of bile flow. The most common cause of cholestasis is extrahepatic obstruction of the biliary tract (obstructive jaundice). The biliary obstruction may be due to a gallstone, stricture, or tumor in the common hepatic duct. Patients with complete or near-complete obstruction present with progressive jaundice, a dark urine with pale stools, and pruritus.

Obstructive jaundice must be differentiated from intrahepatic cholestasis. The latter is due to suppression or obstruction of bile flow at the level of the hepatocyte or bile canaliculus. Intrahepatic cholestasis most commonly results from viral hepatitis or an idiosyncratic drug reaction (most often reactions to phenothiazines or oral contraceptives). The treatment for extrahepatic obstruction is usually surgical, whereas that for intrahepatic cholestasis is medical. Although pruritus (due to retained bile salts) is a prominent feature of intrahepatic cholestasis, correct diagnosis may not be possible based on clinical or laboratory grounds. Both entities produce a predominantly conjugated (> 50%) hyperbilirubinemia and moderate to marked elevations of serum alkaline phosphatase. Imaging studies (ultrasound, cholangiograms, radioisotopic or computed tomographic [CT] scans) are necessary to confirm extrahepatic biliary obstruction.

Gallstone disease (cholelithiasis) limited to the gallbladder is often asymptomatic and may affect 10–20% of the general population. The diagnosis is usually made by abdominal ultrasound. Symptomatic individuals usually present with biliary colic secondary to obstruction of the cystic duct. The triad of sudden right upper quadrant tenderness, fever, and leukocytosis suggests cholecystitis. The diagnosis can be confirmed by failure of the gallbladder to visualize on a radioisotope scan. Passage of a gallstone through the common duct may also produce transient jaundice (above). Concomitant chills or high fever may indicate an ascending bacterial infection of the biliary system (cholangitis). Less commonly, the gallstone can obstruct the pancreatic duct and cause acute pancreatitis. Approximately 75% of episodes of acute cholecystitis resolve within 2–7 days following medical treatment. The remaining 25% have a course complicated by failure to resolve the episode, empyema, perforation, gangrene, hydrops, fistula formation, or gallstone ileus. Five to ten percent of patients with an acute attack have acalculous cholecystitis. The latter typically occurs following or in association with serious trauma, burns, prolonged labor, major surgery, or critical illness. The diagnosis is usually made by ultrasound or CT scan of the abdomen.

Preoperative Considerations

Patients most commonly present to the operating room for cholecystectomy, relief of extrahepatic biliary obstruction, or both. The most common procedure is a cholecystectomy, which is usually performed laparoscopically. Most patients with acute cholecystitis are stabilized medically prior to cholecystectomy. Medical treatment includes nasogastric suction, intravenous fluids, antibiotics, and opioid analgesics. Those in whom the acute attack resolves may defer surgery for a later time, whereas those suffering serious complications may require emergency cholecystectomy. Acalculous cholecystitis usually occurs in critically ill patients, and is associated with a high risk of gangrene and perforation; emergency operation is usually indicated in these patients.

Patients with extrahepatic biliary obstruction from whatever cause readily develop vitamin K deficiency. Vitamin K should be given parenterally but requires 24 h for a full response. Failure of the PT to correct prior to surgery may necessitate administration of FFP. High bilirubin levels may be associated with an increased risk of postoperative renal failure; generous preoperative hydration is advised. Long-standing extrahepatic obstruction (> 1 year) produces secondary biliary cirrhosis and portal hypertension (see above).

Intraoperative Considerations

Laparoscopic cholecystectomy accelerates the patient's recovery but the insufflation of carbon dioxide into the abdomen can complicate anesthetic management (see Case Discussion, Chapter 23). Because all opioids can cause spasm of the sphincter of Oddi to varying degrees, their use has been questioned when an intraoperative cholangiogram is contemplated. Opioid-induced sphincteric spasm may theoretically result in a false-positive intraoperative cholangiogram and needless exploration of the common bile duct. Although this point may have been overemphasized in the past, some clinicians withhold opioids until after the cholangiogram. If opioid-induced sphincter spasm is suspected, naloxone or glucagon can be given.

In patients with biliary tract obstruction, a prolonged duration of action of drugs primarily dependent on biliary excretion should be anticipated. Agents dependent on renal elimination are preferable. Urinary output should be monitored with an indwelling catheter. Maintenance of perioperative diuresis is desirable (see above).

Patients with acalculous cholecystitis and those with severe cholangitis are critically ill and have a high perioperative mortality rate. Invasive hemodynamic monitoring optimizes their anesthetic care.

◼ HEPATIC SURGERY

Common hepatic procedures include repair of lacerations, drainage of abscesses, and resections for tumors (primary or metastatic). Up to 80–85% of the liver can be resected in many patients. Liver transplantation is also performed in many centers. Hepatic surgery can be complicated by large amounts of blood loss. Cirrhosis greatly complicates anesthetic management and increases perioperative mortality. Multiple large-bore intravenous catheters and fluid (blood) warmers are necessary; rapid infusion devices facilitate management when massive blood transfusion is anticipated. Direct arterial and central venous pressure monitoring are also advisable. Some clinicians avoid hypotensive anesthesia because of its potentially deleterious effects on remaining liver tissue, whereas others believe that it can reduce blood loss when used judiciously. Administration of antifibrinolytics such as aprotinin, ε-aminocaproic acid, or tranexamic acid may reduce operative blood loss. Hypoglycemia may occur following large liver resections. Drainage of an abscess or cyst may be complicated by peritoneal contamination. In the case of a hydatid cyst, spillage can cause anaphylaxis due to release of *Echinococcus* antigens.

Postoperative complications include bleeding, sepsis, and hepatic dysfunction. Postoperative mechanical ventilation may be necessary in patients undergoing extensive resections.

CASE DISCUSSION:
LIVER TRANSPLANTATION

A 23-year-old woman develops fulminant hepatic failure after ingesting wild mushrooms. She is not expected to survive without a liver transplant.

What are the indications for liver transplantation?

Orthotopic liver transplantation is usually performed in patients with end-stage liver disease who begin to experience life-threatening compli-

cations. Moreover, the complications become unresponsive to medical or nontransplant surgery. Transplantation is also carried out in patients with fulminant hepatic failure (from viral hepatitis or a hepatotoxin) when survival with medical management alone is judged unlikely.

In order of decreasing frequency, the most common indications for liver transplantation in children are biliary atresia, inborn errors of metabolism (usually α_1-antitrypsin deficiency, Wilson's disease, tyrosinemia, and Crigler–Najjar type I syndrome), and postnecrotic cirrhosis.

The most common indications in adults are postnecrotic (nonalcoholic) cirrhosis, primary biliary cirrhosis, and sclerosing cholangitis, and, less commonly, primary malignant tumors in the liver. Considerable controversy exists over the justification for expenditure of scarce organs in transplanting patients with alcoholic cirrhosis, because of a general impression that a significant number of patients revert to habitual drinking afterward. Some studies, however, suggest the rate of recidivism is as low as 7% in patients who are able to abstain from alcohol for more than 6 months preoperatively.

What factors have contributed to the recent success of liver transplantation?

One-year survival rates for liver transplantations exceed 80–85% in some centers. Currently, 5-year survival rates are 50–60%. The success of this procedure owes much to the use of cyclosporine and tacrolimus (FK-506) for immunosuppressant therapy. The drug selectively suppresses the activities of helper T cells (CD4 lymphocytes) by inhibiting production of interleukin-2 (IL-2) and other cytokines. IL-2 is required for the generation and proliferation of cytotoxic T cells responsible for graft rejection and for activating B cells responsible for T cell-dependent humoral responses. Cyclosporine is usually initially combined with corticosteroids and other agents, eg, mycophenolate and azathioprine. The use of anti-OKT-3, a monoclonal antibody directed against lymphocytes, has been extremely useful in treating steroid-resistant acute rejection. Tacrolimus (FK-506) has proved effective in cyclosporine-resistant rejection and is the preferred alternative to cyclosporine as the primary immunosuppressant agent.

Additional factors may include greater understanding and experience with transplantation, the safe use of venovenous bypass, and the introduction of rapid infusion devices that allow transfusion of up to 2 L/min of warmed blood.

What major problems complicate anesthesia for liver transplantation?

Problems include the multisystem nature of cirrhosis, including the often massive blood loss throughout the procedure, the hemodynamic consequences of clamping and unclamping the inferior vena cava and portal vein, the metabolic consequences of the anhepatic phase, and the risks of air embolism and hyperkalemia when circulation to the new liver is fully established.

Preoperative coagulation defects, thrombocytopenia, and previous abdominal surgery greatly increase blood loss. Extensive venous collaterals between the portal and systemic venous circulations also probably contribute to increased bleeding from the abdominal wall. Hypothermia, coagulopathies, hyperkalemia, citrate intoxication, and the potential transmission of infectious agents complicate massive blood transfusion. Typical transfusion requirements consist of 15–30 U of red blood cells, 15–30 U of FFP, 15–25 U of platelets, and 10–20 U of cryoprecipitate. Blood salvaging techniques can be extremely useful in reducing donor red cell transfusions. Aprotinin or ε-aminocaproic acid infusion may significantly reduce blood loss.

What is adequate venous access for these procedures?

Bleeding is a recurring problem during each phase of liver transplantation. Adequate venous access is paramount in anesthetic management. Several large-bore (14-gauge or larger) intravenous catheters should be placed above the diaphragm. Specialized 8.5F catheters can be placed in antecubital veins and used in conjunction with rapid infusion devices. Catheters should generally not be placed in the arm to be used for venovenous bypass. All transfusion lines should pass through a warming device that heats fluids to normal body temperature to prevent hypothermia; additional measures such as a forced-air surface warming are also necessary. Total blood replacement can range between 1 and 35 blood volumes.

What monitoring techniques are most useful during surgery?

All patients require direct intraarterial pressure monitoring. A central venous or pulmonary artery catheter should be used to guide fluid replacement. The latter is preferred for most adult patients. Urinary output should be monitored *carefully throughout surgery via an indwelling urinary catheter.*

Laboratory measurements constitute an important part of intraoperative monitoring. Serial hematocrit measurements are mandatory to guide red blood cell replacement. Similarly, frequent measurements of arterial blood gases, serum electrolytes, serum ionized calcium, and serum glucose are necessary to detect and appropriately treat metabolic derangements. Coagulation can be monitored by measuring prothrombin time, activated partial thromboplastin time, and fibrinogen and by platelet counts, or by thromboelastography. The latter not only measures overall clotting and platelet function but can also detect fibrinolysis (below).

What anesthetic technique may be used for liver transplantation?

Premedication is usually administered unless the patient is in an advanced stage of hepatic encephalopathy. Intramuscular injections are avoided in patients with coagulopathy. Lorazepam 2–3 mg is preferred in adults, whereas diazepam 0.1–0.2 mg/kg can be used orally for children. Most patients should be considered as having a "full stomach" often because of marked abdominal distention or recent upper gastrointestinal bleeding. General anesthesia is usually induced via a rapid-sequence induction with cricoid pressure. The semiupright position during induction prevents rapid oxygen desaturation and facilitates ventilation until the abdomen is open. Thiopental, 3–5 mg/kg, ketamine, 1–2 mg/kg, or etomidate, 0.1–0.3 mg/kg, may be used. Succinylcholine, 1.5 mg/kg, is usually employed to facilitate rapid intubation. Hyperventilation should be avoided unless there is increased intracranial pressure. Anesthesia is usually maintained with a volatile agent, usually isoflurane, and an intravenous opioid, usually fentanyl or sufentanil. The concentration of the volatile agent should be limited to less than 1 minimum alveolar concentration in patients with severe encephalopathy. Nitrous oxide is usually avoided. The choice of a subsequent nondepolarizing neuromuscular blocking agent is generally at the discretion of the anesthesiologist. At the end of the procedure, many, but not all, patients are routinely transferred to the intensive care unit intubated and mechanically ventilated.

Why are these operations so lengthy?

These procedures usually require an average of 8 h of surgery (range 4–18 h), which can be di-

vided into three phases: a dissection phase, an anhepatic phase, and a revascularization phase.

1. Dissection (preanhepatic) phase: *Through a wide subcostal incision, the liver is dissected so that it remains attached only by the inferior vena cava, portal vein, hepatic artery, and common bile duct. Previous abdominal procedures greatly prolong the duration of and increase the blood loss associated with this phase.*

2. Anhepatic phase: *Once the liver is freed, the inferior vena cava is clamped above and below the liver, as are the hepatic artery, portal vein, and common bile duct. The liver is then completely excised. Venovenous bypass (see below) may or may not be employed during this phase. The donor liver is then anastomosed to the supra- and infrahepatic inferior venae cavae and the portal vein.*

3. Revascularization and biliary reconstruction (neohepatic or postanhepatic) phase: *Following completion of the venous anastomoses, venous clamps are removed and the circulation to the new liver is completed by anastomosing the hepatic artery. Lastly, the common bile duct of the donor liver is then usually connected to the recipient via a choledochocholedochostomy or Roux-en-Y choledochojejunostomy.*

How are the circulatory effects of venous clamping managed?

When the inferior vena cava and portal vein are clamped, marked decreases in cardiac output and hypotension are typically encountered. Moreover, the increase in distal venous pressure can markedly increase bleeding and impair renal perfusion and often promotes edema and ischemia of the intestines. Some patients (usually children) tolerate caval clamping because of extensive transdiaphragmatic collateral venous channels. For patients identified at increased risk with vena cava clamping, some surgeons use the technique of venovenous bypass in adults and in children weighing over 10 kg. This technique involves cannulating the inferior vena cava and the portal vein and diverting their blood flow (1–3 L/min) away from the liver and back to the heart, usually via an axillary vein. The pump and tubing are designed in such a way that heparinization of the patient is not necessary. Venovenous bypass can help minimize severe hypotension, intestinal edema, ischemia, the build-up of acid metabolites, and postoperative renal dysfunction. Prophylactic measures such as mannitol or low-dose dopamine (2–3 µg/kg/min) prior to and during venous clamping may be beneficial in preserving renal function but are unproved. Temporary inotropic support (in addition to blood and fluid replacement) is often required transiently until effective venovenous bypass is established. Technical considerations have prevented the routine use of venovenous bypass for small children. The use of venovenous bypass is not without risk; it increases operative time; can be associated with air embolism, thromboembolic complications, and brachial plexus injuries; and may contribute to hypothermia.

What physiological derangements are associated with the anhepatic phase?

When the liver is removed, the large citrate load from blood products is no longer metabolized and results in hypocalcemia and secondary myocardial depression (see Chapter 29). Periodic calcium chloride administration (200–500 mg) is necessary but should be guided by ionized calcium concentration measurements to avoid hypercalcemia. Electrocardiographic signs are unreliable for hypocalcemia but reliable for hyperkalemia (see Chapter 28). Progressive acidosis is also encountered because acid metabolites from the intestines (and lower body) are not cleared by the liver. Sodium bicarbonate therapy may be necessary and should similarly be guided by arterial blood gas analysis. Excessive NaHCO$_3$ administration results in hypernatremia, hyperosmolality, and accentuation of the metabolic alkalosis that typically follows massive blood transfusions. Tromethamine should be considered when large amounts of alkali therapy are necessary. Although hypoglycemia can occur during the anhepatic phase, hyperglycemia is a more common occurrence. The large amounts of transfused blood products given usually provide a large glucose load. Glucose-containing intravenous solutions are therefore not used unless hypoglycemia is documented.

Pulmonary and systemic (paradoxic) air embolism can occur when the circulation is fully reestablished to the donor liver because air often enters hepatic sinusoids after harvesting. Systemic air embolism probably reflects the fact that many of these patients have extensive arteriovenous communications. Venous air embolism can be detected as a sudden increase in end-expired nitrogen concentration. In addition, after completion of the portal and suprahepatic caval anastomoses but before completion of the infrahepatic caval anastomosis, the portal vein clamp is re-

leased; blood from the portal vein then "flushes out" any air remaining in the liver, which can now escape through the incomplete infrahepatic caval anastomotic site. Marked hypotension is often encountered during this period and requires inotropic support as well as intravenous fluid replacement. After "flushing," venous clamps are reapplied until the infrahepatic caval anastomosis is completed. The anhepatic phase ends when the three venous clamps are removed and the donor liver is perfused. Thromboembolic phenomena are also described following reperfusion.

What problems may be anticipated during the revascularization phase?

Perfusion of the donor liver by the recipient's blood often results in a transient increase in serum potassium concentration of up to 1–2 mEq/L and increased systemic acidosis. Acidosis accentuates the hyperkalemia (see Chapter 28). Reperfusion releases potassium from any remaining preservative solution (115–120 mEq/L of K$^+$) still within the liver as well as potassium released from tissues distal to venous clamps. Unclamping may also release a large acid load from ischemic tissue in the lower body (particularly without venovenous bypass); prophylactic administration of NaHCO$_3$ is advocated by some.

When the circulation to the new liver is established, the sudden increase in blood volume, acidosis, and hyperkalemia can produce either tachyarrhythmias or, more commonly, bradyarrhythmias. In addition to CaCl$_2$ and NaHCO$_3$, inotropic support is also often required. Hyperfibrinolysis is commonly present and appears to be due to a marked increase in tissue plasminogen activator and decrease in plasminogen activator inhibitor and α_2-antiplasmin during the anhepatic phase. Fibrinolysis can be detected by thromboelastography. ε-Aminocaproic acid or tranexamic acid, which inhibit the formation of plasmin, may be indicated in those instances (if not used prophylactically).

What problems are encountered postoperatively?

Patients often have an uncomplicated postoperative course, and after a sufficient period of observation in the postoperative care unit may be transferred directly to the nursing unit designed for liver transplant patients. Problems to be aware of include persistent hemorrhage, fluid overload, metabolic abnormalities (particularly metabolic alkalosis and hypokalemia), respiratory failure, pleural effusions, paralysis of the right hemidiaphragm (secondary to injury of the right phrenic nerve), renal failure, systemic infections, and surgical complications such as bile leaks or stricture, or thrombosis of the hepatic or portal vessels. The last two complications may be suspected during Doppler ultrasound and are confirmed by angiography. Neurological complications include seizures, intracranial hemorrhage, encephalopathy, central pontine myelinolysis, and immunosuppressant neurotoxicity. Renal dysfunction is often multifactorial in origin; contributory factors include periods of hypotension, impaired renal perfusion when the inferior vena cava is clamped (resulting in high pressures in the renal veins), and cyclosporine or antibiotic nephropathy. Measurement of immunosuppressant levels may be helpful in avoiding toxicity.

Prophylactic antibiotics and antifungal agents are routinely given in many centers because of a high incidence of infections. Prophylactic ganciclovir therapy may also be used in patients receiving anti-OKT3. Life-threatening infections include intraabdominal, pulmonary, wound, urinary tract, and catheter-related infections. Pulmonary infections involve common pathogens such as gram-negative bacteria as well as viruses (cytomegalovirus), fungi (Candida and Aspergillus), and parasites (Pneumocystis). Postoperative viral hepatitis may be due to cytomegalovirus, herpesvirus, Epstein–Barr virus, adenovirus (children), as well as hepatitis B and C viruses; de novo infection or viral reactivation may be responsible.

Rejection of the transplant is generally not a problem until 1–6 weeks after surgery. Graft function is usually monitored by the prothrombin time, serum bilirubin, aminotransferase activity, and lactate measurements. Diagnosis requires liver biopsy.

SUGGESTED READING

Cecil RL, Goldman L, Bennett JC: *Cecil Textbook of Medicine,* 21st ed. W.B. Saunders, 2000.

Sharpe MD, Gelb AW: *Anesthesia and Transplantation.* Butterworth-Heinemann, 1999.

Stoelting RK, Dierdorf SF: *Handbook for Anesthesia and Co-existing Disease,* 2nd ed. Churchill Livingstone, 2002.

Wiesner RH, Rakela J, Ishitani MB, et al: Recent advances in liver transplantation. Mayo Clin Proc 2003;78:197.

Anesthesia for Patients with Endocrine Disease

KEY CONCEPTS

 Diabetic autonomic neuropathy may limit the heart's ability to compensate for intravascular volume changes and may predispose patients to cardiovascular instability (eg, postinduction hypotension) and even sudden cardiac death.

 Diabetic patients should be routinely evaluated preoperatively for adequate temporomandibular joint and cervical spine mobility to help anticipate difficult intubations, which occur in approximately 30% of persons with type I diabetes.

 Sulfonylureas and metformin should not be used for 24–48 h before surgery because of their long half-lives. They can be started postoperatively when the patient is taking drugs per os. Metformin is restarted if renal and hepatic function remain adequate.

 Hyperthyroid patients can be chronically hypovolemic and vasodilated and are prone to an exaggerated hypotensive response during induction of anesthesia.

 Hypothyroid patients are more susceptible to the hypotensive effect of anesthetic agents because of their diminished cardiac output, blunted baroreceptor reflexes, and decreased intravascular volume.

 Patients with Cushing's syndrome tend to be volume overloaded and have hypokalemic metabolic alkalosis resulting from the mineralocorticoid activity of glucocorticoids.

 The key to the anesthetic management of patients with glucocorticoid deficiency is to ensure adequate steroid replacement therapy during the perioperative period.

 In patients with a pheochromocytoma anesthetic drugs or techniques that stimulate the sympathetic nervous system (eg, ephedrine, ketamine, hypoventilation), potentiate the arrhythmic effects of catecholamines (eg, halothane), inhibit the parasympathetic nervous system (eg, pancuronium), or release histamine (eg, atracurium, morphine sulfate) may precipitate hypertension and are best avoided.

 Particular attention should be paid to the airway in obese patients because they are often difficult to intubate as a result of limited mobility of the temporomandibular and atlantooccipital joints, a narrowed upper airway, and a shortened distance between the mandible and sternal fat pads.

 The key to anesthetic management of patients with carcinoid syndrome is to avoid anesthetic techniques or agents that could cause the tumor to release vasoactive substances.

The underproduction or overproduction of hormones can have dramatic physiological and pharmacological consequences. Therefore, it is not surprising that endocrinopathies affect anesthetic management. This chapter briefly reviews the normal physiology and discusses the dysfunction of four endocrine organs: the pancreas, the thyroid, the parathyroids, and the adrenal gland. It also considers obesity and carcinoid syndrome.

■ THE PANCREAS

Physiology

Adults normally secrete approximately 50 U of insulin each day from the β cells of the islets of Langerhans in the pancreas. The rate of insulin secretion is primarily determined by the plasma glucose level. Insulin, the most important anabolic hormone, has multiple metabolic effects, including increased glucose and potassium entry into adipose and muscle cells; increased glycogen, protein, and fatty acid synthesis; and decreased glycogenolysis, gluconeogenesis, ketogenesis, lipolysis, and protein catabolism.

In general, insulin stimulates anabolism, whereas lack of insulin is associated with catabolism and a negative nitrogen balance (Table 36–1).

Table 36–1. Endocrinologic effects of insulin.[1]

Effects on liver
  Anabolic
    Promotes glycogenesis
    Increases synthesis of triglycerides, cholesterol, and VLDL[2]
    Increases protein synthesis
    Promotes glycolysis
  Anticatabolic
    Inhibits glycogenolysis
    Inhibits ketogenesis
    Inhibits gluconeogenesis
Effects on muscle
  Promotes protein synthesis
    Increases amino acid transport
    Stimulates ribosomal protein synthesis
  Promotes glycogen synthesis
    Increases glucose transport
    Enhances activity of glycogen synthetase
    Inhibits activity of glycogen phosphorylase
Effects on fat
  Promotes triglyceride storage
    Induces lipoprotein lipase, making fatty acids available for absorption into fat cells
    Increases glucose transport into fat cells, thus increasing availability of α-glycerol phosphate for triglyceride synthesis
    Inhibits intracellular lipolysis

[1]Modified and reprinted, with permission, from Greenspan FS (editor): *Basic & Clinical Endocrinology*, 6th ed. McGraw-Hill, 2001.
[2]VLDL, very low-density lipoprotein.

Table 36–2. Diagnosis and classification of diabetes mellitus.

Diagnosis (based on blood glucose level)

Fasting	126 mg/dL (7.0 mmol/L)
Glucose tolerance test	200 mg/dL (11.1 mmol/L)

Classification

Type I	Absolute insulin deficiency secondary to immune-mediated or idiopathic
II	Adult onset secondary to resistance/relative deficiency
III	Specific types of diabetes mellitus secondary to genetic defects
IV	Gestational

DIABETES MELLITUS

Clinical Manifestations

Diabetes mellitus is characterized by impairment of carbohydrate metabolism caused by an absolute or relative deficiency of insulin or insulin responsiveness, which leads to hyperglycemia and glycosuria. The diagnosis is based on an elevated fasting plasma glucose (> 140 mg/dL) or blood glucose (126 mg/dL). Values are sometimes reported for blood glucose, which runs 12–15% lower than plasma glucose. Even when testing whole blood, newer glucose meters calculate and display plasma glucose. Diabetes has recently been reclassified to include four types (Table 36–2); type I (insulin-dependent) and type II (noninsulin-dependent) diabetes are the most common and well known. Diabetic ketoacidosis (DKA) is associated with type I diabetes mellitus, but there are individuals who present with DKA who phenotypically appear to have type II diabetes mellitus. Furthermore, individuals with an initial diagnosis of type II diabetes mellitus can later develop type I diabetes. Long-term complications of diabetes include hypertension, coronary artery disease, myocardial infarction, congestive heart failure, diastolic dysfunction, peripheral and cerebral vascular disease, peripheral and autonomic neuropathies, and renal failure. There are three life-threatening acute complications: DKA, hyperosmolar nonketotic coma, and hypoglycemia.

Decreased insulin activity allows the catabolism of free fatty acids into ketone bodies (acetoacetate and β-hydroxybutyrate), some of which are weak acids (see Chapter 30). Accumulation of these organic acids results in an anion-gap metabolic acidosis—DKA. DKA can easily be distinguished from lactic acidosis, with which it can coexist; lactic acidosis is identified by elevated plasma lactate (> 6 mmol/L) and the absence of urine and plasma ketones (although they can occur concurrently and starvation ketosis may occur with lactic acidosis). Alcoholic ketoacidosis can be differentiated by a history of recent heavy alcohol consumption (binge drinking) in a nondiabetic patient with a low or slightly elevated blood glucose level. Such patients may also have a disproportionate increase in β-hydroxybutyrate compared with acetoacetate.

Infection is the most common cause of DKA, which in some patients, particularly adolescents, is the first manifestation of type I diabetes mellitus. Clinical manifestations of DKA include tachypnea (attempting to compensate for the metabolic acidosis), abdominal pain mimicking an acute abdomen, nausea and vomiting, and changes in sensorium. The treatment of DKA depends on first correcting the often substantial hypovolemia, the hyperglycemia, and the total body potassium deficit, with a continuous infusion of isotonic fluids and potassium, and an insulin infusion.

The goal for decreasing blood glucose in ketoacidosis should be 75–100 mg/dL/h or 10%/h. Therapy can be begun with an intravenous infusion of 0.1 U/kg/h or the blood glucose value minus 60 times 0.1 U/h. These patients are often quite resistant to insulin therapy, and the rate may need to be increased if glucose levels do not decrease. As glucose moves intracellularly, so does potassium. Although this can quickly lead to a critical level of hypokalemia if not corrected, overaggressive replacement can cause an equally life-threatening hyperkalemia. Potassium, blood glucose, and serum ketones should be monitored no less often than every 2 h and preferably hourly.

Several liters of normal saline (1–2 L the first hour, followed by 200–500 mL/h) is typically required to correct the dehydration. Lactated Ringer's solution should be avoided as the liver eventually converts lactate to bicarbonate; because of potentially poor tissue perfusion, volume expansion with normal saline is safest. When plasma glucose reaches 250 mg/dL, an infusion of D_5W is added to the insulin infusion to decrease the possibility of hypoglycemia and to provide a continuous source of glucose and insulin for eventual normalization of intracellular metabolism. These patients may require a nasogastric tube for gastric decompression and bladder catheterization to monitor urinary output.

Correction of severe acidosis (pH < 7.1) with bicarbonate is seldom necessary, as the acidosis corrects with volume expansion and with normalization of the hyperglycemia.

Ketoacidosis is not a feature of **hyperosmolar nonketotic coma** possibly because enough insulin is available to prevent ketone body formation. Instead, a hyperglycemic diuresis results in dehydration and hyperosmolality. Severe dehydration eventually leads to renal failure, lactic acidosis, and a predisposition to form intravascular thromboses. Hyperosmolality, frequently exceeding 360 mOsm/L, alters cerebral water balance, causing changes in mental status and seizures. Severe hyperglycemia causes a factitious hyponatremia: each 100 mg/dL increase in plasma glucose lowers plasma sodium concentration by 1.6 mEq/L. Treatment includes fluid resuscitation with normal saline, relatively small doses of insulin, and potassium supplementation.

Hypoglycemia in the diabetic patient is the result of an excess of insulin relative to carbohydrate intake. Furthermore, some diabetic patients are unable to counter hypoglycemia by secreting glucagon or epinephrine (counterregulatory failure). The dependence of the brain on glucose as an energy source makes it the organ most susceptible to episodes of hypoglycemia. If hypoglycemia is not treated, mental status changes can progress from lightheadedness or confusion to convulsions and permanent coma. Systemic manifestations of hypoglycemia result from catecholamine discharge and include diaphoresis, tachycardia, and nervousness. Most of the signs and symptoms of hypoglycemia will be masked by general anesthesia. Although normal plasma glucose levels are ill-defined and depend on age and sex, hypoglycemia can generally be considered to be levels of less than 50 mg/dL. The treatment of hypoglycemia is the intravenous administration of 50% glucose (each milliliter of 50% glucose will raise the blood glucose of a 70-kg patient by approximately 2 mg/dL).

Anesthetic Considerations

A. PREOPERATIVE

Hemoglobin A_{1c} levels may help identify those patients who are at greatest risk of perioperative hyperglycemia and, therefore, increased complications and a worse outcome. The perioperative morbidity of diabetic patients is related to preoperative end-organ damage, although one-third to one-half of patients with type II diabetes mellitus may be unaware that they have it. The pulmonary, cardiovascular, and renal systems demand close examination. A preoperative chest radiograph in a diabetic patient is more likely to uncover cardiac enlargement, pulmonary vascular congestion, or pleural effusion. Diabetics also have an increased incidence of ST-segment and T-wave-segment abnormalities on preoperative electrocardiograms (ECGs). Myocardial ischemia may be evident on an ECG despite a negative history (silent myocardial ischemia and infarction). Diabetic patients with hypertension have a 50% likelihood of coexisting **diabetic autonomic neuropathy** (Table 36–3). Reflex dysfunction of the autonomic nervous system may be increased by old age, diabetes of longer than 10 years, coronary artery disease, or β-adrenergic blockade. Diabetic autonomic neuropathy may limit the heart's ability to compensate for intravascular volume changes and may predispose patients to cardiovascular instability (eg, postinduction hypotension) and even sudden cardiac death, the incidence of which may be increased by the concomitant

Table 36–3. Clinical signs of diabetic autonomic neuropathy.

Hypertension
Painless myocardial ischemia
Orthostatic hypotension
Lack of heart rate variability[1]
Reduced heart rate response to atropine and propranolol
Resting tachycardia
Early satiety
Neurogenic bladder
Lack of sweating
Impotence

[1]Normal heart rate variability during voluntary deep breathing (6 breaths/min) is greater than 10 beats/min.

use of angiotensin-converting enzyme inhibitors or angiotensin receptor blockers. Furthermore, autonomic dysfunction contributes to delayed gastric emptying (gastroparesis). Premedication with an antacid and metoclopramide would be particularly prudent in an obese diabetic patient with signs of cardiac autonomic dysfunction. However, autonomic dysfunction can affect the gastrointestinal tract without any signs of cardiac involvement.

Renal dysfunction is manifested first by proteinuria and later by elevated serum creatinine. By these criteria, most type I diabetic patients have evidence of renal failure by 30 years of age. Because of a high incidence of infections related to a compromised immune system, strict attention to aseptic technique must accompany the placement of all intravenous catheters and invasive monitors.

Chronic hyperglycemia can lead to glycosylation of tissue proteins and a limited-mobility joint syndrome. Diabetic patients should be routinely evaluated preoperatively for adequate temporomandibular joint and cervical spine mobility to help anticipate difficult intubations, which occur in approximately 30% of persons with type I diabetes.

B. Intraoperative

The primary goal of intraoperative blood sugar management is to avoid hypoglycemia. Although attempting to maintain euglycemia is imprudent, unacceptably loose blood sugar control (> 180 mg/dL) also carries risk. Hyperglycemia has been associated with hyperosmolarity, infection, and poor wound healing. More important, it may worsen neurological outcome following an episode of cerebral ischemia and compromise outcome following cardiac surgery or after an acute myocardial infarction. Unless hyperglycemia is treated aggressively in type I diabetic patients, metabolic control may be lost, particularly in association with major surgery or

sepsis. Tight control benefits patients undergoing cardiopulmonary bypass by improving cardiac contractility and weaning, and by decreasing infectious and neurological complications. Tight control of the pregnant diabetic patient has been shown to improve fetal outcome. Nonetheless, as noted earlier, the brain's dependence on glucose as an energy supply makes it essential that hypoglycemia be avoided.

There are several perioperative management regimens for diabetic patients. In the most common, the patient receives a fraction—usually half—of the total morning insulin dose in the form of intermediate-acting insulin (Table 36–4). To decrease the risk of hypoglycemia, insulin is administered *after* intravenous access has been established and the morning blood glucose level is checked. For example, a patient who normally takes 30 U of NPH (neutral protamine Hagedorn; intermediate-acting) insulin and 10 U of regular or Lispro (short-acting) insulin or insulin analogue each morning and whose blood sugar is at least 150 mg/dL would receive 15 U (half of 30, half the normal morning dose) of NPH subcutaneously or intramuscularly before surgery along with an infusion of 5% dextrose solution (1.5 mL/kg/h). Absorption of subcutaneous or intramuscular insulin depends on tissue blood flow, however, and can be unpredictable during surgery. Dedication of a small-gauge intravenous line for the dextrose infusion prevents interference with other intraoperative fluids and drugs. Supplemental dextrose can be administered if the patient becomes hypoglycemic (< 100 mg/dL). However, intraoperative hyperglycemia (> 150–180 mg/dL) is treated with intravenous regular insulin according to a sliding scale. One unit of regular insulin given to an adult usually lowers plasma glucose by 25–30 mg/dL. It must be stressed that these doses are approximations and do not apply to patients in catabolic states (eg, sepsis, hyperthermia).

Table 36–4. Two common techniques for perioperative insulin management in diabetes mellitus.

	Bolus Administration	Continuous Infusion
Preoperative	D_5W (1.5 mL/kg/h) NPH[1] insulin (half usual AM dose)	D_5W (1 mL/kg/h) Regular insulin: Units/h = $\dfrac{\text{Plasma glucose}}{150}$
Intraoperative	Regular insulin (as per sliding scale)	Same as preoperative
Postoperative	Same as intraoperative	Same as preoperative

[1]NPH, neutral protamine Hagedorn.

An alternative method is to administer regular insulin as a continuous infusion. The advantage of this technique is more precise control of insulin delivery than can be achieved with a subcutaneous or intramuscular injection of NPH insulin, particularly in conditions associated with poor skin and muscle perfusion. Two hundred and fifty units of regular insulin can be added to 250 mL of normal saline and the infusion begun at 0.1 U/kg/h. As blood sugar fluctuates, the regular insulin infusion can be adjusted according to the following formula:

$$\text{Units per hour} = \frac{\text{Plasma glucose (mg/dL)}}{150}$$

A general target for the intraoperative maintenance of blood glucose is 120–150 mg/dL, although some have an upper target of 120 mg/dL. The tighter control afforded by a continuous intravenous technique may be preferable in type I diabetics. Adding 20 mEq of KCl to each liter of fluid might be prudent, as insulin causes an intracellular potassium shift. The effect of insulin absorption by intravenous tubing can be minimized by flushing the line before beginning the infusion. Some anesthesiologists also suggest placing the insulin infusion in a glass bottle to minimize absorption by a plastic intravenous bag. Because individual insulin needs can vary dramatically, any formula should be considered only as a guideline.

If the patient is taking an oral hypoglycemic agent preoperatively instead of insulin, the drug can be continued until the day of surgery, but sulfonylureas and metformin should not be used for 24–48 h before surgery because of their long half-lives. They can be started postoperatively when the patient is taking drugs per os. Metformin is restarted if renal and hepatic function remain adequate. Because of the long duration of action, a glucose infusion is begun and blood sugars are monitored as though intermediate-acting insulin had been given. The effects of oral hypoglycemic drugs with a short duration of action can be prolonged in the presence of renal failure. Many of these patients may require some exogenous insulin during the intraoperative and postoperative periods. This is because the stress of surgery causes elevations in counterregulatory hormones (eg, catecholamines, glucocorticoids, growth hormone) and inflammatory mediators such as tumor necrosis factor and interleukins. Each of these contributes to stress hyperglycemia, which increases insulin requirements. Nonetheless, some type II diabetics will tolerate minor, brief surgical procedures without any exogenous insulin.

The key to any management regimen is to monitor plasma glucose levels frequently and appreciate the variation between patients. Patients with diabetes vary in their ability to produce endogenous insulin. Patients with brittle type I diabetes may need to have their glucose measured every hour, while every 2 or 3 h is sufficient for many patients with type II diabetes. Likewise, insulin requirements vary with the stress of the surgical procedure. Patients receiving insulin in the morning but not going to surgery until the afternoon are prone to hypoglycemia despite a dextrose infusion. Unless an arterial line is available, drawing multiple blood specimens and sending them to the laboratory is time consuming and expensive, and is traumatic to the patient's veins. Portable spectrophotometers are capable of determining the glucose concentration in a drop of blood obtained from a finger stick within a minute. These devices measure the color conversion of a glucose-oxidase-impregnated strip that has been exposed to the patient's blood for a specified period. Their accuracy depends, to a large extent, on the care with which the measurements are made. Monitoring urine sugar is not accurate enough for intraoperative management.

Patients who take NPH or protamine zinc insulin are at increased risk for allergic reactions to protamine sulfate—including anaphylactic shock and death. Unfortunately, operations that require the use of heparin and subsequent reversal with protamine (eg, cardiopulmonary bypass) are more common in diabetic patients. These patients should receive a small protamine test dose of 1–5 mg over 5–10 min prior to the full reversal dose.

C. POSTOPERATIVE

Close monitoring of the diabetic's blood sugar must continue postoperatively. One reason for this is the individual variation in onset and duration of action of insulin preparations (Table 36–5). For example, the onset of action of regular insulin may be less than 1 h, but its duration of action may exceed 6 h. NPH insulin typically has an onset of action within 2 h, but the action can last longer than 24 h. Another reason for close monitoring is the progression of stress hyperglycemia in the recovery period. If large volumes of lactate-containing intravenous fluids have been administered intraoperatively, blood sugar will tend to rise 24–48 h postoperatively as the liver converts the lactate to glucose. Diabetic outpatients may require admission to the hospital overnight if persistent nausea and vomiting from gastroparesis prevent oral intake.

■ THE THYROID

Physiology

Dietary iodine is absorbed by the gastrointestinal tract, converted to iodide ion, and actively transported into the

Table 36–5. Summary of bioavailability characteristics of the insulins.[1]

	Insulin Type[2]	Onset	Peak Action	Duration
Short-acting	Lispro	10–20 min	30–90 min	4–6 h
	Regular, Actrapid, Velosulin	15–30 min	1–3 h	5–7 h
	Semilente, Semitard	30–60 min	4–6 h	12–16 h
Intermediate-acting	Lente, Lentard, Monotard, NPH, Insulatard	2–4 h	8–10 h	18–24 h
Long-acting	Ultralente, Ultratard, PZI	4–5 h	8–14 h	25–36 h

[1]There is considerable patient-to-patient variation.
[2]NPH, neutral protamine Hagedorn; PZI, protamine zinc insulin.

thyroid gland. Once inside, iodide is oxidized back to iodine, which is bound to the amino acid tyrosine. The end result is two hormones—triiodothyronine (T_3) and thyroxine (T_4)—which are bound to proteins and stored within the thyroid. Although the gland releases more T_4 than T_3, the latter is more potent and less protein bound. Most T_3 is formed peripherally from partial deiodination of T_4. An elaborate feedback mechanism controls thyroid hormone synthesis and involves the hypothalamus (thyrotropin-releasing hormone), the anterior pituitary (thyroid-stimulating hormone, or TSH), and autoregulation (thyroid iodine concentration).

Thyroid hormone increases carbohydrate and fat metabolism and is an important factor in determining growth and metabolic rate. An increase in metabolic rate is accompanied by an increase in oxygen consumption and CO_2 production, indirectly increasing minute ventilation. Heart rate and contractility are also increased, presumably from an alteration in adrenergic-receptor physiology and other internal protein alterations, as opposed to an increase in catecholamine levels.

HYPERTHYROIDISM

Clinical Manifestations

Excess thyroid hormone levels can be caused by Graves' disease, toxic multinodular goiter, thyroiditis, thyroid-stimulating-hormone-secreting pituitary tumors, functioning thyroid adenomas, or overdosage (accidental or intentional) of thyroid replacement hormone. Clinical manifestations of excess thyroid hormones include weight loss, heat intolerance, muscle weakness, diarrhea, hyperactive reflexes, and nervousness. A fine tremor, exophthalmos, or goiter may be noted, particularly when the cause is Graves' disease. Cardiac signs range from sinus tachycardia to atrial fibrillation and congestive heart failure. The diagnosis of hyperthyroidism is confirmed by abnormal thyroid function tests, which may include an elevation in total (bound and unbound) serum T_4, serum T_3, and free (unbound) T_4.

Medical treatment of hyperthyroidism relies on drugs that inhibit hormone synthesis (eg, propylthiouracil, methimazole), prevent hormone release (eg, potassium, sodium iodide), or mask the signs of adrenergic overactivity (eg, propranolol). Although β-adrenergic antagonists do not affect thyroid gland function, they do decrease the peripheral conversion of T_4 to T_3. Radioactive iodine destroys thyroid cell function but is not recommended for pregnant patients and may result in hypothyroidism. Subtotal thyroidectomy is now less commonly used as an alternative to medical therapy. Typically, it is reserved for patients with large toxic multinodular goiters or solitary toxic adenomas. Graves' disease is currently usually treated with thyroid drugs or radioiodine.

Anesthetic Considerations

A. PREOPERATIVE

All elective surgical procedures, including subtotal thyroidectomy, should be postponed until the patient is rendered clinically and chemically euthyroid with medical treatment. The days of a "thyroid steal" induction with covertly administered medications are past. Preoperative assessment should include normal thyroid function tests, and a resting heart rate less than 85 beats/min has been recommended. Benzodiazepines are a good choice for preoperative sedation. Antithyroid medications and β-adrenergic antagonists are continued through the morning of surgery. Administration of propylthiouracil and methimazole is particularly important because of their relatively sort half-lives. If emergency surgery must proceed, the hyperdynamic circulation can be controlled by titration of an esmolol infusion.

B. INTRAOPERATIVE

Cardiovascular function and body temperature should be closely monitored in patients with a history of hyperthyroidism. Patients' eyes should be well protected, as the exophthalmos of Graves' disease increases the risk of corneal abrasion or ulceration. The head of the operating table can be raised 15–20° to aid venous drainage and decrease blood loss, although doing so increases the risk of venous air embolism.

Ketamine, pancuronium, indirect-acting adrenergic agonists, and other drugs that stimulate the sympathetic nervous system are best avoided because of the possibility of exaggerated elevations in blood pressure and heart rate. Thiopental may be the induction agent of choice as it possesses some antithyroid activity at high doses. Hyperthyroid patients can be chronically hypovolemic and vasodilated and are prone to an exaggerated hypotensive response during induction of anesthesia. Adequate anesthetic depth must be obtained, however, before laryngoscopy or surgical stimulation to avoid tachycardia, hypertension, and ventricular arrhythmias.

Neuromuscular blocking agents (NMBAs) should be administered cautiously, because thyrotoxicosis is associated with an increased incidence of myopathies and myasthenia gravis. Hyperthyroidism does not increase anesthetic requirements—ie, there is no change in minimum alveolar concentration.

C. POSTOPERATIVE

The most serious threat to hyperthyroid patients in the postoperative period is **thyroid storm,** which is characterized by hyperpyrexia, tachycardia, altered consciousness (eg, agitation, delirium, coma), and hypotension. The onset is usually 6–24 h after surgery but can occur intraoperatively, mimicking malignant hyperthermia. Unlike malignant hyperthermia, however, thyroid storm is not associated with muscle rigidity, elevated creatine kinase, or a marked degree of metabolic (lactic) and respiratory acidosis. Treatment includes hydration and cooling, an esmolol infusion or intravenous propranolol (0.5-mg increments until the heart rate is < 100/min), propylthiouracil (250–500 mg every 6 h orally or by nasogastric tube) followed by sodium iodide (1 g intravenously over 12 h), and correction of any precipitating cause (eg, infection). Cortisol (100–200 mg every 8 h) is recommended to prevent complications from coexisting adrenal gland suppression. Thyroid storm is a medical emergency that requires aggressive management and monitoring (see Case Discussion, Chapter 48).

Subtotal thyroidectomy is associated with several potential surgical complications. Recurrent laryngeal nerve palsy will result in hoarseness (unilateral) or aphonia and stridor (bilateral). Vocal cord function can be evaluated by laryngoscopy immediately following deep extubation, however, this is rarely necessary. Failure of one or both cords to move may require intubation and exploration of the wound. Hematoma formation may cause airway compromise from collapse of the trachea in patients with tracheomalacia. Dissection into the compressible soft tissues of the neck may make intubation difficult. Immediate treatment includes opening the neck wound and evacuating the clot, then reassessing the need for reintubation.

Hypoparathyroidism from unintentional removal of the parathyroid glands will cause acute hypocalcemia within 12–72 h (see the section on Clinical Manifestations under Hypoparathyroidism, below). Unintentional pneumothorax is a possible complication of neck exploration.

HYPOTHYROIDISM

Clinical Manifestations

Hypothyroidism can be caused by autoimmune disease (eg, Hashimoto's thyroiditis), thyroidectomy, radioactive iodine, antithyroid medications, iodine deficiency, or failure of the hypothalamic–pituitary axis (secondary hypothyroidism). Hypothyroidism during neonatal development results in cretinism, a condition marked by physical and mental retardation. Clinical manifestations in the adult are usually subtle and include weight gain, cold intolerance, muscle fatigue, lethargy, constipation, hypoactive reflexes, dull facial expression, and depression. Subclinical hypothyroidism commonly occurs in elderly patients with severe illnesses. Heart rate, myocardial contractility, stroke volume, and cardiac output decrease, and extremities are cool and mottled because of peripheral vasoconstriction. Pleural, abdominal, and pericardial effusions are common. The diagnosis of hypothyroidism may be confirmed by a low free T_4 level. Primary hypothyroidism is differentiated from secondary disease by an elevation in TSH. The treatment of hypothyroidism consists of oral replacement therapy with a thyroid hormone preparation, which takes several days to produce a physiological effect and several weeks to evoke clear-cut clinical improvement.

Myxedema coma results from extreme hypothyroidism and is characterized by impaired mentation, hypoventilation, hypothermia, hyponatremia (from inappropriate antidiuretic hormone secretion), and congestive heart failure. It is more common in elderly patients and may be precipitated by infection, surgery, or trauma. Myxedema coma is a life-threatening disease that has been successfully treated with intravenous thyroid hormones. A loading dose of T_3 or T_4 (eg, 300–500 mg of levothyroxine sodium in patients without heart disease) is followed by a maintenance infusion (eg, 50 mg of levothyroxine per day). The ECG must be monitored during therapy to detect myocardial ischemia or arrhythmias. Steroid replacement (eg, hydrocortisone, 100 mg intravenously every 8 h) is routinely given in case of coexisting adrenal gland suppression. Some patients may require ventilatory support and external warming.

Anesthetic Considerations

A. PREOPERATIVE

Patients with uncorrected severe hypothyroidism (T_4 < 1 mg/dL) or myxedema coma should not undergo elective surgery and should be treated with thyroid hormone prior to emergency surgery. Although a euthyroid state is ideal, mild to moderate hypothyroidism does not appear to be an absolute contraindication to surgery. In fact, hypothyroid patients with symptomatic coronary artery disease may benefit from a delay in thyroid therapy until after coronary artery bypass surgery.

Hypothyroid patients usually do not require much preoperative sedation and are very prone to drug-induced respiratory depression. In addition, they fail to respond to hypoxia with increased minute ventilation. Consideration should be given to premedicating these patients with histamine H_2 antagonists and metoclopramide because of their decreased gastric-emptying times. Patients who have been rendered euthyroid may receive their usual dose of thyroid medication on the morning of surgery; it must be remembered, however, that most commonly used preparations have long half-lives (the $t_{1/2}$ of T_4 is about 8 days).

B. INTRAOPERATIVE

Hypothyroid patients are more susceptible to the hypotensive effect of anesthetic agents because of their diminished cardiac output, blunted baroreceptor reflexes, and decreased intravascular volume. For this reason, ketamine is often recommended for induction of anesthesia. The possibility of coexistent primary adrenal insufficiency or congestive heart failure should be considered in cases of refractory hypotension. Decreased cardiac output may speed the rate of induction with an inhalation anesthetic, but hypothyroidism does not significantly decrease minimum alveolar concentration. **Other potential problems include hypoglycemia, anemia, hyponatremia, difficulty during intubation because of a large tongue, and hypothermia from a low basal metabolic rate.**

C. POSTOPERATIVE

Recovery from general anesthesia may be delayed in hypothyroid patients by hypothermia, respiratory depression, or slowed drug biotransformation. These patients often require prolonged mechanical ventilation. Patients should remain intubated until awake and normothermic. Because hypothyroidism increases vulnerability to respiratory depression, a nonopioid such as ketorolac would be a good choice for relief of postoperative pain.

■ THE PARATHYROID GLANDS

Physiology

Parathyroid hormone is the principal regulator of calcium homeostasis. It increases serum calcium by promoting bone resorption, limiting renal excretion, and indirectly enhancing gastrointestinal absorption by its effect on vitamin D metabolism. Parathyroid hormone decreases serum phosphate by increasing renal excretion. The effects of parathyroid hormone on calcium serum levels are countered in lower animals by calcitonin, a hormone excreted by parafollicular C-cells in the thyroid, but a physiological calcium-lowering effect for calcitonin has not been demonstrated in humans (Table 36–6). Of total body calcium, 99% is in the skeleton. Of the calcium in the blood, 40% is bound to proteins and 60% is ionized or complexed to organic ions. Unbound ionized calcium is physiologically the more important of the two.

HYPERPARATHYROIDISM

Clinical Manifestations

Causes of primary hyperparathyroidism include adenoma, carcinoma, and hyperplasia of the parathyroid gland. Secondary hyperparathyroidism is an adaptive response to hypocalcemia produced by diseases such as renal failure or intestinal malabsorption syndromes. Ectopic hyperparathyroidism is due to production of parathyroid hormone by rare tumors outside the parathyroid gland. Parathyroid hormone-related peptide may cause significant hypercalcemia when secreted by a carcinoma (eg, hepatoma, bronchogenic carcinoma) and is the most common cause of hypercalcemia of malignancy.

Most of the clinical manifestations of hyperparathyroidism are due to hypercalcemia (Table 36–7). Causes of hypercalcemia (other than hyperparathyroidism) include bone metastases, vitamin D intoxication, milk-alkali syndrome, sarcoidosis, and prolonged immobilization. The treatment of hyperparathyroidism depends on the cause, but surgical removal of all four glands is usually required in the setting of parathyroid hyperplasia. However, removal of a single adenoma cures many patients with sporadic primary hyperparathyroidism.

Anesthetic Considerations

Preoperative evaluation should include an assessment of volume status to avoid hypotension during induction. Hydration with normal saline and diuresis with furo-

Table 36–6. Actions of major calcium-regulating hormones.[1]

	Bone	Kidney	Intestines
Parathyroid hormone	Increases resorption of calcium and phosphate	Increases reabsorption of calcium; decreases reabsorption of phosphate; increases conversion of 25-OHD$_3$ to 1,25 (OH)$_2$ D$_3$;[2] decreases reabsorption of bicarbonate	No direct effects
Calcitonin	Decreases resorption of calcium and phosphate	Decreases reabsorption of calcium and phosphate; questionable effect on vitamin D metabolism	No direct effects
Vitamin D	Maintains Ca^{2+} transport system	Decreases reabsorption of calcium	Increases absorption of calcium and phosphate

[1]Reproduced, with permission, from Greenspan FS (editor): *Basic & Clinical Endocrinology*, 6th ed. McGraw-Hill, 2001.
[2]25-OHD$_3$, 25-hydroxyvitamin D$_3$; 1,25 (OH)$_2$D$_3$, 1,25-dihydroxyvitamin D$_3$.

semide usually decrease serum calcium to acceptable levels (< 14 mg/dL, 7 mEq/L, or 3.5 mmol/L). Rarely, more aggressive therapy with the intravenous bisphosphonates pamidronate (Aredia) or etidronate (Didronel) may be necessary. Plicamycin (Mithramycin), glucocorticoids, calcitonin, or dialysis may be necessary when intravenous bisphosphonates are not sufficient or are contraindicated. Hypoventilation should be avoided, as acidosis increases ionized calcium. Elevated calcium levels can cause cardiac arrhythmias. The response to NMBAs may be altered in patients with preexisting muscle weakness caused by the effects of calcium at the neuromuscular junction. Osteoporosis worsened by hyperparathyroidism predisposes patients to vertebral compression during laryngos-

copy and bone fractures during transport. The postoperative complications of parathyroidectomy are similar to those described above for subtotal thyroidectomy.

HYPOPARATHYROIDISM

Clinical Manifestations

Hypoparathyroidism is usually due to deficiency of parathyroid hormone following parathyroidectomy. Clinical manifestations of hypoparathyroidism are a result of hypocalcemia (Table 36–8), which is also caused by renal failure, hypomagnesemia, vitamin D deficiency, and acute pancreatitis (see Chapter 28). Hypoalbuminemia decreases total serum calcium (a 1 g/dL drop in serum albumin causes a 0.8 mg/dL decrease in total serum calcium), but ionized calcium, the active entity, is unaltered. Neuromuscular irritability can be clinically confirmed by the presence of Chvostek's sign (painful twitching of the facial musculature following tapping

Table 36–7. Effects of hyperparathyroidism.

Organ System	Clinical Manifestations
Cardiovascular	Hypertension, ventricular arrythmias, ECG[1] changes (shortened QT interval)[2]
Renal	Impaired renal concentrating ability, hyperchloremic metabolic acidosis, polyuria, dehydration, polydipsia, renal stones, renal failure
Gastrointestinal	Ileus, nausea and vomiting, peptic ulcer disease, pancreatitis
Musculoskeletal	Muscle weakness, osteoporosis
Neurologic	Mental status change (eg, delirium, psychosis, coma)

[1]ECG, electrocardiogram.
[2]The QT interval may be prolonged at serum calcium levels > 16 mg/dL.

Table 36–8. Effects of hypoparathyroidism.

Organ System	Clinical Manifestations
Cardiovascular	Hypotension, congestive heart failure, ECG[1] changes (prolonged QT interval)
Musculoskeletal	Muscle cramps, weakness
Neurologic	Neuromuscular irritability (eg, laryngospasm, inspiratory stridor, tetany, seizures), perioral paresthesia, mental status changes (eg, dementia, depression, psychosis)

[1]ECG, electrocardiogram.

over the facial nerve) or Trousseau's sign (carpopedal spasm following inflation of a tourniquet above systolic blood pressure for 3 min). These signs are also occasionally present in nonhypocalcemic persons. Treatment of symptomatic hypocalcemia consists of intravenous administration of calcium chloride.

Anesthetic Considerations

Serum calcium should be normalized in any patient with cardiac manifestations of hypocalcemia. Anesthetics that depress the myocardium should be avoided in these patients. Alkalosis from hyperventilation or sodium bicarbonate therapy will further decrease ionized calcium. Although citrate-containing blood products do not usually lower serum calcium significantly, they should not be administered rapidly in patients with preexisting hypocalcemia. Other considerations include avoiding the use of 5% albumin solutions (which might bind and lower ionized calcium) and exploring the possibility of coagulopathy or a sensitivity to nondepolarizing NMBAs.

■ THE ADRENAL GLAND

Physiology

The adrenal gland is divided into two parts. The adrenal cortex secretes androgens, mineralocorticoids (eg, aldosterone), and glucocorticoids (eg, cortisol). The adrenal medulla secretes catecholamines (eg, epinephrine, norepinephrine, dopamine). The adrenal androgens have insignificant relevance for anesthetic management and will not be considered further.

Aldosterone is primarily involved with fluid and electrolyte balance. Aldosterone secretion causes sodium to be reabsorbed in the distal renal tubule in exchange for potassium and hydrogen ions. The net effect is an expansion in extracellular fluid volume caused by fluid retention, a decrease in plasma potassium, and metabolic alkalosis. Aldosterone secretion is stimulated by the renin–angiotensin system (specifically, angiotensin II), pituitary adrenocorticotropic hormone (ACTH), and hyperkalemia. Hypovolemia, hypotension, congestive heart failure, and surgery result in an elevation of aldosterone concentrations.

Glucocorticoids are essential for life and have multiple physiological effects. Metabolic actions include enhanced gluconeogenesis and inhibition of peripheral glucose utilization. These antiinsulin effects tend to raise blood glucose and worsen diabetic control. Glucocorticoids are required for vascular and bronchial smooth muscle to be responsive to catecholamines. Because these hormones are structurally related to aldosterone, they tend to promote sodium retention and potassium excretion (a mineralocorticoid effect). ACTH from the anterior pituitary is the principal regulator of glucocorticoid secretion. Secretion of ACTH and glucocorticoids exhibits a diurnal rhythm, is stimulated by stress, and is inhibited by circulating glucocorticoids. Endogenous production of cortisol, the most important glucocorticoid, averages 20 mg/d.

The structure, biosynthesis, physiological effects, and metabolism of catecholamines are discussed in Chapter 12. Eighty percent of adrenal catecholamine secretion in humans is in the form of epinephrine. Catecholamine release is regulated mainly by cholinergic preganglionic fibers of the sympathetic nervous system that innervate the adrenal medulla. Stimuli include hypotension, hypothermia, hypoglycemia, hypercapnia, hypoxemia, pain, and fear.

MINERALOCORTICOID EXCESS

Clinical Manifestations

Intrinsic hypersecretion of aldosterone by the adrenal cortex (primary aldosteronism and patients with Conn's syndrome) can be due to a unilateral adenoma (aldosteronoma), bilateral hyperplasia, or carcinoma of the adrenal gland. Some diseases stimulate aldosterone secretion by affecting the renin–angiotensin system. For example, congestive heart failure, hepatic cirrhosis with ascites, nephrotic syndrome, and some forms of hypertension (eg, renal artery stenosis) can cause secondary aldosteronism. Although both primary and secondary aldosteronism are characterized by increased levels of aldosterone, only the latter is associated with increased renin activity. Clinical manifestations of mineralocorticoid excess include an elevation in blood pressure, hypervolemia, hypokalemia, muscle weakness, and metabolic alkalosis. Prolonged hypokalemia may lead to a renal concentrating defect and polyuria. Alkalosis will lower ionized calcium levels and can cause tetany. Serum sodium is often normal.

Anesthetic Considerations

Fluid and electrolyte disturbances can be corrected preoperatively with supplemental potassium and spironolactone. This aldosterone antagonist is a potassium-sparing diuretic with antihypertensive properties. Intravascular volume can be assessed preoperatively by testing for orthostatic hypotension or measuring cardiac filling pressures. Correction of plasma potassium, however, does not guarantee normal total body potassium.

MINERALOCORTICOID DEFICIENCY

Clinical Manifestations & Anesthetic Considerations

Atrophy or destruction of both adrenal glands results in a combined deficiency of mineralocorticoids and glucocorticoids (see the section on Glucocorticoid Deficiency, below). Nonetheless, unilateral adrenalectomy, diabetes, or heparin therapy occasionally causes isolated hypoaldosteronism. These patients are hyperkalemic, acidotic, and usually hypotensive (the opposite of mineralocorticoid excess). Preoperative preparation includes treatment with an exogenously administered mineralocorticoid (eg, fludrocortisone).

GLUCOCORTICOID EXCESS

Clinical Manifestations

Glucocorticoid excess may be due to exogenous administration of steroid hormones, intrinsic hyperfunction of the adrenal cortex (eg, adrenocortical adenoma), ACTH production by a nonpituitary tumor (ectopic ACTH syndrome), or hypersecretion by a pituitary adenoma (Cushing's disease). Regardless of the cause, an excess of corticosteroids produces Cushing's syndrome, characterized by muscle wasting and weakness, osteoporosis, central obesity, abdominal striae, glucose intolerance, hypertension, and mental status changes.

Anesthetic Considerations

Patients with Cushing's syndrome tend to be volume overloaded and have hypokalemic metabolic alkalosis resulting from the mineralocorticoid activity of glucocorticoids. These abnormalities should be corrected preoperatively with supplemental potassium and spironolactone. Patients with osteoporosis are at risk for fracture during positioning, whereas preoperative weakness may indicate an increased sensitivity to NMBAs. If the cause of Cushing's syndrome is exogenous glucocorticoids, the patient's adrenal glands may not be able to respond to perioperative stresses, and supplemental steroids are indicated (see the section on Glucocorticoid Deficiency, below). Likewise, patients undergoing adrenalectomy require intraoperative glucocorticoid replacement (intravenous hydrocortisone succinate, 100 mg every 8 h). Other complications of adrenalectomy include significant blood loss during resection of a highly vascularized tumor and unintentional penetration of the pleura, causing pneumothorax.

GLUCOCORTICOID DEFICIENCY

Clinical Manifestations

Primary adrenal insufficiency (Addison's disease) is caused by destruction of the adrenal gland, which results in a combined mineralocorticoid and glucocorticoid deficiency. Clinical manifestations are due to aldosterone deficiency (hyponatremia, hypovolemia, hypotension, hyperkalemia, and metabolic acidosis) and cortisol deficiency (weakness, fatigue, hypoglycemia, hypotension, and weight loss). Etomidate suppresses adrenal function by inhibiting enzymes that are essential for the production of corticosteroid hormones (see Chapter 8); long-term etomidate therapy can lead to significant glucocorticoid deficiency.

Secondary adrenal insufficiency is a result of inadequate ACTH secretion by the pituitary. The most common cause of secondary adrenal insufficiency is iatrogenic, the result of the administration of exogenous glucocorticoids. Because mineralocorticoid secretion is usually adequate in this disease, fluid and electrolyte disturbances are usually not present. Acute adrenal insufficiency (addisonian crisis), however, can be triggered in steroid-dependent patients who do not receive increased doses during periods of stress (eg, infection, trauma, surgery). The clinical features of this medical emergency include circulatory collapse, fever, hypoglycemia, and depressed mentation.

Anesthetic Considerations

The key to the anesthetic management of patients with glucocorticoid deficiency is to ensure adequate steroid replacement therapy during the perioperative period. Because the risk of supplementation is probably low, all patients who have received potentially suppressive doses of steroids (eg, the daily equivalent of 5 mg of prednisone) by any route of administration (topical, inhalational, or oral) for a period of more than 2 weeks any time in the previous 12 months may be unable to respond appropriately to surgical stress.

What represents adequate steroid coverage is controversial. Although adults normally secrete 20 mg of cortisol daily, this may increase to over 300 mg under conditions of maximal stress. Thus, one recommendation is to administer 100 mg of hydrocortisone phosphate every 8 h beginning the evening before or on the morning of surgery. An alternative low-dose regimen (25 mg of hydrocortisone at the time of induction followed by an infusion of 100 mg during the subsequent 24 h) achieves plasma cortisol levels equal to or higher than those reported in healthy patients undergoing similar elective surgery. This second regimen might be particularly appropriate for diabetic patients, in whom glucocorticoid administration often interferes with control of blood glucose.

CATECHOLAMINE EXCESS

Clinical Manifestations

Pheochromocytoma is a catecholamine-secreting tumor that consists of cells originating from the embryonic neural crest (epinephrine tissue) and accounts for 0.1% of all cases of hypertension. Although the tumor is usually benign and localized in a single adrenal gland, 10–15% are malignant, and another 10–15% are bilateral or extraadrenal. The cardinal manifestations of pheochromocytoma are paroxysmal headache, hypertension, sweating, and palpitations. Unexpected intraoperative hypertension and tachycardia are occasionally the first indications of an undiagnosed pheochromocytoma. The pathophysiology, diagnosis, and treatment of these tumors require an understanding of catecholamine metabolism and of the pharmacology of adrenergic agonists and antagonists. The Case Discussion in Chapter 12 examines these aspects of pheochromocytoma management.

Anesthetic Considerations

Preoperative assessment should focus on the adequacy of adrenergic blockade and volume replacement. Specifically, resting arterial blood pressure, orthostatic blood pressure and heart rate, ventricular ectopy, and electrocardiographic evidence of ischemia should be evaluated.

A decrease in red cell mass and plasma volume contributes to the severe chronic hypovolemia seen in these patients. Although the hematocrit is usually elevated or normal, depending on the relative contribution of these two factors, it does not reliably reflect volume status. Preoperative α-adrenergic blockade with phenoxybenzamine helps correct the volume deficit, in addition to correcting hypertension and hyperglycemia. A drop in hematocrit should accompany the expansion of circulatory volume; this often unmasks an underlying anemia.

Potentially life-threatening variations in blood pressure—particularly during induction and manipulation of the tumor—indicate the need for direct arterial pressure monitoring. Large intraoperative fluid-volume shifts underscore the importance of good intravenous access and urinary output monitoring. Young patients with healthy hearts probably need only central venous pressure monitoring, although patients with evidence of catecholamine cardiomyopathy may benefit from the use of a pulmonary artery catheter.

Intubation should not be attempted until a deep level of anesthesia has been established. Intraoperative hypertension can be effectively treated with phentolamine, nitroprusside, or nicardipine. Nitroprusside is favored by some anesthesiologists because of a more rapid onset of action, a shorter duration of action, and increased familiarity with the drug. Phentolamine specifically blocks adrenergic receptors and prevents the effects of excessive circulating catecholamines. Nicardipine is being used more frequently preoperatively and intraoperatively. Anesthetic drugs or techniques that stimulate the sympathetic nervous system (eg, ephedrine, ketamine, hypoventilation), potentiate the arrhythmic effects of catecholamines (eg, hal-

othane), inhibit the parasympathetic nervous system (eg, pancuronium), or release histamine (eg, atracurium, morphine sulfate) may precipitate hypertension and are best avoided.

After tumor ligation and resection, the primary problem frequently becomes *hypotension* from hypovolemia, persistent adrenergic blockade, and prior tolerance to the high levels of endogenous catecholamines that have abruptly ended. Fluid resuscitation should include consideration of surgical bleeding and third-space fluid loss. Assessment of intravascular volume includes urinary output, central venous pressure, arterial blood pressure, and, if available, pulmonary capillary occlusion pressure. Infusions of adrenergic agonists, such as phenylephrine or norepinephrine, may occasionally prove necessary. Postoperative *hypertension* may indicate the presence of occult tumors or volume overload.

■ OBESITY

Overweight and obesity are classified using the body mass index (BMI). Overweight is defined as a BMI of ≥ 24 kg/m², obesity as a BMI ≥ 30, and extreme obesity (old term "morbid obesity") as a BMI of ≥ 40. Health risks increase with the degree of obesity and with increased abdominal distribution of weight. Men with a waist measurement of ≥ 40 in. and women with a waist measurement of ≥ 35 in. are at increased health risk. For a patient 1.8 m tall and weighing 70 kg, the BMI would be as shown in the following formula:

$$BMI = \frac{Weight\ (kg)}{(Height\ [meters])^2} = \frac{70\ kg}{1.8^2} = \frac{70}{3.24} = 21.6\ kg/m^2$$

Clinical Manifestations

Obesity is associated with many diseases, including type II diabetes mellitus, hypertension, coronary artery disease, and cholelithiasis. (The triad of obesity, hypertension, and type II diabetes is known as the metabolic syndrome.) Even in the absence of obvious coexisting disease, however, extreme obesity has profound physiological consequences. Oxygen demand, CO_2 production, and alveolar ventilation are elevated because metabolic rate is proportional to body weight. Excessive adipose tissue over the thorax decreases chest wall compliance even though lung compliance may remain normal. Increased abdominal mass forces the diaphragm cephalad, yielding lung volumes suggestive of restrictive lung disease. Reductions in lung volumes are accentuated by the supine and Trendelenburg positions. In particular, functional residual capacity may fall below closing capacity. If this occurs, some alveoli will close during normal tidal volume ventilation, causing a ventilation/perfusion mismatch.

Whereas obese patients are often found to be hypoxic, only a few are hypercapnic, which should be an alert to impending complications. Obesity-hypoventilation syndrome (old name, Pickwickian syndrome) is a complication of extreme obesity characterized by hypercapnia, cyanosis-induced polycythemia, right-sided heart failure, and somnolence. These patients appear to have blunted respiratory drive and often suffer from loud snoring and upper-airway obstruction during sleep (obstructive sleep apnea syndrome [OSAS]). Patients often report dry mouths and short arousals and bed partners frequently describe apnea pauses. OSAS has also been associated with increased perioperative complications including hypertension, hypoxia, arrhythmias, myocardial infarction, pulmonary edema, and stroke. Difficult airway management during induction and upper airway obstruction during recovery should be anticipated.

Patients are particularly vulnerable during the postoperative period if opioids or other sedatives have been given, and if they are placed supine, making the upper airway even more prone to obstruction. For patients with known or suspected OSAS, a trial of postoperative continuous positive airway pressure (CPAP) should be considered until the anesthesiologist can be sure that the patient can protect his or her airway and maintain spontaneous ventilation without evidence of obstruction.

The heart also has an increased workload, as cardiac output and blood volume rise to perfuse additional fat stores. The elevation in cardiac output (0.1 L/min/kg of adipose tissue) is achieved through an increase in stroke volume—as opposed to heart rate—and frequently results in arterial hypertension and left ventricular hypertrophy. Elevations in pulmonary blood flow and pulmonary artery vasoconstriction from persistent hypoxia can lead to pulmonary hypertension and cor pulmonale.

Obesity is also associated with gastrointestinal pathophysiology, including hiatal hernia, gastroesophageal reflux, poor gastric emptying, and hyperacidic gastric fluid, as well as with an increased risk of gastric cancer. Fatty infiltration of the liver also occurs and may be associated with abnormal liver tests, but the extent of infiltration does not correlate well with the degree of liver test abnormality.

Anesthetic Considerations

A. PREOPERATIVE

For the reasons outlined above, obese patients are at an increased risk for developing aspiration pneumonia. Routine pretreatment with H_2 antagonists and metoclopramide should be considered. Premedication with

respiratory depressant drugs must be avoided in patients with evidence of preoperative hypoxia, hypercapnia, or obstructive sleep apnea. Intramuscular injections are often unreliable due to the thickness of the overlying adipose tissue.

Preoperative evaluation of extremely obese patients undergoing major surgery should attempt to assess cardiopulmonary reserve with a chest radiograph, an ECG, arterial blood gases, and pulmonary function tests. Classic physical signs of cardiac failure (eg, sacral edema) may be difficult to identify. Blood pressures must be taken with the appropriate size cuff. Intravenous and intraarterial access sites should be checked in anticipation of technical difficulties. Obscured landmarks, difficult positioning, and extensive layers of adipose tissue may make regional anesthesia impossible with standard equipment and techniques. Particular attention should be paid to the airway in obese patients because they are often difficult to intubate as a result of limited mobility of the temporomandibular and atlantooccipital joints, a narrowed upper airway, and a shortened distance between the mandible and sternal fat pads.

B. INTRAOPERATIVE

Because of the risk of aspiration, obese patients are usually intubated for all but the shortest of general anesthetics. Furthermore, controlled ventilation with large tidal volumes often provides better oxygenation than shallow, spontaneous breaths. If intubation appears likely to be difficult, keeping the patient awake and intubating with a fiberoptic bronchoscope is strongly recommended. Breath sounds may be difficult to appreciate; confirmation of tracheal intubation requires detection of end-tidal CO_2. Even controlled ventilation may require relatively high-inspired oxygen concentrations to prevent hypoxia, particularly in the lithotomy, Trendelenburg, or prone position. Subdiaphragmatic abdominal laparotomy packs can cause further deterioration of pulmonary function and a reduction of arterial blood pressure by impairing venous return. The addition of positive end-expiratory pressure worsens pulmonary hypertension in some patients with extreme obesity.

Volatile anesthetics may be metabolized more extensively in obese patients. This is of particular concern with respect to the defluorination of halothane. Increased metabolism and a predisposition to hypoxia may explain the increased incidence of halothane hepatitis in obese patients. Volatile anesthetics distribute so slowly to the lipid stores that increasing the fat reservoir has little clinical effect on wake-up time, even during long surgical procedures.

Theoretically, larger fat stores provide an increased volume of distribution for lipid-soluble drugs (eg, benzodiazepines, opioids). Thus, a larger loading dose would be required to produce the same plasma concentration. This is the rationale for basing some drug doses on actual body weight in obese patients. By the same reasoning, maintenance doses should be administered less frequently because clearance would be expected to be slower with a larger volume of distribution. In contrast, water-soluble drugs (eg, NMBAs) have a much more limited volume of distribution, which should not be influenced by fat stores. The dosing of these drugs should therefore be based on ideal body weight to avoid overdosing. In reality, however, clinical practice does not always validate these expectations.

The technical difficulties associated with regional anesthesia have been mentioned. Although dosage requirements for epidural and spinal anesthesia are difficult to predict, obese patients usually require 20–25% less local anesthetic because of epidural fat and distended epidural veins. A high level of blockade can easily result in respiratory compromise. Continuous epidural anesthesia has the advantage of providing pain relief and decreasing respiratory complications in the postoperative period.

C. POSTOPERATIVE

Respiratory failure is the major postoperative problem of extremely obese patients. The risk of postoperative hypoxia is increased by preoperative hypoxia and by surgery involving the thorax or upper abdomen (particularly vertical incisions). Extubation should be delayed until the effects of NMBAs are completely reversed and the patient is fully awake. An obese patient should remain intubated until there is no doubt that an adequate airway and tidal volume will be maintained. This does *not* mean that all obese patients need to remain on ventilators overnight in an intensive care unit. If the patient is extubated in the operating room, supplemental oxygen should be provided during transportation to the recovery room. A 45° modified sitting position will unload the diaphragm and improve ventilation and oxygenation. The risk of hypoxia extends for several days into the postoperative period, and providing supplemental oxygen should be routinely considered. Other common postoperative complications in obese patients include wound infection, deep venous thrombosis, and pulmonary embolism.

■ CARCINOID SYNDROME

Carcinoid syndrome is the complex of symptoms and signs caused by the secretion of vasoactive substances (eg, serotonin, kallikrein, histamine) from enteroepinephrine tumors (carcinoid tumors). Because most of these tumors are located in the gastrointestinal tract, their metabolic products are released into the portal circulation and destroyed by the liver before they can cause systemic effects. However, the products of nonintestinal tumors (eg, pulmonary, ovarian) or hepatic metastases bypass the portal circulation and, therefore, can cause a variety of clinical manifestations.

Clinical Manifestations

The most common manifestations of carcinoid syndrome are cutaneous flushing, bronchospasm, profuse diarrhea, dramatic swings in arterial blood pressure (usually hypotension), and supraventricular arrhythmias (Table 36–9). **Carcinoid syndrome is associated with right-sided heart disease caused by valvular and myocardial plaque formation.** Lung metabolism of serotonin evidently prevents involvement of the left side of the heart. The diagnosis of carcinoid syndrome is confirmed by detection of serotonin metabolites in the urine (5-hydroxyindoleacetic acid) or suggested by elevated plasma levels of chromogranin A. Treatment varies depending on tumor location but may include surgical resection, symptomatic relief, or specific serotonin and histamine antagonists. Somatostatin, an inhibitory peptide, reduces the release of vasoactive tumor products.

Anesthetic Considerations

The key to anesthetic management of patients with carcinoid syndrome is to avoid anesthetic techniques or agents that could cause the tumor to release vasoactive substances. **For example, hypotension, which can itself cause hormone release, should be treated with volume expansion.** Administration of catecholamine has been associated with kallikrein activation. Regional anesthesia may limit perioperative stress and the subsequent release of vasoactive agents. Clearly, histamine-releasing drugs (eg, morphine and atracurium) should be avoided. Surgical manipulation of the tumor can cause a massive release of hormones. Monitoring should include an arterial line and a central venous or pulmonary artery catheter because of the hemodynamic instability and

Table 36–9. Principal mediators of carcinoid syndrome and their clinical manifestations.

Mediator	Clinical Manifestations
Serotonin	Vasoconstriction (coronary artery spasm, hypertension), increased intestinal tone, water and electrolyte imbalance (diarrhea), tryptophan deficiency (hypoproteinemia, pellagra)
Kallikrein	Vasodilation (hypotension, flushing), bronchoconstriction
Histamine	Vasodilation (hypotension, flushing), arrhythmias, bronchoconstriction

intrinsic heart disease caused by carcinoid syndrome. Alterations in carbohydrate metabolism may lead to unsuspected hypoglycemia or hyperglycemia. Consultation with an endocrinologist may help clarify the role of antihistamine, antiserotonin drugs (eg, methysergide), octreotide (a long-acting somatostatin analogue), or antikallikrein drugs (eg, corticosteroids) in specific patients.

CASE DISCUSSION: MULTIPLE ENDOCRINE NEOPLASIA

An isolated thyroid nodule is discovered during physical examination of a 36-year-old woman complaining of diarrhea and headaches. Workup of the tumor reveals hypercalcemia and an elevated calcitonin level, which leads to the diagnosis of medullary cancer of the thyroid. During induction of general anesthesia for total thyroidectomy, the patient's blood pressure rises to 240/140 mm Hg and her heart rate approaches 140 beats/min, with frequent premature ventricular contractions. The operation is canceled, an arterial line is placed, and the patient is treated with intravenous phentolamine, propranolol, lidocaine, and sodium nitroprusside.

What is the probable cause of this patient's hypertensive crisis during induction of general anesthesia?

Multiple endocrine neoplasia (MEN) is characterized by tumor formation in several endocrine organs. MEN type I consists of pancreatic (gastrinomas, insulinomas), pituitary (chromophobes), and parathyroid tumors. MEN type II consists of medullary thyroid carcinoma, pheochromocytoma, and hyperparathyroidism (type IIa) or multiple mucosal neuromas (type IIb or type III). The hypertensive episode in this case may be due to a previously undiagnosed pheochromocytoma. The pheochromocytoma in MEN often consists of small multiple tumors. These patients are typically young adults with strong family histories of MEN. If multiple surgeries are planned, pheochromocytoma resection will usually be scheduled first.

What is calcitonin, and why is it associated with medullary cancer?

Calcitonin is a polypeptide manufactured by the parafollicular cells (C cells) in the thyroid gland. It is secreted in response to increases in plasma ionic calcium and tends to lower calcium levels by affecting kidney and bone function. Therefore, it acts as an antagonist of parathyroid hormone (see Table 36–6).

Why is this patient hypercalcemic if calcitonin lowers serum calcium?

An excess or deficiency of calcitonin has minor effects in humans compared with the effects of parathyroid disorders. This patient's hypercalcemia may be due to coexisting primary hyperparathyroidism (MEN type IIa).

Are headache and diarrhea consistent with the diagnosis of MEN?

The history of headaches suggests the possibility of pheochromocytoma, whereas diarrhea may be due to calcitonin or one of the other peptides often produced by medullary thyroid carcinoma (eg, ACTH, somatostatin, β-endorphin).

What follow-up is required for this patient?

Because of the life-threatening hemodynamic changes associated with pheochromocytoma, this entity must be medically controlled before surgery can be considered (see Case Discussion, Chapter 12). Because MEN syndromes are hereditary, family members should be screened for early signs of pheochromocytoma, thyroid cancer, and hyperparathyroidism.

SUGGESTED READING

Adams JP, Murphy PG: Obesity in anaesthesia and intensive care. Br J Anaesth 2000;85:91.

Arlt W, Allolio B: Adrenal insufficiency. Lancet 2003;361:1881. Outstanding overview of adrenal insufficiency, an increasingly common problem during the perioperative period.

Graham GW, Unger BP, Coursin DB: Perioperative management of selected endocrine disorders. Int Anesthesiol Clin 2000;38:31.

Jones GC, Macklin JP, Alexander WD: Contraindications to the use of metformin. Evidence suggests that it is time to amend the list. BMJ 2003;326:4. The list of contraindications to the use of metformin is growing.

Kirby RR: *Clinical Anesthesia Practice,* 2nd ed. Saunders, 2000.

Prys-Roberts C: Phaeochromocytoma—recent progress in its management. Br J Anaesth 2000;85:44.

McAnulty GR, Hall GM: Anaesthesia for the diabetic patient. Br J Anaesth 2003;90:428. As the incidence of diabetes increases and as the number of complications from intraoperative hyperglycemia is better recognized, this short review is an excellent overview of anesthesia for the diabetic patient.

Stoelting RK, Dierdorf SF: *Handbook of Anesthesia and Co-existing Disease,* 2nd ed. Churchill Livingstone, 2002.

Wilson JD, Foster DW, Kronenberg HM, et al: *Williams Textbook of Endocrinology,* 10th ed. W.B. Saunders, 2003.

Anesthesia for Patients with Neuromuscular Disease

37

KEY CONCEPTS

 1 The weakness associated with myasthenia gravis is thought to be due to autoimmune destruction or inactivation of postsynaptic acetylcholine receptors at the neuromuscular junction, leading to a reduced number of receptors and loss of folds on the postsynaptic membrane.

2 Patients who have myasthenia gravis with respiratory muscle or bulbar involvement are at increased risk for pulmonary aspiration.

 3 Many patients with myasthenia gravis are exquisitely sensitive to nondepolarizing neuromuscular blocking agents (NMBAs).

4 Patients who have myasthenia gravis are at greatest risk for postoperative respiratory failure. Disease duration of more than 6 years, concomitant pulmonary disease, a peak inspiratory pressure of < –25 cm H₂O (ie, –20 cm H₂O), a vital capacity < 4 mL/kg, and a pyridostigmine dose > 750 mg/d are predictive of the need for postoperative ventilation following thymectomy.

 5 Patients with the myasthenic syndrome are very sensitive to both depolarizing and nondepolarizing NMBAs.

 6 Degeneration of the respiratory muscles in patients with muscular dystrophy interferes with an effective coughing mechanism and leads to retention of secretions and frequent pulmonary infections.

 7 Degeneration of cardiac muscle in patients with muscular dystrophy is also common, but results in dilated or hypertrophic cardiomyopathy in only 10% of patients.

 8 Succinylcholine has been used safely in some patients with Duchenne's and Becker's muscular dystrophies but is best avoided because of unpredictable responses and the risks of inducing severe hyperkalemia or triggering malignant hyperthermia.

 9 In patients with periodic paralysis, anesthetic management is directed toward preventing attacks. Careful electrocardiographic monitoring is necessary to detect attacks and arrhythmias during anesthesia.

 10 In patients with periodic paralysis, the response to NMBAs is unpredictable. Increased sensitivity to nondepolarizing NMBAs is particularly apt to be encountered in patients with hypokalemic periodic paralysis.

Although neuromuscular disorders are relatively uncommon, patients present to the operating room with some regularity at tertiary medical centers for diagnostic studies, for treatment of complications, or for surgical management of unrelated disorders. Diminished respiratory muscle strength and enhanced sensitivity to neuromuscular blocking agents (NMBAs) predispose these patients to postoperative ventilatory failure. A basic understanding of the major disorders and their potential interaction with anesthetic agents is necessary to avoid postoperative morbidity of this nature.

MYASTHENIA GRAVIS

Myasthenia gravis is characterized by weakness and easy fatigability of skeletal muscle and is classified according to whether the patient has only ocular or ocular and nonocular muscle weakness (Table 37–1). The lifetime prevalence of myasthenia gravis is anywhere between 5 and 40 per 100,000 people. The incidence is about 4–11 per million and is highest in women during their third decade; in men, it typically presents in the sixth and seventh decades. The weakness associated with myasthenia gravis is thought to be due to autoimmune destruction or inactivation of postsynaptic acetylcholine receptors at the neuromuscular junction, leading to a reduced number of receptors and loss of folds on the postsynaptic membrane. Antibodies (IgG) against the nicotinic acetylcholine receptor in neuromuscular junctions are found in 85–90% of patients with generalized myasthenia gravis and up to 50–70% of patients with ocular myasthenia. Ten to fifteen percent of patients with myasthenia develop a thymoma, whereas 65% have thymic hyperphasia. Other autoimmune disorders (hypothyroidism, hyperthyroidism, rheumatoid arthritis) are also present in 10% of patients.

The course of the disease is marked by exacerbations and remissions. Remissions may be partial or complete. The weakness can be asymmetric, confined to one group of muscles, or generalized. Ocular muscles are most commonly affected, resulting in fluctuating ptosis and diplopia. With bulbar involvement, laryngeal and pharyngeal muscle weakness can result in dysarthria, difficulty in chewing and swallowing, problems clearing secretions, or pulmonary aspiration. Severe disease is usually also associated with proximal muscle weakness (primarily in the neck and shoulders) and involvement of respiratory muscles. Muscle strength characteristically improves with rest but deteriorates rapidly with exertion. Infection, stress, surgery, and pregnancy have unpredictable effects on the disease but often lead to exacerbations.

Table 37–1. Classification of myasthenia.

Class I	Ocular muscle weakness
Class II	Mild nonocular muscle weakness[1]
Class III	Moderate nonocular muscle weakness[2]
Class IV	Severe nonocular muscle weakness[1]
Class V	Tracheal intubation[2] or tracheostomy to protect the airway with or without mechanical ventilation

[1] ± Ocular muscle weakness of any severity.
[2] Except in the perioperative period.

Anticholinesterase drugs are the most commonly used agents to treat muscle weakness. These drugs increase the amount of acetylcholine at the neuromuscular junction through inhibition of end-plate acetylcholinesterase. Pyridostigmine is the most often used agent; when given orally, it has an effective duration of 2–4 h. Excessive administration of an anticholinesterase may precipitate cholinergic crisis, which is characterized by increased weakness and excessive muscarinic effects, including salivation, diarrhea, miosis, and bradycardia. An edrophonium test may help differentiate a cholinergic from a myasthenic crisis. Increased weakness after up to 10 mg of intravenous edrophonium indicates cholinergic crisis, whereas increasing strength implies myasthenic crisis. If this test is equivocal or if the patient clearly has manifestations of cholinergic hyperactivity, all cholinesterase drugs should be discontinued and the patient should be monitored closely (in most cases in an intensive care unit). Anticholinesterase drugs are often the only agents used to treat patients with mild disease. Moderate to severe disease is treated with a combination of an anticholinesterase drug and immunomodulating therapy. Corticosteroids are usually tried first, followed by azathioprine or cyclosporine. Several alternative immunomodulating treatments can also be tried including cyclophosphamide, mycophenolate, mofetil, and intravenous immunoglobulin. Plasmapheresis is reserved for patients with dysphagia or respiratory failure, or to normalize muscle strength preoperatively in patients undergoing a surgical procedure. Up to 85% of patients under 55 years of age show clinical improvement following thymectomy even in the absence of a tumor, but improvement may be delayed up to several years.

Anesthetic Considerations

Patients with myasthenia may present for thymectomy or for unrelated surgical or obstetric procedures. In all cases, patients should be under the best possible medical control prior to operation. Myasthenic patients with respiratory and oropharyngeal weakness should be treated aggressively preoperatively with intravenous immunoglobulin or plasmapheresis. If strength normalizes the incidence of postoperative respiratory complications should be similar to that of a nonmyasthenic patient undergoing a similar surgical procedure. Patients scheduled for thymectomy often have deteriorating muscle strength, whereas those undergoing other elective procedures may be well controlled or in remission. Adjustments in anticholinesterase medication, immunosuppressants, or steroid therapy may be necessary. Management of anticholinesterase therapy in the perioperative period is controversial but should probably be individualized. Potential problems in continuing such therapy include altered patient requirements following surgery, increased vagal reflexes, and the possibility of disrupting bowel anastomoses secondary to hyperperistalsis. Moreover, because these agents also inhibit plasma cholinesterase, they can prolong the duration of ester-type local anesthetics and succinylcholine. Conversely, patients with advanced generalized disease may deteriorate significantly when anticholinesterase agents are withheld.

These medications should be restarted when the patient resumes oral intake. When necessary, cholinesterase inhibitors can also be given parenterally at $1/30$ the oral dose.

Preoperative evaluation should focus on the recent course of the disease, the muscle groups affected, drug therapy, and coexisting illnesses. Patients who have myasthenia gravis with respiratory muscle or bulbar involvement are at increased risk for pulmonary aspiration. Premedication with metoclopramide or an H_2 blocker may decrease this risk, but supporting studies are lacking in this group of patients. Because some patients with myasthenia are often very sensitive to respiratory depressants, premedication with opioids, benzodiazepines, and similar drugs is usually omitted.

With the exception of NMBAs, standard anesthetic agents may be used in patients with myasthenia gravis. Marked respiratory depression, however, may be encountered following even moderate doses of barbiturates or opioids. Propofol may be preferable because of its short duration of action. A volatile agent–based anesthetic is generally most satisfactory. Deep anesthesia with a volatile agent alone in patients with myasthenia may provide sufficient relaxation for tracheal intubation as well as most surgical procedures. Some clinicians routinely try to avoid NMBAs. The response to succinylcholine is unpredictable. Patients may manifest a relative resistance, a prolonged effect, or an unusual response (phase II block; see Chapter 9). The dose of succinylcholine may be increased to 2 mg/kg to overcome any resistance, but a prolonged effect should be anticipated.

Many patients with myasthenia gravis are exquisitely sensitive to nondepolarizing NMBAs. Even a defasciculating dose in some patients can result in nearly complete paralysis. If NMBAs are necessary, small doses of a relatively short-acting nondepolarizing agent (cisatracurium or mivacurium) are preferred. Neuromuscular blockade should be monitored very closely with a nerve stimulator. Ventilatory function should be evaluated carefully prior to extubation.

Patients who have myasthenia gravis are at greatest risk for postoperative respiratory failure. Disease duration of more than 6 years, concomitant pulmonary disease, a peak inspiratory pressure of < -25 cm H_2O (ie, -20 cm H_2O), a vital capacity < 4 mL/kg, and a pyridostigmine dose > 750 mg/d are predictive of the need for postoperative ventilation following thymectomy.

Women with myasthenia can experience increased weakness in the last trimester of pregnancy and the early postpartum period. Epidural anesthesia is generally preferable for these patients because it avoids potential problems with respiratory depression and NMBAs during general anesthesia. Excessively high levels of motor blockade, however, can also result in hypoventilation. Babies of myasthenic mothers may show transient myasthenia for 1–3 weeks, induced by transplacental transfer of acetylcholine receptor antibodies, sometimes necessitating controlled mechanical ventilation.

LAMBERT–EATON MYASTHENIC SYNDROME

The Lambert–Eaton myasthenic syndrome (LEMS) is a paraneoplastic syndrome characterized by proximal muscle weakness that typically begins in the lower extremities, but may spread to involve upper limb, bulbar, and respiratory muscles. Dry mouth, male impotence, and other manifestations of autonomic dysfunction are also very common. LEMS is usually associated with small cell carcinoma of the lung. It may also be seen with other occult malignancies or as an idiopathic autoimmune disease. The disorder results from a presynaptic defect of neuromuscular transmission. Antibodies to voltage-gated calcium channels on the nerve terminal markedly reduce the quantal release of acetylcholine at the motor end-plate. Small cell carcinoma cells express identical voltage-gated calcium channels, serving as a trigger for the autoimmune response in patients with paraneoplastic LEMS.

In contrast to myasthenia gravis, muscle weakness improves with repeated effort and is improved less dramatically by anticholinesterase drugs. Guanidine hydrochloride and 3,4-diaminopyridine (DAP), which increases the release of acetylcholine, often produce significant improvement in LEMS. The use of guanidine hydrochloride is limited by hepatoxicity. DAP is available only on a compassionate-use basis in the United States, but is widely available in other countries. Many patients with LEMS improve with immunosuppression or plasmapheresis.

Patients with the myasthenic syndrome are very sensitive to both depolarizing and nondepolarizing NMBAs. The response to other drugs used in anesthesia is usually normal. Volatile agents alone are often sufficient to provide muscle relaxation for both intubation and most surgical procedures. NMBAs should be given only in small increments and with careful neuromuscular monitoring. The management of autonomic defects is discussed in Chapter 27.

MUSCULAR DYSTROPHIES

Preoperative Considerations

Muscular dystrophies are a heterogeneous group of hereditary disorders characterized by muscle fiber necrosis and regeneration, leading to progressive weakness and degeneration of muscle. Sporadic cases are presumably due to mutations. α-Dystroglycan (α-DG) dysglycosylation is the most common pathophysiology for the congenital muscular dystrophies and one form of limb-girdle muscular dystrophy.

Duchenne's Muscular Dystrophy

Duchenne's muscular dystrophy is the most common and most severe form of muscular dystrophy. Other major variants include Becker's, myotonic facioscapulohumeral, and limb-girdle dystrophies. An X-linked recessive disorder, Duchenne's muscular dystrophy affects males almost exclusively. It has an incidence of approximately one to three cases per 10,000 live male births and most commonly presents between 3 and 5 years of age. Affected individuals produce abnormal dystrophin, a protein found on the sarcolemma of muscle fibers. Patients characteristically develop symmetric proximal muscle weakness that is manifested as a gait disturbance. Fatty infiltration typically causes enlargement (pseudohypertrophy) of muscles, particularly the calves. Progressive weakness and contractures eventually result in kyphoscoliosis. By age 12, most patients are confined to wheelchairs. Disease progression may be delayed by up to 2–3 years with glucocorticoid therapy in some patients. Intellectual impairment is common but generally nonprogressive. Plasma creatine kinase (CK) levels are 10–100 times normal even early in the disease and are thought to reflect an abnormal increase in the permeability of muscle cell membranes. Female carriers often also have high plasma CK levels, variable degrees of muscle weakness, and, rarely, cardiac involvement. Plasma myoglobin concentration may also be elevated. The diagnosis is confirmed by muscle biopsy. Deletions or duplications in the dystrophin gene may be detected by Southern blot analysis or polymerase chain reaction methods in 65% of patients with Duchenne's or Becker's muscular dystrophy.

Degeneration of the respiratory muscles in patients with muscular dystrophy interferes with an effective coughing mechanism and leads to retention of secretions and frequent pulmonary infections. The combination of marked kyphoscoliosis and muscle wasting produces a severe restrictive ventilatory defect. Pulmonary hypertension is common with disease progression. Degeneration of cardiac muscle in patients with muscular dystrophy is also common, but results in dilated or hyper-

trophic cardiomyopathy in only 10% of patients. Mitral regurgitation secondary to papillary muscle dysfunction can also be documented in up to 25% of patients. Electrocardiographic (ECG) abnormalities include P–R interval prolongation, QRS and ST-segment abnormalities, and prominent R waves over the right precordium with deep Q waves over the left precordium. Atrial arrhythmias are common. Death is usually due to recurrent pulmonary infections, respiratory failure, or cardiac failure by the age of 15–25 years.

Becker's Muscular Dystrophy

Becker's muscular dystrophy, a less common disorder (1:30,000 male births), is also an X-linked recessive muscular dystrophy. It is also thought to be due to a deletion or point mutation in the dystrophin gene, leading to a defect in dystrophin production. Manifestations are almost identical to those of Duchenne's muscular dystrophy except that they usually present later in life (adolescence) and progress more slowly. Mental retardation is less common. Patients often reach the fourth or fifth decade, although some may survive into their 80s. Death is usually from respiratory complications. Cardiomyopathy may occur in some cases and may precede severe skeletal weakness.

Myotonic Dystrophy

Myotonic dystrophy (MD) is a multisystem disorder that is the most common cause of myotonia—slowing of relaxation after muscle contraction in response to electrical or percussive stimuli. The disease is transmitted in an autosomal dominant fashion and has an incidence of 1:8000. The most common form is localized to chromosome 19, locus q12.3; the gene codes for a serine/threonine protein kinase. An abnormally long trinucleotide repeat is thought to lead to the disease. MD manifests in the second to third decade of life; however, patients can present from infancy to late life. Myotonia is the principal manifestation early in the disease, but as the disease progresses, muscle weakness and atrophy become more prominent. This weakness and atrophy usually affect cranial muscles (orbicularis oculi and oris, masseter, and sternocleidomastoid) and result in the typical facial appearance. As opposed to most myopathies, distal muscles are more involved than proximal muscles. Plasma CK levels are normal or slightly elevated.

Multiple organ systems are involved in the disease as evidenced by presenile cataracts; premature frontal baldness; hypersomnolence with sleep apnea; and endocrine dysfunction leading to pancreatic, adrenal, thyroid, and gonadal insufficiency. Respiratory involvement leads to decreased vital capacity. Alveolar hypoventilation is caused by either pulmonary or central nervous system dysfunction. Chronic hypoxemia may lead to cor pulmonale. Gastrointestinal hypomotility can predispose patients to pulmonary aspiration. Uterine atony can prolong labor and increases the incidence of retained placenta. Cardiac manifestations, which are often present before other clinical symptoms appear, consist of atrial arrhythmias, varying degrees of heart block, and, less frequently, depression of ventricular function.

The myotonia is usually described by patients as a "stiffness" that may ease with continued activity, the so-called "warm-up" phenomenon. Patients often report that cold temperatures worsen stiffness, although electrophysiological studies have shown improvement in myotonic discharges with cooling. Antimyotonic treatment can be undertaken with membrane-stabilizing medications. Phenytoin, quinine sulfate, and procainamide have all been used in this manner. Phenytoin does not appear to worsen cardiac conduction abnormalities, whereas quinine and procainamide may prolong the P–R interval. Mexiletine and tocainide should not be used in patients with MD. A cardiac pacemaker should be placed in patients with significant conduction defect, even if they are asymptomatic.

Facioscapulohumeral Dystrophy

Facioscapulohumeral dystrophy is an autosomal dominant variant with an incidence of approximately 1–3:100,000, due to a DNA deletion on chromosome 4q35. It affects both males and females, although more females with the gene defect are asymptomatic. Patients usually present in the second or third decade of life with weakness that is confined primarily to the muscles of the face and the shoulder girdle. Muscles in the lower extremities are less commonly affected, and respiratory muscles are usually spared. The disease is slowly progressive and has a variable course. Plasma CK levels are usually normal or only slightly elevated. Cardiac involvement is rare, but atrial paralysis has been reported in a few patients. The latter results in loss of all atrial electrical activity and in an inability to atrially pace the heart; ventricular pacing is still possible. Longevity is minimally affected in most of these patients.

Limb-Girdle Dystrophy

Limb-girdle muscular dystrophy is a heterogeneous entity composed of several variants of neuromuscular diseases, which are further being defined by molecular genetics. Limb-girdle syndromes include severe childhood autosomal recessive muscular dystrophy (SCARMD, chromosome 13), autosomal recessive muscular dystrophy (chromosome 15), and other incompletely defined autosomal recessive syndromes such as Erb's (scapulohumeral type) and Leyden–Mobius (pelvifemoral type). Most patients present in childhood to the second or third decade of life

with muscle weakness that may involve the shoulder girdle, the hip girdle, or both. The disease tends to be very slowly progressive. Plasma CK levels are usually elevated. Cardiac involvement, similar to what occurs in Duchenne's muscular dystrophy, can present as frequent arrhythmias or congestive heart failure but is relatively uncommon. Respiratory complications, such as hypoventilation and recurrent respiratory infections, may occur early in the disease but are more common after longstanding disease (> 30 years).

Anesthetic Considerations

A. Duchenne's and Becker's Muscular Dystrophies

The anesthetic management of these patients is complicated not only by muscle weakness but also by cardiac and pulmonary manifestations. An association with malignant hyperthermia has been suggested but is unproven. Preoperative premedication with sedatives or opioids is best avoided, because patients may be at increased risk for aspiration from respiratory muscle weakness or gastric hypomotility. Intraoperative positioning can be complicated if the patient has kyphoscoliosis or flexion contractures of the extremities or neck.

Succinylcholine has been used safely in some patients with Duchenne's and Becker's muscular dystrophies but is best avoided because of unpredictable responses and the risks of inducing severe hyperkalemia or triggering malignant hyperthermia. Although some patients exhibit a normal response to nondepolarizing NMBAs, others may be very sensitive. Marked respiratory and circulatory depression may be seen with volatile anesthetics in patients with advanced disease. Regional or local anesthesia may therefore be preferable in these patients. Respiratory complications are largely responsible for perioperative morbidity. Patients with vital capacities less than 30% of predicted appear to be at greatest risk and often require temporary postoperative mechanical ventilation.

B. Myotonic Dystrophy

Patients with MD are at high risk for perioperative respiratory and cardiac complications. Surgery with general anesthesia should be avoided, therefore, when not absolutely necessary. Knowledge of the patients' diagnosis of MD is obviously vital to patient care; however, patients with the disease may not volunteer this information, and some patients may be simply presymptomatic and undiagnosed. The diagnosis of MD has been made in some patients only after prolonged apnea after general anesthesia. Most perioperative problems arise in MD patients with severe weakness and in those cases in which surgeons and anesthesiologists are unaware of the diagnosis.

Patients with MD have altered responses to a number of anesthetic medicines. They are often very sensitive to even small doses of opioids, sedatives, and inhalation and intravenous agents, all of which may cause sudden and prolonged apnea. Premedication should therefore be avoided, if possible. Succinylcholine has been relatively contraindicated because it may precipitate intense myotonic contractions; trismus can prevent opening the mouth for intubation. Myotonic contraction of respiratory, chest wall, or laryngeal muscles can make ventilation difficult or impossible. Other drugs that act on the motor end plate, such as decamethonium, neostigmine, and physostigmine, can aggravate myotonia. Regional anesthesia can be employed but does not always prevent myotonic contractions. Troublesome myotonia rarely occurs, but can be reduced by injecting procaine in the muscles or by giving 300–600 mg of quinine hydrochloride intravenously.

The response to nondepolarizing NMBAs is reported to be normal; however, they do not consistently prevent or relieve myotonic contractions. As reversal of nondepolarizing NMBAs can induce myotonic contractions, the use of short-acting nondepolarizing agents (cisatracurium or mivacurium) is recommended. The postoperative shivering commonly associated with volatile agents, particularly when associated with decreased body temperature, can induce myotonic contractions in the recovery room. Small doses of meperidine can often prevent such shivering and perhaps the myotonic contractions.

Induction of anesthesia without complications has been reported for a number of agents including thiopental, inhalation agents, and propofol (with or without ketamine). Neuromuscular blockade, if needed, should be performed with short-acting NMBAs. Nitrous oxide and inhalation agents can be used as maintenance anesthesia. Reversal with anticholinesterases is to be avoided, if possible. There is no association between the type of anesthesia used and any postoperative complications.

The main postoperative complications are pulmonary: prolonged hypoventilation, atelectasis, and pneumonia. Aggressive pulmonary hygiene with physical therapy, incentive spirometry, and careful postoperative monitoring are indicated. Aspiration prophylaxis is also probably indicated. Patients undergoing upper abdominal surgery or those with severe proximal weakness are more likely to experience this type of complication. Perioperative cardiac conduction abnormalities are less likely to occur but still warrant close cardiovascular monitoring.

As association between MD and malignant hyperthermia has been suggested but has not been firmly established. It does not seem, therefore, that patients with MD are at an increased risk for malignant hyperthermia. Interestingly, both disorders map to chromosome 19, albeit in different locations.

C. OTHER FORMS OF MUSCULAR DYSTROPHY

Patients with facioscapulohumeral and limb-girdle muscular dystrophy generally have normal responses to anesthetic agents. Nonetheless, because of the great variability and overlap between the various forms of muscular dystrophy, nondepolarizing NMBAs should be used cautiously, and succinylcholine should probably be avoided.

MYOTONIAS

Myotonia Congenita & Paramyotonia Congenita

Myotonia congenita is a disorder manifested early in life with generalized myotonia. The disease is caused by mutations of a gene on chromosome 7q35 encoding a chloride channel of the skeletal muscle fiber surface membrane. Both autosomal dominant (Thomsen's) and recessive (Becker's) forms exist. The disease is confined to skeletal muscle and produces no, minimal, or nonprogressive weakness. Many patients, in fact, have very well- developed musculature due to near constant muscle contraction. Myotonia is usually more bothersome in patients with myotonia than in those with MD. Antimyotonic therapy includes phenytoin, mexiletine, quinine sulfate, or procainamide. Other medicines that have been used include tocainide, dantrolene, prednisone, acetazolamide, and taurine. There is no cardiac involvement in myotonia congenita, and a normal life span is expected.

Paramyotonia congenita is a very rare autosomal dominant disorder localized to chromosome 17q. Mutations in the α-subunit of the sodium channel are associated with the disease. Symptoms of paramyotonia congenita include transient stiffness (myotonia) and, occasionally, weakness after exposure to cold temperatures. The stiffness worsens with activity, in contrast to true myotonia, thus the term "paramyotonia." Serum potassium concentration may rise following an attack similar to hyperkalemic periodic paralysis (see below). Medicines that have been used to block the cold response include mexiletine and tocainide.

Anesthetic management of patients with myotonia congenita and paramyotonia is complicated by an abnormal response to succinylcholine, troublesome intraoperative myotonic contractions, and the need to avoid hypothermia. NMBAs may paradoxically cause generalized muscle spasms, including trismus, leading to difficulty with intubation and ventilation.

Infiltration of muscles in the operative field with a dilute local anesthetic may alleviate refractory myotonic contraction. No patients with these types of myotonia have been reported with positive *in vitro* tests for malignant hyperthermia. Excised muscle in these patients does, however, display a prolonged myotonic contraction when exposed to a depolarizing NMBA. Excessive muscle contraction during anesthesia, therefore, likely represents aggravation of myotonia and not malignant hyperthermia.

PERIODIC PARALYSIS

This group of disorders is characterized by sudden attacks of transient muscle weakness or paralysis. Symptoms usually begin in childhood. The attacks generally last a few h and typically spare respiratory muscles. The attacks of weakness are due to a loss of muscle fiber excitability because of partial depolarization of the resting potential. The depolarization prevents the generation of action potentials and thereby precipitates the weakness.

These entities are classified into primary genetic channelopathies and secondary acquired forms. The genetic or inherited types are due to dominantly inherited mutations in the voltage-gated sodium, calcium, or potassium ion channels. Classifications have been based on clinical differences, but these have not been shown to relate to specific ion channels. Different defects in the same channel can cause different clinical pictures, whereas mutations in different channels may have similar clinical pictures. However, the clinical classifications remain useful as guides to prognosis and therapy.

There is a dominantly inherited disorder in which there is a defect in voltage-gated, calcium channels. This entity is typically associated with low serum potassium levels during spells of weakness. A dominantly inherited defect in sodium channels, which also results in periodic paralysis, is typically associated with elevated serum potassium levels during episodes of weakness. Both defects result in inexcitable muscle membranes to both direct and indirect stimulation due to either decreased potassium conductance or increased sodium conductance, respectively. Both are associated with fluid and electrolyte shifts. Both disorders are inherited as autosomal dominant traits, but both have a number of allelic variants resulting in different presentations in different families. Paramyotonia with sensitivity to cold is one example of the sodium channelopathies.

The primary forms of these disorders have a number of clinical similarities. They are characterized by sporadic episodes of weakness. Muscle strength and serum potassium concentrations are usually normal between attacks. The disorder is also characterized by worsening induced by hypothermia. The weakness usually lasts less than 1 h, but can last 2 days, and frequent attacks can lead to progressive long-term weakness in some patients. Episodes can be increased by rest after vigorous exercise, but minimized by continued muscle exercise.

1. Voltage-Gated Calcium Channelopathy (Hypokalemic Periodic Paralysis)

The hypokalemic variant often presents in childhood to early adulthood. As time progresses, there is usually an increased frequency of attacks, although they may subside in later life.

The hypokalemic variant is most common and may be inherited, occur sporadically, or be associated with hyperthyroidism. Up to 10% of hyperthyroid men of Latin or Asian descent have episodes of hypokalemic periodic paralysis. The episodes are characterized by weakness or paralysis of limb muscles that lasts 3–4 h, but that may last for days. Episodes are most common in the early morning and can be precipitated by strenuous exertion or high carbohydrate meals. Mild exertion can actually prevent or delay paralysis. Interestingly, local anesthetics with antiphlogistics can precipitate an episode. During an attack, the potassium level is normal to moderately decreased, along with the phosphorus level. The kidneys retain sodium, potassium, chloride, and water, which are associated with increased intracellular fluid volume and decreased extracellular volume. This order may be associated with oliguria, obstipation, and diaphoresis. There may be ECG changes (see Chapter 28) consistent with a low potassium level. As noted, permanent muscle damage can develop as the attacks increase in frequency.

The diagnosis is usually made by a careful family history, the patient's history, and notation of changing potassium myotonia on electromyography. An acute attack is typically treated with 2–10 g of oral potassium without glucose, with mild physical activity being encouraged. Intravenous potassium is no longer recommended because it may lead to hyperkalemia. This disorder may be prevented by the administration of low-dose acetazolamide. Glucose solutions should be avoided, as uptake of glucose by cells, associated with changes in serum potassium, can exacerbate the hypokalemia and weakness.

A secondary form of this same disorder is associated with thyrotoxicosis. It resembles the primary form but is much more common in men than women, particularly in persons of Asiatic descent and in young adults. Once the thyroid condition is treated, the episodes usually cease. The disorder can develop in anywhere from 10 to 25% of hyperthyroid Asian men. The metabolic sequelae and fluid and electrolyte shifts that are seen in the primary form are also seen in secondary hypokalemic periodic paralysis. Treatment involves the management of the hyperthyroidism, avoidance of high carbohydrate and low potassium meals, and potassium chloride for acute attacks.

Secondary hypokalemic paralysis can also develop if there are marked losses of potassium through the kidneys or through the gastrointestinal tract. It is associated with weakness, which is at times episodic. Potassium levels are much lower than in any other variant. There are many causes of this entity. Therapy of the primary disease with potassium replacement as well as treating acidosis or alkalosis is important in preventing attacks.

Persons who consume large amounts of barium salts, because they block potassium channels, can also develop hypokalemic periodic paralysis. This condition is treated by stopping the barium salts and administering oral potassium.

2. Sodium Channelopathy (Hyperkalemic Periodic Paralysis)

Patients with this type of periodic paralysis are prone to shorter (1–2 h) but more frequent attacks. It is a primary hyperkalemic muscle membrane sodium channelopathy. Although it is dominant, there are multiple allelic mutations. The paralysis is triggered by abnormal inactivation of sodium channels by a mild increase in potassium. Sodium and water flow into the cells with prolonged depolarization. There is hemoconcentration associated with the elevation in serum potassium levels.

The clinical presentation is usually during childhood with early morning episodes, which increase in frequency over time. The episodes are more frequent and worse with rest after strenuous exercise. However, mild exercise prevents paralysis in the same muscles. The frequency of the attacks decreases later in life. Hypothermia, pregnancy, the administration of glucocorticoids, and potassium aggravate the condition. During an attack, the potassium levels usually increase to over 6 mEq/L but remain normal between attacks. Because of the shift of sodium and water into cells, it may also be associated with hyponatremia and hemoconcentration. Other electrolyte shifts have been noted. Hypothermia can induce weakness or make it worse.

Normokalemic periodic paralysis resembles hyperkalemic periodic paralysis and often has the same genotype. They differ in the lack of benefit from glucose, because the potassium level is normal during an episode. Even though potassium levels are normal, these patients can also develop persistent myopathy.

A high potassium level between episodes of weakness suggests a secondary form of the disorder. In these circumstances, the diagnosis is made based on a careful review of the family history, clinical documentation of an elevated potassium level between attacks, and an electromyogram demonstrating myotonia associated with vigorous exercise followed by rest. In this circumstance, therapy is with frequent high-carbohydrate meals, maintenance of a low potassium diet if possible, and avoidance of strenuous activity and cold. Acetazolamide may help prevent attacks. Interestingly, paramyotonia congenita is an allelic variant of the sodium channel mutation.

There is a secondary hyperkalemic disorder seen in persons (men more often than women) with potassium levels over 7 mEq/L. Weakness persists between attacks. There are multiple medical causes, but common to all the hyperkalemic disorders is weakness with rest after exercise. Treatment is targeted toward the primary disease and restriction of potassium.

3. Potassium Channelopathy (Andersen's Syndrome)

Andersen's syndrome is a recently defined, dominantly inherited disorder seen in a group of patients with periodic paralysis and ventricular arrhythmias that are independent of serum potassium. A wide range of forms of cardiac arrhythmias can occur, and there may be dysmorphic features, particularly of the face and head.

Anesthetic Considerations

In patients with periodic paralysis, anesthetic management is directed toward preventing attacks. Careful ECG monitoring is necessary to detect attacks and arrhythmias during anesthesia. Frequent intraoperative measurement of plasma potassium concentration is advisable whenever possible. Glucose-containing intravenous fluids should not be used in patients with hypokalemic paralysis, whereas such solutions may benefit patients with hyperkalemic and normokalemic paralysis (see above). Neuromuscular function should be carefully monitored during general anesthesia. In patients with periodic paralysis, the response to NMBAs is unpredictable. Increased sensitivity to nondepolarizing NMBAs is particularly apt to be encountered in patients with hypokalemic periodic paralysis. Succinylcholine is contraindicated in hyperkalemic paralysis and perhaps other variants as well because of the risk of hyperkalemia. Because shivering and hypothermia may trigger attacks, maintenance of core temperature intraoperatively is important (see Chapter 6).

CASE DISCUSSION: ANESTHESIA FOR MUSCLE BIOPSY

A 16-year-old boy with progressive proximal muscle weakness is suspected of having a primary myopathy and is scheduled for biopsy of the quadriceps muscle.

What other potential abnormalities should concern the anesthesiologist?

The diagnosis of myopathy can be difficult to make and the differential diagnosis may include any one of several hereditary, inflammatory, endocrine, metabolic, or toxic disorders. A muscle biopsy may be necessary to supplement clinical, laboratory, nerve conduction, and electromyographic findings and help establish the diagnosis. Although the cause of the myopathy in this case is not yet clear, the clinician must always consider potential problems that can be associated with primary myopathies.

Respiratory muscle involvement should always be suspected in patients with muscle weakness. Pulmonary reserve can be assessed clinically by questions regarding dyspnea and activity level. Pulmonary function tests are indicated if significant dyspnea on exertion is present. An increased risk of pulmonary aspiration is suggested by a history of dysphagia, regurgitation, recurrent pulmonary infections, or abdominal distention. Cardiac abnormalities may be manifested as arrhythmias, mitral valve prolapse, or cardiomyopathy. A 12-lead electrocardiogram is also helpful in excluding conduction abnormalities. A chest radiograph can evaluate inspiratory effort, the pulmonary parenchyma, and cardiac size; gastric distention secondary to smooth muscle or autonomic dysfunction may also be evident. Preoperative laboratory evaluation should have excluded a metabolic cause with measurement of serum sodium, potassium, magnesium, calcium, and phosphate concentrations. Similarly, thyroid, adrenal, and pituitary disorders should have been excluded. Plasma CK measurement may not be helpful, but very high levels (10 times normal) generally suggest a muscular dystrophy or polymyositis.

What anesthetic technique should be used?

The choice of anesthesia should be based on both patient and surgical requirements. Most muscle biopsies can be performed under local or regional anesthesia with supplemental intravenous sedation, using small doses of midazolam. Because most procedures are performed on an outpatient basis, spinal and epidural anesthesia are often avoided. A femoral nerve block can pro-

vide excellent anesthesia for biopsy of the quadriceps muscle; a separate injection may be necessary for the lateral femoral cutaneous nerve to anesthetize the anterolateral thigh. General anesthesia should be reserved for uncooperative patients or for times when local anesthesia proves to be inadequate. The anesthesiologist must therefore always be prepared with a plan for general anesthesia.

What agents may be safely used for general anesthesia?

The same principles discussed in Chapter 36 should be applied. Major goals include preventing pulmonary aspiration, avoiding excessive respiratory or circulatory depression, avoiding NMBAs if possible, and perhaps avoiding agents known to trigger malignant hyperthermia. A normal response to a previous general anesthetic in the patient or a family member may be reassuring but does not guarantee the same response subsequently. General anesthesia may be induced and maintained with a combination of a barbiturate (thiopental or methohexital), benzodiazepine (midazolam), propofol, or opioid (fentanil) and nitrous oxide. Patients at increased risk for aspiration should be intubated (see above). When an NMBA is necessary, a short-acting nondepolarizing agent (cisatracurium or mivacurium) should be used. Succinylcholine should generally be avoided because of the unknown risk of an unusual response (myotonic contractions, prolonged duration, or phase II block), of inducing severe hyperkalemia, or of triggering malignant hyperthermia.

SUGGESTED READING

Booij LH, Vree TB: Skeletal muscle relaxants: pharmacodynamics and pharmacokinetics in different patient groups. Clin Pract 2000;54:526.

Ichizo N, Eijiro O: Muscular dystrophies. Curr Opin Neurol 2002;15:539.

Mathieu J, Allard P, Gobeil G, et al: Anesthetic and surgical complications in 219 cases of myotonic dystrophy. Neurology 1997;49:1646.

Pourmand R: *Neuromuscular Diseases: Expert Clinician's Views.* Butterworth-Heineman, 2001.

Stoelting RK, Dierdorf SF: *Handbook for Anesthesia and Co-existing Disease,* 2nd ed. Churchill Livingstone, 2002.

Anesthesia for Ophthalmic Surgery   **38**

KEY CONCEPTS

 ① Any factor that normally increases intraocular pressure will tend to decrease intraocular volume by causing drainage of aqueous or extrusion of vitreous through the wound. The latter is a serious complication that can permanently worsen vision.

 ② Succinylcholine increases intraocular pressure by 5–10 mm Hg for 5–10 min after administration, principally through prolonged contracture of the extraocular muscles.

 ③ Traction on extraocular muscles or pressure on the eyeball can elicit a wide variety of cardiac dysrhythmias ranging from bradycardia and ventricular ectopy to sinus arrest or ventricular fibrillation.

 ④ Complications involving the intraocular expansion of gas bubbles can be avoided by discontinuing nitrous oxide at least 15 min prior to the injection of air or sulfur hexafluoride.

 ⑤ Topically applied drugs are absorbed at a rate intermediate between absorption following intravenous and subcutaneous injection.

⑥ Echothiophate is an irreversible cholinesterase inhibitor used in the treatment of glaucoma. Topical application leads to systemic absorption and a reduction in plasma cholinesterase activity. Because succinylcholine and mivacurium are metabolized by this enzyme, echothiophate will prolong their duration of action.

⑦ The key to inducing anesthesia in a patient with an open eye injury is controlling intraocular pressure with a smooth induction. Specifically, coughing during intubation must be avoided by achieving a deep level of anesthesia and profound paralysis.

 ⑧ The postretrobulbar apnea syndrome is probably due to injection of local anesthetic into the optic nerve sheath, with spread into the cerebrospinal fluid.

 ⑨ Regardless of the technique employed for intravenous sedation, ventilation and oxygenation must be carefully monitored, and equipment to provide positive-pressure ventilation must be immediately available.

Eye surgery provides several unique challenges for the anesthesiologist, including regulation of intraocular pressure, prevention of the oculocardiac reflex, management of its consequences, control of intraocular gas expansion, and the need to deal with the possible systemic effects of ophthalmic drugs. An understanding of the mechanisms and management of these potential problems can favorably influence surgical outcome. This chapter also considers specific techniques of general and regional anesthesia in ophthalmic surgery.

INTRAOCULAR PRESSURE DYNAMICS

Physiology of Intraocular Pressure

The eye can be considered a hollow sphere with a rigid wall. If the contents of the sphere increase, the **intraocular pressure** (normal: 12–20 mm Hg) must rise. For example, glaucoma is caused by an obstruction to aqueous humor outflow. Similarly, intraocular pressure will rise if the volume of blood within the globe is increased. A rise in venous pressure will increase intraocular pres-

Table 38–1. The effect of cardiac and respiratory variables on intraocular pressure (IOP).[1]

Variable	Effect on IOP
Central venous pressure	
Increase	↑↑↑
Decrease	↓↓↓
Arterial blood pressure	
Increase	↑
Decrease	↓
Pa_{CO_2}	
Increase (hypoventilation)	↑↑
Decrease (hyperventilation)	↓↓
Pa_{O_2}	
Increase	0
Decrease	↑

[1]↓, decrease (mild, moderate, marked); ↑, increase (mild, moderate, marked); 0, no effect.

sure by decreasing aqueous drainage and increasing choroidal blood volume. Extreme changes in arterial blood pressure and ventilation can also affect intraocular pressure (Table 38–1). Any anesthetic event that alters these parameters can affect intraocular pressure (eg, laryngoscopy, intubation, airway obstruction, coughing, Trendelenburg position).

Alternatively, decreasing the size of the globe without a proportional change in the volume of its contents will increase intraocular pressure. Pressure on the eye from a tightly fitted mask, improper prone positioning, or retrobulbar hemorrhage can lead to marked increases in pressure.

Intraocular pressure helps maintain the shape and therefore the optical properties of the eye. Temporary variations in pressure are usually well tolerated in normal eyes. In fact, blinking raises intraocular pressure by

Table 38–2. Open-eye surgical procedures.

Cataract extraction
Corneal laceration repair
Corneal transplant (penetrating keratoplasty)
Peripheral iridectomy
Removal of foreign body
Ruptured globe repair
Secondary intraocular lens implantation
Trabeculectomy (and other filtering procedures)
Vitrectomy (anterior and posterior)
Wound leak repair

5 mm Hg and squinting by 26 mm Hg. Even transient episodes of increased intraocular pressure in patients with low ophthalmic artery pressure (eg, deliberate hypotension, arteriosclerotic involvement of the retinal artery), however, may jeopardize retinal perfusion and cause retinal ischemia.

When the globe is open during certain surgical procedures (Table 38–2) or after traumatic perforation, intraocular pressure approaches atmospheric pressure. Any factor that normally increases intraocular pressure will tend to decrease intraocular volume by causing drainage of aqueous or extrusion of vitreous through the wound. The latter is a serious complication that can permanently worsen vision.

Effect of Anesthetic Drugs on Intraocular Pressure

Most anesthetic drugs either lower or have no effect on intraocular pressure (Table 38–3). Inhalational anesthetics decrease intraocular pressure in proportion to the depth of anesthesia. The decrease has multiple causes: A drop in blood pressure reduces choroidal volume, relaxation of the extraocular muscles lowers wall tension, and pupillary constriction facilitates aqueous outflow. Intravenous anesthetics also decrease intraocular pressure. A possible exception is ketamine, which usually raises arterial blood pressure and does not relax extraocular muscles.

Topically administered anticholinergic drugs result in pupillary dilation (mydriasis), which may precipitate angle-closure glaucoma. Premedication doses of system-

Table 38–3. The effect of anesthetic agents on intraocular pressure (IOP).[1]

Drug	Effect on IOP
Inhaled anesthetics	
Volatile agents	↓↓
Nitrous oxide	↓
Intravenous anesthetics	
Barbiturates	↓↓
Benzodiazepines	↓↓
Ketamine	?
Opioids	↓
Muscle relaxants	
Depolarizers (succinylcholine)	↑↑
Nondepolarizers	0/↓

[1]↓, decrease (mild, moderate); ↑, increase (mild, moderate); 0/↓, no change or mild decrease; ?, conflicting reports.

ically administered atropine are not associated with intraocular hypertension, however, even in patients with glaucoma. The bulky quaternary ammonium structure of glycopyrrolate may provide an even greater margin of safety by preventing its passage into the central nervous system.

Succinylcholine increases intraocular pressure by 5–10 mm Hg for 5–10 min after administration, principally through prolonged contracture of the extraocular muscles. Unlike other skeletal muscle, extraocular muscles contain cells with multiple neuromuscular junctions. Repeated depolarization of these cells by succinylcholine causes the prolonged contracture. The resulting increase in intraocular pressure may have several effects. It will cause spurious measurements of intraocular pressure during examinations under anesthesia in glaucoma patients, potentially leading to unnecessary surgery. Furthermore, a rise in intraocular pressure may cause extrusion of ocular contents through an open surgical or traumatic wound. A final effect of prolonged contracture of the extraocular muscles is shown as an abnormal forced duction test for 20 min. This maneuver evaluates the cause of extraocular muscle imbalance and may influence the type of strabismus surgery performed. Congestion of choroidal vessels may also contribute to the rise in intraocular pressure. Nondepolarizing muscle relaxants do not increase intraocular pressure.

THE OCULOCARDIAC REFLEX

Traction on extraocular muscles or pressure on the eyeball can elicit a wide variety of cardiac dysrhythmias ranging from bradycardia and ventricular ectopy to sinus arrest or ventricular fibrillation. This reflex, originally described in 1908, consists of a trigeminal afferent (V1) and a vagal efferent pathway. The **oculocardiac reflex** is most common in pediatric patients undergoing strabismus surgery. Nonetheless, it can be evoked in all age groups and during a variety of ocular procedures, including cataract extraction, enucleation, and retinal detachment repair. In awake patients, the oculocardiac reflex may be associated with somnolence and nausea.

Anticholinergic medication is often helpful in preventing the oculocardiac reflex. Intravenous atropine or glycopyrrolate immediately prior to surgery is more effective than intramuscular premedication. It should be remembered that anticholinergic medications can be hazardous in elderly patients, who often have some degree of coronary artery disease. Retrobulbar blockade or deep inhalational anesthesia may also be of value, but these procedures impose risks of their own. Retrobulbar blockade can, in fact, elicit the oculocardiac reflex. The need for any routine prophylaxis is controversial.

Management of the oculocardiac reflex when it occurs consists of the following procedures: (1) immediate notification of the surgeon and temporary cessation of surgical stimulation until heart rate increases; (2) confirmation of adequate ventilation, oxygenation, and depth of anesthesia; (3) administration of intravenous atropine (10 µg/kg) if the conduction disturbance persists; and (4) in recalcitrant episodes, infiltration of the rectus muscles with local anesthetic. The reflex eventually fatigues itself (self-extinguishes) with repeated traction on the extraocular muscles.

INTRAOCULAR GAS EXPANSION

A gas bubble may be injected by the ophthalmologist into the posterior chamber during vitreous surgery. Intravitreal air injection will tend to flatten a detached retina and allow anatomically correct healing. The air bubble is absorbed within 5 days by gradual diffusion through adjacent tissue and into the bloodstream. If the patient is breathing nitrous oxide, the bubble will increase in size. This is because nitrous oxide is 35 times more soluble than nitrogen in blood (see Chapter 7). Thus, it tends to diffuse into an air bubble more rapidly than nitrogen (the major component of air) is absorbed by the bloodstream. If the bubble expands after the eye is closed, intraocular pressure will rise.

Sulfur hexafluoride (SF_6) is an inert gas that is less soluble in blood than is nitrogen—and much less soluble than nitrous oxide. Its longer duration of action (up to 10 days) compared with an air bubble can provide an advantage to the ophthalmologist. Bubble size doubles within 24 h after injection because nitrogen from inhaled air enters the bubble more rapidly than the sulfur hexafluoride diffuses into the bloodstream. Even so, unless high volumes of pure sulfur hexafluoride are injected, the slow bubble expansion does not usually raise intraocular pressure. If the patient is breathing nitrous oxide, however, the bubble will rapidly increase in size and may lead to intraocular hypertension. A 70% inspired nitrous oxide concentration will almost triple the size of a 1-mL bubble and may double the pressure in a closed eye within 30 min. Subsequent discontinuation of nitrous oxide will lead to reabsorption of the bubble, which has become a mixture of nitrous oxide and sulfur hexafluoride. The consequent fall in intraocular pressure may precipitate another retinal detachment.

These complications involving the intraocular expansion of gas bubbles can be avoided by discontinuing nitrous oxide at least 15 min prior to the injection of air or sulfur hexafluoride. Obviously, the amount of time required to eliminate nitrous oxide from the blood will depend on several factors, including fresh gas flow rate and adequacy of alveolar ventilation. Depth of anesthesia should be maintained by substitut-

Table 38–4. Systemic effects of ophthalmic medications.

Drug	Mechanism of Action	Effect
Acetylcholine	Cholinergic agonist (miosis)	Bronchospasm, bradycardia, hypotension
Acetazolamide	Carbonic anhydrase inhibitor (decreases IOP[1])	Diuresis, hypokalemic metabolic acidosis
Atropine	Anticholinergic (mydriasis)	Central anticholinergic syndrome[2]
Cyclopentolate	Anticholinergic (mydriasis)	Disorientation, psychosis, convulsions
Echothiophate	Cholinesterase inhibitor (miosis, decreases IOP)	Prolongation of succinylcholine and mivacurium paralysis, bronchospasm
Epinephrine	Sympathetic agonist (mydriasis, decreases IOP)	Hypertension, bradycardia, tachycardia, headache
Phenylephrine	α-Adrenergic agonist (mydriasis, vasoconstriction)	Hypertension, tachycardia, dysrythmias
Scopolamine	Anticholinergic (mydriasis, vasoconstriction)	Central anticholinergic syndrome[2]
Timolol	β-Adrenergic blocking agent (decreases IOP)	Bradycardia, asthma, congestive heart failure

[1]IOP, intraocular pressure.
[2]See Chapter 11 Case Discussion.

ing other anesthetic agents. Nitrous oxide should be avoided until the bubble is absorbed (5 days after air and 10 days after sulfur hexafluoride injection).

SYSTEMIC EFFECTS OF OPHTHALMIC DRUGS

Topically applied eye drops are absorbed by vessels in the conjunctival sac and the nasolacrimal duct mucosa (see Case Discussion, Chapter 11). One drop (typically 1/20 mL) of 10% phenylephrine contains 5 mg of drug. Compare this with the intravenous dose of phenylephrine (0.05–0.1 mg) used to treat an adult patient with hypotension. Topically applied drugs are absorbed at a rate intermediate between absorption following intravenous and subcutaneous injection (the toxic subcutaneous dose of phenylephrine is 10 mg). Children and the elderly are at particular risk for the toxic effects of topically applied medications and should receive at most a 2.5% phenylephrine solution (Table 38–4). Coincidentally, these patients are most apt to require eye surgery.

Echothiophate is an irreversible cholinesterase inhibitor used in the treatment of glaucoma. Topical application leads to systemic absorption and a reduction in plasma cholinesterase activity. **Because succinylcholine and mivacurium are metabolized by this enzyme, echothiophate will prolong their duration of action.** Paralysis usually does not exceed 20 or 30 min, however, and postoperative apnea is unlikely (see Chapter 9). The inhibition of cholinesterase activity lasts for 3–7 weeks after discontinuation of echothiophate drops. Muscarinic side

effects—such as bradycardia during induction—can be prevented with intravenous anticholinergic drugs (eg, atropine, glycopyrrolate).

Epinephrine eye drops can cause hypertension, tachycardia, and ventricular dysrhythmias; the dysrhythmogenic effects are potentiated by halothane. Direct instillation of epinephrine into the anterior chamber of the eye has not been associated with cardiovascular toxicity.

Timolol, a nonselective β-adrenergic antagonist, reduces intraocular pressure by decreasing production of aqueous humor. Topically applied timolol eye drops, commonly used to treat glaucoma, have in rare cases been associated with atropine-resistant bradycardia, hypotension, and bronchospasm during general anesthesia.

GENERAL ANESTHESIA FOR OPHTHALMIC SURGERY

The choice between general and local anesthesia should be made jointly by the patient, anesthesiologist, and surgeon. Some patients refuse to consider local anesthesia due to fear of being awake during a surgical procedure or the recollection of pain during prior regional techniques. Although there is no conclusive evidence that any one form of anesthesia is safer, local anesthesia seems to be less stressful. General anesthesia is indicated in children and uncooperative patients, as even small head movements can prove disastrous during microsurgery. Local-general anesthesia—a technique of deep sedation with questionable airway control—should be avoided because it imposes the combined risks of both local and general anesthesia.

PREMEDICATION

Patients undergoing eye surgery may be apprehensive, particularly if they have undergone multiple procedures and there is a possibility of permanent blindness. Pediatric patients often have associated congenital disorders (eg, rubella syndrome, Goldenhar's syndrome, Down syndrome). Adult patients are usually elderly, with myriad systemic illnesses (eg, hypertension, diabetes mellitus, coronary artery disease). These factors must all be considered when selecting premedication.

INDUCTION

The choice of induction technique for eye surgery usually depends more on the patient's other medical problems than on the patient's eye disease or the type of surgery contemplated. One exception is the patient with a ruptured globe. The key to inducing anesthesia in a patient with an open eye injury is controlling intraocular pressure with a smooth induction. Specifically, coughing during intubation must be avoided by achieving a deep level of anesthesia and profound paralysis. The intraocular pressure response to laryngoscopy and endotracheal intubation can be somewhat blunted by prior administration of intravenous lidocaine (1.5 mg/kg) or an opioid (eg, remifentanil 0.5–1 µg/kg or alfentanil 20 µg/kg). A nondepolarizing muscle relaxant is used instead of succinylcholine because of the latter's influence on intraocular pressure. Most patients with open globe injuries have full stomachs and require a rapid-sequence induction technique (see Case Discussion below).

MONITORING & MAINTENANCE

Eye surgery necessitates positioning the anesthesiologist away from the patient's airway, making close monitoring of pulse oximetry and the capnograph particularly important for all ophthalmological procedures. Kinking of the endotracheal tube, breathing-circuit disconnections, and unintentional extubation may be more likely. Kinking and obstruction can be minimized by using a reinforced or preformed right-angle endotracheal tube (see Figure 39–1). The possibility of arrhythmias caused by the oculocardiac reflex increases the importance of constantly scrutinizing the electrocardiograph and making sure the pulse tone is audible. In contrast to most other types of pediatric surgery, infant body temperature often rises during ophthalmic surgery

because of head-to-toe draping and insignificant body-surface exposure. End-tidal CO_2 analysis helps differentiate this from malignant hyperthermia.

The pain and stress evoked by eye surgery are considerably less than during a major intraabdominal procedure. A lighter level of anesthesia would be satisfactory if the consequences of patient movement were not so catastrophic. The lack of cardiovascular stimulation inherent in most eye procedures combined with the need for adequate anesthetic depth can result in hypotension in elderly individuals. This problem is usually avoided by ensuring adequate intravenous hydration, administering small doses of ephedrine (2–5 mg), or establishing intraoperative paralysis with nondepolarizing muscle relaxants. The latter allows maintenance of a lighter level of anesthesia.

Emesis caused by vagal stimulation is a common postoperative problem, particularly following strabismus surgery. The Valsalva effect and the increase in central venous pressure that accompany vomiting can be detrimental to the surgical result and increase the risk of aspiration. Intraoperative administration of intravenous metoclopramide (10 mg in adults) or a 5-HT$_3$ antagonist (eg, ondansetron 4 mg in adults) decreases the incidence of postoperative nausea and vomiting (PONV). Antiemetics should generally be given to patients receiving opioids and those with a history of PONV. Dexamethasone (4 mg in adults) should also be considered for patients with a strong history of PONV.

EXTUBATION & EMERGENCE

Although modern suture materials and wound-closure techniques decrease the risk of postoperative wound dehiscence, a smooth emergence from general anesthesia is still desirable. Coughing while on the endotracheal tube can be prevented by extubating the patient during a moderately deep level of anesthesia. As the end of the surgical procedure approaches, muscle relaxation is reversed and spontaneous respirations return. Anesthetic agents may be continued during suction of the airway. Nitrous oxide is then discontinued, and intravenous lidocaine (1.5 mg/kg) can be given to blunt cough reflexes temporarily. Extubation proceeds 1–2 min after the lidocaine and during spontaneous respiration of 100% oxygen. Proper airway control is crucial until the patient's cough and swallowing reflexes return. Obviously, this technique is not suitable in patients at increased risk for aspiration (see Case Discussion below).

Severe postoperative pain is unusual following eye surgery. Scleral buckling procedures, enucleation, and ruptured-globe repair are the most painful operations. Small doses of intravenous narcotics (eg, 15–25 mg of meperidine for an adult) are usually sufficient. Severe pain may signal intraocular hypertension, corneal abrasion, or other surgical complications.

Figure 38–1. A: During administration of a retrobulbar block, the patient looks supranasally as a needle is advanced 1.5 cm along the inferotemporal wall of the orbit. ***B:*** The needle is then redirected upward and nasally toward the apex of the orbit and advanced until its tip penetrates the muscle cone.

■ REGIONAL ANESTHESIA FOR OPHTHALMIC SURGERY

Regional anesthesia for eye surgery has traditionally consisted of a **retrobulbar or peribulbar block,** a facial nerve block, and intravenous sedation. Although less invasive than general anesthesia with endotracheal intubation and less likely to be associated with postoperative nausea, local anesthesia is not without possible complications. In addition, the block may not provide adequate akinesia or analgesia of the eye, or the patient may be unable to lie perfectly still for the duration of the surgery. For these reasons, equipment and personnel required to treat the complications of local anesthesia and to induce general anesthesia must be readily available. At one time, the term local-standby described the anesthesiologist's role in these cases. This term has now been replaced by monitored anesthesia care, as the anesthesiologist should be continually monitoring the patient during surgery and not just standing by.

RETROBULBAR BLOCKADE

In this technique, local anesthetic is injected behind the eye into the cone formed by the extraocular muscles (Figure 38–1). A blunt-tipped 25-gauge needle penetrates the lower lid at the junction of the middle and lateral one-third of the orbit (usually 0.5 cm medial to the lateral canthus). The patient is instructed to stare supranasally as the needle is advanced 3.5 cm toward the apex of the muscle cone. After aspiration to preclude intravascular injection, 2–5 mL of local anesthetic is injected and the needle is removed. Choice of local anesthetic varies, but lidocaine 2% and bupivacaine 0.75% are most common. Ropivacaine may be used instead of bupivacaine. Addition of epinephrine (1:200,000 or 1:400,000) may reduce bleeding and prolongs the anesthesia. Hyaluronidase, a hydrolyzer of connective tissue polysaccharides, is frequently added (3–7 U/mL) to enhance the retrobulbar spread of the local anesthetic. A successful retrobulbar block is accompanied by anesthesia, akinesia, and abolishment of the oculocephalic reflex (ie, a blocked eye does not move during head turning).

Complications of retrobulbar injection of local anesthetics include retrobulbar hemorrhage, globe perforation (particularly of eyes with an axial length greater than 26 mm), optic nerve atrophy, frank convulsions, oculocardiac reflex, acute neurogenic pulmonary edema, trigeminal nerve block, and respiratory arrest. Forceful injection of local anesthetic into the ophthalmic artery causes retrograde flow toward the brain and may result in an instantaneous seizure. The postretrobulbar apnea syndrome is probably due to injection of local anesthetic into the optic nerve sheath, with spread into the cerebrospinal fluid. The central nervous system is exposed to high concentrations of local anesthetic, leading to apprehension and unconsciousness. Apnea occurs within 20 min and resolves within an hour. In the meantime, treatment is supportive, with positive-pressure ventilation to prevent hypoxia, bradycardia, and cardiac arrest. Adequacy of ventilation must be constantly monitored in patients who have received retrobulbar anesthesia.

Retrobulbar injection is usually not performed in patients with bleeding disorders (because of the risk of retrobulbar hemorrhage), extreme myopia (the longer globe increases the risk of perforation), or an open eye injury (the pressure from injecting fluid behind the eye may cause extrusion of intraocular contents through the wound).

PERIBULBAR BLOCKADE

In contrast to retrobulbar blockade, with peribulbar blockade the needle does not penetrate the cone formed by the extraocular muscles. Both techniques achieve akinesia of the eye equally well. Advantages of the peribulbar technique may include less risk of eye penetration, optic nerve and artery, and less pain on injection. Disadvantages include a slower onset and an increased likelihood of ecchymosis.

The block is performed with the patient supine and looking directly ahead. After topical anesthesia of the conjunctiva, one or two transconjunctival injections are given. As the eyelid is retracted, an inferotemporal injection is given halfway between the lateral canthus and the lateral limbus. The needle is advanced under the globe parallel to the orbital floor and when it passes the equator of the eye it is directed slightly medial (20°) and cephalad (10°). Five milliliters of anesthetic is injected. To ensure akinesia, a second 5-mL injection may be given through the conjunctiva on the nasal side, medial to the caruncle and directed straight back

parallel to the medial orbital wall pointing slightly cephalad (20°).

Sub-Tenon Block

Tenon's fascia surrounds the globe and extraocular muscles. Local anesthetic injected beneath it diffuses into the retrobulbar space. A special blunt 25-mm or 19-gauge curved cannula is used for a sub-Tenon block. After topical anesthesia, the conjunctiva is lifted along with Tenon's fascia in the inferonasal quadrant with forceps. A small nick is then made with blunt-tipped Westcott scissors, which are then slid underneath to create a path in Tenon's fascia that follows the contour of the globe and extends past the equator. While the eye is still fixed with forceps the cannula is inserted and 3–4 mL of local anesthetic is injected. Complications with the sub-Tenon blocks are significantly less than with retrobulbar and peribulbar techniques, but rare reports of globe perforation, hemorrhage, cellulitis, permanent visual loss, and local anesthetic spread into cerebrospinal fluid exist.

FACIAL NERVE BLOCK

A facial nerve block prevents squinting of the eyelids during surgery and allows placement of a lid speculum. There are several techniques of facial nerve block: van Lint, Atkinson, and O'Brien (Figure 38–2). The major complication of these blocks is subcutaneous hemorrhage. Another procedure, Nadbath's technique, blocks the facial nerve as it exits the stylomastoid foramen under the external auditory canal, in close proximity to the vagus and glossopharyngeal nerves. This block is not recommended because it has been associated with vocal cord paralysis, laryngospasm, dysphagia, and respiratory distress.

TOPICAL ANESTHESIA

Over the past several years, less traumatic local anesthetic techniques have evolved for anterior chamber (eg, cataract) and glaucoma surgeries. An increasing trend has been to eliminate anesthetic injections altogether. After topical instillation of anesthetic drops, 0.5% proparacaine (also known as proxymetacaine chlorhydrate), repeated at 5-min intervals for five applications, an anesthetic gel (lidocaine chlorhydrate plus 2% methylcellulose) is applied with a cotton swab to the inferior and superior conjunctival sacs. Ophthalmic 0.5% tetracaine may also be used. Use of topical anesthesia is not appropriate for posterior chamber surgery (eg, retinal detachment repair with a buckle) and works best for surgeons with a fast but gentle surgical technique who do not require akinesia of the eye.

Figure 38–2. There are many techniques of facial nerve block, including (1) van Lint, (2) Atkinson, and (3) O'Brien.

INTRAVENOUS SEDATION

Several techniques of intravenous sedation are available for eye surgery. The particular drug used is less important than the dose. Deep sedation should be avoided because it increases the risk of apnea and unintentional patient movement during surgery. On the other hand, retrobulbar and facial nerve blocks can be quite uncomfortable. As a compromise, some anesthesiologists administer a small dose of propofol (30–100 mg slowly) or a short-acting barbiturate (eg, 10–20 mg of methohexital or 25–75 mg of thiopental) to produce a brief state of unconsciousness during the regional block. Alternatively, a small bolus of an opioid (remifentanil 0.1–0.5 µg/kg or alfentanil 375–500 µg) allows a brief period of intense analgesia. Other anesthesiologists, believing that the risks of respiratory arrest and aspiration are unacceptable, limit doses to provide only minimal relaxation and amnesia. Midazolam (1–2 mg) with or without fentanyl (12.5–25 µg) or sufentanil (2.5–5 µg) is a common regimen. Doses vary considerably among patients and should be administered in small increments. Moreover, concomitant use of more than one type of drug (benzodiazepine, hypnotic, and opioid) potentiates the effects of other agents; doses must

be reduced accordingly. An antiemetic should probably be administered if an opioid is used. Regardless of the technique employed, ventilation and oxygenation must be carefully monitored, and equipment to provide positive-pressure ventilation must be immediately available.

CASE DISCUSSION: AN APPROACH TO A PATIENT WITH AN OPEN EYE & A FULL STOMACH

A 12-year-old boy arrives at the emergency room after being shot in the eye with a pellet gun. A brief examination by the ophthalmologist reveals intraocular contents presenting at the wound. The boy is scheduled for emergency repair of the ruptured globe.

What should be stressed in the preoperative evaluation of this patient?

Aside from taking a routine history and performing a physical examination, the time of last oral intake before or after the injury should be established as accurately as possible. The patient must be considered to have a full stomach if the injury occurred within 8 h after the last meal, even if the patient did not eat for several hours after the injury: gastric emptying is delayed by the pain and anxiety that follow trauma.

What is the significance of a full stomach in a patient with an open globe injury?

Managing patients who have sustained penetrating eye injuries provides a challenge to anesthesiologists because of the need to develop an anesthetic plan that is consistent with at least two conflicting objectives. One obvious objective is to prevent further damage to the eye by avoiding increases in intraocular pressure. A second important objective is to prevent pulmonary aspiration in a patient with a full stomach.

Many of the common strategies used to achieve these objectives are in direct conflict with one another, however (Tables 38–5 and 38–6). For example, although regional anesthesia (eg, retrobulbar block) minimizes the risk of aspiration pneumonia, it is relatively contraindicated

Table 38–5. Strategies to prevent increases in intraocular pressure (IOP).

Avoid direct pressure on the globe
    Patch eye with Fox shield
    No retrobulbar or peribulbar injections
    Careful face mask technique
Avoid increases in central venous pressure
    Prevent coughing during induction and intubation
    Ensure a deep level of anesthesia and relaxation
        prior to laryngoscopy[1]
    Avoid head-down positions
    Extubate deeply asleep[1]
Avoid pharmacological agents that increase IOP
    Succinylcholine
    Ketamine (?)

---

[1]These strategies are not recommended for patients with full stomachs.

in patients with penetrating eye injuries because injecting local anesthetic behind the globe increases intraocular pressure and may lead to expulsion of intraocular contents. Therefore, these patients require general anesthesia—despite the increased risk of aspiration pneumonia.

What preoperative preparation should be considered in this patient?

The goal of preoperative preparation is to minimize the risk of aspiration pneumonia by decreasing gastric volume and acidity (see Case Discussion, Chapter 15). Aspiration in patients with eye injuries is prevented by proper selection of pharmacological agents and anesthetic techniques. Evacuation of gastric contents with a nasogastric tube may lead to coughing, retching, and other responses that can dramatically increase intraocular pressure.

Metoclopramide increases lower esophageal sphincter tone, speeds gastric emptying, lowers gastric fluid volume, and exerts an antiemetic effect. It should be given intravenously (10 mg) as soon as possible and repeated every 2–4 h until surgery.

Ranitidine (50 mg intravenously), cimetidine (300 mg intravenously), and famotidine (20 mg intravenously) are H_2-histamine–receptor antagonists that inhibit gastric acid secretion. Because they have no effect on the pH of gastric secretions present in the stomach prior to their administration, they have limited value in patients presenting for emergency surgery.

Unlike H_2-receptor antagonists, antacids have an immediate effect. Unfortunately, they increase intragastric volume. Nonparticulate antacids (preparations of sodium citrate, potassium citrate, and citric acid) lose effectiveness within 30–60 min and should be given immediately prior to induction (15–30 mL orally).

Which induction agents are recommended in patients with penetrating eye injuries?

The ideal induction agent for patients with full stomachs would provide a rapid onset of action in order to minimize the risk of regurgitation. Ketamine, thiopental, propofol, and etomidate have essentially equally rapid onsets of action (ie, one-arm-to-brain circulation time).

Furthermore, the ideal induction agent would not increase the risk of ocular expulsion by raising intraocular pressure. (In fact, most intravenous induction agents lower intraocular pressure.) Although investigations of the effects of ketamine on intraocular pressure have provided conflicting results, ketamine is not recommended in penetrating eye injuries owing to the high rate of blepharospasm and nystagmus.

Although etomidate may prove valuable in some patients with cardiac disease, it is associated with an incidence of myoclonus ranging from 10% to 60%. An episode of severe myoclonus may have contributed to complete retinal detachment and vitreous prolapse in one pa-

Table 38–6. Strategies to prevent aspiration pneumonia.

Regional anesthesia with minimal sedation[1]
Premedication
    Metoclopramide
    Histamine H_2-receptor antagonists
    Nonparticulate antacids
Evacuation of gastric contents
    Nasogastric tube[1]
Rapid-sequence induction
    Cricoid pressure
    A rapid-acting induction agent
    Succinylcholine,[1] rocuronium, or rapacuronium
    Avoidance of positive-pressure ventilation
    Intubation as soon as possible
Extubation awake

---

[1]These strategies are not recommended for patients with penetrating eye injuries.

tient with an open globe injury and limited cardiovascular reserve.

Propofol and thiopental have a rapid onset of action and decrease intraocular pressure; however, neither prevents the hypertensive response to laryngoscopy and intubation or prevents the increase in intraocular pressure that accompanies laryngoscopy and intubation. Prior administration of fentanyl (1–3 μg/kg), remifentanil (0.5–1 μg/kg), alfentanil (20 μg/kg), esmolol (0.5–1 mg/kg), or lidocaine (1.5 mg/kg) attenuates this response with varying degrees of success.

How does the choice of muscle relaxant differ between these patients and other patients at risk for aspiration?

The choice of muscle relaxant in patients with penetrating eye injuries has provided controversy for more than three decades. Succinylcholine definitely increases intraocular pressure. Although there is conflicting research, it is probably most prudent to conclude that this rise in pressure is not consistently and reliably prevented by pretreatment with a nondepolarizing agent, self-taming doses of succinylcholine, or lidocaine. Contradictory findings by various investigators using different regimens are probably due to differences in doses and timing of the pretreatment drugs.

Some anesthesiologists argue that the relatively small and transient rise in intraocular pressure caused by succinylcholine is insignificant when compared with changes caused by laryngoscopy and intubation. They claim that a slight rise in intraocular pressure is a small price to pay for two distinct advantages that succinylcholine offers: a rapid onset of action that decreases the risk of aspiration, and profound muscle relaxation that decreases the chance of a Valsalva response during intubation. Furthermore, advocates of succinylcholine usually point to the lack of case reports documenting further eye injury when succinylcholine has been used.

Nondepolarizing muscle relaxants do not increase intraocular pressure. Until the release of rocuronium, however, nondepolarizing agents did not provide a rapid enough onset of action. Regardless of the muscle relaxant chosen, intubation should not be attempted until a level of paralysis is achieved that will definitely prevent coughing on the endotracheal tube.

How do induction strategies vary in pediatric patients without an intravenous line?

A hysterical child with a penetrating eye injury and a full stomach provides an anesthetic challenge for which there is no perfect solution. Once again, the dilemma is due to the need to avoid increases in intraocular pressure yet minimize the risk of aspiration. For example, screaming and crying can lead to tremendous increases in intraocular pressure. Attempting to sedate children with rectal suppositories or intramuscular injections, however, often heightens their state of agitation and may worsen the eye injury. Similarly, although preoperative sedation may increase the risk of aspiration by obtunding airway reflexes, it is often necessary for establishing an intravenous line for a rapid-sequence induction. An ideal strategy would be to administer enough sedation painlessly to allow placement of an intravenous line yet maintain a level of consciousness adequate to protect airway reflexes. Although this solution is currently hard to achieve, the introduction of new drugs and innovative delivery systems, such as opioid-containing lollipops, may provide some acceptable alternatives. In the meantime, the prudent strategy is to do everything possible to avoid aspiration—even at the cost of further eye damage.

Are there special considerations during extubation and emergence?

Patients at risk for aspiration during induction are also at risk during extubation and emergence. Therefore, extubation must be delayed until the patient is awake and has intact airway reflexes (eg, spontaneous swallowing and coughing on the endotracheal tube). Deep extubation increases the risk for vomiting and aspiration. Intraoperative administration of antiemetic medication and nasogastric tube suctioning may decrease the incidence of emesis during emergence, but they do not guarantee an empty stomach.

SUGGESTED READING

Dell R, Williams B: Anaesthesia for strabismus surgery: A regional survey. Br J Anaesth 1999;82:761. This paper deals with the effect of succinylcholine on the forced duction test.

Gomez RS, Andrade LOF, Costa JRR: Brainstem anesthesia after peribulbar anesthesia. Can J Anaesth 1997;44:732. Peribulbar anesthesia may be safer than retrobulbar block, but serious complications can still occur.

Johnson RW: Anatomy for ophthalmic anaesthesia. Br J Anaesth 1995;75:80. A comprehensive review of the orbit and its contents.

Kumar C, Dodds C, Fanning G: *Ophthalmic Anesthesia.* Netherlands: Swetts and Zeitlinger, 2002.

McGoldrick KE (editor): *Anesthesia for Ophthalmic and Otolaryngologic Surgery.* W.B. Saunders, 1992.

Rosenfeld SI, Litinsky SM, Snyder DA, et al: Effectiveness of monitored anesthesia care in cataract surgery. Ophthalmology 1999;106:1256. The presence of anesthesia personnel during monitored anesthesia care for cataract surgery appeared warranted in this study.

Schein OD, Katz J, Bass EB, et al: The value of routine preoperative medical testing before cataract surgery. N Engl J Med 2000;342:168. A review of almost 20,000 cataract surgeries revealed no effect of routine preoperative medical testing on perioperative morbidity or mortality.

Smith GB: *Ophthalmic Anaesthesia: A Practical Handbook,* 2nd ed. Oxford University Press, 1996. An overview from the British perspective.

Anesthesia for Otorhinolaryngological Surgery

39

KEY CONCEPTS

 The anesthetic goals for endoscopy include profound muscle paralysis to provide masseter muscle relaxation for introduction of the suspension laryngoscope and an immobile surgical field, adequate oxygenation and ventilation during surgical manipulation of the airway, and cardiovascular stability during periods of rapidly varying surgical stimulation.

 It is crucial to monitor chest wall motion constantly and to allow sufficient time for exhalation to avoid air trapping and barotrauma.

 The greatest fear during laser airway surgery is a tracheal tube fire. This can be avoided by using a technique of ventilation that does not involve a flammable tube or catheter (eg, intermittent apnea or jet ventilation through the laryngoscope side port).

 Techniques to minimize intraoperative blood loss include supplementation with cocaine or an epinephrine-containing local anesthetic, maintaining a slightly head-up position, and providing a mild degree of controlled hypotension.

 As always, if there is serious doubt regarding potential airway problems, an intravenous induction should be avoided in favor of awake direct or fiberoptic laryngoscopy (cooperative patient) or an inhalational induction, maintaining spontaneous ventilation (uncooperative patient). In any case, the equipment and personnel required for an emergency tracheostomy must be immediately available.

 The surgeon may request the omission of neuromuscular blocking agents during neck dissection or parotidectomy to identify nerves (eg, spinal accessory, facial nerves) by direct stimulation and to preserve them.

 Manipulation of the carotid sinus and stellate ganglion during radical neck dissection (right side more than the left) has been associated with wide swings in blood pressure, bradycardia, dysrhythmias, sinus arrest, and prolonged QT intervals. Infiltration of the carotid sheath with local anesthetic will usually ameliorate these problems. Bilateral neck dissection may result in postoperative hypertension and loss of hypoxic drive because of denervation of the carotid sinuses and bodies.

 Patients undergoing maxillofacial reconstruction or orthognathic surgical procedures often pose the greatest airway challenges to the anesthesiologist. If there are any anticipated signs of problems with mask ventilation or tracheal intubation, the airway should be secured prior to induction.

 If there is a chance of postoperative edema involving structures that could obstruct the airway (eg, tongue), the patient should be carefully observed and perhaps should be left intubated.

 Nitrous oxide is either entirely avoided during tympanoplasty or discontinued prior to graft placement.

Never are cooperation and communication between surgeon and anesthesiologist more important than during head and neck surgery. Establishing, maintaining, and protecting an airway in the face of abnormal anatomy and simultaneous surgical intervention can test the skills and patience of any anesthesiologist. Clearly, a thorough understanding of airway anatomy (see Chapter 5) and an appreciation of common otorhinolaryngological and maxillofacial procedures will prove invaluable in handling these demanding anesthetic challenges.

ENDOSCOPY

Endoscopy includes laryngoscopy (diagnostic and operative), microlaryngoscopy (laryngoscopy aided by an operating microscope), esophagoscopy, and bronchoscopy (discussed in Chapter 24). Endoscopic procedures may be accompanied by laser surgery.

Preoperative Considerations

Patients presenting for endoscopic surgery are often being evaluated for hoarseness, stridor, or hemoptysis. Possible causes include foreign body aspiration, trauma to the aerodigestive tract, papillomatosis, tracheal stenosis, obstructing tumors, or vocal cord dysfunction. Thus, a meticulous preoperative physical examination and medical history, with particular attention to potential airway problems, must precede any decisions regarding the anesthetic plan. In some patients, flow-volume loops (Chapter 6) or special radiographic studies (eg, tomograms, computed tomography, or magnetic resonance imaging) may be available for review. Many patients will have undergone indirect laryngoscopy by the surgeon in clinic, and the importance of discussing the findings and plans with the surgeon preoperatively cannot be overemphasized.

The most important questions that must be answered are whether the patient will be easy to ventilate with a face mask and easy to intubate with direct laryngoscopy. If either is in doubt, the patient's airway should be secured prior to induction by using an alternative technique such as described in the Chapter 5 Case Discussion (eg, use of a fiberoptic bronchoscope or a tracheostomy under local anesthesia). It should be stressed that even securing an airway with tracheotomy does not necessarily prevent intraoperative airway obstruction due to surgical manipulation and techniques.

Sedative premedication is contraindicated in any patient with any significant degree of upper airway obstruction. Administering glycopyrrolate (0.2–0.3 mg intramuscularly) 1 h before surgery may prove helpful by minimizing secretions, thereby facilitating airway visualization.

Intraoperative Management

The anesthetic goals for endoscopy include profound muscle paralysis to provide masseter muscle relaxation for introduction of the suspension laryngoscope and an immobile surgical field, adequate oxygenation and ventilation during surgical manipulation of the airway, and cardiovascular stability during periods of rapidly varying surgical stimulation.

A. MUSCLE RELAXATION

Intraoperative muscle relaxation can be achieved by either a continuous infusion of succinylcholine or intermittent boluses of intermediate-duration nondepolarizing neuromuscular blocking agents (NMBAs) (eg, rocuronium, vecuronium, cisatracurium). A disadvantage of a succinylcholine drip is the potential of developing a phase II block during unexpectedly long procedures (see Chapter 9). On the other hand, an intermediate-duration nondepolarizing block may prove difficult to reverse and may delay return of protective airway reflexes and extubation. These problems may be avoided by administering an intermittent bolus or continuous infusion of mivacurium or cisatracurium, short-acting nondepolarizing NMBAs. It should be noted that although profound relaxation is needed until the very end of the surgery, rapid recovery is important since endoscopy is often an outpatient procedure.

B. OXYGENATION AND VENTILATION

Several methods have successfully been used to provide oxygenation and ventilation during endoscopy. Most commonly, the patient is intubated with a small-diameter (4.0–6.0 mm) tracheal tube through which conventional positive pressure is administered. Standard tracheal tubes of this size, however, are designed for pediatric patients. They therefore tend to be too short for the adult trachea, with a low-volume cuff that will exert high pressure against it. A 4.0-, 5.0-, or 6.0-mm microlaryngeal tracheal (MLT) tube (Mallinckrodt Critical Care) is the same length as an adult tube, has a disproportionately large high-volume low-pressure cuff, and is stiffer and less prone to compression than a regular tracheal tube. The advantages of intubation include protection against aspiration and the ability to administer inhalational anesthetics and to continuously monitor end-tidal CO_2.

In some cases (eg, those involving the posterior commissure), intubation with a tracheal tube may interfere with the surgeon's visualization or performance of the procedure. A simple alternative is insufflation of high flows of oxygen through a small catheter placed in the trachea. Although oxygenation may be maintained for brief periods in patients with good lung function, ventilation is inadequate for longer procedures unless the patient is allowed to breathe spontaneously.

Another possibility is the intermittent-apnea technique, in which periods of ventilation with oxygen by face mask or tracheal tube alternate with periods of apnea, during which the surgery is performed. The duration of apnea, usually 2–3 min, is determined by how well the patient maintains oxygen saturation as measured by a pulse oximeter. Hypoventilation with hypercarbia and pulmonary aspiration are risks of this technique.

A more sophisticated approach involves connecting a manual jet ventilator to a side port of the laryngoscope. During inspiration (1–2 s), a high-pressure (30–50 psi) source of oxygen is directed through the glottic opening and entrains room air into the lungs (Venturi effect). Expiration (4–6 s duration) is passive. It is crucial to monitor chest wall motion constantly and to allow sufficient time for exhalation to avoid air trapping and barotrauma. A variation of this technique is high-frequency jet ventilation, which utilizes a small cannula or tube in the trachea, through which gas is injected 80–300 times per minute (see Chapter 49). High-frequency jet ventilation requires an intravenous anesthetic. Capnography will tend to greatly underestimate the $PaCO_2$ during jet ventilation due to constant and sizable dilution of alveolar gases.

C. CARDIOVASCULAR STABILITY

Blood pressure and heart rate often fluctuate strikingly during endoscopic procedures for two reasons. First, many of these patients have a long history of heavy tobacco and alcohol use that predisposes them to cardiovascular diseases. In addition, the procedure is, in essence, a series of stress-filled laryngoscopies and intubations, separated by varying periods of minimal surgical stimulation. Attempting to maintain a patient at a constant level of anesthesia invariably results in alternating intervals of hypertension and hypotension. Providing a modest baseline level of anesthesia allows supplementation with short-acting anesthetics (eg, propofol, remifentanil) or sympathetic antagonists (eg, esmolol) as needed during periods of increased stimulation. Alternatively, regional nerve block of the glossopharyngeal nerve and superior laryngeal nerve would minimize intraoperative swings in blood pressure (see Chapter 5, Case Discussion). Invasive monitoring of arterial blood pressure should be considered in patients with a history of hypertension or coronary heart disease, even if the surgeon anticipates a short procedure.

Laser Precautions

Laser (light amplification by stimulated emission of radiation) light differs from ordinary light in three ways: it is monochromatic (ie, it possesses one wavelength), coherent (it oscillates in the same phase), and collimated (it exists as a narrow, parallel beam). These characteristics offer the surgeon excellent precision and hemostasis with minimal postoperative edema or pain. Unfortunately, they also introduce some major hazards into the operating room.

The potential uses and side effects of a laser vary with its wavelength, which is determined by the medium in which the laser beam is generated. For example, a medium of CO_2 gas produces a long wavelength laser (the CO_2 laser has a 10,600-nm wavelength), whereas a medium of yttrium–aluminum–garnet (YAG) gem results in a shorter wavelength (the YAG laser can emit at 1064- or 1320-nm wavelength). As wavelength increases, absorption by water increases and tissue penetration decreases. Thus, the effects of the CO_2 laser are much more localized and superficial than those of the YAG laser.

General precautions include evacuation of toxic fumes (laser plume) from tissue vaporization; these may have the potential to transmit microbacterial diseases. Depending on the wavelength of laser being used, all operating room personnel should wear some type of eye protection, and the patient's eyes should be taped shut.

The greatest fear during laser airway surgery is a tracheal tube fire. This can be avoided by using a technique of ventilation that does not involve a flammable tube or catheter (eg, intermittent apnea or jet ventilation through the laryngoscope side port). Some procedures, however, require a tracheal tube because of the expected duration of the case, location of the lesion, or preexisting lung problems in the patient. In these cases, using a tracheal tube that is relatively resistant to laser ignition may be warranted (Table 39–1). In an

Table 39–1. Advantages and disadvantages of various tracheal tubes for laser airway surgery.

Type of Tube	Advantages	Disadvantages
Polyvinyl chloride	Inexpensive, nonreflective	Low melting point, highly combustible[1]
Red rubber	Puncture-resistant, maintains structure, nonreflective	Highly combustible[1]
Silicone rubber	Nonreflective	Combustible,[1] turns to toxic ash
Metal	Combustion-resistant,[1] kink-resistant	Thick-walled flammable cuff, transfers heat, reflects laser, cumbersome

[1]Combustibility depends on fraction of inspired oxygen and laser energy.

Table 39–2. Disadvantages of wrapping a tracheal tube with metallic tape.

No cuff protection
Adds thickness to tube
Not an FDA-approved device
Protection varies with type of metal foil
Adhesive backing may ignite
May reflect laser onto nontargeted tissue
Rough edges may damage mucosal surfaces

effort to protect tracheal tubes from laser ignition, tubes can be wrapped with a variety of metallic tapes; however, they should be used with caution (Table 39–2).

There are commercially available flexible stainless steel tracheal tubes that resist laser strikes. If laser beams hit the tube, they are defocused, decreasing the chance of damage to healthy tissue. There are double cuffs at the distal end to seal the airway. Therefore if the upper cuff is struck by laser and the saline escapes, the lower cuff will continue to seal the airway. The technology for the tube was developed by the National Aeronautics and Space Administration (NASA), another civilian benefit of the space program.

It should be emphasized that no cuffed tracheal tube or any currently available tube protection is completely laser-proof. **Therefore, whenever laser airway surgery is being performed with a tracheal tube in place, the following precautions should be observed:**

- Inspired oxygen concentration should be as low as possible (many patients tolerate an FIO_2 of 21%).

- Nitrous oxide supports combustion and should be replaced with air (nitrogen) or helium.

- The tracheal tube cuffs should be filled with saline dyed with methylene blue to dissipate heat and signal cuff rupture. A cuffed tube will minimize oxygen concentration in the pharynx. The addition of 2% lidocaine jelly (a 1:2 mixture with saline) into the proximal cuff can seal small laser-induced cuff leaks, potentially preventing combustion.

- Laser intensity and duration should be limited as much as possible.

Table 39–3. Airway-fire protocol.

1. Stop ventilation and remove tracheal tube.
2. Turn off oxygen and disconnect circuit from machine.
3. Submerge tube in water.
4. Ventilate with face mask and reintubate.
5. Assess airway damage with bronchoscopy, serial chest x-rays and arterial blood gases.
6. Consider bronchial lavage and steroids.

- Saline-soaked pledgets (completely saturated) should be placed in the airway to limit risk of ignition.

- A source of water (eg, 60-mL syringe) should be immediately available in case of fire.

These precautions limit, but do not eliminate, the risk of an airway fire; anesthesiologists must always be prepared for that eventuality (Table 39–3).

NASAL & SINUS SURGERY

Common nasal and sinus surgeries include polypectomy, endoscopic sinus surgery, maxillary sinusotomy (Caldwell–Luc procedure), rhinoplasty, and septoplasty.

Preoperative Considerations

Patients undergoing nasal or sinus surgery may have a considerable degree of preoperative nasal obstruction caused by polyps, a deviated septum, or mucosal congestion from infection. This may make face mask ventilation difficult, particularly if combined with other causes of difficult ventilation (eg, obesity, maxillofacial deformities).

Nasal polyps are often associated with allergic disorders such as asthma. Patients who also have a history of allergic reactions to aspirin should not be given any nonsteroidal antiinflammatory drugs (eg, ketorolac). Nasal polyps are a common feature of cystic fibrosis.

Because of the rich vascular supply of the nasal mucosa, the preoperative interview should concentrate on questions concerning drug use (eg, aspirin) and any history of bleeding problems.

Intraoperative Management

Many nasal procedures can be satisfactorily performed under local anesthesia with sedation. The anterior ethmoidal nerve and sphenopalatine nerves (see Figure 5–3) provide sensory innervation to the nasal septum and lateral walls. Both can be blocked by packing the nose with gauze or cotton-tipped applicators soaked with local anesthetic. The topical anesthetic should be allowed to remain in place at least 10 min before instrumentation is attempted. Supplementation with submucosal injections of local anesthetic is often required, particularly if scar tissue is present from prior surgery. Use of an epinephrine-containing solution or cocaine (usually a 4% or 10% solution) will shrink the nasal mucosa and potentially decrease intraoperative blood loss. Intranasal cocaine (maximum dose, 3 mg/kg) is rapidly absorbed (reaching peak levels in 30 min) and may cause detrimental cardiovascular effects (see Chapter 14).

General anesthesia is often preferred for nasal surgery because of the discomfort and incomplete block that may accompany topical anesthesia. Special considerations during induction include using an oral airway

Figure 39–1. An oral right-angle endotracheal (RAE) tube has a preformed right-angle bend at the level of the teeth so that it exits the mouth away from the surgical field during ophthalmic or nasal surgery.

during face mask ventilation to mitigate the effects of nasal obstruction, intubation with a reinforced or preformed **right-angle endotracheal** (RAE) tube (eg, an oral RAE tube, Mallinckrodt Critical Care; Figure 39–1), and tucking the patient's padded arms to the side. Because of the proximity of the surgical field, it is important to tape the patient's eyes closed to avoid a **corneal abrasion.** One exception to this is during endoscopic sinus surgery, when the surgeon may wish to periodically check for eye movement during dissec-

tion because of the close proximity of the sinuses and orbit (Figure 39–2). Similarly, NMBAs are strongly suggested because of the potential neurological or ophthalmic complications that might arise if the patient moves during sinus instrumentation.

Techniques to minimize intraoperative blood loss include supplementation with cocaine or an epinephrine-containing local anesthetic, maintaining a slightly head-up position, and providing a mild degree of controlled hypotension. A posterior pharyngeal pack is often placed to limit the risk of aspiration of blood. Despite these precautions, the anesthesiologist must be prepared for significant blood loss, particularly during the resection of vascular tumors (eg, juvenile nasopharyngeal angiofibroma).

Ideally, extubation should be smooth, with a minimum of coughing or straining, as these will increase venous pressure and tend to increase postoperative bleeding. Unfortunately, strategies that accomplish this goal also tend to increase the risk of aspiration (eg, deep extubation).

HEAD & NECK CANCER SURGERY

Surgery for cancer of the head and neck includes laryngectomy, glossectomy, pharyngectomy, parotidectomy, hemimandibulectomy, and radical neck dissection. An endoscopic examination often precedes these procedures, while the timing of a tracheostomy depends on the patient's preoperative airway compromise. Some procedures may include reconstruc-

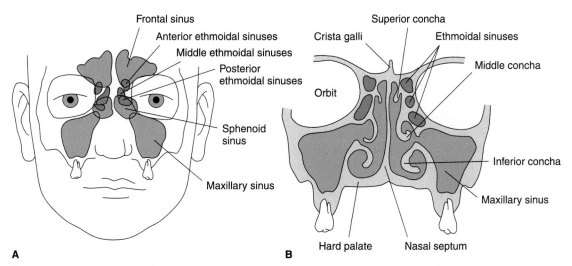

Figure 39–2. The proximity of the sinuses to the orbit (**A,** frontal view; **B,** coronal section) introduces the possibility of orbital fracture during endoscopic sinus surgery. (Reproduced and modified, with permission, from Snell RS, Katz J: *Clinical Anatomy for Anesthesiologists.* Appleton & Lange, 1988.)

tive surgery, such as the transplantation of a free microvascular muscle flap.

Preoperative Considerations

The typical patient presenting for head and neck cancer surgery is elderly and has a long history of heavy tobacco and alcohol use. Preexisting medical conditions that often need preoperative evaluation and optimization include chronic obstructive pulmonary disease, coronary artery disease, chronic alcoholism, aspiration pneumonia, and malnutrition.

Airway management may be complicated by an obstructing lesion or preoperative radiation therapy that has further distorted the patient's anatomy. As always, if there is serious doubt regarding potential airway problems, an intravenous induction should be avoided in favor of awake direct or fiberoptic laryngoscopy (cooperative patient) or an inhalational induction, maintaining spontaneous ventilation (uncooperative patient). In any case, the equipment and personnel required for an emergency tracheostomy must be *immediately* available. Elective tracheostomy under local anesthesia is a prudent option, particularly if indirect laryngoscopy shows that the lesion is susceptible to dislodgment during intubation.

Intraoperative Management

A. Monitoring

Because of the substantial blood loss associated with many of these procedures and the prevalence of coexisting cardiopulmonary disease, these patients often require arterial cannulation for blood pressure, blood gas, and hematocrit monitoring. If a central venous line or pulmonary artery catheter is deemed necessary, antecubital or femoral veins provide the best access. Arterial lines and intravenous cannulas should not be placed in the arms if a radial forearm flap is planned. A minimum of two large-bore intravenous lines should be secured and a urinary catheter (preferably with temperature-monitoring capability) placed. Inspiratory gases should be heated and humidified, and a forced-air warming blanket should be positioned over the lower extremities to help maintain normal body temperature. Intraoperative hypothermia and consequent vasoconstriction can be particularly detrimental for perfusion of a microvascular free flap.

B. Tracheostomy

Intraoperative tracheostomy is often a part of head and neck cancer surgery. During ventilation with 100% oxygen, the tracheal tube and hypopharynx should be thoroughly suctioned to limit the risk of aspiration of blood and secretions. After dissection down to the tra-

chea, the tracheal tube cuff is deflated to avoid perforation by the scalpel. When the tracheal wall is transected, the tracheal tube is withdrawn so that its tip is just cephalad to the incision. Ventilation during this period is difficult because of the large leak through the trachea. A sterile wire-reinforced tracheal tube or J-shaped laryngectomy tube is placed in the trachea, connected to a sterile breathing circuit, and sutured to the chest wall. As soon as correct positioning is confirmed by capnography and chest auscultation, the old tracheal tube may be removed. An increase in peak inspiratory pressure immediately after tracheostomy usually signals a malpositioned tube, bronchospasm, or debris in the trachea.

C. Maintenance of Anesthesia

The surgeon may request the omission of NMBAs during neck dissection or parotidectomy to identify nerves (eg, spinal accessory, facial nerves) by direct stimulation and to preserve them. A mild hypotensive technique may be helpful in limiting blood loss. Cerebral perfusion pressure may be severely compromised, however, when the tumor involves the carotid artery (decreased cerebral arterial pressure) or jugular vein (increased cerebral venous pressure). Furthermore, a head-up tilt may increase the chance of venous air embolism. Following reanastomosis of a microvascular free flap, blood pressure should be maintained at the patient's baseline level. Vasoconstrictive agents (eg, phenylephrine) should be avoided because even though systemic blood pressure increases, flap perfusion decreases due to vasoconstriction of graft vessels. Likewise, vasodilators (eg, sodium nitroprusside or hydralazine) should be avoided due to decreased perfusion pressures.

D. Transfusion

Blood loss can be rapid and substantial. Transfusion decisions must balance the patient's medical problems with the possibility of an increased posttransfusion cancer recurrence rate as a result of immune suppression. Rheological factors make a relatively low hematocrit (eg, 27–30%) desirable when microvascular free flaps are performed. Diuresis should be avoided during microvascular free-flap surgery to allow adequate graft perfusion in the postoperative period.

E. Cardiovascular Instability

Manipulation of the carotid sinus and stellate ganglion during radical neck dissection (the right side more than the left) has been associated with wide swings in blood pressure, bradycardia, arrhythmias, sinus arrest, and prolonged QT intervals. Infiltration of the carotid sheath with local anesthetic will usually ameliorate these problems. Bilateral neck dissection may result in postoperative hypertension and loss of hypoxic drive because of denervation of the carotid sinuses and bodies.

MAXILLOFACIAL RECONSTRUCTION & ORTHOGNATHIC SURGERY

Maxillofacial reconstruction is often required to correct the effects of trauma (eg, LeFort fractures) or developmental malformations, for radical cancer surgeries (eg, mandibulectomy), or for obstructive sleep apnea. Orthognathic procedures (eg, LeFort osteotomies, mandibular osteotomies) for skeletal malocclusion share many of the same surgical and anesthetic techniques.

Preoperative Considerations

Patients undergoing maxillofacial reconstruction or orthognathic surgical procedures often pose the greatest airway challenges to the anesthesiologist. Preoperative airway evaluation must be detailed and thorough. Particular attention should be focused on jaw opening, mask fit, neck mobility, micrognathia, retrognathia, maxillary protrusion (overbite), macroglossia, dental pathology, nasal patency, and the existence of any intraoral lesions or debris. If there are any anticipated signs of problems with mask ventilation or tracheal intubation, the airway should be secured prior to induction. This may involve fiberoptic nasal intubation, fiberoptic oral intubation, or tracheostomy. Nasal intubation with a preformed tube (nasal RAE) or a straight tube with a flexible angle connector (Figure 39–3) is usually preferred in dental and oral surgery. The tracheal tube can then be directed cephalad and connected to breathing tubes coming over the patient's head. On the other hand, nasal intubation should be carefully considered in LeFort II and III fractures because of the possibility of a coexisting basilar skull fracture and cerebrospinal fluid rhinorrhea (Figure 39–4).

Intraoperative Management

Reconstructive and orthognathic surgeries can be associated with substantial blood loss. Strategies to minimize bleeding include a slight head-up position, controlled hypotension, and local infiltration with epinephrine solutions. Because patients' arms are typically tucked at their sides, at least two intravenous lines should be established prior to surgery. This is particularly important if one line is used for delivery of an intravenous anesthetic or hypotensive agent. An arterial line can be helpful during high-blood-loss cases, particularly as a surgeon leaning against the patient's arm may interfere with noninvasive blood pressure cuff readings. An oropharyngeal pack is often placed to minimize the amount of blood and other debris reaching the larynx and trachea.

A

B

Figure 39–3. **A:** A nasal right-angle endotracheal (RAE) tube has a preformed right-angle bend at the level of the nose so that the tube is directed over the forehead. **B:** Alternatively, a regular straight tracheal tube can be cut at the level of the nares and a flexible connector attached.

Because of the proximity of the airway to the surgical field, the anesthesiologist's location is more remote than usual. This increases the likelihood of serious intraoperative airway problems such as tracheal tube kinking, disconnection, or perforation by a surgical instrument. Airway monitoring of end-tidal CO_2, peak inspiratory pressures, and esophageal stethoscope breath sounds assumes increased importance in such cases.

At the end of surgery, the oropharyngeal pack must be removed and the pharynx suctioned. Although it is not unusual for there to be some bloody debris during initial suctioning, repeat efforts should be less produc-

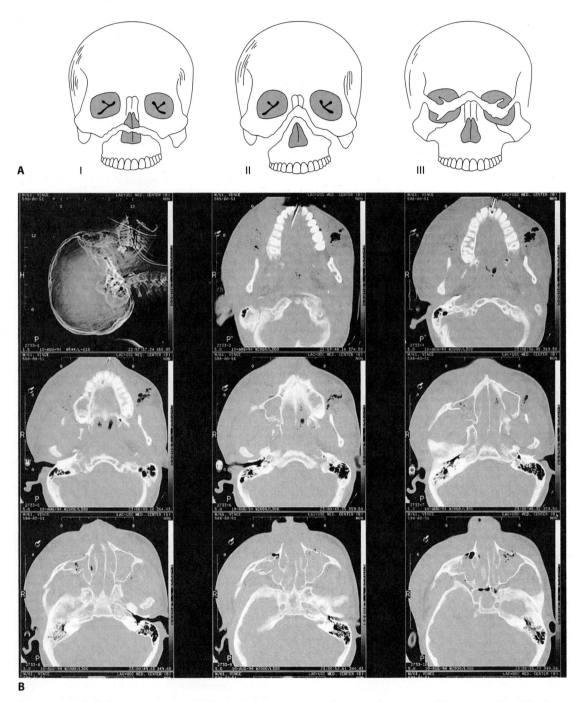

Figure 39–4. **A:** Diagrammatic representation of LeFort I, II, and III fractures. LeFort II and III may coexist with a basilar skull fracture, a contraindication to nasal intubation. **B:** CT scan demonstrating evidence of LeFort II fracture. There is no evidence of basilar skull fracture on these slices.

tive. If there is a chance of postoperative edema involving structures that could potentially obstruct the airway (eg, tongue), the patient should be carefully observed and perhaps should be left intubated. Otherwise, extubation can be attempted once the patient is fully awake and there are no signs of continued bleeding. Patients with intermaxillary fixation (eg, maxillomandibular wiring) should have appropriate cutting tools at their bedside in case of vomiting or other airway emergencies.

EAR SURGERY

Frequently performed ear surgeries include stapedectomy (usually under local anesthesia), tympanoplasty, and mastoidectomy. Myringotomy with insertion of tympanostomy tubes is the most common pediatric surgical procedure and is discussed in Chapter 44.

Intraoperative Management

A. NITROUS OXIDE

Because nitrous oxide is more soluble than nitrogen in blood, it diffuses into air-containing cavities more rapidly than nitrogen (the major component of air) can be absorbed by the bloodstream (see Chapter 7). Normally, changes in middle ear pressures caused by nitrous oxide are well tolerated as a result of passive venting through the eustachian tube. Patients with a history of chronic ear problems (eg, otitis media, sinusitis), however, often suffer from obstructed eustachian tubes and may rarely experience hearing loss or tympanic membrane rupture during nitrous oxide anesthesia.

During tympanoplasty, the middle ear is open to the atmosphere and there is no pressure build-up. Once the surgeon has placed a tympanic membrane graft, the middle ear becomes a closed space. If nitrous oxide is allowed to diffuse into this space, middle ear pressure will rise, and the graft may be displaced. Conversely, discontinuing nitrous oxide after graft placement will create a negative middle ear pressure that could also cause graft dislodgment. Therefore, nitrous oxide is either entirely avoided during tympanoplasty or discontinued prior to graft placement. Obviously, the exact amount of time required to wash out the nitrous oxide depends on many factors, including alveolar ventilation and fresh gas flows (see Chapter 7), but 15–30 min is usually recommended.

B. HEMOSTASIS

As with any form of microsurgery, even small amounts of blood can obscure the operating field. Techniques to minimize blood loss during ear surgery include mild (15°) head elevation, infiltration or topical application of epinephrine (1:50,000–1:200,000), and controlled

hypotension. The use of controlled hypotension in ear surgery is somewhat controversial because of its inherent risks and questionable necessity. Because coughing on a tracheal tube during awakening (particularly during head bandaging) will increase venous pressure and may cause bleeding, a deep extubation may prove helpful.

C. FACIAL NERVE IDENTIFICATION

Preservation of the facial nerve is an important consideration during some types of ear surgery (eg, resection of a glomus tumor or acoustic neuroma). During these cases, intraoperative paralysis with NMBAs may confuse the interpretation of facial nerve stimulation and should be avoided.

D. POSTOPERATIVE NAUSEA AND VOMITING

Because the inner ear is intimately involved with the sense of balance, ear surgery may cause postoperative dizziness (vertigo), nausea, and vomiting. Induction and maintenance with propofol have been shown to decrease postoperative nausea and vomiting in patients undergoing middle ear surgery. Prophylaxis with decadron prior to induction, with administration of a 5-HT$_3$ blocker prior to emergence, should be considered.

Oral Surgical Procedures

Most minor oral surgical procedures are performed under local anesthesia, augmented with varying degrees of intravenous sedation, in a clinic or office setting. If sedation is required or if the procedure is complex, an anesthesiologist can help provide safe, optimal care. For the oral surgeon and anesthesiologist to provide such care, considerable cooperation is required. Typically, a bite block and an oropharyngeal throat pack protect the airway. For light to moderate levels of sedation, the oropharyngeal pack keeps irrigating fluids and dental fragments from entering the airway. Obviously, deep sedation and general anesthesia, if anticipated, require an increased level of airway control by the anesthesiologist. Because the oral surgeon operates in the mouth, thereby limiting access to the airway by the anesthesiologist, the preoperative plan must be adjusted.

Minor oral surgical procedures, such as exodontias, typically last no more than 1 h. The surgical field is amenable to a nerve block or infiltration by a local anesthetic. In adults most oral surgeons use 2% lidocaine with 1/100,000 epinephrine and 0.5% bupivacaine with 1/200,000 epinephrine in quantities no greater than 12 mL and 8 mL, respectively. The anesthesiologist must be informed of the amount of local anesthesia injected by the surgeon so that the allowed dosage based on weight is not exceeded. Pediatric patients, in particular, are at risk for local anesthesia toxicity due to an actual overdose or an inadvertent intravascular injection.

Intravenous sedation during oral surgical procedures greatly increases the patient's comfort and helps create a more favorable operative field. A combination of fentanyl (2–3 µg/kg) and midazolam (20–50 µg/kg) is usually adequate as a loading dose prior to injection of the local anesthetic. The sedation can be further augmented by additional small dosages of fentanyl, midazolam, and propofol. Propofol (20–30 mg is a typical incremental dose for an adult) is a good standby drug if the surgeon requires a brief episode of unconsciousness.

These techniques require a high level of cooperation and participation by both the surgeon and anesthesiologist; if questionable, the patient is probably safer having the procedure performed in a hospital setting with general anesthesia and protection of the airway.

CASE DISCUSSION: BLEEDING FOLLOWING SINUS SURGERY

A 50-year-old man has a paroxysm of coughing in the recovery room while awakening following uneventful endoscopic sinus surgery. Immediately afterward, his respirations appear labored with a loud inspiratory stridor.

What is the differential diagnosis of inspiratory stridor?

The acute onset of inspiratory stridor in a postoperative patient may be due to laryngospasm, laryngeal edema, foreign body aspiration, or vocal cord dysfunction. Laryngospasm, an involuntary spasm of the laryngeal musculature, may be triggered by blood or secretions stimulating the superior laryngeal nerve (see Chapter 5). Laryngeal edema may be caused by an allergic drug reaction, hereditary or iatrogenic angioedema, or a traumatic intubation. Vocal cord dysfunction could be due to residual muscle relaxant effect, hypocalcemic alkalotic tetany, intubation trauma, or paradoxical vocal cord motion (ie, hysterical stridor).

Another paroxysm of coughing is accompanied by hemoptysis. What is your immediate management?

Bleeding after nose or throat surgery can be very serious. Patients who are not fully awake may continue to gag and cough on the secretions, increasing venous pressure and worsening the bleeding. Furthermore, they may aspirate blood and other secretions. Fortunately, because of its physiological pH, aspiration of blood is not as serious as aspiration of acidic gastric contents. Nonetheless, the airway should be immediately secured in the obtunded patient. This may be accomplished with an awake intubation or a rapid-sequence induction.

If the patient is awake and alert enough to cough and swallow and does not appear to be aspirating blood, the first priority should be to decrease the bleeding as quickly as possible. Immediate measures that should be considered include raising the head of the bed to decrease venous and arterial pressures at the site of bleeding and aggressively treating any degree of systolic hypertension with intravenous antihypertensive agents. Sedation should be avoided so that airway reflexes are not compromised.

Despite these measures the bleeding continues, and surgical intervention appears necessary. Describe your strategy for induction of anesthesia in this patient.

Before induction of general anesthesia in a bleeding patient, hypovolemia should be corrected with isotonic crystalloid, or colloid if the patient does not respond to crystalloid. The degree of hypovolemia is difficult to assess because much of the blood may be swallowed, but it may be estimated by changes in vital signs, postural hypotension, and hematocrit. Cross-matched blood should be readily available, and a second large-bore intravenous line secured. It must be appreciated that from an anesthetic standpoint, this is an entirely different patient than the one who presented for surgery initially: the patient now has a full stomach, is hypovolemic, and may prove to be a more difficult intubation.

The preferred technique in this patient is a rapid-sequence induction with cricoid pressure. Drug choice (eg, ketamine, etomidate) and dosage should anticipate the possibility of hypotension from persistent hypovolemia. Personnel and equipment for an emergency tracheostomy should be readily available. An orogastric tube should be passed to decompress the stomach.

Which arteries supply blood to the nose?

The arterial supply of the nose is provided by the internal maxillary artery and the anterior ethmoid artery. These may have to be ligated in uncontrollable epistaxis.

Describe extubation.

Because this patient is still at risk for aspiration, extubation should not be attempted until the patient has fully awakened and regained airway reflexes. Although it is desirable to limit coughing and "bucking" on the tracheal tube during emergence, these are difficult to achieve in the awakening patient. Some authorities suggest the intravenous administration of lidocaine (1.5 mg/kg) during this period.

SUGGESTED READING

Banic A, Krejci V, Erni D, et al: Effects of sodium nitroprusside and phenylephrine on blood flow in free musculocutaneous flaps during general anesthesia. Anesthesiology 1999;90:147. Free flap survival can be greatly influenced by anesthetic management.

Brooker CR, Hunsaker DH, Zimmerman AA: A new anesthetic system for microlaryngeal surgery. Otolaryngol Head Neck Surg 1998;118:55. This system combines a nonflammable tube and a subglottic jet ventilator with special safety features.

Fujii Y, Toyooka H, Tanaka H: Prophylactic antiemetic therapy with a combination of granisetron and dexamethasone in patients undergoing middle ear surgery. Br J Anaesth 1998;81:754. The high incidence of nausea and vomiting following middle ear surgery requires combination antiemetic therapy.

Magnusson L, Lang FJW, Monnier P, Ravussin P: Anaesthesia for tracheal resection: report of 17 cases. Can J Anaesth 1997;44:1282. This paper describes the use of high-frequency jet ventilation for tracheal resection surgery.

McGoldrick KE (editor): *Anesthesia for Ophthalmic and Otolaryngologic Surgery.* W.B. Saunders, 1992. The first 12 chapters of this book are devoted to anesthetic considerations in otolaryngological surgery, including airway anatomy, management of difficult intubations, laser surgery, and emergency surgery.

Rampil IJ: Anesthetic considerations for laser surgery. Anesth Analg 1992;74:424. This article reviews the physics of laser light, clinical applications of laser hardware, laser hazards, and strategies to avoid tracheal tube fires.

Sosis MB (editor): *Anesthesia for Otolaryngologic and Head and Neck Surgery.* Volume 11, No. 3 of Anesth Clin N Am. W.B. Saunders, 1993.

Webster AC, Morley-Forster PK, Janzen V: Anesthesia for intranasal surgery: A comparison between tracheal intubation and the flexible reinforced laryngeal mask airway. Anesth Analg 1999;88:421. The authors demonstrate a lower incidence of laryngospasm, hemoglobin desaturation, and hoarseness following the use of a laryngeal mask airway for intranasal surgery.

Anesthesia for Orthopedic Surgery

Julio Raya, MD, & Maged Mikhail, MD

KEY CONCEPTS

 1 Clinical manifestations of bone cement implantation syndrome include hypoxia (increased pulmonary shunt), hypotension, dysrhythmias (including heart block and sinus arrest), pulmonary hypertension (increased pulmonary vascular resistance), and decreased cardiac output.

2 Pneumatic tourniquets are often used in knee arthroscopic surgeries because they create a bloodless field, which greatly facilitates the procedure. However, tourniquets are associated with potential problems of their own, including hemodynamic changes, pain, metabolic alterations, arterial thromboembolus, and even pulmonary embolism.

 3 Fat embolism syndrome classically presents within 72 h following long-bone or pelvic fracture, with the triad of dyspnea, confusion, and petechiae.

4 Deep vein thrombosis and pulmonary embolism can be major causes of morbidity and mortality following orthopedic operations on the pelvis and lower extremities.

 5 Neuraxial anesthesia alone or when combined with general anesthesia may reduce thromboembolic complications by several mechanisms, including sympathectomy-induced increases in lower-extremity venous blood flow, systemic antiinflammatory effects of local anesthetics, decreased platelet reactivity, attenuated postoperative increase in factor VIII and von Willebrand factor, attenuated postoperative decrease in antithrombin III, and alterations in stress hormone release.

 6 Placement of an epidural needle or catheter (or removal) should generally not be undertaken within 6–8 h of a subcutaneous "minidose" of unfractionated heparin, or within 12–24 h of low-molecular-weight heparin. Although potentially less traumatic, spinal anesthesia may represent a similar risk.

 7 Flexion and extension lateral radiographs of the cervical spine should be obtained preoperatively in all patients with rheumatoid arthritis severe enough to require steroids or methotrexate. If atlantoaxial instability exceeds 5 mm, intubation should be performed with neck stabilization and an awake fiberoptic technique.

 8 Pulmonary artery monitoring in patients undergoing bilateral hip arthroplasties reliably signals embolization by a rise in pulmonary vascular resistance. If pulmonary artery pressures rise above normal ($200 \, dyn \times s \times cm^{-5}$) during the first hip arthroplasty, the contralateral surgery should be postponed.

 9 Like bilateral cemented hip replacement, monitoring during bilateral knee replacement should include pulmonary artery and pulmonary artery occlusion pressure measurements.

 10 Effective postoperative analgesia is essential for early physical rehabilitation to maximize postoperative range of motion and prevent joint adhesions following knee replacement.

 11 The interscalene technique of brachial plexus blockade is ideally suited for shoulder procedures. Even when general anesthesia is employed, an interscalene block can supplement anesthesia and provide good postoperative analgesia.

Orthopedic surgery challenges the anesthesiologist with its diversity. The degree of surgical trespass varies from minor finger surgery to hemipelvectomy. Orthopedic patients range from neonates with congenital anomalies to healthy young athletes to immobile geriatric patients with end-stage multiorgan failure. Long bone fractures predispose to fat embolism syndrome. Patients may be at high risk for venous thromboembolism, particularly following pelvic, hip, and knee operations. Use of bone cement during arthroplasties can cause hemodynamic instability. Limb tourniquets limit blood loss but introduce additional risks. Neuraxial and other regional anesthetic techniques play an important role in decreasing the incidence of perioperative thromboembolic complications, providing postoperative analgesia, and facilitating early rehabilitation and hospital discharges. Advances in surgical techniques, such as minimally invasive approaches to hip replacement utilizing computer-assisted surgery, are necessitating modifications in anesthetic management to allow for overnight or even same day discharge of patients undergoing procedures that used to require a week or more in the hospital. After reviewing problems that are frequently encountered in orthopedic surgery, this chapter discusses the anesthetic management of patients undergoing some common orthopedic operations. Anesthesia for surgery on the spine is discussed in Chapter 26.

SPECIAL CONSIDERATIONS IN ORTHOPEDIC SURGERY

Bone Cement

Bone cement, polymethylmethacrylate, is frequently required for joint arthroplasties. The cement interdigitates within the interstices of cancellous bone and strongly binds the prosthetic device to the patient's bone. Mixing polymerized methylmethacrylate powder with liquid methylmethacrylate monomer causes polymerization and cross-linking of the polymer chains. This exothermic reaction leads to hardening of the cement and expansion against the prosthetic components. The resultant intramedullary hypertension (> 500 mm Hg) causes embolization of fat, bone marrow, cement, and air into the femoral venous channels. Residual methylmethacrylate monomer can produce vasodilation and a decrease in systemic vascular resistance. The release of tissue thromboplastin may trigger platelet aggregation, microthrombus formation in the lungs, and cardiovascular instability as a result of the circulation of vasoactive substances.

The clinical manifestations of bone cement implantation syndrome include hypoxia (increased pulmonary shunt), hypotension, dysrhythmias (including heart block and sinus arrest), pulmonary hypertension (increased pulmonary vascular resistance), and decreased cardiac output. Emboli most frequently occur during insertion of a femoral prosthesis. Strategies to minimize the effects of this complication include increasing inspired oxygen concentration prior to cementing, maintaining euvolemia by monitoring central venous pressure, creating a vent hole in the distal femur to relieve intramedullary pressure, performing high-pressure lavage of the femoral shaft to remove debris (potential microemboli), or using an uncemented femoral component.

Another major disadvantage of cement is the potential for gradual loosening of the prosthesis resulting from breakage of small pieces of cement over the years. Components of cementless implants are made of a porous material that allows the natural bone to grow into them. Cementless prostheses generally last longer and may be advantageous for younger, active patients, even though full recovery may be longer compared to cemented joint replacements. Unfortunately, cementless implants require healthy active bone formation. Therefore cemented prosthesis are still preferred for older (> 80 years) and less active patients who often have osteoporosis and/or thin bone (cortex). Practices continue to evolve regarding selection of cemented versus cementless joint replacements, depending on the joint replaced, patient, and surgical technique. In many cases cemented and cementless components are used in the same patient (eg, total hip arthroplasty). Articular surfaces on modern prostheses may be metal, plastic, or ceramic.

Pneumatic Tourniquets

Use of a pneumatic tourniquet on the upper or lower extremity creates a bloodless field that greatly facilitates surgery. Unfortunately, tourniquets are associated with potential problems of their own, including hemodynamic changes, pain, metabolic alterations, arterial thromboembolism, and even pulmonary embolism. Inflation pressure is usually about 100 mm Hg over systolic blood pressure. Prolonged inflation (> 2 h) routinely leads to transient muscle dysfunction and may be associated with permanent peripheral nerve injury or even rhabdomyolysis. Tourniquet inflation has also been associated with increases in body temperature in pediatric patients undergoing leg surgery.

Exsanguination of a lower extremity and tourniquet inflation cause a shift of blood volume into the central circulation. Although this is usually not clinically significant, bilateral Esmarch bandage exsanguination can cause a rise in central venous pressure and arterial blood pressure that may not be well tolerated in patients with left ventricular dysfunction.

Anyone who has had a tourniquet on the thigh inflated to 100 mm Hg above systolic blood pressure for more than a few minutes appreciates tourniquet pain. Although the mechanism and neural pathways for this severe aching and burning sensation defy precise explanation, unmyelinated, slow-conduction C fibers, which are relatively resistant to local anesthetic blockade, probably play a critical role. **Tourniquet pain gradually becomes so severe over time that patients may require substantial supplemental analgesia, if not general anesthesia, despite a regional block that is adequate for surgical incision.** Even during general anesthesia, tourniquet pain is often manifested as a gradually increasing mean arterial blood pressure beginning about $^3/_4$ to 1 h after cuff inflation. Signs of progressive sympathetic activation include marked hypertension, tachycardia, and diaphoresis. The likelihood of tourniquet pain and its accompanying hypertension may be influenced by many factors, including anesthetic technique (intravenous regional > epidural > spinal > general anesthesia), intensity and level of regional anesthetic block, choice of local anesthetic (hyperbaric spinal with tetracaine > isobaric bupivacaine), and supplementation of the block with opioids.

Cuff deflation invariably and immediately relieves the sensation of tourniquet pain and its hypertension. In fact, cuff deflation can be accompanied by a significant fall in central venous pressure and arterial blood pressure. Heart rate usually increases and core temperature decreases. Washout of accumulated metabolic wastes in the ischemic extremity increases $PaCO_2$, $ETCO_2$, and serum lactate and potassium levels. **These metabolic alterations can cause an increase in minute ventilation in the spontaneously breathing patient and, rarely, dysrhythmias.** Ironically, cuff deflation and blood reoxygenation have been demonstrated to worsen ischemic tissue injury due to the formation of lipid peroxides. This reperfusion injury may be attenuated by propofol, which has been reported to limit superoxide generation.

Tourniquet-induced ischemia of a lower extremity may lead to the development of deep venous thrombosis. Transesophageal echocardiography has detected subclinical pulmonary embolism (miliary emboli) following tourniquet deflation in cases as minor as diagnostic knee arthroscopy. Rare episodes of massive pulmonary embolism during total knee arthroplasty have been reported during leg exsanguination, after tourniquet inflation, and following tourniquet deflation. Tourniquets are generally contraindicated in patients with significant calcific arterial disease. They have been safely used in patients with sickle cell disease, although particular attention should be paid to maintaining oxygenation, normocarbia or hypocarbia, hydration, and normothermia.

Fat Embolism Syndrome

Although some degree of fat embolism probably occurs in all cases of long-bone fracture, **fat embolism syndrome** is a less frequent but potentially fatal (10–20%

mortality) event that can complicate anesthetic management. Fat embolism syndrome classically presents within 72 h following long-bone or pelvic fracture, with the triad of dyspnea, confusion, and petechiae. This syndrome can also be seen following cardiopulmonary resuscitation, parental feeding with lipid infusion, and liposuction. Two theories have been proposed for its pathogenesis. The most popular theory holds that fat globules are released by the disruption of fat cells in the fractured bone and enter the circulation through tears in medullary vessels. An alternative theory proposes that the fat globules are chylomicrons resulting from the aggregation of circulating free fatty acids caused by changes in fatty acid metabolism. Regardless of their source, the increased free fatty acid levels can have a toxic effect on the capillary–alveolar membrane leading to the release of vasoactive amines and prostaglandins and the development of acute respiratory distress syndrome (see Chapter 49). Neurological manifestations (agitation, confusion, stupor, or coma) probably represent capillary damage to the cerebral circulation and cerebral edema and may be exacerbated by hypoxia.

The diagnosis of fat embolism syndrome is suggested by petechiae on the chest, upper extremities, axillae, and conjunctiva. Fat globules may be found in the retina, urine, or sputum. Coagulation abnormalities such as thrombocytopenia or prolonged clotting times are occasionally present. Serum lipase activity may be elevated, but bears no relationship to disease severity. Pulmonary involvement typically progresses from mild hypoxia and a normal chest radiograph to severe hypoxia and a chest film showing diffuse patchy pulmonary infiltrates. Most of the classic signs and symptoms of fat embolism syndrome occur 1–3 days after the precipitant event. Signs during general anesthesia may include a decline in $ETCO_2$ and arterial oxygen saturation or a rise in pulmonary artery pressures. Electrocardiography may show ischemic-appearing ST-segment changes and right-sided heart strain.

Treatment is 2-fold: prophylactic and supportive. Early stabilization of the fracture decreases the incidence of fat embolism syndrome. Supportive treatment consists of oxygen therapy with continuous positive airway pressure ventilation. Treatment with heparin or alcohol has generally been disappointing. High-dose corticosteroid therapy may be beneficial, particularly in the presence of cerebral edema.

Deep Venous Thrombosis & Thromboembolism

Deep vein thrombosis (DVT) and pulmonary embolism (PE) can be major causes of morbidity and mortality following orthopedic operations on the pelvis and lower extremities. Additional risk factors include obesity, age > 60 years, procedures lasting > 30 min, use of a tourniquet, lower extremity fracture, and immobilization for more than 4 days (see Chapter 23). Patients at highest risk are those undergoing hip surgery and knee reconstruction, where DVT rates in older studies were as high as 50%. The incidence of clinically significant pulmonary embolism following hip surgery in some studies was reported to be as high as 20%, whereas that of fatal pulmonary embolism was as much as 1–3%. Major pathophysiological mechanisms likely include venous stasis and a hypercoagulable state due to localized and systemic inflammatory responses to surgery. Prophylactic anticoagulation and use of intermittent pneumatic (leg) compression (IPC) devices have been shown to significantly decrease the incidence of DVT and PE. For high-risk patients, low-dose heparin, 5000 U every 8 h, IPC, warfarin, or low-dose molecular weight heparin (LMWH) is recommended. Unless patients pose an exceptionally high risk, anticoagulants are often started several hours after surgery to reduce intraoperative surgical bleeding. Indeed, more recent data suggest that the overall incidence of DVT following total hip or knee arthroplasty may in fact be as low as 1.5% and that of PE as low as 0.7%, both still being highest in patients over 70 years old. This major reduction in thromboembolic complications likely reflects implementation of contemporary surgical and anesthetic management strategies, eg, routine DVT prophylaxis, early rehabilitation, and more frequent use of regional anesthesia.

Neuraxial anesthesia alone or when combined with general anesthesia may reduce thromboembolic complications by several mechanisms. These include sympathectomy-induced increases in lower-extremity venous blood flow, systemic antiinflammatory effects of local anesthetics, decreased platelet reactivity, attenuated postoperative increases in factor VIII and von Willebrand factor, attenuated postoperative decreases in antithrombin III, and alterations in stress hormone release. Intravenous lidocaine has been shown to prevent thrombosis, enhance fibrinolysis, and decrease platelet aggregation.

Although most clinicians agree that full anticoagulation or fibrinolytic therapy (eg, urokinase) represents an unacceptable risk for spinal or epidural hematoma following neuraxial anesthesia, the danger for patients already receiving low-dose anticoagulation preoperatively is somewhat controversial. Placement of an epidural needle or catheter (or removal) should generally not be undertaken within 6–8 h of a subcutaneous "minidose" of unfractionated heparin, or within 12–24 h of LMWH. Although potentially less traumatic, spinal anesthesia may represent a similar risk. Concomitant administration of an antiplatelet agent may further increase the risk of a spinal hematoma. Another major concern is that a regional anesthetic could mask the hallmarks of an expanding hematoma and spinal cord compression (eg, lower back pain and lower extremity weakness), thus delaying diagnosis and treatment.

HIP SURGERY

Common hip procedures encountered in adult patients include repair of hip fracture, total hip arthroplasty, and closed reduction of hip dislocation.

FRACTURE OF THE HIP

Preoperative Considerations

Most patients presenting for hip surgery are frail and elderly, particularly those with hip fractures. An exception is the occasional young patients who sustain major trauma to the femur or pelvis. Some studies have reported mortality rates following hip fracture of 10% during the initial hospitalization and over 25% within 1 year. Many of these patients have concomitant diseases such as coronary artery disease, cerebral vascular disease, chronic obstructive pulmonary disease, or diabetes.

Patients presenting with hip fractures are frequently dehydrated because of inadequate oral intake. Depending on the site of the hip fracture, occult blood loss may be significant and further compromise intravascular volume. In general, intracapsular (subcapital, transcervical) fractures are associated with less blood loss than extracapsular (base of the femoral neck, intertrochanteric, subtrochanteric) fractures (Figure 40–1). A normal or borderline to low preoperative hematocrit may represent hemoconcentration due to occult blood loss.

Another characteristic of hip fracture patients is the frequent presence of preoperative hypoxia that may, at least in part, be due to fat embolism; other factors can include bibasilar atelectasis from bed rest, pulmonary congestion (and effusion) from congestive heart failure, or consolidation due to infection.

Intraoperative Management

The choice between regional (spinal or epidural) and general anesthesia has been extensively evaluated for hip fracture surgery. Many studies have found a lower mortality in the early postoperative period following regional anesthesia, presumably because of a decrease in thromboembolic disease. After 2 months, however, the mortality rates for regional and general anesthesia have not been consistently different. Postoperative delirium and cognitive impairment may also decrease following regional anesthesia, if sedation can be avoided (see Chapter 45).

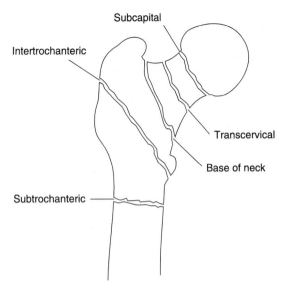

Figure 40–1. Blood loss from hip fracture depends on the location of the fracture (subtrochanteric, intertrochanteric > base of femoral neck > transcervical, subcapital) because the capsule restricts blood loss by acting like a tourniquet.

A continuous epidural technique, with or without concomitant general anesthesia, provides the additional advantage of postoperative pain control. If a spinal anesthetic is planned, a hypobaric technique allows easier positioning because the patient does not have to lie on the fractured hip and can remain in the same position for the surgery. Intrathecal morphine can also be used for postoperative analgesia but the potential for an increased risk of delayed respiratory depression in elderly patients warrants dose reduction (0.1–0.2 mg) and vigilant postoperative monitoring (see Chapter 18).

Consideration should also be given to the type of open reduction and internal fixation to be used. This is dependent on the fracture site, degree of displacement, preoperative functional status of the patient, and surgeon preference. Undisplaced intracapsular fractures are usually treated with cannulated screw fixation. Displaced intracapsular fractures may be treated either with internal fixation, hemiarthroplasty, or total hip replacement (Figure 40–2). A hemiarthroplasty may be cemented or uncemented. Surgical treatment of extracapsular hip fractures is accomplished with either an extramedullary implant (eg, sliding screw and plate) or intramedullary implant (eg, Gamma nail). A hip compression screw and side plate are most often employed for intertrochanteric fractures.

Hemiarthroplasty and total hip replacement are longer, more invasive operations than other procedures.

They are usually performed in the lateral decubitus position, are associated with greater blood loss, and, potentially, result in greater hemodynamic changes, particularly if cement is used. Consideration should be given to direct arterial pressure monitoring, securing large-bore venous access for transfusion, and even full hemodynamic monitoring in frail elderly patients.

TOTAL HIP ARTHROPLASTY

Preoperative Considerations

Most patients undergoing total hip replacement suffer from osteoarthritis, rheumatoid arthritis, or osteonecrosis (avascular necrosis). Osteoarthritis is a degenerative disease affecting the articular surface of one or more joints (most commonly the hip and knee). The etiology of osteoarthritis appears to involve repetitive joint trauma (eg, morbid obesity). Because the spine is often involved, neck positioning during intubation should be as gentle as possible to avoid nerve root compression or nucleus pulposus protrusion.

Rheumatoid arthritis differs from osteoarthritis in three key aspects. First, it is characterized by an immune-mediated joint destruction with chronic and progressive inflammation of synovial membranes, as opposed to articular wear and tear. Second, but very important to the anesthesiologist, is the systemic involvement that can

Figure 40–2. Uncemented total hip arthroplasty.

Table 40–1. Systemic manifestations of rheumatoid arthritis.

Organ System	Abnormalities
Cardiovascular	Pericardial thickening and effusion, myocarditis, coronary arteritis, conduction defects, vasculitis, cardiac valve fibrosis (aortic regurgitation)
Pulmonary	Pleural effusion, pulmonary nodules, interstitial pulmonary fibrosis
Hematopoietic	Anemia, eosinophilia, platelet dysfunction (from aspirin therapy), thrombocytopenia
Endocrine	Adrenal insufficiency (from glucocorticoid therapy), impaired immune system
Dermatological	Thin and atrophic skin from the disease and immunosuppressive drugs

accompany rheumatoid arthritis (Table 40–1). In addition, rheumatoid arthritis typically involves multiple joints, including the small joints of the hands, wrists, and feet, in a symmetric fashion. Inserting invasive catheters and even gaining intravenous access are a challenge in patients with severe deformities.

Debilitation and limited joint mobility prohibit assessment of exercise tolerance, potentially masking underlying coronary artery disease and pulmonary dysfunction. The cardiovascular status of patients unable to exercise, yet at risk for coronary artery disease (eg, a history of angina, diabetes, congestive heart failure, myocardial infarction), can be evaluated with dipyridamole thallium scanning or dobutamine echocardiography (Chapter 20).

Extreme cases of rheumatoid arthritis can involve almost all synovial membranes, including those in the cervical spine and temporomandibular joint. Atlantoaxial subluxation, which can be diagnosed radiologically, may lead to protrusion of the odontoid process into the foramen magnum during intubation, compromising vertebral blood flow and compressing the spinal cord or brain stem (Figure 40–3). Flexion and extension lateral radiographs of the cervical spine should be obtained preoperatively in all patients with rheumatoid arthritis severe enough to require steroids or methotrexate. If atlantoaxial instability exceeds 5 mm, intubation should be performed with neck stabilization and an awake fiberoptic technique. Involvement of the temporomandibular joint can limit jaw mobility and range of motion to such a degree that successful

A   **B**

Figure 40–3. Because instability of the cervical spine may be asymptomatic, lateral radiographs are mandatory in patients with severe rheumatoid arthritis. **A:** A radiograph of a normal lateral cervical spine. **B:** The lateral cervical spine of a patient with rheumatoid arthritis; note the severe C1–C2 instability.

intubation will require a nasal fiberoptic technique. Hoarseness or inspiratory stridor may signal a narrowing of the glottic opening caused by cricoarytenoid arthritis. Despite the use of a smaller-diameter endotracheal tube, this condition may lead to postextubation airway obstruction.

Patients with rheumatoid arthritis or osteoarthritis commonly receive nonsteroidal antiinflammatory drugs (NSAIDs) for management of pain. These drugs can have serious side effects such as life-threatening gastrointestinal bleeding, renal toxicity, and platelet dysfunction. The mechanism of action of NSAIDs has been related to their inhibition of the synthesis of prostaglandins by the cyclooxygenase (COX) enzyme, of which there are two isoforms (COX-1 and COX-2). **It appears that the pain relief and antiinflammatory properties are related to COX-2 inhibition, whereas most of the side effects are principally due to COX-1 inhibition (renal toxicity may be an exception).** Thus, drugs that specifically inhibit COX-2 (eg, celecoxib, parecoxib, valdecoxib) would be expected to have a lower risk of side effects than nonspecific NSAIDs. On the other hand, COX-2 inhibitors would not be expected to confer the benefits of long-term platelet inhibition (ie, prevention of myocardial infarction and stroke). In fact, patients taking some (and possibly all) COX-2 inhibitors appear to have an increase in cardiovascular mortality, prompting withdrawal of at least one COX-2 inhibitor (rofecoxib). Because of their greater cost, COX-2 agents are typically reserved for patients at increased risk for side effects (eg, prior history of gastrointestinal bleeding or reflux, coagulopathy, concurrent steroid use). Likewise, the perioperative period may be a rational time to choose COX-2 drugs to decrease the risk of wound bleeding or epidural hematoma.

Intraoperative Management

Total hip replacement (THR) involves several surgical steps including positioning of the patient (usually in the lateral decubitus position), dislocation and removal of the femoral head, reaming of the acetabulum and insertion of a prosthetic acetabular cup (with or without cement), and reaming of the femur and insertion of a femoral component (femoral head and stem) into the femoral shaft (with or without cement). THR is also associated with three potentially life-threatening complications: bone cement implantation syndrome, intra- and postoperative hemorrhage, and venous thromboembolism. Thus, there are many reasons why invasive arterial monitoring is generally recommended for these procedures. Embolic phenomena most frequently occur during insertion of the femoral prosthesis. Some clinicians increase inspired oxygen concentration prior to cementing. The surgeon may also create a vent hole in the dis-

tal femur to relieve intramedullary pressure, perform high-pressure lavage of the femoral shaft to remove debris (potential microemboli), or use an uncemented femoral component.

Venous thromboembolism is a significant cause of morbidity and mortality following hip replacement surgery. As discussed earlier, use of regional anesthesia decreases the incidence of deep venous thrombosis and pulmonary embolism. Most centers therefore utilize neuraxial anesthesia either alone or in conjunction with general anesthesia, whenever possible. Epidural or spinal (usually isobaric or hypobaric) anesthesia may be used. Some centers routinely administer spinal opioids at the end of the procedure, whereas others rely on parenteral and oral opioids for postoperative analgesia. Other preventative measures against DVT include intermittent leg-compression devices and low-dose anticoagulant prophylaxis.

A. BILATERAL ARTHROPLASTIES

Bilateral hip arthroplasties can be safely performed during one anesthetic, assuming the absence of significant pulmonary embolization after insertion of the first femoral component. Pulmonary artery monitoring reliably signals embolization by a rise in pulmonary vascular resistance (PVR). This is usually indicated by a rise in pulmonary artery pressures (PAP) concurrent with unchanged pulmonary artery occlusion pressure (PAOP) and falling cardiac output:

$$PVR = \frac{\overline{PA} - PAOP}{Cardiac\ output} \times 80$$

If pulmonary artery pressures rise above normal (200 $dyn \times s \times cm^{-5}$) during the first hip arthroplasty, the contralateral surgery should be postponed. New cementless prosthetic systems help avoid the adverse effects of cement. Bilateral uncemented hip arthroplasties do not require pulmonary artery pressure monitoring. Preoperative insertion of an epidural catheter greatly facilitates postoperative pain management. A dilute local anesthetic solution with or without an opiate may be utilized for 24–72 h postoperatively.

B. REVISION ARTHROPLASTY

Hip replacement surgery, particularly revision of a prior hip arthroplasty, may be associated with significant surgical blood loss. Blood loss depends on many factors, including the experience and skill of the surgeon, the surgical technique used, and the type of prosthesis chosen. **Controlled hypotension** (see Chapter 13, Case Discussion) can decrease intraoperative bleeding. Some studies have suggested that blood loss may be decreased during hip surgery if a regional technique is used (eg, spinal or epidural anesthesia) than with general anesthesia even at similar mean arterial blood pressures. The reasons for this dichotomy remain uncertain but may include differences in the resulting vasodilation of the venous and arterial vascular systems, leading to a redistribution of blood flow. By providing a dry bone surface, controlled hypotension also improves prosthetic cementing and shortens the duration of surgery. Because a relatively large number of revision hip replacement patients require perioperative blood transfusions, preoperative autologous blood donation and intraoperative blood salvage should be considered (see Chapter 29). High-dose aprotinin, a proteinase inhibitor of fibrinolytic activity and the intrinsic coagulation pathway by decreasing activation of plasminogen, may reduce intraoperative blood loss in patients undergoing revision surgery. It is usually reserved for high-risk cases (eg, coagulopathies), however, because of its propensity to produce immunological sensitization. Use of aprotinin does not appear to increase the incidence of DVT or PE. Preoperative administration of recombinant human erythropoietin (600 IU/kg subcutaneously weekly beginning 21 days before surgery and ending on the day of surgery) represents another alternative for decreasing the need for perioperative allogeneic blood transfusion. Erythropoietin increases red blood cell production by stimulating the division and differentiation of erythroid progenitors in the bone marrow. Maintaining normal body temperature during hip replacement surgery has been shown to reduce blood loss.

C. MINIMALLY INVASIVE ARTHROPLASTY

The advent of computer-assisted surgery (CAS) has facilitated the development of minimally invasive techniques for cementless hip replacement. CAS allows preoperative planning, intraoperative surgical navigation, and, with some systems, robotic surgery. CAS greatly improves surgical outcomes with minimally invasive arthroplasties. Computer software can accurately reconstruct three-dimensional images of bone and soft tissue based on radiographs, fluoroscopy, computed tomography, or magnetic resonance imaging. Implant-specific software can simulate the procedure and facilitates preoperative planning better than older techniques using translucent prosthesis templates on plain radiographs. Moreover, CAS can make use of surgical navigation systems and image-guided surgical devices. By a process called registration, the computer matches preoperative images or planning information to the position of the patient on the operating room table. Tracking devices are attached to the target bones (Figure 40–4) and to tools during surgery, with the computer using optical cameras and infrared light-emitting diodes to sense their position. CAS thus allows very accurate and optimal placement of implants through very small incisions; this greatly reduces tissue and muscle damage resulting in less pain, early hospital discharge, and faster recovery. The lateral approach utilizes a single 3-in incision with the patient in the lateral decubitus position (Figure 40–4); an anterior approach utilizes two separate 2-in incisions (one for the acetabular component and another for the femoral component) with the patient supine. Minimally invasive techniques can reduce hospitalization to 24 h or less. Anesthetic techniques have evolved to accommodate these radical changes in surgical management.

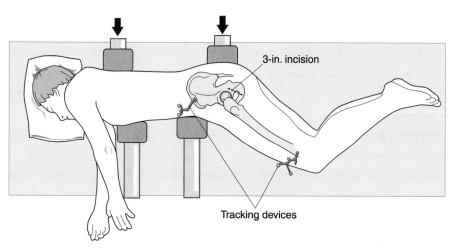

Figure 40–4. Minimally invasive total hip arthroplasty: lateral approach. Note the small 3-in. incision and tracking devices for the CAS navigation system.

Epidural anesthesia with a propofol infusion and a laryngeal mask airway is most often used. Using this technique some centers have largely eliminated the need for parenteral opioids, relying only on oral opioids in the pre- and postoperative periods. Premedication includes multimodal analgesia, consisting of oxycodone 10 mg, valdecoxib 20 mg, and acetaminophen 500 mg. Midazolam 1–2 mg is also administered for sedation immediately prior to surgery. Antiemetic prophylaxis is routinely administered. Surgical anesthesia is usually provided by epidural lidocaine 2% (4 mL test dose) and ropivacaine 1% (8 mL total); this amount of local anesthetic is adequate for most patients and lasts 2–3 h. Use of an epidural catheter allows additional administration of local anesthetic when necessary. Sedation or light general anesthesia is provided with propofol 75–150 μg/kg/min. Most surgeons also inject ropivacaine or bupivacaine (80–100 mg with methylprednisolone 80 mg and morphine 4 mg) into the joint and wound. The epidural catheter is withdrawn at the end of the surgery. Postoperative analgesia is provided with hydrocodone and acetaminophen (or propoxyphene and acetaminophen) and NSAIDs (valdecoxib).

CLOSED REDUCTION HIP DISLOCATION

There is a 3% incidence of hip dislocation following primary hip arthroplasty and a 20% incidence following total hip revision. This incidence appears to be significantly reduced with the used of CAS. Because less force is required to dislocate a prosthetic hip, patients with hip implants require special precautions during positioning for subsequent surgical procedures. Extremes of hip flexion (> 90°), internal rotation (> 20°), and adduction (> 20°) increase the risk of dislocation and should be avoided. Hip dislocations are usually correctable with closed reduction. General anesthesia with a face mask or laryngeal mask airway is usually sufficient for this very brief procedure. Profound paralysis can be provided by succinylcholine or mivacurium and will facilitate the surgeon's manipulations by relaxing the hip musculature. Successful reduction may need to be confirmed radiologically prior to the patient's awakening.

■ KNEE SURGERY

The two most frequently performed knee surgeries are arthroscopy and total or partial joint replacement.

KNEE ARTHROSCOPY

Preoperative Considerations

Arthroscopy has revolutionized surgery of many joints, including the knee, shoulder, ankle, and wrist. Joint arthroscopies are usually outpatient procedures. Although the typical patient undergoing knee arthroscopy is often thought of as being a healthy young athlete, knee arthroscopies are frequently performed in elderly patients with multiple medical problems.

Intraoperative Management

A bloodless field greatly facilitates arthroscopic surgery. Fortunately, knee surgery lends itself to the use of a pneumatic tourniquet (see above). The procedure is performed as an outpatient procedure with the patient in a supine position and in a majority of patients is performed under general anesthesia with a laryngeal mask airway. Some centers routinely utilize neuraxial anesthesia. Alternative regional techniques include a three-in-one femoral nerve and lateral femoral cutaneous nerve blocks (with or without sciatic nerve block), psoas compartment block, and local infiltration (all with sedation—see Chapter 17).

Success and patient satisfaction appear to be equal with both epidural anesthesia (3% 2-chloroprocaine) and spinal anesthesia (lidocaine 25 mg or bupivacaine 6 mg plus fentanyl 15–20 μg). Of note is that even with mini-dose spinal lidocaine the incidence of transient neurological syndrome exceeds 10% (see Chapter 16). Also about 30% of patients complain of back pain following spinal or epidural anesthesia. Time of discharge following general and neuraxial anesthesia appear to be similar.

Postoperative Pain Relief

Successful outpatient recovery depends on early ambulation, adequate pain relief, and minimal nausea and vomiting. Techniques that avoid large doses of systemic opioids have obvious appeal. Intraarticular bupivacaine (15–30 mL of 0.25–0.5% bupivacaine or ropivacaine with 1:200,000 epinephrine) often provides satisfactory analgesia for a few hours postoperatively. The addition of 1–5 mg of morphine may prolong analgesia for several hours in some patients. The presumed mechanism of this somewhat controversial effect involves interactions with peripheral opioid receptors in the joint. Other pain-control strategies include systemic ketorolac, intraarticular corticosteroid injection (eg, 10 mg triamcinolone acetonide in 20 mL saline), a three-in-one nerve block, or the placement during wound closure of a multiorifice catheter connected to a portable pump (eg, Pain Buster).

TOTAL KNEE REPLACEMENT

Preoperative Considerations

Patients presenting for total knee replacement (Figure 40–5) closely resemble those undergoing total hip replacement (eg, rheumatoid arthritis, osteoarthritis).

A   B

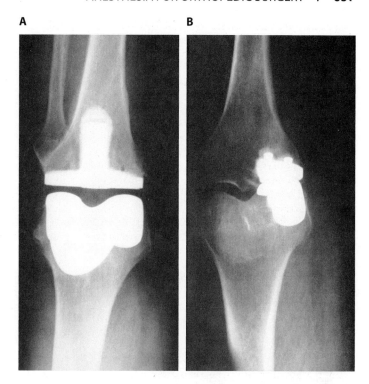

Figure 40–5. Total (**A**) and partial (**B**) knee replacement.

Intraoperative Management

The duration of total knee arthroplasty tends to be shorter than hip replacement; patients remain in a supine position, and blood loss is limited by the use of a tourniquet. Cooperative patients usually tolerate a regional technique with intravenous sedation. Bone cement implantation syndrome following insertion of a femoral prosthesis is possible, but is less likely than during hip arthroplasty. Subsequent release of emboli into the systemic circulation may exaggerate any tendency for hypotension following tourniquet release. As with bilateral cemented hip replacement, monitoring during bilateral knee replacement should include pulmonary artery and PAOP measurements.

Preoperative placement of an epidural catheter can be very helpful in managing postoperative pain, which is typically more severe than pain following hip replacement surgery. Effective postoperative analgesia is essential for early physical rehabilitation to maximize postoperative range of motion and prevent joint adhesions following knee replacement. It is important to balance pain control with the need for a cooperative patient for early rehabilitation. Epidural analgesia is particularly useful in bilateral knee replacements. Epidural ropivacaine 0.2% at 5–10 mL/h provides good analgesia with minimal motor blockade for 48–72 h. Alternatively, an indwelling femoral sheath catheter may be used to provide postoperative analgesia

for 48 h (Figure 40–6). Twenty milliliters of ropivacaine 0.5% (or bupivacaine 0.25%) is used for initial activation at the end of surgery, followed by a ropivacaine 0.2% (or bupivacaine 0.25%) infusion at 5 mL/h. The indwelling femoral sheath catheter technique appears to provide excellent postoperative analgesia, possibly with fewer side effects than epidural analgesia.

Partial knee replacement (unicompartmental or patellofemoral) may be used for selected patients. This limited approach reduces muscle damage, facilitates early ambulation, and may allow for early discharge on the following day. Again, anesthetic management should accommodate the accelerated recovery schedule. The same technique described for minimally invasive total hip arthroplasty can be utilized, with addition of an indwelling femoral catheter for postoperative analgesia.

SURGERY ON THE UPPER EXTREMITY

Procedures on the upper extremities include those for disorders of the shoulder (eg, subacromial impingement or rotator cuff tears), traumatic fractures, nerve entrapment syndromes (eg, carpal tunnel syndrome), and joint arthroplasties (eg, rheumatoid arthritis).

Shoulder Surgery

Shoulder operations may be open or arthroscopic. These procedures are performed either in a sitting

A

B

C

D

Figure 40–6. Placement of an in-dwelling femoral catheter for postoperative analgesia. ***A:*** Equipment: an insulated needle, an 18-gauge introducer catheter, and a nerve stimulator are required. (Note the injection tubing and wire attachment for the nerve stimulator on the insulated needle.) ***B:*** Preparation: the insulated needle is placed inside the introducer catheter and a 20-gauge epidural catheter is prepared for insertion. ***C:*** Introducer-needle placement: the femoral arterial pulse is palpated just beneath the inguinal ligament and the needle-introducer unit is inserted lateral to it and advanced with the nerve stimulator on. Correct placement is indicated by contraction of the patella with 1.5 mA current or less. ***D:*** Catheter insertion: the insulated needle is removed and the epidural catheter is inserted into the introducer and advanced 2–4 cm inside the femoral sheath before the introducer catheter is removed and the indwelling catheter is secured to the skin.

("beach chair") or, less commonly, a lateral decubitus position. The interscalene technique of brachial plexus blockade is ideally suited for shoulder procedures (see Chapter 17). Even when general anesthesia is employed, an interscalene block can supplement anesthesia and provide good postoperative analgesia. Intense muscle relaxation is usually required during general anesthesia, particularly when not combined with a brachial plexus block. Mild controlled hypotension may be requested to improve visualization during arthroscopic procedures.

Use of an indwelling interscalene catheter allows postoperative analgesia for 48 h following major shoulder operations. Infusion of a dilute local anesthetic solution for the latter can allow assessment of neurological problems in the immediate postoperative period. Ropivacaine 0.2% may be infused at 4–8 mL/h. Alternatively, some surgeons implant a small multiorifice catheter in the wound for slow postoperative infusion of local anesthetic (eg, Pain Buster). Administration of ketorolac at the end of the procedure and in the first 24 h can help reduce postoperative opioid requirements.

Hand Surgery

One of the most common operations in anesthetic practice is carpal tunnel release. Intravenous regional anesthesia, or Bier block (see Chapter 17), is ideally suited for this procedure. The availability of very short-acting anesthetics (eg, propofol and desflurane) together with laryngeal mask airways has facilitated general anesthesia for hand surgery and allows comparable early discharge.

Operations lasting more than 1 h may be performed under a brachial plexus block. The axillary approach is generally preferred for surgery below the elbow (see Chapter 17). Use of a pneumatic tourniquet requires a field block in the subcutaneous tissue over the axillary artery because the medial brachial cutaneous nerve leaves the plexus sheath just below the clavicle and is missed along with the intercostobrachial nerve during an axillary block.

CASE DISCUSSION: MANAGING BLOOD LOSS IN JEHOVAH'S WITNESSES

A 58-year-old Jehovah's Witness presents for hemipelvectomy because of a malignant bone tumor (osteogenic sarcoma). The patient has received chemotherapy over the last 2 months with multiple drugs, including doxorubicin. The patient has no other medical problems and the preoperative hematocrit is 47%.

How does the care of Jehovah's Witnesses particularly challenge the anesthesiologist?

Jehovah's Witnesses, a fellowship of more than 1 million Americans, object to the administration of blood for any indication. This objection stems from their interpretation of the Bible ("to keep abstaining from...blood," Acts 15:28,29), not for medical reasons (eg, the fear of hepatitis). Physicians are obliged to honor the principle of bodily integrity, which states that patients have final authority over what is done to them. Witnesses sign a waiver that relieves physicians of responsibility for any consequences of blood refusal.

Which intravenous fluids will Witnesses accept?

Witnesses abstain from blood and blood products (eg, packed red blood cells, fresh frozen plasma, platelets) but not non–blood-containing solutions. They accept crystalloids, hetastarch, and dextran replacement solutions. Witnesses view albumin, erythropoietin (because of the use of albumin), immune globulins, and hemophiliac preparations as a gray area that requires a personal decision by the believer.

Do they allow the use of autologous blood?

According to their religion, any blood that is removed from the body should be discarded ("You should pour it out upon the ground as water," Deuteronomy 12:24) and not stored. Thus, the usual practice of autologous preoperative collection and storage would not be allowed. Techniques of acute normovolemic hemodilution and intraoperative blood salvaging have been accepted by some Witnesses, however, as long as their blood maintains continuity with their circulatory systems at all times. For example, up to 4 U of blood could be drawn from the patient immediately before surgery and kept in anticoagulant-containing bags that maintain a constant link to the patient's body. The blood would be replaced by an acceptable colloid or crystalloid solution, and reinfused as needed during the surgery.

How would the inability to transfuse blood affect intraoperative monitoring decisions?

Hemipelvectomy involves radical resection that can lead to massive blood loss. This is particularly true for large tumors and if an internal approach, rather than the classic external hemipelvectomy, is planned. Invasive arterial blood pressure and central venous pressure monitors would probably be indicated in most patients undergoing this procedure. Techniques that minimize intraoperative blood loss (eg, controlled hypotension, aprotinin) should be considered. In a Jehovah's Witness, the management of life-threatening anemia (Hb < 5 g/dL) may be improved by monitoring cardiac output, oxygen delivery, and oxygen consumption. Thus, a pulmonary artery catheter with continuous mixed venous oxygen saturation monitoring capability might prove useful. Continuous electrocardiograph ST-segment analysis may signal myocardial ischemia. Hypoventilation-induced decreases in cerebral blood flow can be prevented by continuous $E_{TO_{2}}$ monitoring.

What physiological effects result from severe anemia?

Assuming the maintenance of normovolemia and the absence of preexisting major end-organ dysfunction, most patients tolerate severe anemia surprisingly well. Decreased blood viscosity and vasodilation lower systemic vascular resistance and increase blood flow. Augmentation of stroke volume increases cardiac output, allowing arterial blood pressure and heart rate to remain relatively unchanged. Coronary and cerebral blood flows increase in the absence of coronary artery disease and carotid artery stenosis. A decrease in venous oxygen saturation reflects an increase in tissue oxygen extraction. Oozing from surgical wounds as a result of dilutional coagulopathy may accompany extreme degrees of anemia.

What are some of the anesthetic implications of preoperative doxorubicin therapy?

This anthracycline antibiotic has well-recognized cardiac side effects, ranging from transient dysrhythmias and electrocardiograph changes (eg, ST-segment and T-wave abnormalities) to irreversible cardiomyopathy and congestive heart failure. The risk of cardiomyopathy appears to increase with a cumulative dose greater than 550 mg/m^{-2}, prior radiotherapy, and concurrent cyclophosphamide treatment. Mild degrees of cardiomyopathy can be detected preoperatively with endomyocardial biopsy, echocardiography, or exercise radionuclide angiography. Doxorubicin's other important toxicity is myelosuppression (eg, thrombocytopenia, leukopenia, anemia).

Are there any special considerations regarding postoperative pain management in the Jehovah's Witness?

Witnesses generally refrain from any mind-altering drugs or medications, although opioids prescribed by a physician for severe pain are accepted by some believers. Insertion of an epidural catheter could provide pain relief with local anesthetics, with or without opioids.

SUGGESTED READING

Capdevila X, Biboulet P, Bouregba M: Comparison of the three-in-one and fascia iliaca compartment blocks in adults: Clinical and radiographic analysis. Anesth Analg 1998;86:1039. These blocks can provide very effective anesthesia for lower limb surgery.

Capdevila X, Barthelet Y, Biboulet P, et al: Effects of perioperative analgesic technique on the surgical outcome and duration of rehabilitation after major knee surgery. Anesthesiology 1999;91:8. Continuous femoral block shortened the hospital stay compared with patient-controlled analgesia, and resulted in fewer side effects than continuous epidural infusion.

Chelly JE, Ben-David B, Williams BA, Kentor ML: Anesthesia and postoperative analgesia: Outcomes following orthopedic surgery. Orthopedics 2003;26:s865.

Connolly D: Orthopaedic anaesthesia. Anaesthesia 2003;58:1189.

Ereth MH, Weber JG, Abel MD, et al: Cemented versus noncemented total hip arthroplasty—embolism, hemodynamics, and intrapulmonary shunting. Mayo Clin Proc 1992;67:1066. A classic prospective study using transesophageal echocardiography and pulmonary artery monitoring.

Horlocker TT, Wedel DJ, Benzon H, et al: Regional anesthesia in the anticoagulated patient: Defining the risks. Reg Anesth Pain Med 2004;29:1.

Lafont ND, Kalonji MK, Barre J, et al: Clinical features and echocardiography of embolism during cemented hip arthroplasty. Can J Anaesth 1997;44:112.

Mantilla CB, Horlocker TT, Schroeder DR, et al: Frequency of myocardial infarction, pulmonary embolism, deep venous thrombosis, and death following primary hip or knee arthroplasty. Anesthesiology 2002;96:1140.

Pietak S, Holmes J, Matthews R, et al: Cardiovascular collapse after femoral prosthesis surgery for acute hip fracture. Can J Anaesth 1997;444:198. Two cases of fatal hemodynamic collapse coinciding with femoral reaming and placement of prosthesis.

Pollock JE, Mulroy MF, Bent E, Polissar NL: A comparison of two regional anesthetic techniques for outpatient knee arthroscopy. Anesth Analg 2003;97:397.

Rathmell JP, Pino CA, Taylor R, et al: Intrathecal morphine for postoperative analgesia: A randomized, controlled, dose-ranging study after hip and knee arthroplasty. Anesth Analg 2003;97:1452.

Samama CM, Langeron O, Rosencher N, et al: Aprotinin versus placebo in major orthopedic surgery: A randomized, double-blinded, dose-ranging study. Anesth Analg 2002;95:287.

Schmied H, Schiferer A, Sessler DI: The effects of red-cell scavenging, hemodilution, and active warming on allogenic blood requirements in patients undergoing hip or knee arthroplasty. Anesth Analg 1998;86:387. All three techniques effectively reduce transfusion requirements.

Stratmann G, Gregory GA: Neurogenic and humoral vasoconstriction in acute pulmonary thromboembolism. Anesth Analg 2003;97:341.

Sulek CA, Davies LK, Enneking FK: Cerebral microembolism diagnosed by transcranial Doppler during total knee arthroplasty: Correlation with transesophageal echocardiography. Anesthesiology 1999;91:672. Over 50% of the patients studied had evidence of cerebral fat emboli following tourniquet deflation, with a higher average number of emboli following bilateral versus unilateral knee arthroplasty.

Tenholder M, Cushner FD: Intraoperative blood management in joint replacement surgery. Orthopedics 2004;27:s663.

Anesthesia for the Trauma Patient   41

KEY CONCEPTS

 The initial assessment of the trauma patient can be divided into primary, secondary, and tertiary surveys. The primary survey should take 2–5 min and consists of the ABCDE sequence of trauma: Airway, Breathing, Circulation, Disability, and Exposure. Resuscitation and assessment proceed simultaneously. Trauma resuscitation includes two additional phases: control of hemorrhage and definitive repair of the injury. More comprehensive secondary and tertiary surveys of the patient follow the primary survey.

 Five criteria increase the risk for potential instability of the cervical spine: (1) neck pain, (2) severe distracting pain, (3) any neurological signs or symptoms, (4) intoxication, and (5) loss of consciousness at the scene. A cervical spine fracture must be assumed if any one of these criteria is present. Even with these criteria, the incidence of cervical spine trauma is approximately 2%. The incidence of cervical spine instability increases up to 10% in the presence of a severe head injury.

 Neck hyperextension and excessive axial traction must be avoided whenever cervical spine instability is suspected. Manual immobilization of the head and neck by an assistant should be used to stabilize the cervical spine during laryngoscopy ("manual in-line stabilization" or MILS).

 The mainstay of therapy of hemorrhagic shock is intravenous fluid resuscitation and transfusion. Multiple short (1.5–2 in), large-bore (14–16 gauge or 7–8.5F) catheters are placed in whichever veins are easily accessible.

 Rapid-infusion systems that use large-bore tubing and rapidly warm fluids are invaluable during massive transfusions. A convection forced-air warming blanket and heated humidifier will also help maintain body temperature. Hypothermia worsens acid–base disorders, coagulopathy, and myocardial dysfunction.

 Hypotension in patients with hypovolemic shock should be aggressively treated with intravenous fluids and blood products, not vasopressors unless there is profound hypotension that is unresponsive to fluid therapy, coexisting cardiogenic shock, or cardiac arrest.

 Commonly used induction agents for trauma patients include ketamine and etomidate. Even after adequate fluid resuscitation, the induction dose requirements for propofol are greatly (80–90%) reduced in patients with major trauma. Even drugs such as ketamine and nitrous oxide that normally indirectly stimulate cardiac function can display cardiodepressant properties in patients who are in shock and already have maximal sympathetic stimulation. Hypotension may also be encountered following etomidate.

 Invasive monitoring (direct arterial, central venous, and pulmonary artery pressure monitoring) can be extremely helpful in guiding fluid resuscitation but insertion of these monitors should not detract from the resuscitation itself. Serial hematocrits (or hemoglobin), arterial blood gas measurement, and serum electrolytes (particularly K$^+$) are invaluable in protracted resuscitations.

 Any trauma victim with altered consciousness must be considered to have a brain injury. The level of consciousness is assessed by serial Glasgow Coma Scale evaluations.

Trauma is the leading cause of death in Americans from the first to the thirty-fifth year of age. Up to one-third of all hospital admissions in the United States are directly related to trauma. Fifty percent of trauma deaths occur immediately, with another 30% occurring within a few hours of injury (the "golden hour"). Because many trauma victims require immediate surgery, anesthesiologists can directly affect their survival. In fact, the role of the anesthesiologist is often that of primary resuscitator, with provision of anesthesia a secondary activity. It is important for the anesthesiologist to remember that these patients may have an increased likelihood of being drug abusers, acutely intoxicated, and carriers of hepatitis or human immunodeficiency virus (HIV). This chapter presents a framework for the initial assessment of the trauma victim and anesthetic considerations in the treatment of patients with injuries of the head and spine, chest, abdomen, and extremities. The Case Discussion at the end of the chapter considers burn trauma.

■ INITIAL ASSESSMENT

The initial assessment of the trauma patient can be divided into primary, secondary, and tertiary surveys. The primary survey should take 2–5 min and consists of the ABCDE sequence of trauma: Airway, Breathing, Circulation, Disability, and Exposure. If the function of any of the first three systems is impaired, resuscitation must be initiated immediately. In critically ill patients, resuscitation and assessment proceed simultaneously by a team of trauma practitioners. Basic monitoring including the electroencephalograph (ECG), noninvasive blood pressure, and pulse oximetry can often be initiated in the field and is continued during treatment. Principles of cardiopulmonary resuscitation are presented in detail in Chapter 47. Trauma resuscitation includes two additional phases: control of hemorrhage and definitive repair of the injury. More comprehensive secondary and tertiary surveys of the patient follow the primary survey.

PRIMARY SURVEY

Airway

Establishing and maintaining an airway is always the first priority. If a patient can talk the airway is usually clear, but if unconscious the patient will likely require airway and ventilatory assistance. Important signs of obstruction include snoring or gurgling, stridor, and paradoxical chest movements. The presence of a foreign body should be considered in unconscious patients. Advanced airway management (such as endotracheal intubation, cricothyrotomy, or tracheostomy) is indicated if there is apnea, persistent obstruction, severe head injury, maxillofacial trauma, a penetrating neck injury with an expanding hematoma, or major chest injuries.

Cervical spine injury is unlikely in alert patients without neck pain or tenderness. Five criteria increase the risk for potential instability of the cervical spine: (1) neck pain, (2) severe distracting pain, (3) any neurological signs or symptoms, (4) intoxication, and (5) loss of consciousness at the scene. A cervical spine fracture must be assumed if any one of these criteria is present, even if there is no known injury above the level of the clavicle. Even with these criteria, the incidence of cervical spine trauma is approximately 2%. The incidence of cervical spine instability increases up to 10% in the presence of a severe head injury. To avoid neck hyperextension, the jaw-thrust maneuver is the preferred means of establishing an airway. Oral and nasal airways may help maintain airway patency. Unconscious patients with major trauma are always considered to be at increased risk for aspiration, and the airway must be secured as soon as possible with an endotracheal tube or tracheostomy. Neck hyperextension and excessive axial traction must be avoided, and manual immobilization of the head and neck by an assistant should be used to stabilize the cervical spine during laryngoscopy ("manual in-line stabilization" or MILS). The assistant places his or her hands on either side of the head, holding down the occiput and preventing any head rotation. Studies have demonstrated neck movement, however, particularly at C1 and C2, during mask ventilation and direct laryngoscopy despite attempts at stabilization (eg, MILS, axial traction, sandbags, forehead tape, soft collar, Philadelphia [hard] collar). Of all these techniques, MILS may be most effective, but it also makes direct laryngoscopy more difficult. For this reason, some clinicians prefer nasal intubation (blind or fiberoptic) in spontaneously breathing patients with suspected cervical spine injury, although this technique may be associated with a higher risk of pulmonary aspiration. Others advocate use of a lightwand, Bullard laryngoscope, WuScope, or an intubating laryngeal mask airway. Clearly, the expertise and preferences of individual clinicians affect the choice of technique, together with the need for expediency and risks of complications in a given patient. Most practitioners have greater familiarity with oral intubation, and this technique should be considered in patients who are apneic and require immediate intubation. Furthermore, nasal intubation should be avoided in patients with midface or basilar skull fractures. If an esophageal obturator airway has been placed in the field, it should not be removed until the trachea has been intubated because of the likelihood of regurgitation (see Chapter 47).

Laryngeal trauma makes a complicated situation worse. Open injuries may be associated with bleeding from major neck vessels, obstruction from hematoma or edema, subcutaneous emphysema, and cervical spine injuries. Closed laryngeal trauma is less obvious but can present as neck crepitations, hematoma, dysphagia, hemoptysis, or poor phonation. An awake intubation with a small endotracheal tube (6.0 in adults) under direct laryngoscopy or fiberoptic bronchoscopy with topical anesthesia can be attempted if the larynx can be well visualized. If facial or neck injuries preclude endotracheal intubation, tracheostomy under local anesthesia should be considered. Acute obstruction from upper airway trauma may require emergency cricothyrotomy or percutaneous or surgical tracheostomy (see Case Discussion, Chapter 5).

Breathing

Assessment of ventilation is best accomplished by the look, listen, and feel approach. Look for cyanosis, use of accessory muscles, flail chest, and penetrating or sucking chest injuries. Listen for the presence, absence, or diminution of breath sounds. Feel for subcutaneous emphysema, tracheal shift, and broken ribs. The clinician should have a high index of suspicion for tension pneumothorax and hemothorax (see below), particularly in patients with respiratory distress. Pleural drainage may be necessary before the chest X-ray can be obtained.

Most critically ill trauma patients require assisted— if not controlled—ventilation. Bag-valve devices (eg, a self-inflating bag with a nonrebreathing valve) usually provide adequate ventilation immediately after intubation and during periods of patient transport. A 100% oxygen concentration is delivered until oxygenation is assessed by arterial blood gases.

Circulation

Adequacy of circulation is based on pulse rate, pulse fullness, blood pressure, and signs of peripheral perfusion. Signs of inadequate circulation include tachycardia, weak or unpalpable peripheral pulses, hypotension, and pale, cool, or cyanotic extremities. The first priority in restoring adequate circulation is to stop bleeding; the second priority is to replace intravascular volume. Cardiac arrest during transport to the hospital or shortly after arrival following penetrating chest injuries and possibly blunt chest is an indication for emergency room thoracotomy (ERT). The latter, which is also called resuscitative thoracotomy, allows rapid control of

obvious bleeding, opens the pericardium, and allows suturing of cardiac injuries and cross-clamping of the aorta above the diaphragm. Some trauma surgeons also advocate ERT for cardiac arrest during transport or shortly after arrival at the hospital following penetrating or blunt injuries to the abdomen. Pregnant patients at term who are in cardiac arrest or shock often can be resuscitated properly only after delivery of the baby.

A. HEMORRHAGE

Obvious sites of hemorrhage should be identified and controlled with direct pressure on the wound. Bleeding from the extremities is easily controlled with pressure dressings and packs; tourniquets can cause reperfusion injuries. Bleeding due to chest trauma is usually from intercostal arteries and often slows or stops when the lung is expanded following chest tube drainage. Bleeding due to intraabdominal injuries, depending on its severity, may tamponade itself, allowing a variable period of fluid and blood resuscitation while surgical evaluation is completed. Pneumatic antishock garments can decrease bleeding in the abdomen and lower extremities, increase peripheral vascular resistance, and augment perfusion of the heart and brain. Bleeding wounds above the level of the suit (eg thorax or head) contraindicate the use of these garments because of the risk of increasing hemorrhage.

The term shock denotes circulatory failure leading to inadequate vital organ perfusion and oxygen delivery. Although there are many causes of shock (Table 41–1), in the trauma patient it is usually due to hypovolemia. Physiological responses to hemorrhage range from tachycardia, poor capillary perfusion, and a decrease in pulse pressure to hypotension, tachypnea, and delirium (Table 41–2). Serum hematocrit and hemoglobin concentrations are often not accurate indicators of acute blood loss. Peripheral somatic nerve stimulation and massive tissue injury appear to exacerbate the reductions in cardiac output and stroke volume seen in hypovolemic shock. The hemodynamic lability of these patients demands invasive arterial blood pressure monitoring. In severe hypovolemia, the pulse waveform can almost disappear during the inspiratory phase of mechanical ventilation. The degree of hypotension on presentation to the emergency room and operating room correlates strongly with the mortality rate.

The mainstay of therapy of hemorrhagic shock is intravenous fluid resuscitation and transfusion. Multiple short (1.5–2 in), large-bore (14–16 gauge or 7–8.5F) catheters are placed in whichever veins are easily accessible. Patients with possible vena caval or hepatic injury should have intravenous access established in both caval systems in case cross-clamping becomes necessary during vascular repair. Although central lines may provide useful infor-

Table 41–1. Classification of shock by mechanism and common causes.[1]

Hypovolemic shock
Loss of blood (hemorrhagic shock)
    External hemorrhage
        Trauma
        Gastrointestinal tract bleeding
    Internal hemorrhage
        Hematoma
        Hemothorax or hemoperitoneum
Loss of plasma
    Burns
    Exfoliative dermatitis
Loss of fluid and electrolytes
    External
        Vomiting
        Diarrhea
        Excessive sweating
        Hyperosmolar states (diabetic ketoacidosis, hyperos-
           molar nonketotic coma)
    Internal ("third-spacing")
        Pancreatitis
        Ascites
        Bowel obstruction
Cardiogenic shock
Dysrhythmia
    Tachyarrhythmia
    Bradyarrhythmia
Pump failure (secondary to myocardial infarction or other
    cardiomyopathy)
Acute valvular dysfunction (especially regurgitant lesions)
Rupture of ventricular septum or free ventricular wall
Obstructive shock
Tension pneumothorax
Pericardial disease (tamponade, constriction)
Disease of pulmonary vasculature (massive pulmonary em-
    boli, pulmonary hypertension)
Cardiac tumor (atrial myxoma)
Left atrial mural thrombus
Obstructive valvular disease (aortic or mitral stenosis)
Distributive shock
Septic shock
Anaphylactic shock
Neurogenic shock
Vasodilator drugs
Acute adrenal insufficiency

[1]Reproduced, with permission, from Ho MT, Saunders CE: *Current Emergency Diagnosis & Treatment,* 4th ed. Appleton & Lange, 1992.

mation regarding volume status, they may be time-consuming and introduce the possibility of life-threatening complications (eg, pneumothorax). Peripheral lines are usually sufficient for initial resuscitation.

Massive hemorrhage depletes the intravascular fluid compartment. Fluid shifts intravascularly from the interstitial compartment to maintain cardiovascular integrity, and interstitial fluid also moves into cells. Anaerobic metabolism leads to depletion of adenosine triphosphate (ATP), dysfunction of the ATP-dependent Na^+–K^+ pump, and progressive cellular edema.

B. Fluid Therapy

The choice of initial fluid therapy is determined primarily by availability. Although fully cross-matched whole blood is ideal, typing and cross-matching take 45–60 min. Type-specific blood (preferably type and screen blood) may cause minor antibody reactions but is appropriate therapy as soon as it is available (5–10 min). Uncrossed O-negative packed red blood cells should be reserved for life-threatening blood loss that cannot be adequately replaced by other fluids (eg, exsanguination). Complications associated with massive blood transfusions are discussed in Chapter 29.

Crystalloid solutions are readily available and inexpensive. Resuscitation requires large quantities, however, because most crystalloid solution does not remain in the intravascular compartment. Lactated Ringer's injection is less likely to cause hyperchloremic acidosis than is normal saline, although calcium in the former makes it less compatible with blood transfusions. Dextrose-containing solutions may exacerbate ischemic brain damage and should be avoided in the absence of documented hypoglycemia. Even lactated Ringer's solution is slightly hypotonic and when administered in large volumes can aggravate cerebral edema. Hypertonic solutions such as 3% or 7.5% saline are effective for volume resuscitation and appear to be associated with less cerebral edema than lactated Ringer's solution or normal saline in the presence of brain injury. Although small volumes of hypertonic saline rapidly expand plasma volume, its use is limited by progressive hypernatremia (see Chapters 28 and 29). Transient vasodilation and hypotension may also be observed.

Colloid solutions are far more expensive than crystalloids, but they are more effective in rapidly restoring intravascular volume. Nonetheless, the interstitial fluid deficit associated with hypovolemic shock may be better treated with a crystalloid solution or a combination of colloids and crystalloids. Albumin is usually selected over dextran or hetastarch solutions because of the fear of inducing a coagulopathy (see Chapter 29).

Whichever fluid is chosen, it must be warmed prior to administration. Rapid-infusion systems that use large-bore tubing and rapidly warm fluids are invaluable during massive transfusions. A convection forced-air warming blanket and heated humidifier will also help maintain body temperature. Hypothermia worsens acid–base disorders, coagulopathy, and myocardial dysfunction (see Table 6–7). It also shifts the oxygen–

Table 41–2. Clinical classification of shock.[1,2]

	Pathophysiology	Clinical Manifestations
Mild (< 20% of blood volume lost)	Decreased peripheral perfusion only of organs able to withstand prolonged ischemia (skin, fat, muscle, and bone). Arterial pH normal.	Patient complains of feeling cold. Postural hypotension and tachycardia. Cool pale moist skin; collapsed neck veins; concentrated urine.
Moderate (20–40% of blood volume lost)	Decreased central perfusion of organs able to tolerate only brief ischemia (liver, gut, kidneys). Metabolic acidosis present.	Thirst. Supine hypotension and tachycardia (variable). Oliguria and anuria.
Severe (> 40% of blood volume lost)	Decreased perfusion of heart and brain. Severe metabolic acidosis. Respiratory acidosis possibly present.	Agitation, confusion, or obtundation. Supine hypotension and tachycardia invariably present. Rapid, deep respiration.

[1]Modified and reprinted, with permission, from Ho MT, Saunders CE: *Current Emergency Diagnosis & Treatment,* 4th ed. Appleton & Lange, 1992.
[2]These clinical findings are most consistently observed in hemorrhagic shock but apply to other types of shock as well.

hemoglobin curve to the left and decreases the metabolism of lactate, citrate, and some anesthetic drugs. The amount of fluid administered is based on improvement of clinical signs, particularly blood pressure, pulse pressure, and heart rate.

Central venous pressure and urinary output also provide indications of restoration of vital organ perfusion.

Inadequate organ perfusion interferes with aerobic metabolism, producing lactic acid and metabolic acidosis. Sodium bicarbonate, which dissociates into bicarbonate ion and CO_2, may temporarily worsen intracellular acidosis because cell membranes are relatively insoluble to bicarbonate compared with CO_2. Acid–base imbalances will eventually resolve with hydration and improved organ perfusion. Lactate will be metabolized in the liver to bicarbonate, and H^+ will be excreted by the kidneys.

Hypotension in patients with hypovolemic shock should be aggressively treated with intravenous fluids and blood products, not vasopressors, unless there is profound hypotension that is unresponsive to fluid therapy, coexisting cardiogenic shock, or cardiac arrest.

Shock that is refractory to aggressive fluid therapy may be due to uncontrolled hemorrhage that exceeds the rate of transfusion or to cardiogenic shock (eg, pericardial tamponade, myocardial contusion, myocardial infarction), neurogenic shock (eg, brain stem dysfunction, spinal cord transection), septic shock (a late complication), pulmonary failure (eg, pneumothorax, hemothorax), or severe acidosis or hypothermia.

Disability

Evaluation for disability consists of a rapid neurological assessment. Because there is usually no time for a Glas-

gow Coma Scale (Table 26–1), the AVPU system is used: *a*wake, *v*erbal response, *p*ainful response, and *u*nresponsive.

Exposure

The patient should be undressed to allow examination for injuries. In-line immobilization should be used if a neck or spinal cord injury is suspected.

SECONDARY SURVEY

The secondary survey begins only when the ABCs are stabilized. In the secondary survey, the patient is evaluated from head to toe and the indicated studies (eg, radiographs, laboratory tests, invasive diagnostic procedures) are obtained. Head examination includes looking for injuries to the scalp, eyes, and ears. Neurological examination includes the Glasgow Coma Scale (Table 26–1) and evaluation of motor and sensory functions as well as reflexes. Fixed dilated pupils do not necessarily imply irreversible brain damage. The chest is auscultated and inspected again for fractures and functional integrity (flail chest). Diminished breath sounds may reveal a delayed or enlarging **pneumothorax** that requires chest tube placement. Similarly, distant heart sounds, a narrow pulse pressure, and distended neck veins may signal **pericardial tamponade,** calling for pericardiocentesis. A normal initial examination does not definitively eliminate the possibility of these problems. Examination of the abdomen should consist of inspection, auscultation, and palpation. The extremities are examined for fractures, dislocations, and peripheral pulses. A urinary catheter and nasogastric tube are also normally inserted.

Basic laboratory analysis includes a complete blood count (or hematocrit or hemoglobin), electrolytes, glucose, blood urea nitrogen (BUN), and creatinine. Arterial blood gases may also be extremely helpful. A chest X-ray should be obtained in all patients with major trauma. The possibility of cervical spine injury is evaluated by examining all seven vertebrae in a cross-table lateral radiograph and a swimmer's view. Although these studies detect 80–90% of fractures, only a normal computed tomographic scan reliably rules out significant cervical spine trauma. Additional radiographic studies may include skull, pelvic, and long bone films. A focused assessment with sonography for trauma (FAST) scan is a rapid, bedside, ultrasound examination performed to identify intraperitoneal hemorrhage or pericardial tamponade. The FAST scan, which has become an extension of the physical examination of the trauma patient, examines four areas for free fluid: perihepatic/hepatorenal space; perisplenic space; pelvis; and pericardium. Depending on the injuries and the hemodynamic status of the patient, other imaging techniques (eg, chest computed tomography [CT] or angiography) or diagnostic tests such as diagnostic peritoneal lavage (DPL) may also be indicated.

TERTIARY SURVEY

Many trauma centers also advocate a tertiary trauma survey (TTS) to avoid missed injuries. Between 2% and 50% of traumatic injuries may be missed by primary and secondary surveys, particularly following blunt multiple trauma (eg, car accident). A tertiary survey is defined as a patient evaluation that identifies and catalogues all injuries after initial resuscitation and operative interventions. It typically occurs within 24 h of injuries. This delayed evaluation normally results in a more awake patient who is able to fully communicate all complaints, more detailed information on the mechanism of injury, and a detailed examination of the medical record to determine preexisting comorbidities.

The tertiary survey occurs prior to discharge to reassess and confirm known injuries and identify occult ones. It includes another "head-to-toe examination" and a review of all laboratory and imaging studies. Missed injuries can include extremity and pelvic fractures, spinal cord and head injuries, and abdominal and peripheral nerve injuries.

◼ ANESTHETIC CONSIDERATIONS

GENERAL CONSIDERATIONS

Regional anesthesia is usually impractical and inappropriate in hemodynamically unstable patients with life-threatening injuries.

If the patient arrives in the operating room already intubated, correct positioning of the endotracheal tube must be verified. Patients with suspected head trauma are hyperventilated to decrease intracranial pressure. Ventilation may be compromised by pneumothorax, flail chest, obstruction of the endotracheal tube, or direct pulmonary injury.

If the patient is not intubated the same principles of airway management described above should be followed in the operating room. If time permits, hypovolemia should be at least partially corrected prior to induction of general anesthesia. Fluid resuscitation and transfusion should continue throughout induction and maintenance of anesthesia. Commonly used induction agents for trauma patients include ketamine and etomidate (see Chapter 8). Studies suggest that even after adequate fluid resuscitation, the induction dose requirements for propofol are greatly (80–90%) reduced in patients with major trauma. Even drugs such as ketamine and nitrous oxide, which normally indirectly stimulate cardiac function, can display cardiodepressant properties in patients who are in shock and already have maximal sympathetic stimulation. Hypotension may also be encountered following etomidate induction.

Maintenance of anesthesia in unstable patients may consist primarily of the use of muscle relaxants (also called neuromuscular blocking agents), with general anesthetic agents titrated as tolerated (mean arterial pressure > 50–60 mm Hg) in an effort to provide at least amnesia. Intermittent small doses of ketamine (25 mg every 15 min) are often well tolerated and may help reduce the incidence of recall, particularly when used with low concentrations of a volatile agent (< 0.5 minimum alveolar concentration). Other adjuncts that may be useful in preventing recall include midazolam (intermittent 1 mg) or scopolamine (0.3 mg). Many clinicians avoid nitrous oxide entirely in these patients because of the possibility of a pneumothorax and because it limits inspired oxygen concentration. Obviously, drugs that tend to lower blood pressure (eg, histamine release from atracurium and mivacurium) should generally be avoided in patients in hypovolemic shock. The rate of rise of the alveolar concentration of inhalational anesthetics is greater in shock because of lower cardiac output and increased ventilation (see Chapter 7). Higher alveolar anesthetic partial pressures lead to higher arterial partial pressures and greater myocardial depression. Similarly, the effects of intravenous anesthetics are exaggerated as they are injected into a smaller intravascular volume. The key to the safe anesthetic management of shock patients is to administer small incremental doses of whichever agents are selected.

 Invasive monitoring (direct arterial, central venous, and pulmonary artery pressure monitoring) can be extremely helpful in guiding fluid resuscitation, but insertion of these monitors should not detract from the resuscitation itself. Serial hematocrits (or hemoglobin), arterial blood gas measurement, and serum electrolytes (particularly K^+) are invaluable in protracted resuscitations.

HEAD & SPINAL CORD TRAUMA

 Any trauma victim with altered consciousness must be considered to have a brain injury (also see Chapter 26). The level of consciousness is assessed by serial Glasgow Coma Scale evaluations (Table 26–1).

Common injuries requiring immediate surgical intervention include epidural hematoma, acute subdural hematoma, and some penetrating brain injuries and depressed skull fractures. Other injuries that may be managed conservatively include basilar skull fracture and intracerebral hematoma. Basilar skull fractures are often associated with bruising on the eyelids ("raccoon eyes") or over the mastoid process (Battle's sign), and cerebrospinal fluid (CSF) leaks from the ear or nose (CSF rhinorrhea). Other signs of brain damage include restlessness, convulsions, and cranial nerve dysfunction (eg, a nonreactive pupil). The classic Cushing triad (hypertension, bradycardia, and respiratory disturbances) is a late and unreliable sign that usually just precedes brain herniation (Chapter 25). Hypotension is rarely due to head injury alone. Patients suspected of sustaining head trauma should not receive any premedication that will alter their mental status (eg, sedatives, analgesics) or neurological examination (eg, anticholinergic-induced pupillary dilation).

Brain injuries are often accompanied by increased intracranial pressure from cerebral hemorrhage or edema. Intracranial hypertension is controlled by a combination of fluid restriction (except in the presence of hypovolemic shock), diuretics (eg, mannitol, 0.5 g/kg), barbiturates, and deliberate hypocapnia ($PaCO_2$ of 28–32 mm Hg). The latter two require endotracheal intubation, which also protects against aspiration caused by altered airway reflexes. Hypertension or tachycardia during intubation can be attenuated with intravenous lidocaine or fentanyl. Awake intubations cause a precipitous rise in intracranial pressure. Nasal passage of an endotracheal tube or nasogastric tube in patients with basal skull fractures risks cribriform plate perforation and CSF infection. A slight elevation of the head will improve venous drainage and decrease intracranial pressure. The role of corticosteroids in head injury is controversial; most studies have shown either an adverse effect or no benefit. Anesthetic agents that increase intracranial pressure should be avoided (eg, ketamine). Hyperglycemia should also be avoided and treated with insulin if present. Mild hypothermia may prove beneficial in a patient with a head injury because of its proven value in preventing ischemia-induced injury.

Because autoregulation of cerebral blood flow is usually impaired in areas of brain injury, arterial hypertension can worsen cerebral edema and increase intracranial pressure. In addition, episodes of arterial hypotension will cause regional cerebral ischemia. In general, cerebral perfusion pressure (the difference between mean arterial pressure at the level of the brain and the larger of central venous pressure or intracranial pressure) should be maintained above 60 mm Hg.

Patients with severe head injuries are more prone to arterial hypoxemia from pulmonary shunting and ventilation/perfusion mismatching. These changes may be due to aspiration, atelectasis, or direct neural effects on the pulmonary vasculature. Intracranial hypertension may predispose patients to pulmonary edema because of an increase in sympathetic outflow.

The degree of physiological derangement following spinal cord injury is proportional to the level of the lesion. Great care must be taken to prevent further injury during transportation and intubation. Lesions of the cervical spine may involve the phrenic nerves (C3–C5) and cause apnea. Loss of intercostal function limits pulmonary reserve and the ability to cough. High thoracic injuries will eliminate sympathetic innervation of the heart (T1–T4), leading to bradycardia. Acute high spinal cord injury can cause **spinal shock,** a condition characterized by loss of sympathetic tone in the capacitance and resistance vessels below the level of the lesion, resulting in hypotension, bradycardia, areflexia, and gastrointestinal atony. In fact, venous distention in the legs is a sign of spinal cord injury. Hypotension in these patients requires aggressive fluid therapy—tempered by the possibility of pulmonary edema after the acute phase has resolved. Succinylcholine is reportedly safe during the first 48 h following the injury but is associated with life-threatening hyperkalemia afterward. Short-term high-dose corticosteroid therapy with methylprednisolone (30 mg/kg followed by 5.4 mg/kg/h for 23 h) improves the neurological outcome of patients with spinal cord trauma. **Autonomic hyperreflexia** is associated with lesions above T5 but is not a problem during acute management.

CHEST TRAUMA

Trauma to the chest may severely compromise the function of the heart or lungs, leading to cardiogenic shock or hypoxia. A simple pneumothorax is an accumulation of air between the parietal and visceral pleura. The ipsilateral collapse of lung tissue results in a severe ventilation/perfusion abnormality and hypoxia. The overlying chest wall is hyperresonant to percussion, breath sounds are decreased or absent, and a chest film confirms lung collapse. Nitrous oxide will expand a pneumothorax and is contraindicated in these patients. Treatment includes placement of a chest tube in the fourth or fifth intercostal space, anterior to the midaxillary line. A persistent air leak following chest tube placement may indicate injury to a major bronchus.

A tension pneumothorax develops from air entering the pleural space through a one-way valve in the lung or chest wall. In either case, air is forced into the thorax with inspiration but cannot escape during expiration. As a result, the ipsilateral lung completely collapses and the mediastinum and trachea are shifted to the contralateral side. A simple pneumothorax may develop into a tension pneumothorax when positive-pressure ventilation is instituted. Venous return and expansion of the contralateral lung are impaired. Clinical signs include ipsilateral absence of breath sounds and hyperresonance to percussion, contralateral tracheal shift, and distended neck veins. Insertion of a 14-gauge over-the-needle catheter (3–6 cm long) into the second intercostal space at the midclavicular line will convert a tension pneumothorax to an open pneumothorax. Definitive treatment includes chest tube placement as described above.

Multiple rib fractures may compromise the functional integrity of the thorax, resulting in flail chest. Hypoxia is often worsened in these patients by underlying pulmonary contusion or hemothorax. Pulmonary contusion results in worsening respiratory failure over time. Hemothorax is differentiated from pneumothorax by dullness to percussion over silent lung fields. Hemomediastinum, like hemothorax, can also result in hemorrhagic shock. Massive hemoptysis may require isolation of the affected lung with a double-lumen tube (DLT) to prevent blood from entering the healthy lung. Use of a single-lumen endotracheal tube with a bronchial blocker may be safer whenever laryngoscopy is difficult or problems are encountered with the DLT. A large bronchial injury also requires lung separation and ventilation of the unaffected side only (see Chapter 24). High-frequency jet ventilation may alternately be used to ventilate at lower airway pressures and help minimize the bronchial air leak when the bronchial leak is bilateral or the lung separation is not possible. Air leakage from traumatized bronchi can track an open pulmonary vein causing pulmonary and systemic air embolism. The source of the leak must be quickly identified and controlled. Most bronchial ruptures are within 2.5 cm of the carina.

Cardiac tamponade is a life-threatening chest injury that must be recognized early. When a FAST scan or bedside echocardiography is not available, the presence of Beck's triad (neck vein distention, hypotension, and muffled heart tones), **pulsus paradoxus** (a > 10 mm Hg decline in blood pressure during spontaneous inspiration), and a high index of suspicion will help make the diagnosis.

Pericardiocentesis provides temporary relief. This is performed by directing a 16-gauge over-the-needle catheter (at least 15 cm long) from the xiphochondral junction toward the tip of the left scapula at a 45° angle, under the guidance of transthoracic echocardiography or the electrocardiogram. Electrocardiographic changes during pericardiocentesis indicate overadvancement of the needle into the myocardium. Definitive treatment of pericardial tamponade requires thoracotomy. Anesthetic management of these patients should maximize cardiac inotropism, chronotropism, and preload (Chapter 21). For these reasons, ketamine is a favored induction agent. Penetrating injuries to the heart or great vessels require immediate exploration without delay. Repeated manipulation of the heart often results in intermittent episodes of bradycardia and profound hypotension.

Myocardial contusion is usually diagnosed by electrocardiographic changes consistent with ischemia (ST-segment elevation), cardiac enzyme elevations (creatine kinase MB or troponin levels), or an abnormal echocardiogram. Wall motion abnormalities may be observed with transthoracic echocardiography. Patients are at increased risk for dysrhythmias, such as heart block and ventricular fibrillation. Elective surgery should be postponed until all signs of heart injury resolve.

Other possible injuries following chest trauma include aortic transection or aortic dissection, avulsion of the left subclavian artery, aortic or mitral valve disruption, traumatic diaphragmatic herniation, and esophageal rupture. Aortic transection usually occurs just distal to the left subclavian artery following a severe deceleration injury; it classically presents as wide mediastinum on the chest radiograph and may be associated with a fracture of the first rib.

Acute respiratory distress syndrome (ARDS) is usually a delayed pulmonary complication of trauma that has multiple causes: sepsis, direct thoracic injury, aspiration, head injury, fat embolism, massive transfusion, and oxygen toxicity. Clearly, the trauma patient is often at risk for several of these factors. Even with advances in technology, the mortality rate of ARDS approaches 50%. In some cases, ARDS may present early in the operating room. Similarly, aspiration pneumonia, following aspiration in the field prior to intubation, may first present in the operating room and could be confused with ARDS. Mechanical ventilators on anesthesia machines are often incapable of sustaining adequate gas flows in patients who rapidly develop poor lung compliance; use of an intensive care unit ventilator capable of sustaining adequate gas flows at high airway pressure may be necessary.

ABDOMINAL TRAUMA

Patients involved in major trauma should be considered to have an abdominal injury until proved otherwise. Up to 20% of patients with intraabdominal injuries do not have pain or signs of peritoneal irritation (muscle guarding, percussion tenderness, or ileus) on first examination. Large quantities of blood (acute hemoperitoneum) may be present in the abdomen (eg, hepatic or splenic injury) with minimal signs. Abdominal trauma is usually divided into penetrating (eg, gunshot or stabbing) and nonpenetrating (eg, deceleration, crush, or compression injuries).

Penetrating abdominal injuries are usually obvious with entry marks on the abdomen or lower chest. The most commonly injured organ is the liver. Patients tend to fall into three subgroups: (1) pulseless, (2) hemodynamically unstable, and (3) stable. Pulseless and hemodynamically unstable patients (those who fail to maintain a systolic blood pressure of 80–90 mm Hg with 1–2 L of fluid resuscitation should be rushed for immediate laparotomy. They usually have either major vascular or solid organ injury. Stable patients with clinical signs of peritonitis or evisceration should also undergo laparotomy as soon as possible. In contrast, hemodynamically stable patients with penetrating injuries who do not have clinical peritonitis require close evaluation to avoid unnecessary laparotomy. Signs of significant intraabdominal injuries may include free air under the diaphragm on the chest X-ray, blood from the nasogastric tube, hematuria, and rectal blood. Further evaluation of hemodynamically stable patients may include serial physical examinations, local wound exploration, diagnostic peritoneal lavage (DPL), FAST scans, abdominal CT scan, or diagnostic laparoscopy. The use of FAST scans and abdominal CT has reduced the need for DPLs.

Blunt abdominal trauma is the leading cause of morbidity and mortality in trauma, and the leading cause of intraabdominal injuries. Splenic tears or ruptures are most common. A positive FAST scan in a hemodynamically unstable patient with blunt abdominal trauma is an indication for immediate surgery. If the FAST scan is negative or equivocal in an unstable patient, particularly without peritoneal signs, a search is indicated for other sites of blood loss or causes of nonhemorrhagic shock. Management of hemodynamically stable patients with blunt abdominal trauma is based on the FAST scan. If the FAST scan is positive, the decision to proceed to laparoscopy or laparotomy is usually based on an abdominal CT. If the FAST scan is negative, continued observation with serial examinations and repeat FAST scans is usually indicated.

Profound hypotension may follow opening of the abdomen as the tamponading effect of extravasated blood (and bowel distention) is lost. Whenever time permits, preparations for immediate fluid and blood resuscitation with a rapid infusion device should be completed prior to the laparotomy. Nitrous oxide is avoided to prevent worsening of bowel distention. A nasogastric tube (if not already present) will help prevent gastric dilation but should be placed orally if a cribriform plate fracture is suspected. The potential for massive blood transfusion (see Chapter 29) should be anticipated, particularly when abdominal trauma is associated with vascular, hepatic, splenic, or renal injuries, pelvic fractures, or retroperitoneal hemorrhage. Transfusion-induced hyperkalemia is equally as lethal as exsanguination and must be treated aggressively (see Chapters 28 and 29).

Massive abdominal hemorrhage may require packing of bleeding areas and/or clamping of the abdominal aorta until bleeding sites are identified and the resuscitation can catch up with the blood loss. Prolonged aortic clamping leads to ischemic injury to the liver, kidneys, intestines, and, in some instances, a compartment syndrome of the lower extremities; the latter can produce rhabdomyolysis and acute renal failure. The use of a mannitol infusion and a loop diuretic (prior to aortic cross-clamping), along with resuscitation fluid may prevent renal failure in such instances but is controversial. Rapid resuscitation with fluids and blood products via a rapid transfusion device, together with control of the bleeding, shortens cross-clamp time and likely reduces the incidence of such complications.

Progressive bowel edema from injuries and fluid resuscitation may preclude abdominal closure at the end of the procedure. Tight abdominal closures markedly increase intraabdominal pressure, resulting in an abdominal compartment syndrome that can produce renal and splanchnic ischemia. Oxygenation and ventilation are often severely compromised, even with complete muscle paralysis. Oliguria and renal shutdown follow. In such cases, the abdomen should be left open (but sterilely covered—often with intravenous bag plastic) for 48–72 h until the edema subsides and secondary closure can be undertaken.

EXTREMITY TRAUMA

Extremity injuries can be life-threatening because of associated vascular injuries and secondary infectious complications. Vascular injuries can lead to massive hemorrhage and threaten extremity viability. For example, a femoral fracture can be associated with 2–3 units of occult blood loss, and closed pelvic fractures can cause even more occult blood loss resulting in hypovolemic shock. Delay of treatment or indiscriminate positioning can worsen dislocations and further compromise neurovascular bundles. **Fat emboli** are associated with pelvic and long-bone fractures and may cause pulmonary insufficiency, dysrhythmias, skin petechiae, and mental deterioration within 1–3 days after the traumatic event (see Chapter 40). The laboratory diagnosis of fat embolism depends on elevation of serum lipase, fat in the urine, and thrombocytopenia.

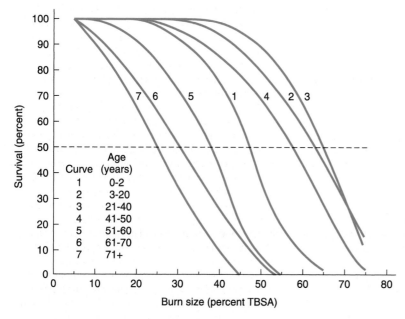

Figure 41–1. Sigmoid curves showing survival of humans as a function of total percentage of body surface burned and age. Survival curves are estimated by probit analysis for seven age categories. (Reproduced, with permission, from Merrell SW et al: Increased survival after major thermal injury. Am J Surg 1987;154:623.)

A compartment syndrome can also occur following large intramuscular hematomas, crush injuries, fractures, and amputation injuries. An increase in internal fascial pressure together with a reduced arterial pressure results in ischemia, tissue hypoxia, and progressive swelling. As previously discussed, rhabdomyolysis and renal failure may result. Reperfusion when blood pressure is restored can aggravate the injury and edema. The forearm and lower leg are most at risk. The diagnosis may be made clinically or based on direct measurement of compartment pressures: greater than 45 mm Hg or within 10–30 mm Hg of diastolic blood pressure. Early fasciotomy to save the limb is recommended.

Modern surgical techniques frequently allow the reimplantation of severed extremities and digits (see Chapter 40). A cooled, amputated, limb part may be reimplanted up to 20 h following amputation; a noncooled part has to be implanted within 6 h. If the injury is isolated, a regional technique (eg, brachial or interscalene plexus block) is often recommended to increase peripheral blood flow by interrupting sympathetic innervation. During general anesthesia, the patient should be kept warm, and emergence shivering must be avoided to maximize perfusion.

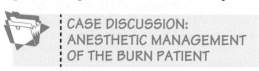

CASE DISCUSSION: ANESTHETIC MANAGEMENT OF THE BURN PATIENT

A 43-year-old man who suffered a major thermal burn 7 days previously is scheduled for excision and grafting under general anesthesia.

How are burn injuries classified?

Burn injuries are described according to the percentage of body surface area involved and the depth of the skin destroyed. Survival is influenced by the percentage surface area involved and the age of the patient (Figure 41–1). The rule of nines divides the body's surface area into areas of 9% or multiples of 9% (Figure 41–2). The surface area of one side of the patient's hand represents 1% of total body surface area.

First-degree burns are limited to the epithelium, second-degree burns extend into the dermis, and third-degree burns destroy the entire skin thickness. It is ironic that because third-degree burns devastate nerve endings, they are not as painful as second-degree burns. A major thermal burn is considered to be a second-degree burn involving at least 25% of the body surface area or a third-degree burn of at least 10% of the body surface area. Electrical burns are typically more serious than superficial inspection would indicate because of underlying tissue damage. Pulmonary involvement, particularly with an underlying pneumonia, adds dramatically to the mortality rate.

How should the pulmonary pathophysiology associated with major burn injuries be described?

Pulmonary function can be directly or indirectly affected. Direct inhalational injury is usually limit-

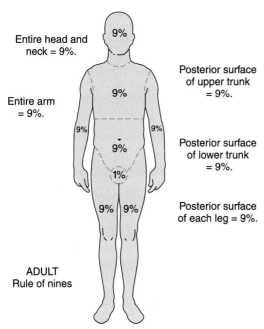

Entire head and
neck = 9%.

9%

Posterior surface
of upper trunk
= 9%.

Entire arm
= 9%.

9%

9%

9%

Posterior surface
of lower trunk
= 9%.

9%

1%

9% 9%

Posterior surface
of each leg = 9%.

ADULT
Rule of nines

Figure 41–2. Estimation of body surface area in burns. (Modified and reproduced, with permission, from Tierney LM Jr et al: *Current Medical Diagnosis & Treatment 2002.* McGraw-Hill, 2002.)

ed to upper airway edema that can lead to life-threatening airway obstruction. Nonetheless, lower airways can also be subjected to direct thermal insult (eg, steam) or can be injured by exposure to smoke and toxic products of combustion. Deactivation of surfactant can lead to atelectasis and pulmonary shunting. Indications of inhalational injury include stridor, hoarseness, facial burns, singed nasal hair or eyebrows, soot in sputum or in the oropharynx, respiratory distress, or a history of combustion in a closed space. Many patients with inhalational injury, however, do not demonstrate any signs until several hours postexposure.

Major burns can alter pulmonary function even in the absence of direct lung injury. For example, permeability can be increased throughout the entire microvascular system and may contribute to the development of pulmonary edema and acute respiratory distress syndrome. Circumferential burns of the thorax may decrease chest wall compliance and further increase peak inspiratory pressures.

Carbon monoxide inhalation shifts the oxygen–hemoglobin curve to the left (interfering with the unloading of oxygen at tissues) and decreases oxyhemoglobin saturation. Pao_2 and skin color may remain normal, but carboxyhemoglobin (COHb) concentration will be increased (normal COHb < 1.5% in nonsmokers and < 10% in smokers). As opposed to laboratory cooximeters, pulse oximeters using two wavelengths cannot detect COHb (see Chapter 6). Carbon monoxide's affinity for hemoglobin is 200 times greater than that of oxygen. Administration of 100% oxygen will shorten the half-life of COHb from 4 h in room air to less than 1 h. The use of hyperbaric oxygen is controversial, but it should be considered if available. Hydrogen cyanide released from synthetic materials will further limit oxygen availability and utilization (the normal blood cyanide level is < 0.2 μg/mL) and may provide another indication for hyperbaric oxygen therapy.

Metabolism is markedly increased during the healing phase of a burn injury. This hypermetabolic state is reflected by increased oxygen consumption and CO_2 production. Therefore, alveolar ventilation must be proportionately increased and supplemental oxygen supplied.

What cardiovascular effects are associated with major burn injuries?

Increases in permeability at the site of injury and throughout the microvasculature cause a tremendous shift of fluid from the plasma volume to the interstitial space. Despite red blood cell destruction, hematocrit may rise as a result of the contraction of intravascular volume. This decrease in intravascular volume is most pronounced during the first 24 h and is typically replaced with crystalloid solutions (eg, lactated Ringer's injection, 2–4 mL/kg per percentage of body surface burned). Cardiac output declines as a result of the contraction of plasma volume and a circulating myocardial depressant factor. Perfusion of vital organs is monitored by measurement of urinary output through a Foley catheter. If volume replacement does not provide an adequate diuresis (1 mL/kg/h), inotropic support with dopamine may be beneficial.

After 24–48 h, capillary integrity returns to normal, and colloid solutions will remain intravascular. Interstitial fluid reabsorption, increased metabolic demands, and high levels of circulating catecholamines may lead to high-output failure. Blood pressure and heart rate are typically elevated.

What electrolyte derangements can be found in burn patients?

Hyperkalemia from tissue destruction may complicate management during the acute resuscitation phase. Later, renal wasting and gastric losses may result in hypokalemia. Topical antibiotic therapy may also cause electrolyte imbalances. Mafenide acetate inhibits carbonic anhydrase, causing hyperchloremic acidosis. Another topical medication, silver nitrate, decreases serum sodium, chloride, and potassium levels. Significant methemoglobinemia is a rare complication of topical silver nitrate therapy. Electrical burns are associated with such severe muscle cell damage that myoglobinuria can lead to renal failure.

Which monitors would be useful during this excision and grafting procedure?

Excision of dead tissue after a major burn injury is usually associated with significant blood loss. This is particularly true if surgery is delayed more than a few days after the burn or if the burn is not limited to areas that can be isolated with tourniquets. In these situations, at least two large-bore intravenous lines, an arterial line, and often a central venous catheter or pulmonary artery catheter are indicated. A central triple-lumen catheter can be helpful in patients with difficult intravenous access. If possible, a noninvasive blood pressure unit should be used as a backup to the arterial line, which may malfunction if the patient is frequently repositioned.

Electrocardiograph skin electrodes will not stick to burned areas, and they interfere with chest wall excision. As an alternative, needle electrodes are often sutured in place. Patients with respiratory insufficiency should be monitored with pulse oximetry if a suitable probe location is available.

Heat loss through denuded skin is a serious problem in the burn patient and should be closely monitored. Hypothermia can be minimized by using warming blankets and heat lamps, increasing operating room temperature, humidifying inspired gases, and warming intravenous fluids.

Are there any special intubation considerations in these patients?

Burn victims with inhalational injury will often be intubated prior to surgery. Indications for early intubation include hypoxia not correctable with a face mask, upper airway edema that may progress to obstruction, or the presence of copious secretions. If in doubt, or if periods of questionable airway monitoring are anticipated (eg, during transport), intubate before edema develops and before intubation becomes technically difficult. This is particularly important if the patient is being stabilized prior to transfer to another hospital. Impending airway obstruction or severe facial contractures call for an awake fiberoptic intubation. Precautions to prevent emesis and aspiration should be considered in the acute resuscitation phase, during episodes of sepsis, or if the patient is receiving large doses of narcotics. Tracheostomies have been associated with increased morbidity in burn patients because of pulmonary sepsis.

How does a burn injury affect the pharmacology of anesthetic drugs?

Succinylcholine is contraindicated in burn patients after the first 24 h. Its administration has caused cardiac arrest because of dramatic increases in serum potassium levels. Prolonged muscle depolarization following succinylcholine appears to be related to an increase in postjunctional acetylcholine receptors. This response has even been documented in patients with less than a 10% body surface area burn. In contrast, burn patients require higher than normal doses of nondepolarizing muscle relaxants. This resistance is due to altered protein binding and an increased number of extrajunctional acetylcholine receptors, which bind nondepolarizing drug without causing a neuromuscular effect.

Volatile anesthetics will exacerbate myocardial depression but are useful after the acute phase. Because of the potential for serious dysrhythmias, halothane is best avoided if epinephrine-soaked bandages are being used to decrease blood loss.

SUGGESTED READING

Boffard KD, Brooks AJ: Pancreatic trauma—injuries to the pancreas and pancreatic duct. Eur J Surg 2000;166:4.

Brooks AJ, Rowlands BJ: Blunt abdominal injuries. Br Med Bull 1999;55:844.

Dabrowski GP, Steinberg SM, Ferrara JJ, Flint LM: A critical assessment of endpoints of shock resuscitation. Surg Clin North Am 2000;80:825.

Dutton RP, Sharrar SR: Trauma. Int Anesth Clin 2002:40:1.

Dykes EH: Paediatric trauma. Br J Anaesth 1999;83:130.

Ferrada R, Birolini D: New concepts in the management of patients with penetrating abdominal wounds. Surg Clin North Am 1999;79:1331.

Ho AM, Ling E: Systemic air embolism after lung trauma. Anesthesiology 1999;90:564.

Kao CC, Garner WL: Acute burns. Plastic Reconstruct Surg 2000;105:2482.

King BS, Gupta R, Narayan RK: The early assessment and intensive care unit management of patients with severe traumatic brain and spinal cord injuries. Surg Clin North Am 2000;80:855.

Kirkpatrick AW, Sirois M, Bali CG, et al: The hand-held ultrasound examination for penetrating abdominal trauma. Am J Surg 2004;187:660.

Parks RW, Chrysos E, Diamond T: Management of liver trauma. Br J Surg 1999;86:1121.

Peach SE, Trunkey D: Blunt injury of the thoracic aorta. Eur J Surg 1999;165:1110.

Resources for Optimal Care of the Injured Patient: 1999 Committee on Trauma, American College of Surgeons, 1998.

Rosenberg AD, Grande C, Bernstein RL: *Pain Management and Regional Anesthesia in Trauma.* W.B. Saunders, 1999.

Slater MDJ, Mullins RJ: Crush injury and rhabdomyolysis. Crit Care Clin 2004;20:171.

Strong RW: The management of blunt liver injuries. Aust NZ J Surg 1999;69:609.

Trunkey DD, Lewis FR: *Current Therapy of Trauma,* 4th ed. Mosby-Yearbook, 1999.

WEB SITES

http://www.trauma.org/

This web site provides educational information, useful references, and links for professionals in trauma and critical care.

Maternal & Fetal Physiology & Anesthesia

42

KEY CONCEPTS

 The minimal alveolar concentration (MAC) progressively decreases during pregnancy—at term, by as much as 40%—for all general anesthetic agents; MAC returns to normal by the third day after delivery.

 Pregnant patients display enhanced sensitivity to local anesthetics during regional anesthesia; dose requirements may be reduced as much as 30%.

 Obstruction of the inferior vena cava by the enlarging uterus distends the epidural venous plexus and increases the risk of intravascular injection during epidural anesthesia.

 Up to 20% of women at term develop the supine hypotension syndrome, which is characterized by hypotension associated with pallor, sweating, or nausea and vomiting.

 The reduction in gastric motility and the tone of the gastroesophageal sphincter as well as hypersecretion of gastric acid place the parturient at high risk for regurgitation and pulmonary aspiration.

 Ephedrine, which has predominantly β-adrenergic activity, has traditionally been considered the vasopressor of choice for hypotension during pregnancy. However, clinical studies suggest that α-adrenergic agonists such as phenylephrine and

metaraminol are just as effective in treating hypotension in pregnant patients and are associated with less fetal acidosis than ephedrine.

 Volatile inhalational anesthetics decrease blood pressure and, potentially, uteroplacental blood flow. In concentrations of less than 1 MAC, however, their effects are generally minor, consisting of dose-dependent uterine relaxation and minor reductions in uterine blood flow.

 The greatest strain on the parturient's heart occurs immediately after delivery, when intense uterine contraction and involution suddenly relieve inferior vena caval obstruction and increase cardiac output as much as 80% above prelabor values.

 Current techniques employing very dilute combinations of a local anesthetic (eg bupivacaine 0.125% or less) and an opioid (eg, fentanyl 5 μg/mL or less) for epidural or combined spinal–epidural (CSE) analgesia do not appear to prolong labor or increase the likelihood of a cesarean section.

  Because the maturation of the lungs occurs later in fetal development, extrauterine life is not possible until after 24–25 weeks of gestation, when pulmonary capillaries are formed and come to lie in close approximation to an immature alveolar epithelium.

Pregnancy produces profound physiological changes that alter the usual responses to anesthesia. Moreover, anesthetic care of the pregnant patient is unique in that two patients are cared for simultaneously: the parturi-

ent and the fetus. Failure to take these facts into consideration can have disastrous consequences.

This chapter reviews the normal physiological changes associated with pregnancy, labor, and delivery.

Uteroplacental physiology and its response to common anesthetic agents are also discussed. Much of this knowledge forms the basis for current anesthetic practices for labor and delivery (see Chapter 43). Lastly, care of the neonate in the obstetric suite or the intensive care unit requires an understanding of the physiological transition from fetal to neonatal life.

PHYSIOLOGICAL CHANGES DURING PREGNANCY

Pregnancy affects virtually every organ system (Table 42–1). Many of these physiological changes appear to be adaptive and useful to the mother in tolerating the stresses of pregnancy, labor, and delivery. Other changes lack obvious benefits but nonetheless require special consideration in caring for the parturient.

Central Nervous System Effects

The minimal alveolar concentration (MAC) progressively decreases during pregnancy—at term, by as much as 40%—for all general anesthetic agents; MAC returns to normal by the third day after delivery. Changes in maternal hormonal and endogenous opioid levels have been implicated. Progesterone, which is sedating when given in pharmacological doses, increases up to 20 times normal at term and is probably at least partly responsible for this observation. A surge in β-endorphin levels during labor and delivery also likely plays a major role.

At term, pregnant patients also display enhanced sensitivity to local anesthetics during regional anesthesia; dose requirements may be reduced as much as 30%. This phenomenon appears to be hormonally mediated but may also be related to engorgement of the epidural venous plexus. Neural blockade occurs at lower concentrations of local anesthetics. The minimum local analgesic concentration (MLAC) is used in obstetric anesthesia to compare the relative potencies of local anesthetics and the effects of additives; MLAC is defined as the median effective analgesic concentration (EC_{50}) in a 20 mL volume for epidural analgesia in the first stage of labor. Contrary to previous studies, more recent data suggest that pregnancy does not increase susceptibility to local anesthetic toxicity. Obstruction of the inferior vena cava by the enlarging uterus distends the epidural venous plexus and increases epidural blood volume. The latter has three major effects: (1) decreased spinal cerebrospinal fluid volume, (2) decreased potential volume of the epidural space, and (3) increased epidural (space) pressure. The first two effects enhance the cephalad spread of local anesthetic solutions during spinal and epidural anesthesia, respectively, whereas the

Table 42–1. Average maximum physiological changes associated with pregnancy.[1]

Parameter	Change
Neurological	
MAC	−40%
Respiratory	
Oxygen consumption	+20 to 50%
Airway resistance	−35%
FRC	−20%
Minute ventilation	+50%
Tidal volume	+40%
Respiratory rate	+15%
PaO_2	+10%
$PaCO_2$	−15%
HCO_3	−15%
Cardiovascular	
Blood volume	+35%
Plasma volume	+45%
Cardiac output	+40%
Stroke volume	+30%
Heart rate	+20%
Systolic blood pressure	−5%
Diastolic blood pressure	−15%
Peripheral resistance	−15%
Pulmonary resistance	−30%
Hematologic	
Hemoglobin	−20%
Platelets	−10%
Clotting factors[2]	+30 to 250%
Renal	
GFR	+50%

[1]MAC, minimum alveolar concentration; FRC, functional residual capacity; GFR, glomerular filtration rate.
[2]Varies with each factor.

last may predispose to a higher incidence of dural puncture with epidural anesthesia (see Chapter 16). Bearing down during labor further accentuates all these effects. Positive epidural pressures have been recorded in parturients and complicate identification of the epidural space without dural puncture. Engorgement of the epidural veins also increases the likelihood of placing an epidural catheter in a vein, resulting in an unintentional intravascular injection (see Chapter 16).

Respiratory Effects

Oxygen consumption and minute ventilation progressively increase during pregnancy. Both tidal volume and, to a lesser extent, respiratory rate increase. By term, oxygen consumption has increased about 20–50% and minute ventilation has increased up to 50%. $PaCO_2$ decreases to 28–32 mm Hg; significant respiratory alkalosis is prevented by a compensatory decrease in plasma bicarbonate concentration. Hyperventilation may also increase PaO_2 slightly. Elevated levels of 2,3-diphosphoglycerate offset the effect of hyperventilation on hemoglobin's affinity for oxygen (see Chapter 22). The P-50 for hemoglobin increases from 27 to 30 mm Hg; the combination of the latter with an increase in cardiac output (see section on Cardiovascular Effects below) enhances oxygen delivery to tissues.

The maternal respiratory pattern changes as the uterus enlarges. In the third trimester, elevation of the diaphragm is compensated by an increase in the anteroposterior diameter of the chest; diaphragmatic motion, however, is not restricted. Thoracic breathing is favored over abdominal breathing. Both vital capacity and closing capacity are minimally affected but functional residual capacity (FRC) decreases up to 20% at term; FRC returns to normal within 48 h of delivery. This decrease is principally due to a reduction in expiratory reserve volume as a result of larger than normal tidal volumes (see Chapter 22). Flow–volume loops are unaffected, and airway resistance decreases. Physiological dead space decreases but intrapulmonary shunting increases toward term. A chest film often shows prominent vascular markings due to increased pulmonary blood volume and an elevated diaphragm. Pulmonary vasodilatation prevents pulmonary pressures from rising.

The combination of decreased FRC and increased oxygen consumption promotes rapid oxygen desaturation during periods of apnea (see Chapter 22). Preoxygenation prior to induction of general anesthesia is therefore mandatory to avoid hypoxemia in pregnant patients. Closing volume exceeds FRC in up to 50% of all pregnant women when they are supine at term. Under these conditions, atelectasis and hypoxemia readily occur. Parturients should generally not lie completely flat without supplemental oxygen. The decrease in FRC coupled with the increase in minute ventilation accelerates the uptake of all inhalational anesthetics. The reduction in dead space narrows the arterial end-tidal CO_2 gradient.

Capillary engorgement of the respiratory mucosa during pregnancy predisposes the upper airways to trauma, bleeding, and obstruction. Gentle laryngoscopy and the use of small endotracheal tubes (6–6.5 mm) should be employed during general anesthesia.

Cardiovascular Effects

Cardiac output and blood volume increase to meet accelerated maternal and fetal metabolic demands. An increase (45%) in plasma volume in excess of an increase in red cell mass produces dilutional anemia and reduces blood viscosity. Hemoglobin concentration, however, usually remains greater than 11 g/dL. Moreover, in terms of tissue oxygen delivery, the reduction in hemoglobin concentration is offset by the increase in cardiac output and the rightward shift of the hemoglobin dissociation curve (see the section on Respiratory Effects). A decrease in systemic vascular resistance by the second trimester decreases both diastolic and, to a lesser degree, systolic blood pressure. The response to adrenergic agents and vasoconstrictors is blunted.

At term, blood volume has increased by 1000–1500 mL in most women, allowing them to easily tolerate the blood loss associated with delivery; total blood volume reaches 90 mL/kg. Average blood loss during vaginal delivery is 400–500 mL, compared with 800–1000 mL for a cesarean section. Blood volume does not return to normal until 1–2 weeks after delivery.

The increase in cardiac output (40% at term) is due to increases in both heart rate (15–20%) as well as stroke volume (30%). Cardiac chambers enlarge and myocardial hypertrophy is often noted on echocardiography. Pulmonary artery, central venous, and pulmonary artery wedge pressures, however, remain unchanged. Most of these effects are observed in the first and, to a lesser extent, the second trimester. In the third trimester, cardiac output does not appreciably rise, except during labor. The greatest increases in cardiac output are seen during labor and immediately after delivery (see the section on Effect of Labor on Maternal Physiology). Cardiac output often does not return to normal until 2 weeks after delivery.

Decreases in cardiac output can occur in the supine position after week 28 of pregnancy. (Some authors suggest even earlier.) Such decreases have been shown to be secondary to impeded venous return to the heart as the enlarging uterus compresses the inferior vena cava. Up to 20% of women at term develop the supine hypotension syndrome, which is characterized by hypotension associated with pallor, sweating, or nausea and vomiting. The cause of this syndrome appears to be complete or near-complete occlusion of the inferior vena cava by the gravid uterus. Turning the patient on her side typically restores venous return from the lower body and corrects the hypotension in such instances. The Trendelenburg position may exacerbate caval compression. The gravid uterus also compresses the aorta in most parturients when they are supine. This latter effect decreases blood flow to the lower extremities and, more importantly, to the uteroplacental circulation. Uterine contraction relieves caval compression but exacerbates aortic compression.

Aortocaval compression is an important but preventable cause of fetal distress. The combination of systemic hypotension (due to decreased venous return), increased uterine venous pressure, and uterine arterial hypoperfusion severely compromises uterine and placental blood flows. When combined with the hypotensive effects of regional or general anesthesia, **aortocaval compression** can readily produce fetal asphyxia. Parturients with a 28-week or longer gestation should not be placed supine without left uterine displacement. This maneuver is most readily accomplished by placing a wedge (> 15°) under the right hip.

Chronic partial caval obstruction in the third trimester predisposes to venous stasis, phlebitis, and edema in the lower extremities. Moreover, compression of the inferior vena cava below the diaphragm distends and increases blood flow through collateral venous drainage, ie, the paravertebral venous plexus (including the epidural veins) and to a minor degree the abdominal wall.

Lastly, elevation of the diaphragm shifts the heart's position in the chest, resulting in the appearance of an enlarged heart on a plain chest film and in left axis deviation and T wave changes on the electrocardiogram (ECG). Physical examination often reveals a systolic ejection flow murmur (grade I or II) and exaggerated splitting of the first heart sound (S_1); a third heart sound (S_3) may be audible. A few patients develop small, asymptomatic pericardial effusions.

Renal Effects

Renal vasodilatation increases renal blood flow early during pregnancy but autoregulation is preserved. The kidneys often enlarge. Increased renin and aldosterone levels promote sodium retention. Renal plasma flow and the glomerular filtration rate increase as much as 50% during the first trimester; glomerular filtration declines toward normal in the third trimester. Serum creatinine and blood urea nitrogen may decrease to 0.5–0.6 mg/dL and 8–9 mg/dL, respectively. A decreased renal tubular threshold for glucose and amino acids is common and often results in mild glycosuria (1–10 g/d) or proteinuria (< 300 mg/d). Plasma osmolality decreases by 8–10 mOsm/kg.

Gastrointestinal Effects

Gastroesophageal reflux and esophagitis are common during pregnancy. Upward and anterior displacement of the stomach by the uterus promotes incompetence of the gastroesophageal sphincter. Elevated progesterone levels reduce the tone of the gastroesophageal sphincter, whereas placental gastrin secretion causes hypersecretion of gastric acid. These factors place the parturient at high risk for regurgitation and pulmonary aspiration. Intragastric pressure is unchanged. Data with regard to gastric emptying are conflicting; some studies suggest normal gastric empty-

ing is preserved until the onset of labor. Nonetheless, nearly all parturients have a gastric pH under 2.5, and over 60% of them have gastric volumes greater than 25 mL. Both factors have been associated with an increased risk of severe aspiration pneumonitis. Opioids and anticholinergics reduce lower esophageal sphincter pressure, may facilitate gastroesophageal reflux, and delay gastric emptying. These physiological effects, together with recent food ingestion just prior to labor and any delayed gastric emptying associated with labor pains, predispose parturients to nausea and vomiting.

Hepatic Effects

Overall hepatic function and blood flow are unchanged; minor elevations in serum transaminases and lactic dehydrogenase levels may be observed in the third trimester. Elevations in serum alkaline phosphatase are due to its secretion by the placenta (see Chapter 34). A mild decrease in serum albumin is due to an expanded plasma volume; as a result, colloid oncotic pressure is reduced. A 25–30% decrease in serum pseudocholinesterase activity is also present at term but rarely produces significant prolongation of succinylcholine's action. The breakdown of mivacurium and ester-type local anesthetics is not appreciably altered. Pseudocholinesterase activity may not return to normal until up to 6 weeks postpartum. High progesterone levels appear to inhibit the release of cholecystokinin, resulting in incomplete emptying of the gallbladder. The latter, together with altered bile acid composition, can predispose to the formation of cholesterol gallstones during pregnancy.

Hematological Effects

Pregnancy is associated with a hypercoagulable state that may be beneficial in limiting blood loss at delivery. Fibrinogen and factors VII, VIII, IX, X, and XII concentrations all increase; only factor XI levels may decrease. Accelerated fibrinolysis can be observed late in the third trimester. In addition to the dilutional anemia (see the section on Cardiovascular Effects), leukocytosis (up to 21,000/μL) and a 10% decrease in platelet count may be encountered during the third trimester. Because of fetal utilization, iron and folate deficiency anemias readily develop if supplements of these nutrients are not taken. Cell-mediated immunity is markedly depressed and may increase susceptibility to viral infections.

Metabolic Effects

Complex metabolic and hormonal changes occur during pregnancy. Altered carbohydrate, fat, and protein metabolism favors fetal growth and development. These changes resemble starvation, because blood glucose and amino acid levels are low whereas free fatty acids, ketones, and triglyceride levels are high. Nonetheless, pregnancy is a diabetogenic state; insulin levels steadily rise during pregnancy. Secretion of human placental lactogen, also called human chorionic somatomammotropin, by the placenta is probably responsible for the relative insulin resistance associated with pregnancy. Pancreatic B cell hyperplasia occurs in response to an increased demand for insulin secretion.

Secretion of human chorionic gonadotropin and elevated levels of estrogens promote hypertrophy of the thyroid gland and increase thyroid-binding globulin; although T_4 and T_3 levels are elevated, free T_4, free T_3, and thyrotropin (thyroid-stimulating hormone) remain normal. Serum calcium levels decrease, but ionized calcium concentration remains normal.

Musculoskeletal Effects

Elevated levels of relaxin throughout pregnancy help prepare for delivery by softening the cervix, inhibiting uterine contractions, and relaxing the pubic symphysis and pelvic joints. Ligamentous laxity of the spine increases the risk of back injury. The latter may contribute to the relatively high incidence of back pain during pregnancy.

UTEROPLACENTAL CIRCULATION

A normal uteroplacental circulation (Figure 42–1) is critical in the development and maintenance of a healthy fetus. Uteroplacental insufficiency is an important cause of intrauterine fetal growth retardation and when severe can result in fetal demise. The integrity of

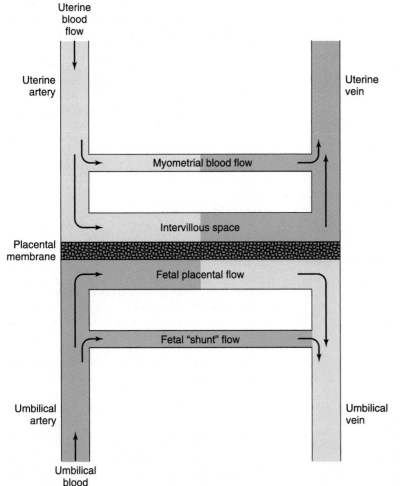

Figure 42–1. The uteroplacental circulation. (Modified and reproduced, with permission, from Schnider S, Levinson G: *Anesthesia for Obstetrics*, 2nd ed. Williams & Wilkins, 1987.)

this circulation is, in turn, dependent on both adequate uterine blood flow and normal placental function.

Uterine Blood Flow

At term, **uterine blood flow** represents about 10% of the cardiac output, or 600–700 mL/min (compared with 50 mL/min in the nonpregnant uterus). Eighty percent of uterine blood flow normally supplies the placenta; the remainder goes to the myometrium. Pregnancy maximally dilates the uterine vasculature, so that autoregulation is absent, but it remains sensitive to α-adrenergic agonists. Uterine blood flow is not usually significantly affected by respiratory gas tensions, but extreme hypocapnia ($PaCO_2$ < 20 mm Hg) can reduce uterine blood flow and causes fetal hypoxemia and acidosis.

Blood flow is directly proportionate to the difference between uterine arterial and venous pressures but inversely proportionate to uterine vascular resistance. Although not under appreciable neural control, the uterine vasculature has α-adrenergic and possibly some β-adrenergic receptors.

Three major factors decrease uterine blood flow during pregnancy: (1) systemic hypotension, (2) uterine vasoconstriction, and (3) uterine contractions. Common causes of hypotension during pregnancy include aortocaval compression, hypovolemia, and sympathetic blockade following regional anesthesia. Stress-induced release of endogenous catecholamines (sympathoadrenal activation) during labor causes uterine arterial vasoconstriction. Any drug with α-adrenergic activity (eg, phenylephrine) potentially is capable of decreasing uterine blood flow by vasoconstriction. Ephedrine, which has predominantly β-adrenergic activity, has traditionally been considered the vasopressor of choice for hypotension during pregnancy. However, clinical studies suggest that α-adrenergic agonists such as phenylephrine and metaraminol are just as effective in treating hypotension in pregnant patients and are associated with *less* fetal acidosis than ephedrine.

Paradoxically, hypertensive disorders are often associated with decreased uterine blood flow due to generalized vasoconstriction. **Uterine contractions decrease blood flow by elevating uterine venous pressure and, when intense, compressing arterial vessels as they traverse the myometrium.** Hypertonic contractions during labor or during oxytocin infusions can critically compromise uterine blood flow.

Placental Function

The fetus is dependent on the placenta for respiratory gas exchange, nutrition, and waste elimination. The placenta is formed by both maternal and fetal tissues

and derives a blood supply from each. The resulting exchange membrane has a functional area of about 1.8 m².

A. PHYSIOLOGICAL ANATOMY

The placenta (Figure 42–2) is composed of projections of fetal tissue (villi) that lie in maternal vascular spaces (intervillous spaces). As a result of this arrangement, the fetal capillaries within villi readily exchange substances with the maternal blood that bathes them. Maternal blood in the intervillous spaces is derived from spiral branches of the uterine artery and drains into the uterine veins. Fetal blood within villi is derived from the umbilical cord via two umbilical arteries and returns to the fetus via a single umbilical vein.

B. PLACENTAL EXCHANGE

Placental exchange can occur by one of five mechanisms:

1. Diffusion—Respiratory gases and small ions are transported by diffusion. Most drugs used in anesthesia have molecular weights well under 1000 and consequently can diffuse across the placenta.

2. Bulk flow—Water moves across by bulk flow.

3. Active transport—Amino acids, vitamins, and some ions (calcium and iron) utilize this mechanism.

4. Pinocytosis—Large molecules, such as immunoglobulins, are transported by pinocytosis.

5. Breaks—Breaks in the placental membrane and mixing of maternal and fetal blood are probably responsible for Rh sensitization (see Chapter 29).

Respiratory Gas Exchange

Of all the substances exchanged across the placenta, oxygen has the lowest storage-to-utilization ratio. At term, fetal oxygen consumption averages about 21 mL/min, yet fetal oxygen stores are normally estimated to be only 42 mL. Fortunately, because of multiple adaptive mechanisms, the normal fetus at term can survive 10 min or longer instead of the expected 2 min of total oxygen deprivation. Partial or complete oxygen deprivation can result from umbilical cord compression, umbilical cord prolapse, placental abruption, severe maternal hypoxemia, or hypotension. Compensatory mechanisms include redistribution of fetal blood flow primarily to the brain, heart, placenta, and adrenal gland; decreased oxygen consumption; and anaerobic metabolism.

Transfer of oxygen across the placenta is dependent on the ratio of maternal uterine blood flow to fetal umbilical blood flow. Animal studies suggest that the reserve for oxygen transfer is small even during normal pregnancy. Well-oxygenated fetal blood from the pla-

Figure 42–2. The placenta.

centa has a PaO$_2$ of only 40 mm Hg. To aid oxygen transfer, the fetal hemoglobin oxygen dissociation curve is shifted to the left such that fetal hemoglobin has greater affinity for oxygen than does maternal hemoglobin (whose curve is already shifted to the right; see the section on Respiratory Effects). In addition, fetal hemoglobin concentration is usually 15 g/dL (compared with approximately 12 g/dL in the mother).

Carbon dioxide readily diffuses across the placenta. Maternal hyperventilation (see the section on Respiratory Effects) increases the gradient for the transfer of carbon dioxide from the fetus into the maternal circulation. Fetal hemoglobin also appears to have less affinity for carbon dioxide than does maternal hemoglobin.

Placental Transfer of Anesthetic Agents

Transfer of a drug across the placenta is reflected by the ratio of its fetal umbilical vein to maternal venous con-

centrations (UV/MV), whereas its uptake by fetal tissues can be correlated with the ratio of its fetal umbilical artery to umbilical vein concentrations (UA/UV). Fetal effects of drugs administered to parturients depend on multiple factors including route of administration (intramuscular, intravenous, epidural, or intrathecal), dose, timing of administration (both relative to delivery as well as contractions), and maturity of the fetal organs (brain and liver). Thus, giving a drug hours before delivery or as a single intravenous bolus during a uterine contraction just prior to delivery (when uterine blood flow is maximally reduced) is least likely to produce high fetal levels. Effects on the fetus can be evaluated intrapartum by changes in fetal heart rate pattern or acid–base status, or postpartum by Apgar scores or neurobehavioral examinations (see Chapter 43). Fortunately, current anesthetic techniques for labor and delivery (see Chapter 43) generally have minimal fetal effects despite significant placental transfer of anesthetic agents and adjuncts.

All inhalational agents and most intravenous agents freely cross the placenta. Inhalational agents generally produce little fetal depression when they are given in limited doses (< 1 MAC) and delivery occurs within 10 min of induction. Thiopental, ketamine, propofol, and benzodiazepines readily cross the placenta and can be detected in the fetal circulation. Fortunately, when these agents, with the exception of benzodiazepines, are used in usual induction doses, drug distribution, metabolism, and possibly placental uptake may limit fetal effects. Although most opiates readily cross the placenta, their effects on neonates at delivery vary considerably. Newborns appear to be more sensitive to the respiratory depressant effect of morphine compared with that of other opioids. Although respiratory depression is significant with meperidine, peaking 1–3 h after administration, it is still less than morphine; butorphanol and nalbuphine produce even less respiratory depression, but still may have significant neurobehavioral depressant effects. Although fentanyl readily crosses the placenta, it appears to have minimal neonatal effects unless large intravenous doses (> 1 μg/kg) are given immediately before delivery. Epidural or intrathecal fentanyl, sufentanil, and, to a lesser extent, morphine (see Chapter 43) generally produce minimal neonatal effects. Alfentanil causes neonatal depression similar to meperidine. Remifentanil also readily crosses the placenta and has the potential to produce respiratory depression in newborns. Fetal blood concentrations of remifentanil are generally about half those of the mother just prior to delivery. The UA/UV ratio is about 30%, suggesting fairly rapid metabolism of remifentanil in the neonate. The highly ionized property of muscle relaxants impedes placental transfer, resulting in minimal effects on the fetus.

Local anesthetics are weakly basic drugs that are principally bound to α_1-acid glycoprotein. Placental transfer depends on three factors: (1) pK_a (see Chapter 14), (2) maternal and fetal pH, and (3) degree of protein binding. Except for chloroprocaine, fetal acidosis produces higher fetal-to-maternal drug ratios because binding of hydrogen ions to the nonionized form causes trapping of the local anesthetic in the fetal circulation. Highly protein-bound agents diffuse poorly across the placenta; thus, greater protein binding of bupivacaine and ropivacaine, compared with that of lidocaine, likely accounts for their lower fetal blood levels. Chloroprocaine has the least placental transfer because it is rapidly broken down by plasma cholinesterase in the maternal circulation.

Most commonly used anesthetic adjuncts also readily cross the placenta. Thus, maternally administered ephedrine, β-adrenergic blockers (such as labetalol and esmolol), vasodilators, phenothiazines, antihistamines (H_1 and H_2), and metoclopramide are transferred to the fetus. Atropine and scopolamine, but not glycopyrrolate, cross the placenta; the latter's quaternary ammonium (ionized) structure results in only limited transfer.

Effect of Anesthetic Agents on Uteroplacental Blood Flow

Intravenous anesthetic agents have variable effects on uteroplacental blood flow. Barbiturates and propofol are typically associated with small reductions in uterine blood flow due to mild to moderate, dose-dependent decreases in maternal blood pressure. A small induction dose, however, can produce greater reductions in blood flow as a result of sympathoadrenal activation (due to light anesthesia). Ketamine, in doses < 1.5 mg/kg, does not appreciably alter uteroplacental blood flow; its hypertensive effect typically counteracts any vasoconstriction. Uterine hypertonus may occur with ketamine at doses > 2 mg/kg. Compared with thiopental and propofol, midazolam may be more likely to produce transient systemic hypotension when used as an induction agent. Etomidate likely has minimal effects, but its actions on uteroplacental circulation are not well described.

 Volatile inhalational anesthetics decrease blood pressure and, potentially, uteroplacental blood flow. In concentrations of less than 1 MAC, however, their effects are generally minor, consisting of dose-dependent uterine relaxation and minor reductions in uterine blood flow. Nitrous oxide has minimal effects when administered with a volatile agent. In animal studies, nitrous oxide alone can vasoconstrict the uterine arteries.

High blood levels of local anesthetics—particularly lidocaine—cause uterine arterial vasoconstriction. Such levels are seen only with unintentional intravascular injections and occasionally following paracervical blocks (in which the injection site is in close proximity to the uterine arteries). Spinal and epidural anesthesia typically do not decrease uterine blood flow, provided arterial hypotension is avoided. Moreover, uterine blood flow during labor may actually improve in preeclamptic patients following epidural anesthesia; a reduction in circulating endogenous catecholamines likely decreases uterine vasoconstriction. The addition of dilute concentrations of epinephrine to local anesthetic solutions does not appreciably alter uterine blood flow. Intravascular uptake of the epinephrine from the epidural space may result in only minor systemic β-adrenergic effects.

THE PHYSIOLOGY OF NORMAL LABOR

On average, labor commences 40 ± 2 weeks following the last menstrual period. The factors involved in the initia-

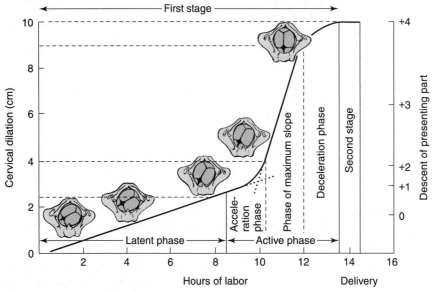

Figure 42–3. The course of normal labor. (Reproduced, with permission, from DeCherney AH, Pernoll ML [editors]: *Current Obstetric & Gynecologic Diagnosis & Treatment,* 9th ed. McGraw-Hill, 2001.)

tion of labor are as yet not entirely elucidated but likely involve overdistention of the uterus, enhanced myometrial sensitivity to oxytocin, and altered prostaglandin synthesis by fetal membranes and decidual tissues. Although circulating oxytocin levels often do not increase at the beginning of labor, the number of myometrial oxytocin receptors rapidly increases. Several prodromal events also usually precede true labor about 2–4 weeks prior to delivery: the fetal presenting part settles into the pelvis (lightening); patients develop uterine (Braxton Hicks) contractions that are characteristically irregular in frequency, duration, and intensity; and the cervix softens and thins out (cervical effacement). Approximately 1 week to 1 h before true labor, the cervical mucous plug (which is often bloody) breaks free (bloody show).

True labor begins when the sporadic and haphazard Braxton Hicks contractions increase in strength (25–60 mm Hg), coordination, and frequency (15–20 min apart). Amniotic membranes may rupture spontaneously prior or subsequent to the onset of true labor. Following progressive cervical dilatation, the contractions propel first the fetus and then the placenta through the pelvis and perineum. By convention, labor is divided into three stages. The first stage is defined by the onset of true labor and ends with complete cervical dilatation. The second stage begins with full cervical dilatation, is characterized by fetal descent, and ends with complete delivery of the fetus. Finally, the third stage extends from the birth of the baby to the delivery of the placenta.

Based on the rate of cervical dilatation, the first stage is further divided into a slow latent phase followed by a faster active phase (Figure 42–3). The latent phase is characterized by progressive cervical effacement and minor dilatation (2–4 cm). The subsequent active phase is characterized by more frequent contractions (3–5 min apart) and progressive cervical dilatation up to 10 cm. The first stage usually lasts 8–12 h in nulliparous patients and about 5–8 h in multiparous patients.

Contractions during the second stage occur 1.5–2 min apart and last 1–1.5 min. Although contraction intensity does not appreciably change, the parturient, by bearing down, can greatly augment intrauterine pressure and facilitate expulsion of the fetus. The second stage usually lasts 15–120 min and the third stage typically 15–30 min.

The course of labor is monitored by uterine activity, cervical dilatation, and fetal descent. Uterine activity refers to the frequency and magnitude of uterine contractions. The latter may be measured directly, with a catheter inserted through the cervix, or indirectly, with a tocodynamometer applied externally around the abdomen. Cervical dilatation and fetal descent are assessed by pelvic examination. Fetal station refers to the level of descent (in centimeters) of the presenting part relative to the ischial spines (eg, –1 or +1).

Effect of Labor on Maternal Physiology

During intense painful contractions, maternal minute ventilation may increase up to 300%. Oxygen consumption also increases another 60% above third-trimester values. With excessive hyperventilation, $PaCO_2$ falls below 20 mm Hg. Marked hypocapnia can cause periods of hypoventilation and transient maternal and fetal hypoxemia between contractions. Excessive maternal hyperventilation also reduces uterine blood flow and promotes fetal acidosis.

Each contraction places an additional burden on the heart by displacing 300–500 mL of blood from the uterus into the central circulation (analogous to an autotransfusion). Cardiac output rises 45% over third-trimester values. The greatest strain on the heart, however, occurs immediately after delivery, when intense uterine contraction and involution suddenly relieve inferior vena caval obstruction and increase cardiac output as much as 80% above prelabor values.

Effect of Anesthetic Agents on Uterine Activity & Labor

A. INHALATIONAL AGENTS

Halothane, enflurane, isoflurane, sevoflurane, and desflurane depress uterine activity equally at equipotent doses; all cause dose-dependent uterine relaxation. Low doses (< 0.75 MAC) of these agents, however, do not interfere with the effect of oxytocin on the uterus. Higher doses can result in uterine atony and increase blood loss at delivery. Nitrous oxide has minimal if any effects.

B. PARENTERAL AGENTS

Opioids minimally decrease the progression of labor, whereas ketamine in doses < 2 mg/kg appears to have little effect.

C. REGIONAL ANESTHESIA

Does the use of epidural analgesia for labor increase the likelihood of a cesarean section or forceps delivery? Older dogma suggested that regional anesthesia administered early in the course of labor prolongs it, whereas a regional block given once labor is well established (eg, 4–5 cm cervical dilation) has little effect. Recent evidence has cast serious doubts on this view. Current techniques employing very dilute combinations of a local anesthetic (eg, bupivacaine 0.125% or less) and an opioid (eg, fentanyl 5 μg/mL or less) for epidural or combined spinal–epidural (CSE) analgesia do not appear to prolong labor or increase the likelihood of a cesarean section.

The administration of epidural analgesia is normally based on the patient's choice. Therefore there is a natural bias toward epidural analgesia being most often administered to patients who have maternal or fetal factors that increase the likelihood of cesarean section or prolong labor (Table 42–2). Moreover, in studies of

Table 42–2. Factors that prolong labor, increase the likelihood of cesarean section, and often cause patients to request an epidural.

Primigravida
Prolonged labor
High parenteral analgesic requirements
Use of oxytocin
Large baby
Small pelvis
Fetal malpresentation

patients *not* receiving epidural analgesia, women who experienced more severe pain (eg, requiring > 50 mg meperidine, and would have been more likely to request epidural analgesia) had up to a 10-fold increase in cesarean section rate.

The specific effects of regional anesthesia are complex and predominantly indirect. Direct effects are observed only with toxic systemic levels of local anesthetics, producing tetanic contractions. Indirect effects mostly relate to local anesthetic and opioid concentrations, intravenous fluid boluses, and the use of epinephrine. In the past, when higher concentrations of local anesthetic (eg, bupivacaine 0.25%) were used, regional anesthesia increased the incidence of low forceps deliveries. Intense regional analgesia/anesthesia can remove the urge to bear down during the second stage (Ferguson reflex) and motor weakness can impair expulsive efforts, often prolonging the second stage of delivery. Use of dilute local anesthetic/opioid mixtures (see Chapter 43) can preserve motor function and allows more effective pushing. Intravenous fluid loading (crystalloid boluses) is often use to prevent or reduce the severity of hypotension following an epidural injection. This practice has been shown to reduce endogenous oxytocin secretion from the pituitary and can transiently decrease uterine activity. Epinephrine-containing local anesthetic solutions can theoretically prolong the first stage of labor if absorption of epinephrine from the epidural space results in significant systemic β-adrenergic effects. Although somewhat controversial, prolongation of labor is generally not clinically observed with very dilute (eg, 1:400,000) epinephrine-containing local anesthetics.

D. VASOPRESSORS

Uterine muscle has both α- and β-receptors. α_1-Receptor stimulation causes uterine contraction, whereas β_2-receptor stimulation produces relaxation. Large doses of α-adrenergic agents, such as metaraminol and phenylephrine, in addition to causing uterine arterial constriction, can produce tetanic uterine contractions. Small doses of phenylephrine (50 μg) may increase uterine blood flow in normal parturients by raising arterial blood pressure. In contrast, ephedrine has little effect on uterine contractions.

E. Oxytocin

Oxytocin (Pitocin) is usually administered intravenously to induce or augment uterine contractions or to maintain uterine tone postpartum. It has a half-life of 3–5 min. Induction doses for labor are 0.5–8 mU/min. **Complications include fetal distress due to hyperstimulation, uterine tetany, and, less commonly, maternal water intoxication. Rapid intravenous infusion can also cause transient systemic hypotension due to relaxation of vascular smooth muscle; reflex tachycardia may also be noted.**

F. Ergot Alkaloids

Methylergonovine (Methergine) causes intense and prolonged uterine contractions. It is therefore given only after delivery (postpartum) to treat uterine atony. Moreover, because it also constricts vascular smooth muscle and can cause severe hypertension, it is usually administered only as a single 0.2 mg dose intramuscularly.

G. Carboprost

Carboprost tromethamine (Hemabate) is a synthetic analogue of prostaglandin F_2 that stimulates uterine contractions. It is often used to treat refractory postpartum hemorrhage. As with methergine, it should be administered only intramuscularly. An initial dose of 0.25 mg may be repeated every 15–90 min to a maximum of 2 mg. Common side effects include nausea, vomiting, and diarrhea.

H. Magnesium

Magnesium is used in obstetrics both to stop premature labor (tocolysis) and to prevent eclamptic seizures (see Chapter 43). It is usually administered as a 4 g intravenous loading dose (over 20 min) followed by a 2 g/h infusion. Therapeutic serum levels are considered to be 6–8 mg/dL. Serious side effects include hypotension, heart block muscle weakness, and sedation (see Chapter 28).

H. β₂-Agonists

The β_2-adrenergic agonists ritodrine and terbutaline inhibit uterine contractions and are used to treat premature labor (see Chapter 43).

FETAL PHYSIOLOGY

The placenta, which receives nearly one-half of the fetal cardiac output, is responsible for respiratory gas exchange. As a result, the lungs receive little blood flow and the pulmonary and systemic circulations are parallel instead of in series, as in the adult (Figures 42–4 and 42–5). This arrangement is made possible by two cardiac shunts—the **foramen ovale** and the **ductus arteriosus:**

1. Well-oxygenated blood from the placenta (approximately 80% oxygen saturation) mixes with venous blood returning from the lower body (25% oxygen saturation) and flows via the inferior vena cava into the right atrium.
2. Right atrial anatomy preferentially directs blood flow from the inferior vena cava (67% oxygen saturation) through the foramen ovale into the left atrium.
3. Left atrial blood is then pumped by the left ventricle to the upper body (mainly the brain and the heart).
4. Poorly oxygenated blood from the upper body returns via the superior vena cava to the right atrium.
5. Right atrial anatomy preferentially directs flow from the superior vena cava into the right ventricle.
6. Right ventricular blood is pumped into the pulmonary artery.
7. Because of high pulmonary vascular resistance, 95% of the blood ejected from the right ventricle (60% oxygen saturation) is shunted across the ductus arteriosus, into the descending aorta, and back to the placenta and lower body.

The parallel circulation results in unequal ventricular flows; the right ventricle ejects two-thirds of the combined ventricular outputs, whereas the left ventricle ejects only one-third.

Up to 50% of the well-oxygenated blood in the umbilical vein can pass directly to the heart via the ductus venosus, bypassing the liver. The remainder of the blood flow from the placenta mixes with blood from the portal vein (via the portal sinus) and passes through the liver before reaching the heart. The latter may be important in allowing relatively rapid hepatic degradation of drugs (or toxins) that are absorbed from the maternal circulation.

In contrast to the fetal circulation, which is established very early during intrauterine life, maturation of the lungs lags behind. Extrauterine life is not possible until after 24–25 weeks of gestation, when pulmonary capillaries are formed and come to lie in close approximation to an immature alveolar epithelium. At 30 weeks, the cuboidal alveolar epithelium flattens out and begins to produce pulmonary surfactant. This substance provides alveolar stability and is necessary to maintain normal lung expansion after birth (see Chapter 22). Sufficient pulmonary surfactant is usually present after 34 weeks of gestation. Administration of glucocorticoids to the mother can accelerate fetal surfactant production.

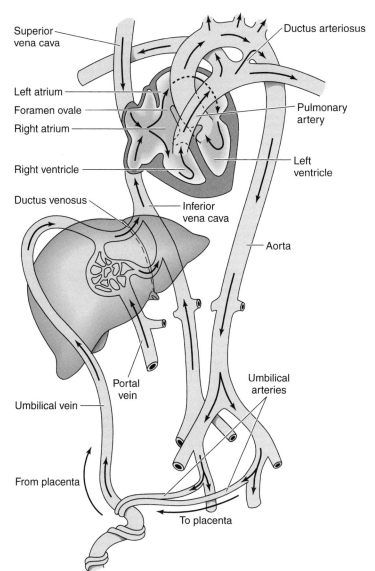

Superior vena cava

Ductus arteriosus

Left atrium

Foramen ovale

Right atrium

Pulmonary artery

Right ventricle

Left ventricle

Ductus venosus

Inferior vena cava

Aorta

Portal vein

Umbilical arteries

Umbilical vein

From placenta

To placenta

Figure 42–4. The fetal circulation before and after birth. (Reproduced, with permission, from Ganong WF: *Review of Medical Physiology,* 20th ed. McGraw-Hill, 2001.)

PHYSIOLOGICAL TRANSITION OF THE FETUS AT BIRTH

The most profound adaptive changes at birth involve the circulatory and respiratory systems. Failure to make this transition successfully results in fetal death or permanent neurological damage.

At term, the fetal lungs are developed but contain about 90 mL of a plasma ultrafiltrate. During expulsion of the fetus at delivery, this fluid is normally squeezed from the lungs by the forces of the pelvic muscles and the vagina acting on the baby (the vaginal squeeze). Any remaining fluid is reabsorbed by the pulmonary capillaries and lymphatics. Catecholamine in the neonate during labor may augment release of surfactant from type II pneumocytes. Small (preterm) neonates and neonates delivered via cesarean section do not benefit from the vaginal squeeze and thus typically have greater difficulty in maintaining respirations (transient tachypnea of the newborn). Respiratory efforts are normally initiated within 30 s after birth and become sustained within 90 s. Mild hypoxia and acidosis as well as sensory stimulation—cord clamping, pain, touch, and noise—help initiate and sustain respirations, whereas the outward recoil of the chest at delivery aids in filling the lungs with air.

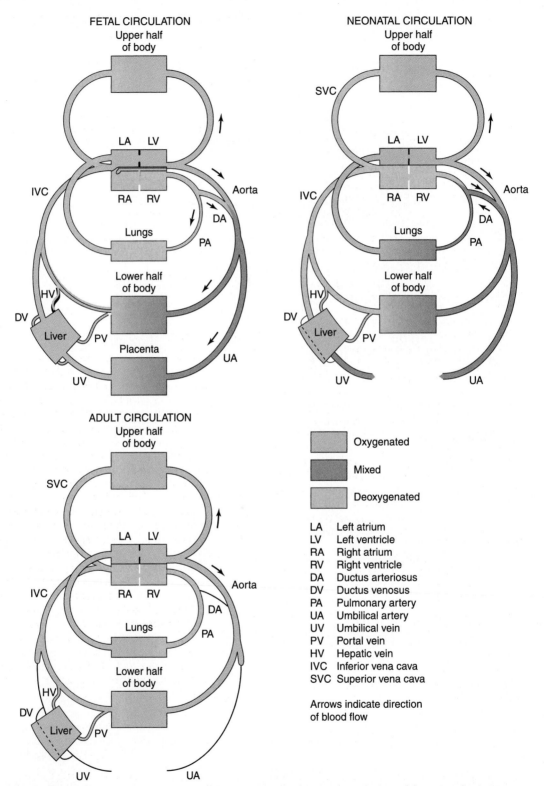

Figure 42–5. A schematic comparison of fetal and neonatal circulation. (Adapted from Danforth DN, Scott JR: *Obstetrics and Gynecology,* 5th ed. Lippincott, 1986.)

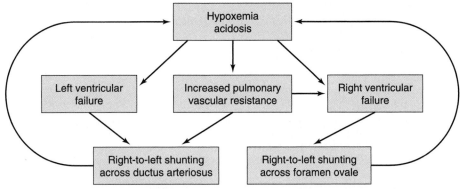

Figure 42–6. Pathophysiology of persistent pulmonary hypertension of the newborn (persistent fetal circulation). (Modified and reproduced, with permission, from Gregory GA: *Pediatric Anesthesia,* 2nd ed. Churchill Livingstone, 1989.)

Lung expansion increases both alveolar and arterial oxygen tensions and decreases pulmonary vascular resistance. The increase in oxygen tension is a potent stimulus for pulmonary arterial vasodilatation. The resultant increase in pulmonary blood flow and augmented flow to the left heart elevates left atrial pressure and functionally closes the foramen ovale. The increase in arterial oxygen tension also causes the ductus arteriosus to contract and functionally close. Other chemical mediators that may play a role in ductal closure include acetylcholine, bradykinin, and prostaglandins. The overall result is elimination of right-to-left shunting and establishment of the adult circulation (Figure 42–5). Anatomic closure of the ductus arteriosus does not usually occur until about 2–3 weeks, whereas closure of the foramen ovale takes months if it occurs at all.

Hypoxia or acidosis during the first few days of life can prevent or reverse these physiological changes, resulting in persistence of (or return to) the fetal circulation, or persistent pulmonary hypertension of the newborn (PPHN). A vicious circle is established where the right-to-left shunting promotes hypoxemia and acidosis, which in turn promote more shunting (Figure 42–6). Right-to-left shunting may occur across the foramen ovale, the ductus arteriosus, or both. Unless this circle is broken, neonatal demise can occur rapidly.

CASE DISCUSSION:
POSTPARTUM TUBAL LIGATION

A 36-year-old woman is scheduled for bilateral tubal ligation 12 h after delivery of a healthy baby.

Is this patient still at increased risk for pulmonary aspiration?

Controversy exists over when the increased risk for pulmonary aspiration diminishes following pregnancy. Certainly, many factors contributing to delayed gastric emptying are alleviated shortly after delivery: mechanical distortion of the stomach is relieved, labor pains cease, and the circulating progesterone level rapidly declines. In addition, a period of 8–12 h of elective fasting is possible. Some studies suggest that the risk of pulmonary aspiration as judged by gastric volume and gastric fluid pH (see the section on Gastrointestinal Effects) normalizes within 24 h. Unfortunately, even these studies report up to a 30–60% incidence of either a gastric volume greater than 25 mL or a gastric fluid pH less than 2.5. Therefore, most clinicians still consider the postpartum patient at increased risk for pulmonary aspiration and take appropriate precautions (see Chapters 15 and 43). It is not known when the risk returns to that associated with elective surgical patients. Although some physiological changes associated with pregnancy may require up to 6 weeks for resolution, the increased risk of pulmonary aspiration probably returns to "normal" well before that time.

Other than aspiration risk, what factors determine the "optimal" time for postpartum sterilization?

The decision when to perform postpartum tubal ligation (or laparoscopic fulguration) is complex and varies according to patient and obstetrician preferences as well as local practices. In addition, the decision may be based on whether the patient had a vaginal delivery or cesarean section and whether an anesthetic was administered for labor (epidural anesthesia) or delivery (epidural or general anesthesia).

Postpartum tubal ligation or fulguration may be (1) performed immediately following delivery of the baby and repair of the uterus during a cesarean section, (2) delayed 8–48 h following delivery to allow an elective fasting period, or (3) deferred until after the postpartum period (generally 6 weeks). Many obstetricians are reluctant to do immediate postpartum sterilizations because the patient may change her mind later, particularly if something untoward happens to the baby. Furthermore, they want to ensure that the patient is stable, particularly after a complicated delivery. On the other hand, sterilization is technically much easier to perform in the immediate postpartum period because of the enlargement of the uterus and tubes. Postpartum sterilizations following natural vaginal delivery are generally performed within 48 h of delivery, because bacterial colonization of the reproductive tract thereafter is thought to increase the risk of postoperative infection.

What factors determine selection of an anesthetic technique for postpartum sterilization?

When continuous epidural anesthesia is administered for labor and vaginal delivery, the epidural catheter may be left in place up to 48 h for subsequent tubal ligation. The delay allows a period of elective fasting. A T4–5 sensory level with regional anesthesia is usually necessary to ensure a pain-free anesthetic experience. Lower sensory levels (as low as T10) may be adequate but sometimes fail to prevent pain during surgical traction on viscera.

When the patient has not had anesthesia for delivery, postpartum sterilization may be performed under either regional or general anesthesia. Because of the increased risk of pulmonary aspiration, regional anesthesia usually is preferred for bilateral tubal ligation via a minilaparotomy. Many clinicians prefer spinal over epidural anesthesia in this setting because of the risk of unintentional intravascular or intrathecal injections with the latter (see Chapter 16). Moreover, the risk of a precipitous decrease in blood pressure following spinal anesthesia may be significantly diminished following delivery (particularly when preceded by an intravenous fluid

bolus). In addition, the incidence of postdural puncture headache is as low as 1% when a 25-gauge or smaller pencil-point needle is used. Dosage requirements for regional anesthesia generally return to normal within 24–36 h after delivery. Tetracaine, 7–10 mg, bupivacaine, 8–12 mg, or lidocaine, 60–75 mg, may be used for spinal anesthesia. For epidural anesthesia, 15–20 mL of lidocaine 1.5–2% or chloroprocaine 3% is most commonly used.

In contrast, when laparoscopic tubal fulguration is planned, general endotracheal anesthesia is usually preferred. Insufflation of gas during laparoscopy impairs pulmonary gas exchange and predisposes the patient to nausea, vomiting, and possibly pulmonary aspiration. Endotracheal intubation generally ensures adequate ventilation and protects the airway.

What considerations are important for postpartum patients undergoing general anesthesia?

Preoperative concerns include a decreased blood hemoglobin concentration and the persistent increased risk of pulmonary aspiration. Anemia is nearly always present as a result of the physiological effects of pregnancy combined with blood loss during and following delivery. Hemoglobin concentrations are usually greater than 9 g/dL, but levels as low as 7 g/dL are generally considered safe. Fortunately, sterilization procedures are rarely associated with significant blood loss.

The risk of pulmonary aspiration is diminished by a minimum of 8 h of fasting, premedication with an H_2 histamine blocker (ranitidine), a clear antacid (sodium citrate), or metoclopramide (see Chapters 15 and 43). In addition, induction of anesthesia should employ a rapid-sequence technique with cricoid pressure prior to endotracheal intubation, and the patient should be extubated only when she is awake. Decreased plasma cholinesterase levels persist after delivery (see the section on Hepatic Effects) and generally modestly prolong the effect of succinylcholine and mivacurium. The duration of vecuronium but not atracurium (or cisatracurium) has also been reported to be prolonged in postpartum women. High concentrations of volatile agents should be avoided because of the at least theoretical risk of increasing uterine blood loss or inducing postpartum hemorrhage secondary to uterine relaxation. Intravenous opioids may be used to supplement inhalational agents. Intravenous drugs administered intraoperatively to mothers *who are breast-feeding appear to have minimal if any effects on their neonates. Nonetheless, it may be prudent to avoid breast-feeding 12–24 h following general anesthesia.*

SUGGESTED READING

Birnbach DJ, Datta S, Gatt SP: *Textbook of Obstetric Anesthesia.* Churchill Livingstone, 2000.

Bucklin BA, Smith CV: Postpartum tubal ligation: safety, timing, and other implications for anesthesia. Anesth Analg 1999;89: 1269.

Chestnut DH: *Obstetric Anesthesia,* 3rd ed. Mosby, 2004.

Holdcroft TT: *Principles and Practice of Obstetric Anaesthesia.* Blackwell, 2000.

Hughes SC, Levinson G, Rosen MA: *Shnider and Levinson's Anesthesia for Obstetrics,* 4th ed. Lippincott, Williams & Wilkins, 2002.

Koren G, Pastuszak A, Ito S: Drugs in pregnancy. N Engl J Med 1998;338:1128.

Rosen MA: Management of anesthesia for the pregnant surgical patient. Anesthesiology 1999;91:1159.

Segal S. Epidural analgesia and the progress and outcome of labor and delivery. Int Anesthesiol Clin 2002;40:13.

Zhang J, Yancey MK, Klebanoff MA, et al: Does epidural analgesia prolong labor and increase risk of cesarean delivery? A natural experiment. Am J Obstet Gynecol 2001;185:128.

Obstetric Anesthesia

43

KEY CONCEPTS

 The most common morbidities encountered in obstetrics are severe hemorrhage and severe preeclampsia.

 Regardless of the time of last oral intake, all obstetric patients are considered to have a full stomach and to be at risk for pulmonary aspiration.

 Nearly all parenteral opioid analgesics and sedatives readily cross the placenta and can affect the fetus. Regional anesthetic techniques are preferred for management of labor pain.

 Using a local anesthetic–opioid mixture for lumbar epidural analgesia during labor significantly reduces drug requirements, compared with using either agent alone.

 Optimal analgesia for labor requires neural blockade at T10–L1 in the first stage of labor and T10–S4 in the second stage.

 Continuous lumbar epidural analgesia is the most versatile and most commonly employed technique, because it can be used for pain relief for the first stage of labor as well as analgesia/anesthesia for subsequent vaginal delivery or cesarean section, if necessary.

 When dilute mixtures of a local anesthetic and an opioid are used epidural analgesia has little if any effect on the progress of labor.

 Even when aspiration does not yield blood or cerebrospinal fluid, unintentional intravascular or intrathecal placement of an epidural needle or catheter is possible.

 Hypotension is the most common side effect of regional anesthetic techniques and must be treated aggressively with ephedrine and intravenous fluid boluses to prevent fetal compromise.

 Techniques using combined spinal epidural analgesia and anesthesia may particularly benefit patients with severe pain early in labor and those who receive analgesia/anesthesia just prior to delivery.

 Spinal or epidural anesthesia is preferred to general anesthesia for cesarean section because regional anesthesia is associated with lower maternal mortality.

 Spinal anesthesia for cesarean section is easier to perform and results in more rapid and intense neural blockade than epidural anesthesia. Epidural anesthesia allows greater control over sensory level and results in a more gradual fall in arterial blood pressure.

Systemic, local anesthetic toxicity during epidural anesthesia may be best avoided by slowly administering dilute solutions for labor pain and fractionating the total dose for cesarean section into 5-mL increments.

(continued on next page)

(continued from previous page)

 In general anesthesia for cesarean section, if endotracheal intubation fails, the life of the mother takes priority over delivery of the fetus.

 Maternal hemorrhage is one of the most common severe morbidities complicating obstetric anesthesia. Causes include placenta previa, abruptio placentae, and uterine rupture.

 Pregnancy-induced hypertension describes one of three syndromes: preeclampsia, eclampsia, and the HELLP syndrome.

 Common causes of postpartum hemorrhage include uterine atony, a retained placenta, obstetric lacerations, uterine inversion, and use of tocolytic agents prior to delivery.

 Intrauterine asphyxia during labor is the most common cause of neonatal depression. Fetal monitoring throughout labor is helpful in identifying which babies may be at risk, detecting fetal distress, and evaluating the effect of acute interventions.

Obstetric anesthesia is a demanding but gratifying subspecialty of anesthesiology. The widespread acceptance and use of regional anesthesia for labor has made obstetric anesthesia a major part of most anesthetic practices. The guidelines of the American College of Obstetricians and Gynecologists and American Society of Anesthesiologists require that anesthesia service be readily available continuously and that cesarean section be started within 30 min of the recognition for its need. Moreover, high-risk patients, such as those undergoing a trial of vaginal birth after a previous cesarean delivery (VBAC), may require the immediate availability of anesthesia services.

Although most parturients are young and healthy, they nonetheless represent a high-risk group of patients for all the reasons discussed in the preceding chapter.

This chapter focuses on the practice of obstetric anesthesia; techniques for analgesia and anesthesia during labor, vaginal delivery, and cesarean section are presented. The chapter ends with a review of neonatal resuscitation. The suggested procedures are intended to serve only as guidelines consistent with our current understanding of maternal and fetal physiology.

ANESTHETIC RISK IN OBSTETRIC PATIENTS

To understand anesthetic risk in obstetric patients it is important first to fully appreciate obstetric risk in general. Although the majority of women of childbearing age are healthy and would be considered to be at very good operative surgical risk, pregnancy, certain maternal/fetal factors, and preexisting medical conditions significantly increase surgical and obstetric risks.

Pregnancy-Related Mortality

Pregnancy-related mortality is usually calculated as the number of pregnancy-related deaths divided by the number of live births. Although this number has decreased nearly 100-fold since 1900, it has not changed appreciably since 1982. In fact, perhaps due to better reporting, it has risen slightly in the United States to 11.8 deaths per 100,000 live births in the period 1991–1999. Roughly similar rates (between 6.1 and 12 per 100,000) have been reported from Canada and the United Kingdom. Figure 43–1A shows cause of death based on the Pregnancy Mortality Surveillance System of the Centers for Disease Control. Overall mortality was higher for women > 35 years old, black patients, and patients without prenatal care. The leading causes of death associated with a live birth were pulmonary embolism (21%), pregnancy-induced hypertension (19%), and other medical conditions (17%). Major causes of death associated with a stillbirth were hemorrhage (21%), pregnancy-induced hypertension (20%), and sepsis (19%). Only 34% of patients died within 24 h of delivery, whereas 55% died between 1 and 42 days, and another 11% died between 43 days and 1 year.

Direct causes of maternal deaths are more clearly detailed from Canadian data (Figure 43–1B). In addition to pulmonary embolism and preeclampsia/pregnancy-induced hypertension, amniotic fluid embolism and intracranial hemorrhage emerge as important additional causes of death.

Some investigators have examined the incidence of severe obstetric morbidity and its relationship to mortality as a more sensitive measure of outcome. Data from the United Kingdom suggest that incidence of severe obstetric morbidity is 12 per 1000 delivery, or 100 times more

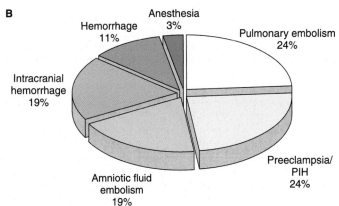

Figure 43–1. A: Causes of pregnancy-related mortality, based on data from the Centers for Disease Control and Prevention. Medical conditions exacerbated by pregnancy were primarily cardiovascular, pulmonary, and neurological diseases. (Deaths associated with undelivered, ectopic, and molar pregnancies as well as abortions are excluded.) **B:** Direct causes of maternal deaths, based on Maternal and Infant Health Section–PPHB–Health Canada from http://www.hc-sc.gc.ca/ (Excludes Quebec). Data for ectopic pregnancy and septic abortion have been excluded. PIH, pregnancy-induced hypertension.

Table 43–1. Incidence of severe obstetric morbidity.[1,2]

Morbidity	Incidence per 1000
Severe hemorrhage	6.7
Severe preeclampsia	3.9
HELLP syndrome[3]	0.5
Severe sepsis	0.4
Eclampsia	0.2
Uterine rupture	0.2

[1]Adapted from Waterstone M, Bewley S, Wolfe C: Incidence and predictors of severe obstetric morbidity: case-control study. BMJ 2001;322:1089.

[2]Note thromboembolic disease was excluded.

[3]HELLP syndrome consists of hemolysis, elevated liver enzymes, and low platelet count.

common that mortality. Risk factors included age > 34 years, nonwhite ethnic group, multiple pregnancy, history of hypertension, previous postpartum hemorrhage, and emergency cesarean delivery. Table 43–1 lists the estimated incidence of the most common causes of severe morbidity; thromboembolic disease was deliberately excluded because of the difficulty in making the diagnosis in nonfatal cases. By far the most common morbidities encountered in obstetrics are severe hemorrhage and severe preeclampsia.

Anesthetic Mortality

Anesthesia accounts for approximately 2–3% of maternal deaths. Data collected between 1985 and 1990 suggest a maternal mortality of 32 deaths per 1,000,000 live births due to general anesthesia and 1.9 deaths per 1,000,000 live births due to regional anesthesia. More

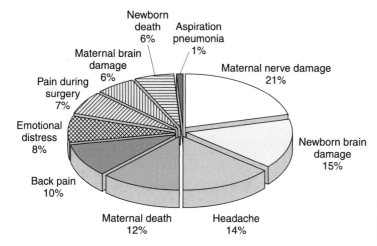

Figure 43–2. Obstetric anesthesia malpractice claims, based on ASA Closed Claims Data. (American Society of Anesthesiologists Newsletter 2004;68:12.)

recent data between 1991 and 1999 suggest a lower overall maternal mortality from anesthesia (about 1.6 deaths per 1,000,000 live births), possibly due to greater use of regional anesthesia for labor and cesarean section. Most deaths occur during or after cesarean section. Moreover, the risk of an adverse outcome appears to be much greater with emergency than with elective cesarean sections.

Obstetric Anesthesia Closed Claims

Obstetric anesthesia care accounts for approximately 12% of the American Society of Anesthesiologists (ASA) Closed Claims database. Claims involving general anesthesia have dropped in proportion to its decreasing use in obstetrics; previously, maternal death was the most frequent claim (30%). The proportion of claims associated with regional anesthesia has risen steadily, with the majority of claims in the 1990s associated with less severe injury (Figure 43–2). Maternal nerve injury was the most common claim in the 1990s, followed by newborn brain damage and headache.

■ GENERAL APPROACH TO THE OBSTETRIC PATIENT

All patients entering the obstetric suite potentially require anesthesia, whether planned or emergent. The anesthesiologist should therefore be aware of the presence and relevant history of all patients in the suite. Pertinent historic items include age, parity, duration

of the pregnancy, and any complicating factors. Patients definitely requiring anesthetic care (for labor or cesarean section) should undergo a focused preanesthetic evaluation as early as possible. This should consist of a maternal health history, anesthesia-related obstetric history, blood pressure measurement, airway assessment, and back examination for regional anesthesia.

All women in true labor should be managed with intravenous fluids (usually lactated Ringer's injection with dextrose) to prevent dehydration. An 18-gauge or larger intravenous catheter is employed in case rapid transfusion should become necessary. Blood should be sent for typing and screening in patients at high risk for hemorrhage or with a borderline acceptable hematocrit. Regardless of the time of last oral intake, all patients are considered to have a full stomach and to be at risk for pulmonary aspiration. Because the duration of labor is often prolonged, guidelines usually allow small amounts of clear liquid for uncomplicated labor. In contrast, patients at high risk for an operative delivery should take nothing by mouth. The minimum fasting period for elective cesarean section should be 6 h. Prophylactic administration of a clear antacid (15–30 mL of 0.3 M sodium citrate orally) every 3 h can help maintain gastric pH greater than 2.5 and may decrease the likelihood of severe aspiration pneumonitis. An H_2-blocking drug (ranitidine, 100–150 mg orally or 50 mg intravenously) or metoclopramide, 10 mg orally or intravenously, should also be considered in high-risk patients and in those expected to receive general anesthesia. H_2-blockers reduce both gastric volume and pH but have no effect on the gastric contents already present. Metoclopramide accelerates gastric emptying, decreases gastric volume, and increases lower esophageal sphincter tone. All patients should ideally have a tocodyna-mometer and fetal heart rate monitor. The supine position should be avoided unless a left uterine displacement device (> 15° wedge) is placed under the right hip. Uterine contractions can be directly measured via a catheter in patients with ruptured membranes, particularly those receiving oxytocin or those undergoing a trial of VBAC.

ANESTHESIA FOR LABOR & VAGINAL DELIVERY

PAIN PATHWAYS DURING LABOR

The pain of labor arises from contraction of the myometrium against the resistance of the cervix and perineum, progressive dilatation of the cervix and lower uterine segment, as well as stretching and compression of pelvic and perineal structures.

Pain during the first stage of labor is mostly visceral pain resulting from uterine contractions and cervical dilatation. It is usually initially confined to the T11–T12 dermatomes during the latent phase but eventually involves the T10–L1 dermatomes as the labor enters the active phase. The visceral afferent fibers responsible for labor pain travel with sympathetic nerve fibers first to the uterine and cervical plexuses, then through the hypogastric and aortic plexuses before entering the spinal cord with the T10–L1 nerve roots (see Chapter 18). The pain is primarily in the lower abdomen but may increasingly be referred to the lumbosacral area, gluteal region, and thighs as labor progresses. Pain intensity also increases with progressive cervical dilatation and the increasing intensity and frequency of uterine contractions. Nulliparous women and those with a history of dysmenorrhea appear to experience greater pain during the first stage of labor. Studies also suggest that women who experience more intense pain during the latent phase of labor have longer labors and are more likely to require cesarean section.

The onset of perineal pain at the end of the first stage signals the beginning of fetal descent and the second stage of labor. Stretching and compression of pelvic and perineal structures intensify the pain. Sensory innervation of the perineum is provided by the pudendal nerve (S2–4) so pain during the second stage of labor involves the T10–S4 dermatomes. Studies suggest that the more rapid fetal descent in multiparous women is associated with more intense pain than the more gradual fetal descent in nulliparous patients.

PSYCHOLOGICAL & NONPHARMACOLOGICAL TECHNIQUES

Psychological and nonpharmacological techniques are based on the premise that the pain of labor can be suppressed by reorganizing one's thoughts. Patient education and positive conditioning about the birthing process are central to such techniques. Pain during labor tends to be accentuated by fear of the unknown or previous unpleasant experiences. Techniques include those of Bradley, Dick-Read, Lamaze, Duola, and LeBoyer. The Lamaze technique, one of the most popular, coaches the parturient to take a deep breath at the beginning of each contraction followed by rapid shallow breathing for the duration of the contraction. The parturient also concentrates on an object in the room and attempts to focus her thoughts away from the pain. Less common nonpharmacological techniques include hypnosis, transcutaneous electrical nerve stimulation, biofeedback, and acupuncture (see Chapter 18). The success of all these techniques varies considerably from patient to patient, but most patients require additional forms of pain relief.

PARENTERAL AGENTS

Nearly all parenteral opioid analgesics and sedatives readily cross the placenta and can affect the fetus. Concern over fetal depression limits the use of these agents to the early stages of labor or to situations in which regional anesthetic techniques are not available. Central nervous system depression in the neonate may be manifested by a prolonged time to sustain respirations, respiratory acidosis, or an abnormal neurobehavioral examination. Moreover, loss of beat-to-beat variability in the fetal heart rate (seen with most central nervous system depressants) and decreased fetal movements (due to sedation of fetus) complicate the evaluation of fetal well-being during labor. Long-term fetal heart variability is affected more than short-term variability. The degree and significance of these effects depend on the specific agent, the dose, the time elapsed between its administration and delivery, and fetal maturity. Premature neonates exhibit the greatest sensitivity. In addition to maternal respiratory depression, opioids can also induce maternal nausea and vomiting and delay gastric emptying. Some clinicians have advocated use of opioids via patient-controlled analgesia devices (see Chapter 18) early in labor because this technique appears to reduce total opioid requirements.

Meperidine, the most commonly used opioid, can be given in doses of 10–25 mg intravenously or 25–50 mg intramuscularly, usually up to a total of 100 mg. Maximal maternal and fetal respiratory depression is seen in 10–20 min following intravenous administration and in 1–3 h following intramuscular administration. Consequently, meperidine is usually administered early in labor when delivery is not expected for at least 4 h. Intravenous fentanyl, 25–100 µg/h, has also been used for labor. Fentanyl in 25–100 µg doses has a 3- to 10-min analgesic onset that initially lasts about 60 min, and lasts longer following multiple doses. However, *maternal respiratory depression outlasts the analgesia.* Lower doses of fentanyl may be associated with little or no neonatal respiratory depression and are reported to have no effect on Apgar scores. Morphine is not used because in equianalgesic doses it appears to cause greater respiratory depression in the fetus than meperidine and fentanyl. Agents with mixed agonist–antagonist activity (butorphanol 1–2 mg and nalbuphine 10–20 mg intravenously or intramuscularly) are effective and are associated with little or no cumulative respiratory depression (ceiling effect), but excessive sedation with repeat doses can be problematic.

Promethazine (25–50 mg intramuscularly) and hydroxyzine (50–100 mg intramuscularly) can be useful alone or in combination with meperidine. Both drugs reduce anxiety, opioid requirements, and the incidence of nausea but do not add appreciably to neonatal depression. A significant disadvantage of hydroxyzine is pain at the injection site following intramuscular administration. Nonsteroidal antiinflammatory agents, such as ketorolac, are not recommended because they suppress uterine contractions and promote closure of the fetal ductus arteriosus.

Benzodiazepines, particularly longer acting agents such as diazepam, are not used during labor because of their potential to cause prolonged neonatal depression. The amnestic properties of benzodiazepines make them undesirable agents for parturients because they usually want to remember the experience of delivery.

Low-dose intravenous ketamine is a powerful analgesic. In doses of 10–15 mg intravenously, good analgesia can be obtained in 2–5 min without loss of consciousness. Unfortunately, fetal depression with low Apgar scores is associated with doses greater than 1 mg/kg. Large boluses of ketamine (> 1 mg/kg) can be associated with hypertonic uterine contractions. Low-dose ketamine is most useful just prior to delivery or as an adjuvant to regional anesthesia. Some clinicians avoid use of ketamine because it may produce unpleasant psychotomimetic effects (see Chapter 8).

PUDENDAL NERVE BLOCK

Pudendal nerve blocks are often combined with perineal infiltration of local anesthetic to provide perineal anesthesia during the second stage of labor when other forms of anesthesia are not employed or prove to be inadequate. Paracervical plexus blocks are no longer used because of their association with a relatively high rate of fetal bradycardia; the close proximity of the injection site (paracervical plexus or Frankenhäuser's ganglia) to the uterine artery can result in uterine arterial vasoconstriction, uteroplacental insufficiency, and high levels of the local anesthetic in the fetal blood.

During a pudendal nerve block, a special needle (Koback) or guide (Iowa trumpet) is used to place the needle transvaginally underneath the ischial spine on each side (see Chapter 18); the needle is advanced 1–1.5 cm through the sacrospinous ligament, and 10 mL of 1% lidocaine or 2% chloroprocaine is injected following careful aspiration. The needle guide is used to limit the depth of injection and protect the fetus and vagina from the needle. Other potential complications include intravascular injection, retroperitoneal hematoma, and retropsoas or subgluteal abscess.

REGIONAL ANESTHETIC TECHNIQUES

Regional techniques employing the epidural or intrathecal route (see Chapter 16), alone or in combination, are currently the most popular methods of pain relief during labor and delivery. They can provide excellent pain relief, yet allow the mother to be awake and cooperative during labor. Although spinal opioids or local anesthetics alone can provide satisfactory analgesia, techniques that combine the two have proved to be the most satisfactory in most parturients. Moreover, the apparent synergy between the two types of agents decreases dose requirements and provides excellent analgesia with few maternal side effects and little or no neonatal depression.

1. Spinal Opioids Alone

Preservative-free opioids may be given intraspinally as a single injection or intermittently via an epidural or intrathecal catheter (Table 43–2). Relatively high doses are required for analgesia during labor when spinal opioids

Table 43–2. Spinal opioid dosages for labor and delivery.

Agent	Intrathecal	Epidural
Morphine	0.25–0.5 mg	5 mg
Meperidine	10–15 mg	50–100 mg
Fentanyl	12.5–25 µg	50–150 µg
Sufentanil	3–10 µg	10–20 µg

are used alone. For example, the ED_{50} during labor is 124 µg for epidural fentanyl and 21 µg for epidural sufentanil. The higher doses may be associated with a high risk of side effects, most importantly respiratory depression. For that reason combinations of local anesthetics and opioids are most commonly used (see below). Pure opioid techniques are therefore most useful for high-risk patients who may not tolerate the functional sympathectomy associated with spinal or epidural anesthesia (see Chapter 16). This group includes patients with hypovolemia or significant cardiovascular disease such as aortic stenosis, tetralogy of Fallot, Eisenmenger's syndrome, or pulmonary hypertension. With the exception of meperidine, which has local anesthetic properties, spinal opioids alone do not produce motor blockade or maternal hypotension (sympathectomy). Thus, they do not impair the ability of the parturient to push the baby out. Disadvantages include less complete analgesia, lack of perineal relaxation, and side effects such as pruritus, nausea, vomiting, sedation, and respiratory depression (see Chapter 18). Side effects may improve with low doses of naloxone (0.1–0.2 mg/h intravenously).

Intrathecal Opioids

Intrathecal morphine in doses of 0.25–0.5 mg may produce satisfactory and prolonged (4–6 h) analgesia during the first stage of labor. Unfortunately, the onset of analgesia is slow (45–60 min), and these doses may not be sufficient in many patients. Higher doses are associated with a relatively high incidence of side effects. Morphine is therefore rarely used alone. The combination of morphine, 0.25 mg, and fentanyl, 12.5 µg, (or sufentanil, 5 µg) may result in a more rapid onset of analgesia (5 min). Intermittent boluses of 10–15 mg of meperidine, 12.5–25 µg of fentanyl, or 3–10 µg of sufentanil via an intrathecal catheter can also provide satisfactory analgesia for labor. Early reports of fetal bradycardia following intrathecal opioid injections (eg, sufentanil) are not supported by subsequent studies. Spinal meperidine has some weak local anesthetic properties and therefore can decrease blood pressure. Hypotension following intrathecal sufentanil for labor is likely related to the analgesia and decreased circulating catecholamine levels.

Epidural Opioids

Again relatively high doses (≥ 7.5 mg) of morphine are required for satisfactory analgesia during labor, but doses larger than 5 mg are not recommended because of the increased risk of delayed respiratory depression and because the analgesia is effective only in the early first stage of labor. The onset of analgesia may take 30–60 min but lasts up to 12–24 h (as will the risk of delayed

respiratory depression). Epidural meperidine, 50–100 mg, provides consistently good but relatively brief analgesia (1–3 h). Epidural fentanyl, 50–150 µg, or sufentanil, 10–20 µg, usually produces analgesia within 5–10 min with few side effects, but it has a short duration (1–2 h). Although "single-shot" epidural opioids do not appear to cause significant neonatal depression, caution should be exercised following repeated administrations. Combinations of a lower dose of morphine, 2.5 mg, with fentanyl, 25–50 µg (or sufentanil, 7.5–10 µg), may result in a more rapid onset and prolongation of analgesia (4–5 h) with fewer side effects.

2. Local Anesthetic/Local Anesthetic–Opioid Mixtures

Epidural and spinal (intrathecal) analgesia more commonly utilizes local anesthetics either alone or with opioids for labor and delivery. Pain relief during the first stage of labor requires neural blockade at the T10–L1 sensory level, whereas pain relief during the second stage of labor requires neural blockade at T10–S4. Continuous lumbar epidural analgesia is the most versatile and most commonly employed technique, because it can be used for pain relief for the first stage of labor as well as analgesia/anesthesia for subsequent vaginal delivery or cesarean section, if necessary. "Single-shot" epidural, spinal, or combined spinal epidural analgesia may be appropriate when pain relief is initiated just prior to vaginal delivery (the second stage). Obstetric caudal injections have largely been abandoned because of less versatility (they are most effective for perineal analgesia/anesthesia), the need for large volumes of local anesthetic, early paralysis of the pelvic muscles that may interfere with normal rotation of the fetal head, and a small risk of accidental puncture of the fetus.

Absolute contraindications to regional anesthesia include infection over the injection site, coagulopathy, thrombocytopenia, marked hypovolemia, true allergies to local anesthetics, and the patient's refusal or inability to cooperate for regional anesthesia. Preexisting neurological disease, back disorders, and some forms of heart disease (see Chapter 20) are relative contraindications. Neuraxial anesthesia is contraindicated in the setting of anticoagulation (see Chapter 16). The use of regional anesthesia in patients on "minidose" heparin is controversial, but an epidural should generally not be performed within 6–8 h of a subcutaneous minidose of unfractionated heparin or 12–24 h of low-molecular-weight heparin (LMWH). Concomitant administration of an antiplatelet agent increases the risk of spinal hematoma. A previous VBAC is not considered a contraindication to regional anesthesia during labor. Concern that the anesthesia masks the pain associated with uterine rupture may not be justified, because dehiscence of a lower segment scar frequently does not cause pain even without epidural anesthesia; moreover, changes in uterine tone and contraction pattern may be more reliable signs.

Before performing any regional block, appropriate equipment and supplies for resuscitation should be checked and made immediately available. Minimum supplies include oxygen, suction, a mask with a positive-pressure device for ventilation, a functioning laryngoscope, endotracheal tubes (6 or 6.5 mm), oral or nasal airways, intravenous fluids, ephedrine, atropine, thiopental (or propofol), and succinylcholine. The ability to frequently monitor blood pressure and heart rate is mandatory. A pulse oximeter and capnograph should also be readily available.

Lumbar Epidural Anaglesia

As discussed in Chapter 42, traditionally epidural analgesia for labor is administered only when labor is well established. However, recent studies suggest that *when dilute mixtures of a local anesthetic and an opioid are used* epidural analgesia has little if any effect on the progress of labor. Concerns about increasing the likelihood of an oxytocin augmentation, operative (eg, forceps) delivery, or cesarean sections appear to be unjustified. It is often advantageous to place an epidural catheter early, when the patient is comfortable and can be positioned easily. Moreover, should emergent cesarean section become necessary the presence of a well-functioning epidural catheter makes it possible to avoid general anesthesia.

Epidural analgesia should generally be initiated when the parturient wants it (on demand) and the obstetrician approves it. A more conservative approach is to wait until labor is well established. Although exact criteria vary, commonly accepted conservative criteria include no fetal distress; good regular contractions 3–4 min apart and lasting about 1 min; adequate cervical dilatation, ie, 3–4 cm; and engagement of the fetal head. Even with a conservative approach, epidural anesthesia is often administered earlier to parturients who are committed to labor, eg, ruptured membranes and receiving an oxytocin infusion once a good contraction pattern is achieved.

A. Technique

The technique of epidural analgesia/anesthesia is described in Chapter 16. Parturients may be positioned on their sides or in the sitting position for the block. The sitting position is often more useful for identifying the midline in obese patients. When epidural anesthesia is being given for vaginal delivery (second stage), the sitting position helps ensure good sacral spread.

Because the epidural space pressure may be positive in some parturients, correct identification of the epidural space may be difficult, and unintentional dural puncture can readily occur; the incidence of wet taps in obstetric patients is 0.25–9%, depending on clinician experience. Some clinicians advocate the midline approach, whereas others favor the paramedian approach. If air is used for detecting loss of resistance, the amount injected should be limited as much as possible; injection of excessive amounts of air (> 2–3 mL) in the epidural space has been associated with patchy or unilateral analgesia and headache. The average depth of the epidural space in obstetric patients is reported to be 5 cm from the skin. Placement of the epidural catheter at the L3–4 or L4–5 interspace is generally optimal for achieving a T10–S5 neural blockade. If unintentional dural puncture occurs, the anesthetist has two choices: (1) place the epidural catheter in the subarachnoid space for continuous spinal analgesia and anesthesia (see below), or (2) remove the needle and attempt placement at a higher spinal level.

B. Choice of Epidural Catheter

Many clinicians advocate use of a multiholed catheter instead of a single-holed catheter for obstetric anesthesia. Use of a multiholed catheter appears to be associated with fewer unilateral blocks, and greatly reduces the incidence of false-negative aspiration for intravascular catheter placement. Advancing a multiholed catheter 7–8 cm into the epidural space appears to be optimal for obtaining adequate sensory levels. A single-hole catheter need only be advanced 3–5 cm into the epidural space. Shorter insertion depths (< 5 cm), however, may favor dislodgment of the catheter out of the epidural space in obese patients following flexion/extension movements of the spine. Spiral wire-reinforced catheters are very resistant to kinking. A spiral or spring tip, particularly when used without a stylet, is associated with fewer, less intense paresthesias and may also be associated with a lower incidence of inadvertent intravascular insertion.

C. Choice of Local Anesthetic Solutions

The addition of opioids to local anesthetic solutions for epidural anesthesia has dramatically changed the practice of obstetric anesthesia. The synergy between epidural opioids and local anesthetic solutions appears to reflect separate sites of action, namely, opiate receptors and neuronal axons, respectively. When the two are combined, very low concentrations of both local anesthetic and opioid can be used. More importantly, the incidence of adverse side effects, such as hypotension and drug toxicity, is likely reduced. Although local anesthetics can be used alone, there is rarely a reason to do so. Moreover, when an opioid is omitted, the higher concentration of local anesthetic required (eg, bupivacaine 0.25% and ropivacaine 0.2%) can impair the parturient's ability to push effectively as the labor progresses. Bupivacaine or ropivacaine in concentrations of 0.0625–0.125% with either fentanyl 2–3 μg/mL or sufentanil 0.3–0.5 μg/mL is most often used. In general, the lower the concentration of the local anesthetic the higher the concentration of opioid that is required. Very dilute local anesthetic mixtures (0.0625%) generally do not produce motor blockade and may allow some patients to ambulate ("walking" or "mobile" epidural). The long duration of action of bupivacaine makes it a popular agent for labor. Ropivacaine may be preferable because of possibly less motor blockade and its reduced potential for cardiotoxicity (see Chapter 14). Systemic absorption of the opioid can decrease fetal heart rate variability due to transient sedation of the fetus.

The effect of epinephrine-containing solutions on the course of labor is somewhat controversial. Many clinicians use epinephrine-containing solutions only for intravascular test doses because of concern that the solutions may slow the progression of labor (see Chapter 42) or adversely affect the fetus; others use only very dilute concentrations of epinephrine such as 1:800,000 or 1:400,000. Studies comparing these various agents have failed to find any differences in neonatal Apgar scores, acid–base status, or neurobehavioral evaluations.

D. Epidural Activation for the First Stage of Labor

Epidural injections may be done either before or after the catheter is placed. Activation through the needle can facilitate catheter placement, whereas activation through the catheter ensures proper function of the catheter. The following sequence is suggested for epidural activation:

1. Administer a 500- to 1000-mL intravenous bolus of lactated Ringer's injection while the epidural catheter is being placed. The value of crystalloid fluid boluses in preventing hypotension following activation has been questioned because of their modest efficacy (see below). Moreover, rapid infusion of intravenous fluids can transiently decrease uterine activity. Glucose-free intravenous fluid boluses are used to avoid maternal hyperglycemia and hypersecretion of insulin by the fetus. When placental transfer of glucose ceases abruptly following delivery, persistent high circulating levels of insulin in the neonate can result in transient hypoglycemia.

2. Test for unintentional subarachnoid or intravascular placement of the needle or catheter with a 3-mL test dose of a local anesthetic with 1:200,000 epinephrine (controversial; see the section on Prevention of Unintentional Intravascular and Intrathecal Injections). Many clinicians test with lidocaine 1.5% because of less toxicity following unintentional intravascular injection and a more rapid onset of spinal anesthesia than with bupivacaine and ropivacaine. The test dose should be injected between contractions to help reduce false positive signs of an intravascular injection, ie, tachycardia due to a painful contraction.

3. If after 5 min signs of intravascular or intrathecal injection are absent, with the patient supine and left uterine displacement, give 10 mL of the local anesthetic–opioid mixture in 5 mL increments, waiting 1–2 min between doses, to achieve a T10–L1 sensory level. The initial bolus is usually 0.1–0.2% of ropivacaine or 0.0625–0.125% of bupivacaine combined with either 50–100 μg of fentanyl or 10–20 μg of sufentanil.

4. Monitor with frequent blood pressure measurements for 20–30 min or until the patient is stable. Pulse oximetry should also be used. Oxygen is administered via face mask if there are any significant drops in blood pressure or oxygen saturation readings.

5. Repeat steps 3 and 4 when pain recurs until the first stage of labor is completed. Alternatively, a continuous epidural infusion technique may be employed using bupivacaine or ropivacaine in concentrations of 0.0625–0.125% with either fentanyl 1–5 μg/mL or sufentanil 0.2–0.5 μg/mL 10 mL/h, subsequently adjusted according to the patient's needs (range 5–15 mL/h). A third choice would be to use patient-controlled epidural analgesia (PCEA). Some studies suggest that total drug requirements may be less and patient satisfaction is greater with PCEA compared to other epidural techniques. PCEA settings are typically a 5 mL bolus dose with a 5–10 min lockout and 0–5 mL/h basal rate; a 1 h limit of 15–20 mL may used. Migration of the epidural catheter into a blood vessel during a continuous infusion technique may be heralded by loss of effective analgesia; a high index of suspicion is required because overt signs of systemic toxicity may be absent. Erosion of the catheter through the dura results in a slowly progressive motor blockade of the lower extremities and a rising sensory level.

E. Epidural Activation During the Second Stage of Labor

Activation for the second stage of labor extends the block to include the S2–4 dermatomes. Whether a catheter is already in place or epidural anesthesia is just being initiated, the following steps should be undertaken:

1. Give a 500- to 1000-mL intravenous bolus of lactated Ringer's injection.

2. If the patient does not already have a catheter in place, identify the epidural space while the patient is in a sitting position. A patient who already has an epidural catheter in place should be placed in a semiupright or sitting position prior to injection.

3. Give a 3-mL test dose of local anesthetic (eg, lidocaine 1.5%) with 1:200,000 epinephrine. Again the injection should be between contractions.

4. If after 5 min signs of an intravascular or intrathecal injection are absent, give 10–15 mL of additional local anesthetic–opioid mixture at a rate not faster than 5 mL every 1–2 min.

5. Administer oxygen by face mask and lay the patient supine with left uterine displacement and monitor blood pressure every 1–2 min for the first 15 min, then every 5 min thereafter.

F. PREVENTION OF UNINTENTIONAL INTRAVASCULAR AND INTRATHECAL INJECTIONS

Safe administration of epidural anesthesia is critically dependent on avoiding unintentional intrathecal or intravascular injections. Unintentional intravascular or intrathecal placement of an epidural needle or catheter is possible even when aspiration fails to yield blood or cerebrospinal fluid (CSF). The incidence of unintentional intravascular or intrathecal placement of an epidural catheter is 5–15% and 0.5–2.5%, respectively. Even a properly placed catheter can subsequently erode into an epidural vein or an intrathecal position. This possibility should be excluded each time local anesthetic is injected through an epidural catheter.

Test doses of lidocaine, 45–60 mg, bupivacaine, 7.5–10 mg, ropivacaine, 6–8 mg, or chloroprocaine, 100 mg, can be given to exclude unintentional intrathecal placement. Signs of sensory and motor blockade usually become apparent within 2–3 min and 3–5 min, respectively, if the injection is intrathecal.

Test dose techniques for unintentional intravascular injections may not be reliable in parturients. The best method for detecting intravascular injections is controversial in obstetric anesthesia. In patients not receiving β-adrenergic antagonists, the intravascular injection of a local anesthetic solution with 15–20 μg of epinephrine consistently increases the heart rate by 20–30 beats/min within 30–60 s if the catheter (or epidural needle) is intravascular. This technique is not always reliable in parturients because they often have marked spontaneous baseline variations in heart rate with contractions. In fact, bradycardia has been reported in a parturient following intravenous injection of 15 μg of epinephrine. Moreover, in animal studies, 15 μg of epinephrine intravenously reduces uterine blood flow, and the dose has been associated with

fetal distress in humans. Alternative methods of detecting unintentional intravascular catheter placement include eliciting tinnitus or perioral numbness following a 100-mg test dose of lidocaine, eliciting a chronotropic effect following injection of 5 μg of isoproterenol, or injecting 1 mL of air while monitoring the patient with a precordial Doppler. With the possible exception of the precordial Doppler, false-negative responses may be encountered with all methods; false-positive responses can also be observed. The use of dilute local anesthetic solutions and slow injection rates of no more than 5 mL at a time may also enhance detection of unintentional intravascular injections before catastrophic complications develop.

G. MANAGEMENT OF COMPLICATIONS

1. Hypotension—Generally defined as a 20–30% decrease in blood pressure or a systolic pressure less than 100 mm Hg, hypotension is the most common side effect of regional anesthesia. It is primarily due to decreased sympathetic tone and is greatly accentuated by aortocaval compression and an upright or semiupright position. Treatment should be aggressive in obstetric patients and consists of intravenous boluses of ephedrine (5–15 mg) or phenylephrine (25–50 μg), supplemental oxygen, left uterine displacement, and an intravenous fluid bolus. Use of the head-down (Trendelenburg) position is controversial because of its potentially detrimental effects on pulmonary gas exchange.

2. Unintentional intravascular injections—Early recognition of intravascular injections, detected by the use of small incremental doses of local anesthetic, may prevent more serious local anesthetic toxicity, such as seizures or cardiovascular collapse. Intravascular injections of toxic doses of lidocaine or chloroprocaine usually present as seizures. Thiopental, 50–100 mg, will cease frank seizure activity. Small doses of propofol may also terminate seizures but experience with it is more limited for this purpose. Maintenance of a patent airway and adequate oxygenation are of paramount importance. Immediate endotracheal intubation with succinylcholine and cricoid pressure should be considered. Intravascular injections of bupivacaine can cause rapid and profound cardiovascular collapse as well as seizure activity. Cardiac resuscitation may be exceedingly difficult and is particularly aggravated by acidosis and hypoxia. Amiodarone appears to be particularly useful in reversing bupivacaine-induced decreases in the threshold for ventricular tachycardia.

3. Unintentional intrathecal injection—If dural puncture is recognized immediately after injection of local anesthetic, an attempt to aspirate the local anesthetic may be tried but is usually unsuccessful. The patient should be gently placed supine with left uterine displacement. Head elevation accentuates hypotension and should be avoided. The hypotension should be treated aggressively with ephedrine and intravenous fluids. A high spinal level can also result in diaphragmatic paralysis, which necessitates intubation and ventilation with 100% oxygen. Delayed onset of a very high and often patchy or unilateral block may be due to unrecognized subdural injection (see Chapter 16), which is managed similarly.

4. Postdural puncture headache (PDPH)—Headache frequently follows unintentional dural puncture in parturients. A self-limited headache may occur without dural puncture; in such instances injection of significant amounts of air into the epidural space during a loss of resistance technique may be responsible. PDPH is due to decreased intracranial pressure with compensatory cerebral vasodilatation (see Chapter 16). Bed rest, hydration, oral analgesics, epidural saline injection (50 mL), and caffeine sodium benzoate (500 mg intravenously) may be effective in patients with mild headaches. Patients with moderate to severe headaches usually require an epidural blood patch (15–20 mL) (see Chapter 16). Prophylactic epidural blood patches are generally not recommended; 25–50% of patients may not require a blood patch following dural puncture. Some clinicians believe that delaying a blood patch for 24 h increases its efficacy, but this practice is controversial. Subdural hematoma has been reported as a rare complication 1–6 weeks following unintentional dural puncture in obstetric patients.

5. Maternal fever—Epidural analgesia for labor is associated with a higher incidence of temperature elevation in parturients compared with those delivering without the benefit of epidural analgesia. Maternal fever is often interpreted as chorioamnionitis and may trigger an invasive neonatal sepsis evaluation. There is no evidence, however, that neonatal sepsis is actually increased with epidural analgesia. This elevation in temperature may result from epidural-induced shivering or inhibition of sweating and hyperventilation; it is most commonly encountered in nulliparous women, who often have prolonged labor and are more likely to receive epidural analgesia.

Combined Spinal & Epidural (CSE) Analgesia

Techniques using CSE analgesia and anesthesia (see Chapter 16) may particularly benefit patients with severe pain early in labor and those who receive analgesia/anesthesia just prior to delivery. Intrathecal opioid and local anesthetic are injected and an epidural catheter is left in place. The intrathecal drugs provide almost immediate pain control and have minimal effects on the early progress of labor, whereas the epidural catheter provides a route for subsequent analgesia for labor and delivery or anesthesia for cesarean section. Addition of small doses of local anesthetic agents to intrathecal opioid injection greatly potentiates their analgesia and can significantly reduce opioid requirements. Thus, many clinicians will inject 2.5 mg of preservative-free bupivacaine or 3–4 mg of ropivacaine with intrathecal opioids for analgesia in the first stage of labor. Intrathecal doses for CSE are fentanyl 4–5 μg or sufentanil 2–3 μg. Addition of 0.1 mg of epinephrine prolongs the analgesia with such mixtures but not for intrathecal opioids alone. Some studies suggest that CSE techniques may be associated with greater patient satisfaction than epidural analgesia alone. A 24- to 27-gauge pencil-point spinal needle (Whitacre, Sprotte, or Gertie Marx) is used to minimize the incidence of PDPH.

The spinal and epidural needles may be placed at different interspaces, but most clinicians use the same interspace. Use of saline for identification for the epidural space (see Chapter 16) is best avoided because of potential confusion of saline for CSF. With the needle-through-needle technique, the epidural needle is placed in the epidural space and a long spinal needle is then introduced through it and advanced further into the subarachnoid space. A distinct pop is felt as the needle penetrates the dura. The needle-beside-needle technique typically employs a specially designed epidural needle that has a channel for the spinal needle. After the intrathecal injection and withdrawal of the spinal needle, the epidural catheter is threaded into position and the epidural needle is withdrawn. The risk of advancing the epidural catheter through the dural hole created by the spinal needle appears to be very small when a 25-gauge or smaller needle is used. The epidural catheter, however, should be aspirated carefully and local anesthetic should always be given slowly and in small increments to avoid unintentional intrathecal injections. Moreover, epidural drugs should be administered and titrated carefully because the dural hole may increase the flux of epidural drugs into CSF and enhance their effects. Some studies suggest that the incidence of dural puncture from an epidural needle is less with CSE than with an epidural technique alone.

Spinal Anesthesia

Spinal anesthesia given just prior to delivery—also known as saddle block—provides profound anesthesia for operative vaginal delivery. A 500- to 1000-mL fluid bolus is given prior to the procedure, which is performed with the patient in the sitting position. Use of a 22-gauge or smaller, pencil-point spinal needle (Whitacre, Sprotte, or Gertie Marx) decreases the likelihood of PDPH. Hyperbaric tetracaine (3–4 mg), bupivacaine (6–7 mg), or lidocaine (20–40 mg) usually provides excellent perineal anesthesia. Addition of fentanyl 12.5–25 μg or sufentanil 5–7.5 μg significantly potentiates the block. A T10 sensory level can be obtained with slightly larger amounts of local anesthetic. The intrathecal injec-

Table 43–3. Possible indications for general anesthesia during vaginal delivery.

Fetal distress during the second stage
Tetanic uterine contractions
Breech extraction
Version and extraction
Manual removal of a retained placenta
Replacement of an inverted uterus
Psychiatric patients who become uncontrollable

tion should be given slowly over 30 s and between contractions to minimize excessive cephalad spread. Three minutes after injection, the patient is placed in the lithotomy position with left uterine displacement.

GENERAL ANESTHESIA

Because of the increased risk of aspiration, general anesthesia for vaginal delivery is avoided except for a true emergency. If an epidural catheter is already in place and time permits, rapid-onset regional anesthesia can often be obtained with alkalinized lidocaine 2% or chloroprocaine 3%. Table 43–3 lists indications for general anesthesia during vaginal delivery. Many of these indications share the need for uterine relaxation. Intravenous nitroglycerin, 50–100 μg, has been shown to be effective in inducing uterine relaxation and may obviate the need for general anesthesia in these cases.

Suggested Technique for Vaginal Delivery

(1) Place a wedge under the right hip for left uterine displacement.

(2) Preoxygenate the patient for 3–5 min as monitors are applied. Defasciculation with a nondepolarizing muscle relaxant is usually not necessary, because most pregnant patients do not fasciculate following succinylcholine. Moreover, fasciculations do not appear to promote regurgitation, because any increase in intragastric pressure is matched by a similar increase in the lower esophageal sphincter.

(3) Once all monitors are applied and the obstetrician is ready, proceed with a rapid-sequence induction while cricoid pressure is applied and intubate with a 6- to 6.5-mm endotracheal tube. Propofol, 2 mg/kg, or thiopental, 4 mg/kg, and succinylcholine, 1.5 mg/kg, are most commonly used unless the patient is hypovolemic or hypotensive, in which case ketamine, 1 mg/kg, is used as the induction agent.

(4) After successful intubation, use 1–2 minimum alveolar concentration (MAC) of any potent volatile inhalational agent (see Chapter 7) in 100% oxygen while carefully monitoring blood pressure.

(5) If skeletal muscle relaxation is necessary, a short- to intermediate-acting, nondepolarizing muscle relaxant (eg, mivacurium or atracurium) is used.

(6) Once the fetus and placenta are delivered, the volatile agent is decreased to less than 0.5 MAC or discontinued, an oxytocin infusion is started (20–40 U/L of intravenous fluid), and a nitrous oxide–opioid technique or propofol infusion can be used to avoid recall.

(7) An attempt to aspirate gastric contents may be made via an orogastric tube to decrease the likelihood of pulmonary aspiration on emergence.

(8) At the end of the procedure, the skeletal nondepolarizing muscle relaxant is reversed, the gastric tube (if placed) is removed, and the patient is extubated while awake.

■ ANESTHESIA FOR CESAREAN SECTION

Common indications for cesarean section are listed in Table 43–4. The choice of anesthesia for cesarean section

Table 43–4. Major indications for cesarean section.

Labor unsafe for mother and fetus
  Increased risk of uterine rupture
    Previous classic cesarean section
    Previous extensive myomectomy or uterine
      reconstruction
  Increased risk of maternal hemorrhage
    Central or partial placenta previa
    Abruptio placentae
    Previous vaginal reconstruction
Dystocia
  Abnormal fetopelvic relations
    Fetopelvic disproportion
    Abnormal fetal presentation
      Transverse or oblique lie
      Breech presentation
  Dysfunctional uterine activity
Immediate or emergent delivery necessary
  Fetal distress
  Umbilical cord prolapse
  Maternal hemorrhage
  Amnionitis
  Genital herpes with ruptured membranes
  Impending maternal death

is determined by multiple factors, including the indication for operating, its urgency, patient and obstetrician preferences, and the skills of the anesthetist. Cesarean section rates between institutions generally vary between 15 and 25%. In the United States approximately 80–90% are performed under regional anesthesia, nearly evenly split between spinal and epidural anesthesia. Regional anesthesia has become the preferred technique because general anesthesia has been associated with higher maternal mortality. Deaths associated with general anesthesia are generally related to airway problems, such as inability to intubate, inability to ventilate, or aspiration pneumonitis, whereas deaths associated with regional anesthesia are generally related to excessively high neural blockade or local anesthetic toxicity.

Other advantages of regional anesthesia include (1) less neonatal exposure to potentially depressant drugs, (2) a decreased risk of maternal pulmonary aspiration, (3) an awake mother at the birth of her child, with the father also present if desired, and (4) the option of using spinal opioids for postoperative pain relief. The choice between spinal and epidural anesthesia is often based on physician preferences. Epidural anesthesia is preferred over spinal anesthesia by some clinicians because of the more gradual decrease in blood pressure associated with epidural anesthesia. Continuous epidural anesthesia also allows better control over the sensory level. Conversely, spinal anesthesia is easier to perform, has a more rapid, predictable onset, may produce a more intense (complete) block, and does not have the potential for serious systemic drug toxicity (because of the smaller dose of local anesthetic employed). Regardless of the regional technique chosen, the ability to administer a general anesthetic at any time during the procedure is mandatory. Moreover, administration of a nonparticulate antacid 1 h prior to surgery should also be considered.

General anesthesia offers (1) a very rapid and reliable onset, (2) control over the airway and ventilation, and (3) potentially less hypotension than regional anesthesia. General anesthesia also facilitates management in the event of severe hemorrhagic complications such as placenta accreta. Its principal disadvantages are the risk of pulmonary aspiration, the potential inability to intubate or ventilate the patient, and drug-induced fetal depression. Present anesthetic techniques, however, limit the dose of intravenous agents such that fetal depression is usually not clinically significant with general anesthesia when delivery occurs within 10 min of induction of anesthesia. Regardless of the type of anesthesia, neonates delivered more than 3 min after uterine incision have lower Apgar scores and acidotic blood gases.

REGIONAL ANESTHESIA

Cesarean section requires a T4 sensory level. Because of the associated high sympathetic blockade, all patients should receive a 1000- to 1500-mL bolus of lactated Ringer's injection prior to neural blockade. Crystalloid boluses do not consistently prevent hypotension but can be helpful in some patients. Smaller volumes (250–500 mL) of colloid solutions, such as albumin or hetastarch, are more effective. After injection of the anesthetic, the patient is placed supine with left uterine displacement; supplemental oxygen (40–50%) is given; blood pressure is measured every 1–2 min until it stabilizes. Intravenous ephedrine, 10 mg, should be used to maintain systolic blood pressure > 100 mm Hg. Small intravenous doses of phenylephrine, 25–100 μg, or an infusion up to 100 μg/min may also be used safely. Some studies suggest less neonatal acidosis with phenylephrine compared to ephedrine. Prophylactic administration of ephedrine (5 mg intravenous or 25 mg intramuscular) has been advocated by some clinicians for spinal anesthesia, as precipitous hypotension may be seen but is not recommended for most patients because of a risk of inducing excessive hypertension. Hypotension following epidural anesthesia typically has a slower onset. Slight Trendelenburg positioning facilitates achieving a T4 sensory level and may also help prevent severe hypotension. Extreme degrees of Trendelenburg may interfere with pulmonary gas exchange.

1. Spinal Anesthesia

The patient is usually placed in the lateral decubitus or sitting position, and a hyperbaric solution of tetracaine (7–10 mg), lidocaine (50–60 mg), or bupivacaine (10–15 mg) is injected. Epinephrine 0.1 mg can enhance the quality of the block and may prolong its duration of tetracaine and bupivacaine (see Chapter 16). Use of a 22-gauge or smaller, pencil-point spinal needle (Whitacre, Sprotte, or Gertie Marx) decreases the incidence of PDPH. Adding 12.5–25 μg of fentanyl or 5–10 μg of sufentanil to the local anesthetic solution enhances the intensity of the block and prolongs its duration without adversely affecting neonatal outcome. Addition of preservative-free morphine, 0.2–0.3 mg, can prolong postoperative analgesia up to 24 h but requires special monitoring for delayed postoperative respiratory depression. Regardless of the anesthetic agents used, considerable variability in the maximum sensory level should be expected (see Chapter 16).

Continuous spinal anesthesia is also a reasonable option following unintentional dural puncture while placing an epidural catheter for cesarean section. After the catheter is advanced 2–2.5 cm into the lumbar subarachnoid space and secured, it can be used to inject anesthetic agents; moreover, it allows later supplementation of the anesthesia if necessary.

2. Epidural Anesthesia

Epidural anesthesia for cesarean section is generally most satisfactory when an epidural catheter is used. The catheter facilitates achieving an initial T4 sensory level, allows supplementation if necessary, and provides an excellent route for postoperative opioid administration. After a negative test dose, a total of 15–25 mL of local anesthetic is injected slowly in 5-mL increments. Lidocaine 2% (with or without 1:200,000 epinephrine) or chloroprocaine 3% is most commonly used. Addition of fentanyl, 50–100 μg, or sufentanil, 10–20 μg, greatly enhances the intensity of the block and prolongs its duration without adversely affecting neonatal outcome. Some practitioners also add sodium bicarbonate (7.5% or 8.4% solution) to local anesthetic solutions (1 mEq/10 mL of lidocaine and 0.05 mEq/10 mL of bupivacaine or ropivacaine) to increase the concentration of the nonionized free base and produce a faster onset and more rapid spread of epidural anesthesia. If pain develops as the sensory level recedes, additional local anesthetic is given in 5-mL increments to maintain a T4 sensory level. "Patchy" anesthesia prior to delivery of the baby can be treated with 10–20 mg of intravenous ketamine or 30% nitrous oxide. After delivery, intravenous opioid supplementation may also be used, provided excessive sedation and loss of consciousness are avoided. Pain that remains intolerable in spite of a seemingly adequate sensory level and that proves unresponsive to these measures necessitates general anesthesia with endotracheal intubation. Nausea can be treated intravenously with ondansetron 4 mg or metoclopramide 10 mg.

Epidural morphine, 5 mg, at the end of surgery provides good to excellent pain relief postoperatively for 6–24 h. An increased incidence (3.5–30%) of recurrent herpes simplex labialis infection has been reported 2–5 days following epidural morphine in some studies. Postoperative analgesia can also be provided by continuous epidural infusions of fentanyl, 25–75 μg/h, or sufentanil, 5–10 μg/h, at a volume rate of approximately 10 mL/h. Epidural butorphanol, 2 mg, can also provide effective postoperative pain relief, but marked somnolence is often a troublesome side effect.

3. CSE Anesthesia

The technique for CSE is described in the above section on combined spinal epidural analgesia. For cesarean section, it combines the benefit of rapid, reliable, intense blockade of spinal anesthesia with the flexibility of an epidural catheter. The catheter also allows supplementation of anesthesia and can be used for postoperative analgesia. As mentioned previously, drugs given epidurally should be administered and titrated carefully because the dural hole created by the spinal needle increases the flux of epidural drugs into CSF and enhances their effects.

GENERAL ANESTHESIA

Pulmonary aspiration of gastric contents (incidence: 1:500–400 for obstetric patients versus 1:2000 for all patients) and failed endotracheal intubation (incidence: 1:300 versus 1:2000 for all patients) during general anesthesia are the major causes of maternal morbidity and mortality. Every effort should be made to ensure optimal conditions prior to the start of anesthesia and to follow measures aimed at preventing these complications.

All patients should possibly receive prophylaxis against severe nonparticulate aspiration pneumonia with 30 mL of 0.3 M sodium citrate 30–45 min prior to induction. Patients with additional risk factors predisposing them to aspiration should also receive intravenous ranitidine, 50 mg, and/or metoclopramide, 10 mg, 1–2 h prior to induction; such factors include morbid obesity, symptoms of gastroesophageal reflux, a potentially difficult airway, or emergent surgical delivery without an elective fasting period. Premedication with oral omeprazole, 40 mg, at night and in the morning also appears to be highly effective in high-risk patients undergoing elective cesarean section. Although anticholinergics theoretically may reduce lower esophageal sphincter tone, premedication with a small dose of glycopyrrolate (0.1 mg) helps reduce airway secretions and should be considered in patients with a potentially difficult airway.

Anticipation of a difficult endotracheal intubation may help reduce the incidence of failed intubations. Examination of the neck, mandible, dentition, and oropharynx often helps predict which patients may have problems. Useful predictors of a difficult intubation include Mallampati classification, short neck, receding mandible, and prominent maxillary incisors (see Chapter 5). The higher incidence of failed intubations in pregnant patients compared with nonpregnant surgical patients may be due to airway edema, a full dentition, or large breasts that can obstruct the handle of the laryngoscope in patients with short necks. Proper positioning of the head and neck may facilitate endotracheal intubation in obese patients: elevation of the shoulders, flexion of the cervical spine, and extension of the atlantooccipital joint (Figure 43–3). A variety of laryngoscope blades, a short laryngoscope handle, at least one extra styletted endotracheal tube (6 mm), Magill forceps (for nasal intu-

A

B

Figure 43–3. Optimal positioning for obese patients with a short neck. *A:* The normal supine position often prevents extension of the head and makes endotracheal intubation difficult. *B:* Elevation of the shoulder allows some neck flexion with more optimal extension of the head at the atlantooccipital joint, facilitating intubation.

bation), a laryngeal mask airway (LMA), an intubating LMA (Fastrach), a fiberoptic bronchoscope, the capability for transtracheal jet ventilation, and possibly an esophageal-tracheal Combitube should be readily available (see Chapter 5). When difficulty in securing the airway is suspected, alternatives to the standard rapid-sequence induction, such as regional anesthesia or awake fiberoptic techniques, should be considered. Moreover, a clear plan should be formulated for a failed endotracheal intubation following induction of anesthesia (Figure 43–4). Note that the life of the mother takes priority over delivery of the fetus. In the absence of fetal distress, the patient should be awakened, and an awake intubation, with regional or local (infiltration) anesthesia, may be tried. In the presence of fetal distress, if spontaneous or positive ventilation (by mask

or LMA) with cricoid pressure is possible, delivery of the fetus may be attempted. In such instances, a potent volatile agent in oxygen is employed for anesthesia, but once the fetus is delivered, nitrous oxide can be added to reduce the concentration of the volatile agent; sevoflurane may be the best volatile agent because it may be least likely to depress ventilation. The inability to ventilate the patient at any time mandates immediate cricothyrotomy or tracheostomy.

Suggested Technique for Cesarean Section

(1) The patient is placed supine with a wedge under the right hip for left uterine displacement.

(2) Preoxygenation is accomplished with 100% oxygen for 3–5 min while monitors are applied. Defasciculation is generally not necessary (see the section on Suggested Technique for Vaginal Delivery).

(3) The patient is prepared and draped for surgery.

(4) When the surgeons are ready, a rapid-sequence induction with cricoid pressure is performed using propofol, 2 mg/kg (or thiopental 4 mg/kg) and succinylcholine, 1.5 mg/kg. Ketamine, 1 mg/kg, is used instead of thiopental in hypovolemic or asthmatic patients. Other agents, including methohexital, etomidate, and midazolam, offer little benefit in obstetric patients. In fact, midazolam may be more likely to produce maternal hypotension and neonatal depression.

(5) Surgery is begun only after proper placement of the endotracheal tube is confirmed by capnography. Excessive hyperventilation ($PaCO_2$, 25 mm Hg) should be avoided because it can reduce uterine blood flow and has been associated with fetal acidosis.

(6) Fifty percent nitrous oxide in oxygen with up to 0.75 MAC of a low concentration of a volatile agent (eg, 1% sevoflurane, 0.75% isoflurane, or 3% desflurane) is used for maintenance. The low dose of volatile agent helps ensure amnesia but is generally not enough to cause excessive uterine relaxation or prevent uterine contraction following oxytocin. A muscle relaxant of intermediate duration (mivacurium, atracurium, cisatracurium, or rocuronium) is used for relaxation.

(7) After the neonate and placenta are delivered, 20–30 U of oxytocin is added to each liter of intravenous fluid. The nitrous oxide concentration may then be increased to 70% and/or additional intravenous agents, such as additional propofol, an opioid or benzodiazepine, can be given to ensure amnesia.

(8) If the uterus does not contract readily, an opioid should be given, and the halogenated agent should be discontinued. Methylergonovine (Methergine),

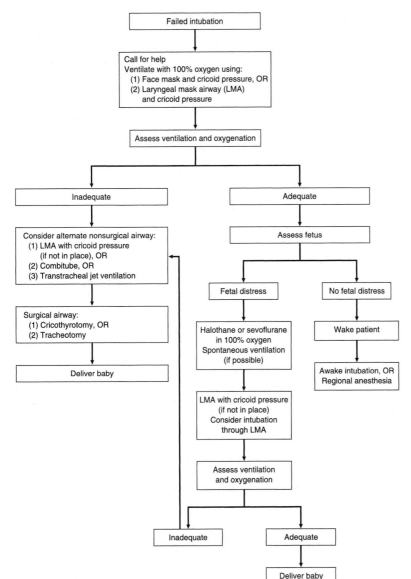

Figure 43–4. An algorithm for a difficult intubation in obstetric patients.

0.2 mg intramuscularly, may also be given but can increase arterial blood pressure (see Chapter 42). 15-Methylprostaglandin $F_{2\alpha}$ (Hemabate), 0.25 mg intramuscularly, may also be used.

(9) An attempt to aspirate gastric contents may be made via an oral gastric tube to decrease the likelihood of pulmonary aspiration on emergence.

(10) At the end of surgery, muscle relaxants are completely reversed, the gastric tube (if placed) is removed, and the patient is extubated while awake to reduce the risk of aspiration.

ANESTHESIA FOR EMERGENCY CESAREAN SECTION

Indications for emergency cesarean section include massive bleeding (placenta previa or accreta, abruptio placentae, or uterine rupture), umbilical cord prolapse, and severe fetal distress. A distinction must be made between a true emergency requiring immediate delivery (previous referred to as "crash") and one in which some delay is possible. Close communication with the obstetrician is necessary to determine whether fetus, mother,

Table 43–5. Signs of fetal distress.

Nonreassuring fetal heart rate pattern
Repetitive late decelerations
Loss of fetal beat-to-beat variability associated with late
or deep decelerations
Sustained fetal heart rate < 80 beats/min
Fetal scalp pH < 7.20
Meconium-stained amniotic fluid
Oligohydramnios
Intrauterine growth restriction

or both are in immediate jeopardy requiring general anesthesia or there is time to safely administer regional anesthesia. In the first instance, even if the patient has an epidural catheter in place, the delay in establishing adequate epidural anesthesia may prohibit its use. Moreover, regional anesthesia is contraindicated in severely hypovolemic or hypotensive patients. Adequate preoxygenation may be achieved rapidly with four maximal breaths of 100% oxygen while monitors are being applied. Ketamine, 1 mg/kg, should be substituted for thiopental in hypotensive or hypovolemic patients.

Table 43–5 lists commonly accepted signs of fetal distress, an imprecise and poorly defined term. In most instances the diagnosis is primarily based on monitoring of fetal heart rate (see below). Because worrisome fetal heart rate patterns have a relatively high incidence of false-positive results, careful interpretation of other parameters, such as fetal scalp pH or fetal pulse oximetry, may also be necessary. Moreover, continuation of fetal monitoring in the operating room may help avoid unnecessary induction of general anesthesia for fetal distress when additional time for use of regional anesthesia is possible. In selected instances where immediate delivery is not absolutely mandatory, epidural anesthesia (with 3% chloroprocaine or alkalinized 2% lidocaine) or spinal anesthesia may be appropriate.

■ ANESTHESIA FOR THE COMPLICATED PREGNANCY

UMBILICAL CORD PROLAPSE

Prolapse of the umbilical cord complicates 0.2–0.6% of deliveries. Umbilical cord compression following prolapse can rapidly lead to fetal asphyxia. Predisposing factors include excessive cord length, malpresentation, low birth weight, grand parity (more than five pregnan-

cies), multiple gestations, and artificial rupture of membranes. The diagnosis is suspected after sudden fetal bradycardia or profound decelerations and is confirmed by physical examination. Treatment includes immediate steep Trendelenburg or knee-chest position and manual pushing of the presenting fetal part back up into the pelvis until immediate cesarean section under general anesthesia. If the fetus is not viable, vaginal delivery is allowed to continue.

DYSTOCIA & ABNORMAL FETAL PRESENTATIONS & POSITIONS

Dystocia, or difficult labor, may be due to ineffective uterine contractions; abnormal lie, position, or presentation; or cephalopelvic disproportion that is either due to a large fetus or a small maternal pelvis. Abnormal fetal positions and presentations increase maternal and fetal morbidity and mortality. They also increase the likelihood that anesthesia will be required.

The fetus may lie longitudinally, transversely, or obliquely in the uterus. Fetal presentation refers to the body part that overlies the pelvic inlet. Spontaneous vaginal delivery can occur only with a longitudinal lie, in which either the head (vertex) or buttocks or legs (breech) descend first. The posture (attitude) of the fetus is normally flexion but may be extension. A vertex presentation with flexion together with rotation of the head into an occiput anterior position allows for optimal passage of the fetal skull through the pelvis.

Primary Dysfunctional Labor

Failure of labor to progress normally (see Chapter 42) may be due to inadequate or ineffective uterine contractions, referred to as primary dysfunctional labor. Although in most instances abnormal uterine contractility is responsible, anatomic abnormalities may also play a major role (see the section on Abnormal Vertex Presentations).

A prolonged latent phase by definition exceeds 20 h in a nulliparous parturient and 14 h in a multiparous patient. The cervix usually remains at 4 cm or less but is completely effaced. The etiology is likely ineffective contractions without a dominant myometrial pacemaker. Arrest of dilatation is present when the cervix undergoes no further change after 2 h in the active phase of labor. A protracted active phase refers to slower than normal cervical dilatation, defined as < 1.2 cm/h in a nulliparous patient and < 1.5 cm/h in a multiparous parturient. A prolonged deceleration phase occurs when cervical dilatation slows markedly after 8 cm. The cervix becomes very edematous and appears to lose effacement. A prolonged second stage (disorder of descent) is defined as a descent of less than 1 cm/h and 2 cm/h in nulliparous and multiparous parturients, respectively. Failure of the head to descend 1 cm in station after adequate pushing is referred to as arrest of descent.

Oxytocin (see Chapter 42) is generally the treatment of choice for uterine contractile abnormalities. The drug is given intravenously at 1–6 mU/min and increased in increments of 1–6 mU/min every 15–40 min, depending on the protocol. Use of amniotomy is controversial. Treatment is usually expectant management, as long as the fetus and mother are tolerating the prolonged labor. When a trial of oxytocin is unsuccessful or when malpresentation or cephalopelvic disproportion is also present, operative vaginal delivery or cesarean section is indicated.

Breech Presentation

Breech presentations complicate 3–4% of deliveries and significantly increase both maternal and fetal morbidity and mortality rates. The most common cause is prematurity. Breech presentations increase neonatal mortality more than 5-fold. The incidence of cord prolapse is up to 10%. External cephalic version may be attempted after 36–38 weeks gestation and prior to the onset of labor; the procedure attempts to reverse the fetal lie and guide the head into the pelvis. Some obstetricians may also administer a tocolytic agent at the same time. In some centers, epidural anesthesia is used; the epidural catheter can then be used for analgesia after induction of labor. Although an external version is successful in 75% of patients it can cause placental abruption and umbilical cord compression necessitating immediate cesarean section.

Because the shoulders or head can become trapped after vaginal delivery of the body, some obstetricians employ cesarean section for all breech presentations. The cesarean section rate for breech is 80–100%. Manual or forceps-assisted partial breech extraction is usually necessary with vaginal delivery. The need for breech extraction does not appear to be increased when epidural anesthesia is used for labor—if labor is well established prior to epidural activation. Moreover, epidural anesthesia may decrease the likelihood of a trapped head, because the former relaxes the perineum. Nonetheless, the fetal head can become trapped in the uterus even during cesarean section under regional anesthesia; rapid induction of general endotracheal anesthesia and administration of a volatile agent are necessary in such instances to relax the uterus. Alternatively, nitroglycerin 50–100 μg intravenously can be tried.

Abnormal Vertex Presentations

When the fetal occiput fails to spontaneously rotate anteriorly, a persistent occiput posterior presentation results in a more prolonged and painful labor. Manual, vacuum, or forceps rotation is usually necessary but increases the likelihood of maternal and fetal injuries. Regional anesthesia can be used to provide perineal analgesia and pelvic relaxation, allowing manual or forceps rotation followed by forceps delivery.

A face presentation occurs when the fetal head is hyperextended and generally requires cesarean section. Vaginal delivery of a face presentation is possible only if the chin is directed anteriorly (mentum anterior). Persistent mentum posterior requires cesarean section. Brow presentation is often associated with prolonged and dysfunctional labor. Vaginal delivery can occur only if the head extends into a face presentation or flexes into a normal vertex presentation. Shoulder presentations occur with an oblique lie or transverse lie. Vaginal delivery is impossible. It typically leads to dysfunctional labor and predisposes to cord prolapse when the membranes rupture. Delivery requires cesarean section. A compound presentation occurs when an extremity enters the pelvis along with either the head or the buttocks. Vaginal delivery is usually still possible as the extremity often withdraws as the labor progresses.

Impaction of a shoulder against the pubic symphysis, or shoulder dystocia, complicates 0.2–2% of deliveries and is one of the major causes of birth injuries. The most important risk factor is fetal macrosomia. Shoulder dystocias are often difficult to predict. Several obstetric maneuvers can be used to relieve it, but a prolonged delay in the delivery could result in fetal asphyxia. Induction of general anesthesia may be necessary, if an epidural catheter is not already in place.

MULTIPLE GESTATIONS

Multiple gestations account for 1 birth in 90 and are commonly associated with two complications: breech presentation and prematurity. Anesthesia may be necessary for version, extraction, or cesarean section. The second baby (and any subsequent ones) is often more depressed and asphyxiated than the first. Regional anesthesia provides effective pain relief during labor, minimizes the need for central nervous system depressants, and may shorten the interval between the birth of the first and second baby. Some studies suggest that the acid–base status of the second twin is better when epidural anesthesia is used. Patients with multiple gestations, however, are more prone to develop hypotension from aortocaval compression, particularly after regional anesthesia. Left lateral uterine displacement and intravenous fluid loading are mandatory prior to regional anesthesia. Either regional or general anesthesia may be used for cesarean section; regional anesthesia may be associated with less neonatal depression.

PARTUM HEMORRHAGE

 Maternal hemorrhage is one of the most common severe morbidities complicating obstetric anesthesia. Causes include placenta previa, abruptio placentae, and uterine rupture.

Placenta Previa

The incidence of placenta previa is 0.5% of pregnancies. Placenta previa often occurs in patients who have had a previous cesarean section or uterine myomectomy; other risk factors include multiparity, advanced maternal age, and a large placenta. The placenta may completely cover the internal cervical os (central or complete placenta previa), may partially cover the os (partial placenta previa), or may be close to the internal cervical os without extending beyond its edge (low-lying or marginal placenta). An anterior lying placenta previa increases the risk of excessive bleeding for cesarean section.

Placenta previa usually presents as painless vaginal bleeding. Although the bleeding often stops spontaneously, severe hemorrhage can occur at any time. When the gestation is less than 37 weeks in duration and the bleeding is mild to moderate, the patient is usually treated with bed rest and observation. After 37 weeks of gestation, delivery is usually accomplished via cesarean section. Patients with low-lying placenta may be allowed—although rarely—to deliver vaginally if the bleeding is mild.

All parturients with vaginal bleeding are assumed to have placenta previa until proved otherwise. An abdominal ultrasound examination can localize the placenta and establishes the diagnosis. If the patient is stable and fluid resuscitation has already taken place, regional anesthesia may be considered. Active bleeding or an unstable patient requires immediate cesarean section under general anesthesia. The patient should have two large-bore intravenous catheters in place, intravascular volume deficits must be vigorously replaced, and blood must be available for transfusion. A central venous line may be useful in monitoring and provides excellent access for rapid transfusion. The bleeding can continue after delivery because the placental implantation site in the lower uterine segment often does not contract well as does the rest of the uterus.

A history of a previous placenta previa or cesarean section increases the risk of placenta accreta, placenta increta, and placenta percreta in subsequent pregnancies. In these conditions, the placenta becomes adherent to the surface, invades the muscle, or completely penetrates the myometrium and surrounding tissues, respectively. The placenta becomes difficult or impossible to separate from the uterus. Moreover, these conditions regularly produce life-threatening maternal hemorrhage. Hysterectomy after delivery of the fetus is usually required to control profuse bleeding following separation of the placenta. Coagulopa-thy is common and requires correction with blood components.

Abruptio Placentae

Premature separation of a normal placenta complicates approximately 1–2% of pregnancies; it is said to be the most common cause of intrapartum fetal death. Bleeding into the basal layers of the decidua causes placental separation. Expansion of the hematoma can progressively extend the separation. The blood occasionally may extend into the myometrium (Couvelaire uterus). Most abruptions are mild (grade I), but up to 25% are severe (grade III). Risk factors include hypertension, trauma, a short umbilical cord, multiparity, a prolonged premature rupture of membranes, alcohol abuse, cocaine use, and an abnormal uterus. Patients usually experience painful vaginal bleeding with uterine contraction and tenderness. The diagnosis is made by excluding placenta previa on abdominal ultrasound. Amniotic fluid is port wine colored. Mild to moderate abruptions may be managed with vaginal delivery if the fetus is over 37 weeks of gestational age, but immediate cesarean section should be carried out after any signs of fetal distress. The choice between regional and general anesthesia must factor in the urgency for delivery, maternal hemodynamic stability, and any coagulopathy. The bleeding may remain concealed inside the uterus and cause underestimation of blood loss. Severe abruptio placentae can cause coagulopathy, particularly following fetal demise. Fibrinogen levels are mildly reduced (150–250 mg/dL) with moderate abruptions but are typically less than 150 mg/dL with fetal demise. The coagulopathy is thought to be due to activation of circulating plasminogen (fibrinolysis) and the release of tissue thromboplastins that precipitate disseminated intravascular coagulation (DIC). Platelet count and factors V and VIII are low, and fibrin split products are elevated. Severe abruption is a life-threatening emergency that necessitates a crash emergency cesarean section under general anesthesia. Massive blood transfusion, including replacement of coagulation factors and platelets, is necessary.

Uterine Rupture

Uterine rupture is relatively uncommon (1:1000–3000 deliveries) but can occur during labor as a result of (1) dehiscence of a scar from a previous (usually classic) cesarean section (VBAC), extensive myomectomy, or uterine reconstruction; (2) intrauterine manipulations or use of forceps (iatrogenic); or (3) spontaneous rupture following prolonged labor in patients with hypertonic contractions (particularly with oxytocin infusions), fetopelvic disproportion, or a very large, thin, and weakened uterus. Uterine rupture can present as frank hemorrhage, fetal distress, loss of uterine tone, and/or hypotension with occult bleeding into the abdomen. Even when epidural anesthesia is employed for labor, uterine rupture is often heralded by the abrupt onset of continuous abdominal pain and hypotension. The use of dilute concentrations of local anesthetics for epidural anesthesia during labor may facilitate early recognition. Treatment requires volume resuscitation and immediate laparotomy under general anesthesia. Ligation of the internal iliac (hypogastric) arteries, with or without hysterectomy, may be necessary to control intraoperative bleeding.

PREMATURE RUPTURE OF MEMBRANES & CHORIOAMNIONITIS

Premature rupture of membranes (PROM) is present when leakage of amniotic fluid occurs before the onset of labor. The pH of amniotic fluid causes nitrazine paper to change color from blue to yellow. PROM complicates 10% of all pregnancies and up to 35% of premature deliveries. Predisposing factors include a short cervix, prior history of PROM or preterm delivery, infection, multiple gestations, polyhydramnios, and smoking. Spontaneous labor commences within 24 h of ruptured membranes in 90% of patients. Management of PROM balances the risk of infection with the risk of fetal prematurity. Delivery is usually indicated sometime after 34 weeks gestation. Patients with a gestation of less than 34 weeks can be managed expectantly with prophylactic antibiotics and tocolytics for 5–7 days to allow some additional maturation of fetal organs. The longer the interval between rupture and the onset of labor, the higher the incidence of chorioamnionitis. PROM also predisposes to placental abruption and postpartum endometritis.

Chorioamnionitis represents infection of the chorionic and amnionic membranes, and may involve the placenta, uterus, umbilical cord, and fetus. It complicates up to 1–2% of pregnancies and is usually but not always associated with ruptured membranes. The contents of the amniotic cavity are normally sterile, but become vulnerable to ascending bacterial infection from the vagina when the cervix dilates or the membranes rupture. Intraamniotic infections are less commonly caused by hematogenous spread of bacteria or retrograde seeding through the fallopian tubes. The principal maternal complications of chorioamnionitis are dysfunctional labor, often leading to cesarean section, intraabdominal infection, septicemia, and postpartum hemorrhage. Fetal complications include premature labor, acidosis, hypoxia, and septicemia.

Diagnosis of chorioamnionitis requires a high index of suspicion. Clinical signs include fever (> 38°C),

maternal and fetal tachycardia, uterine tenderness, and foul smelling or purulent amniotic fluid. Blood leukocyte count is useful only if markedly elevated because it normally increases during labor (normal average 15,000/ μL). C-reactive protein levels are usually elevated (> 2 mg/dL). Gram stain of amniotic fluid obtained by amniocentesis is helpful in ruling out infection.

The use of regional anesthesia in patients with chorioamnionitis is controversial because of the theoretical risk of promoting the development of meningitis or an epidural abscess. Available evidence suggests that this risk is very low and that concerns may be unjustified. Moreover, antepartum antibiotic therapy appears to reduce maternal and fetal morbidity. Nonetheless, concerns over hemodynamic stability following sympathectomy are justified, particularly in patients with chills, high fever, tachypnea, changes in mental status, or borderline hypotension. Therefore, in the absence of overt signs of septicemia, thrombocytopenia, or coagulopathy, most clinicians offer regional anesthesia to patients with chorioamnionitis following antibiotic therapy. When general anesthesia is being considered, the relative risks of failed intubation and aspiration must be weighed against those of a spinal infection following regional anesthesia.

PRETERM LABOR

Preterm labor by definition occurs between weeks 20 and 37 of gestation and is the most common complication of the third trimester. Approximately 8% of liveborn infants in the United States are delivered before term. Important contributory maternal factors include extremes of age, inadequate prenatal care, unusual body habitus, increased physical activity, infections, prior preterm labor, multiple gestation, and other medical illnesses or complications during pregnancy.

Because of their small size and incomplete development, preterm infants—particularly those under 30 weeks of gestational age or weighing less than 1500 g— experience a greater number of complications than term infants. Premature rupture of membranes complicates a third of premature deliveries; the combination of premature rupture of membranes and premature labor increases the likelihood of umbilical cord compression resulting in fetal hypoxemia and asphyxia. Preterm infants with a breech presentation are particularly prone to prolapse of the umbilical cord during labor. Moreover, inadequate production of pulmonary surfactant frequently leads to the idiopathic respiratory distress syndrome (hyaline membrane disease) after delivery. Surfactant levels are generally adequate only after week 35 of gestation. Lastly, a soft, poorly calcified cranium predisposes these neonates to intracranial hemorrhage during vaginal delivery.

When preterm labor occurs before 35 weeks of gestation, bed rest and tocolytic therapy are usually initiated. Treatment is successful in 75% of patients. Labor is inhibited until the lungs mature and sufficient pulmonary surfactant is produced, as judged by amniocentesis. The risk of respiratory distress syndrome is markedly reduced when the amniotic fluid lecithin/sphingomyelin ratio is greater than 2. Glucocorticoid (betamethasone) may be given to induce production of pulmonary surfactant, which requires a minimum of 24–48 h. Prophylactic antibiotics (penicillins) are given to patients until cultures for group B streptococcus are determined to be negative. The most commonly used tocolytics are β_2-adrenergic agonists (ritodrine or terbutaline) and magnesium (6 g intravenously over 30 min followed by 2–4 g/h); intravenous alcohol is no longer used. Ritodrine (given intravenously as 100–350 µg/min) and terbutaline (given orally as 2.5–5 mg every 4–6 h) also have some β_1-adrenergic receptor activity, which accounts for some of their side effects. Maternal side effects include tachycardia, arrhythmias, myocardial ischemia, mild hypotension, hyperglycemia, hypokalemia, and, rarely, pulmonary edema. Other tocolytic agents include calcium channel blockers (nifedipine), prostaglandin synthetase inhibitors, oxytocin antagonists (atosiban), and possibly nitric oxide. Fetal ductal constriction can occur after 32 weeks gestation with nonsteroidal antiinflammatory drugs, such as indomethacin, but it is usually transient and resolves after discontinuation of the drug; renal impairment in the fetus may also cause oligohydramnios.

When tocolytic therapy fails to stop labor, anesthesia often becomes necessary. The goal during vaginal delivery of a preterm fetus is a slow controlled delivery with minimal pushing by the mother. A large episiotomy and low forceps are often employed. Spinal or epidural anesthesia allows complete pelvic relaxation. Cesarean section is performed for fetal distress, breech presentation, intrauterine growth retardation, or failure of labor to progress. Regional or general anesthesia may be employed, but because preterm infants may be more sensitive to all central nervous system depressants, regional anesthesia may be preferable. Residual effects from β-adrenergic agonists may complicate general anesthesia. The half-life of ritodrine may be as long as 3 h. Halothane, pancuronium, ketamine, and ephedrine should be used cautiously (if at all). Hypokalemia is usually due to an intracellular uptake of potassium and rarely requires treatment; however, it may increase sensitivity to muscle relaxants. Magnesium therapy potentiates muscle relaxants and may predispose to hypotension (secondary to vasodilatation). Residual effects from tocolytics interfere with uterine contraction following delivery. Lastly, preterm newborns are often depressed at delivery and frequently need resuscitation.

Preparations for resuscitation should be completed prior to delivery.

PREGNANCY-INDUCED HYPERTENSION

Hypertension during pregnancy can be classified as pregnancy-induced hypertension (PIH, often also referred to as preeclampsia), chronic hypertension that preceded pregnancy, or chronic hypertension with superimposed preeclampsia. **PIH is usually defined as a systolic blood pressure greater than 140 mm Hg or diastolic pressure greater than 90 mm Hg, or, alternatively, as a consistent increase in systolic or diastolic pressure by 30 mm Hg and 15 mm Hg, respectively, above the patient's normal baseline.** PIH more accurately describes one of three syndromes: preeclampsia, eclampsia, and the HELLP syndrome. Preeclampsia (or toxemia) refers to the triad of hypertension, proteinuria (> 500 mg/d), and edema (hand and face) occurring after week 20 of gestation and resolving within 48 h after delivery. When seizures occur, the syndrome is termed eclampsia. The HELLP syndrome describes PIH associated with *h*emolysis, *e*levated *l*iver enzymes, and a *l*ow *p*latelet count. In the United States, preeclampsia complicates approximately 7–10% of pregnancies; eclampsia is much more uncommon, occurring in one of 10,000–15,000 pregnancies. Severe PIH causes or contributes to 20–40% of maternal deaths and 20% of perinatal deaths. Maternal deaths are usually due to stroke, pulmonary edema, and hepatic necrosis or rupture.

Pathophysiology & Manifestations

PIH primarily affects primigravidas, but it can occur in multiparous women, particularly those with vascular disorders. Some evidence suggests that it may have an immunogenetic basis. The pathophysiology of this multisystem disease remains obscure but appears to be related to abnormal prostaglandin metabolism and endothelial dysfunction that lead to vascular hyperreactivity. Patients with PIH have elevated levels of thromboxane A_2 (TXA_2) production and decreased prostacyclin (PGI_2) production. TXA_2 is a potent vasoconstrictor and promoter of platelet aggregation, whereas PGI_2 is a potent vasodilator and inhibitor of platelet aggregation. Endothelial dysfunction may reduce production of nitric oxide and increase production of endothelin-1. The latter is also a potent vasoconstrictor and activator of platelets. Abnormal regulation of oxygen-derived free radical and lipid peroxidation may also play an important role. Marked vascular reactivity and endothelial injury reduce placental perfusion and can lead to widespread systemic manifestations.

Other major manifestations of PIH include (1) generalized vasospasm, (2) reduced intravascular volume, (3) decreased glomerular filtration, and (4) generalized edema (Table 43–6). Severe PIH substantially increases both maternal and fetal morbidity and mortality and is defined by a blood pressure greater than 160/110 mm Hg, proteinuria in excess of 5 g/d, oliguria (< 500 mL/d), pulmonary edema, central nervous system manifestations (headache, visual disturbances, or seizures), hepatic tenderness, or the HELLP syndrome. Hepatic rupture may also occur in patients with the HELLP syndrome.

Patients with severe preeclampsia or eclampsia have widely differing hemodynamic profiles. Most patients have low-normal cardiac filling pressures with high systemic vascular resistance, but cardiac output may be low, normal, or high.

Treatment

Treatment consists of bed rest, sedation, antihypertensive drugs (usually labetalol 5–10 mg intravenously, hydralazine 5 mg intravenously, or methyldopa 250–500 mg orally), and magnesium sulfate (4 g intravenous loading, followed by 1–3 g/h) to treat hyperreflexia and prevent convulsions. Therapeutic magnesium levels are 4–6 mEq/L. Unlike labetalol, esmolol can have significant, potentially adverse fetal effects. Calcium channel blockers are generally not used because of their tocolytic action and potentiation of magnesium-induced circulatory depression.

Invasive arterial, central venous, and possibly pulmonary artery monitoring are probably indicated in patients with severe hypertension, pulmonary edema, or refractory oliguria; an intravenous vasodilator (nitroglycerin or nitroprusside) is often necessary. Nitroprusside in large doses (> 10 µg/kg/min) or for prolonged periods increases the risk of cyanide toxicity in the fetus. Definitive treatment of PIH is delivery of the fetus and placenta.

Anesthetic Management

Patients with mild PIH generally require only extra caution during anesthesia; standard anesthetic practices may be used. Spinal and epidural anesthesia are associated with similar decreases in arterial blood pressure in these patients. Patients with severe disease, however, are critically ill and require stabilization prior to administration of any anesthetic. Hypertension should be controlled and hypovolemia corrected before anesthesia. In the absence of coagulopathy, continuous epidural anesthesia is the first choice for most patients with PIH during labor, vaginal delivery, and cesarean section. Moreover, continuous epidural anesthesia avoids the increased risk of a failed intubation due to severe edema of the upper airway.

Table 43–6. Complications of pregnancy-induced hypertension.

Neurological
Headache
Visual disturbances
Hyperexcitability
Seizures
Intracranial hemorrhage
Cerebral edema
Pulmonary
Upper airway edema
Pulmonary edema
Cardiovascular
Decreased intravascular volume
Increased arteriolar resistance
Hypertension
Heart failure
Hepatic
Impaired function
Elevated enzymes
Hematoma
Rupture
Renal
Proteinuria
Sodium retention
Decreased glomerular filtration
Renal failure
Hematological
Coagulopathy
Thrombocytopenia
Platelet dysfunction
Prolonged partial thromboplastin time
Microangiopathic hemolysis

A platelet count and coagulation profile should be checked prior to the institution of regional anesthesia in patients with severe PIH. It has been recommended that regional anesthesia be avoided if the platelet count is less than 100,000/µL, but a platelet count as low as 70,000/µL may be acceptable. Although some patients have a qualitative platelet defect, the usefulness of a bleeding time is questionable. Continuous epidural anesthesia has been shown to decrease catecholamine secretion and improve uteroplacental perfusion up to 75% in these patients, provided hypotension is avoided. Judicious colloid fluid boluses (250–500 mL) before epidural activation may be more effective than crystalloids in correcting the hypovolemia and preventing profound hypotension. A central venous line may be used to guide volume replacement; however, a pulmonary artery catheter should be used in severe cases (such as marked hypertension, refractory oliguria, hypoxemia, or frank pulmonary edema). Use of an epinephrine-containing test dose for epidural anesthesia is controversial because of questions about its reliability (see the above section on Prevention of Unintentional Intravascular and Intrathecal Injection) and the risk of exacerbating hypertension. Hypotension should be treated with small doses of vasopressors (ephedrine, 5 mg) because patients tend to be very sensitive to these agents.

Intraarterial blood pressure monitoring is indicated in patients with severe hypertension during both general and regional anesthesia. Intravenous nitroprusside, trimethaphan, or nitroglycerin is usually necessary to control blood pressure during general anesthesia. Intravenous labetalol (5–10 mg increments) can also be effective in controlling the hypertensive response to intubation and does not appear to alter placental blood flow. Because magnesium potentiates muscle relaxants, doses of nondepolarizing muscle relaxants should be reduced in patients receiving magnesium therapy and guided by a peripheral nerve stimulator.

HEART DISEASE

The marked cardiovascular changes associated with pregnancy, labor, and delivery often cause pregnant patients with heart disease (2% of parturients) to decompensate during this period. Although most patients have rheumatic heart disease, an increasing number of parturients are presenting with congenital heart lesions. Anesthetic management is directed toward employing techniques that minimize the added stresses of labor and delivery. Specific management of the various lesions is discussed elsewhere. Most patients can be divided into one of two groups. Patients in the first group include those with mitral valve disease, aortic insufficiency, or congenital lesions with left-to-right shunting. These patients benefit from regional techniques, particularly continuous epidural anesthesia. The induced sympathectomy reduces both preload and afterload, relieves pulmonary congestion, and in some cases increases forward flow (cardiac output).

Patients in the second group include those with aortic stenosis, congenital lesions with right-to-left or bidirectional shunting, or primary pulmonary hypertension. Regional anesthesia is generally detrimental in this group. Reductions in venous return (preload) or afterload are usually poorly tolerated. These patients are better managed with intraspinal opioids alone, systemic medications, pudendal nerve blocks, and, if necessary, general anesthesia.

AMNIOTIC FLUID EMBOLISM

Amniotic fluid embolism is a rare (1:20,000 deliveries) but potentially lethal complication (86% mortality rate in some series) that can occur during labor, delivery, cesarean section, or postpartum. The mortality exceeds 50% in the first hour. Entry of amniotic fluid into the maternal circulation can occur through any break in the uteroplacental membranes. Such breaks may occur during normal delivery or cesarean section or following placental abruption, placenta previa, or uterine rupture. In addition to desquamated fetal debris, amniotic fluid contains various prostaglandin and leukotrienes, which appear to play an important role in the genesis of this syndrome. The alternate term "anaphylactoid syndrome of pregnancy" has been suggested to emphasize the role of chemical mediators in this syndrome.

Patients typically present with sudden tachypnea, cyanosis, shock, and generalized bleeding. Three major pathophysiological manifestations are responsible: (1) acute pulmonary embolism, (2) DIC, and (3) uterine atony. Seizures and pulmonary edema may develop; the latter has both cardiogenic and noncardiogenic components. Acute left ventricular dysfunction appears to be a common feature. Although the diagnosis can be firmly established only by demonstrating fetal elements in the maternal circulation (usually at autopsy or less commonly by aspirating amniotic fluid from a central venous catheter), amniotic fluid embolism should always be suggested by sudden respiratory distress and circulatory collapse. The presentation may initially mimic acute pulmonary thromboembolism, venous air embolism, overwhelming septicemia, or hepatic rupture or cerebral hemorrhage in a patient with toxemia.

Treatment consists of aggressive cardiopulmonary resuscitation, stabilization, and supportive care. When cardiac arrest occurs prior to delivery of the fetus, the efficacy of closed-chest compressions appears to be marginal at best. Aortocaval compression impairs resuscitation in the supine position, whereas chest compressions are less effective in a lateral tilt position. Moreover, expeditious delivery appears to improve maternal and fetal outcome; immediate (cesarean) delivery should therefore be carried out. Once the patient is resuscitated, stabilization with mechanical ventilation, fluids, and inotropes is best carried out with full invasive hemodynamic monitoring. Uterine atony is treated with oxytocin, methylergonovine, and prostaglandin $F_{2\alpha}$, whereas significant coagulopathies are treated with platelets and coagulation factors based on laboratory findings.

POSTPARTUM HEMORRHAGE

Postpartum hemorrhage is usually considered present when the postpartum blood loss exceeds 500 mL. Up to 4% of parturients may experience postpartum hemorrhage, which is often associated with a prolonged third stage of labor, preeclampsia, multiple gestations, forceps delivery, and mediolateral episiotomy. Common causes include uterine atony, a retained placenta, obstetric lacerations, uterine inversion, and use of tocolytic agents prior to delivery. Atony is often associated with uterine overdistention (multiple gestation and polyhydramnios). Less commonly, a clotting defect may be responsible.

The anesthesiologist may be consulted to assist in venous access or fluid (and blood) resuscitation, as well as to provide anesthesia for careful examination of the vagina, cervix, and uterus. Perineal lacerations can usually be repaired with local infiltration of anesthetic or pudendal nerve blocks. Residual anesthesia from prior institution of epidural or spinal anesthesia facilitates examination of the patient; however, supplementation with an opioid, nitrous oxide, or both may be required. Induction of spinal or epidural anesthesia in the presence of hypovolemia is contraindicated. **General anesthesia is usually required for bimanual massage of the uterus, manual extraction of a retained placenta, reversion of an inverted uterus, or repair of a major laceration.** Uterine atony should be treated with oxytocin (20–30 U/L of intravenous fluid), methylergonovine (0.2 mg intramuscularly), and carboprost (0.25 mg intramuscularly). Emergency laparotomy and hysterectomy may be necessary in rare instances. Early ligation of the internal iliac (hypogastric) arteries may help avoid hysterectomy or reduce blood loss.

■ FETAL & NEONATAL RESUSCITATION

FETAL RESUSCITATION

Resuscitation of the neonate starts during labor. Any compromise of the uteroplacental circulation readily produces fetal asphyxia. Intrauterine asphyxia during labor is the most common cause of neonatal depression. Fetal monitoring throughout labor is helpful in identifying which babies may be at risk, detecting fetal distress, and evaluating the effect of acute interventions. These include correcting hypotension with fluids or vasopressors, supplemental oxygen, and decreasing uterine contraction (stopping oxytocin or administering tocolytics). Some studies suggest that the normal fetus can compensate for up to 45 min of fetal hypoxia, a period termed "fetal stress"; the latter is associated with a marked redistribution of blood flow primarily to the heart, brain, and adrenal glands. With

time, however, progressive lactic acidosis and asphyxia produce increasing fetal distress that necessitates immediate delivery.

1. Fetal Heart Rate Monitoring

Monitoring of fetal heart rate (FHR) is presently the most useful technique in assessing fetal well being. Alone it has a 35–50% false-positive rate of predicting fetal compromise. Because of this, the term "fetal distress" in the context of FHR monitoring has been largely replaced with "nonreassuring" FHR. Correct interpretation of heart rate patterns is crucial. Three parameters are evaluated: baseline heart rate, baseline variability, and the relationship to uterine contractions (deceleration patterns). Monitoring of heart rate is most accurate when fetal scalp electrodes are used, but this may require rupture of the membranes and is not without complications (ie, amnionitis or fetal injury).

Baseline Heart Rate

The mature fetus normally has a baseline heart rate of 110–160 beats/min. An increased baseline heart rate may be due to prematurity, mild fetal hypoxia, chorioamnionitis, maternal fever, maternally administered drugs (anticholinergics or β-agonists), or, rarely, hyperthyroidism. A decreased baseline heart rate may be due to a postterm pregnancy, fetal heart block, or fetal asphyxia.

Baseline Variability

The healthy mature fetus normally displays a baseline beat-to-beat (R wave to R wave) variability that can be classified as minimal (< 5 beats/min), moderate (6–25 beats/min), or marked (> 25 beats/min). Baseline variability, which is best assessed with scalp electrodes, has become an important sign of fetal well-being and represents a normally functioning autonomic system. **Sustained decreased baseline variability is a prominent sign of fetal asphyxia.** Central nervous system depressants (opioids, barbiturates, benzodiazepines, or magnesium sulfate) and parasympatholytics (atropine) also decrease baseline variability, as do prematurity, fetal dysrhythmias, and anencephaly. A sinusoidal pattern that resembles a smooth sine wave is associated with fetal depression (hypoxia, drugs, and anemia secondary to Rh isoimmunization).

Accelerations

Accelerations of FHR are defined as increases of 15 beats/min or more lasting for more than 15 s. Periodic accelerations in FHR reflect normal oxygenation and are usually related to fetal movements and responses to

Figure 43–5. Periodic changes in fetal heart rate related to uterine contraction. **A:** Early (type I) decelerations. **B:** Late (type II) decelerations. **C:** Variable (type III) decelerations. (Modified and reproduced, with permission, from Danforth DN, Scott JR: *Obstetrics and Gynecology,* 5th ed. Lippincott, 1986.)

uterine pressure. Such accelerations are generally considered reassuring. By 32 weeks, fetuses display periodic increases in baseline heart rate that are associated with fetal movements. Normal fetuses have 15–40 accelerations/h. The mechanism is thought to be increases in catecholamine secretion with decreases in vagal tone. Accelerations diminish with fetal sleep, some drugs (opioids, magnesium, and atropine), as well as fetal hypoxia. Accelerations to fetal scalp or vibroacoustic stimulation are considered a reassuring sign of fetal well-being. **The absence of both baseline variability and accelerations is "nonreassuring" and may be important signs of fetal compromise.**

Deceleration Patterns

A. EARLY (TYPE I) DECELERATIONS

Early deceleration (usually 10–40 beats/min) (Figure 43–5A) is thought to be a vagal response to compression of the fetal head or stretching of the neck during uterine contractions. The heart rate forms a smooth mirror image of the contraction. Early decelerations are generally not associated with fetal distress and occur during descent of the head.

B. LATE (TYPE II) DECELERATIONS

Late decelerations (Figure 43–5B) are associated with fetal compromise and are characterized by a decrease in heart rate at or following the peak of uterine contractions. Late decelerations may be as few as 5 beats/min and are thought to be due to the effect of a decrease in arterial oxygen tension on chemoreceptors or the sinoatrial node. Late decelerations with normal variability may be observed following acute insults (maternal hypotension or hypoxemia) and are usually reversible with treatment. Late decelerations with decreased variability are associated with prolonged asphyxia and may be an indication for fetal scalp sampling (see the section below on Other Monitoring). Complete abolition of variability in this setting is an ominous sign signifying severe decompensation and the need for immediate delivery.

C. VARIABLE (TYPE III) DECELERATIONS

The most common type of decelerations are of the variable type (Figure 43–5C). These decelerations are variable in onset, duration, and magnitude (often > 30 beats/min). They are typically abrupt in onset and are thought to be related to umbilical cord compression and acute intermittent decreases in umbilical blood flow. Variable decelerations are typically associated with fetal asphyxia when they are greater than 60 beats/min, last more than 60 s, or occur in a pattern that persists for more than 30 min.

2. Other Monitoring

Other less commonly used monitors include fetal scalp pH measurements, scalp lactate concentration, fetal pulse oximetry, and fetal ST-segment analysis. Experience is limited with all except fetal scalp pH measurements. Unfortunately the latter is associated with a small but significant incidence of false negatives and false positives. Fetal blood can be obtained and analyzed via a small scalp puncture once the membranes are ruptured. **A fetal scalp pH higher than 7.20 is usually associated with a vigorous neonate, whereas a pH less than 7.20 is often but not always associated with a depressed neonate.** Because of wide overlap, fetal blood sampling can be interpreted correctly only in conjunction with heart rate monitoring.

3. Treatment of the Fetus

Aggressive treatment of intrauterine fetal asphyxia is necessary to prevent fetal demise or permanent neurological damage. All interventions are directed at restoring an adequate uteroplacental circulation. Aortocaval compression, maternal hypoxemia or hypotension, or excessive uterine activity (during oxytocin infusions) must be corrected. Changes in maternal position, supplemental oxygen, and intravenous ephedrine or fluid, or adjustments in an oxytocin infusion often correct the problem. Failure to relieve fetal stress as well as progressive acidosis and asphyxia necessitate immediate delivery.

NEONATAL RESUSCITATION

1. General Care of the Neonate

One person whose sole responsibility is to care for the neonate and is capable of providing resuscitation should attend every delivery. As the head is delivered, the nose, mouth, and pharynx are suctioned with a bulb syringe. After the remainder of the body is delivered, the skin is dried with a sterile towel. Once the umbilical cord stops pulsating or breathing is initiated, the cord is then clamped and the neonate is placed in a radiant warmer with the bed tilted in a slight Trendelenburg position.

Evaluation and treatment are carried out simultaneously (Figure 43–6). If the neonate is obviously depressed, the cord is clamped early and resuscitation is initiated immediately. Breathing normally begins within 30 s and is sustained within 90 s. Respirations should be 30–60 breaths/min and the heart rate 120–160 beats/min. Respirations are assessed by auscultation of the chest, whereas heart rate is determined by palpation of the pulse at the base of the umbilical cord or auscultation of the precordium. It is critically important to keep the neonate warm.

In addition to respirations and heart rate, color, tone, and reflex irritability should be evaluated. The Apgar score (Table 43–7), recorded at 1 min and again at 5 min after delivery, remains the most valuable assessment of the neonate. The 1-min score correlates with survival, whereas the 5-min score is related to neurological outcome.

Neonates with Apgar scores of 8–10 are vigorous and may require only gentle stimulation (flicking the foot, rubbing the back, and additional drying). A catheter should first be gently passed through each nostril to rule out choanal atresia, and then through the mouth to suction the stomach and rule out esophageal atresia.

2. Meconium-Stained Neonates

The presence or absence of meconium in the amniotic fluid (about 10–12% of deliveries) dictates the immediate management of the neonate at birth. Fetal distress, particularly after 42 weeks of gestation, is often associated with release of thick meconium into the fluid. Fetal gasping during stress results in entry of a large amount of

Figure 43–6. An algorithm for resuscitation of the newly born infant. (Reproduced, with permission, from the American Heart Association.)

meconium-tainted amniotic fluid into the lungs. When the neonate initiates respiration at birth, the meconium moves from the trachea and large airways down toward the periphery of the lung. Thick or particulate meconium obstructs small airways and causes severe respiratory distress in 15% of meconium-stained neonates. Moreover, these infants can develop persistent fetal circulation (see Chapter 42). Amnioinfusion prior to delivery can reduce the severity of meconium aspiration syndrome.

Unless the neonate has absent or depressed respirations, thin watery meconium does not require suctioning beyond careful bulb suctioning of the oropharynx when the head emerges from the perineum (or from the uterus at cesarean section). When thick (pea soup) meconium is present in the amniotic fluid, however, some clinicians intubate and suction the trachea immediately after delivery but before the first breath is taken. If the baby is not vigorous, tracheal suctioning is recommended when meconium is present. Tracheal suctioning of the thick meconium is accomplished by a special suctioning device attached to the endotracheal tube as the tube is withdrawn. If meconium is aspirated

from the trachea, the procedure should be repeated until no meconium is obtained—but no more than

Table 43–7. Apgar score.

Sign	Points		
	0	1	2
Heart rate (beats/min)	Absent	< 100	> 100
Respiratory effort	Absent	Slow, irregular	Good, crying
Muscle tone	Flaccid	Some flexion	Active motion
Reflex irritability	No response	Grimace	Crying
Color	Blue or pale	Body pink, extremities blue	All pink

three times, after which it is usually of no further benefit. The infant should then be given supplemental oxygen by face mask and observed closely. The stomach should also be suctioned to prevent passive regurgitation of any meconium. Newborns with meconium aspiration have an increased incidence of pneumothorax (10% compared with 1% for all vaginal deliveries).

3. Care of the Depressed Neonate

Approximately 6% of newborns, most of whom weigh less than 1500 g, require some form of advanced life support. Resuscitation of the depressed neonate requires two or more persons—one to manage the airway and ventilation and another to perform chest compressions, if necessary. A third person greatly facilitates the placement of intravascular catheters and the administration of fluids or drugs. The anesthesiologist caring for the mother can render only brief assistance and only when it does not jeopardize the mother; other personnel are, therefore, generally responsible for neonatal resuscitation.

Because the most common cause of neonatal depression is intrauterine asphyxia, the emphasis in resuscitation is on respiration. Hypovolemia is also a contributing factor in a significant number of neonates. Factors associated with hypovolemia include early clamping of the umbilical cord, holding the neonate above the introitus prior to clamping, prematurity, maternal hemorrhage, placental transection during cesarean section, sepsis, and twin-to-twin transfusion.

Failure of the neonate to quickly respond to respiratory resuscitative efforts mandates vascular access and blood gas analysis; pneumothorax (1% incidence) and congenital anomalies of the airway, including tracheoesophageal fistula (1:3000–5000 live births), and congenital diaphragmatic hernia (1:2000–4000) should also be considered.

Grouping by the 1-min Apgar score greatly facilitates resuscitation: (1) mildly asphyxiated neonates (Apgar score of 5–7) usually need only stimulation while 100% oxygen is blown across the face; (2) moderately asphyxiated neonates (Apgar score of 3–4) require temporary assisted positive-pressure ventilation with mask and bag; and (3) severely depressed neonates (Apgar score of 0–2) should be immediately intubated, and chest compressions may be required.

Guidelines for Ventilation

Indications for positive-pressure ventilation include (1) apnea, (2) gasping respirations, (3) persistent central cyanosis with 100% oxygen, and (4) heart rate less than 100 beats/min. Excessive flexion or extension of the neck can cause airway obstruction. A 1-in.-high towel under the shoulders may be helpful in maintaining

Figure 43–7. Intubation of the neonate. The head is placed in a neutral position, and the laryngoscope handle is held with the thumb and index finger as the chin is supported with the remaining fingers. Pressure applied over the hyoid bone with the little finger will bring the larynx into view. A straight blade such as a Miller 0 or 1 usually provides the best view.

proper head position. Assisted ventilation by bag and mask should be at a rate of 30–60 breaths/min with 100% oxygen. Initial breaths may require peak pressures of up to 40 cm H_2O, but pressures should not exceed 30 cm H_2O subsequently. Adequacy of ventilation should be checked by auscultation and chest excursions. Gastric decompression with an 8F tube often facilitates ventilation. If after 30 s the heart rate is over 100 beats/min and spontaneous ventilations become adequate, assisted ventilation is no longer necessary. If the heart rate is less than 60 beats/min or is 60–80 beats/min and not rising, the neonate is intubated and chest compressions are started. If the heart rate is 60–80 beats/min and rising, assisted ventilation is continued and the neonate is observed. Failure of the heart rate to rise above 80 beats/min is an indication for chest compressions. Indications for endotracheal intubation include ineffective ventilation, prolonged mask ventilation, and the need to administer medications.

Intubation (Figure 43–7) is performed with a Miller 00, 0, or 1 laryngoscope blade, using a 2.5-, 3-, or 3.5-mm endotracheal tube (for neonates < 1 kg, 1–2 kg, and > 2 kg, respectively). Correct endotracheal tube size is indicated by a small leak with 20 cm H_2O pressure. Right endobronchial intubation should be excluded by chest auscultation. The correct depth of the endotracheal tube ("tip to lip") is usually 6 cm plus the weight in kilograms. Oxygen saturation can

Figure 43–8. Chest compressions in the neonate. The neonate is held with both hands as each thumb is placed just beneath a line connecting the nipples and the remaining fingers encircle the chest. The sternum is compressed $^{1}/_{3}$ to $^{3}/_{4}$ in. (1 cm) at a rate of 120/min. (Reproduced, with permission, from the American Heart Association.)

usually be measured by a pulse oximeter probe applied to the palm. Capnography is also very useful in confirming endotracheal intubation. Transcutaneous oxygen sensors are useful for measuring tissue oxygenation but unfortunately require time for initial equilibration. Use of a laryngeal mask airway (LMA#1) has been reported in neonates > 2.5 kg and may be useful if endotracheal intubation is difficult (eg, Pierre Robin syndrome).

Guidelines for Chest Compressions

Indications for chest compressions are a heart rate that is less than 60 beats/min or 60–80 beats/min and not rising after 30 s of adequate ventilation with 100% oxygen.

Cardiac compressions should be provided at a rate of 120/min. The two thumb-encircling hands (Figure 43–8) technique is generally preferred because it appears to generate higher peak systolic and coronary perfusion pressures. Alternatively, the two-finger technique can be used (Figure 43–9). The depth of compressions should be approximately one-third of the anterior–posterior diameter of the chest and enough to generate a palpable pulse.

Compressions should be interposed with ventilation in a 3:1 ratio, such that 90 compressions and 30 ventilations are given per minute. The heart rate should be checked periodically. Chest compressions should be stopped when the spontaneous heart rate exceeds 80 beats/min.

Vascular Access

Cannulation of the umbilical vein with a 3.5F or 5F umbilical catheter is easiest and the preferred technique. The tip of the catheter should be just below skin level and allow free backflow of blood; further advancement may result in infusion of hypertonic solutions directly into the liver. A peripheral vein or even the endotracheal tube can be used as an alternate route for drug administration.

Figure 43–9. The alternative technique for neonatal chest compressions: two fingers are placed on the lower third of the sternum at right angles to the chest. The chest is compressed approximately 1 cm at a rate of 120/min.

Cannulation of one of the two umbilical arteries allows measurement of blood pressure and facilitates blood gas measurements but may be more difficult. Specially designed umbilical artery catheters allow continuous PaO_2 or oxygen saturation monitoring as well as blood pressure. Care must be taken not to introduce any air into either the artery or the vein.

Volume Resuscitation

Some neonates at term and nearly two-thirds of premature infants requiring resuscitation are hypovolemic at birth. Diagnosis is based on physical examination (low blood pressure and pallor) and a poor response to resuscitation. Neonatal blood pressure generally correlates with intravascular volume, and should therefore routinely be measured. Normal blood pressure depends on birth weight and varies from 50/25 mm Hg for neonates weighing 1–2 kg to 70/40 mm Hg for those weighing over 3 kg. A low blood pressure suggests hypovolemia. Volume expansion may be accomplished with 10 mL/kg of either lactated Ringer's injection, normal saline, or type O-negative blood cross-matched with maternal blood. Less common causes of hypotension include hypocalcemia, hypermagnesemia, and hypoglycemia.

Drug Therapy

A. EPINEPHRINE

Epinephrine, 0.01–0.03 mg/kg (0.1–0.3 mL/kg of a 1:10,000 solution), should be given for asystole or a spontaneous heart rate of less than 60 beats/min in spite of adequate ventilation and chest compressions. It may be repeated every 3–5 min. Epinephrine may be given in 1 mL of saline down the endotracheal tube if venous access is not available.

B. NALOXONE

Naloxone, 0.1 mg/kg intravenously or 0.2 mg/kg intramuscularly, is given to reverse the respiratory depressant effect of opioids given to the mother in the last 4 h of labor. Withdrawal symptoms may be precipitated in babies of opioid addicts.

C. OTHER DRUGS

Other drugs may be indicated only in specific settings. Sodium bicarbonate (2 mEq/kg of a 0.5 mEq/mL 4.2% solution) should generally be given only for a severe metabolic acidosis documented by blood gas measurements and when ventilation is adequate. It may also be administered during prolonged resuscitation (> 5 min)—particularly if blood gas measurements are not readily available. The infusion rate should not exceed 1 mEq/kg/min to avoid hypertonicity and intracranial hemorrhage. Moreover, to prevent hypertonicity-induced

hepatic injury, the catheter tip should not be in the liver. Calcium gluconate 100 mg/kg ($CaCl_2$, 30 mg/kg) should be given only to neonates with documented hypocalcemia or those with suspected magnesium intoxication (from maternal magnesium therapy); these neonates are usually hypotensive, hypotonic, and appear vasodilated. Glucose (8 mg/kg/min of a 10% solution) is given only for documented hypoglycemia because hyperglycemia worsens hypoxic neurological deficits. Blood glucose should be measured because up to 10% of neonates may have hypoglycemia (glucose < 35 mg/dL), particularly those delivered by cesarean section. Dopamine may be started at 5 µg/kg/min to support arterial blood pressure. Lastly, surfactant may be given through the endotracheal tube to premature neonates with respiratory distress syndrome.

CASE DISCUSSION: APPENDICITIS IN A PREGNANT WOMAN

A 31-year-old woman with a 24-week gestation presents for an appendectomy.

How does pregnancy complicate the management of this patient?

Nearly 1–2% of pregnant patients require surgery during their pregnancy. The most common procedure during the first trimester is laparoscopy; appendectomy (1:1500 pregnancies) and cholecystectomy (1:2000–10,000 pregnancies) are the most commonly performed open abdominal procedures. Cervical cerclage may be necessary in some patients for cervical incompetence. The physiological effects of pregnancy can alter the manifestations of the disease process and make diagnosis difficult. Patients may therefore present with advanced or complicated disease. The physiological changes associated with pregnancy (see Chapter 42) further predispose the patient to increased morbidity and mortality. Moreover, both the surgery and the anesthesia can adversely affect the fetus.

What are the potentially detrimental effects of surgery and anesthesia on the fetus?

The procedure can have both immediate and long-term undesirable effects on the fetus. Hypotension, hypovolemia, severe anemia, hypoxemia, and marked increases in sympathetic tone can seriously compromise the transfer of oxygen and other nutrients across the uteroplacental circu-

lation and promote intrauterine fetal asphyxia. The stress of the procedure and the underlying process may also precipitate preterm labor, which often follows intraabdominal surgery near the uterus. Laparoscopy may be safely performed but the CO_2 insufflation has the potential to cause fetal respiratory acidosis. Mild to moderate maternal hyperventilation and limiting both insufflation pressure and duration of the procedure limit the degree of acidosis. Long-term detrimental effects relate to possible teratogenic effects on the developing fetus.

When is the fetus most sensitive to teratogenic influences?

Three stages of susceptibility are generally recognized. In the first 2 weeks of intrauterine life, teratogens have either a lethal effect or no effect on the embryo. The third to eighth weeks are the most critical period, when organogenesis takes place; drug exposure during this period can produce major developmental abnormalities. From the eighth week onward, organogenesis is complete, and organ growth takes place. Teratogen exposure during this last period usually results in only minor morphological abnormalities but can produce significant physiological abnormalities and growth retardation. Although the teratogenic influences of anesthetic agents have been extensively studied in animals, retrospective human studies have been inconclusive. Past concerns about possible teratogenic effects of nitrous oxide and benzodiazepines do not appear to be justified. Nonetheless, as with all drugs, exposure to anesthetic agents should be kept to a minimum in terms of the number of agents, dosage, and duration of exposure.

What would be the ideal anesthetic technique in this patient?

Toward the end of the second trimester (after 20–24 weeks gestation), most of the physiological changes associated with pregnancy have taken place. Regional anesthesia is preferable to general anesthesia to decrease the risks of pulmonary aspiration and failed intubation and to minimize drug exposure to the fetus. The patient should be transported and maintained with left lateral uterine displacement when supine. Drug exposure is least (probably negligible) with spinal anesthesia. Moreover, spinal anesthesia may be preferable to epidural anesthesia because it is not associated with unintentional intravascular injections or potentially large intrathecal doses of local anesthetic. On the other hand, general anesthesia guarantees patient comfort and, when a volatile agent is used, may even suppress preterm labor (see Chapter 42). Nitrous oxide without concomitant administration of a halogenated anesthetic is reported to reduce uterine blood flow.

Although regional anesthesia is preferable in most instances, the choice between regional and general anesthesia must be individualized according to the patient, the anesthesiologist, and the type of surgery. Spinal anesthesia is usually satisfactory for appendectomies, whereas general anesthesia is more satisfactory for cholecystectomies. The same techniques and doses used for the parturient should be followed.

Are any special monitors indicated perioperatively?

In addition to standard monitors, fetal heart rate and uterine activity should be monitored with a Doppler and tocodynamometer during induction of anesthesia, emergence, and recovery, and, whenever possible, during surgery in a woman who is 24 weeks or more pregnant. When regular organized uterine activity is detected, early treatment with a β-adrenergic agonist such as ritodrine usually aborts the preterm labor. Magnesium sulfate and oral or rectal indomethacin may also be used as tocolytics.

When should elective operations be performed during pregnancy?

All elective operations should be postponed until 6 weeks after delivery. Only emergency procedures that pose an immediate threat to the mother or fetus should be routinely performed. The timing of semielective procedures, such as those for cancer, valvular heart disease, or intracranial aneurysms, must be individualized and must balance the threat to maternal health versus fetal well-being. Controlled (deliberate) hypotensive anesthesia may be necessary to reduce blood loss during extensive cancer operations; nitroprusside, nitroglycerin, and hydralazine have been used during pregnancy without apparent fetal compromise. Nonetheless, large doses and prolonged infusions of nitroprusside should be avoided because the immature liver of the fetus may have a limited ability to metabolize the cyanide breakdown product. Cardiopulmonary bypass has been employed in pregnant patients successfully without adverse fetal outcome, but should probably be carried out only with continuous fetal echocardiography. Circulatory arrest during pregnancy is not recommended.

SUGGESTED READING

American Heart Association: Neonatal resuscitation. Circulation 2000;102(8)Supplement:I-343.

Birnbach DJ, Datta S, Gatt SP: *Textbook of Obstetric Anesthesia.* Churchill Livingstone, 2000.

Chang J, Elam-Evans LD, Berg CJ, et al: Pregnancy-related mortality surveillance—United States, 1991–1999. MMWR 2003;52:1.

Chestnut DH: *Obstetric Anesthesia,* 3rd ed. Mosby, 2004.

Comparative Obstetric Mobile Epidural Trial Study Group UK: Randomized controlled trial comparing traditional with two "mobile" epidural techniques. Anesthesiology 2002;97:1567.

Cooper DW, Carpenter M, Mowbray P, et al: Fetal and maternal effects of phenylephrine and ephedrine during spinal anesthesia for cesarean delivery. Anesthesiology 202;97:1582.

Crochetiere C: Obstetric emergencies. Anesth Clin North Am 2003;21:111.

Dahl JB, Jeppesen IS, Jørgensen H, et al: Intraoperative and postoperative analgesic efficacy and adverse effects of intrathecal opioids in patients undergoing cesarean section with spinal anesthesia: a qualitative and quantitative systematic review of randomized controlled trials. Anesthesiology 1999;91:1919.

Datta S: *The Obstetric Anesthesia Handbook,* 3rd ed. Mosby, 2000.

Eisenach JC: Combined spinal-epidural analgesia in obstetrics. Anesthesiology 1999;91:299.

Eltzschig HK, Lieberman ES, Camann WR: Regional anesthesia and analgesia for labor and delivery. N Engl J Med 2003;348:319.

Gambling DR, Douglas MJ: *Obstetric Anesthesia and Uncommon Disorders.* W.B. Saunders, 1998.

Gei AF, Vadhera RB, Hankins GDV: Embolism during pregnancy: thrombus, air, and amniotic fluid. Anesth Clin North Am 2003;21:165.

Halpern SH, Walsh V: Epidural ropivacaine versus bupivacaine for labor: a meta-analysis. Anesth Analg 2003;96:1473.

Hawkins JL, Koonin LM, Palmer SK, Gibbs CP: Anesthesia-related deaths during obstetric delivery in the United States, 1979–1990. Anesthesiology 1997;86:277.

Hawthorne L, Wilson R, Lyons G, Dresser M: Failed intubation revisited: 17 year experience in a teaching maternal unit. Br J Anaesth 1996;76:680.

Holdcroft TT: *Principles and Practice of Obstetric Anaesthesia.* Blackwell, 2000.

Hughes SC, Levinson G, Rosen MA: *Shnider and Levinson's Anesthesia for Obstetrics,* 4th ed. Lippincott, Williams & Wilkins, 2002.

Koren G: Drugs in pregnancy. N Engl J Med 1998;338:1128.

Lapinsky SE, Kruczynski K, Seaward GR, et al: Critical care management of the obstetric patient. Can J Anaesth 1997;44:325.

Lee A, Ngan Kee WD, Gin T: A quantitative systematic review of randomized controlled trials of ephedrine versus phenylephrine for the management of hypotension during spinal anesthesia for cesarean delivery. Anesth Analg 2002;94:920.

Macario A, Scibettaa WC, Navarro J, Riley E: Analgesia for labor pain. A cost model. Anesthesiology 2000;92:841.

Norris MC: *Handbook of Obstetric Anesthesia.* Lippincott, Williams & Wilkins, 2000.

Paech M: Newer techniques of labor analgesia. Anesth Clin North Am 2003;21:1. Practice guidelines for obstetric anesthesia. A report by the American Society of Anesthesiologists Task Force on Obstetrical Anesthesia. Anesthesiology 1999;90:600.

Ramanathan J, Bennett K: Pre-eclampsia: fluids, drugs, and anesthetic management. Anesth Clin North Am 2003;21:145.

Rawal N, Van Zundert A, Holmstrom B, Crowhurst JA: Combined spinal-epidural technique. Regional Anesth 1997;22:406.

Rosen MA: Management of anesthesia for the pregnant surgical patient. Anesthesiology 1999;91:1159.

Ross BK: ASA closed claims in obstetrics: lessons learned. Anesth Clin North Am 2003;21:183.

Santos AC, Birnbach DJ: Spinal anesthesia in the parturient with severe preeclampsia: time for reconsideration. Anesth Analg 2003;97:621.

Segal S: Epidural analgesia and the progress and outcome of labor and delivery. Int Anesthesiol Clin 2002;40:13.

Sharma Sk, Alexander JM, Messick G, et al: Cesarean delivery. A randomized trial of epidural analgesia versus intravenous meperidine analgesia during labor in nulliparous women. Anesthesiology 2002;96:946.

Thomas TA, Cooper GM: Maternal deaths from anaesthesia. An extract from *Why Mothers Die 1997–1999,* the confidential enquiries into maternal deaths in the United Kingdom. Br J Anaesth 2002;89:499.

Walker JJ: Pre-eclampsia. Lancet 2000;356:1260.

Watersone M, Bewley, Wolfe C: Incidence and predictors of severe obstetric morbidity: case-control study. BMJ 2001;322:1089.

Williams KP, Galerneau F: Intrapartum fetal heart rate patterns in the prediction of neonatal acidemia. Am J Obstet Gynecol 2003;188:820.

Zhang J, Yancey MK, Klebanoff MA, et al: Does epidural analgesia prolong labor and increase risk of cesarean delivery? A natural experiment. Am J Obstet Gynecol 2001;185:128.

Pediatric Anesthesia

44

KEY CONCEPTS

 The small and limited number of alveoli in neonates and infants reduces lung compliance; in contrast, their cartilaginous rib cage makes their chest wall very compliant. The combination of these two characteristics promotes chest wall collapse during inspiration and relatively low residual lung volumes at expiration. The resulting decrease in functional residual capacity (FRC) is important because it limits oxygen reserves during periods of apnea (eg, intubation) and readily predisposes them to atelectasis and hypoxemia.

 Neonates and infants have a proportionately larger head and tongue, narrow nasal passages, an anterior and cephalad larynx, a long epiglottis, and a short trachea and neck. These anatomic features make neonates and most young infants obligate nasal breathers until about 5 months of age. The cricoid cartilage is the narrowest point of the airway in children younger than 5 years of age.

 Stroke volume is relatively fixed by a noncompliant and poorly developed left ventricle in neonates and infants. The cardiac output is therefore very dependent on heart rate.

 Thin skin, low fat content, and a higher surface relative to weight allow greater heat loss to the environment in neonates. This problem is compounded by cold operating rooms, wound exposure, intravenous fluid administration, dry anesthetic gases, and the direct effect of anesthetic agents on temperature regulation. Hypothermia has been associated with delayed awakening from anesthesia, cardiac irritability, respiratory depression, increased pulmonary vascular resistance, and altered drug responses.

 Neonates, infants, and young children have relatively higher alveolar ventilation and lower FRC compared with older children and adults. This higher minute ventilation-to-FRC ratio with relatively higher blood flow to vessel-rich organs contributes to a rapid rise in alveolar anesthetic concentration and speeds inhalation induction.

 Minimum alveolar concentration (MAC) is higher in infants than in neonates and adults for halogenated agents. Unlike other agents, sevoflurane has the same MAC in neonates and infants. Sevoflurane appears to have a greater therapeutic index than halothane and has become a preferred induction agent in pediatric anesthesia.

 Children are more susceptible than adults to cardiac arrhythmias, hyperkalemia, rhabdomyolysis, myoglobinemia, masseter spasm, and malignant hyperthermia (MH) after administration of succinylcholine. If a child unexpectedly experiences cardiac arrest following administration of succinylcholine, immediate treatment for hyperkalemia should be instituted.

(continued on next page)

(continued from previous page)

 Unlike in adult patients, profound bradycardia and sinus node arrest can develop in pediatric patients following the first dose of succinylcholine without atropine pretreatment.

 A viral infection within 2–4 weeks before general anesthesia and endotracheal intubation appears to place the child at an increased risk for perioperative pulmonary complications, such as wheezing, laryngospasm, hypoxemia, and atelectasis.

 Temperature must be closely monitored in pediatric patients because of their higher risk for MH and the potential for both iatrogenic hypothermia and hyperthermia.

Meticulous fluid management is required in small pediatric patients because of extremely limited

margins of error. A programmable infusion pump or a buret with a microdrip chamber should be used for accurate measurements. Drugs are flushed through low dead-space tubing to minimize unnecessary fluid administration.

 Laryngospasm can usually be avoided by extubating the patient either awake or while deeply anesthetized; both techniques have advocates. Extubation during the interval between these extremes, however, is generally recognized as hazardous.

 Patients with scoliosis due to muscular dystrophy are predisposed to MH, cardiac dysrhythmias, and untoward effects of succinylcholine (hyperkalemia, myoglobinuria, and sustained muscular contractures).

Pediatric patients are not small adults. Neonates (0–1 months), infants (1–12 months), toddlers (1–3 years), and small children (4–12 years of age) have differing anesthetic requirements. Safe anesthetic management depends on full appreciation of the physiological, anatomic, and pharmacological characteristics of each group (Table 44–1). These characteristics, which differentiate them from each other and adults, necessitate modification of anesthetic equipment and techniques. Indeed infants are at much greater risk of anesthetic morbidity and mortality than are older children; risk is generally inversely proportional to age, neonates being at highest risk. In addition, pediatric patients are prone to illnesses that require unique surgical and anesthetic strategies.

ANATOMIC & PHYSIOLOGICAL DEVELOPMENT

Respiratory System

The transition from fetal to neonatal physiology is reviewed in Chapter 42. Compared with older children and adults, neonates and infants have less efficient ventilation because of weak intercostal and diaphragmatic musculature (due to a paucity of type I fibers), horizontal and more pliable ribs, and a protuberant abdomen.

Respiratory rate is elevated in neonates and gradually falls to adult levels by adolescence. Tidal volume and dead space per kilogram remain constant during development. A relative paucity of small airways increases airway resistance. Alveolar maturation is not complete until late childhood (about 8 years of age). The work of breathing is increased and respiratory muscles easily fatigue. The small and limited number of alveoli in neonates and infants reduces lung compliance; in contrast, their cartilaginous rib cage makes their chest wall very compliant. The combination of these two characteristics promotes chest wall collapse during inspiration and relatively low residual lung volumes at expiration. The resulting decrease in functional residual capacity (FRC) is important because it limits oxygen reserves during periods of apnea (eg, intubation) and readily predisposes neonates and infants to atelectasis and hypoxemia. This may be exaggerated by their relatively higher rate of oxygen consumption. Moreover, hypoxic and hypercapnic ventilatory drives are not well developed in neonates and infants. In fact, unlike in adults, hypoxia and hypercapnia depress respiration in these patients.

Neonates and infants have a proportionately larger head and tongue, narrow nasal passages, an anterior and cephalad larynx (at a vertebral level of C4 versus C6 in adults), a long epiglottis, and a

Table 44–1. Characteristics of neonates and infants that differentiate them from adult patients.[1]

Physiological
  Heart-rate-dependent cardiac output
  Faster heart rate
  Lower blood pressure
  Faster respiratory rate
  Lower lung compliance
  Greater chest wall compliance
  Lower functional residual capacity
  Higher ratio of body surface area to body weight
  Higher total body water content
Anatomic
  Noncompliant left ventricle
  Residual fetal circulation
  Difficult venous and arterial cannulation
  Large head and tongue
  Narrow nasal passages
  Anterior and cephalad larynx
  Long epiglottis
  Short trachea and neck
  Prominent adenoids and tonsils
  Weak intercostal and diaphragmatic muscles
  High resistance to airflow
Pharmacological
  Immature hepatic biotransformation
  Decreased protein binding
  Rapid rise in F_A/F_I
  Rapid induction and recovery
  Increased minimum alveolar concentration
  Larger volume of distribution for water-soluble drugs
  Immature neuromuscular junction

[1]F_A/F_I, Fractional alveolar concentration/fractional inspired concentration.

short trachea and neck (Figure 44–1). These anatomic features make neonates and most young infants obligate nasal breathers until about 5 months of age. **The cricoid cartilage is the narrowest point of the airway in children younger than 5 years of age; in adults, the narrowest point is the glottis.** One millimeter of edema will have a proportionately greater effect in children because of their smaller tracheal diameters.

Cardiovascular System

Stroke volume is relatively fixed by a noncompliant and poorly developed left ventricle in neonates and infants. The cardiac output is therefore very dependent on heart rate (see Chapter 19). Although basal heart rate is higher than in adults (Table 44–2), activation of the parasympathetic nervous system, anesthetic overdose, or hypoxia can cause bradycardia and profound reductions in cardiac output. Sick infants undergoing emergency or prolonged surgical procedures appear particularly prone to episodes of bradycardia that can lead to hypotension, asystole, and intraoperative death. The sympathetic nervous system and baroreceptor reflexes are not fully mature. The infant cardiovascular system maintains lower catecholamine stores and displays a blunted response to exogenous catecholamines. The immature heart is more sensitive to the calcium channel blocking properties of volatile anesthetics and opioid-induced bradycardia. The vascular tree is less able to respond to hypovolemia with vasoconstriction. The hallmark of intravascular fluid depletion in neonates and infants is therefore hypotension without tachycardia.

Metabolism & Temperature Regulation

Pediatric patients have a larger surface area per kilogram than adults (increased surface area/weight ratio). Metabolism and its associated parameters (oxygen consumption, CO_2 production, cardiac output, and alveolar ventilation) correlate better with surface area than with weight.

Thin skin, low fat content, and a higher surface relative to weight allow greater heat loss to the environment in neonates. This problem is compounded by cold operating rooms, wound exposure, intravenous fluid administration, dry anesthetic gases, and the direct effect of anesthetic agents on temperature regulation. Hypothermia is a serious problem that has been associated with delayed awakening from anesthesia, cardiac irritability, respiratory depression, increased pulmonary vascular resistance, and altered drug responses. The major mechanisms for heat production in neonates are nonshivering thermogenesis by metabolism of brown fat and shunting of hepatic oxidative phosphorylation to the thermogenic proton leak pathway. Metabolism of brown fat is severely limited in premature infants and in sick neonates who are deficient in fat stores. Furthermore, volatile anesthetics inhibit thermogenesis in brown adipocytes.

Renal & Gastrointestinal Function

Normal kidney function is not present until 6 months of age; renal function may not achieve adult levels until the child is 2 years old. Premature neonates often possess multiple renal defects, including decreased creatinine clearance; impaired sodium retention, glucose excretion, and bicarbonate reabsorption; and poor diluting and concentrating ability. These abnormalities increase the importance of meticulous attention to fluid administration in the early days of life.

Neonates also have a relatively high incidence of gastroesophageal reflux. A relatively immature liver causes impaired hepatic conjugation early in life.

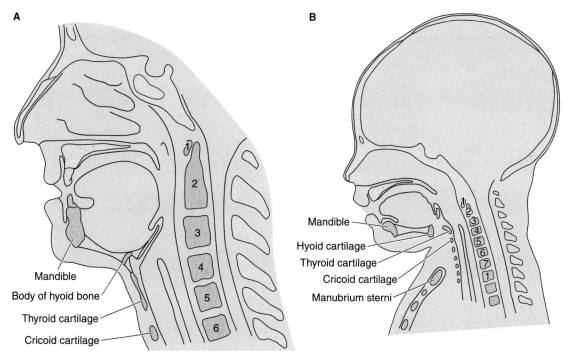

Figure 44–1. Sagittal section of the adult (*A*) and infant (*B*) airway. (Reproduced, with permission, from Snell RS, Katz J: *Clinical Anatomy for Anesthesiologists.* Appleton & Lange, 1988.)

Glucose Homeostasis

Neonates have low glycogen stores that predispose them to hypoglycemia. Impaired glucose excretion by the kidneys may partially offset this tendency. Neonates at greatest risk for hypoglycemia are premature or small for gestational age, have been receiving hyperalimentation, and were born to diabetic mothers.

PHARMACOLOGICAL DIFFERENCES

Pediatric drug dosing is typically based on a per-kilogram recommendation (Table 44–3). A child's weight can be roughly estimated based on age:

$$\text{50th percentile weight (kg)} = (\text{Age} \times 2) + 9$$

Weight, however, does not take into account the disproportionately larger pediatric intravascular and extracellular fluid compartments, the immaturity of hepatic biotransformation pathways, increased organ blood flow, decreased protein binding, or higher metabolic rate. These variables must be considered on an individual basis.

Neonates and infants have a proportionately higher total water content (70–75%) than adults (50–60%). Total body water content decreases as fat and muscle content increase with age. As a direct result, the volume of distribution for most intravenous drugs is disproportionately higher in neonates, infants, and young children, and the dose (per kilogram) is usually higher than in older children and adults. A disproportionately smaller muscle mass in neonates prolongs the clinical termination of action by redistribution to muscle for drugs such as thiopental

Table 44–2. Age-related changes in vital signs.[1]

| | | | Arterial Blood Pressure | |
Age	Respiratory Rate	Heart Rate	Systolic	Diastolic
Neonate	40	140	65	40
12 months	30	120	95	65
3 years	25	100	100	70
12 years	20	80	110	60

[1]Values are mean averages derived from numerous sources. Normal ranges vary by as much as 25–50%.

Table 44–3. Pediatric drug dosages.

Drug	Comment	Dosage
Acetaminophen	Rectal	40 mg/kg
	PO	10–20 mg/kg
	Maximum (per day)	60 mg/kg
Adenosine	Rapid IV bolus	0.1 mg/kg
	Repeat dose	0.2 mg/kg
	Maximum dose	12 mg
Albuterol	Nebulized	1.25–2.5 mg in 2 mL saline
Alfentanil	Anesthetic supplement (IV)	20–25 µg/kg
	Maintenance infusion	1–3 µg/kg/min
Amiodarone	Loading dose (IV)	5 mg/kg
	Repeat dose (slowly)	5 mg/kg
	Infusion	5–10 µg/kg/min
	Maximum dose	20 mg/kg/day
Aminophylline	Loading dose administered over 20 min (IV)	5–6 mg/kg
	Maintenance dose (therapeutic level: 10–20 mg/mL)	0.5–0.9 mg/kg/h
Amoxicillin	PO	50 mg/kg
Ampicillin	IV	50 mg/kg
Ampicillin/sulbactam	IV	25–50 mg/kg
Amrinone	Loading (IV)	0.75–1 mg/kg
	Maintenance	5–10 µg/kg/min
Atropine	IV	0.01–0.02 mg/kg
	IM	0.02 mg/kg
	Minimum dose	0.1 mg
	Premedication (PO)	0.03–0.05 mg/kg
Atracurium	Intubation (IV)	0.5 mg/kg
Bretylium	Loading dose (IV)	5 mg/kg
Caffeine	IV	10 mg/kg
Calcium chloride	IV (slowly)	5–20 mg/kg
Calcium gluconate	IV (slowly)	15–100 mg/kg
Cardioversion	See Table 43–3	0.5–2 J/kg
Cefazolin	IV	25 mg/kg
Cefotaxime	IV	25–50 mg/kg
Cefotetan	IV	20–40 mg/kg
Cefoxitin	IV	30–40 mg/kg
Ceftazidime	IV	30–50 mg/kg
Ceftriaxone	IV	25–50 mg/kg
Cefuroxime	IV	25 mg/kg
Chloral hydrate	PO	25–100 mg/kg
	Rectal	50 mg/kg
Cimetidine	IV or PO	5–10 mg/kg
Cisatracurium	Intubation (IV)	0.15 mg/kg
Clindamycin	IV	20 mg/kg
Dantrolene	Initial dose (IV)	2.5 mg/kg
	Maximum dose	10 mg/kg
Defibrillation	First attempt	2 J/kg
	Subsequent attempts	4 J/kg
Desmopressin	IV	0.2–0.4 µg/kg
Dexamethasone	IV	0.1–0.5 mg/kg
Dextrose	$D_{25}W$ or $D_{50}W$ (IV)	0.5–1 g/kg
Diazepam	Sedation (IV)	0.1–0.2 mg/kg
Digoxin	Three divided doses over 24 h (IV)	15–30 µg/kg
Diltiazem	IV over 2 min	0.25 mg/kg

(continued)

Table 44–3. Pediatric drug dosages. (continued)

Drug	Comment	Dosage
Diphenhydramine	IV, IM, or PO	1 mg/kg
Dobutamine	Infusion	2–20 µg/kg/min
Dolasetron	IV	0.35 mg/kg
Dopamine	Infusion	2–20 µg/kg/min
Droperidol	IV	50–75 µg/kg
Edrophonium	Depends on degree of paralysis (IV)	0.5–1 mg/kg
Ephedrine	IV	0.1–0.3 mg/kg
Epinephrine	IV bolus	0.01 mg/kg
	Endotracheal dose	0.1 mg/kg
	Infusion	0.1–1.0 µg/kg/min
Epinephrine, 2.25% racemic	Nebulized	0.05 mL/kg in 3 mL saline
Esmolol (bolus)	IV	0.1–0.5 mg/kg
Esmolol (infusion)	IV	25–200 µg/kg/min
Famotidine	IV	0.15 mg/kg
Fentanyl	Pain relief (IV)	1–2 µg/kg
	Pain relief (Intranasal)	2 µg/kg
	Premedication (Actiq)	10–15 µg/kg
	Anesthetic adjunct (IV)	1–5 µg/kg
	Maintenance infusion	2–4 µg/kg/h
	Main anesthetic (IV)	50–100 µg/kg
Flumazinil	IV	0.01 mg/kg
Fosphenytoin	IV	15–20 mg/kg
Furosemide	IV	0.2–1 mg/kg
Gentamicin	IV	2 mg/kg
Glucose	IV	0.5–1 g/kg
Glucagon	IV	0.5–1 mg
Glycopyrrolate	IV	0.01 mg/kg
Granisetron	IV	0.04 mg/kg
Heparin	IV	100 U/kg
Hydrocortisone	IV	1 mg/kg
Hydromorphone	IV	15–20 µg/kg
Ibuprofen	PO	4–10 mg/kg
Imipenem	IV	15–25 mg/kg
Insulin	Infusion	0.02–0.1 U/kg/h
Isoproterenol	Infusion	0.1–1 µg/kg/min
Ketamine	Induction (IV)	1–2 mg/kg
	Induction (IM)	6–10 mg/kg
	Induction (per rectum)	10 mg/kg
	Maintenance infusion	25–75 µg/kg/min
	Premedication (PO)	6–10 mg/kg
	Sedation (IV)	2–3 mg/kg
	Sedation (IV)	0.5–1 mg/kg
Ketorolac	IV	0.5–0.75 mg/kg
Labetalol	IV	0.25 mg/kg
Lidocaine	Loading	1 mg/kg
	Maintenance	20–50 µg/kg/min
Magnesium	IV (slowly)	25–50 mg/kg
	Maximum single dose	2 g
Mannitol	IV	0.25–1 g/kg
Meperidine	Pain relief (IV)	0.2–0.5 mg/kg
	Premedication (IM)	1 mg/kg

(continued)

Table 44–3. Pediatric drug dosages. (continued)

Drug	Comment	Dosage
Methohexital	Induction (IV)	1–2 mg/kg
	Induction (per rectum)	25–30 mg/kg
	Induction (IM)	10 mg/kg
Methylprednisolone	IV	2–4 mg/kg
Metoclopramide	IV	0.15 mg/kg
Metronidazole	IV	7.5 mg/kg
Midazolam	Premedication (PO)	0.5 mg/kg
	Maximum dose (PO)	20 mg
	Sedation (IM)	0.1–0.15 mg/kg
	Maximum dose (IM)	7.5 mg
	Sedation (IV)	0.05 mg/kg
Milrinone	Loading (IV)	50–70 µg/kg
	Maintenance	0.375–0.75 µg/kg/min
Mivacurium	Intubation (IV)	0.2–0.3 mg/kg
	Infusion	3–24 µg/kg/min
Morphine	Pain relief (IV)	0.025–0.1 mg/kg
	Premedication (IM)	0.1 mg/kg
Naloxone	IV	0.01 mg/kg
Neostigmine	Depends on degree of paralysis (IV)	0.04–0.07 mg/kg
Nitroglycerin	IV	0.5–3 µg/kg/min
Nitroprusside	Infusion	0.5–8 µg/kg/min
Norepinephrine	Infusion	0.1–2 µg/kg/min
Ondansetron	IV	0.1 mg/kg
Oxacillin	IV	50 mg/kg
Pancuronium	IV	0.1 mg/kg
Penicillin G	IV	50,000 U/kg
Pentobarbital	Premedication (IM)	4–6 mg/kg
Phenobarbital	Sedation (IV or IM)	1–3 mg/kg
	Anticonvulsant dose (IV)	5–20 mg/kg
Phentolamine	IV	30 µg/kg
Phenylephrine	IV	1–10 µg/kg
Phenytoin	Slowly IV	5–20 mg/kg
Physostigmine	IV	0.01–0.03 mg/kg
Prednisone	PO	1 mg/kg
Protamine	IV	1 mg/100 U heparin
Procainamide	Loading dose (IV)	15 mg/kg
Propanolol	IV	10–25 µg/kg
Propofol	Induction (IV)	2–3 mg/kg
	Maintenance infusion	60–250 µg/kg/min
Prostaglandin E$_1$	Infusion	0.05–0.1 µg/kg/min
Ranitidine	IV	0.25–1.0 mg/kg
Remifentanil (bolus)	IV	0.25–1 µg/kg
Remifentanil (infusion)	IV	0.05–2 µg/kg/min
Rocuronium	Intubation (IV)	0.6–1.2 mg/kg
Scopolamine	IV	0.01 mg/kg
Sodium bicarbonate	IV	1 mEq/kg
Succinylcholine	Intubation (IV)	2–3 mg/kg
	Intubation (IM)	4–6 mg/kg
Sufentanil	Premedication (Intranasal)	2 µg/kg
	Anesthetic adjunct (IV)	0.5–1 µg/kg
	Maintenance infusion	0.5–2 µg/kg/h
	Main anesthetic (IV)	10–15 µg/kg

(continued)

Table 44–3. Pediatric drug dosages. (continued)

Drug	Comment	Dosage
Thipental	Induction (IV)	5–6 mg/kg
	(per rectum)	25–30 mg/kg
Trimethoprim/sulfamethoxazole	IV	4–5 mg/kg
Vancomycin	IV	20 mg/kg
Vecuronium	IV	0.1 mg/kg
Verapamil	IV	0.1–0.3 mg/kg

and fentanyl. Neonates also have a relatively lower glomerular filtration rate and hepatic blood flow, as well as immature renal tubular function and immature hepatic enzyme systems. Increased intraabdominal pressure and abdominal surgery further reduce hepatic blood flow. All these factors impair renal drug handling, hepatic metabolism, or biliary excretion of many drugs in neonates and young infants. Neonates also have decreased or impaired protein binding for some drugs, most notably thiopental, bupivacaine, and many antibiotics. In the first instance, increased free drug enhances potency and reduces the induction dose compared to older children. In the second instance, an increase in free bupivacaine may enhance systemic toxicity.

Inhalational Anesthetics

 Neonates, infants, and young children have relatively higher alveolar ventilation and lower FRC compared with older children and adults. This higher minute ventilation-to-FRC ratio with relatively higher blood flow to vessel-rich organs contributes to a rapid rise in alveolar anesthetic concentration and speeds inhalation induction. Furthermore, the blood/gas coefficients of volatile anesthetics are lower in neonates than in adults, resulting in even faster induction times and potentially increasing the risk of overdosing.

 The minimum alveolar concentration (MAC) for halogenated agents is higher in infants than in neonates and adults (Table 44–4). Unlike other agents, sevoflurane has the same MAC in neonates and infants. For unknown reasons, use of nitrous oxide in children does not augment the effects (lower MAC requirements) of desflurane and to some extent sevoflurane as it does for other agents.

The blood pressure of neonates and infants tends to be more sensitive to volatile anesthetics, probably because of not fully developed compensatory mechanisms (eg, vasoconstriction, tachycardia) and an immature myocardium that is very sensitive to myocardial depressants. As with adults, halothane also sensitizes the heart to catecholamines; the maximum recommended dose of epinephrine in local anesthetic solutions during halothane anesthesia is 10 μg/kg. Cardiovascular

depression, bradycardia, and arrhythmias are significantly less with sevoflurane than with halothane. Halothane and sevoflurane are least likely to irritate the airway and cause breath holding or laryngospasm during induction (see Chapter 7). Volatile anesthetics appear to depress ventilation more in infants than in older children. Sevoflurane is associated with the least respiratory depression. Prepubertal children are at much less risk for halothane-induced hepatic dysfunction than are adults. There are no reported instances of renal toxicity from inorganic fluoride production during sevoflurane anesthesia in children. Overall, sevoflurane appears to have a greater therapeutic index than halothane and has become a preferred induction agent in pediatric anesthesia.

The rate of emergence is fastest following desflurane and sevoflurane anesthesia, but both agents are associated with an increased incidence of agitation or delirium upon emergence, particularly in young children. Because of the latter, many clinicians switch to either isoflurane or halothane for maintenance anesthesia following a sevoflurane induction (see below). The speed of emergence from halothane and isoflurane anesthesia appears to be similar for procedures lasting less than 1 h.

Nonvolatile Anesthetics

Based on weight, infants and young children require larger doses of propofol because of a larger volume of distribution compared to adults. Children also have a

Table 44–4. Approximate MAC[1] values for pediatric patients.[2]

Agent	Neonates	Infants	Small Children	Adults
Halothane	0.87	1.1–1.2	0.87	0.75
Sevoflurane	3.2	3.2	2.5	2.0
Isoflurane	1.60	1.8–1.9	1.3–1.6	1.2
Desflurane	8–9	9–10	7–8	6.0

[1]MAC, minimum alveolar concentration.
[2]Values are derived from various sources.

shorter elimination half-life and higher plasma clearance for propofol. Whereas recovery from a single bolus is not appreciably different from adults, recovery following a continuous infusion may be more rapid. For the same reasons, children may require higher rates of infusion for maintenance of anesthesia (up to 250 µg/kg/min). Propofol is not recommended for sedation of critically ill pediatric patients in the intensive care unit (ICU). The drug has been associated with higher mortality compared to other agents, and a controversial "propofol infusion syndrome" has been described. Its essential features are metabolic acidosis, hemodynamic instability, hepatomegaly, rhabdomyolysis, and multiorgan failure. Although appearing primarily in critically ill children, this rare syndrome has been reported in adults and in patients undergoing long-term propofol infusion (> 48 h) for sedation at high doses (> 5 mg/kg/h).

Children require relatively higher doses of thiopental compared to adults. The elimination half-life is shorter and the plasma clearance is greater than in adults. In contrast, neonates, particularly those depressed at birth, appear to be more sensitive to barbiturates and have less protein binding, a longer half-life, and impaired clearance. The thiopental induction dose for neonates is 3–4 mg/kg compared to 5–6 mg/kg for infants.

Opioids appear to be more potent in neonates than in older children and adults. Possible explanations include easier entry across the blood–brain barrier, decreased metabolic capability, or increased sensitivity of the respiratory centers. Morphine sulfate should be used with caution in neonates because hepatic conjugation is reduced and renal clearance of morphine metabolites is decreased. The cytochrome P-450 pathways mature at the end of the neonatal period. Older pediatric patients have relatively high rates of biotransformation and elimination as a result of high hepatic blood flow. Sufentanil, alfentanil, and, possibly, fentanyl clearances may be higher in children than in adults. Remifentanil clearance is increased in neonates and infants but elimination half-life is unaltered compared to adults. Neonates and infants may be more resistant to the hypnotic effects of ketamine, requiring slightly higher doses than adults; pharmacokinetics do not appear to be significantly different from adults. The combination of ketamine and fentanyl is more likely to cause hypotension in neonates and young infants than ketamine and midazolam. Etomidate has not been studied adequately in pediatric patients less than 10 years old; its profile in older children is similar to adults. Midazolam has the fastest clearance of all the benzodiazepines; however, midazolam clearance is significantly less in neonates than in older children. Moreover, the combination of midazolam and fentanyl can cause profound hypotension.

Muscle Relaxants

All muscle relaxants generally have a shorter onset (up to 50% less) in pediatric patients because of shorter circulation times than adults. Nonetheless, intravenous succinylcholine (1–1.5 mg/kg) has the fastest onset (see Chapter 9). Infants require significantly higher doses of succinylcholine (2–3 mg/kg) than older children and adults because of the relatively larger volume of distribution (extracellular space). This discrepancy disappears if dosage is based on body surface area. Table 44–5 lists commonly used muscle relaxants and their ED_{95} (effective dose in 95% of patients). With the notable exclusion of succinylcholine, mivacurium, and possibly cisatracurium, infants require significantly less muscle relaxant than older children. Moreover, based on weight, older children require higher doses than adults for some neuromuscular blocking agents (eg, mivacurium and atracurium, see Chapter 9). As with adults, a more rapid intubation can be achieved with a muscle relaxant dose that is 1.5–2 times the ED_{95} dose at the expense of prolonging the duration of action.

The response of neonates to nondepolarizing muscle relaxants is quite variable. Immaturity of the neuromuscular junction (particularly in premature neonates) tends to increase sensitivity, whereas a disproportionately large extracellular compartment dilutes drug concentration. The relative immaturity of neonatal hepatic function prolongs the duration of action for drugs that depend primarily on hepatic metabolism (eg, pancuronium, vecuronium, and rocuronium). In contrast, atracurium and cisatracurium, which do not depend on hepatic biotransformation, reliably behave as intermediate acting muscle relaxants. Breakdown

Table 44–5. Approximate ED_{95} for muscle relaxants in infants and children.[1]

Agents	Infants ED_{95} (mg/kg)	Children ED_{95} (mg/kg)
Succinylcholine	0.7	0.4
Mivacurium	0.15	0.15
Atracurium	0.25	0.35
Cisatracurium	0.05	0.06
Rocuronium	0.25	0.4
Vecuronium	0.05	0.08
Pancuronium	0.07	0.09

[1]Average values during nitrous oxide/oxygen anesthesia.

of mivacurium also does not appear to be significantly altered in neonates.

Children are more susceptible than adults to cardiac arrhythmias, hyperkalemia, rhabdomyolysis, myoglobinemia, masseter spasm, and malignant hyperthermia after administration of succinylcholine. If a child unexpectedly experiences cardiac arrest following administration of succinylcholine, immediate treatment for hyperkalemia should be instituted. Prolonged and heroic (eg, cardiopulmonary bypass) resuscitative efforts may be required. For this reason, succinylcholine is best avoided for routine elective surgery in children and adolescents. Unlike in adult patients, profound bradycardia and sinus node arrest can develop in pediatric patients following the first dose of succinylcholine without atropine pretreatment. Atropine (0.1 mg minimum) must therefore always be administered prior to succinylcholine in children. Generally accepted indications for succinylcholine in children are rapid sequence induction with a full stomach, laryngospasm, and rapid muscle relaxation prior to intravenous access (eg, regurgitation). Intramuscular succinylcholine (4–6 mg/kg) can be used for the latter; in this situation, atropine (0.02 mg/kg intramuscularly) should be administered at the same time to prevent bradycardia. Some clinicians advocate intralingual administration (2 mg/kg in the mid-line to avoid hematoma formation) as an emergency alternate route.

Some clinicians consider rocuronium (0.6 mg/kg) to be the drug of choice for routine intubation in pediatric patients with intravenous access because it has the fastest onset of nondepolarizing neuromuscular blocking agents (see Chapter 9). Higher doses of rocuronium (0.9–1.2 mg/kg) may be used for rapid sequence induction but a prolonged duration (up to 90 min) should be expected. Rocuronium is the only nondepolarizing neuromuscular blocker that can be given intramuscularly (1.0–1.5 mg/kg) but requires 3–4 min for onset.

Mivacurium, atracurium, or cisatracurium may be preferred agents in young infants, particularly for short procedures, because these three drugs consistently display short to intermediate duration. Mivacurium is typically used for procedures lasting 10–15 min, whereas atracurium or cisatracurium is usually used for procedures lasting more than 30 min.

As with adults, the effect of incremental doses of muscle relaxants (usually 25–30% of the initial dose) should be monitored with a peripheral nerve stimulator. Sensitivity can vary significantly between patients. Nondepolarizing blockade can be reversed with neostigmine (0.03–0.07 mg/kg) or edrophonium (0.5–1 mg/kg) along with an anticholinergic agent (glycopyrrolate 0.01 mg/kg or atropine 0.01–0.02 mg/kg).

PEDIATRIC ANESTHETIC RISK

Perhaps the most current database for assessing pediatric anesthetic risk is the Pediatric Perioperative Cardiac Arrest (POCA) Registry. This registry includes reports based on approximately one million pediatric anesthetic cases administered since 1994. All cardiac arrests and deaths of pediatric patients during the administration of or recovery from anesthesia were analyzed to investigate the possible relationship of anesthesia to these incidents. Nearly all patients received general anesthesia alone or combined with regional anesthesia. In a preliminary analysis of the data that included 289 cases of cardiac arrest, 150 arrests were judged to be related to anesthesia. Thus the risk of cardiac arrest in pediatric anesthetic cases would appear to be approximately 1.4 in 10,000. Moreover, an overall mortality of 26% was reported following cardiac arrest. Approximately 6% suffered permanent injury, with the majority (68%) having either no or temporary injury. Mortality was 4% in American Society of Anesthesiologists (ASA) physical status 1 and 2 patients compared to 37% in ASA physical status 3–5 patients. It is important to note that 33% of patients who suffered a cardiac arrest were ASA physical status 1–2. Moreover, infants accounted for 55% of all anesthesia-related arrests with those less than 1 month (ie, neonates) having the highest risk. As with adults, two major predictors of mortality were ASA physical status 3–5 and emergency surgery.

Most (82%) arrests occurred during induction of anesthesia; bradycardia, hypotension, and a low SpO_2 were frequent preceding events. The most common mechanism of cardiac arrest was judged to be medication related (Figure 44–2). Cardiovascular depression from halothane, alone or in combination with other drugs, was believed to be responsible in 66% of all medication-related arrests. Another 9% was due to intravascular injection of a local anesthetic, most often following a negative aspiration test during a caudal injection. A presumed cardiovascular mechanism was most often of unclear etiology, but in more than 50% of those cases the patient had congenital heart disease. Where a cardiovascular mechanism could be identified, it was most often related to hemorrhage, transfusion, or inadequate/inappropriate fluid therapy.

A respiratory mechanism was most often due to laryngospasm, airway obstruction, and difficult intubation (in decreasing order). In most cases the laryngospasm occurred during induction. Nearly all patients who had airway obstruction or were difficult to intubate had significant underlying disease.

The most common equipment-related mechanism that led to a cardiac arrest was complications from

Figure 44–2. Mechanisms of cardiac arrest in pediatric patients, based on POCA Registry Data.

placement of a central venous catheter (eg, pneumothorax, hemothorax, or cardiac tamponade).

PEDIATRIC ANESTHETIC TECHNIQUES

Preoperative Considerations

A. Preoperative Interview

Depending on age, past surgical experiences, and maturity, children suffer from varying degrees of terror when faced with the prospect of surgery. In contrast to adults, who are usually most concerned about the possibility of death, children are principally worried about pain and separation from their parents. Presurgical preparation programs—such as brochures, videos, or tours—can be very helpful in preparing many children and parents. Unfortunately, outpatient and morning-of-admission surgery together with a busy operating room schedule often make it difficult for an anesthesiologist to have enough time to break through the barriers erected by pediatric patients. For this reason, premedication (below) can be extremely helpful. A key strategy is to demystify the process of anesthesia and surgery by explaining in age-appropriate terms what lies ahead. For example, the anesthesiologist might bring an anesthesia mask for the child to play with during the interview and describe it as something the astronauts use. Alternatively, in some centers, someone who the child trusts (eg, a parent, nurse, other physician) may be allowed to be in attendance during preanesthetic preparations and induction of anesthesia. This can have a particularly calming influence on children undergoing repeated procedures (eg, examination under anesthesia following glaucoma surgery).

B. Recent Upper Respiratory Tract Infection

Children frequently present for surgery with evidence—a runny nose with fever, cough, or sore throat—of a coincidental viral upper respiratory tract infection (URTI).

Attempts should be made to differentiate between an infectious cause of rhinorrhea and an allergic or vasomotor cause. A viral infection within 2–4 weeks before general anesthesia and endotracheal intubation appears to place the child at an increased risk for perioperative pulmonary complications, such as wheezing (10-fold), laryngospasm (5-fold), hypoxemia, and atelectasis. This is particularly likely if the child has a severe cough, high fever, or a family history of reactive airway disease. The decision to anesthetize children with URTIs remains controversial and depends on the presence of other coexisting illnesses, the severity of URTI symptoms, and the urgency of the surgery. If surgery cannot be deferred, consideration should be given to an anticholinergic premedication, mask ventilation, humidification of inspired gases, and a longer-than-usual stay in the recovery room.

C. Laboratory Tests

Few, if any, preoperative laboratory results have been deemed cost effective. Some pediatric centers require *no* preoperative laboratory tests in *healthy* children undergoing *minor* procedures. Obviously, this places more responsibility on the anesthesiologist, surgeon, and pediatrician to correctly identify those patients who should have preoperative testing for specific surgical procedures.

Most asymptomatic patients with murmurs do not have significant cardiac pathology. Innocent murmurs may occur in more than 30% of normal children. They are usually soft, short systolic ejection murmurs that are best heard along the left upper or left lower sternal border without significant radiation. Innocent murmurs at the left upper sternal border are due to flow across the pulmonic valve (pulmonic ejection) whereas those at the lower left border are due to flow from the left ventricle to the aorta (Still's vibratory murmur). The pediatrician and possibly a cardiologist should carefully evaluate patients with a newly diagnosed murmur, particularly in infancy. An echocardiogram should be obtained if the patient is symptomatic (eg, poor feeding, failure to thrive, or easy fatigability); the murmur is harsh, loud, holosystolic, diastolic, or radiates widely; or pulses are either bounding (eg, with aortic runoff lesions) or markedly diminished.

D. PREOPERATIVE FASTING

Because pediatric patients are more prone to dehydration, their preoperative fluid restriction has always been more lenient. Several studies, however, have documented low gastric pH (< 2.5) and relatively high residual volumes in pediatric patients scheduled for surgery, suggesting that children may be at a higher risk for aspiration than previously thought. The incidence of aspiration is reported to be approximately 1:1000. Prolonged fasting does not necessarily decrease this risk. In fact, several studies have demonstrated lower residual volumes and higher gastric pH in pediatric patients who received clear fluids a few h before induction. **Depending on age, regular formula feedings or solid foods are continued until 4–8 h before surgery.** More specifically, infants younger than 6 months are fed formula up to 4 h before induction, whereas infants 6–36 months of age can be given formula or solids up to 6 h before induction. Clear fluids are offered until 2–3 h before induction. These recommendations are for healthy neonates, infants, and children without risk factors for decreased gastric emptying or aspiration.

E. PREMEDICATION

There is great variation in the recommendations for premedication of pediatric patients. Sedative premedication is generally omitted for neonates and sick infants. Children who appear likely to exhibit uncontrollable separation anxiety can be given a sedative, such as midazolam (0.3–0.5 mg/kg, 15 mg maximum). The oral route is generally preferred because it is less traumatic than intramuscular injection, but it requires 20–45 min for effect. Smaller doses of midazolam may be used with the addition of oral ketamine (4–6 mg/kg), but the combination may not be suitable for outpatients. For uncooperative patients, intramuscular midazolam (0.1–0.15 mg/kg, 10 mg maximum) and/or ketamine (2–3 mg/kg) with atropine (0.02 mg/kg) may be helpful. Rectal midazolam (0.5–1 mg/kg, 20 mg maximum) or rectal methohexital (25–30 mg/kg of 10% solution) may also be administered in such cases while the child is in the parent's arms. The nasal route can be used with some drugs but is unpleasant, and some concerns exist over potential neurotoxicity of nasal midazolam. Fentanyl can also be administered as a lollipop (Actiq 5–15 µg/kg); fentanyl levels continue to rise intraoperatively and can contribute to postoperative analgesia. Older agents such as chloral hydrate and pentobarbital are rarely used. Other premedication considerations are discussed in the case study presented in Chapter 8.

Some anesthesiologists routinely premedicate young children with anticholinergic drugs (eg, atropine 0.02 mg/kg intramuscularly) to decrease the likelihood of bradycardia during induction. Atropine reduces the incidence of hypotension during induction in neonates and in infants less than 3 months. Atropine can also prevent accumulation of secretions that can block small airways and endotracheal tubes. Secretions can be particularly problematic for patients with URTIs or those who have been given ketamine. Atropine is often administered orally (0.05 mg/kg), intramuscularly, or occasionally rectally. Many anesthesiologists prefer to give atropine intravenously at or shortly after induction.

Monitoring

Monitoring requirements for infants and children are generally similar to adults with some minor modifications. Alarm limits should be appropriately adjusted. Smaller electrocardiographic electrode pads may be necessary so that they do not encroach on sterile surgical areas. Blood pressure cuffs must be properly fitted (see Figure 6–8). Noninvasive blood pressure monitors have proved to very reliable. A precordial stethoscope provides an inexpensive means of monitoring heart rate, quality of heart sounds, and airway patency.

Small pediatric patients have a smaller allowable margin of error. Pulse oximetry and capnography assume an even greater monitoring role in pediatric patients because hypoxia from inadequate ventilation is a major cause of perioperative morbidity and mortality. In neonates, the pulse oximeter probe should preferably be placed on the right hand or earlobe to measure preductal oxygen saturation. End-tidal CO_2 analysis allows assessment of the adequacy of ventilation, confirmation of endotracheal tube placement, and early warning of malignant hyperthermia. Nonetheless, the small tidal volumes and rapid respiratory rates of small infants can present difficulties with some capnograph models. Flow-through (mainstream) analyzers are usually less accurate in patients weighing less than 10 kg. Even with aspiration (sidestream) capnographs, the inspired (baseline) CO_2 can appear falsely elevated and the expired (peak) CO_2 can be falsely low. The degree of error depends on many factors but can be minimized by placing the sampling site as close as possible to the tip of the endotracheal tube, using a short length of sampling line, and lowering gas-sampling flow rates (100–150 mL/min). Furthermore, the size of some flow-through sensors may lead to kinking of the endotracheal tube or hypercapnia as a result of increased equipment dead space.

Temperature must be closely monitored in pediatric patients because of a higher risk for malignant hyperthermia and the potential for both iatrogenic hypothermia and hyperthermia. Hypothermia can be prevented by maintaining a warm operating room environment (26°C or higher), warming and humidifying inspired gases, using a warming blanket and warming lights, and warming all intravenous fluids. The room temperature required for a neutral thermal environment varies with age; it is highest in premature newborns. Note that care must be taken to prevent unintentional skin burns and iatrogenic hyperthermia from overzealous warming efforts.

Invasive monitoring (eg, arterial cannulation, central venous catheterization) requires considerable expertise and extreme caution. All air bubbles should be removed from pressure tubing and only small volume flushes should be used to prevent air embolism, inadvertent heparinization, and fluid overload. Pulmonary artery catheters are usually not used in pediatric patients because of the predictable relationship between right- and left-sided filling pressures. The right radial artery is often chosen for cannulation in the neonate because its preductal location mirrors the oxygen content of the carotid and retinal arteries. A femoral artery catheter may be a suitable alternative in very small neonates. Critically ill neonates may still have an umbilical artery catheter in place. Urinary output is an important measure of volume status.

Neonates who are premature or small for gestational age, who have received hyperalimentation, or whose mothers are diabetic may be prone to hypoglycemia. These infants should have frequent serum glucose determinations: levels < 30 mg/dL in the neonate and < 40 mg/dL in older children indicate hypoglycemia. Blood sampling (from an arterial or central venous catheter) for arterial blood gases, hemoglobin, potassium, and ionized calcium concentration can be invaluable in critically ill patients, particularly when transfusion is necessary.

Induction

General anesthesia is usually induced by an intravenous or inhalational technique. Induction with intramuscular ketamine (5–10 mg/kg) is reserved for specific situations, such as those involving combative children. Intravenous induction is preferred if the patient comes to the operating room with an intravenous catheter or is cooperative enough to allow awake venous cannulation. Prior application of EMLA (eutectic [easily melted] mixture of local anesthetic) cream (see Chapter 14) may make intravenous cannulation less stressful for the patient, parent, and anesthesiologist. EMLA cream is not a perfect solution, however. Some children become very anxious at the sight of a needle, particularly those who have had multiple needle punctures in the past. Furthermore, it can be difficult to anticipate in which extremity intravenous cannulation will prove to be successful. Finally, to be effective, EMLA cream must remain in contact with the skin for at least 30–60 min. Awake or sedated-awake intubation with topical anes-

thesia should be considered for emergency procedures in neonates and small infants when they are critically ill or a potential difficult airway is present.

Intravenous Induction

The same induction sequence can be used as in adults: a rapid-acting barbiturate (eg, thiopental, 3 mg/kg in neonates, 5–6 mg/kg in infants and children) or propofol (2–3 mg/kg) followed by a nondepolarizing muscle relaxant (eg, rocuronium, cisatracurium, atracurium, mivacurium, or succinylcholine). Atropine should be given intravenously prior to succinylcholine. Propofol may be associated with less hypertension during intubation, faster awakening, and less postoperative nausea and vomiting. The advantages of an intravenous technique include familiarity with the agents, availability of intravenous access if emergency drugs need to be administered, and rapidity of induction in the child at risk for aspiration.

Inhalational Induction

Most children do not arrive in the operating room with an intravenous line in place and dread the prospect of being stuck with a needle. Fortunately, modern potent volatile anesthetics can render small children unconscious within minutes. This is usually easier in children who have been sedated prior to entering the operating room and who are sleepy enough to be anesthetized without ever knowing what has happened (steal induction). Alternatives to frightening a child with a black mask include insufflation of the anesthetic gases over the face, substituting a clear face mask, placing a drop of food flavoring on the inside of the mask (eg, oil of orange), and allowing the child to sit during the early stages of induction. Specially contoured masks minimize dead space (see Figure 5–6).

There are many differences between adult and pediatric anatomy that affect mask ventilation and intubation. Equipment appropriate for age and size should be selected (Table 44–6). Neonates and most young infants are obligate nasal breathers and obstruct easily. Oral airways often help displace an oversized tongue, whereas nasal airways can traumatize small nares or prominent adenoids. Compression of submandibular soft tissues should be avoided during mask ventilation to prevent upper airway obstruction.

Typically, the child is coaxed into breathing an odorless mixture of nitrous oxide (70%) and oxygen (30%). Sevoflurane or halothane is added to the anesthetic gas mixture in 0.5% increments every three to five breaths. As previously discussed, sevoflurane has a wider therapeutic index in terms of cardiovascular depression and depression of ventilatory drive. Many if not most pediatric anesthesiologists consider sevoflu-

Table 44–6. Airway equipment for pediatric patients.

	Premature	Neonate	Infant	Toddler	Small Child	Large Child
Age	0–1 month	0–1 month	1–12 months	1–3 years	3–8 years	8–12 years
Weight (kg)	0.5–3	3–5	4–10	8–16	14–30	25–50
Tracheal (ET)[1] tube (mm i.d.)	2.5–3	3–3.5	3.5–4	4–4.5	4.5–5.5	5.5–6 (cuffed)
ET depth (cm at lips)	6–9	9–10	10–12	12–14	14–16	16–18
Suction catheter (F)	6	6	8	8	10	12
Laryngoscope blade	00	0	1	1.5	2	3
Mask size	00	0	0	1	2	3
Oral airway	000–00	00	0 (40 mm)	1 (50 mm)	2 (70 mm)	3 (80 mm)
Laryngeal mask airway (LMA#)	—	1	1	2	2.5	3

[1]ET, endotracheal tube.

rane the agent of choice for inhalation induction. Desflurane and isoflurane are not used for induction because they are more pungent and are associated with more coughing, breath-holding, and laryngospasm during an inhalational induction. Some clinicians use a single breath induction technique with sevoflurane (7–8% sevoflurane in 60% nitrous oxide) to speed up induction. After an adequate depth of anesthesia has been achieved, an intravenous line can be started and a muscle relaxant administered. Patients typically pass through an excitement stage during which any stimulation can induce laryngospasm. Breath holding must be distinguished from laryngospasm. Steady application of 10 cm of positive end-expiratory pressure can help overcome laryngospasm.

Alternatively, the anesthesiologist can deepen the level of anesthesia by increasing the concentration of volatile anesthetic, and place a laryngeal mask airway (LMA) or, less commonly, intubating the patient without a muscle relaxant. Because greater anesthetic depth is required for tracheal intubation with the latter technique, the possibility of severe cardiac depression, bradycardia, or laryngospasm occurring without intravenous access detracts from this technique. Intramuscular succinylcholine (4–6 mg/kg, not to exceed 150 mg) and atropine (0.02 mg/kg, not to exceed 0.4 mg) should be available if laryngospasm or bradycardia occurs before an intravenous line is established; intralingual succinylcholine may be an alterative route (see above).

Positive-pressure ventilation during mask induction and prior to intubation sometimes causes gastric distention, resulting in impairment of lung expansion. Suctioning with an orogastric or nasogastric tube will decompress the stomach, but it must be done without traumatizing fragile mucous membranes.

Intravenous Access

Cannulation of tiny pediatric veins can be a trying ordeal. This is particularly true for infants who have spent weeks in a neonatal intensive care unit and have few veins left unscarred. Even healthy 1-year-old children can prove a challenge because of extensive subcutaneous fat. Veins usually become more accessible after 2 years of age. The saphenous vein has a consistent location at the ankle and, with experience, the practitioner can usually cannulate it even if it is not visible or palpable. Twenty-four-gauge over-the-needle catheters are adequate in neonates and infants when blood transfusions are not anticipated. All air bubbles should be removed from the intravenous line, as a high incidence of patent foramen ovale increases the risk of paradoxical air embolism. In emergency situations where intravenous access is impossible, fluids can be effectively infused through an 18-gauge needle inserted into the medullary sinusoids within the tibial bone. This intraosseous infusion can be used for all medications normally given intravenously with almost as rapid results (see Chapter 47).

Tracheal Intubation

Following inhalational induction, nitrous oxide should be discontinued prior to intubation so that the patient's lungs will contain a high inspired oxygen concentration that allows adequate arterial oxygen saturation during this period of apnea. The choice of muscle relaxant is discussed above. In the case of an awake intubation in a neonate or young infant, adequate preoxygenation and use of oxygen insufflation during laryngoscopy (eg, Oxyscope) may help prevent hypoxemia.

A prominent occiput tends to place the head in a flexed position prior to intubation. This is easily corrected by slightly elevating the shoulders with towels and placing the head on a doughnut-shaped pillow. In older children, prominent tonsillar tissue can obstruct visualization of the larynx. Straight laryngoscope blades aid intubation of the anterior larynx in neonates, infants, and young children (Table 44–6). Endotracheal tubes that pass through the glottis may still impinge upon the cricoid cartilage, which is the narrowest point of the airway in children younger than 5 years of age. Mucosal trauma from trying to force a tube through the cricoid cartilage can cause postoperative edema, stridor, croup, and airway obstruction.

The appropriate diameter inside the endotracheal tube can be estimated by a formula based on age:

$$4 + \text{Age}/4 = \text{Tube diameter (in mm)}$$

For example, a 4-year-old child would be predicted to require a 5-mm tube. This formula provides only a rough guideline, however. Exceptions include premature neonates (a 2.5–3 mm tube) and full-term neonates (a 3–3.5 mm tube). Endotracheal tubes 0.5 mm larger and smaller than predicted should be readily available. Uncuffed endotracheal tubes are usually selected for children up to 8–10 years old to decrease the risk of postintubation croup and to provide a leak to minimize the risk of accidental barotrauma. Correct tube size is confirmed by easy passage into the larynx and the development of a gas leak at 15–20 cm H_2O pressure for an uncuffed tube. No leak indicates an oversized tube that should be replaced to prevent postoperative edema, whereas an excessive leak may preclude adequate ventilation and contaminate the operating room with anesthetic gases. Many clinicians, however, use a down-sized cuffed tube with the cuff completely deflated in younger patients at high risk for aspiration; minimal inflation of the cuff can stop any air leak. There is also a formula to estimate endotracheal length:

$$12 + \text{Age}/2 = \text{Length of tube (in cm)}$$

Again, this formula provides only a guideline, and the result must be confirmed by auscultation and clinical judgment. To avoid endobronchial intubation, the tip of the endotracheal tube should pass only 1–2 cm beyond an infant's glottis. An alternative technique is to intentionally place the tip of the endotracheal tube into the right mainstem bronchus and then withdraw it until breath sounds are equal.

Maintenance

Ventilation is usually controlled during anesthesia of neonates and infants. During spontaneous ventilation, even the low resistance of a circle system can become a significant obstacle for a sick neonate to overcome. Unidirectional valves, breathing tubes, and absorbers account for most of this resistance. For patients weighing less than 10 kg, some anesthesiologists prefer the Mapleson D circuit or the Bain system because of their low resistance and light

weight (see Chapter 3). Nonetheless, because breathing-circuit resistance is easily overcome by positive-pressure ventilation, the circle system can be safely used in patients of all ages if ventilation is controlled. Monitoring of airway pressure may provide early evidence of obstruction caused by a kinked endotracheal tube or advancement of the tube into a mainstem bronchus.

Many anesthesia ventilators on older machines are designed for adult patients and cannot reliably provide the low tidal volumes and rapid rates required by neonates and infants. Unintentional delivery of large tidal volumes to a small child can generate enormous peak airway pressures and cause extensive barotrauma. The pressure-limited mode, which is found on all newer anesthesia ventilators and some older models, should be used for neonates, infants, and toddlers. Small tidal volumes can also be manually delivered with greater sensitivity with a 1-L breathing bag than with a 3-L adult bag. For children < 10 kg, adequate tidal volumes are achieved with peak inspiratory pressures of 15–18 cm H_2O. For larger children the volume control ventilation may be used and tidal volumes may be set at 8–10 mL/kg. Many spirometers are less accurate at lower tidal volumes. In addition, the gas lost in long, highly compliant breathing circuits becomes quite significant relative to a child's small tidal volume. For this reason, pediatric tubing is usually shorter and stiffer (less compliant). Equipment dead space, a critical determinant of rebreathing in children, is minimized by a septum that divides the inspiratory and expiratory gas in the Y-piece. Condenser humidifiers or heat and moisture exchangers (HME) can add considerable dead space; depending on the size of the patient, they either should not be used or an appropriately sized, pediatric HME should be employed.

Anesthesia can be maintained in pediatric patients with the same agents as in adults. Many clinicians switch to either isoflurane or halothane following a sevoflurane induction to help reduce the likelihood of postoperative delirium or agitation on emergence (see above). If sevoflurane is continued for maintenance, administration of an opioid (eg, fentanyl 1–1.5 μg/kg) 15–20 min before the end of the procedure can reduce the incidence of emergence delirium and agitation. Although the MAC is higher in children than in adults (see Table 44–4), neonates may be particularly susceptible to the cardiodepressant effects of general anesthetics. Nondepolarizing muscle relaxants are often required for optimal surgical conditions; this is particularly true in neonates and sick infants who may not tolerate higher doses of volatile agents.

Perioperative Fluid Requirements

Meticulous fluid management is required in small pediatric patients because of extremely limited margins of error. A programmable infusion pump or a buret with a microdrip chamber should be used for accurate measurements. Drugs are flushed through low dead-space tubing to minimize unnecessary fluid administration. Fluid overload is diagnosed by prominent veins, flushed skin, increased blood pressure, decreased serum sodium, and a loss of the folds in the upper eyelids. Fluid therapy can be divided into maintenance, deficit, and replacement requirements.

A. MAINTENANCE FLUID REQUIREMENTS

Maintenance requirements for pediatric patients can be determined by the formula presented in Chapter 29, the 4:2:1 rule: 4 mL/kg/h for the first 10 kg of weight, 2 mL/kg/h for the second 10 kg, and 1 mL/kg/h for each remaining kilogram. The choice of maintenance fluid remains controversial. A solution such as $D_5{}^1/_2NS$ with 20 mEq/L of potassium chloride provides adequate dextrose and electrolytes at these maintenance infusion rates. $D_5{}^1/_4NS$ may be a better choice in neonates because of their limited ability to handle sodium loads. Neonates require 3–5 mg/kg/min of a glucose infusion to maintain euglycemia (40–125 mg/dL); premature neonates require 5–6 mg/kg/min.

B. DEFICITS

In addition to a maintenance infusion, any preoperative fluid deficits must be replaced. For example, if a 5-kg infant has not received oral or intravenous fluids for 4 h prior to surgery, a deficit of 80 mL has accrued (5 kg × 4 mL/kg/h × 4 h). In contrast to adults, infants respond to dehydration with decreased blood pressure but without increased heart rate. Preoperative fluid deficits are typically administered with hourly maintenance requirements in aliquots of 50% in the first hour and 25% in the second and third hours. In the example above, a total of 60 mL would be given in the first hour (80/2 + 20) and 40 mL in the second and third hours (80/4 + 20). Large quantities of dextrose-containing solutions are avoided to prevent hyperglycemia. Preoperative fluid deficits are usually replaced with a balanced salt solution (eg, lactated Ringer's injection) or $^1/_2$ normal saline. Compared with lactated Ringer's injection, normal saline has the disadvantage of promoting hyperchloremic acidosis.

C. REPLACEMENT REQUIREMENTS

Replacement can be subdivided into blood loss and third-space loss.

1. Blood loss—The blood volume of premature neonates (100 mL/kg), full-term neonates (85–90 mL/kg), and infants (80 mL/kg) is proportionately higher than that of adults (65–75 mL/kg). An initial hematocrit of 55% in the healthy full-term neonate gradually falls to as low as 30% in the 3-month-old infant before rising to 35% by 6 months. Hemoglobin (Hb) type is also changing during this period: from a 75% concentration of HbF (high oxygen affinity, low PaO_2, poor tissue

unloading) at birth to almost 100% HbA (low oxygen affinity, high PaO_2, good tissue unloading) by 6 months.

Blood loss is typically replaced with non-glucose-containing crystalloid (eg, 3 mL of lactated Ringer's injection for each milliliter of blood lost) or colloid solutions (eg, 1 mL of 5% albumin for each milliliter of blood lost) until the patient's hematocrit reaches a predetermined lower limit. In premature and sick neonates, this may be as high as 40% or 50%, whereas in healthy older children a hematocrit of 20–26% is generally well tolerated. Because of their small intravascular volume, neonates and infants are at an increased risk for electrolyte disturbances (eg, hyperglycemia, hyperkalemia, and hypocalcemia) that can accompany rapid blood transfusion. Dosing of packed red blood cell transfusions is discussed in Chapter 29. Platelets and fresh frozen plasma 10–15 mL/kg should be given when blood loss exceeds 1–2 blood volumes. One unit of platelets per 10 kg weight raises the platelet count by about $50,000/\mu L$. The pediatric dose of cryoprecipitate is 1 U/10 kg weight.

2. Third-space loss—These losses are impossible to measure and must be estimated by the extent of the surgical procedure. One popular guideline is 0–2 mL/kg/h for relatively atraumatic surgery (eg, strabismus correction) and up to 6–10 mL/kg/h for traumatic procedures (eg, abdominal abscess). Third-space loss is usually replaced with lactated Ringer's injection (see Chapter 29).

Regional Anesthesia

The primary uses of regional techniques in pediatric anesthesia have been to supplement and lower general anesthetic requirements and provide good postoperative pain relief. Blocks range in complexity from the relatively simple peripheral nerve blocks described in Chapter 17 (eg, penile block, ilioinguinal block) to major conduction blocks (eg, spinal anesthesia).

Caudal blocks have proved useful in a variety of surgeries, including circumcision, inguinal herniorrhaphy, hypospadias repair, anal surgery, clubfoot repair, and other subumbilical procedures. Contraindications include infection around the sacral hiatus, coagulopathy, or anatomic abnormalities. The patient is usually lightly anesthetized or sedated and placed in the lateral position.

The technique of caudal anesthesia for adults is described in Chapter 16. For pediatric caudal anesthesia, a short bevel 22-gauge needle can be used. Loss of resistance should be assessed with saline, not air, because of the latter's possible association with hemodynamically significant air embolism. After the characteristic "pop" that signals penetration of the sacrococcygeal membrane, the needle is lowered and advanced only a few more millimeters to avoid entering the dural sac or the anterior body of the sacrum. Aspiration is used to check for blood or cerebrospinal fluid; local anesthetic can then be slowly injected; a 2-mL test dose of local anesthetic with epinephrine (1:200,000) helps exclude intravascular placement.

Many anesthetic agents have been used for caudal anesthesia in pediatric patients, with 1% lidocaine (up to 7 mg/kg for an epinephrine-containing solution) and 0.125–0.25% bupivacaine (up to 2.5 mg/kg) being most common. Ropivacaine 0.2% (up to 2 mg/kg) can provide analgesia similar to bupivacaine but with less motor blockade. Morphine sulfate (25 μg/kg) or hydromorphone (6 μg/kg) may be added to the local anesthetic solution to prolong postoperative analgesia for inpatients, but it increases the risk of delayed postoperative respiratory depression. The volume of local anesthetic required depends on the level of blockade desired, ranging from 0.5 mL/kg for a sacral block to 1.25 mL/kg for a midthoracic block. Single-shot injections generally last 4–12 h. Placement of 20-gauge caudal catheters with continuous infusion of local anesthetic (eg, 0.125% bupivacaine or 0.1% ropivacaine at 0.2–0.4 mg/kg/h) or an opioid (eg, fentanyl 2 μg/mL at 0.6 μg/kg/h) allows prolonged anesthesia and postoperative analgesia. Complications are rare but include local anesthetic toxicity from prolonged continuous infusions or intravascular injection (eg, seizures, hypotension, dysrhythmias), spinal blockade, and respiratory depression. Postoperative urinary retention does not appear to be a problem following single-dose caudal anesthesia.

Sedation for Procedures in and out of the Operating Room

Sedation is often requested for pediatric patients inside and outside the operating room for nonsurgical procedures. Cooperation and motionlessness may be required for imaging studies, bronchoscopy, gastrointestinal (GI) endoscopy, cardiac catheterization, dressing changes, and minor procedures (eg, casts and bone marrow aspiration). Requirements vary depending on the patient and the procedure, ranging from anxiolysis (minimal sedation), to conscious sedation (moderate sedation and analgesia), to deep sedation/analgesia, and finally to general anesthesia. For all practical purposes, the same standards and guidelines that are provided for general anesthesia are also applied to moderate and deep sedation. This includes preoperative preparation (eg, fasting), assessment, monitoring, and postoperative care. Airway obstruction and hypoventilation are the most commonly encountered problems. With deep sedation and general anesthesia, cardiovascular depression can also be a problem.

Table 44–3 includes doses of sedatives/hypnotic drugs. One of the most commonly used sedatives, particularly by nonanesthesiologists, is chloral hydrate, 25–

100 mg/kg orally or rectally. It has a slow onset of up to 60 min and a long half-life (8–11 h) that results in prolonged somnolence. Although it generally has little effect on ventilation, it can cause fatal airway obstruction in patients with sleep apnea and in frail children. Like chloral hydrate, pentobarbital 1–3 mg/kg intramuscularly is an excellent long-acting sedative with a low incidence of respiratory depression when used alone. Midazolam, 0.5 mg/kg orally or 0.1–0.15 mg/kg intramuscularly, is particularly useful because its effects can be readily reversed with flumazenil. Doses should be reduced whenever more than one agent is used because of the potential for synergistic respiratory and cardiovascular depression.

By far the most useful sedative/hypnotic is propofol. Although the drug is not approved for sedation of pediatric ICU patients, it can be used safely for most procedures in doses up to 250 μg/kg/min. Supplemental oxygen and close monitoring of the airway, ventilation, and other vital signs are mandatory (as with other agents). A laryngeal mask airway is usually well tolerated at higher doses.

Emergence & Recovery

Pediatric patients are particularly vulnerable to two postanesthetic complications: laryngospasm and postintubation croup. As with adult patients, postoperative pain should be aggressively managed.

A. LARYNGOSPASM

Laryngospasm is a forceful, involuntary spasm of the laryngeal musculature caused by stimulation of the superior laryngeal nerve (see Chapter 5). It may occur at induction, emergence, or any time in between without an endotracheal tube. Laryngospasm is more common in young pediatric patients (almost 1 in 50) than in adults, being highest in infants 1–3 months old. Laryngospasm at the end of a procedure can usually be avoided by extubating the patient either awake (opening the eyes) or while deeply anesthetized (spontaneously breathing but not swallowing or coughing); both techniques have advocates. Extubation during the interval between these extremes, however, is generally recognized as hazardous. A recent URTI or exposure to secondhand tobacco smoke predisposes patients to laryngospasm on emergence. Treatment of laryngospasm includes gentle positive- pressure ventilation, forward jaw thrust, intravenous lidocaine (1–1.5 mg/kg), or paralysis with intravenous succinylcholine (0.5–1 mg/kg) or rocuronium (0.4 mg/kg) and controlled ventilation. Intramuscular succinylcholine (4–6 mg/kg) remains an acceptable alternative in patients without intravenous access and in whom more conservative measures have failed. Laryngospasm is usually an immediate postoperative event but may occur in the recovery room as the patient wakes up and chokes on pharyngeal secretions. For this reason, recovering pediatric patients should be positioned in the lateral position so that oral secretions pool and drain away from the vocal cords. As the child begins to regain consciousness, it is comforting to have the parents at the bedside.

B. POSTINTUBATION CROUP

Croup is due to glottic or tracheal edema. Because the narrowest part of the pediatric airway is the cricoid cartilage, this is the most susceptible area. Croup is less common with endotracheal tubes that are uncuffed and small enough to allow a slight gas leak at 10–25 cm H_2O. Postintubation croup is associated with early childhood (age 1–4 years), repeated intubation attempts, large endotracheal tubes, prolonged surgery, head and neck procedures, and excessive movement of the tube (eg, coughing with the tube in place, moving the patient's head). Intravenous dexamethasone (0.25–0.5 mg/kg) may prevent formation of edema, and inhalation of nebulized racemic epinephrine (0.25–0.5 mL of a 2.25% solution in 2.5 mL normal saline) is an effective treatment. Although postintubation croup is a complication that occurs later than laryngospasm, it almost always appears within 3 h after extubation.

C. POSTOPERATIVE PAIN MANAGEMENT

Pain in pediatric patients has received considerable attention in recent years, particularly the use of regional anesthetic techniques (above). Commonly used parenteral opioids include fentanyl 1–2 μg/kg, morphine 0.05–0.1 mg/kg, hydromorphone 0.015 mg/kg, and meperidine 0.5 mg/kg. Ketorolac (0.5–0.75 mg/kg) significantly lowers opioid requirements. Rectal acetaminophen (40 mg/kg) may also be helpful.

Patient-controlled analgesia (see Chapter 18) can also be successfully used in patients as young as 6–7 years old, depending on their maturity and on preoperative preparation. The most commonly used opioids are morphine and hydromorphone. With a 10-min lockout interval, the recommended interval dose is either morphine 20 μg/kg or hydromorphone 5 μg/kg. As with adults, continuous infusions increase the risk of respiratory depression; recommended continuous infusion doses are morphine 0–12 μg/kg/h or hydromorphone 0-3 μg/kg/h. The subcutaneous route may be used with morphine.

As with adults, epidural infusions for postoperative analgesia usually consist of a local anesthetic plus an opioid. Bupivacaine 0.1–0.125% or ropivacaine 0.1–0.2% are used with fentanyl 2–2.5 μg/mL. Recommended infusion rates depend on the size of the patient, the final drug concentration, and the location of the epidural catheter, and range from 0.1 to 0.4 mL/kg/h.

■ PATHOPHYSIOLOGY & ANESTHETIC CONSIDERATIONS IN SPECIFIC PEDIATRIC DISORDERS

PREMATURITY

Pathophysiology

Prematurity is defined as birth before 37 weeks of gestation. This is in contrast to "small for gestational age," which describes an infant (full-term or premature) whose age-adjusted weight is less than the fifth percentile. The multiple medical problems of premature neonates are usually due to immaturity of major organ systems or to intrauterine asphyxia. Pulmonary complications include hyaline membrane disease, apneic spells, and bronchopulmonary dysplasia. Exogenous pulmonary surfactant has proved to be an effective treatment for respiratory distress syndrome in premature infants. A patent ductus arteriosus leads to shunting, pulmonary edema, and congestive heart failure. Persistent hypoxia or shock may result in an ischemic gut and necrotizing enterocolitis. Prematurity increases susceptibility to infection, hypothermia, intracranial hemorrhage, and kernicterus. Premature neonates also have an increased incidence of congenital anomalies.

Anesthetic Considerations

The small size (often less than 1000 g) and fragile medical condition of premature neonates demand meticulous anesthetic technique. Obviously, special attention must be paid to airway control, fluid management, and temperature regulation. The problem of the retinopathy of prematurity, a fibrovascular proliferation overlying the retina that leads to progressive visual loss, deserves special consideration. While hyperoxia is associated with this blinding disease, the presence of fetal hemoglobin and treatment with vitamin E may be protective. Recent evidence suggests that fluctuating oxygen levels may be more damaging than high oxygen tensions. Moreover, other major risk factors, such as respiratory distress, apnea, mechanical ventilation, hypoxia, hypercarbia, acidosis, heart disease, bradycardia, infection, parenteral nutrition, anemia, and multiple blood transfusions, must be present. Nonetheless, oxygenation should be continuously monitored with pulse oximetry or transcutaneous oxygen analysis, with particular attention given to infants younger than 44 weeks postconception. Normal PaO_2 is 60–80 mm Hg in neonates. Excessive inspired oxygen concentrations are avoided by blending oxygen with air or nitrous oxide. High inspired oxygen tensions can also predispose to chronic lung disease.

Anesthetic requirements of premature neonates are reduced. Opioid agonists, such as fentanyl, are often favored over volatile anesthetics because of the tendency of the latter to cause myocardial depression. Even nitrous oxide can cause significant cardiovascular depression. Muscle relaxants provide good surgical conditions, and ventilation is controlled.

Premature infants who are less than 50 (some authorities would say 60) weeks postconceptional age at the time of surgery are prone to postoperative episodes of obstructive and central apnea for up to 24 h. In fact, even term infants can experience—albeit rarely—apneic spells following general anesthesia. **Risk factors for postanesthetic apnea include a low gestational age at birth, anemia (< 30%), hypothermia, sepsis, and neurological abnormalities.** The risk of postanesthetic apnea may be decreased by intravenous administration of caffeine (10 mg/kg) or aminophylline.

Nonetheless, elective or outpatient procedures should be deferred until the preterm infant reaches the age of at least 50 weeks postconception. A 6-month symptom-free interval has been suggested for infants with a history of apneic episodes or bronchopulmonary dysplasia. If surgery must be performed earlier, monitoring with pulse oximetry for 12–24 h postoperatively is mandatory for infants less than 50 weeks postconception; infants between 50 and 60 weeks postconception should be closely observed in the postanesthesia recovery unit for at least 2 h.

Sick, premature neonates often receive multiple aliquots of blood during their stay in the pediatric intensive care unit. Their immunocompromised status predisposes them to clinically significant cytomegalovirus infection following transfusion. Signs of infection include generalized lymphadenopathy, fever, pneumonia, hepatitis, hemolytic anemia, and thrombocytopenia. Preventive measures include using cytomegalovirus-seronegative donor blood or frozen blood cells.

INTESTINAL MALROTATION & VOLVULUS

Pathophysiology

Malrotation of the intestines is a developmental abnormality that permits spontaneous abnormal rotation of the midgut around the mesentery (superior mesenteric artery). The incidence of malrotation is estimated to be about 1:500 live births. The majority of patients with malrotation of the midgut present during infancy with symptoms of acute or chronic bowel obstruction. Coiling of the duodenum with the ascending colon can produce complete or partial duodenal obstruction. The most serious complication of malrotation, a midgut volvulus, can rapidly compromise intestinal blood supply. Midgut volvulus is a true surgical emergency that most commonly occurs in infancy, with up to one-third occurring in the first week of life. Patients typically present with bilious vomiting, progressive abdominal distention and tenderness, metabolic acidosis, and hemodynamic instability. Bloody diarrhea may be indicative of bowel infarction. Abdominal ultrasonography or upper gastrointestinal imaging confirms the diagnosis.

Anesthetic Considerations

Definitive treatment of malrotation and midgut volvulus is surgical correction. If obstruction is present but obvious volvulus has not yet occurred, preoperative preparation may include stabilization of any coexisting conditions, insertion of a nasogastric (or orogastric tube) to help decompress the abdomen, broad-spectrum antibiotics, fluid and electrolyte replacement, and expedition of transport to the operating room.

Patients are at high risk for pulmonary aspiration. Depending on the size of the patient, after adequate preoxygenation, awake intubation or rapid sequence induction should be employed. Patients with volvulus are usually hypovolemic and acidotic, and often tolerate anesthesia poorly. In such instances ketamine may be the preferred anesthetic agent. An opioid-based anesthetic is also recommended as postoperative ventilation is usually necessary. Aggressive fluid resuscitation, including blood products, and sodium bicarbonate therapy are also usually necessary. Invasive monitoring is very helpful. Surgical treatment involves reducing the volvulus, freeing the obstruction, widening the base of mesenteric attachments, and resecting the obviously necrotic bowel. Bowel edema can complicate abdominal closure and has the potential to produce an abdominal compartment syndrome. The latter can impair ventilation, hinder venous return, and produce renal compromise; temporary closure with a Silastic silo may be necessary. A second-look laparotomy may be required 24–48 h later to ensure viability of the remaining bowel. Mortality of volvulus is high (up to 25%).

CONGENITAL DIAPHRAGMATIC HERNIA

Pathophysiology

During fetal development, the gut can herniate into the thorax through one of three possible diaphragmatic defects: the left or right posterolateral foramen of Bochdalek or the anterior foramen of Morgagni. The reported incidence of diaphragmatic hernia is 1 in 3000–5000 live births. Left-sided herniation is the most common type (90%). Hallmarks of **diaphragmatic herniation** include hypoxia, a scaphoid abdomen, and evidence of bowel in the thorax by auscultation or radiography. Congenital diaphragmatic hernia is often diagnosed antenatally as a result of a routine ultrasound examination. A reduction in alveoli and bronchioli (pulmonary hypoplasia) and malrotation of the intestines are almost always present. The ipsilateral lung is particularly impaired and the herniated gut can compress and retard the maturation of both lungs. Diaphragmatic hernia is often accompanied by marked pulmonary hypertension and is associated with 40–50% mortality. Cardiopulmonary compromise is generally thought to be primarily due to pulmonary hypoplasia and pulmonary hypertension rather than to the mass effect of the herniated viscera.

Treatment is aimed at immediate stabilization with sedation, paralysis, and moderate hyperventilation. Pressure-limited ventilation is used. Some centers employ permissive hypercapnia (postductal $PaCO_2$ < 65 mm Hg) and accept mild hypoxemia (preductal SpO_2 > 85%) in an effort to reduce pulmonary barotrauma. High-frequency oscillatory ventilation (HFOV) can improve ventilation and oxygenation with less barotrauma. Inhaled nitric oxide may be used to lower pulmonary artery pressures but does not appear to improve survival. If the pulmonary hypertension stabilizes and there is little right-to-left shunting, early surgical repair may be undertaken. If the patient fails to stabilize, extracorporeal membrane oxygenation (ECMO) may be undertaken in some centers. ECMO usually involves pumping blood from the right atrium through a membrane oxygenator and countercurrent heat exchanger before returning it to the ascending aorta (venoarterial ECMO). Alternatively, blood can be returned to the femoral vein (venovenous ECMO). Timing of the repair following ECMO is controversial. Treatment with prenatal intrauterine surgery appears promising.

Anesthetic Considerations

Gastric distention must be minimized by placement of a nasogastric tube and avoidance of high levels of positive-pressure ventilation. The neonate is preoxygenated and intubated awake, or without the aid of muscle relaxants. Anesthesia is maintained with low concentrations of volatile agents or opioids, muscle relaxants, and air as tolerated. Hypoxia and expansion of air in the bowel contraindicate the use of nitrous oxide. If possible, peak inspiratory airway pressures should be less than 30 cm H_2O. **A sudden fall in lung compliance, blood pressure, or oxygenation may signal a *contralateral* (usually right-sided) pneumothorax and necessitate placement of a chest tube.** Arterial blood gases are preferably monitored by sampling a preductal artery if an umbilical artery catheter is not already in place. Surgical repair is performed via a subcostal incision of the affected side; the bowel is reduced into the abdomen and the diaphragm is closed. Aggressive attempts at expansion of the ipsilateral lung following surgical decompression are detrimental. Postoperative prognosis parallels the extent of pulmonary hypoplasia and the presence of other congenital defects.

TRACHEOESOPHAGEAL FISTULA

Pathophysiology

There are several types of tracheoesophageal fistula (Figure 44–3). The most common (type IIIB) is the combination of an upper esophagus that ends in a blind pouch and a lower esophagus that connects to the trachea. Breathing results in gastric distention, whereas feeding leads to choking, coughing, and cyanosis (three Cs). The diagnosis is suspected by failure to pass a catheter into the

Figure 44–3. Of the five types of tracheoesophageal fistula, type IIIB represents 90% of cases.

stomach and confirmed by visualization of the catheter coiled in a blind, upper esophageal pouch. Aspiration pneumonia and the coexistence of other congenital anomalies (eg, cardiac) are common. These may also include the nonrandom association of *v*ertebral defects, *a*nal atresia, *t*racheoesophageal fistula with *e*sophageal atresia, and *r*adial dysplasia, known as the VATER syndrome. The VACTERL variant also includes *c*ardiac and *l*imb anomalies. Preoperative management is directed at identifying all congenital anomalies and preventing aspiration pneumonia. This may include nursing in a head-up position, an oral-esophageal tube, and avoiding feedings. In some instances a gastrostomy may be performed under local anesthesia. Definitive surgical treatment is usually postponed until any pneumonia clears or improves with antibiotic therapy.

Anesthetic Considerations

These neonates tend to have copious pharyngeal secretions that require frequent suctioning before and during surgery. Positive-pressure ventilation is avoided prior to intubation, as the resulting gastric distention may interfere with lung expansion. Intubation is often performed awake and without muscle relaxants. These neonates are often dehydrated and malnourished due to poor oral intake.

The key to successful management is correct endotracheal tube position. Ideally, the tip of the tube lies between the fistula and the carina, so that anesthetic gases pass into the lungs instead of the stomach. This is impossible if the fistula connects to the carina or a mainstem bronchus. In these situations, intermittent venting of a gastrostomy tube that has been placed preoperatively may permit positive-pressure ventilation without excessive gastric distention. Suctioning of the gastrostomy tube and upper esophageal pouch tube helps prevent aspiration pneumonia. Surgical division of the fistula and esophageal anastomosis is performed via a right extrapleural thoracotomy with the patient in the left lateral position. A precordial stethoscope should be placed in the dependent (left) axilla, since obstruction of the mainstem bronchus during surgical retraction is not uncommon. A drop in oxygen saturation indicates that the retracted lung needs to be reexpanded. Surgical retraction can also compress the great vessels, trachea, heart, and vagus nerve. Blood pressure should be continuously monitored with an arterial line. These infants usually require ventilation with 100% oxygen, despite the risk of the retinopathy of prematurity. Blood should be immediately available for transfusion. Postoperative complications include gastroesophageal reflux, aspiration pneumonia, tracheal compression, and anastomotic leakage. Most patients continue to require intubation and positive-pressure ventilation in the immediate postoperative period. Neck extension and instrumentation (eg, suctioning) of the esophagus may disrupt the surgical repair and should be avoided.

GASTROSCHISIS & OMPHALOCELE

Pathophysiology

Gastroschisis and omphalocele are congenital disorders characterized by defects in the abdominal wall that allow external herniation of viscera. Omphaloceles occur at the base of the umbilicus, have a hernia sac, and are often associated with other congenital anomalies such as trisomy 21, diaphragmatic hernia, and cardiac and bladder malformations. In contrast, the gastroschisis defect is usually lateral to the umbilicus, does not have a hernia sac, and is often an isolated finding. Antenatal diagnosis by ultrasound can be followed by elective cesarean section at 38 weeks and immediate surgical repair. Perioperative management centers around preventing hypothermia, infection, and dehydration. These problems are usually more serious in gastroschisis, as the protective hernial sac is absent.

Anesthetic Considerations

The stomach is decompressed with a nasogastric tube before induction. Intubation can be accomplished with the patient awake or asleep and with or without muscle relaxation. Nitrous oxide should be avoided to prevent further bowel distention. Muscle relaxation is required for replacing the bowel into the abdominal cavity. A one-stage closure (primary repair) is not always advisable, as it can cause an abdominal compartment syndrome. A staged closure with a temporary Dacron-reinforced Silastic silo may be initially necessary, followed by a second procedure a few days later for complete closure. Suggested criteria for a staged closure include intragastric or intravesical pressure > 20 cm H_2O, peak inspiratory pressure > 35 cm H_2O, or an end-tidal carbon dioxide > 50 mm Hg. **Third-space fluid losses are aggressively replaced with a balanced salt solution and 5% albumin.** The neonate remains intubated after the procedure and is weaned from the ventilator over the next 1–2 days in the intensive care unit.

HYPERTROPHIC PYLORIC STENOSIS

Pathophysiology

Hypertrophic pyloric stenosis interferes with emptying of gastric contents. **Persistent vomiting depletes sodium, potassium, chloride, and hydrogen ions, causing hypochloremic metabolic alkalosis.** Initially, the kidney tries to compensate for the alkalosis by excreting sodium bicarbonate in the urine. Later, as hyponatremia and dehydration worsen, the kidneys must conserve sodium even at the expense of hydrogen ion excretion (paradoxic aciduria). Correction of the volume deficit and metabolic alkalosis requires hydration with a sodium chloride solution supplemented with potassium. Because lactate is metabolized to bicarbonate, lactated Ringer's injection should not be used.

Anesthetic Considerations

Surgery should be postponed until fluid and electrolyte abnormalities have been corrected. The stomach should be emptied with a large nasogastric or orogastric tube; the tube should be suctioned with the patient in the supine, lateral, and prone positions. Techniques of intubation and induction vary, but in all cases the patient's high risk of aspiration must be considered. Experienced clinicians have advocated awake intubation, rapid sequence induction, and even careful inhalation induction in selected patients. Pyloromyotomy is a short procedure that requires muscle relaxation. These neonates may be at increased risk for respiratory depression and hypoventilation in the recovery room because of persistent metabolic or cerebrospinal fluid alkalosis.

INFECTIOUS CROUP, FOREIGN BODY ASPIRATION, & ACUTE EPIGLOTTITIS

Pathophysiology

Croup is obstruction of the airway characterized by a barking cough. One type of croup, postintubation croup, has already been discussed. Another type is due to viral infection. **Infectious croup** usually follows a viral URTI in children aged 3 months to 3 years. The airway *below* the epiglottis is involved (laryngotracheobronchitis). Infectious croup progresses slowly and rarely requires intubation. Foreign body aspiration is typically encountered in children aged 6 months to 5 years. Commonly aspirated objects include peanuts, coins, and small pieces of toys. Onset is typically acute and the obstruction may be supraglottic, glottic, or subglottic. Stridor is prominent with the first two, whereas wheezing is more common with the latter. A clear history of an aspiration may be absent. **Acute epiglottitis** is a bacterial infection (most commonly *Haemophilus influenzae* type B) classically affecting 2- to 6-year-old children. It rapidly progresses from a sore throat to dysphagia and complete airway obstruction. The term supraglottitis has been suggested because the inflammation typically involves all supraglottic structures. Endotracheal intubation and antibiotic therapy can be lifesaving. Epiglottitis has increasingly become a disease of adults because of the widespread use of *H influenza* vaccines in children.

Anesthetic Considerations

Patients with croup are managed conservatively with oxygen and mist therapy. Nebulized racemic epinephrine (0.5 mL of a 2.25% solution in 2.5 mL normal saline) and intravenous dexamethasone (0.25–0.5 mg/kg) are used. Indications for intubation include progressive intercostal retractions, obvious respiratory fatigue, and central cyanosis.

Anesthetic management of a foreign body aspiration is challenging, particularly with supraglottic and glottic obstruction. Minor manipulation of the airway can convert partial into complete obstruction. Experts recommend careful inhalational induction for a supraglottic object and gentle upper airway endoscopy to remove the object and/or secure the airway. When the object is subglottic, a rapid-sequence or inhalational induction is usually followed by rigid bronchoscopy by the surgeon or endotracheal intubation and flexible bronchoscopy. Surgical preferences may vary according to the size of the patient and the nature and location of the foreign body. Communication and close cooperation between the surgeon and anesthesiologist are essential.

Children with impending airway obstruction from epiglottitis present in the operating room for definitive diagnosis by laryngoscopy followed by intubation. A preoperative lateral neck radiograph may show a characteristic thumblike epiglottic shadow, which is very specific but often absent. The radiograph is also helpful in revealing other causes of obstruction, such as foreign bodies. Stridor, drooling, hoarseness, rapid onset and progression, tachypnea, chest retractions, and a preference for the upright position are predictive of airway obstruction. Total obstruction can occur at any moment, and adequate preparations for a possible tracheostomy must be made prior to induction of general anesthesia. Laryngoscopy should not be performed before induction of anesthesia because of the possibility of laryngospasm. In most cases, an inhalational induction is performed with the patient in the sitting position, using a volatile anesthetic and a high concentration of oxygen. Oral intubation with an endotracheal tube one-half to one size smaller than usual is attempted as soon as an adequate depth of anesthesia is established. The oral tube may be replaced with a well-secured nasal endotracheal tube at the end of the procedure, as the latter is better tolerated in the postoperative period. If intubation is impossible, rigid bronchoscopy or emergency tracheostomy must be performed.

TONSILLECTOMY & ADENOIDECTOMY

Pathophysiology

Lymphoid hyperplasia can lead to upper airway obstruction, obligate mouth breathing, and even pulmonary hypertension with cor pulmonale. Although these extremes of pathology are unusual, all children undergoing tonsillectomy or adenoidectomy should be considered to be at increased risk for perioperative airway problems.

Anesthetic Considerations

Surgery should be postponed if there is evidence of acute infection or suspicion of a clotting dysfunction (eg, recent aspirin ingestion). Preoperative administration of an anticholinergic will decrease pharyngeal secretions. A history of airway obstruction or apnea suggests an inhalational induction without paralysis until the ability to ventilate with positive pressure is established. A reinforced or preformed endotracheal tube (eg, RAE tube) may decrease the risk of kinking by the surgeon's self-retaining mouth gag. Blood transfusion is usually not necessary, but the anesthesiologist must be wary of occult blood loss. Meticulous but gentle inspection and suctioning of the pharynx precede extubation. Although deep extubation decreases the chance of laryngospasm and may prevent blood clot dislodgment from coughing, most anesthesiologists prefer an awake extubation because of the risks of aspiration. Postoperative vomiting is common. The anesthesiologist must be alert in the recovery room for postoperative bleeding, which may be evidenced by restlessness, pallor, tachycardia, or hypotension. If reoperation is necessary to control bleeding, intravascular volume must first be restored. Evacuation of stomach contents with a nasogastric tube is followed by a rapid-sequence induction with cricoid pressure. Because of the possibility of bleeding and airway obstruction, children younger than 3 years old may be hospitalized for the first postoperative night. Sleep apnea and recent infection increase the risk of postoperative complications.

MYRINGOTOMY & INSERTION OF TYMPANOSTOMY TUBES

Pathophysiology

Children presenting for myringotomy and insertion of tympanostomy tubes have a long history of upper respiratory infections that have spread through the eustachian tube, causing episodes of otitis media. Causative organisms are usually bacterial and include *Pneumococcus, H influenza, Streptococcus,* and *Mycoplasma pneumoniae.* Myringotomy, a radial incision in the tympanic membrane, releases any fluid that has accumulated in the middle ear. Tympanostomy tubes provide long-term ventilation and drainage. Because of the chronic and recurring nature of this illness, it is not surprising that these patients often have symptoms of a URTI on the day of scheduled surgery (see Recent Upper Respiratory Tract Infection, above).

Anesthetic Considerations

These are typically very short (10–15 min) outpatient procedures. An inhalational induction with nitrous oxide, oxygen, and halothane is a common technique. Unlike tympanoplasty surgery, nitrous oxide diffusion into the middle ear is not a problem during myringotomy because of the brief period of anesthetic exposure before the middle ear is vented. Because most of these patients are otherwise healthy and there is no blood loss, intravenous access is usually not necessary. Ventilation with a face mask or LMA minimizes the risk of perioperative respiratory complications (eg, laryngospasm) associated with intubation.

TRISOMY 21 SYNDROME (DOWN SYNDROME)

Pathophysiology

An additional chromosome 21—part or whole—results in the most common congenital pattern of human malformation: Down syndrome. Characteristic abnormalities of interest to the anesthesiologist include a short neck, irregular dentition, mental retardation, hypotonia, and a large tongue. Associated abnormalities include congenital heart disease in 40% of patients (particularly endocardial cushion defects and ventricular septal defect), subglottic stenosis, tracheoesophageal fistula, chronic pulmonary infections, and seizures. These neonates are often premature and small for their gestational age. Later in life many patients with Down syndrome often require multiple procedures requiring general anesthesia.

Anesthetic Considerations

Because of anatomic differences, these patients often have difficult airways, particularly during infancy. The size of the endotracheal tube required is typically smaller than that predicted by age. Respiratory complications such as postoperative stridor and apnea are common. Neck flexion during laryngoscopy and intubation may result in atlantooccipital dislocation because of the congenital laxity of these ligaments. The possibility of associated congenital diseases must always be considered. As in all pediatric patients, care must be taken to avoid air bubbles in the intravenous line because of possible right-to-left shunts (paradoxic air embolus).

CYSTIC FIBROSIS

Pathophysiology

Cystic fibrosis is a hereditary disease of the exocrine glands primarily affecting the pulmonary and gastrointestinal systems. Abnormally thick and viscous secretions coupled with decreased ciliary activity lead to pneumonia, wheezing, and bronchiectasis. Pulmonary function studies reveal increased residual volume and airway resistance with decreased vital capacity and expiratory flow rate. Malabsorption syndrome may lead to dehydration and electrolyte abnormalities.

Anesthetic Considerations

Premedication should not include respiratory depressants. Anticholinergic drugs are controversial, but they have been used in large series without ill effects. Induction with inhalational anesthetics may be prolonged in patients with severe pulmonary disease. Intubation should not be performed until the patient is deeply anesthetized to avoid coughing and stimulation of mucus secretions. Aggressive suctioning throughout the anesthesia and before extubation minimizes the accumulation of pulmonary secretions. Intraoperative hyperventilation will cause shallow respirations postoperatively and should be avoided. Outcome is favorably influenced by aggressive preoperative and postoperative respiratory therapy that includes bronchodilators, incentive spirometry, postural drainage, and pathogen-specific antibiotic therapy.

SCOLIOSIS

Pathophysiology

Scoliosis is lateral rotation and curvature of the vertebrae and a deformity of the rib cage. It is classified by etiology: idiopathic, congenital, neuromuscular, traumatic, and so on. Scoliosis can affect cardiac and respiratory function. Elevated pulmonary vascular resistance from chronic hypoxia causes pulmonary hypertension and right ventricular hypertrophy. Respiratory abnormalities include reduced lung volumes and chest wall compliance. PaO_2 is reduced as a result of ventilation/perfusion mismatching, whereas an increased $PaCO_2$ signals severe disease.

Anesthetic Considerations

Preoperative evaluation should include pulmonary function tests, arterial blood gases, and electrocardiography. Corrective surgery is complicated by the prone position, significant blood loss, and the possibility of paraplegia. Spinal cord function can be assessed by neurophysiological monitoring (somatosensory and motor evoked potentials, see Chapter 6) or by waking the patient intraoperatively to test lower limb muscle strength. Patients with severe respiratory disease are often left intubated postoperatively. Patients with scoliosis due to muscular dystrophy are predisposed to malignant hyperthermia, cardiac dysrhythmias, and untoward effects of succinylcholine (hyperkalemia, myoglobinuria, and sustained muscular contractures).

CASE DISCUSSION:
MASSETER SPASM
& MALIGNANT HYPERTHERMIA

A 4-year-old boy is scheduled for correction of strabismus. Inhalational induction with nitrous oxide and halothane is followed by the intravenous administration of atropine and succinylcholine. Rigidity of the masseter muscle prevents mouth opening and intubation.

What is malignant hyperthermia?

Malignant hyperthermia (MH) is a rare (1:15,000 in pediatric patients and 1:40,000 adult patients) myopathy, characterized by an acute hypermetabolic state within muscle tissue following induction of general anesthesia. It can also present in the postoperative period more than an hour after anesthesia and even without exposure to known triggering agents, albeit rarely. Although most cases are reported in pediatric patients, all ages can be affected. The earliest signs reported during anesthesia are masseter muscle rigidity (MMR), tachycardia, and hypercarbia due to increased CO_2 production (Table 44–7). Two or more of these signs greatly increase the likelihood of MH. Tachypnea is prominent when muscle relaxants are not used. Sympathetic system overactivity produces tachycardia, arrhythmias, hypertension, and mottled cyanosis. Hyperthermia may be a late sign, but when it occurs, core temperature can rise as much as 1°C every 5 min. Generalized muscle rigidity is not consistently present. Hypertension may be rapidly followed by hypotension as cardiac depression occurs.

Table 44–7. Signs of malignant hyperthermia.

Hypermetabolism
Increased carbon dioxide production
Increased oxygen consumption
Low mixed venous oxygen tension
Metabolic acidosis
Cyanosis
Mottling
Increased sympathetic activity
Tachycardia
Initial hypertension
Arrhythmias
Muscle damage
Masseter spasm
Generalized rigidity
Elevated serum creatine kinase
Hyperkalemia
Hypernatremia
Hyperphosphatemia
Myoglobinemia
Myglobinuria
Hyperthermia
Fever
Sweating

Dark colored urine reflects myoglobinemia and myoglobinuria.

Laboratory evaluation reveals a mixed metabolic and respiratory acidosis, a marked base deficit, hyperkalemia, hypermagnesemia, and a very low mixed venous oxygen saturation. Serum ionized calcium concentration may initially increase before it falls. Patients also typically have increased serum myoglobin, creatine kinase (CK), lactic dehydrogenase, and aldolase levels. Serum CK levels usually exceed 20,000 IU/L. It should be noted that both serum myoglobin and CK levels can increase markedly in some normal patients after succinylcholine administration without MH.

Part of the problem in diagnosing MH is its variable presentation during or after an anesthetic. For instance, fever is an inconsistent and often late sign. The unanticipated doubling or tripling of end-tidal carbon dioxide is one of the earliest and most sensitive indicators of MH. Ventricular fibrillation can follow the onset of MH within minutes and is the most common cause of death. If the patient survives the first few minutes acute renal failure and disseminated intravascular coagulation can develop rapidly. Other complications of hyperthermia include cerebral edema with seizures and hepatic failure.

What is the pathophysiology of MH?

Succinylcholine or a halogenated anesthetic agent alone may trigger an episode of MH (Table 44–8). In 80% of reported cases, both succinylcholine and a halogenated anesthetic agent were used. Nearly 50% of patients with an episode of MH have had a previous uneventful anesthetic where they were exposed to a triggering agent. Why MH does not occur after every exposure to a triggering agent is unclear. Although the precise cellular origin of MH

remains poorly understood, investigations reveal an uncontrolled increase in intracellular calcium in skeletal muscle. The sudden release of calcium from sarcoplasmic reticulum removes the inhibition of troponin, resulting in intense muscle contractions. Markedly enhanced and sustained adenosine triphosphatase activity results in an uncontrolled increase in aerobic and anaerobic metabolism. The hypermetabolic state rapidly progresses, markedly increasing oxygen consumption and CO_2 production and producing severe lactic acidosis and hyperthermia. As muscle membranes break down, an efflux of potassium from muscle cells together with systemic acidosis produces hyperkalemia. Increased sympathetic tone, acidosis, and hyperkalemia all predispose patients to ventricular fibrillation and sudden death, which may occur in as little as 15 min.

The initial focus of investigations was on an abnormal ryanodine Ryr_1 receptor in patients with MH. This calcium channel receptor is responsible for calcium release from the sarcoplasmic reticulum and plays a critical role in muscle depolarization. However, further studies have revealed that many MH patients have a normal ryanodine receptor and that abnormalities in secondary messengers and modulators of calcium release, such as fatty acids and phosphatidylinositol, may be present. An abnormal sodium channel in skeletal muscle may also play a role in some patients.

How should an episode of MH be treated?

Treatment is directed at terminating the episode and treating complications such as acidosis and hyperkalemia. The triggering agent must be stopped and dantrolene must be given immediately. The mortality of MH even with prompt treatment may still be as high as 5–30%.

Because succinylcholine and volatile anesthetics are considered to be the principal triggering agents, they should be discontinued immediately. Even trace amounts of anesthetics absorbed by soda lime, breathing tubes, and breathing bags may be detrimental. The patient should be aggressively ventilated with 100% oxygen to minimize the effects of hypercapnia, metabolic acidosis, and increased oxygen consumption. If fever is present, cooling measures should also be instituted immediately. Surface cooling with ice packs over major arteries, cold air convection, and cooling blankets are used. Iced saline lavage of the stomach and body cavities (whenever possible) should also be instituted. Cold dialysis and cardiopulmonary bypass may also be appropriate if other measures fail.

Table 44–8. Drugs known to trigger malignant hyperthermia.

Halogenated general anesthetics
Ether
Cyclopropane
Halothane
Methoxyflurane
Enflurane
Isoflurane
Desflurane
Sevoflurane
Nondepolarizing muscle relaxants
Succinylcholine

MALIGNANT HYPERTHERMIA PROTOCOL

1. Discontinue volatile anesthetic and succinylcholine. *Call for help!*

2. Hyperventilate with 100% O_2 at high flows.

3. Administer sodium bicarbonate, 1–2 mEq/kg intravenously.

4. Mix dantrolene sodium with sterile distilled water and administer 2.5 mg/kg intravenously *as soon as possible*.

5. Institute cooling measures (lavage, cooling blanket, cold intravenous solutions).

6. Administer inotropes and antiarrhythmic agents as necessary.

7. Administer additional doses of dantrolene if needed.

8. Change anesthetic tubing and soda lime.

9. Monitor urinary output, K^+, Ca^{2+}, blood gases, end-tidal carbon dioxide; perform clotting studies.

10. Treat severe hyperkalemia with dextrose, 25–50 g intravenously, and regular insulin, 10–20 U intravenously (adult dose).

11. Consider invasive monitoring of arterial blood pressure and central venous pressure.

12. If necessary, consult on-call physicians at the 24-hour MHAUS hotline, **1-800-MH-HYPER**.

An arterial line will provide precise blood pressure monitoring and access to serial arterial blood gas measurements. Acidosis should be treated aggressively with intravenous sodium bicarbonate 1–2 mEq/kg. Hyperkalemia should be treated with insulin and glucose and with diuresis. Intravenous calcium should be used cautiously, if at all. Antiarrhythmic agents and catecholamine vasopressors and inotropes are considered safe if used appropriately. Calcium channel blockers should not be used with dantrolene because this combination appears to promote hyperkalemia. Mannitol infusion 0.5 g/kg and/or furosemide should be used to establish a diuresis and prevent acute renal failure from myoglobinuria. Nonetheless, the mainstay of therapy for an MH crisis is immediate administration of intravenous dantrolene.

Describe the mechanism of action of dantrolene, its recommended dosage, and its possible side effects.

Dantrolene, a hydantoin derivative, directly interferes with muscle contraction by binding the Ryr_1 receptor calcium channel and inhibiting calcium ion release from the sarcoplasmic reticulum. This intracellular dissociation of excitation–contraction coupling contrasts with the depolarizing and nondepolarizing muscle relaxants that antagonize the extracellular neuromuscular junction. The dose is 2.5 mg/kg intravenously every 5 min until the episode is terminated. The upper limit of dantrolene therapy is generally 10 mg/kg. Dantrolene is packaged as 20 mg of lyophilized powder to be dissolved in 60 mL of sterile water. Depending on the dose required, reconstitution can be time consuming. The effective half-life of dantrolene is about 6 h. After initial control, dantrolene 1 mg/kg intravenously is recommended every 6 h for 24–48 h to prevent relapse because MH can recur within 24 h. It should be noted that dantrolene is not specific for MH; it also decreases temperature in thyroid storm and neuroleptic malignant syndrome. Dantrolene is a relatively safe drug. Although chronic therapy for spastic disorders has been associated with hepatic dysfunction, the most serious complication following acute administration is generalized muscle weakness that may result in respiratory insufficiency or aspiration pneumonia. Dantrolene can cause phlebitis in small peripheral veins and should be given through a central venous line if one is available. The safety and efficacy of dantrolene call for its immediate use in this potentially life-threatening disease.

What is the differential diagnosis of masseter spasm during intubation?

Masseter muscle spasm, also known as MMR, or trismus, is a forceful contraction of the jaw musculature that prevents full mouth opening. This contrasts with incomplete jaw relaxation, which is a fairly common finding. Both myotonia and MH can cause masseter spasm. The two disorders can be differentiated by the medical history, neurological examination, and electromyography. The incidence of masseter spasm following administration of succinylcholine in pediatric patients at some medical centers may be higher than 1%. Isolated MMR occurs in only 15–30% of true MH episodes. Moreover, less than 50% of patients in whom MMR develops prove to be susceptible to MH by muscle testing. The safest course is to assume that masseter spasm is due to MH and to postpone elective surgery. However, if there are no other signs of MH, and if monitoring and treatment capabilities are readily available, some anesthesiologists will allow surgery to continue and use a safe (nontriggering) anesthetic. Serum CK levels should be followed for 24 h after an episode of MMR, because an elevation of this enzyme may indicate an underlying myopathy.

Which patients should be considered at increased risk for developing MH?

Several musculoskeletal diseases are associated with a relatively high incidence of MH. These include Duchenne's muscular dystrophy, central-core disease, and osteogenesis imperfecta. King–Denborough syndrome is consistently associated with MH. This syndrome is seen primarily in young boys who exhibit short stature, mental retardation, cryptorchidism, kyphoscoliosis, pectus deformity, slanted eyes, low-set ears, webbed neck, and winged scapulae.

Operations associated with an increased incidence of MH include orthopedic cases (joint-dislocation repair), ophthalmic surgery (ptosis and strabismus correction), and head and neck procedures (cleft palate repair, tonsillectomy and adenoidectomy, dental surgery). Other possible clues to susceptibility include a family history of anesthetic complications, intolerance to caffeine-containing foods, or a history of unexplained fevers or muscular cramps. Prior uneventful anesthesia and absence of a positive family history are notoriously unreliable predictors of susceptibility to MH, however. As previously mentioned, any patient in whom trismus develops during induction of anesthesia should be considered to be susceptible to MH.

What type of hereditary pattern does MH follow?

Although sporadic cases are described, most patients with an episode of MH have a history of relatives with a similar episode or an abnormal halothane–caffeine contracture test. An autosomal pattern of dominance with variable penetrance occurs in about 50% of susceptible families. The complexity of genetic inheritance patterns in families reflects the fact that MH is a heterogeneous genetic disorder; it can be caused by mutations of one or more genes on more than one chromosome. Thus, genes on chromosomes 1, 3, 7, 17, and 19 have been linked with MH in different families. The earliest reports linked MH with mutations in the gene for the skeletal muscle, ryanodine (Ryr_1) receptor, calcium release channel on chromosome 19 in humans. Subsequent reports on other families linked MH with mutations in the adult muscle, sodium channel, α-subunit gene on chromosome 17. An autosomal recessive form of MH has been associated with the King–Denborough syndrome. Reports of MH vary greatly from country to country and even in different geographic localities within a country, reflecting varying gene pools. The Midwest appears to have the highest incidence of MH in the United States.

How is susceptibility to MH confirmed?

Patients who have survived an unequivocal episode of MH are considered susceptible. If the diagnosis remains in doubt postoperatively, a biopsy of a fresh section of living skeletal muscle is obtained and exposed to a caffeine, halothane, or combination caffeine–halothane bath. The halothane–caffeine contracture test may have a 10–20% false-positive rate, but the false-negative rate is close to zero. Because of the relative complexity of this test, only a few centers worldwide perform it. Both European and North American MH registries have been established to help physicians identify and treat patients with suspected MH, as well as provide standardization between testing centers. The Malignant Hyperthermia Association of the United States (MHAUS, telephone 1-800-98-MHAUS) operates a 24-hour hotline (1-800-MH-HYPER), an on-demand fax service (1-800-440-9990), and a Web site (http://www.mhaus.org). If the halothane–caffeine contracture test is positive, genetic counseling and testing of family members are appropriate. Baseline CK may be elevated chronically in 50–70% of people at risk for MH, but the only reliable way to diagnose MH susceptibility is by muscle testing.

How does MH differ from neuroleptic malignant syndrome?

Neuroleptic malignant syndrome (NMS) is characterized by hyperthermia, muscle rigidity with extrapyramidal signs (dyskinesia), altered consciousness, and autonomic lability in patients receiving antidopaminergic agents. The syndrome is caused by an imbalance of neurotransmitters in the central nervous system. A functional dopamine deficiency results in hyperactivity of excitatory amino acids in the basal ganglia and hypothalamus. It can occur either during drug therapy with antidopaminergic agents (phenothiazines, butyrophenones, thioxanthines, dibenzoxapines, or metoclopramide) or less commonly following the withdrawal of dopaminergic agonists (levodopa or amantadine) in patients with Parkinson's disease. Thus, it appears to involve abnormal central dopaminergic activity, as opposed to the altered peripheral calcium release seen in MH. These differing mechanisms probably explain why nondepolarizing relaxants reverse the rigidity of NMS, but not the rigidity associated with MH. NMS does not appear to be inherited and typically takes hours to weeks to develop; the majority of episodes develop within 2 weeks of a dose adjustment. Hyperthermia generally tends to be mild, and appears to be proportional to the amount of rigidity. Autonomic dysfunction results in tachycardia, labile blood pressure, diaphoresis, dyspnea, increased secretions, and urinary incontinence. Muscle rigidity can produce respiratory distress and, together with the increased secretions, can promote aspiration pneumonia. CK levels are typically elevated; some patients may develop rhabdomyolysis resulting in myoglobinemia, myoglobinuria, and renal failure.

Mild forms of the NMS promptly resolve after withdrawal of the causative drug (or reinstitution of antiparkinsonian therapy). Initial treatment of more severe forms of NMS should include oxygen therapy and endotracheal intubation for respiratory distress or altered consciousness. Marked muscle rigidity can be controlled with muscle paralysis, dantrolene, or a dopaminergic agonist (amantadine, bromocriptine, or levodopa), depending on the severity and acuity of the syndrome. Resolution of the muscle rigidity usually decreases body temperature.

Although this syndrome is considered a separate entity from MH, many clinicians believe that NMS may predispose patients to MH. Patients with NMS should probably not receive succinylcholine or a volatile anesthetic; however, patients susceptible to MH can safely receive phenothiazines.

What other diseases can present like MH?

A number of other disorders may resemble MH (Table 44–9). Surgery and anesthesia can precipitate **thyroid storm** in undiagnosed or poorly controlled hyperthyroid patients. Its signs include tachycardia, tachyarrhythmias (particularly atrial fibrillation), hyperthermia (often $\geq 40°C$), hypotension, and in some cases congestive heart failure. In contrast to MH, hypokalemia is very common. Also unlike the typical intraoperative presentation of MH, thyroid storm generally develops postoperatively (see Chapter 36 and Case Discussion, Chapter 48). Pheochromocytoma is associated with dramatic increases in heart rate and blood pressure but not end-tidal CO_2 (see Chapter 36) or temperature. Cardiac manifestations such as arrhythmias, ischemia, or congestive heart failure may also be prominent. Rarely, some patients may present with significant hyperthermia ($> 38°C$), which is generally thought to be due to increased heat production from catecholamine-mediated increases in metabolic rate together with decreased heat elimination from intense vasoconstriction. Sepsis shares several characteristics with MH, including fever, tachypnea, tachycardia, and metabolic acidosis (see Chapter 49). This can be a difficult differential diagnosis if there is no obvious primary site of infection. Less commonly, drug-induced hyperthermia may be encountered in the perioperative period with some drug combinations as well as in patients who have been taking certain illicit drugs. These drugs appear to markedly increase serotonin activity in the brain, causing hyperthermia, confusion, shivering, diaphoresis, hyperreflexia, and myoclonus. Combinations associated with this "serotonin syndrome" include monoamine oxidase inhibitors (MAOIs) and meperidine, and MAOIs and selective serotonin reuptake inhibitors (SSRIs). Hyperthermia can also be caused by some illicit drugs, including 3,4-methylenedioxymethamphetamine (MDMA or "ecstasy"), "crack" cocaine, amphetamines, phenylcyclidine (PCP), and lysergic acid diethylamine (LSD). Iatrogenic hyperthermia is not uncommon, particularly in pediatric patients. Common sources of excessive heat in the operating room include humidifiers on ventilators, warming blankets, heat lamps, as well as ambient temperature. Brain stem or hypothalamic injury near the hypothalamus and brain stem can be associated with marked hyperthermia, but this diagnosis requires exclusion of all other causes.

MH, however, is associated with more dramatic degrees of metabolic acidosis and venous desaturation than are any of these diseases.

What constitutes a safe anesthetic in patients who are susceptible to MH?

Thiopental and pancuronium appear to be protective, as they raise the triggering threshold for MH. Other safe drugs include nitrous oxide,

Table 44–9. Differential diagnosis of hyperthermia in the intraoperative and immediate postoperative periods.

Malignant hyperthermia
Neuroleptic malignant syndrome
Thyroid storm
Pheochromocytoma
Drug-induced hyperthermia
    Serotonin syndrome
Iatrogenic hyperthermia
Brain stem/hypothalamic injury
Sepsis
Transfusion reaction

---

propofol, etomidate, benzodiazepines, ketamine, opiates, droperidol, and all local anesthetics. An adequate supply of dantrolene should always be available wherever general anesthesia is provided. Prophylactic use of intravenous dantrolene prior to induction of general anesthesia in susceptible patients is probably not necessary if a safe anesthetic is administered. A minimum recovery room stay of 4 h has been recommended for patients who are susceptible to MH.

SUGGESTED READING

American Academy of Pediatrics—Section on Anesthesiology: Guidelines for the pediatric anesthesia environment. Pediatrics 1999;103:512.

American Society of Anesthesiologists Task Force on Preoperative Fasting: Practice Guidelines for preoperative fasting and the use of pharmacological agents to reduce the risk of pulmonary aspiration: application to healthy patient undergoing elective procedures. Anesthesiology 1999;90:896.

Bissonnette B, Dalens B: *Principles & Practice of Pediatric Anesthesia.* McGraw-Hill, 2002.

Brandom BW, Fine GF: Neuromuscular blocking drugs in pediatric anesthesia. Anesth Clin North Am 2002;20:45.

Butler MG, Hayes BG, Hathaway MM, Begleiter ML: Specific genetic diseases at risk for sedation/anesthesia complications. Anesth Analg 2000;91:837.

Cote CJ, Todres ID, Goudsouzian NG, Ryan JF. *A Practice of Anesthesia for Infants and Children,* 3rd ed. W.B. Saunders, 2001.

De Beer DAH, Thomas ML: Caudal additives in children—solutions or problems? Br J Anaesth 2003;90:487.

Fishkin S, Litman RS: Current issues in pediatric ambulatory anesthesia. Anesth Clin North Am 2003;21:305.

Gregory GA (editor): *Pediatric Anesthesia,* 4th ed. Churchill Livingstone, 2001.

Hatch DJ, Hunter JM (editors): The paediatric patient. Br J Anaesth 1999;83:1.

Hopkins PM: Malignant hyperthermia: advances in clinical management and diagnosis. Br J Anaesth 2000;85:118.

Kaplan RF, Yang CI: Sedation and analgesia in pediatric patients for procedures outside the operating room. Anesth Clin North Am 2002;20:181.

Mazurek AJ, Rae B, Hann S, et al: Rocuronium versus succinylcholine: are they equally effective during rapid sequence induction of anesthesia? Anesth Analg 1998;87:1259.

Morray JP: Anesthesia-related cardiac arrest in children: an update. Anesth Clin North Am 2002;20:1.

Peutrell JM: *Regional Anaesthesia for Babies and Children.* Oxford University Press, 1997.

Ross AK, Eck JB, Tobias JD: Pediatric regional anesthesia: beyond the caudal. Anesth Analg 2000;91:16.

Salvo I, Vidyasagar D: *Anaesthesia and Intensive Care in Neonates and Children.* Springer-Verlag, 1999.

Skoulakis CE, Doxas PG, Papadakis CE, et al: Bronchoscopy for foreign body removal in children. A review and analysis of 210 cases. Int J Pediatr Otorhinolaryngol 2000;53:143.

Steward DJ, Lerman J: *Manual of Pediatric Anesthesia,* 5th ed. Churchill Livingstone, 2001.

Suresh S, Wheeler M: Practical pediatric regional anesthesia. Anesth Clin North Am 2002;20:83.

Geriatric Anesthesia

45

KEY CONCEPTS

1 In the absence of coexisting disease, resting systolic cardiac function appears to be preserved even in octogenarians. Increased vagal tone and decreased sensitivity of adrenergic receptors lead to a decline in heart rate.

2 Elderly patients undergoing evaluation for surgery have a high incidence of diastolic dysfunction that can be detected with Doppler echocardiography.

3 Diminished cardiac reserve in many elderly patients may be manifested as exaggerated drops in blood pressure during induction of general anesthesia. A prolonged circulation time delays the onset of intravenous drugs but speeds induction with inhalational agents.

4 Elasticity is decreased in lung tissue, allowing overdistention of alveoli and collapse of small airways. Airway collapse increases residual volume and closing capacity. Even in normal persons, closing capacity exceeds functional residual capacity at age 45 in the supine position and age 65 in the sitting position. When this happens, some airways close during part of normal tidal breathing, resulting in a mismatch of ventilation and perfusion.

5 Aging is associated with a decreasing response to β-adrenergic agents ("endogenous β-blockade").

6 Impairment of sodium handling, concentrating ability, and diluting capacity predisposes elderly patients to dehydration or fluid overload. As renal function declines, so does the kidney's ability to excrete drugs.

7 Hepatic function (reserves) declines in proportion to the decrease in liver mass.

8 Dosage requirements for local (minimum anesthetic concentration) and general (minimum alveolar concentration) anesthetics are reduced. Administration of a given volume of epidural anesthetic tends to result in more extensive cephalad spread in elderly patients, but with a shorter duration of analgesia and motor block. A longer duration of action should be expected from a spinal anesthetic.

9 Many elderly patients experience varying degrees of an acute confusional state, delirium, or cognitive dysfunction postoperatively.

10 Aging produces both pharmacokinetic and pharmacodynamic changes. Disease-related changes and wide interindividual variations even in similar populations lead to inconsistent generalizations.

11 Elderly patients display a lower dose requirement for propofol, etomidate, barbiturates, opioids, and benzodiazepines.

By the year 2040, people aged 65 or older are expected to make up 24% of the population and account for 50% of health care expenditures. Of these individuals half will require surgery before they die, despite being at a 3-fold increased risk for perioperative death compared with younger patients. Emergency surgery, surgical site, and physical status defined by the American Society of Anesthesiologists increase anesthetic risk (see Chapter 1). Operations associated with increased risk of perioperative mortality and morbidity for elderly patients

Table 45–1. Similarities between elderly people and infants, compared with the general population.

Decreased ability to increase heart rate in response to hypovolemia, hypotension, or hypoxia
Decreased lung compliance
Decreased arterial oxygen tension
Impaired ability to cough
Decreased renal tubular function
Increased susceptibility to hypothermia

include thoracic, intraperitoneal (particularly colon surgery), and major vascular procedures.

As with pediatric patients, optimal anesthetic management of geriatric patients depends on an understanding of the normal changes in physiology, anatomy, and response to pharmacological agents that accompany aging. In fact, there are many similarities between elderly and pediatric patients (Table 45–1). Compared with pediatric patients, however, older people show a wider range of variation in these parameters. The relatively high frequency of serious physiological abnormalities in elderly patients demands a particularly careful preoperative evaluation.

■ AGE-RELATED ANATOMIC & PHYSIOLOGICAL CHANGES

CARDIOVASCULAR SYSTEM

It is important to distinguish between changes in physiology that normally accompany aging and the pathophysiology of diseases common in the geriatric population (Table 45–2). For example, atherosclerosis is pathological—it is not present in healthy elderly patients. On the other hand, a reduction in arterial elasticity caused by fibrosis of the media is part of the normal aging process. Reduced arterial compliance results in increased afterload, elevated systolic blood pressure, and left ventricular hypertrophy. The left ventricular wall thickens at the expense of the left ventricular cavity. Some myocardial fibrosis and calcification of the valves are common. In the absence of coexisting disease, diastolic blood pressure remains unchanged or decreases. Baroreceptor function is depressed. Similarly, whereas cardiac output typically declines with age, it appears to be maintained in well-conditioned healthy individuals. In the absence of disease, resting systolic cardiac function appears to be preserved even in octogenarians. Increased vagal tone and decreased sensitivity of adrenergic receptors lead to a decline in heart rate; maximal heart rate declines by approximately one beat per minute per year of age over 50. Fibrosis of the conduction system and loss of sinoatrial node cells increase the incidence of dysrhythmias, particularly atrial fibrillation and flutter.

Elderly patients undergoing evaluation for surgery have a high incidence of diastolic dysfunction that can be detected with Doppler echocardiography. Marked diastolic dysfunction may be seen with systemic hypertension, coronary artery disease, cardiomyopathies, and valvular heart disease, particularly aortic stenosis. Patients may be asymptomatic or complain of exercise intolerance, dyspnea, cough, or fatigue. Diastolic dysfunction results in relatively large increases in ventricular end-diastolic pressure with small changes of left ventricular volume; the atrial contribution to ventricular filling becomes even more important than in younger patients (see Chapter 19). Atrial enlargement predisposes patients to atrial fibrillation and flutter. Patients are at increased risk for developing congestive heart failure.

Diminished cardiac reserve in many elderly patients may be manifested as exaggerated drops in blood pressure during induction of general anesthesia. A prolonged circulation time delays the onset of intravenous drugs but speeds induction with inhalational agents. Like infants, elderly patients have less ability to respond to hypovolemia, hypotension, or hypoxia with an increase in heart rate.

RESPIRATORY SYSTEM

Elasticity is decreased in lung tissue also, allowing overdistention of alveoli and collapse of small airways. The former reduces the alveolar surface area, which decreases the efficiency of gas exchange. Airway collapse increases residual volume (the volume of air remaining in the lungs at the end of a forced expiration) and closing capacity (the volume of air in the lungs at which small airways begin to close). Even in normal persons, closing capacity exceeds functional residual capacity (the volume of air remaining in the lungs at the end of a normal expiration) at age 45 years in the supine position and age 65 in the sitting position. When this happens, some airways close during part of normal tidal breathing, resulting in a mismatch of ventilation and perfusion. The additive effect of these emphysema-like changes is said to decrease arterial oxygen tension by an average rate of 0.35 mm Hg per year. There is a wide range of arterial oxygen tensions in elderly preoperative patients, however (Figure 45–1). Both anatomic and physiological dead space increase. Other pulmonary effects of aging are summarized in Table 45–2.

Table 45–2. Age-related physiological changes and common diseases of the elderly.

Normal Physiological Changes	Common Pathophysiology
Cardiovascular	
Decreased arterial elasticity	Atherosclerosis
Elevated afterload	Coronary artery disease
Elevated systolic blood pressure	Essential hypertension
Left ventricular hypertrophy	Congestive heart failure
Decreased adrenergic activity	Cardiac arrhythmias
Decreased resting heart rate	Aortic stenosis
Decreased maximal heart rate	
Decreased baroreceptor reflex	
Respiratory	
Decreased pulmonary elasticity	Emphysema
Decreased alveolar surface area	Chronic bronchitis
Increased residual volume	Pneumonia
Increased closing capacity	
Ventilation/perfusion mismatching	
Decreased arterial oxygen tension	
Increased chest wall rigidity	
Decreased muscle strength	
Decreased cough	
Decreased maximal breathing capacity	
Blunted response to hypercapnia and hypoxia	
Renal	
Decreased renal blood flow	Diabetic nephropathy
Decreased renal plasma flow	Hypertensive nephropathy
Decreased glomerular filtration rate	Prostatic obstruction
Decreased renal mass	Congestive heart failure
Decreased tubular function	
Impaired sodium handling	
Decreased concentrating ability	
Decreased diluting capacity	
Impaired fluid handling	
Decreased drug excretion	
Decreased renin–aldosterone responsiveness	
Impaired potassium excretion	

Mask ventilation may be more difficult in edentulous patients, whereas arthritis of the temporomandibular joint or cervical spine may make intubation challenging. On the other hand, the absence of upper teeth often improves visualization of the vocal cords during laryngoscopy.

Prevention of perioperative hypoxia includes a longer preoxygenation period prior to induction, a higher inspired oxygen concentrations during anesthesia, small increments of positive end-expiratory pressure, and aggressive pulmonary toilet. Aspiration pneumonia is a common and potentially life-threatening complication in elderly patients. One reason for this predisposition is a progressive decrease in protective laryngeal reflexes with age. Ventilatory impairment in the recovery room is more common in elderly patients. Therefore, patients with severe preexisting respiratory disease and those who have just had major abdominal surgery should generally be left intubated postoperatively. In addition, pain control techniques that facilitate postoperative pulmonary function should be seriously considered (eg, epidural local anesthetics and opioids, intercostal nerve blocks).

METABOLIC & ENDOCRINE FUNCTION

Basal and maximal oxygen consumption declines with age. After reaching peak weight at about age 60, most men and women begin losing weight; the average elderly man and woman weigh less than younger counterparts.

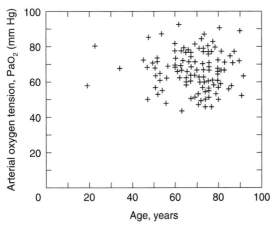

Figure 45–1. There is a wide range of arterial oxygen tensions in elderly preoperative patients. (Redrawn and reproduced, with permission, from Del Guercio LRM, Cohn JD: Monitoring operative risk in elderly. JAMA 1980;243:1350.)

Heat production decreases, heat loss increases, and hypothalamic temperature-regulating centers may reset at a lower level. Increasing insulin resistance leads to a progressive decrease in the ability to handle glucose loads. The neuroendocrine response to stress appears to be preserved or slightly decreased in most healthy elderly patients. Aging is associated with a decreasing response to β-adrenergic agents ("endogenous β-blockade"). Circulating norepinephrine levels are reported to be elevated in elderly patients.

RENAL FUNCTION

Renal blood flow and kidney mass (eg, glomerular number and tubular length) decrease with age. These changes are particularly prominent in the renal cortex where they are replaced by fat and fibrotic tissue. Renal function as determined by glomerular filtration rate and creatinine clearance is reduced (Table 45–2). The serum creatinine level is unchanged because of a decrease in muscle mass and creatinine production, whereas blood urea nitrogen gradually increases (0.2 mg/dL per year). Impairment of sodium handling, concentrating ability, and diluting capacity predisposes elderly patients to dehydration or fluid overload. The response to antidiuretic hormone and aldosterone is reduced. The ability to reabsorb glucose is decreased. The combination of reduced renal blood flow and decreased nephron mass increases the risk of elderly patients for acute renal failure in the postoperative period.

As renal function declines, so does the kidney's ability to excrete drugs. The decreased capacity to handle water and electrolyte loads makes proper fluid management more critical; elderly patients are more predisposed to developing hypokalemia and hyperkalemia. This is further complicated by the common use of diuretics in the elderly population. To this end, serum electrolytes, cardiac filling pressures, and urinary output are more frequently monitored.

GASTROINTESTINAL FUNCTION

Liver mass declines as a person ages, with a corresponding decrease in hepatic blood flow. Hepatic function (reserves) declines in proportion to the decrease in liver mass. Thus, the rate of biotransformation and albumin production decreases. Plasma cholinesterase levels are reduced in elderly men. Gastric pH tends to rise, whereas gastric emptying is prolonged, although some studies suggest elderly patients have lower gastric volumes than younger patients.

NERVOUS SYSTEM

Brain mass decreases with age; neuronal loss is prominent in the cerebral cortex, particularly the frontal lobes. Cerebral blood flow also decreases about 10–20% in proportion to neuronal losses. It remains tightly coupled to metabolic rate; autoregulation is intact. Neurons decrease in size and lose some complexity of their dendritic tree and number of synapses. The synthesis of some neurotransmitters, such as dopamine, and the number of their receptors are reduced. Serotonergic, adrenergic, and γ-aminobutyric acid (GABA) binding sites are also reduced. Astrocytes and microglial cells increase in number.

Degeneration of peripheral nerve cells results in prolonged conduction velocity and skeletal muscle atrophy.

Aging is associated with an increasing threshold for nearly all sensory modalities, including touch, temperature sensation, proprioception, hearing, and vision. Changes in pain perception are complex and poorly understood; central and peripheral processing mechanisms are likely altered. Dosage requirements for local (C_m: minimum anesthetic concentration) and general (MAC: minimum alveolar concentration) anesthetics are reduced. Administration of a given volume of epidural anesthetic tends to result in more extensive cephalad spread in elderly patients, but with a shorter duration of analgesia and motor block. In contrast, a longer duration of action should be expected from a spinal anesthetic.

In the absence of disease, decreases in cognitive function are normally modest but variable. Short-term memory appears to be most affected. Continued physical and intellectual activity appears to have a positive effect on preservation of cognitive functions.

Elderly patients often take more time to recover completely from the central nervous system effects of general anesthesia, particularly if they were confused or disoriented preoperatively. This is important in geriatric outpatient surgery, where socioeconomic factors such as the lack of a caretaker at home necessitate a higher level of self-care. Many elderly patients experience varying degrees of an acute confusional state, delirium, or cognitive dysfunction postoperatively. The etiology of postoperative cognitive dysfunction (POCD) is likely multifactorial and includes drug effects, pain, underlying dementia, hypothermia, and metabolic disturbances. Low levels of certain neurotransmitters, such as acetylcholine, may be contributory. Elderly patients are particularly sensitive to centrally acting anticholinergic agents such as scopolamine and atropine. Interestingly, the incidence of postoperative delirium appears similar with both regional and general anesthesia; it may be less following regional anesthesia without any sedation. Some patients suffer from prolonged or permanent POCD after surgery and anesthesia. Some studies suggest that POCD can be detected in 10–15% of patients > 60 years of age up to 3 months following major surgery. In some settings, eg, following cardiac and major orthopedic procedures, intraoperative arterial emboli may be contributory. Animal studies suggest that anesthesia without surgery can impair learning for weeks, particularly in older animals. Elderly inpatients appear to have a significantly higher risk for POCD than elderly outpatients. Although the etiology remains unclear, both anesthetic and nonanesthetic factors are likely responsible for POCD.

MUSCULOSKELETAL

Muscle mass is reduced. At the microscopic level, neuromuscular junctions thicken. There also appears to be some extrajunctional spread of acetylcholine receptors. Skin atrophies with age and is prone to trauma from adhesive tape, electrocautery pads, and electrocardiographic electrodes. Veins are often frail and easily ruptured by intravenous infusions. Arthritic joints may interfere with positioning (eg, lithotomy) or regional anesthesia (eg, subarachnoid block). Degenerative cervical spine disease can limit neck extension potentially making intubation difficult.

■ AGE-RELATED PHARMACOLOGICAL CHANGES

Aging produces both pharmacokinetic (the relationship between drug dose and plasma concentration) and pharmacodynamic (the relationship between plasma concentration and clinical effect) changes. Unfortunately, disease-related changes and wide interindividual variations even in similar populations lead to inconsistent generalizations.

A progressive decrease in muscle mass and increase in body fat (more pronounced in older women) results in decreased total body water. The reduced volume of distribution for water-soluble drugs can lead to higher plasma concentrations; conversely, an increased volume of distribution for lipid-soluble drugs can lower their plasma concentration. These changes in volume of distribution may affect elimination half-life. If a drug's volume of distribution expands, its elimination half-life will be prolonged unless the rate of clearance is also increased. However, because renal and hepatic functions decline with age, reductions in clearance prolong the duration of action for many drugs. Studies suggest that unlike those who are ill, healthy, active, elderly patients have little or no change in plasma volume.

Distribution and elimination are also affected by altered plasma protein binding (see Chapter 8). Albumin, which tends to bind acidic drugs (eg, barbiturates, benzodiazepines, opioid agonists), typically decreases with age. α_1-Acid glycoprotein, which binds basic drugs (eg, local anesthetics), is increased. Protein-bound drugs cannot interact with end-organ receptors and are unavailable for metabolism or excretion.

The principal pharmacodynamic change associated with aging is a reduced anesthetic requirement, represented by a lower MAC. Careful titration of anesthetic agents helps to avoid adverse side effects and prolonged duration; short-acting agents such as propofol, desflurane, remifentanil, and succinylcholine may be particularly useful in elderly patients. Drugs that are not significantly dependent on hepatic or renal function or blood flow, such as mivacurium, atracurium, and cisatracurium, are also useful.

INHALATIONAL ANESTHETICS

The MAC for inhalational agents is reduced by 4% per decade of age over 40 years. For example, the MAC of halothane in an 80-year-old person would be expected to be 0.65 (0.77 – [0.77 × 4% × 4]). Onset of action will be more rapid if cardiac output is depressed, whereas it will be delayed if there is a significant ventilation/perfusion abnormality (see Chapter 7). The myocardial depressant effects of volatile anesthetics are exaggerated in elderly patients, whereas the tachycardiac tendencies of isoflurane and desflurane are attenuated. Thus, in contrast to its effects on younger patients, isoflurane reduces cardiac output and heart rate in elderly patients. Recovery from anesthesia with a volatile anesthetic may be prolonged because of an increased volume of distribution (increased body fat), decreased hepatic function (decreased halothane metabolism), and decreased pulmonary gas exchange. The rapid elimination of desflurane may make it the inhalation anesthetic of choice for elderly patients.

NONVOLATILE ANESTHETIC AGENTS

 In general, elderly patients display a lower dose requirement for propofol, etomidate, barbiturates, opioids, and benzodiazepines. For example, the typical octogenarian may require less than half the induction dose of propofol or thiopental than that required by a 20-year-old patient.

Although propofol may be close to an ideal induction agent for elderly patients because of its rapid elimination, it is more likely to cause apnea and hypotension than in younger patients. Concomitant administration of midazolam, opioids, or ketamine further decreases propofol requirements. Both pharmacokinetic and pharmacodynamic factors are responsible for this enhanced sensitivity. Elderly patients require nearly 50% lower blood levels of propofol for anesthesia than younger patients. Moreover, both the rapidly equilibrating peripheral compartment and systemic clearance for propofol are significantly reduced in elderly patients. In the case of thiopental, enhanced sensitivity appears to be primarily due to pharmacokinetics factors. The typical 40–50% reduction in induction dose may be the result of peak levels not decreasing as rapidly in geriatric patients because of a slower distribution from the central compartment to the rapidly equilibrating compartment. The initial volume of distribution for etomidate significantly decreases with aging: lower doses are required to achieve the same electroencephalographic (EEG) end point in elderly patients (compared to young patients).

Enhanced sensitivity to fentanyl, alfentanil, and sufentanil is primarily pharmacodynamic. Pharmacokinetics for these opioids are not significantly affected by age. Dose requirements for the same EEG end point using fentanyl and alfentanil are 50% lower in elderly patients. In contrast, the volume of the central compartment and clearance are reduced for remifentanil; thus both pharmacodynamic and pharmacokinetic factors are important. The pharmacokinetics of other opioids have not been studied as well in elderly patients, but enhanced sensitivity should be expected.

Aging increases the volume of distribution for all benzodiazepines, which effectively prolongs their elimination half-lives. In the case of diazepam, the elimination half-life can be as long as 36–72 h. Enhanced pharmacodynamic sensitivity to benzodiazepines is also observed. Midazolam requirements are generally 50% less in elderly patients; its elimination half-life is prolonged from about 2.5 to 4 h.

MUSCLE RELAXANTS

The response to succinylcholine and nondepolarizing agents is unaltered with aging. Decreased cardiac output and slow muscle blood flow, however, may cause up to a 2-fold prolongation in onset of neuromuscular blockade in elderly patients. Recovery from nondepolarizing muscle relaxants that depend on renal excretion (eg, metocurine, pancuronium, doxacurium, tubocurarine) may be delayed due to decreased drug clearance. Likewise, decreased hepatic excretion from a loss of liver mass prolongs the elimination half-life and duration of action of rocuronium and vecuronium. The pharmacological profiles of atracurium and pipecuronium are not significantly affected by age. Elderly men—but not elderly women—may display a slightly prolonged effect from succinylcholine due to lower plasma cholinesterase levels.

CASE DISCUSSION: THE ELDERLY PATIENT WITH A FRACTURED HIP

An 86-year-old nursing home patient is scheduled for open reduction and internal fixation of a subtrochanteric fracture of the femur.

How should this patient be evaluated for the risk of perioperative morbidity?

Anesthetic risk correlates much better with the presence of coexisting disease than chronological age. Therefore, preanesthetic evaluation should concentrate on the identification of age-related diseases (Table 45–2) and an estimation of physiological reserve. There is a tremendous physiological difference between a patient who walks three blocks to a grocery store on a regular basis and one who is bedridden, even though both may be the same age. Obviously, any condition that may be amenable to preoperative therapy (eg, bronchodilator administration) must be identified and addressed. At the same time, lengthy delays may compromise surgical repair and increase overall morbidity.

What are some of the considerations in selection of premedication for this patient?

In general, elderly patients require lower doses of premedication. Nonetheless, hip fractures are painful, particularly during movement to the operating room. Unless contraindicated by severe concomitant disease, an opioid premedication may be valuable. Anticholinergic medication is rarely needed, as aging is accompanied by atrophy of the salivary glands. These patients may be at risk for aspiration, as opioid premedication and pain from the injury will decrease gastric emptying. Therefore, pretreatment with an H_2 antagonist should be considered (see Chapter 15). Metoclopramide can also be used to promote gastric emptying, but elderly patients may be at increased risk for extrapyramidal side effects, such as rigidity.

What factors might influence the choice between regional and general anesthesia?

Advancing age is not a contraindication for either regional or general anesthesia. Each technique, however, has its advantages and disadvantages in the elderly population. For hip surgery, regional anesthesia can be achieved with a subarachnoid or epidural block extending to the T8 sensory level. Both these blocks require patient cooperation and the ability to lie still for the duration of the surgery. A paramedian approach is helpful when optimal positioning is not possible (see Chapter 16). Unless regional anesthesia is accompanied by heavy sedation, postoperative confusion and disorientation are less troublesome than after general anesthesia. Cardiovascular changes are usually limited to a fall in arterial blood pressure as sympathetic block is established. Although this fall can be minimized by prophylactic fluid loading, a patient with borderline heart function may develop congestive heart failure when the block dissipates and sympathetic tone returns. Reduced afterload can result in profound hypotension in patients with aortic stenosis, a common valvular lesion in the elderly population. Patients with coronary artery disease may experience an increase in myocardial oxygen demand as a result of reflex tachycardia or a decrease in supply caused by lower coronary artery perfusion.

Are there any specific advantages or disadvantages to a regional technique in elderly patients having hip surgery?

A major advantage in regional anesthesia—particularly for hip surgery—is a lower incidence of postoperative thromboembolism (see Chapter 40). This is presumably due to peripheral vasodilation and maintenance of venous blood flow in the lower extremities. In addition, local anesthetics inhibit platelet aggregation and stabilize endothelial cells. Many anesthesiologists believe that regional anesthesia maintains respiratory function better than general anesthesia. Unless the anesthetic level involves the intercostal mus-

culature, ventilation and the cough reflex are well maintained.

Technical problems associated with regional anesthesia in the elderly include altered landmarks as a result of degeneration of the vertebral column and the difficulty of obtaining adequate patient positioning. To avoid having the patient lie on the fracture, a hypobaric solution can be injected intrathecally. Postpuncture headache is less of a problem in the elderly population.

If the patient refuses regional anesthesia, is general anesthesia acceptable?

General anesthesia is an acceptable alternative to regional block. One advantage is that the patient can be induced in bed and moved to the operating room table after intubation, avoiding the pain of positioning. A disadvantage is that the patient is unable to provide feedback regarding pressure points on the unpadded orthopedic table.

What specific factors should be considered during induction and maintenance of general anesthesia with this patient?

Intravenous induction agents should be administered slowly, as slow blood circulation will delay the onset of action. It is important to remember that because a subtrochanteric fracture can be associated with more than 1 L of occult blood loss, induction with sodium thiopental or propofol may lead to an exaggerated drop in arterial blood pressure. Thus, although the patient may be at risk for aspiration, the usual rapid-sequence induction should be modified to minimize cardiovascular changes. An acceptable compromise allows slower drug administration and gentle mask ventilation but maintains firm cricoid pressure until satisfactory endotracheal tube position is confirmed. Initial hypotension may be replaced by hypertension and tachycardia during laryngoscopy and intubation. This roller-coaster volatility in blood pressure increases the risk of myocardial ischemia and can be avoided by preceding airway instrumentation with lidocaine (1.5 mg/kg), esmolol (0.3 mg/kg), or alfentanil (5–15 μg/kg).

Intraoperative paralysis with a nondepolarizing muscle relaxant improves surgical conditions and allows maintenance of a lighter plane of anesthesia. Deliberate hypotension may decrease intraoperative blood loss and is not contraindica-

ted solely on the basis of age (see Case Discussion, Chapter 13).

SUGGESTED READING

Dodds C, Allison J: Postoperative cognitive deficit in the elderly surgical patient. Br J Anaesth 1998;81:449.

Ferrell BR, Ferrell BA (editors): *Pain in the Elderly.* IASP Press, 1996.

Jin F, Chung F: Minimizing perioperative adverse events in the elderly. Br J Anaesth 2001;87:608.

McLeskey CH (editor): *Geriatric Anesthesiology.* Williams & Wilkins, 1997.

Muravchick S: *Geroanesthesia. Principles for Management of the Elderly Patient.* Mosby-Year Book, 1997.

O'Keeffe ST, Chonchubhair AN: Postoperative delirium in the elderly. Br J Anaesth 1994;73:673.

Parikh SS, Chung F: Postoperative delirium in the elderly. Anesth Analg 1995;80:1223.

Priebe H-J: The aged cardiovascular risk patient. Br J Anaesth 2000;85:763.

Smith RB, Gurkowski MA, Bracken CA (editors): *Anesthesia and Pain Control in the Geriatric Patient.* McGraw-Hill, 1995.

Wright PMC: Population based pharmacokinetic analysis: why do we need it; what is it; and what has it told us about anaesthetics? Br J Anaesth 1998;80:488.

SECTION V
Special Problems

Anesthetic Complications

Joseph T. Nitti, MD, & Gary J. Nitti, MD

KEY CONCEPTS

 Complications related to the delivery of anesthesia care are inevitable. Even the most experienced, diligent, and careful practitioners will have to manage complications despite acting well within the standard of care.

 Anesthetic mishaps can be categorized as preventable or unpreventable. Of the preventable incidents, most involve human error, as opposed to equipment malfunctions.

 Death and permanent neurological damage were just as often associated with adverse cardiovascular as adverse respiratory events. A reduction in adverse respiratory events was believed to be due to widespread adoption of pulse oximetry and capnography as standard monitors.

 Many anesthetic fatalities occur only after a series of coincidental circumstances, misjudgments, and technical errors (mishap chain).

 Although the mechanisms differ, anaphylactic and anaphylactoid reactions can be clinically indistinguishable and equally life-threatening. Cardiovascular and cutaneous manifestations are more common features of anaphylaxis than bronchospasm during anesthesia.

 True anaphylaxis due to anesthetic agents is rare; anaphylactoid reactions are much more common. Muscle relaxants have emerged as the most common cause of anaphylaxis during anesthesia. Latex allergy is the second most common.

 Patients with spina bifida, spinal cord injury, and congenital abnormalities of the genitourinary tract have a very high incidence of latex allergy.

 Although there is no clear evidence that exposure to trace amounts of anesthetic agents presents a health hazard to operating room personnel, the U.S. Occupational Health and Safety Administration continues to set maximum acceptable trace concentrations of less than 25 ppm for nitrous oxide and 0.5 ppm for halogenated anesthetics (2 ppm if the halogenated agent is used alone).

 Hollow (hypodermic) needles pose a greater risk than solid (surgical) needles because of the potentially larger inoculum. The use of gloves, needleless systems, or protected needle devices may decrease the incidence of some (but not all) types of injury.

 Anesthesiology is a high-risk medical specialty for drug addiction.

 The two most important methods of minimizing radiation exposure are using proper barriers and maximizing one's distance from the source of radiation.

Complications related to the delivery of anesthesia care are inevitable. Even the most experienced, diligent, and careful practitioners will have to manage complications despite acting well within the standard of care. These complications will range from minor (eg, infiltrated intravenous line) to catastrophic (hypoxic brain injury or death).

When complications do occur, appropriate evaluation, management, and documentation are critical in minimizing or eliminating negative outcomes. A good example is the unanticipated difficult airway. Although a comprehensive preanesthetic airway evaluation will help the clinician anticipate and prepare for most difficult intubations, it will still fail to predict problems in a few patients who cannot be intubated except by specialized techniques (see Chapter 6). In these cases, despite preoxygenation and cricoid pressure (if appropriate), the risk of aspiration, airway obstruction, and hypoxia is high and extraordinary measures to secure the airway (cricothyrotomy or surgical tracheostomy) may become necessary. Although establishing a surgical airway is a lifesaving procedure, it will inevitably be considered a "complication." Also, the patient will require postoperative mechanical ventilation, may require a second surgical procedure, and might be left with a small but unsightly scar. Yet another example is the laryngeal granuloma that follows an easy routine endotracheal intubation. These "complications" will trigger institutional review, peer review, and potential legal action.

Litigation may occur despite the best efforts to communicate with the patient and family about the intraoperative events, management decisions, and avoidance of catastrophic complications. It is essential to document the preoperative airway examination, to record maneuvers such as preoxygenation and cricoid pressure and details of laryngoscopy, and to write a complete postanesthesia note so that the actions of the anesthesiologist can be defended should litigation occur.

Earlier chapters have discussed the risks and alternative anesthetic techniques associated with specific procedures. This chapter reviews the incidences, causes, and prevention of both common and catastrophic anesthetic complications. The discussion includes important aspects of documentation that may make perioperative management and decision-making processes clearer to consultants when they review the medical record following complications. Documentation is also discussed in Chapter 1. After a discussion of hypersensitivity reactions, anaphylaxis, and latex allergy, the chapter concludes with an examination of occupational hazards in anesthesiology, including trace exposure to anesthetic agents, infections, substance abuse, and radiation exposure.

ADVERSE ANESTHETIC OUTCOMES

Incidence

There are several reasons why it is difficult to accurately measure the incidence of adverse anesthesia-related outcomes, also referred to as anesthetic mishaps. First, it is often impossible to assign the responsibility for a poor outcome to the patient's inherent disease, the surgical procedure, or the anesthetic management. In fact, all three can contribute to a poor outcome. It is also difficult to define a measurable event. Death is a clear end point, but because anesthesia-related perioperative death is rare, a very large series of patients must be studied to assemble conclusions that have statistical significance.

Nonetheless, many studies have attempted to determine the incidence of complications due to anesthesia. Unfortunately, studies vary in criteria for defining an anesthesia-related adverse outcome and are limited by retrospective analysis. Finally, medicolegal fears hinder accurate reporting.

Perioperative mortality is usually defined as death within 48 h of surgery. It is clear that most perioperative fatalities are due to the patient's preoperative disease or the surgical procedure. The mortality rate attributable primarily to anesthesia *appears* to have dropped during the past 30 years from one or two deaths per 3000 anesthetic experiences to a current rate of one or two deaths per 20,000 experiences. However, these statistics should be viewed with considerable skepticism, as they are derived from different countries using different methodologies. Recent studies indicate that the anesthetic mortality rate in some institutions may be even less than 1:20,000. This decline may be due to the availability and utilization of new monitoring equipment, greater knowledge of anesthetic physiology and pharmacology, and improved surgical and medical care. Indeed, in one large study, the mortality rate attributed solely to anesthesia was 1 in 185,000.

American Society of Anesthesiologists (ASA) Closed Claims Project

The goal of the ASA Closed Claims Project is to identify major areas of loss in anesthesia, patterns of injury, and strategies for prevention. It is a collection of completed malpractice claims that provides a "snapshot" of anesthesia liability rather than a study of the incidence of anesthetic complications. The most recent analysis spans more than four decades (1970–2003) and includes 5803 claims. These claims are grouped by subject area (eg, awareness and eye injury) and were independently reviewed to determine patterns of causation and liability. Claims for dental injury as well as those in which the sequence of events or nature of injury could not be reconstructed were excluded.

Causes

Anesthetic mishaps can be categorized as preventable or unpreventable. Examples of the latter include sudden death syndrome, fatal idiosyncratic drug reactions, or any poor outcome that occurs despite proper management. However, studies of anesthetic-related deaths or near misses suggest that most accidents are preventable. Of these preventable incidents, most involve human error (Table 46–1), as opposed to equipment malfunctions (Table 46–2). Unfortunately, some rate of human error is inevitable, and a preventable accident is not synonymous with incompetence. During the 1990s, the top three causes for claims in the ASA Closed Claims Project were death (22%), nerve injury (18%), and brain damage (9%).

Adverse respiratory events were previously more than twice as likely as adverse cardiovascular events to be associated with death or permanent brain damage. However, in a recent analysis of the ASA Closed Claims database limited to 1990s claims, death and permanent neurological damage were just as often associated with adverse cardiovascular events as with adverse respiratory events. A reduction in adverse respiratory events was believed to be due to widespread adoption of pulse oximetry and capnography as standard monitors. Although the number of claims associated with inadequate ventilation and esophageal intubation decreased, those involving difficult intubation remained unchanged. The cause for the increase in the proportion of adverse cardiovascular events associated with death and permanent injury is not clear. In fact the largest category of cardiovascular events in such cases was listed as "unexplained/other." This category included pulmonary embolism, stroke, myocardial infarction, arrhythmias, and previously undiagnosed conditions such as cardiomyopathy. A large scale study on anesthetic-related cardiac arrest at a single teaching institution reported that medication-related errors (see below) and problems with central venous access (eg, arrhythmias and bleeding) are the most common causes.

"Equipment problems" is perhaps a misnomer; the Closed Claims Project review of 72 claims involving gas delivery systems found that equipment misuse was

Table 46–1. Common human errors leading to preventable anesthetic accidents.

Unrecognized breathing circuit disconnection
Mistaken drug administration
Airway mismanagement
Anesthesia machine misuse
Fluid mismanagement
Intravenous line disconnection

Table 46–2. Common equipment malfunctions leading to preventable anesthetic accidents.

Breathing circuit
Monitoring device
Ventilator
Anesthesia machine
Laryngoscope

three times more common than equipment malfunction (Chapter 4). Moreover, the majority (76%) of adverse outcomes associated with gas delivery problems led to death or permanent neurological damage.

Errors in drug administration also primarily involve human error. It has been suggested that as much as 20% of the drug doses given to hospitalized patients are incorrect. Errors in drug administration account for 4% of cases in the ASA Closed Claims Project, which found that errors resulting in claims were most frequently due to either incorrect dosage or unintentional administration of the wrong drug (syringe swap). In the latter category, incorrect use of epinephrine proved to be particularly dangerous.

Another type of human error occurs when the most critical problem is ignored because attention is inappropriately focused on a less important problem or an incorrect solution (fixation error). Serious anesthetic mishaps are usually associated with other factors (Table 46–3). For instance, the impact of most equipment failures is decreased or avoided by routine preoperative checkouts and personnel training. Many anesthetic fatalities occur only after a series of coincidental circumstances, misjudgments, and technical errors (mishap chain).

Table 46–3. Factors associated with human errors and equipment misuse.

Factor	Example
Inadequate preparation	No machine checkout or preoperative evaluation; haste and carelessness
Inadequate experience and training	Unfamiliarity with anesthetic technique or equipment
Environmental limitations	Inability to visualize surgical field: poor communication with surgeons
Physical and emotional factors	Fatigue; personal problems

Prevention

Strategies to reduce the incidence of serious anesthetic complications include better monitoring and anesthetic technique, improved education, more comprehensive protocols and standards of practice, and active risk management programs. Better monitoring and anesthetic techniques imply closer patient contact, more comprehensive monitoring equipment, and better designed anesthesia machines and workspaces. The fact that most accidents occur during the maintenance phase of anesthesia—rather than during induction or emergence—implies a failure of vigilance. Inspection, auscultation, and palpation of the patient provide important information. Instruments should supplement but never replace the anesthesiologist's own senses. To minimize errors in drug administration, drug syringes and ampules in the work area should be restricted to only those needed for the current, specific case. They should be consistently diluted to the same concentration for each use and clearly labeled. Computer systems for scanning bar-coded drug labels are being developed to help reduce medication errors.

A major goal of the Society for Education in Anesthesia is to improve resident training. Of course, education must continue beyond residency as new drugs, techniques, and equipment are continually being developed. Part of this continuing education requirement includes awareness of the most current monitoring standards, familiarity with new equipment, and utilization techniques that have been shown to improve anesthetic outcomes.

Risk management and continuous quality improvement programs at the departmental level may reduce anesthetic morbidity and mortality rates by addressing monitoring standards, equipment, practice guidelines, continuing education, and staffing issues. Specific responsibilities of peer-review committees include identifying and preventing potential problems, formulating and periodically revising departmental policies, ensuring the availability of properly functioning anesthetic equipment, enforcing standards required for clinical privileges, and evaluating the appropriateness of patient care. A quality improvement system impartially reviews complications, ensures physician compliance, and continuously monitors quality indicators.

AIRWAY INJURY

Injury to airway structures is a constant concern to practicing anesthesiologists. The daily insertion of endotracheal tubes, laryngeal mask airways, oral/nasal airways, gastric tubes, transesophageal echocardiogram (TEE) probes, esophageal (boogie) dilators, and emergency airways all involve the risk of airway structure damage.

Common morbidities such as sore throat and dysphagia are usually self-limiting but may also be nonspecific symptoms of more ominous complications.

The most common permanent airway injury is dental trauma. In a retrospective study of 600,000 surgical cases, the incidence of injury requiring dental intervention and repair was approximately 1 in 4500. In most cases, laryngoscopy and endotracheal intubation were involved, and the upper incisors were the most frequently injured. Dental trauma may occur less commonly from oral airways. Major risk factors for dental trauma included tracheal intubation, preexisting poor dentition, and patient characteristics associated with difficult airway management (including limited neck motion, previous head and neck surgery, craniofacial abnormalities, and a history of difficult intubation).

Other types of airway trauma are rare. Although there are scattered case reports in the literature, the most comprehensive analysis is the ASA Closed Claims project. This report describes 266 claims, which were grouped by the site of injury. In general, the least serious were temporomandibular joint (TMJ) injuries, which were all associated with otherwise uncomplicated intubations and occurred mostly in females younger than 60 years. Approximately 25% of these patients had previous TMJ disease. Laryngeal injuries primarily included vocal cord paralysis, granuloma, and arytenoid dislocation. Most tracheal injuries were associated with emergency surgical tracheotomy, but a few were related to endotracheal intubation. Some injuries occurred during seemingly easy, routine intubations. Proposed mechanisms include excessive tube movement in the trachea, pressure necrosis, and inadequate relaxation. Esophageal perforations contributed to death in 5 of 13 patients, who most often presented with delayed-onset subcutaneous emphysema or pneumothorax. Finally, pharyngoesophageal perforation was clearly associated with difficult intubation, age over 60 years, and female gender. As in tracheal perforation, obvious signs were often delayed in onset. Instead, initial sore throat, cervical pain, and cough often progress to fever, dysphagia, and dyspnea as mediastinitis, abscess, or pneumonia develop. Mortality rates of 25–50% after esophageal perforation have been reported, with the lower percentage attributable to rapid detection and treatment.

Minimizing the risk of airway injury begins with the preoperative assessment. A thorough airway examination will help determine the risk for difficulty (see Chapter 5). Documentation of current dentition (including dental work) should be included. Many practitioners believe preoperative consent should include a discussion of the risk of dental, oral, vocal cord, and esophageal trauma in every patient who could potentially need any airway manipulation. If a difficult airway is suspected, a more detailed discussion of risks (eg, emergency tracheostomy) is appropriate. In such cases, emergency airway supplies and experienced help should be immediately available, and the ASA algorithm for difficult airway management should be utilized. Follow-up should occur to assess for latent signs of perforation if there is suspicion of airway trauma. If intubation cannot be accomplished by conventional means, the patient or guardian should be informed in case of future airway intervention.

PERIPHERAL NERVE INJURY

Perioperative nerve injury is a known complication of both regional and general anesthesia. Neuraxial (spinal cord or spinal root) injury is discussed in Chapter 16. Peripheral nerve injury, however, is a more frequent and often debilitating problem. In most cases, these injuries resolve within 6–12 weeks, but some persist for months or even years. Because peripheral neuropathies are commonly associated (sometimes incorrectly!) with patient positioning, a review of mechanisms and prevention is necessary.

The most common peripheral nerve injury is ulnar neuropathy. In a retrospective study of over 1 million patients, persistent ulnar neuropathy (greater than 3 months duration) occurred in approximately 1 in 2700 patients. Interestingly, initial symptoms were most frequently noted more than 24 h after a surgical procedure and may have occurred while the patient was on the hospital ward sleeping. Risk factors included male gender, hospital stay greater than 14 days, and very thin or obese body habitus. More than 50% of these patients regained full sensory and motor function within 1 year. Anesthetic technique was not implicated as a risk factor; 25% of patients with ulnar neuropathy underwent monitored care or lower extremity regional technique. This casts doubt that a stretch or compression mechanism caused the injury, because awake patients would likely respond to discomfort. The ASA Closed Claims Project findings support most of these results, particularly the delayed onset of symptoms and the lack of relationship between anesthesia technique and injury. This study also noted that many neuropathies occurred despite notation of extra padding over the elbow area, further negating compression as a possible mechanism of injury.

The Role of Positioning

Other peripheral nerve injuries appear to be more closely related to positioning or surgical procedure. They may involve the peroneal nerve, the brachial plexus, or the femoral and sciatic nerves. External pressure on a nerve could compromise its perfusion, disrupt its cellular integrity, and eventually result in edema, ischemia, and necrosis. Pressure injuries are particularly likely when nerves pass through closed compartments formed by dense osseofascial membranes or take a superficial course (eg, the perineal nerve around the fibula). Lower extremity neuropathies, particularly those involving the peroneal nerve, have been associated with improper, extreme (high), and prolonged (greater than 2 h) maintenance of the lithotomy position. Patient risk factors for this complication include hypotension; thin body habitus; old age; and history of vascular disease, diabetes, or smoking. Ulnar nerve injuries are associated with cardiac surgery because rib retraction may promote stretch on the brachial plexus. Similarly, the long thoracic nerve may be severed during pneumonectomy or axillary lymph node dissection, resulting in paralysis of the serratus anterior muscle and winging of the scapula. Some brachial plexus injuries following lateral decubitus positioning may be related to improper positioning of the axillary roll. This roll should be caudad to the axilla to prevent direct pressure on the brachial plexus, and large enough to relieve any pressure from the mattress on the lower shoulder.

The data suggest that some peripheral nerve injury is not preventable. Patient, procedure, and position factors contribute a significant amount of risk. Although the risk of peripheral neuropathy should be discussed during informed consent, particularly in patients to be placed in a nonsupine position, other practices may be helpful. When reasonable, patients can be positioned before induction of anesthesia to check for discomfort. Final positioning should be evaluated carefully prior to draping. In most circumstances the head and neck should be kept in a neutral position to minimize neural or vascular compromise. Shoulder braces to support a Trendelenburg position should be avoided if possible, and shoulder abduction and lateral rotation should be minimized to reduce the chance of brachial plexus injury. The upper extremities should not be extended greater than 90° at any joint and should be supinated to protect the ulnar tunnel. Prolonged pronation of the forearm can compress the ulnar nerve in the cubital tunnel (Figure 46–1). Lower extremities should not have any obvious pressure points. Although injuries can occur despite the presence of padding, additional padding may be helpful in vulnerable areas. Documentation should include information on positioning, including the presence of padding. Finally, patients who complain of sensory or motor dysfunction in the postoperative period should be reassured that this is frequently a temporary condition. Motor and sensory function should be documented and the patient should be referred for neurological evaluation and physiological testing, such as nerve conduction and electromyographic studies.

Complications Related to Positioning

Changes of body position have physiological consequences that can be exaggerated in disease states.

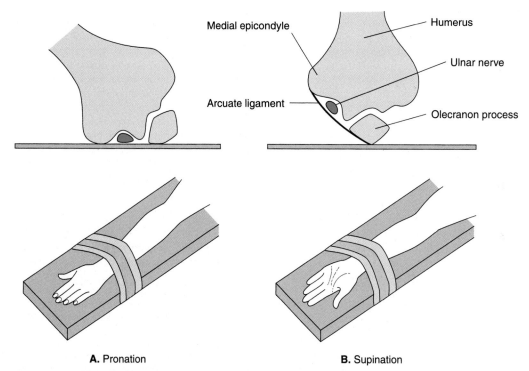

Figure 46–1. Pronation of the forearm can cause external compression of the ulnar nerve in the cubital tunnel (**A**). Forearm supination avoids this problem (**B**). (Modified and reproduced, with permission, from Wadsworth TG: The cubital tunnel and the external compression syndrome. Anesth Analg 1974;53:303.)

General and regional anesthesia may limit the cardiovascular response to such a change. Even positions that are safe for short periods may eventually lead to complications in persons who are not able to move in response to pain. For example, the alcoholic patient who passes out on a hard floor may waken with a brachial plexus injury. Similarly, regional and general anesthesia abolish protective reflexes and predispose patients to injury.

Postural hypotension, the most common physiological consequence of positioning, can be minimized by avoiding abrupt or extreme position changes (eg, sitting up quickly), reversing the position if vital signs deteriorate, keeping the patient as well hydrated as possible, and having drugs available to counter any anticipated reaction. Whereas maintaining a minimal level of anesthesia will decrease the likelihood of hypotension, coincidental movement of the endotracheal tube during positioning may cause the patient to cough and become hypertensive. Table 46–4 summarizes the major physiological effects of common patient positions. Note that these effects are generalizations that can vary with the patient's volume status and cardiac reserve.

Many complications, including air embolism caused by the physiological changes described above, nerve damage as a result of ischemic injury, and the need for finger amputation following a crush injury, have been associated with improper patient positioning (Table 46–5). These complications are best prevented by evaluating the patient's postural limitations during the preanesthetic visit; padding pressure points, susceptible nerves, and any area of the body that will *possibly* be in contact with the operating table or its attachments; avoiding flexion or extension of a joint to its limit; having an awake patient assume the position to ensure comfort; and understanding the potential complications of each position. Periods of patient transport pose a particular threat if monitoring is interrupted for any reason. Similarly, monitors often must be disconnected during patient repositioning.

Compartment syndromes can result from hemorrhage into a closed space following a vascular puncture or prolonged venous outflow obstruction, particularly when associated with hypotension. In severe cases, this may lead to muscle necrosis, myoglobinuria, and renal damage unless the pressure within the compartment is relieved by surgical decompression (fasciotomy).

Table 46–4. Physiological effects of common patient positions.

Position	Organ System	Effects
Supine		
Horizontal[1]	Cardiac	Equalization of pressures throughout the arterial system; increased right-sided filling and cardiac output; decreased heart rate and peripheral vascular resistance.
	Respiratory	Gravity increases perfusion of dependent (posterior) lung segments; abdominal viscera displace diaphragm cephalad. Spontaneous ventilation favors dependent lung segments, while controlled ventilation favors independent (anterior) segments. Functional residual capacity decreases and may fall below closing volume in older patients.
Trendelenburg	Cardiac	Activation of baroreceptors, generally causing decreased cardiac output, peripheral vascular resistance, heart rate, and blood pressure.
	Respiratory	Marked decreases in lung capacities from shift of abdominal viscera; increased ventilation/perfusion mismatching and atelectasis; increased likelihood of regurgitation.
	Other	Increase in intracranial pressure and decrease in cerebral blood flow because of cerebral venous congestion; increased intraocular pressure in patients with glaucoma.
Reverse Trendelenburg	Cardiac	Preload, cardiac output, and arterial pressure decrease. Baroreflexes increase sympathetic tone, heart rate, and peripheral vascular resistance.
	Respiratory	Spontaneous respiration requires less work; functional residual capacity increases.
	Other	Cerebral perfusion pressure and blood flow may decrease.
Lithotomy	Cardiac	Autotransfusion from leg vessels increases circulating blood volume and preload; lowering legs has opposite effect. Effect on blood pressure and cardiac output depends on volume status.
	Respiratory	Decreases vital capacity; increases likelihood of aspiration.
Prone	Cardiac	Pooling of blood in extremities and compression of abdominal muscles may decrease preload, cardiac output, and blood pressure.[2]
	Respiratory	Compression of abdomen and thorax decreases total lung compliance and increases work of breathing.
	Other	Extreme head rotation may decrease cerebral venous drainage and cerebral blood flow.
Lateral decubitus	Cardiac	Cardiac output unchanged unless venous return obstructed (eg, kidney rest). Arterial blood pressure may fall as a result of decreased vascular resistance (right side > left side).
	Respiratory	Decreased volume of dependent lung; increased perfusion of dependent lung. Increased ventilation of dependent lung in awake patients (no $\dot{V}/\dot{Q}$ mismatch); decreased ventilation of dependent lung in anesthetized patients $\dot{V}/\dot{Q}$ mismatch). Further decreases in dependent lung ventilation with paralysis and an open chest (see Chapter 24).
Sitting	Cardiac	Pooling blood in lower body decreases central blood volume. Cardiac output and arterial blood pressure fall despite rise in heart rate and systemic vascular resistance.
	Respiratory	Lung volumes and functional residual capacity increase; work of breathing increases.
	Other	Cerebral blood flow decreases.

[1]The effects described for the horizontal position are in comparison with a patient standing erect. All other positions are compared with the horizontal position.

[2]Changes associated with the prone position are exaggerated by the convex saddle frame used in posterior spinal surgery and minimized by the prone jackknife position.

Table 46–5. Complications associated with patient positioning.

Complication	Position	Prevention
Air embolism	Sitting, prone, reverse Trendelenburg	Maintain venous pressure above 0 at the wound (see Chapter 26).
Alopecia	Supine, lithotomy, Trendelenburg	Normotension, padding, and occasional head turning.
Backache	Any	Lumbar support, padding, and slight hip flexion.
Compartment syndrome	Especially lithotomy	Maintain perfusion pressure and avoid external compression.
Corneal abrasion	Especially prone	Taping and/or lubricating eye.
Digit amputation	Any	Check for protruding digits before changing table configuration.
Nerve palsies		
Brachial plexus	Any	Avoid stretching or direct compression at neck or axilla.
Common peroneal	Lithotomy, lateral decubitus	Pad lateral aspect of upper fibula.
Radial	Any	Avoid compression of lateral humerus.
Ulnar	Any	Padding at elbow, forearm supination.
Retinal ischemia	Prone, sitting	Avoid pressure on globe.
Skin necrosis	Any	Padding over bony prominences.

AWARENESS

A series of media reports have imprinted the fear of awareness under anesthesia into the psyche of the general population. Accounts of recall and helplessness while paralyzed have made unconsciousness a primary concern of patients undergoing general anesthesia. Some reports may appear overdramatized; however, when awareness does occur, patients may exhibit symptoms ranging from mild anxiety to posttraumatic stress disorder (eg, sleep disturbances, nightmares, and social difficulties).

Although the incidence is difficult to document, certain patterns are clear. Evidence of awareness under general anesthesia was found to be 0.2–0.4% in the most quoted studies. Certain types of surgical settings are most frequently associated with awareness, including major trauma, obstetrics, and cardiac surgery. In many instances, awareness may be related to the depth of anesthesia that can be tolerated. In early studies, recall rates for intraoperative events during major trauma surgery have been reported to be as high as 43%; the incidence of awareness during cardiac surgery and cesarean sections is 1.5% and 0.4%, respectively. As of 1999, the ASA Closed Claims Project reported 79 awareness claims; approximately 20% were for awake paralysis and the remainder for recall under general anesthesia. Most claims for awake paralysis were thought to be due to errors in drug labeling and administration. Recall under general anesthesia was found to be more likely in women and when anesthesia relying on opioids and muscle relaxants without volatile anesthetic was used. Poor tolerance of anesthesia, medication errors, younger age, smoking, and long-term use of certain drugs (alcohol, opiates, or amphetamines) may increase the anesthetic requirements for unconsciousness.

The studies referenced above provide clues on how to minimize the chance of awareness and how to deal with it should it occur. Some clinicians routinely discuss recall and the steps that will be taken to minimize it as part of the informed consent for general anesthesia. It is advisable to also remind patients who are undergoing monitored anesthesia care with sedation that awareness is a strong possibility. Volatile anesthetics should be used at a level consistent with amnesia (at least 0.6 minimum alveolar concentration [MAC] when combined with opioids and nitrous oxide or 0.8–1.0 MAC when used alone). If this is not possible, benzodiazepines (and/or scopolamine) can be used. Movement of a patient may be indicative of inadequate anesthetic depth. Documentation should include end-tidal concentrations of anesthetic gases (when available) and accurate dosages of amnesic drugs. Use of a Bispectral Index Scale (BIS) monitor or similar monitors may be helpful (see Chapter 6). Finally, if there is evidence of intraoperative awareness during follow-up, the practitioner should obtain a detailed account of the experience, be very sympathetic, answer patient questions, and refer the patient for psychological counseling if appropriate.

EYE INJURY

A wide range of conditions from simple corneal abrasion to blindness has been reported. Corneal abrasion is by far the most common and transient eye injury. The ASA Closed Claims Project identified a small number of claims for abrasion, in which the cause was rarely identified (20%) and the incidence of permanent injury was low (16%). It also identified a subset of claims concerning blindness that resulted from patient movement during ophthalmological surgery. Both general anesthesia and monitored anesthesia care were used in those instances.

The causation and implications of each subset are quite different. Although the cause of corneal abrasion may not be obvious, properly securing the eyes with tape after loss of consciousness but prior to intubation during general anesthesia and avoiding any direct contact with oxygen masks, drapes, lines, and pillows (particularly during monitored anesthesia care, in transport, and in nonsupine positions) can help minimize the possibility of injury. Paralysis and/or adequate anesthetic depth should be maintained to prevent movement during ophthalmological surgery under general anesthesia. A clear understanding should be reached with the patient that movement under monitored care is hazardous, and minimal sedation to facilitate patient motor control should be considered.

Recently, a devastating eye injury called ischemic optic neuropathy (ION) has been described. ION is now the most common cause of postoperative loss of vision. This syndrome results from optic nerve infarction due to decreased oxygen delivery via one or more small arterioles supplying the nerve head. It is most commonly reported after cardiopulmonary bypass, radical neck dissection, abdominal and hip procedures, and spinal surgeries in the prone position. Both preoperative and intraoperative factors may be contributory. Many of the case reports implicate preexisting hypertension, diabetes, coronary artery disease, and smoking, suggesting that preoperative vascular abnormalities may play a role. Intraoperative deliberate hypotension and anemia have also been implicated, perhaps because of their potential to reduce oxygen delivery. Finally, prolonged surgical time in positions that compromise venous outflow (prone, head down, compressed abdomen) have also been found to be factors. Symptoms, which are usually immediate but have been reported up to 12 days postoperatively, range from decreased visual acuity to complete blindness. Recommendations to prevent this complication are difficult because risk factors for ION are often unavoidable due to the nature of the surgery. Steps that might be taken include (1) enhancing venous outflow by positioning the patient head up and minimizing abdominal constriction, (2) monitoring blood pressure carefully with an arterial line, (3) limiting the degree and duration of hypotension during controlled (deliberate) hypotension, (4) administering a transfusion to anemic patients who appear at risk for ION early enough to avoid severe anemia, and (5) discussing with the surgeon the

possibility of staged operations in high-risk patients to limit prolonged procedures.

CARDIOPULMONARY ARREST DURING SPINAL ANESTHESIA

Sudden cardiac arrest during an otherwise routine administration of spinal anesthetic is an uncommon but catastrophic complication. The initial published report was a closed claims analysis of 14 patients who experienced cardiac arrest during spinal anesthesia. The cases primarily involved young (average age 36 years), relatively healthy (ASA physical status I–II) patients who were given appropriate doses of local anesthetic with a high level of block prior to arrest (T4 level). Subclinical respiratory insufficiency with hypercarbia due to sedatives was thought to be a potential contributing factor. The average time from spinal administration to arrest was 36 ± 18 min, and in all cases arrest was preceded by a gradual decline in heart rate and blood pressure to 20% below baseline values. Just prior to arrest the most common signs were bradycardia, hypotension, and cyanosis. Treatment consisted of ventilatory support, ephedrine, atropine, cardiopulmonary resuscitation (average duration 10.9 min), and finally epinephrine (on average given 5 min into the arrest period). Despite these interventions, 10 patients remained comatose and 4 regained consciousness with significant neurological deficits. A subsequent study concluded that such arrests had little relationship to sedation but were related more to high sympathetic blockade, leading to high vagal tone and profound bradycardia. Rapid, aggressive treatment of bradycardia and hypotension is essential to minimize the risk of arrest. Early, rapid reversal of volume deficits and prophylactic treatment of bradycardia with atropine may prevent a downward spiral. Stepwise doses of ephedrine should be given to treat hypotension. Moreover, practitioners should not hesitate to use epinephrine in small doses (5–10 µg) for bradycardia or hypotension that is unresponsive to atropine and ephedrine and in larger doses if necessary. If cardiopulmonary arrest occurs, ventilatory support, cardiopulmonary resuscitation, and full resuscitation doses of atropine and epinephrine should be administered without delay.

α-AGONIST/β-BLOCKER INTERACTION LEADING TO CARDIAC ARREST

The anesthesia literature from the 1980s describes several instances of severe hypertension leading to congestive heart failure and cardiac arrest in adult patients receiving long-term β-blocker therapy and undergoing ear, nose, and throat procedures. Patients were generally middle aged and all received 8–40 mL of local anesthetic containing 1:100,000 to 1:200,000 epinephrine. A hypertensive/bradycardic response ensued almost immediately and up to 15 min postinjection. The initial recommendation was for treatment with an α-blocker or hydralazine during the acute crisis phase. Subsequently, an editorial in *Archives of Otolaryngology* postulated that in patients being treated with nonselective β-blockers, the primary effect of epinephrine would be α-receptor activation. This would result in profound hypertension and bradycardia due to activation of the carotid baroreceptors and secondary increase in parasympathetic tone. Because β_1-cardiac receptors are blocked, the tachycardia normally induced by epinephrine is not seen, and β_2-receptor blockade of peripheral vasodilation results in an unopposed α-constrictor response.

Since that time, physicians have substituted other topical vasoconstrictors to improve the conditions of the surgical field in various procedures. In March 2000, the Phenylephrine Advisory Committee of New York State reported on the mirror image of this problem—patients receiving vasoconstrictors who were treated for secondary hypertension with β-blockers. A review of 22 cases indicated a recurring pattern: topical vasoconstrictor caused profound hypertension, which was treated with a β-blocker that resulted in pulmonary edema and cardiac arrest. The report strongly implied that the use of β-blockers was responsible for poor patient outcome.

Treatment of hypertension secondary to α-agonists depends on the severity of the patient response. Mild to moderate hypertension may be left untreated, because it is well understood that the hypertension is transient. Severe hypertension, however, can lead to rapid end-organ damage, particularly myocardial ischemia, and as such should be treated immediately with α-blocking agents, such as phentolamine, or a direct vasodilator, such as nitroprusside. The immediate use of β-blockers in this setting is not indicated and may be potentially catastrophic.

HEARING LOSS

Perioperative hearing loss is usually transient and subclinical and often goes unrecognized. The incidence of low-frequency hearing loss following dural puncture may be as high as 50%. It appears to be due to cerebrospinal fluid (CSF) leak and if persistent can be relieved with an epidural blood patch (Chapter 16). Hearing loss following general anesthesia can be due to a variety of causes and is much less predictable. Mechanisms include surgical manipulation, middle ear barotrauma, vascular injury, and ototoxicity of drugs (aminoglycosides, loop diuretics, nonsteroidal antiinflammatory drugs, and antineoplastic agents). Hearing loss following cardiopulmonary bypass is usually unilateral and is thought to be due to embolism and ischemic injury to the organ of Corti.

DOCUMENTATION ISSUES

All anesthesia documentation regarding preoperative evaluation, intraoperative management, invasive procedures, and postoperative care is "patient driven." It will differ with each patient and may change significantly for the same patient within a short period of time due to different surgical procedures and changes in patient status. For example, a 55-year-old patient (status, ASA I) who comes in for an elective laparoscopic cholecystectomy will require an evaluation and anesthetic plan entirely different than what would be needed if he returns 15 h later with an acute abdomen, suspected hepatic bleeding, severe anemia, and new onset of unstable angina with electrocardiographic changes. It is important to customize the evaluation to each patient's particular medical problems and anesthetic needs. However, some general aspects of documentation are important to review. It is critical for clinicians to clearly and legibly document their actions in these areas so that other specialists can understand the rationale for anesthetic management and how it was carried out.

The preoperative anesthesia evaluation should indicate that an airway examination was performed and document its results, such as the Mallampati score, thyromental distance, neck extension, or dentition examination findings. Other evaluation systems are acceptable, but writing or checking "normal" may leave doubt in the mind of malpractice attorneys that a rigorous evaluation was performed. The airway management process should also be outlined in as much detail as possible; "intubation × 2" does not provide the same level of detail as

"Pre-O₂, smooth IV induction, eyes taped, easy mask, laryngoscopy w/MAC 3, grade III view, change head position, Miller 2, grade II view, 7.0 oral endotracheal tube first pass, no blood or trauma noted, cuff up, +ETCO₂, cuff position checked."

Similarly, at extubation, instead of "ETT out" more informative documentation is provided by

"Patient suctioned, cuff down, extubated, no evidence trauma, good airway."

If a patient subsequently developed problems such as dental trauma, altered voice, vocal cord trauma, granuloma, or pharyngoesophageal laceration, the more detailed documentation would better indicate that the standard-of-care for anesthetic management was met (see Chapter 1).

Eye trauma during surgery may be caused by a variety of factors (see above). Because it is assumed that the unsedated/unanesthetized patient retains protective reflexes, eye trauma is frequently, but by no means appropriately, attributed to defects in management of anesthesia. Although awakening patients in the recovery room are far more likely to suffer a corneal abrasion while scratching their noses and pushing the oxygen mask into their eye than to have the same trauma occur when their eyes are taped shut, the anesthesiologist will be called to assess purported "intraoperative eye trauma." It is important to document when the eyes were taped during anesthesia (as noted above, eyes were taped before intubation attempts to rule out corneal abrasion during laryngoscopy), and how the eyes were protected from pressure when the patient is positioned prone or lateral:

"Patient's head in Richard's headrest, eyes/nose/ETT checked, no pressure points."

Neuraxial and peripheral nerve blocks, even with atraumatic placement, have the potential for serious complications including high spinal, subdural injection, epidural hematoma, cauda equina syndrome, radiculopathies, neuropathies, and arachnoiditis. Without adequate documentation, a retrospective review of the chart may attribute these complications to a substandard technique. The written record should include notation of sterile technique, needle type, interspace or approach, number of passes, the presence or absence of blood/paresthesia/CSF, and the type and effect of any test dose given. For example,

"Spinal in lateral position, back prepped/draped, L3–L4 interspace approximated, 1% lidocaine local/25 g Whitacre, 1st pass +CSF, no blood or paresthesia, tetracaine 1% 10 mg plus 1 mL D_{10}, clear CSF aspirated before and after administration, block to T6 at 15 min."

and

"Lumbar epidural in lateral position, back prepped/draped, L3–L4 interspace approximated, 1% lidocaine local/17 g Tuohy, 1st pass LOR w/NS, no blood, CSF, or paresthesia, catheter threaded 4 cm space/7 cm skin, no paresthesia, test dose lidocaine 2% w/epinephrine 3 mL, no evidence subarachnoid placement" (LOR, loss of resistance).

The eventual highest level of the block and length of time it took to achieve it should be recorded.

Placement of central venous lines, arterial lines, nasogastric or orogastric tubes, and TEE probes should also be well documented. With pulmonary artery catheters and central venous lines, sterile technique, number of passes, and lack of pulsatile flow through the needle and respiratory variation of a column of blood in intravenous tubing open to air before the wire is passed all serve to reaffirm proper positioning. The arterial line should be documented with the number of sticks and quality of waveform after the catheter is placed. When placing gastric tubes and TEE probes, use of lubricant, ease of placement, and presence of gastric aspirate (for gastric tubes) or adequate image (TEE) should be noted. If studies such as chest films are ordered, device location and lack of possible complications should be documented. It is very important that a

legible, detailed, and accurate record be completed for every case. Sudden hemodynamic changes in catastrophes, such as pulmonary embolism (thrombus, air, or amniotic fluid) and cardiac arrhythmias, are often not preceded by warning signs. A well-documented record of stable hemodynamics with normal physiological variations may be the only indication of adequate anesthesia care prior to these events and can substantiate the contention that these type of events were not anesthetic mishaps.

Table 46–6 lists eight of the most common errors of documentation in anesthetic practice. It is important to remember that the anesthesia record and any subsequent notes are the only information that will be available should litigation occur. In some instances, the clinician may not be aware of an adverse outcome (or perceived adverse outcome) until weeks or months later. Although it can save time, writing an entry in the anesthesia record *before* the event (eg, "patient extubated to recovery, vitals stable") *severely* compromises the practitioner's credibility if the patient subsequently suffers an adverse event. Events and procedures should be recorded only after they occur. Moreover, notations should be sufficiently descriptive to make it clear that anesthetic management was within the accepted standard of care. *Patient care always supersedes recordkeeping,* but it is important to note times for critical events. Even in the middle of a crisis, hemodynamic variables and time of event should be periodically recorded so that treatment modalities can be accurately reconstructed later. In the event of cardiac arrest, one person (the anesthesiologist) should decide which clock or watch is to be used for all records. *Records, such as cardiopulmonary resuscitation ("code") sheets, should not be signed before they are read and verified for accuracy.* Whenever feasible, save and retrieve important information, such as vital signs, before monitors are turned off. If possible, review the sequence of care with present personnel immediately after the event to ensure accurate documentation in all records. Following an adverse event, it is

Table 46–6. Common documentation pitfalls to avoid.

1. Completing entries for events prior to when they occur.
2. Incomplete descriptions of procedures or management.
3. Inaccurate or conflicting times between different records.
4. Lost critical patient data.
5. Incomplete or poorly thought-out notes following an adverse event.
6. Signing inaccurate documents or documents without reading them.
7. Failure to document meetings with the patient/family, leaving open the possibility of conflicting recollections.
8. Failure to obtain supporting documentation from others.

important to take the time to write a well thought-out note that describes relevant issues and conveys the thought processes and actions involved in the management of the patient. In the emotional atmosphere that occurs after a critical adverse event, a well-intentioned visit to explain events and to comfort a patient's family may be misunderstood and mistakenly recollected 2 years later as an admission of liability or substandard care. It is always important to discuss events openly and answer questions, but it is prudent to have a witness present. Moreover, such meetings should be documented in the medical record and the witness should cosign the note.

ALLERGIC REACTIONS

Hypersensitivity (or allergic) reactions are exaggerated immunological responses to antigenic stimulation in previously sensitized persons. The antigen, or allergen, may be a protein, polypeptide, or smaller molecule that is covalently bound to a carrier protein. Moreover, the allergen may be the substance itself, a metabolite, or a breakdown product. Patients may be exposed to antigens through the nose, lungs, eyes, skin, and gastrointestinal tract, as well as parenterally (intravenously or intramuscularly) and transperitoneally. Specialized classes of monocytes/macrophages process antigens and present them on their cell membrane surface protein to CD4⁺ helper T lymphocytes. The latter can induce a TH1 delayed hypersensitivity, TH2 immediate hypersensitivity, or TH0 anergic (no) response.

Depending on the antigen and the immune system components involved, hypersensitivity reactions are classically divided into four types (Table 46–7). In many cases an allergen, eg, latex, may cause more than one type of hypersensitivity reaction. Type I reactions involve

Table 46–7. Hypersensitivity reactions.

Type I (immediate)
    Atopy
    Urticaria—angioedema
    Anaphylaxis
Type II (cytotoxic)
    Hemolytic transfusion reactions
    Autoimmune hemolytic anemia
    Heparin-induced thrombocytopenia
Type III (immune complex)
    Arthus reaction
    Serum sickness
    Acute hypersensitivity pneumonitis
Type IV (delayed, cell-mediated)
    Contact dermatitis
    Tuberculin-type hypersensitivity
    Chronic hypersensitivity pneumonitis

antigens that cross-link immunoglobulin (Ig) E antibodies triggering the release of inflammatory mediators from mast cells. In type II reactions, complement-fixing (C1-binding) IgG antibodies bind to antigens on cell surfaces, activating the classic complement pathway and lysing the cells. Examples of type II reactions include hemolytic transfusion reactions (see Chapter 29) and heparin-induced thrombocytopenia (see Chapter 21). Type III reactions occur when antigen–antibody (IgG or IgM) immune complexes are deposited in tissues, activating complement and generating chemotactic factors that attract neutrophils to the area. The activated neutrophils cause tissue injury by releasing lysosomal enzymes and toxic products. Type III reactions include serum sickness reactions and acute hypersensitivity pneumonitis. Type IV reactions, often referred to as delayed hypersensitivity, are mediated by CD4⁺ T lymphocytes that have been sensitized to a specific antigen by prior exposure. Prior TH1 response causes expression of a T cell receptor protein that is specific for the antigen. Reexposure to the antigen causes these lymphocytes to produce lymphokines—interleukins (IL), interferon (IFN), and tumor necrosis factor-γ (TNF-γ)—that attract and activate inflammatory mononuclear cells over 48–72 h. Production of IL-1 and IL-6 by antigen-processing cells amplifies clonal expression of the specific sensitized T cells and attracts other types of T cells. IL-2 secretion transforms CD8⁺ cytotoxic T cells into killer cells; IL-4 and IFN-γ cause macrophages to undergo epithelioid transformation, often producing granuloma. Examples of type IV reactions are those associated with tuberculosis, histoplasmosis, schistosomiasis, and hypersensitivity pneumonitis as well as some autoimmune disorders such as rheumatoid arthritis and Wegener's granulomatosis.

1. Immediate Hypersensitivity Reactions

Initial exposure of a susceptible person to an antigen induces CD4⁺ T cells to produce IL-4, IL-5, IL-6, IL-10, and granulocyte–macrophage colony-stimulating factor (GM-CSF). These lymphokines activate and transform specific B lymphocytes into plasma cells, which produce allergen-specific IgE antibodies (Figure 46–2). The Fc portion of these antibodies then associates with high affinity receptors on the cell surface of tissue mast cells and circulating basophils. During subsequent reexposure to the antigen, it binds the Fab portion of adjacent IgE antibodies on the mast cell surface, inducing degranulation and release of inflammatory lipid mediators and additional cytokines from the mast cell. The end result is an increase in intracellular calcium that causes degranulation of the mast cells, releasing histamine, tryptase, proteoglycans (heparin and chondroitin sulfate), and carboxypeptidases. The increase in intracellular calcium also activates prostaglandin (mainly prostaglandin D₂) and

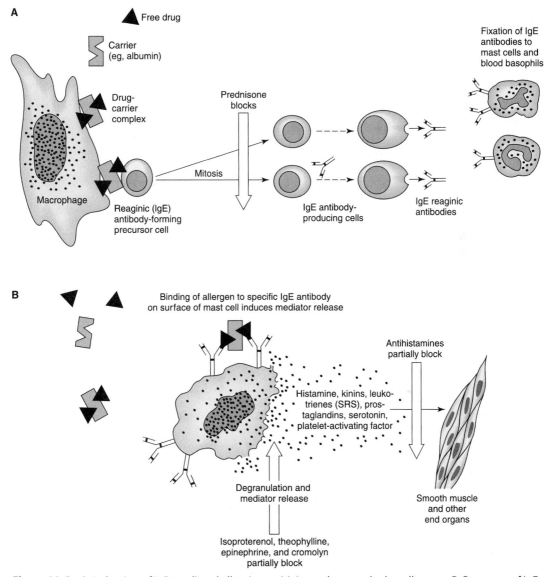

Figure 46–2. *A:* Induction of IgE-mediated allergic sensitivity to drugs and other allergens. ***B:*** Response of IgE-sensitized cells to subsequent exposure to allergens. Ig, immunoglobulin. (Reproduced, with permission, from Katzung BG [editor]: *Basic & Clinical Pharmacology,* 8th ed. McGraw-Hill, 2001.)

leukotriene (B_4, C_4, D_4, E_4, and platelet-activating factor) synthesis. Leukotrienes were previously referred to as slow reacting substance of anaphylaxis. Additional mediators include neutrophil chemotactic factors (NCF), eosinophil chemotactic factor of anaphylaxis (ECF-A), and basophil kallikrein of anaphylaxis (BK-A). Mast cells may also release IL-3, IL-4, IL-5, IL-6, IFN-γ, TNF-α, and GM-CSF. The combined effects of these mediators can produce arteriolar vasodilatation, increased vascular

permeability, increased mucus secretion, smooth muscle contraction, and other clinical manifestations of type I reactions.

Type I hypersensitivity reactions are classified as atopic or nonatopic. Atopic disorders typically affect the skin or respiratory tract and include allergic rhinitis, atopic dermatitis, and allergic asthma. Nonatopic hypersensitivity disorders include urticaria, angioedema, and anaphylaxis; when these reactions are mild they are confined to the skin (urticaria) or subcutaneous tissue (angioedema), but when they are severe, they become generalized and a life-threatening medical emergency (anaphylaxis). Urticarial lesions are characteristically well-circumscribed skin wheals with raised erythematous borders and blanched centers; they are intensely pruritic and may be localized or generalized. Angioedema presents as deep nonpitting cutaneous edema resulting from marked vasodilation and increased permeability of subcutaneous blood vessels. When angioedema is extensive, it can be associated with large fluid shifts; when it is localized to the pharyngeal or laryngeal mucosa, it can rapidly compromise the airway.

2. Anaphylactic Reactions

Anaphylaxis is an exaggerated response to an allergen (eg, antibiotic) that is mediated by a type I hypersensitivity reaction. The syndrome appears within minutes following exposure to a specific antigen in a sensitized person and characteristically presents as acute respiratory distress, circulatory shock, or both. Death usually occurs from asphyxiation or irreversible circulatory shock. The incidence of anaphylactic reactions during anesthesia has been estimated at a rate of 1:5000 to 1:25,000 anesthetics. Antibiotics are the most common cause of anaphylactic reactions, but latex has also become an increasingly important cause.

The most important mediators of anaphylaxis are histamine, leukotrienes, BK-A, and platelet-activating factor. They increase vascular permeability and contract smooth muscle. H_1-receptor activation contracts bronchial smooth muscle, whereas H_2-receptor activation causes vasodilation, enhanced mucus secretion, tachycardia, and increased myocardial contractility. BK-A cleaves bradykinin from kininogen; bradykinin increases vascular permeability and vasodilation and contracts smooth muscle. Activation of Hageman factor can initiate intravascular coagulation in some patients. ECF-A, NCF, and leukotriene B_4 attract inflammatory cells that mediate additional tissue injury. Angioedema of the pharynx, larynx, and trachea produce upper airway obstruction, whereas bronchospasm and mucosal edema result in lower airway obstruction. Histamine may preferentially constrict large airways, whereas leukotrienes primarily affect smaller peripheral airways. Transudation of fluid into the skin (angioedema) and viscera produces hypovolemia and shock, whereas arteriolar vasodilation decreases systemic vascular resistance. Coronary hypoperfusion and hypoxemia promote arrhythmias and myocardial ischemia. Leukotriene and prostaglandin mediators may also cause coronary vasospasm. Prolonged circulatory shock results in progressive lactic acidosis and ischemic damage to other vital organs. Table 46–8 summarizes important manifestations of anaphylactic reactions. It is important to note that cardiovascular and cuta-

Table 46–8. Clinical manifestations of anaphylaxis.

Organ System	Signs and Symptoms
Cardiovascular	Hypotension,[1] tachycardia, arrhythmias
Pulmonary	Bronchospasm,[1] cough, dyspnea, pulmonary edema, laryngeal edema, hypoxia
Dermatological	Urticaria,[1] facial edema, pruritus

[1]Key signs during general anesthesia.

neous manifestations are more common features of anaphylaxis than bronchospasm during anesthesia.

Anaphylactoid reactions resemble anaphylaxis but do not depend on IgE antibody interaction with antigen. A drug can directly release histamine from mast cells (eg, urticaria following high-dose morphine sulfate) or activate complement. Although the mechanisms differ, anaphylactic and anaphylactoid reactions can be clinically indistinguishable and equally life-threatening. Table 46–9 lists common causes of anaphylactic and anaphylactoid reactions. The incidence of anaphylaxis and anaphylactoid reactions under anesthesia is estimated to be between 1 in 3500 to 1 in 13,000.

Factors that may predispose patients to these reactions include youth, pregnancy, known atopy, and previous drug exposure. Laboratory identification of patients who have experienced an adverse allergic reaction or who may be particularly susceptible is often aided by intradermal skin testing, leukocyte or basophil degranulation testing (histamine release test), or radioallergosorbent testing (RAST). The latter is capable of measuring the level of drug-specific IgE antibody in the serum. Serum tryptase measurement is helpful in confirming the diagnosis of an anaphylactic reaction. Prophylactic pretreatment with histamine receptor antagonists and corticosteroids decreases the severity of the reaction. **Treatment must be immediate and tailored to the severity of the reaction (Table 46–10).**

3. Allergic Reactions to Anesthetic Agents

True anaphylaxis due to anesthetic agents is rare; anaphylactoid reactions are much more common (see Table 46–9). Risk factors associated with hypersensitivity to anesthetics include female gender, atopic history, preexisting allergies, and previous anesthetic exposures. Muscle relaxants have emerged as the most common cause of anaphylaxis during anesthesia with an estimated incidence of 1 in 6500 patients. They account for almost 70% of anaphylactic reactions perioperatively. The mechanism involves IgE antibodies directed against tertiary or quaternary ion epitopes. In

Table 46–9. Causes of anaphylactic and anaphylactoid reactions.[1]

Anaphylactic reactions against polypeptides	Venoms (Hymenoptera, fire ant, snake, jellyfish)
	Airborne allergens (pollen, molds, danders)
	Foods (peanuts, milk, egg, seafood, grain)
	Enzymes (trypsin, streptokinase, chymopapain, asparaginase)
	Heterologous serum (tetanus antitoxin, antilymphocyte globulin, antivenin)
	Human proteins (insulin, corticotropin, vasopressin, serum and seminal proteins)
	Latex
Anaphylactic reactions against hapten carrier	Antibiotics (penicillin, cephalosporins, sulfonamides)
	Disinfectants (ethylene oxide, chlorhexidine)
	Local anesthetics (procaine)
Anaphylactoid reactions	Polyionic solutions (radiocontrast medium, polymyxin B)
	Opioids (morphine, meperidine)
	Hypnotics (thiopental, propofol)
	Muscle relaxants (curare, succinylcholine, atracurium)
	Synthetic membranes (dialysis)
	Nonsteroidal antiinflammatory drugs
	Preservatives (sulfites, benzoates)
	Protamine
	Dextran
	Steroids
	Exercise
	Idiopathic

[1]Adapted, with permission, from Bochner BS, Lichtenstein LM: N Engl J Med 1991;324:1786.

many instances, there was no previous exposure to muscle relaxants. Investigators suggest that over-the-counter drugs, cosmetics, and food products, many of which contain tertiary or quaternary ammonium ions, can sensitize susceptible individuals. A French study found that, in decreasing order of frequency, rocuronium, succinylcholine, and atracurium were most often responsible; this likely reflects the propensity to cause anaphylaxis together with frequency of use.

Although rarer, hypnotic agents can also be responsible for some allergic reactions. The incidence of anaphylaxis for thiopental and propofol is 1 in 30,000 and 1 in 60,000, respectively. Allergic reactions to etomidate, ketamine, and benzodiazepines are exceedingly rare. True anaphylactic reactions due to opioids are far less common than nonimmune histamine release. Similarly, anaphylactic reactions to local anesthetics are much less common than vasovagal reactions, toxic reactions, and side effects from epinephrine. IgE-mediated reactions to ester-type local anesthetics, however, are well described. Because they all share common antigenicity with *p*-aminobenzoic acid, cross-reactivity should be expected between ester-type local anesthetics. In contrast, anaphylaxis due to amide-type local anesthetics is very rare; in most instances, the preservative (paraben or methylparaben) was believed to be responsible; moreover, the cross-reactivity between amide-type local anesthetics appears to be low. There are no reports of anaphylaxis to volatile anesthetics.

4. Latex Allergy

The severity of allergic reactions to latex-containing products ranges from mild contact dermatitis to life-threatening anaphylaxis. Latex allergy is the second most common cause of anaphylaxis during anesthesia. Most serious reactions appear to involve a direct IgE-mediated immune response to polypeptides in natural latex, although some cases of contact dermatitis may be due to a type IV sensitivity reaction to chemicals introduced in the manufacturing process. Nonetheless, a relationship between the occurrence of contact dermatitis and the probability of future anaphylaxis has been suggested. Chronic exposure to latex and a history of atopy increases the risk of sensitization. Health care workers and patients undergoing frequent procedures with latex items (eg, repeated urinary bladder catheterization, barium enema examinations) should therefore be considered at increased risk. Between 5% and 17% of health care workers are estimated to be allergic to latex. Patients with spina bifida, spinal cord injury, and congenital abnormalities of the genitourinary tract have a very high incidence of latex allergy. The incidence of latex anaphylaxis in chil-

Table 46–10. Treatment of anaphylactic and anaphylactoid reactions.

Discontinue drug administration
Administer 100% oxygen
Epinephrine (0.01–0.5 mg IV or IM)[1]
Consider intubation or tracheostomy
Intravenous fluids (1–2 L lactated Ringer's injection)
Diphenhydramine (50–75 mg IV)
Ranitidine (150 mg IV)
Hydrocortisone (up to 200 mg IV) or methylprednisolone (1–2 mg/kg)

[1]The dose and route of epinephrine depend on the severity of the reaction. An infusion of 0.001 mg/min may be necessary.

dren is estimated to be 1 in 10,000. A history of allergic symptoms to latex should be sought in all patients during the preanesthetic interview. Foods that cross-react with latex include mango, kiwi, chestnut, avacado, passion fruit, and banana.

Anaphylactic reactions to latex may be confused with reactions to other substances (eg, drugs, blood products) because the onset of symptoms can be delayed for more than 1 h after initial exposure. Treatment is the same as for other forms of anaphylactic reactions. Skin-prick tests, intradermal tests, basophil histamine-release tests, and RAST have been used to evaluate high-risk patients. Preventing a reaction in sensitized patients includes pharmacological prophylaxis and absolute avoidance of latex. Preoperative administration of H_1 and H_2 histamine antagonists (see Chapter 15) and steroids may provide some protection, although their use is controversial. Although many pieces of anesthetic equipment are increasingly latex-free, some may still contain latex, eg, gloves, tourniquets, some ventilator bellows, intravenous injection ports, and older reusable face masks. An allergic reaction has even been documented from inhalation of latex antigen contained within aerosolized glove powder. Manufacturers of latex-containing medical products must label their products accordingly. **Only devices specifically known not to contain latex (eg, polyvinyl or neoprene gloves, silicone endotracheal tubes or laryngeal masks, plastic face masks) can be used in these patients.** Rubber stoppers should be removed from drug vials prior to use and injections should be made through plastic stopcocks.

5. Allergies to Antibiotics

Many true drug allergies in surgical patients are due to antibiotics, mainly β-lactam antibiotics, such as penicillins and cephalosporins. Although 1–4% of β-lactams administrations result in allergic reactions, only 0.004–0.015% of these reactions produce anaphylaxis. To put things in perspective, up to 2% of the general population is allergic to penicillin, but only 0.01% of penicillin administrations result in anaphylaxis. Cephalosporin cross-sensitivity in patients with penicillin allergy is estimated to be 2–7%, but a history of an anaphylactic reaction to penicillin increases the cross-reactivity rate up to 50%. Patients with a prior history of an anaphylactic reaction to penicillin should therefore not receive a cephalosporin. Although imipenem exhibits similar cross-sensitivity, aztreonam appears to be antigenically distinct and reportedly does not cross-react with other β-lactams. Sulfonamide allergy is also relatively common in surgical patients. Sulfa drugs include sulfonamide antibiotics, furosemide, hydrochlorothiazide, and captopril. Fortunately, the frequency of cross-reactivity between these agents is low.

Like cephalosporins, vancomycin is commonly used for antibiotic prophylaxis in surgical patients. Unfortunately, it is commonly associated with adverse reactions. An anaphylactoid-type reaction, "red man's syndrome," consists of intense pruritus, flushing, and erythema of the head and upper torso, often with arterial hypotension; this syndrome may be related more to a rapid rate of administration than to dose or a true allergy. Isolated systemic hypotension is a much more frequent side effect and appears to be primarily mediated by histamine release because pretreatment with H_1 and H_2 antihistamines can prevent hypotension even with rapid rates of administration.

OCCUPATIONAL HAZARDS IN ANESTHESIOLOGY

1. Chronic Exposure to Anesthetic Gases

Chapter 2 began with the statement that anesthesiologists spend more time in operating rooms than do any other group of physicians. This results in greater exposure to the risks of the operating room environment, such as the potential long-term effects of trace anesthetic gases. Fortunately, there is no clear evidence that exposure to trace amounts of anesthetic agents presents a health hazard to operating room personnel. However, because previous studies examining this issue have been flawed or have produced conflicting results, the U.S. Occupational Health and Safety Administration continues to set maximum acceptable trace concentrations of less than 25 ppm for nitrous oxide and 0.5 ppm for halogenated anesthetics (2 ppm if the halogenated agent is used alone). Achieving these low levels depends on efficient scavenging equipment, adequate operating room ventilation, and conscientious anesthetic technique. Most people cannot detect the odor of volatile agents at a concentration of less than 30 ppm (nitrous oxide is essentially odorless). Without a properly functioning scavenging system, anesthetic gas concentrations are about 3000 ppm for nitrous oxide and 50 ppm for volatile agents.

2. Infectious Diseases

Hospital workers are exposed to many infectious diseases prevalent in the community (eg, respiratory viral infections, rubella, and tuberculosis).

Herpetic whitlow is an infection of the finger with herpes simplex virus type 1 or 2 and usually involves direct contact of previously traumatized skin with contaminated oral secretions. Painful vesicles appear at the site of infection. The diagnosis is confirmed by the appearance of giant epithelial cells or nuclear inclusion bodies in a smear taken from the base of a vesicle, the presence of a rise in herpes simplex virus titer, or identi-fication of the virus with antiserum. Treatment is con-servative and includes topical application of 5% acyclo-vir ointment. Prevention involves wearing gloves when contacting oral secretions. Patients at risk for harboring the virus include those suffering from other infections, immunosuppression, cancer, and malnutrition.

Viral DNA has been identified in the smoke plume generated during laser treatment of condyloma. The theoretical possibility of viral transmission from this source can be minimized by using smoke evacuators, gloves, and high-efficiency masks.

More disturbing is the potential of acquiring serious blood-borne infections such as hepatitis B, hepatitis C, or human immunodeficiency virus (HIV). Although parenteral transmission of these diseases can occur fol-lowing mucous membrane, cutaneous, or percutaneous exposure to infected body fluids, accidental injury with a needle contaminated with infected blood represents the most common occupational mechanism. The risk of transmission can be estimated if three factors are known: the prevalence of the infection within the patient population, the incidence of exposure (eg, fre-quency of needlestick), and the rate of seroconversion after a single exposure. The seroconversion rate after a specific exposure depends on several factors, including the infectivity of the organism, the stage of the patient's disease (extent of viremia), the size of the inoculum, and the immune status of the health care provider. Rates of seroconversion following a single needlestick are estimated to range between 0.3% and 30%. It should be noted that hollow (hypodermic) nee-dles pose a greater risk than solid (surgical) nee-dles because of the potentially larger inoculum. The use of gloves, needleless systems, or protected nee-dle devices may decrease the incidence of some (but not all) types of injury.

Initial management of needlesticks involves clean-ing the wound and notifying the appropriate authority within the health care facility. The serological status of the health care worker and, if possible, the source patient should be established. Ig may be partially effective in preventing hepatitis B. Prophylactic IFN (with or without ribavirin) following a high-risk inoc-ulation from a hepatitis C patient is highly controver-sial because of considerable drug side effects. Although prophylactic administration of zidovudine alone reduces the risk of HIV infection following a contaminated needlestick, concerns over rising drug resistance have caused many experts to recommend multidrug pro-phylaxis regimens.

The prevalence of hepatitis B serological markers is several times higher in anesthesia personnel (15–50%) than in the general population (3–5%). The risk of infection is proportional to the number of years in prac-tice. Fulminant hepatitis (1% of acute infections) car-ries a 60% mortality rate. Chronic active hepatitis (< 5% of all cases) is associated with an increased inci-dence of cirrhosis of the liver and hepatocellular carci-noma. Transmission of the virus is primarily through contact with blood products or body fluids. The diag-nosis is confirmed by detection of hepatitis B surface antigen (HBsAg). Uncomplicated recovery is signaled by the disappearance of HBsAg and the appearance of antibody to the surface antigen (anti-HBs). A hepatitis vaccine is available and is strongly recommended pro-phylactically for anesthesia personnel. The appearance of anti-HBs after a three-dose regimen indicates suc-cessful immunization.

Hepatitis C is another important occupational haz-ard in anesthesiology; 4–8% of hepatitis C infections occur in health care workers. Most (50–90%) of these infections lead to chronic hepatitis, which, although often asymptomatic, can progress to liver failure and death. In fact, hepatitis C is the most common cause of nonalcoholic cirrhosis in the United States. There is currently no vaccine to protect against hepatitis C infection. Screening donor blood for antibodies to hep-atitis C has decreased but not eliminated the incidence of hepatitis C infections following blood transfusion.

Anesthesia personnel appear to be at a low but real risk for the occupational contraction of AIDS. The risk of acquiring HIV infection following a single needle-stick contaminated with blood from an HIV-infected patient has been estimated at 0.4–0.5%. Because there are documented reports of transmission of HIV from infected patients to health care workers (including anes-thesiologists), the Centers for Disease Control and Pre-vention has proposed guidelines that apply to all cate-gories of patient contact. These universal precautions, which are equally valid for protection against hepatitis B or C infection, are as follows:

- Needle precautions, including no recapping and im-mediate disposal of contaminated needles.

- Use of gloves and other barriers during contact with open wounds and body fluids.

- Frequent hand-washing.

- Proper techniques for disinfection or disposal of con-taminated materials.

- Particular caution by pregnant health care workers, and no contact with patients by workers who have exudative or weeping dermatitis.

3. Substance Abuse

Anesthesiology is a high-risk medical specialty for drug addiction. Reasons for this include the stress of anesthetic practice, the easy availability of drugs with addiction potential, and curiosity aroused by a patient's euphoria after receiving opioids and sedatives. The likelihood of developing a substance abuse problem is increased by coexisting personal problems (eg, marital, financial difficulties) and a family history of alcoholism or drug addiction.

The voluntary use of mood-altering drugs is a disease. If left untreated, substance abuse often leads to death from drug overdose—intentional or unintentional. One of the greatest challenges in treating this illness is identifying the afflicted individual, since denial is a consistent feature. Unfortunately, changes evident to an outside observer are often both vague and late: reduced involvement in social activities, subtle changes in appearance, extreme mood swings, and altered work habits. Treatment begins with an intervention plan of enrolling the individual in a formal rehabilitation program. The possibility of retaining one's medical license and reentering the mainstream of practice provides powerful motivation. Some diversion programs report a success rate of approximately 70%. Long-term compliance often involves continued participation in support groups (eg, Narcotics Anonymous), random urine testing, and oral naltrexone therapy (a long-acting opioid antagonist). Effective prevention strategies are difficult to formulate but may include better control of drug availability and education about the severe consequences of substance abuse.

4. Radiation Exposure

The intraoperative use of imaging equipment (eg, fluoroscopy) and attendance during radiological procedures (eg, interventional radiology) expose the anesthesiologist to the potential risks of ionizing radiation. The two most important methods of minimizing exposure are using proper barriers and maximizing the distance from the source of radiation. Lead glass partitions or lead aprons with thyroid shields are mandatory protection for all personnel working in an imaging environment. The inverse square law states that the amount of radiation changes inversely with the square of the distance. Thus, the exposure at 4 m will be one-sixteenth that at 1 m. The maximum recommended occupational whole-body exposure to radiation is 5 rem/year. This can be monitored by wearing an exposure badge.

> ### CASE DISCUSSION:
> ### UNEXPLAINED INTRAOPERATIVE
> ### TACHYCARDIA & HYPERTENSION

A 73-year-old man is scheduled for emergency relief of an intestinal obstruction with strangulation from a volvulus at midnight. The patient had a myocardial infarction 1 month ago that was complicated by intermittent congestive heart fail-

ure. His blood pressure is 160/90 mm Hg, pulse 110 beats/min, respiratory rate 22/min, and temperature 38.8°C.

Why is this case an emergency?

Strangulation of the bowel begins with venous obstruction but can quickly progress to arterial occlusion, ischemia, infarction, and perforation. Acute peritonitis could lead to severe dehydration, sepsis, shock, and multiorgan failure—obviously a poor prognosis in this elderly patient. Nonetheless, a few hours could be well spent optimizing the patient's fluid status and cardiovascular parameters before rushing to the operating room. Furthermore, a complex and high-risk case such as this requires extra operating room setup time in preparing medications, monitors, and other anesthetic equipment.

The patient is immediately rushed to an available operating room that has been set up for possible open-heart surgery.

What special monitoring is appropriate for this patient?

Because of the history of recent myocardial infarction and congestive heart failure, an arterial line and a pulmonary artery catheter would be useful. Large fluid shifts should be anticipated, and a beat-to-beat monitor of blood pressure is needed. Furthermore, information regarding myocardial supply (diastolic blood pressure) and demand (systolic blood pressure, left ventricular wall stress, and heart rate) should be continuously available. A central venous pressure may give misleading information because of the potential discrepancy between right- and left-sided pressures in a patient with significant left ventricular dysfunction. Further monitoring might include transesophageal echocardiography for early detection of myocardial ischemia and assessment of ventricular wall motion.

An arterial line is easily placed, but the pulmonary artery catheter gives only an intermittent pulmonary artery tracing.

What cardiovascular medications might be useful during induction and maintenance of general anesthesia?

A continuous intravenous infusion of nitroglycerin could beneficially alter the myocardial supply/demand balance. Esmolol might be useful in decreasing the heart rate, but caution is suggested by the history of congestive heart fail-

ure. Drugs causing tachycardia or extremes in arterial blood pressure should obviously be avoided.

A nitroglycerin drip is begun, and the patient's vital signs remain stable throughout a standard thiopental induction. During the laparotomy, gradual increases in heart rate and blood pressure are noted. The rate of administration of nitroglycerin is increased, and ST-segment elevations appear on the electrocardiogram (ECG). The heart rate is now 130/min and the blood pressure 220/140 mm Hg. The pulmonary artery catheter tracing is consistent with a right ventricular location. The concentration of volatile anesthetic is increased, and propranolol is administered intravenously in 1-mg increments. This results in a decline in heart rate to 115 beats/min but a rise in blood pressure to 250/160 mm Hg. Suddenly, the rhythm converts to ventricular tachycardia, with a profound drop in blood pressure. As lidocaine is being administered and the defibrillation unit prepared, the rhythm degenerates into ventricular fibrillation.

What can explain this series of events?

A differential diagnosis of pronounced tachycardia and hypertension might include pheochromocytoma, malignant hyperthermia, or thyroid storm. In this case, further inspection of the nitroglycerin infusion reveals that the intravenous tubing had been mislabeled. In fact, although the tubing was labeled nitroglycerin, the infusion bag was labeled epinephrine.

How does this explain the paradoxic response to propranolol?

Propranolol is a nonselective β-adrenergic antagonist. It blocks the tachycardia because of epinephrine's β_1-stimulation and the dilatation of blood vessels as a result of β_2-stimulation, but it does not affect α-induced vasoconstriction. The net result is a decrease in heart rate but an increase in blood pressure.

Why wasn't the patient hypotensive during induction?

It was surprising that a standard thiopental induction would not result in profound hypotension in this dehydrated elderly patient with a history of heart disease. The epinephrine infusion may have masked the hypotensive effects of induction, resulting in relatively stable vital signs.

What is the cause of the ventricular tachycardia?

An overdose of epinephrine can cause life-threatening ventricular dysrhythmias. A high concentration of volatile anesthetic could have further sensitized the myocardium to the dysrhythmogenic effects of epinephrine. In addition, the malpositioned tip of the pulmonary artery catheter could have irritated the endothelium and conduction pathways in the right ventricle.

What other factors may have contributed to this anesthetic mishap?

Many factors may have indirectly contributed to this end result, including the midnight timing of the case (eg, physician fatigue), the lack of preparation (eg, patient fine-tuning), the use of drugs prepared by another anesthesiologist, and the decision to proceed with induction and surgery despite unsatisfactory positioning of the pulmonary artery catheter. The end result of this chain of coincidence, misjudgment, and an unhealthy patient was a poor outcome.

SUGGESTED READING

Atlee AL: *Complications in Anesthesia.* W.B. Saunders, 1999.

Benumof JL, Saidman LJ: *Anesthesia & Perioperative Complications,* 2nd ed. Mosby, 1999.

Bogner MS: *Human Error in Medicine.* Lawrence Erlbaum, 1994.

Bowdle TA: Drug administration errors from the ASA closed claims project. ASA Newslett 2003;67(6):11.

Brown RH, Schauble JF, Miller NR: Anemia and hypotension as contributors to perioperative loss of vision. Anesthesiology 1994;80:222.

Caplan RA: Informed consent: patterns of liability from the ASA Closed Claims Project. ASA Newslett 2000;64(6):7.

Caplan RA, Ward RJ, Posner K, Cheney FW: Unexpected cardiac arrest during spinal anesthesia: a closed claims analysis of predisposing factors. Anesthesiology 1988;68:5.

Caplan RA, Vistica MF, Posner KL, Cheney FW: Adverse anesthetic outcomes arising from gas delivery equipment: a closed claims analysis. Anesthesiology 1997;87:741.

Chadwick HS: An analysis of obstetric anesthesia cases from the American Society of Anesthesiologists closed claims project database. Int J Obstet Anesth 1996;5:258.

Chadwick HS: Obstetric anesthesia closed claims update II. ASA Newslett 2003;67(6):6.

Cheney FW: The American Society of Anesthesiologists closed claims project: what have we learned, how has it affected practice, and how will it affect practice in the future? Anesthesiology 1999;91:552.

Cheney FW, Posner KL, Caplan RA, Gild WM: Burns from warming devices in anesthesia. Anesthesiology 1994;80:806.

Cheney FW, Domino KB, Caplan RA, Posner KL: Nerve injury associated with anesthesia: a closed claims analysis. Anesthesiology 1999;90:1062.

Cheney FW: Changing trends in anesthesia-related death and permanent brain damage. ASA Newslett 2002;66:6.

Coppieters MW, Van De Velde M, Stappaerts KH: Positioning in anesthesiology. Toward a better understanding of stretch-induced perioperative neuropathies. Anesthesiology 2002;97:75.

Domino KB, Posner Kl, Caplan RA, Cheney FW: Awareness during anesthesia: a closed claims analysis. Anesthesiology 1999;90:1053.

Domino KB, Posner KL, Caplan RA, Cheney FW: Airway injury during anesthesia: a closed claims analysis. Anesthesiology 1999;91:1703.

Edbril SD, Lagasse RS: Relationship between malpractice litigation and human errors. Anesthesiology 1999;91:848.

Finucane BT: Complications of Regional Anesthesia. Churchill Livingstone, 1999.

Fisher DM: New York State guidelines on the topical use of phenylephrine in operating rooms. Anesthesiology 2000;92:858.

Fitzgibbon DR, Posner KL, Domino KB, et al: Chronic pain management: American Society of Anesthesiologists Closed Claims Project. Anesthesiology. 2004;100:98.

Ghoneim MM: Awareness during anesthesia. Anesthesiology 2000;92:597.

Gild WM, Posner KL, Caplan RA, Cheney FW: Eye injuries associated with anesthesia. Anesthesiology 1992;76:204.

Hepner DL, Castells MC: Anaphylaxis during the perioperative period. Anesth Analg 2003;97:1381.

Lee LA: Postoperative visual loss data gathered and analyzed. ASA Newslett 2000;64(9):25.

Lesser, JB, Sanborn KV, Valskys R, Kuroda M: Severe bradycardia during spinal and epidural anesthesia recorded by an anesthesia information management system. Anesthesiology 2003;99:859.

Martin JT: Compartment syndromes: concept and perspectives for the anesthesiologist. Anesth Analg 1992;75:275.

Martin JT: *Positioning in Anesthesia & Surgery,* 3rd ed. W.B. Saunders, 1997.

McLeskey CH: Awareness during anesthesia. Can J Anaesth 1999;46:R80.

Mertes PM, Laxenaire MC, Alla F: Anaphylactic and anaphylactoid reactions occurring during anesthesia in France in 1999–2000. Anesthesiology 2003;99:536.

Miller CG: Management of the difficult intubation in closed malpractice claims. ASA Newslett 2000;64(6).

Morray JP, Geiduschek JM, Caplan RA: A comparison of pediatric and adult anesthesia closed malpractice claims. Anesthesiology 1993;78:461.

Newland MC, Ellis SJ, Lydiatt CA, et al: Anesthetic-related cardiac arrest and its mortality. Anesthesiology 2002;97:108.

Pollard JB: Cardiac arrest during spinal anesthesia: common mechanisms and strategies for prevention. Anesth Analg 2001;92:252.

Posner KL: Liability profile of ambulatory anesthesia. ASA Newslett 2000;64(6).

Practice advisory for the prevention of perioperative peripheral neuropathies: a report by the American Society of Anesthesiologists Task Force on prevention of peripheral neuropathies. Anesthesiology 2000;92:1168.

Ranta SOV, Lauila R, Saario J, et al: Awareness with recall during general anesthesia: incidence and risk factors. Anesth Analg 1998;86:1084.

Sharma AD, Parmley CL, Sreeram G, Grocott HP: Peripheral nerve injuries during cardiac surgery: risk factors, diagnosis, prognosis, and prevention. Anesth Analg 2000;91:1358.

Silverstein JH, Silva DA, Iberti TJ: Opioid addiction in anesthesiology. Anesthesiology 1993;79:354.

Sprung J, Bourke DL, Contreras MG, et al: Perioperative hearing impairment. Anesthesiology 2003;98:241.

Tait AR: Occupational transmission of tuberculosis: implications for anesthesiologists. Anesth Analg 1997;85:444.

Warner MA, Warner ME, Martin JT: Ulnar neuropathy. Incidence, outcome, and risk factors in sedated or anesthetized patients. Anesthesiology 1994;81:1332.

Warner MA, Warner DO, Harper CM: Lower extremity neuropathies associated with lithotomy positions. Anesthesiology 2000;93:938.

Warner ME, Benenfeld SM, Warner MA, et al: Perianesthetic dental injuries. Anesthesiology 1999;90:1302.

Weinger MB, Englund CE: Ergonomic and human factors affecting anesthetic vigilance and monitoring performance in the operating room environment. Anesthesiology 1990;73:995.

Williams EL, Hart WM Jr, Tempelhoff R: Postoperative ischemic optic neuropathy. Anesth Analg 1995;80:1018.

Cardiopulmonary Resuscitation

47

KEY CONCEPTS

 1 Cardiopulmonary resuscitation and emergency cardiac care should be considered any time an individual cannot adequately oxygenate or perfuse vital organs—not only following cardiac or respiratory arrest.

2 Regardless of which transtracheal jet ventilation system is chosen, it must be readily available, use low-compliance tubing, and have secure connections.

3 Ventilation (and chest compressions) should not be delayed for intubation if a patent airway is established by a jaw-thrust maneuver.

4 Attempts at intubation should not interrupt ventilation for more than 30 s.

5 Chest compressions should be immediately initiated in the pulseless patient.

6 Whether adult resuscitation is performed by a single rescuer or by two rescuers, two breaths are administered every 15 compressions (15:2), allowing 2 s for each breath. The cardiac compression rate should be 100/min regardless of the number of rescuers.

7 Health care personnel working in hospitals and ambulatory care facilities must be able to provide early defibrillation to collapsed patients with ventricular fibrillation as soon as possible. Shock should be delivered within 3 min (± 1 min) of arrest.

8 Lidocaine, epinephrine, atropine, and vasopressin but not sodium bicarbonate can be delivered down a catheter whose tip extends past the tracheal tube. Dosages 2–2½ times higher than recommended for intravenous use, diluted in 10 mL of normal saline or distilled water, are recommended for adult patients.

9 If intravenous cannulation is difficult, an intraosseous infusion can provide emergency vascular access in children.

10 Because carbon dioxide, but not bicarbonate, readily crosses cell membranes and the blood–brain barrier, the resulting arterial hypercapnia will cause intracellular tissue acidosis.

11 A wide QRS complex following a pacing spike signals electrical capture, but mechanical (ventricular) capture must be confirmed by an improving pulse or blood pressure.

One goal of anesthesiology is to maintain the function of vital organ systems during surgery. It is not surprising, therefore, that anesthesiologists have played a major role in the development of cardiopulmonary resuscitation techniques outside the operating room. Cardiopulmonary resuscitation and emergency cardiac care (CPR-ECC) should be considered any time an individual cannot adequately oxygenate or per-fuse vital organs–not only following cardiac or respiratory arrest.

This chapter presents an overview of the American Heart Association and the International Liaison Committee on Resuscitation (ILCOR) Year 2000 recommendations for establishing and maintaining the ABCDs of cardiopulmonary resuscitation: Airway, Breathing, Circulation, and Defibrillation. The

Table 47–1. Emergency cardiac care (ECC).

1. Recognition of impending event
2. Activation of emergency response system
3. Basic life support
4. Defibrillation
5. Ventilation
6. Pharmacotherapy

best outcomes, however, come from instituting ECC (Table 47–1, Figures 47–1 and 47–2). The guidelines have been updated for 2000 with new guidelines planned for 2006, and they are now more than ever evidence based and international. Major changes for the layperson are that the pulse should not be checked, and chest compression without ventilation may be as effective as compression with ventilation for the first several minutes. If a lay-bystander is unwilling to perform mouth-to-mouth ventilation, chest compressions alone are preferred to doing nothing. For the health care provider, defibrillation using biphasic electrical current works best, tracheal tube (TT) placement should be confirmed with a qualitative end-tidal CO_2 device, bretylium is no longer recommended but vasopressin has been added to the algorithms, and amiodarone has gained new emphasis in these newest guidelines. This chapter is not, however, intended as a substitute for a formal course in either life support without the use of special equipment (Basic Life Support [BLS]) or with the use of special equipment and drugs (Advanced Cardiac Life Support [ACLS]).

Resuscitation of neonates is discussed in Chapter 43.

AIRWAY

Although the *A* of the mnemonic *ABC* stands for *airway,* it should also stand for the initial *a*ssessment of the patient. Before CPR is initiated, unresponsiveness is established and the emergency response system activated.

The airway is then evaluated. The patient is positioned supine on a firm surface. The airway is most commonly obstructed by posterior displacement of the tongue or epiglottis. If there is no evidence of cervical spine instability, a head-tilt chin-lift should be tried first (Figure 47–3). One hand (palm) is placed on the patient's forehead applying pressure to tilt the head back while lifting the chin with the forefinger and index finger of the opposite hand. The jaw-thrust may be more effective in opening the airway and is executed by placing both hands on either side of the patient's head, grasping the angles of the jaw, and lifting. Basic airway management is discussed in detail in

Chapter 5, and the trauma patient is considered in Chapter 41.

If vomitus or a foreign body is visible in the mouth of an unconscious patient, it should be swept out with a hooked index finger. If the patient is conscious or if the foreign body cannot be removed by a finger sweep, the Heimlich maneuver is recommended. This subdiaphragmatic abdominal thrust elevates the diaphragm, expelling a blast of air from the lungs that displaces the foreign body (Figure 47–4). Complications of the Heimlich maneuver include rib fracture, trauma to the internal viscera, and regurgitation. A combination of back blows and chest thrusts is recommended to clear foreign body obstruction in infants (Table 47–2).

If after opening the airway there is no evidence of adequate breathing, the rescuer should initiate assisted ventilation, by inflating the victim's lungs with each breath by mouth-to-mouth, mouth-to-nose, mouth-to-stoma, mouth-to-barrier device, mouth-to-face shield, or mouth-to-mask rescue breathing or by using a bag-mask device (see Chapter 5). Breaths are delivered slowly (inspiratory time of $^1/_2$–1 s) with a smaller tidal volume [VT] (approximately 700–1000 mL, smaller [400–600 mL] if supplemental O_2 is used) than was recommended in the past.

With positive-pressure ventilation, even with a small VT, gastric inflation with subsequent regurgitation and aspiration are possible. Therefore, as soon as it is feasible, the airway should be secured with a TT or, if that is not possible, an alternative airway should be inserted. Alternative airways include the esophageal–tracheal Combitube (ETC), the laryngeal mask airway (LMA), the pharyngotracheal lumen airway, and the cuffed oropharyngeal airway. The ETC and LMA along with the oral and nasopharyngeal airways, face masks, laryngoscopes, and TTs are discussed in Chapter 5. Of these, the LMA is increasingly used as the preferred device for in-hospital arrests. The new 2000 CPR-ECC guidelines recommend a TT as the airway adjunct of choice if personnel skilled in placing it are available.

Independent of which airway adjunct is used, the guidelines state that rescuers must confirm TT placement with an end-tidal CO_2 detector—an indicator, a capnograph, or a capnometric device. Once an artificial airway is successfully placed, *it must be* carefully secured with a tie or tape (25% of airways are displaced during transportation).

Some causes of airway obstruction, however, may not be relieved by conventional methods. Furthermore, tracheal intubation may be technically impossible to perform (eg, severe facial trauma), or repeated attempts may be unwise (cervical spine trauma). In these circumstances, cricothyrotomy or tracheotomy may be necessary. Cricothyrotomy involves placing a large intravenous catheter or a commercially available cannula into the trachea through

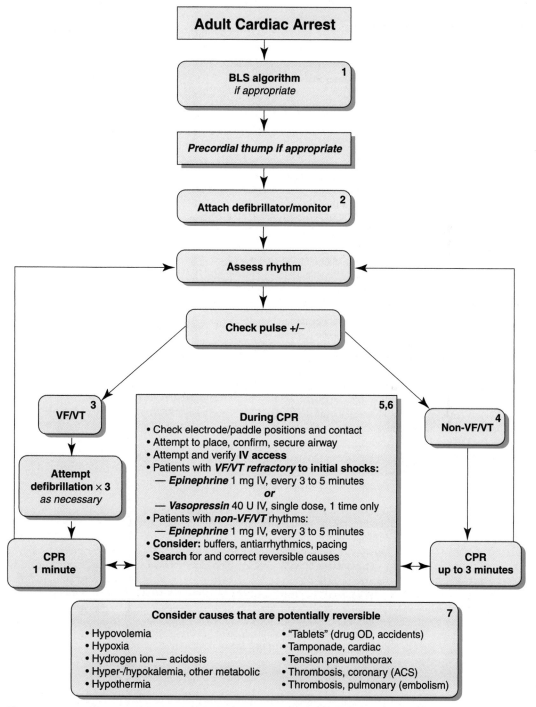

Figure 47–1. Universal algorithm for adult emergency cardiac care. BLS, basic life support; VF/VT, ventricular fibrillation and pulseless ventricular tachycardia; CPR, cardiopulmonary resuscitation. (Reproduced, with permission, from The American Heart Association in Collaboration with the International Liaison Committee on Resuscitation [ILCOR]: Guidelines 2000 for cardiopulmonary resuscitation and emergency cardiovascular care. Circulation 2000;102:1.)

Figure 47–2. Comprehensive emergency cardiac care algorithm. BLS, basic life support; VF/VT, ventricular fibrillation and pulseless ventricular tachycardia; PEA, pulseless electrical activity; CPR, cardiopulmonary resuscitation. (Reproduced, with permission, from The American Heart Association in Collaboration with the International Liaison Committee on Resuscitation [ILCOR]: Guidelines 2000 for cardiopulmonary resuscitation and emergency cardiovascular care. Circulation 2000;102:1.)

Figure 47–3. Loss of consciousness is often accompanied by loss of submandibular muscle tone (**A**). Occlusion of the airway by the tongue can be relieved by a head-tilt chin-lift (**B**) or a jaw thrust (**C**). In patients with possible cervical spine injury, the angles of the jaw should be lifted anteriorly without hyperextending the neck. (Courtesy American Heart Association.)

the midline of the cricothyroid membrane (Figure 47–5). Proper location is confirmed by aspiration of air. A 12- or 14-gauge catheter requires a driving pressure of 50 psi to generate sufficient gas flow (transtracheal jet ventilation).

Various systems are available that connect a high-pressure source of oxygen (eg, central wall oxygen, tank oxygen, or the anesthesia machine fresh gas outlet) to the catheter (Figure 47–6). A hand-operated jet injector or the oxygen flush valve of an anesthesia machine controls ventilation. The addition of a pressure regulator minimizes the risk of barotrauma.

Regardless of which transtracheal jet ventilation system is chosen, it must be readily available, use low-compliance tubing, and have secure connections. Direct connection of a 12- or 14-gauge intravenous catheter to the anesthesia circle system does not allow adequate ventilation because of the high compliance of the corrugated breathing tubing and breathing bag. It is also impossible to reliably deliver acceptable ventilation through a 12- or 14-gauge catheter with a self-inflating resuscitation bag.

Adequacy of ventilation—particularly expiration—is judged by observation of chest wall movement and auscultation of breath sounds. Acute complications include pneumothorax, subcutaneous emphysema, mediastinal emphysema, bleeding, esophageal puncture, aspiration, and respiratory acidosis. Long-term complications include tracheomalacia, subglottic stenosis, and vocal cord changes. Cricothyrotomy is not generally recommended in children under 10 years of age.

Tracheotomy can be performed in a more controlled environment after oxygenation has been secured by cri-

A **B**

Figure 47–4. The Heimlich maneuver can be performed with the victim standing (**A**) or lying down (**B**). The hands are positioned slightly above the navel and well below the xiphoid process and then pressed into the abdomen with a quick upward thrust. The maneuver may need to be repeated. (Courtesy American Heart Association.)

cothyrotomy. A detailed description of tracheotomy, however, is beyond the scope of this text.

BREATHING

Assessment of spontaneous breathing should immediately follow the opening or the establishment of the airway. Ventilation (and chest compressions) should not be delayed for intubation if a patent airway is established by a jaw-thrust

maneuver. Apnea is confirmed by lack of chest movement, absence of breath sounds, and lack of airflow. Regardless of the airway and breathing methods employed, a specific regimen of ventilation has been proposed for the apneic patient. Initially, two breaths are slowly administered (2 s per breath in adults, 1–$1\frac{1}{2}$ s in infants and children). If these breaths cannot be delivered, either the airway is still obstructed and the head and neck need repositioning or a foreign body is present that must be removed.

Table 47–2. Summary of recommended basic life support techniques.

	Infant (1–12 mo)	Child (> 12 mo)	Adult
Breathing rate	20 breaths/min	20 breaths/min	10–12 breaths/min
Pulse check	Brachial	Carotid	Carotid
Compression rate	> 100/min	100/min	100/min
Compression method	Two or three fingers	Heel of one hand	Hands interlaced
Compression/ventilation ratio	5:1	5:1	15:2[1]
Foreign body obstruction	Back blows and chest thrusts	Heimlich maneuver	Heimlich maneuver

[1]Decrease to 5:1 if the airway is secured with a tracheal tube.

A Locate the cricothyroid membrane.

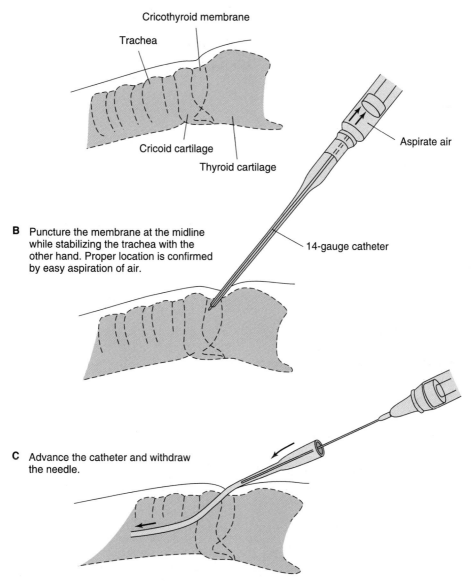

B Puncture the membrane at the midline while stabilizing the trachea with the other hand. Proper location is confirmed by easy aspiration of air.

C Advance the catheter and withdraw the needle.

Figure 47–5. Percutaneous cricothyrotomy with a 14-gauge over-the-needle intravenous catheter.

Mouth-to-mouth or mouth-to-mask (mouth-to-barrier-device) rescue breathing should be instituted in the breathless patient, even in the hospital setting when the crash cart is on its way. Pinching the nose allows formation of an airtight seal between the rescuer's lips and the outside of the victim's mouth. Successful rescue breathing (700–1000 mL V_T, 10–12 times per minute in an adult) is confirmed by observing the chest rising and falling with each breath and hearing and feeling the escape of air during expiration. The most common cause of inadequate mouth-to-mouth ventilation is insufficient airway control. Mouth-to-mouth-and-nose breathing is more effective in infants and small children than in adults.

A rescuer's exhaled air has an oxygen concentration of only 16–17% and contains significant CO_2; new evidence suggests that this method of ventilation may be

A

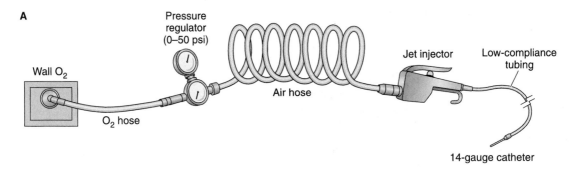

Wall O₂

Pressure regulator (0–50 psi)

O₂ hose

Air hose

Jet injector

Low-compliance tubing

14-gauge catheter

B

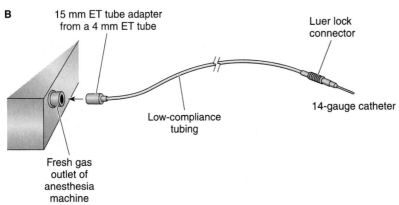

15 mm ET tube adapter from a 4 mm ET tube

Luer lock connector

Low-compliance tubing

14-gauge catheter

Fresh gas outlet of anesthesia machine

Figure 47–6. **A,B:** Two systems for transtracheal jet ventilation after cricothyrotomy (see Figure 47–5). A jet ventilator and pressure regulator (as shown in **A**) provide better control of the inspiratory cycle. Both systems use low-compliance tubing and a high-pressure source of oxygen.

deleterious. Low inspired oxygen concentration and hypercarbia, combined with low cardiac output and intrapulmonary shunting during resuscitation, invariably results in hypoxia. Supplemental oxygen, preferably 100%, should always be used if available. If supplemental oxygen is used, a smaller VT of 400–700 mL is recommended.

Mouth-to-mask or barrier device breathing has a hygienic advantage over mouth-to-mouth breathing as the rescuer's lips form a seal with an intervening device. Devices that avoid mouth-to-mouth contact should be immediately available everywhere in the hospital. Ventilation with a mask may be performed more easily in some patients because the rescuer may be able to adjust the airway or make an airtight seal more effectively. Furthermore, some mouth-to-mask devices allow the delivery of supplemental oxygen.

A self-inflating bag-valve-mask device is described in Chapter 3 (see the section on Resuscitation Breathing Systems). These devices can be less effective than mouth-to-mask or bag-valve-tracheal tube ventilation because of the difficulty inexperienced personnel may have in maintaining an airway and seal with one hand and simultaneously

delivering an adequate VT with the other. If additional personnel are available, cricoid pressure should be considered to prevent regurgitation.

Tracheal intubation should be attempted as soon as practical. Attempts at intubation should not interrupt ventilation for more than 30 s. Cricoid pressure decreases the possibility of regurgitation and aspiration during intubation. After intubation, the patient can be ventilated with a self-inflating bag capable of delivering high oxygen concentrations. Because two hands are now available to squeeze the bag, ventilation should be satisfactory.

Automatic transport ventilators, used in Europe since the 1980s, are now recommended in the United States for prehospital care and transport of intubated patients. When choosing a ventilator for a hospitalized patient undergoing CPR-ECC, avoid pressure-cycled ventilator modes in favor of volume- or time-cycled ventilators.

The ratio of physiological dead space to tidal volume (VD/VT) reflects the efficiency of CO_2 elimination. VD/VT increases during CPR as a result of low pulmonary blood flow and high alveolar pressures. Thus, minute ventilation may need to be increased by 50–100% once circulation is restored as CO_2 from the periphery is brought back to the lungs.

CIRCULATION

After successful delivery of two initial breaths (each 2 s in duration), the circulation must be rapidly assessed—health care providers are advised to continue to check for a pulse (the lay rescuer should not). If the patient has an adequate pulse (carotid artery in an adult or child, brachial or femoral artery in an infant) or blood pressure, breathing is continued at 10–12 breaths/min for an adult or a child older than 8 years, and 20 breaths/min for an infant or a child younger than 8 years of age (Table 47–2). If the patient is pulseless or severely hypotensive, the circulatory system must be supported by a combination of external chest compressions, intravenous drug administration, and defibrillation when appropriate. Initiation of chest compressions is mandated by the inadequacy of peripheral perfusion, and drug choices and defibrillation energy levels often depend on electrocardiographic diagnosis of arrhythmias.

External Chest Compression

Chest compressions should be immediately initiated in the pulseless patient. The xiphoid process is located and the heel of the rescuer's hand is placed over the lower half of the sternum. The other hand is placed over the hand on the sternum with the fingers either interlaced or extended, but off the chest. The rescuer's shoulders should be positioned directly over the hands with the elbows locked into position and arms extended, so that the weight of the upper body is used for compressions. With a straight downward thrust, the sternum is depressed $1^1/_2$–2 in. (4–5 cm) in adults, 1–$1^1/_2$ in. (2–4 cm) in children, and then allowed to return to its normal position. For an infant, compressions $1/_2$–1 in. ($1^1/_2$–$2^1/_2$ cm) in depth are made with the middle and ring fingers on the sternum one finger-breadth below the nipple line. Compression and release times should be equal.

Whether adult resuscitation is performed by a single rescuer or by two rescuers, two breaths are administered every 15 compressions (15:2), allowing 2 s for each breath. The cardiac compression rate should be 100/min regardless of the number of rescuers. A slightly higher compression rate of > 100/min is suggested for infants, with one breath delivered every five compressions. Note that the compression rate refers to the speed of compression (slightly less than 2/s) and not the number of compressions delivered in 1 min. The number of compressions per minute may be less if there is a single rescuer who pauses to ventilate the patient during BLS maneuvers. The adequacy of cardiac output can be estimated by monitoring end-tidal CO_2 or arterial pulsations.

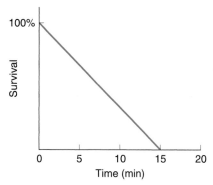

Figure 47–7. Success of defibrillation versus time. The chance of successful defibrillation of a patient in ventricular fibrillation decreases 7–10% per minute.

Chest compressions force blood to flow either by increasing intrathoracic pressure (thoracic pump) or by directly compressing the heart (cardiac pump). During CPR of short duration, blood flow is created more by the cardiac pump mechanism; as CPR continues, the heart becomes less compliant and the thoracic pump mechanism becomes more important. As important as the rate and force of compression are for maintaining blood flow, effective perfusion of the heart and brain is best achieved when chest compression consumes 50% of the duty cycle, with the remaining 50% devoted to the relaxation phase (allowing blood to flow into the chest and heart).

DEFIBRILLATION

Ventricular fibrillation is found most commonly in adults who experience nontraumatic cardiac arrest. The time from collapse to defibrillation is the most important determinant of survival. The chances for survival decline 7–10% for every minute without defibrillation (Figure 47–7). Therefore, patients who have cardiac arrest should be defibrillated at the earliest possible moment. Health care personnel working in hospitals and ambulatory care facilities must be able to provide early defibrillation to collapsed patients with ventricular fibrillation as soon as possible. Shock should be delivered within 3 min (± 1 min) of arrest.

There is no definite relationship between the energy requirement for successful defibrillation and body size; a shock with too low an energy (current) level will not successfully defibrillate; conversely, too high an energy level may result in functional and morphological injury.

Defibrillators deliver energy in either monophasic or biphasic waveforms. Increasingly, biphasic waveforms are recommended for cardioversion as they achieve the same degree of success but with less energy and theoretically less myocardial damage.

In many institutions, automated external defibrillators (AEDs) are available. Such devices are increasingly being used throughout the community by police, firefighters, security personnel, sports marshalls, ski patrol members, airline flight attendants, etc. They are placed in any public place when 20,000 people or more pass by every day. AEDs are technologically advanced, microprocessor-based devices that are capable of electrocardiographic analysis with very high specificity and sensitivity in differentiating shockable from nonshockable rhythms. All AEDs manufactured today deliver some type of biphasic waveform shock. Compared with monophasic shocks, biphasic shocks deliver energy in two directions with equivalent efficacy at lower energy levels and possibly with less myocardial injury. These devices deliver impedance-compensating shocks employing either biphasic truncated exponential (BTE) or rectilinear (RBW) morphology. Biphasic shocks delivering low energy for defibrillation (150–200 joule [J]) have been found to be as effective as 200–360 J monophasic damped sine (MDS) waveform shocks. When using AEDs, one electrode pad is placed beside the upper right sternal border, just below the clavicle, and the other pad is placed just lateral to the left nipple, with the top of the pad a few inches below the axilla.

For cardioversion of atrial fibrillation (Table 47–3), 50–100 J can be used initially with escalation if needed. For atrial flutter or paroxysmal supraventricular tachycardia (PSVT), an initial energy level of 30–50 J is often adequate.

Ventricular tachycardia, particularly monomorphic ventricular tachycardia, responds well to shocks at initial energy levels of 100 J. For polymorphic ventricular tachycardia or for ventricular fibrillation, initial energy can be set at 120–200 J, depending upon the type of biphasic waveform being used. Stepwise increases in energy levels should be used if the first shock fails, although some AEDs operate with a fixed-energy protocol of 150 J with very high success in terminating ventricular fibrillation (Table 47–3).

Cardioversion should be synchronized with the QRS complex and is recommended for hemodynamically stable, wide complex tachycardia requiring cardioversion, PSVT, atrial fibrillation, and atrial flutter.

Invasive Cardiopulmonary Resuscitation

Thoracotomy and open-chest cardiac massage are not part of routine CPR because of the high incidence of severe complications. Nonetheless, these invasive techniques can be helpful in specific life-threatening circumstances that preclude effective closed-chest massage. Possible indications include cardiac arrest associated with penetrating or blunt chest trauma, penetrating abdominal trauma, severe chest deformity, pericardial tamponade, or pulmonary embolism.

Intravenous Access

Some resuscitation drugs are fairly well absorbed following administration through a TT. Lidocaine, epinephrine, atropine, and vasopressin (but *not* sodium bicarbonate) can be delivered down a catheter whose tip extends past the tracheal tube. Dosages 2–2$^1/_2$ times higher than recommended for intravenous use, diluted in 10 mL of normal saline or distilled water, are recommended for adult patients. Even though establishing reliable intravenous access is a high priority, it *should not take precedence* over initial airway management, chest compressions, or defibrillation. A preexisting internal jugular or subclavian line is ideal for venous access during resuscitation. If there is no central line access, an attempt should be made to establish peripheral intravenous access, either in the antecubital or external jugular vein. Peripheral intravenous sites are associated with a significant delay of between 1 and 2 min between drug administration and delivery to the heart, as peripheral blood flow is drastically reduced during resuscitation. Administration of drugs given through a peripheral intravenous line should be followed by an intravenous flush (eg, a 20-mL fluid bolus in adults) and elevation of the extremity for 10–20 s. Cardiac chest compressions may have to be briefly interrupted to establish an internal jugular line if the response to peripherally administered drugs is inadequate.

If intravenous cannulation is difficult, an intraosseous infusion can provide emergency vascular access in children. The success rate is lower in older children, but even in adults intraosseous cannulas have been successfully placed in the tibia and in the distal radius and ulna. A rigid 18-gauge spinal needle with a stylet or a small bone marrow trephine needle can be inserted into the distal femur or proximal tibia. If the tibia is chosen, a needle is inserted 2–3 cm below the tibial tuberosity at a 45° angle away from the epiphyseal plate (Figure 47–8). Once the needle is advanced through the cortex, it should stand upright without support. Proper placement is confirmed by the

Table 47–3. Energy requirements for cardioversion using biphasic truncated exponential (BTE) or rectilinear morphology.[1]

Indications	Shocks (J)
Unstable atrial fibrillation	50–100
Unstable atrial flutter/tachycardia	30–50
Monomorphic ventricular tachycardia	100
Polymorphic ventricular tachycardia or ventricular fibrillation	120–200

[1]Step with increase in energy level if initial shock fails.

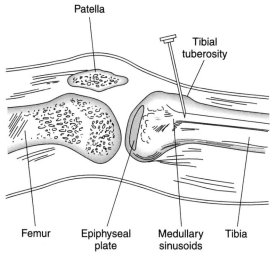

Patella

Tibial tuberosity

Femur   Epiphyseal plate   Medullary sinusoids   Tibia

Figure 47–8. Intraosseous infusions provide emergency access to the venous circulation in pediatric patients by way of the large medullary venous channels. The needle is directed away from the epiphyseal plate to minimize the risk of injury.

ability to aspirate marrow through the needle and a smooth infusion of fluid. A network of venous sinusoids within the medullary cavity of long bones drains into the systemic circulation by way of nutrient or emissary veins. This route is very effective for administration of drugs, crystalloids, colloids, and blood and can achieve flow rates exceeding 100 mL/h under gravity. Much higher flow rates are possible if the fluid is placed under pressure (eg, 300 mm Hg) with an infusion bag. The onset of drug action will be slightly delayed compared with intravenous or tracheal administration. The interosseous route may require a higher dose of some drugs (eg, epinephrine) than recommended for intravenous administration. The use of intraosseous infusion for induction and maintenance of general anesthesia, antibiotic therapy, seizure control, and inotropic support has been described. Because of the risks of osteomyelitis and compartment syndrome, however, intraosseous infusions should be replaced by a conventional intravenous route as soon as possible. In addition, because of the theoretical risk of bone marrow or fat emboli, intraosseous infusions should be avoided in patients with right-to-left shunts, pulmonary hypertension, or severe pulmonary insufficiency.

Arrhythmia Recognition

Successful pharmacological and electrical treatment of cardiac arrest (Figure 47–9) depends on definitive iden-

tification of the underlying arrhythmia. Interpreting rhythm strips in the midst of a resuscitation situation is complicated by artifacts and variations in monitoring techniques (eg, lead systems, equipment).

Drug Administration

Many of the drugs administered during CPR have been described elsewhere in this text. Table 47–4 summarizes the cardiovascular actions, indications, and dosages of drugs commonly used during resuscitation.

Calcium chloride, sodium bicarbonate, and bretylium are conspicuously absent from this table. Calcium (2–4 mg/kg of the chloride salt) is helpful in the treatment of documented hypocalcemia, hyperkalemia, hypermagnesemia, or a calcium channel blocker overdose. When used, 10% calcium chloride can be given at 2–4 mg/kg every 10 min. Sodium bicarbonate (0.5–1 mEq/kg) is not recommended in the ACLS guidelines and should be considered only in specific situations such as preexisting metabolic acidosis or hyperkalemia, or in the treatment of tricyclic antidepressant or barbiturate overdose. Sodium bicarbonate elevates plasma pH by combining with hydrogen ions to form carbonic acid, which readily dissociates into carbon dioxide and water. Because carbon dioxide, but not bicarbonate, readily crosses cell membranes and the blood–brain barrier, the resulting arterial hypercapnia will cause intracellular tissue acidosis. Although successful defibrillation is not related to *arterial* pH, increased *intramyocardial* carbon dioxide may reduce the possibility of cardiac resuscitation. Furthermore, bicarbonate administration can lead to detrimental alterations in osmolality and the oxygen–hemoglobin dissociation curve. Therefore, effective alveolar ventilation and adequate tissue perfusion are the treatments of choice for the respiratory and metabolic acidosis that accompany resuscitation.

Bretylium tosylate is a quaternary compound used to treat ventricular tachycardia and fibrillation. A national shortage stimulated an assessment of its role in managing these rhythms. Based on this review, bretylium was removed from the ACLS guidelines because of a high incidence of serious adverse events associated with its use, the availability of equally effective drugs, and its national shortage.

Intravenous fluid therapy with either colloid or balanced salt solutions (eg, normal saline) is indicated in patients with intravascular volume depletion (eg, acute blood loss, diabetic ketoacidosis, thermal burns). Dextrose-containing solutions may lead to a hyperosmotic diuresis and may worsen neurological outcome. They should be avoided unless hypoglycemia is suspected. Likewise, administration of free water (eg, D_5W) may lead to cerebral edema.

Figure 47–9. Algorithm for treating ventricular fibrillation and pulseless ventricular tachycardia (VF/VT). Pulseless ventricular tachycardia should be treated in the same way as ventricular fibrillation. Note: This figure (and Figures 47–1 and 47–2) emphasize the concept that rescuers and health care providers must assume that all unmonitored adult cardiac arrests are due to VF/VT. In each figure, the flow of the algorithm assumes that the arrhythmia is continuing. In the primary survey, ABCD = airway, breathing, circulation, and defibrillation. In the secondary survey, A = airway with tracheal intubation; B = breathing effectively, verify tracheal tube placement; C = circulation with vital signs and electrocardiographic monitoring, intravenous access, appropriate drugs; and D = differential diagnosis. (Reproduced, with permission, from The American Heart Association in Collaboration with the International Liaison Committee on Resuscitation [ILCOR]: Guidelines 2000 for cardiopulmonary resuscitation and emergency cardiovascular care. Circulation 2000;102:1.)

Table 47–4. Cardiovascular effects, indications, and dosages of resuscitation drugs.[1]

Drug	Cardiovascular Effects	Indications	Initial Dose Adult	Initial Dose Pediatric	Comments
Adenosine	Slows AV nodal conduction	Narrow complex tachycardias, stable supraventricular tachycardia and wide complex tachycardias if supraventricular in origin	6 mg over 1–3 sc; 12 mg repeat dose	Initial dose 0.1–0.2 mg/kg; subsequent doses doubled to maximum single dose of 12 mg	Recommended as diagnostic or therapeutic maneuver for supraventricular tachycardias; give as rapid IV bolus. Vasodilates, BP may decrease. Theoretetcal risk of angina, bronchospasm, proarrhythmic action. Drug–drug interaction with theophylline, dipyridamole.
Atropine	Anticholinergic (parasympampatholytic). Increases sinoatrial node rate and automaticity; increases AV node conduction	Symptomatic brachycardia, AV block	0.5–1.0 mg repeated every 3–5 min	0.02 mg/kg	Repeat atropine doses every 5 min to a total dose of 3 mg in adults or 0.5 mg in children, 1.0 mg in adolescents. The minimum pediatric dose is 0.1 mg. Do not use for infranodal (Mobitz II) block.
		Ventricular asystole	1 mg	0.02 mg/kg	
Epinephrine	α-Adrenergic effects increase myocardial and cerebral blood flow. β-Adrenergic effects may increase myocardial work and decrease subendocardial perfusion and cerebral blood flow	VF/VT, electromechanical dissociation, ventricular asystole, severe bradycardia unresponsive to atropine or pacing	1 mg IV	Initial dose 0.01 mg/kg IV; repeat same for subsequent doses or up to 0.1–0.2 mg/kg IV	Repeat doses every 3–5 min as necessary. An infusion of epinephrine (eg, 1 mg in 250 mL D_5W or NS, 4 µg/mL) can be titrated to effect in adults (1–4 µg/min) or children (0.1–1 µg/kg/min). Administration down a tracheal tube requires higher doses (2–2.5 mg in adults, 0.1 mg/kg in children). High-dose epinephrine (0.1 mg/kg) in adults is recommended only after standard therapy has failed.
		Severe hypotension	1 µg/min in an infusion increased to effect	1 µg/kg	
Lidocaine	Decreases rate of phase 4 depolarization (decreases automaticity); depresses conduction in re-entry pathways. Elevates VF threshold. Reduces disparity in action potential duration between normal and ischemic tissue. Reduces action potential and effective refractory period duration	VT that has not responded to defibrillation; premature ventricular contractions.	1–1.5 mg/kg	1 mg/kg	Doses of 0.5 to 1.5 mg/kg can be repeated every 5–10 min to a total dose of 3 mg/kg. After infarction or successful resuscitation, a continuous infusion (eg, 1 g in 500 mL D_5W, 2 mg/mL) should be run at a rate of 20–50 µg/kg/min (2–4 mg/min in most adults). Therapeutic blood levels are usually 1.5–6 µg/mL.

(continued)

Table 47–4. Cardiovascular effects, indications, and dosages of resuscitation drugs.[1] (continued)

Drug	Cardiovascular Effects	Indications	Initial Dose		Comments
			Adult	Pediatric	
Lidocaine (continued)		Postinfarction arrhythmia prophylaxis	1.5 mg/kg	Not applicable	
Vasopressin	Nonadrenergic peripheral vasoconstrictor; direct stimulation of V_1 receptors	Bleeding esophageal varices; adult shock-refractory VF; hemodynamic support in vasodilatory (septic) shock	40 U IV, single dose, 1 time only	Not recommended	Newly recommended as equivalent to epinephrine in ventricular fibrillation and PEA; may be more effective in asystole; used only one time; has a 10- to 20-min half-life.
Procainamide	Suppresses both atrial and ventricular arrhythmias	AF/flutter; preexcited atrial arrhythmias with rapid ventricular response; wide complex tachycardia that cannot be distinguished as SVT or VT	20 mg/min until arrhythmia suppressed, hypotension develops, QRS complex increases by > 50%, or total dose of 17 mg/kg has infused. In urgent situation, 50 mg/min may be used to maximum of 17 mg/kg. Maintenance infusion, 1–4 mg/min	Loading dose: 15 mg/kg; infusion over 30–60 min; routine use in combination with drugs that prolong QTs is not recommended	Contraindicated in overdose of tricyclic antidepressants or other antiarrhythmic drugs. Bolus doses can result in toxicity. Should not be used in preexisting QT prolongation or torsades de pointes. Blood levels should be monitored in patients with impaired renal function and when constant infusion > 3 mg/min for > 24 h.
Amiodarone	Complex drug with effects on sodium, potassium, and calcium channels as well as α- and β-adrenergic blocking properties	SVT with accessory pathway conduction; unstable VT and VF; stable VT, polymorphic VT, wide-complex tachycardia of uncertain origin; AF/flutter with CHF; preexcited AF/flutter; adjunct to electrical cardioversion in refractory PSVTs, atrial tachycardia, and AF	150 mg over 10 min, followed by 1 mg/min for 6 h, then 0.5 mg/min, with supplementary infusion of 150 mg as necessary up to 2 g. For pulseless VT or VF, initial administration is 300 mg rapid infusion diluted in 20–30 mL of saline or dextrose in water	5 mg/kg for pulseless VT/VF; for perfusing tachycardia loading dose, 5 mg/kg IV/IO; maximum dose, 15 mg/kg/d	Antiarrhythmic of choice if cardiac function is impaired, EF < 40%, or CHF. Routine use in combination with drugs prolonging QT interval is *not* recommended. Most frequent side effects are hypotension and bradycardia.
Verapamil	Calcium channel blocking agent used to slow conduction and increase refractoriness in AV node, terminating reentrant arrhythmias that require AV nodal conduction for continuation	Controls ventricular response rate in AF/flutter and MAT; rate control in AF; terminating narrow-complex PSVT	2.5–5 mg IV over 2 min; without response, repeat dose with 5–10 mg every 15–30 min to a max of 20 mg		Use only in patients with narrow-complex PSVT or supraventricular arrhythmia. Do not use in presence of impaired ventricular function or CHF

Drug				
Diltiazem	Calcium channel blocking agent used to slow conduction and increase refractoriness in AV node, terminating reentrant arrhythmias that require AV nodal conduction for continuation	Slows conduction and increases refractoriness in AV node. May terminate reentrant arrhythmias. Controls ventricular response rate in AF/flutter and MAT	0.25 mg/kg, followed by second dose of 35 mg/kg if necessary; maintenance infusion of 5–15 mg/h in AF/flutter	May exacerbate CHF in severe LV dysfunction; may decrease myocardial contractility, but less so than verapamil.
Dobutamine	Synthetic catecholamine and potent inotropic agent with predominant β-adrenergic receptor-stimulating effects that increase cardiac contractility in a dose-dependent manner, accompanied by a decrease in LV filling pressures.	Severe systolic heart failure	5–20 μg/kg/min	Hemodynamic end points rather than specific dose is goal. Elderly have significantly reduced response. May induce or exacerbate myocardial ischemia with doses > 20 μg/kg/min with increases in heart rate > 10%.
Flecainide	Potent sodium channel blocker with significant conduction-slowing effects	AF/flutter, ventricular arrhythmias and supraventricular arrhythmias with structural heart disease, ectopic atrial heart disease, AV nodal reentrant tachycardia, SVTs associated with an accessory pathway, including pre-excited AF	2 mg/kg at 10 mg/min (IV use not approved in the United States)	Should not be used in patients with impaired LV function, or when coronary artery disease is suspected.
Ibutilide	Short-acting antiarrhythmic, prolongs the action potential duration and increases refractory period	Acute conversion or adjunct to electrical cardioversion of AF/flutter of short duration	In patients > 60 kg, 1 mg (10 mL) over 10 min; a second similar dose may be repeated in 10 min. In patients < 60 kg, initial dose is 0.01 mg/kg	Patients should be monitored for arrhythmias for 4–6 h, and longer in those with hepatic dysfunction.
Magnesium	Hypomagnesemia associated with arrhythmias, cardiac insufficiency, and sudden death; can precipitate refractory VF; can hinder K+ replacement	Torsades de pointes even with normal serum levels of magnesium	1–2 g in 50–100 mL, D$_5$W over 50–60 min, follow with infusion of 0.5–1 g/h 500 mg/mL–IV/IO; 25–50 mg/kg; maximum dose: 2 g per dose	Rapid IV infusion for torsades de pointes or suspected hypomagnesemia not recommended in cardiac arrest except when arrhythmia suspected; 10- to 20-min infusion for asthma poorly responsive to β-adrenergic blockers.

(continued)

Table 47–4. Cardiovascular effects, indications, and dosages of resuscitation drugs.[1] (continued)

Drug	Cardiovascular Effects	Indications	Initial Dose		Comments
			Adult	Pediatric	
Propafenone	Significant conduction slowing and negative inotropic effects. Nonselective β-adrenergic blocking properties	AF/flutter, ventricular arrhythmias and supraventricular arrhythmias with structural heart disease, ectopic atrial heart disease, AV nodal reentrant tachycardia, SVTs associated with an accessory pathway	2.0 mg/kg at 10 mg/min (IV use not approved in the United States)		Should be avoided with impaired LV function or when CAD suspected.
Sotalol	Prolongs action potential duration and increases cardiac tissue refractoriness. Nonselective β-adrenergic blocking properties	Preexcited AF/flutter, ventricular and supraventricular arrhythmias	1.0–1.5 mg/kg at a rate of 10 mg/min (IV use not approved in the United States)		Limited by need to be infused slowly.

[1]AV, atrioventricular; BP, blood pressure; VF, ventricular fibrillation; VT, ventricular tachycardia; PEA, pulseless electrical activity; AF, atrial fibrillation; SVT, supraventricular tachycardia; CHF, congestive heart failure; PSVT, paroxysmal supraventricular tachycardia; IV/IO, intravenous/intraosseous; EF, ejection fraction; MAT, multifocal atrial tachycardia; LV, left ventricular; CAD, coronary artery disease.

Emergency Pacemaker Therapy

Transcutaneous cardiac pacing (TCP) is a noninvasive method of rapidly treating arrhythmias caused by conduction disorders or abnormal impulse. These may include asystole, bradycardia caused by heart block, or tachycardia from a reentrant mechanism. If there is concern about the use of atropine in high-grade block, TCP is always appropriate. If the patient is unstable with marked bradycardia, TCP should be implemented immediately. The pacer unit has become a built-in feature of some defibrillator models. Disposable pacing electrodes are usually positioned on the patient in an anterior–posterior manner. The placement of the negative electrode corresponds to a V_2 electrocardiograph position, whereas the positive electrode is placed on the left posterior chest beneath the scapula and lateral to the spine. Note that this positioning does not interfere with paddle placement during defibrillation. Failure to capture may be due to electrode misplacement, poor electrode-to-skin contact, or increased transthoracic impedance (eg, barrel-shaped chest, pericardial effusion). Current output is slowly increased until the pacing stimuli obtain electrical and mechanical capture. A wide QRS complex following a pacing spike signals *electrical* capture, but *mechanical* (ventricular) capture must be confirmed by an improving pulse or blood pressure. Conscious patients may require sedation to tolerate the discomfort of skeletal muscle contractions. Transcutaneous pacing can provide effective temporizing therapy until transvenous pacing or other definitive treatment can be initiated. TCP has many advantages over transvenous pacing because it can be used by almost all electrocardiogram providers and can be started quickly and conveniently at the bedside.

RECOMMENDED RESUSCITATION PROTOCOLS

A resuscitation team leader integrates the assessment of the patient, including electrocardiographic diagnosis, with the electrical and pharmacological therapy (Table 47–5). This person must have a firm grasp of the guidelines for cardiac arrest presented in the ACLS algorithms (Figures 47–9 to 47–13).

Table 47–5. Steps for synchronized cardioversion.[1]

1. Consider sedation.
2. Turn on defibrillator (monophasic or biphasic).
3. Attach monitor leads to the patient ("white to right, red to ribs, what's left over to the left shoulder") and ensure proper display of the patient's rhythm.
4. Engage the synchronization mode by pressing the "sync" control button.
5. Look for markers on R waves indicating sync mode.
6. If necessary, adjust monitor gain until sync markers occur with each R wave.
7. Select appropriate energy level.
8. Position conductor pads on patient (or apply gel to paddles).
9. Position paddle on patient (sternum-apex).
10. Announce to team members: "Charging defibrillator— stand clear!"
11. Press "charge" button on apex paddle (right hand).
12. When the defibrillator is charged, begin the final clearing chant. State firmly in a forceful voice the following chant before each shock:
    - *"I am going to shock on three. One, I'm clear."* (Check to make sure you are clear of contact with the patient, the stretcher, and the equipment.)
    - *"Two, you are clear."* (Make a visual check to ensure that no one continues to touch the patient or stretcher. In particular, do not forget about the person providing ventilation. That person's hands should not be touching the ventilatory adjuncts, including the tracheal tube!).
    - *"Three, everybody's clear."* (Check yourself one more time before pressing the "shock" buttons.)
13. Apply 25 lb pressure on both paddles.
14. Press the "discharge" buttons simultaneously.
15. Check the monitor. If tachycardia persists, increase the joules according to the electrical cardioversion algorithm.
16. Reset the sync mode after each synchronized cardioversion because most defibrillators default back to unsynchronized mode. This default allows an immediate defibrillation if the cardioversion produces ventricular fibrillation.

[1]Reproduced, with permission, from The American Heart Association in Collaboration with the International Liaison Committee on Resuscitation (ILCOR): Guidelines 2000 for cardiopulmonary resuscitation and emergency cardiovascular care. Circulation 2000;102:1.

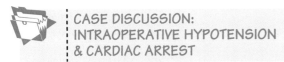

CASE DISCUSSION: INTRAOPERATIVE HYPOTENSION & CARDIAC ARREST

A 16-year-old boy is rushed to the operating room for emergency laparotomy and thoracotomy after suffering multiple abdominal and thoracic stab wounds. In the field, paramedics intubated the patient, started two large-bore intravenous lines, began fluid resuscitation, and inflated a pneumatic anti-

shock garment. Upon arrival in the operating room, the patient's blood pressure is unobtainable, heart rate is 128 beats/min (sinus tachycardia), and respirations are being controlled by a bag-valve device.

What should be done immediately?

Cardiopulmonary resuscitation must be initiated immediately: external chest compressions should be started as soon as the arterial blood pressure is

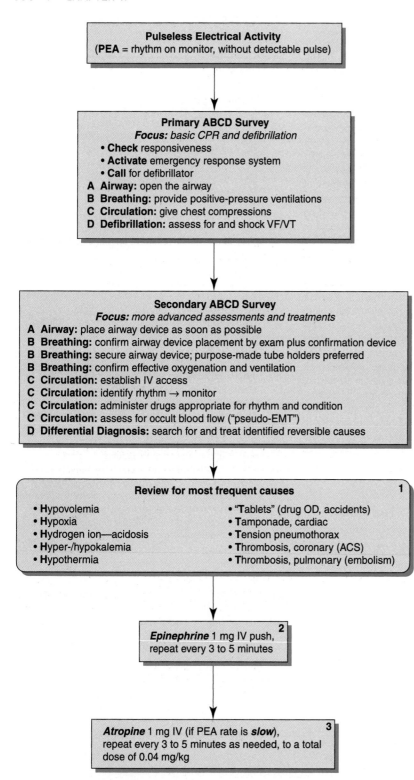

Pulseless Electrical Activity
(**PEA** = rhythm on monitor, without detectable pulse)

Primary ABCD Survey
Focus: basic CPR and defibrillation
- **Check** responsiveness
- **Activate** emergency response system
- **Call** for defibrillator
A **Airway:** open the airway
B **Breathing:** provide positive-pressure ventilations
C **Circulation:** give chest compressions
D **Defibrillation:** assess for and shock VF/VT

Secondary ABCD Survey
Focus: more advanced assessments and treatments
A **Airway:** place airway device as soon as possible
B **Breathing:** confirm airway device placement by exam plus confirmation device
B **Breathing:** secure airway device; purpose-made tube holders preferred
B **Breathing:** confirm effective oxygenation and ventilation
C **Circulation:** establish IV access
C **Circulation:** identify rhythm → monitor
C **Circulation:** administer drugs appropriate for rhythm and condition
C **Circulation:** assess for occult blood flow ("pseudo-EMT")
D **Differential Diagnosis:** search for and treat identified reversible causes

Review for most frequent causes   1
- Hypovolemia
- Hypoxia
- Hydrogen ion—acidosis
- Hyper-/hypokalemia
- Hypothermia
- "Tablets" (drug OD, accidents)
- Tamponade, cardiac
- Tension pneumothorax
- Thrombosis, coronary (ACS)
- Thrombosis, pulmonary (embolism)

Epinephrine 1 mg IV push,   2
repeat every 3 to 5 minutes

Atropine 1 mg IV (if PEA rate is *slow*),   3
repeat every 3 to 5 minutes as needed, to a total
dose of 0.04 mg/kg

Figure 47–10. Pulseless electrical activity algorithm. VF/VT, ventricular fibrillation and pulseless ventricular tachycardia. (Reproduced, with permission, from The American Heart Association in Collaboration with the International Liaison Committee on Resuscitation [ILCOR]: Guidelines 2000 for cardiopulmonary resuscitation and emergency cardiovascular care. Circulation 2000;102:1.)

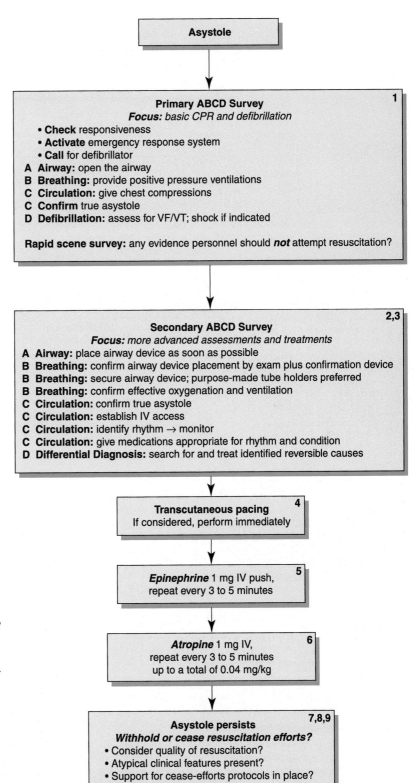

Figure 47–11. Asystole: The silent heart algorithm. CPR, cardiopulmonary resuscitation; VF/VT, ventricular fibrillation and pulseless ventricular tachycardia. (Reproduced, with permission, from The American Heart Association in Collaboration with the International Liaison Committee on Resuscitation [ILCOR]: Guidelines 2000 for cardiopulmonary resuscitation and emergency cardiovascular care. Circulation 2000;102:1.)

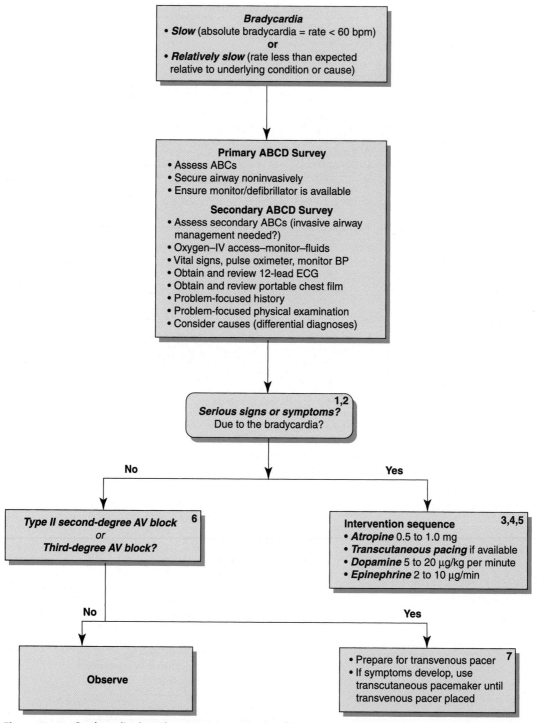

Figure 47–12. **Bradycardia algorithm. AV, atrioventricular.** (Reproduced, with permission, from The American Heart Association in Collaboration with the International Liaison Committee on Resuscitation [ILCOR]: Guidelines 2000 for cardiopulmonary resuscitation and emergency cardiovascular care. Circulation 2000;102:1.)

Figure 47–13. Tachycardia overview algorithm. VT, ventricular tachycardia; CHF, congestive heart failure. (Reproduced, with permission, from The American Heart Association in Collaboration with the International Liaison Committee on Resuscitation [ILCOR]: Guidelines 2000 for cardiopulmonary resuscitation and emergency cardiovascular care. Circulation 2000;102:1.)

found to be inadequate for vital organ perfusion. Because the patient is already intubated, the location of the tracheal tube should be confirmed with chest auscultation, and 100% oxygen should be delivered.

Which cardiopulmonary resuscitation sequence best fits this situation?

Pulselessness in the presence of sinus rhythm suggests severe hypovolemia, cardiac tamponade, ventricular rupture, dissecting aortic aneurysm, tension pneumothorax, profound hypoxemia and acidosis, or pulmonary embolism. Epinephrine, 1 mg, should be administered intravenously.

What is the most likely cause of this patient's profound hypotension?

The presence of multiple stab wounds strongly suggests hypovolemia. Fluids, preferably warmed, should be rapidly administered. Additional venous access can be sought as other members of the operating room team administer fluid through blood pumps or other rapid infusion devices. Five percent albumin or lactated Ringer's solution is acceptable until blood products are available.

What are the signs of tension pneumothorax and pericardial tamponade?

*The signs of **tension pneumothorax**—the presence of air under pressure in the pleural space—include increasing peak inspiratory pressures, tachycardia and hypotension (decreased venous return), hypoxia (atelectasis), distended neck veins, unequal breath sounds, tracheal deviation, and mediastinal shift away from the pneumothorax.*

***Pericardial tamponade**—cardiac compression from pericardial contents—should be suspected in any patient with narrow pulse pressure; pulsus paradoxus (a > 10 mm Hg drop in systolic blood pressure with inspiration); elevated central venous pressure with neck vein distention; equalization of central venous pressure, atrial pressures, and ventricular end-diastolic pressures; distant heart sounds; tachycardia; and hypotension. Many of these signs may be masked by concurrent hypovolemic shock.*

Aggressive fluid administration and properly performed external cardiac compressions do not result in satisfactory carotid or femoral pulsations. What else should be done?

Because external chest compressions are often ineffective in trauma patients, an emergency tho-racotomy should be performed as soon as possible to clamp the thoracic aorta, relieve a tension pneumothorax or pericardial tamponade, identify possible intrathoracic hemorrhage, and perform open-chest cardiac compressions. Cross-clamping of the thoracic aorta increases brain and heart perfusion and decreases subdiaphragmatic hemorrhage. Lack of response to cross-clamping is a good predictor of demise. Direct cardiac massage is more effective than external chest compressions, particularly in the presence of pericardial tamponade.

What is the function of the pneumatic antishock garment, and how should it be removed?

Inflation of the bladders within a pneumatic antishock garment increases arterial blood pressure by elevating peripheral vascular resistance. Functionally, the suit has the same effect as thoracic aorta cross-clamping by decreasing blood flow and hemorrhage in the lower half of the body. Complications of inflating the abdominal section of the pneumatic antishock garment include renal dysfunction, altered lung volumes, and visceral injury during external chest compressions. The suit should be deflated only after restoration of hemodynamic parameters. Even then, deflation should be gradual, as it may be accompanied by marked hypotension and metabolic acidosis caused by reperfusion of ischemic tissues.

SUGGESTED READING

The American Heart Association in Collaboration with the International Liaison Committee on Resuscitation (ILCOR): Guidelines 2000 for cardiopulmonary resuscitation and emergency cardiovascular care. Circulation 2000;102:1.

Kern KB, Halperin RH, Field J: New guidelines for cardiopulmonary resuscitation and emergency cardiac care. Changes in the management of cardiac arrest. JAMA 2001;285:1267.

Otto CW: Current concepts in cardiopulmonary resuscitation. In: *Critical Care Medicine: Perioperative Management,* 2nd ed. Murray MJ, Coursin DB, Pearl RG, Prough DS (editors). Lippincott, Williams & Wilkins, 2002.

Wenzel V, Krismer AC, Arntz HR, et al: A comparison of vasopressin and epinephrine for out-of-hospital cardiopulmonary resuscitation. N Engl J Med 2004;350:105.

White RD: Acute therapy in patients with cardiac arrhythmias. In: *Critical Care Medicine: Perioperative Management,* 2nd ed. Murray MJ, Coursin DB, Pearl RG, Prough DS (editors). Lippincott, Williams & Wilkins, 2002.

Postanesthesia Care

48

KEY CONCEPTS

 Patients should not leave the operating room unless they have a stable and patent airway, have adequate ventilation and oxygenation, and are hemodynamically stable.

 Before the patient is fully responsive, pain is often manifested as postoperative restlessness. Serious systemic disturbances (such as hypoxemia, acidosis, or hypotension), bladder distention, or a surgical complication (such as occult intraabdominal hemorrhage) should always be considered as well.

Intense shivering causes precipitous rises in oxygen consumption, CO_2 production, and cardiac output. These physiological effects are often poorly tolerated by patients with preexisting cardiac or pulmonary impairment.

Respiratory problems are the most frequently encountered serious complications in the postanesthesia care unit (PACU). The overwhelming majority are related to airway obstruction, hypoventilation, or hypoxemia.

 Hypoventilation in the PACU is most commonly due to the residual depressant effects of anesthetic agents on respiratory drive.

 Obtundation, circulatory depression, or severe acidosis (arterial blood pH < 7.15) is an indication for immediate endotracheal intubation in patients suffering from hypoventilation.

Following administration of naloxone to increase respiration, patients should be watched carefully for recurrence of opioid-induced respiratory depression (renarcotization), as naloxone has a shorter duration than most opioids.

 Increased intrapulmonary shunting from a decreased functional residual capacity relative to closing capacity is the most common cause of hypoxemia following general anesthesia.

 The possibility of a postoperative pneumothorax should always be considered following central line placement, intercostal blocks, rib fractures, neck dissections, tracheostomy, nephrectomies, or other retroperitoneal or intraabdominal procedures (including laparoscopy), particularly when the diaphragm might be penetrated.

 Hypovolemia is by far the most common cause of hypotension in the PACU.

 Noxious stimulation from incisional pain, endotracheal intubation, or bladder distention is usually responsible for cases of postoperative hypertension.

Recovery rooms have been in existence for less than 50 years in most medical centers. Prior to that time, many early postoperative deaths occurred immediately after anesthesia and surgery. The realization that many of these deaths were preventable emphasized the need for specialized nursing care immediately following surgery. A nursing shortage in the United States following World War II may also have contributed to centralization of this care in the form of recovery rooms where one or more nurses could pay close attention to several patients at one time. As surgical procedures became increasingly complex and were performed on sicker patients, recovery room care was often extended beyond the first few hours after surgery, and some critically ill patients were kept in the recovery room overnight. The success of these early recovery rooms was a major factor in the evolution of modern surgical intensive care units (ICU, see Chapter 49). Ironically, the recovery rooms received intensive care status relatively recently in most hospitals, where they are referred to as postanesthesia care units (PACUs). In some centers the PACU may function as overflow ICU beds (overnight) when the ICUs are full.

One of the most dramatic transformations in health care delivery during the past two decades has been a shift from inpatient to outpatient surgery (also called *ambulatory surgery*). It is estimated that 60–70% of all surgical procedures in the United States are done on an outpatient basis. The primary impetus for this change was the economic savings afforded by not admitting patients the night before surgery or keeping them in the hospital the night after surgery. Other advantages of outpatient surgery include earlier ambulation, patient convenience, and a decreased risk of nosocomial infection.

At the conclusion of any procedure requiring anesthesia, anesthetic agents are discontinued, monitors are disconnected, and the patient (often still anesthetized) is taken to the PACU. Following general anesthesia, if the patient was intubated and if ventilation was judged adequate, the endotracheal tube is also usually removed prior to transport. Patients are also routinely observed in the PACU following regional anesthesia, and in most instances following monitored anesthesia care (local anesthesia with sedation). Most procedure guidelines require that a patient be admitted to the PACU following any type of anesthesia, except by specific order of the attending anesthesiologist. After a brief verbal report to the PACU nurse, the patient is left in the PACU until the major effects of anesthesia are judged to have worn off. This period is characterized by a relatively high incidence of potentially life-threatening respiratory and circulatory complications.

In some centers, outpatients are discharged home directly from the PACU; other centers have a separate PACU and outpatient area. The latter may also function as a preoperative holding area and second level postanesthesia recovery (predischarge) area. Thus, two phases of recovery may be recognized for outpatient surgery. *Phase 1* is the immediate intensive care level recovery that cares for patients during emergence and awakening from anesthesia and continues until standard PACU criteria are met (see Discharge Criteria below); *Phase 2* is a lower level care that ensures the patient is ready to go home. "Fast-tracking" of selected outpatients may allow them to safely bypass phase 1 recovery and go directly to the phase 2 area.

This chapter discusses the essential components of a modern PACU, the general care of patients recovering from anesthesia, and the most commonly encountered respiratory and circulatory complications.

THE POSTANESTHESIA CARE UNIT

Design

The PACU should be located near the operating rooms. A central location in the operating room area itself is desirable, as it ensures that the patient can be rushed back to surgery if needed or that members of the operating room staff can quickly attend to patients. Proximity to radiographic, laboratory, and other intensive care facilities on the same floor is also highly desirable. The transfer of critically ill patients in elevators or through long corridors can jeopardize their care, because emergencies may arise along the way.

An open ward design facilitates observation of all patients simultaneously. At least one enclosed patient space is desirable for patients needing isolation for infection control. A ratio of 1.5 PACU beds per operating room is customary. Each patient space should be well lighted and large enough to allow easy access to patients in spite of poles for intravenous infusion pumps, a ventilator, or radiographic equipment; construction guidelines dictate a minimum of 7 feet between beds and 120 square feet/patient. Multiple electrical outlets and at least one outlet for oxygen, air, and suction should be present at each space.

Equipment

Pulse oximetry (SpO_2), electrocardiogram (ECG), and automated noninvasive blood pressure (NIBP) monitors for each space are desirable but not mandatory. However, all three monitors should be immediately available for every patient. *Some* PACUs monitor only SpO_2 and NIBP for every patient in the initial phase of recovery from anesthesia (phase 1 care); the ECG is used only for patients with a history of cardiac problems or who exhibit ECG abnormalities intraoperatively. Decreased monitoring may be appropriate subsequently. Most PACU incidents leading to serious morbidity or mortality are related to inadequate monitoring. Monitors with the ability to transduce at least two pressures simultaneously should be available for direct arterial, central venous, pulmonary artery, or intracranial pressure monitoring. Capnography may be useful for intubated patients. Temperature-sensitive strips may be used to measure temperature in the PACU but are generally not sufficiently accurate to follow hypothermia or hyperthermia; mercury or electronic thermometers should be used if an abnormality in temperature is suspected. A forced-air warming device, heating lamps, and warming/cooling blanket should be available.

The PACU should have its own supplies of basic and emergency equipment, separate from that of the operating room. This includes oxygen cannulas, a selection of masks, oral and nasal airways, laryngoscopes, endotracheal tubes, laryngeal mask airways, and self-inflating bags for ventilation. An ample supply of catheters for vascular cannulation (venous, arterial, central venous, or pulmonary artery) is mandatory. Transvenous pacing catheters and a generator should also be available. A defibrillation device with transcutaneous pacing capabilities and an emergency cart with drugs and supplies for advanced life support (see Chapter 47) and infusion pumps should be present and periodically inspected. Tracheostomy, chest tube, and vascular cutdown trays are also important.

Respiratory therapy equipment for aerosol bronchodilator treatments, continuous positive airway pressure (CPAP), and ventilators should be in close proximity to the recovery room. A bronchoscope for the PACU is desirable but not mandatory.

Staffing

The PACU should be staffed only by nurses specifically trained in the care of patients emerging from anesthesia. They should have expertise in airway management and advanced cardiac life support as well as problems commonly encountered in surgical patients relating to wound care, drainage catheters, and postoperative bleeding.

The PACU should be under the medical direction of an anesthesiologist. A physician assigned full-time to the PACU is desirable in busy centers but is not mandatory in smaller facilities. The management of the patient in the PACU should not differ from management in the operating room and should reflect a coordinated effort among the anesthesiologist, surgeon, and any consultants. The anesthesiologist still manages the analgesia as well as airway, cardiac, pulmonary, and metabolic problems, whereas the surgeon manages any problems directly related to the surgical procedure itself. Based on the assumptions that the average PACU stay is 1 h and the average procedure lasts 2 h, a ratio of one recovery nurse for two patients is generally satisfactory. Staffing for nursing care should be tailored to the unique requirements of each facility. A minimum of two nurses generally ensures that if one patient requires continuous nursing care, other patients will still be cared for adequately. The latter is also important medicolegally, because inadequate staffing is often cited as a major contributing factor to mishaps in the PACU. When the operating room schedule regularly includes pediatric patients or frequent short procedures, a ratio of one nurse to one patient is often needed. A charge nurse should be assigned to ensure optimal staffing at all times.

CARE OF THE PATIENT

EMERGENCE FROM GENERAL ANESTHESIA

Recovery from general or regional anesthesia is a time of great physiological stress for many patients. Emergence from general anesthesia should ideally be a smooth and gradual awakening in a controlled environment. Unfortunately, it often begins in the operating room or during transport to the recovery room and is frequently characterized by airway obstruction, shivering, agitation, delirium, pain, nausea and vomiting, hypothermia, and autonomic lability. Even patients receiving spinal or epidural anesthesia can experience marked decreases in blood pressure during transport or recovery; the sympatholytic effects of regional blocks prevent compensatory reflex vasoconstriction when patients are moved or when they sit up.

Following an inhalational-based anesthetic, the speed of emergence is directly proportionate to alveolar ventilation but inversely proportionate to the agent's blood solubility (see Chapter 7). As the duration of anesthesia increases, emergence also becomes increasingly dependent on total tissue uptake, which is a function of agent solubility, the average concentration used, and the duration of exposure to the anesthetic. Recovery is therefore fastest with desflurane and nitrous oxide and slowest from prolonged deep anesthesia with halothane and enflurane. Hypoventilation delays emergence from inhalational anesthesia.

Emergence from an intravenous anesthetic is a function of its pharmacokinetics. Recovery from most intravenous anesthetic agents is dependent primarily on redistribution rather than on elimination half-life. As the total administered dose increases, however, cumulative effects become apparent in the form of prolonged emergence; the termination of action becomes increasingly dependent on the elimination or metabolic half-life. Under these conditions, advanced age or renal or hepatic disease can prolong emergence (see Chapter 8). Use of short and ultra- short-acting anesthetic agents such as propofol and remifentanil significantly shortens emergence, time to awakening, and discharge. Moreover, the use of a Bispectral Index Scale (BIS) monitor (and presumably patient state index [PSI] monitor, see Chapter 6) reduces total drug dosage and shortens recovery and time to discharge. The use of laryngeal mask airways may also allow lighter levels of anesthesia that could speed emergence.

The speed of emergence can also be influenced by preoperative medications. Premedication with agents that outlast the procedure may be expected to prolong emergence. The short duration of action of midazolam makes it a suitable premedication agent for short procedures. The effects of preoperative sleep deprivation or drug ingestion (alcohol, sedatives) can also be additive to those of anesthetic agents and can prolong emergence.

Delayed Emergence

The most frequent cause of delayed emergence (when the patient fails to regain consciousness 30–60 min after general anesthesia) is residual anesthetic, sedative, and analgesic drug effect. Delayed emergence might occur as a result of absolute or relative drug overdose or potentiation of anesthetic agents by prior drug ingestion (alcohol). Administration of naloxone (0.04 mg increments) and flumazenil (0.2 mg increments) readily reverses and can exclude the effects of an opioid and benzodiazepine, respectively. Physostigmine 1–2 mg may partially reverse the effect of other agents. A nerve stimulator can be used to exclude significant neuromuscular blockade in patients on a mechanical ventilator who have inadequate spontaneous tidal volumes.

Less common causes of delayed emergence include hypothermia, marked metabolic disturbances, and perioperative stroke. Core temperatures less than 33°C have an anesthetic effect and greatly potentiate the effects of central nervous system depressants. Forced-air warming devices are most effective in raising body temperature. Hypoxemia and hypercarbia are readily excluded by blood gas analysis. Hypercalcemia, hypermagnesemia, hyponatremia, and hypoglycemia and hyperglycemia are rare causes that require laboratory measurements for diagnosis. Perioperative stroke is rare except after neurological, cardiac, and cerebrovascular surgery (see Chapter 27); diagnosis requires neurological consultation and radiological imaging.

TRANSPORT FROM THE OPERATING ROOM

This period is usually complicated by the lack of adequate monitors, access to drugs, or resuscitative equipment. Patients should not leave the operating room unless they have a stable and patent airway, have adequate ventilation and oxygenation, and are hemodynamically stable. Supplemental oxygen should be administered during transport to patients at risk for hypoxemia. Some studies suggest that transient hypoxemia ($SpO_2 < 90\%$) may develop in as many as 30–50% of otherwise "normal" patients during transport while breathing room air; supplemental oxygen may therefore by advisable in all patients if the PACU is not in immediate proximity to the operating room. Unstable patients should be left intubated and transported with a portable monitor (ECG, SpO_2, and blood pressure) and a supply of emergency drugs.

All patients should be taken to the PACU on a bed or gurney that can be placed in either the head-down (Trendelenburg) or head-up position. The head-down position is useful for hypovolemic patients, whereas the head-up position is useful for patients with underlying pulmonary dysfunction (see Chapter 22). Patients at high risk for vomiting or upper airway bleeding (eg, following tonsillectomy) should be transported in the lateral position. This position also helps prevent airway obstruction and facilitates drainage of secretions.

ROUTINE RECOVERY

General Anesthesia

Airway patency, vital signs, and oxygenation should be checked immediately on arrival. Subsequent blood pressure, pulse rate, and respiratory rate measurements are routinely made at least every 5 min for 15 min or until stable, and every 15 min thereafter. Pulse oximetry should be monitored continuously in all patients recovering from general anesthesia, at least until they regain consciousness. The occurrence of hypoxemia does not necessarily correlate with the level of consciousness. Neuromuscular function should be assessed clinically, eg, head-lift. At least one temperature measurement should also be obtained. Additional monitoring includes pain assessment (eg, numerical or descriptive scales), the presence or absence of nausea or vomiting, and fluid input and output including urine flow, drainage, and bleeding. After initial vital signs have been recorded, the anesthesiologist should give a brief report to the PACU nurse that includes the preoperative history (including mental status and any communication problems such as language barriers, deafness, blindness, or mental retardation), pertinent intraoperative events (type of anesthesia, the surgical procedure, blood loss, fluid replacement, and any complications), expected postoperative problems, and postanesthesia orders (epidural catheter care, transfusion, postoperative ventilation, etc).

All patients recovering from general anesthesia should receive 30–40% oxygen during emergence because transient hypoxemia can develop even in healthy patients. Patients at increased risk for hypoxemia, such as those with underlying pulmonary dysfunction or those undergoing upper abdominal or thoracic procedures, should continue to be monitored with a pulse oximeter even after emergence and may need oxygen supplementation for longer periods. A rational decision regarding continuing supplemental oxygen therapy at the time of discharge from the PACU can be made based on SpO_2 readings on room air. Arterial blood gas measurements can be obtained to confirm abnormal oximetry readings. Oxygen therapy should be carefully controlled in patients with chronic obstructive pulmonary disease and a history of CO_2 retention. Patients should generally be nursed in the head-up position whenever possible to optimize oxygenation. However, elevating the head of the bed before the patient is responsive can lead to airway obstruction. In such cases, the oral or nasal airway should be left in place until the patient is awake. Deep breathing and coughing should be encouraged periodically.

Regional Anesthesia

Patients who are heavily sedated or hemodynamically unstable following regional anesthesia should also receive supplemental oxygen in the PACU. Sensory and motor levels should be periodically recorded following regional anesthesia to document dissipation of the block. Precautions in the form of padding or repeated warning may be necessary to prevent self-injury from uncoordinated arm movements following brachial plexus blocks. Blood pressure should be closely monitored following spinal and epidural anesthesia. Bladder catheterization may be necessary in patients who have had spinal or epidural anesthesia for longer than 4 h.

Pain Control

Preoperative administration of nonsteroidal antiinflammatory drugs (NSAIDs) alone or with acetaminophen can significantly reduce postoperative opioid requirements for selected procedures. Use of selective cyclooxygenase-2 inhibitors (eg, rofecoxib and parecoxib) reduces any potential adverse effects on platelet function and gastrointestinal complications. Similarly, intraoperative wound infiltration and nerve blocks (eg, ilioinguinal and caudal) for selected procedures can also reduce operative analgesic requirements.

Mild to moderate pain can be treated orally with acetaminophen plus codeine, hydrocodone, or oxycodone (see Chapter 18). Alternatively, an opioid agonist–antagonist (butorphanol, 1–2 mg, or nalbuphine, 5–10 mg) or ketorolac tromethamine, 30 mg, may be used intravenously. The latter is particularly useful following orthopedic and gynecological procedures.

Moderate to severe postoperative pain in the PACU can be managed with parenteral or intraspinal opioids, regional anesthesia, or specific nerve blocks (see Chapter 18). When opioids are used, titration of small intravenous doses is generally safest. Although considerable variability may be encountered, most patients are quite sensitive to opioids within the first hour after general anesthesia. Adequate analgesia must be balanced against excessive sedation. Opioids of intermediate to long duration, such as meperidine, 10–20 mg (0.25–0.5 mg/kg in children), hydromorphone 0.25–0.5 mg (0.015–0.02 mg/kg in children), or morphine, 2–4 mg (0.025–0.05 mg/kg in children), are most commonly used.

Analgesic effects usually peak within 4–5 min. Maximal respiratory depression, particularly with morphine and hydromorphone, may not be seen until 20–30 min later. When the patient is fully awake, patient-controlled analgesia (PCA) can be instituted for inpatients (see Chapter 18). Intramuscular administration of opioids has the disadvantage of delayed and variable onset (10–20 min) and delayed respiratory depression (up to 1 h).

When an epidural catheter has been left in place, epidural administration of fentanyl, 50–100 µg, sufentanil, 20–30 µg, or morphine, 3–5 mg, can provide excellent pain relief in adults; however, the risk of delayed respiratory depression with morphine mandates special monitoring precautions for 12–24 h afterward (see Chapter 18). Intercostal, interscalene, femoral, epidural, or caudal anesthesia is often helpful when opioid analgesia alone is unsatisfactory (see Chapter 18).

Agitation

Before the patient is fully responsive, pain is often manifested as postoperative restlessness. Serious systemic disturbances (such as hypoxemia, acidosis, or hypotension), bladder distention, or a surgical complication (such as occult intraabdominal hemorrhage) should always be considered as well. Marked agitation may necessitate arm and leg restraints to avoid self-injury, particularly in children. When serious physiological disturbances have been excluded in children, cuddling and kind words from a sympathetic attendant or the parents (if they are allowed in the PACU) often calm the pediatric patient. Other contributory factors include marked preoperative anxiety and fear as well as adverse drug effects (large doses of central anticholinergic agents, phenothiazines, or ketamine). Physostigmine, 1–2 mg intravenously (0.05 mg/kg in children), is most effective in treating delirium due to atropine and scopolamine but may also be useful in other cases. If serious systemic disturbances and pain can be excluded, persistent agitation may require sedation with intermittent intravenous doses of midazolam, 0.5–1 mg (0.05 mg/kg in children).

Nausea & Vomiting

Postoperative nausea and vomiting (PONV) are a common problem following general anesthesia, occurring in 20–30% of all patients. Moreover, PONV may occur only at home within 24 h of an uneventful discharge (postdischarge nausea and vomiting) in a significant number of additional patients. The etiology of PONV is usually multifactorial, involving anesthetic agents, the type of procedure, and patient factors. It is important to recognize that nausea is a common complaint that is reported at the onset of hypotension, particularly following spinal or epidural anesthesia.

Patricia Kapur, MD

PREOPERATIVE SELECTION OF PATIENTS FOR AMBULATORY SURGERY

Ambulatory surgeries as a percentage of total surgeries are now approaching 70% or greater in the United States, with ever advancing surgical techniques and presumed safety of anesthesia care. It is ever more important that appropriate criteria be applied to identify not only those patients who can benefit from the efficiency and particular attention of ambulatory perioperative care, but those for whom the risks of early discharge and home care in the early postoperative period may be too high. Additional limitations are dictated by the physical distance of the ambulatory surgical facility to a full-service hospital should complications arise. Free-standing centers may lack an extensive laboratory, comprehensive pharmacy, advanced radiology support, blood bank, respiratory therapy support, and specialty consultants. The excellent cost-containment and patient satisfaction outcomes of ambulatory surgical care may result in a high demand for services that must be provided with an ever vigilant eye to safety concerns. Underlying assumptions are that all patients are as well prepared for anesthesia and surgery as possible, that the anesthesiologist is prepared and capable of caring for all

patient outcomes, and that the facility is equipped and staffed to stabilize the patient with complications prior to transport to a facility that can provide a higher level of care. Ambulatory perioperative care is routinely being provided for American Society of Anesthesiologists (ASA) physical status 3 patients with appropriate selection criteria.

Extremes of age pose a common challenge for patient selection. In facilities that accept infants and young children, a careful perinatal history is done to evaluate for prematurity and/or a history of apnea or bradycardia spells. Full-term infants without any such history may be accepted at greater than 44 weeks postconceptual age if the facility is otherwise staffed and equipped for their care. Ex-prematures may be denied access if they are less than 52 weeks postconceptual age or longer if complications were present. Of equal concern are the old elderly, particularly those greater than 85 years of age, after which age perioperative complications arise at a greater frequency than predicted based upon disease comorbidities and severity of the surgery. A careful social history must also be taken for the elderly to determine whether a qualified care giver will be available to accompany the patient home and to provide postoperative care. Perioperatively, judicious reduction of medication doses should be undertaken, in view of diminished organ function as well as diminished clearance and metabolic capacity in the elderly, to permit return of a preoperative level of functioning at the earliest.

Obese patients must be carefully evaluated because of the concomitant pulmonary, cardiac, and airway changes that may occur. Such patients must be able to use the available equipment in the facility, lay supine, and be evaluated for the presence of obstructive sleep apnea (OSA). Based on age, sex, type of surgery, and weight-matched controls, Sabers et al[1] were not able to find any difference in unanticipated hospital admission or in other adverse events among diagnosed and well-treated OSA patients undergoing outpatient surgical procedures in a tertiary referral

Table 48–1 lists commonly recognized risk factors for PONV. An increased incidence of nausea is reported following opioid administration during anesthesia, intraperitoneal surgery (particularly laparoscopy), and strabismus surgery. The highest incidence appears to be in young women; studies suggest nausea is more common during menstruation. Increased vagal tone manifested as sudden bradycardia commonly precedes or coincides with emesis. Propofol anesthesia decreases the incidence of PONV, as does a preoperative history of smoking. Selective 5-hydroxytryptamine (serotonin) receptor 3 (5-HT$_3$) antagonists such as ondansetron 4 center. However, the study did not include airway surgeries and found more frequent use of endotracheal intubation and less use of laryngeal mask airways in the OSA patients compared to the controls.

Of common comorbidities in potential ambulatory surgical patients, diabetes mellitus is often encountered. Stable diabetic patients on oral hypoglycemics, intermittent insulin therapy, and implanted insulin pumps may be safely anesthetized on an ambulatory basis, provided they do not have serious cardiovascular complications and are having procedures that are not likely to result in prolonged postoperative nausea or emesis. With implanted insulin pumps, a quick and clear-headed wake-up can result in patients programming their pumps early after surgery to adjust to anticipated oral intake. Patients with renal failure may come for surgery for shunt replacement and other procedures. Their intravascular volume status should be stable, their laboratory values including serum potassium level must be current, their blood pressure should be controlled, and no untoward fluid shifts should be anticipated from the surgery.

Stable cardiovascular patients may be cared for if their symptoms are controlled, their ventricular function is adequate, and their cardiac rhythm is stable. It is unlikely that patients with severe pulmonary dysfunction, marginal myocardial function, severe coronary disease, brittle diabetes, an unusually challenging airway, or severe sleep apnea[1] would be considered for anesthesia on an ambulatory basis. On the other hand, post-organ transplant patients may be considered if there are no signs of organ rejection and their immunosuppressive regimen can be maintained. Blood-borne infected patients are acceptable, eg, hepatitis and HIV, since universal precautions should be in place for all patients. However, patients with severe respiratory infections, such as active tuberculosis, may be turned away because of the generally close quarters in ambulatory centers and lack of isolation rooms. Mentally challenged patients with behavioral disruptions also may not be able to be suitably accommodated in every ambulatory setting.

Key components to an effective preoperative screening paradigm include development of a definition of suitable patients for the facility, preoperative workup expectations from referring physicians, preoperative testing guidelines, and guidelines for handling chronic medications preoperatively. In addition, the facility needs reliable information gathering and tracking systems as well as clear roles and expectations for all of the staff participating in presurgery and day of surgery preoperative activities.

An additional selection component to minimize outcome risk is the complexity of surgery to be undertaken at an ambulatory surgical venue. If the patients are well-screened with regard to their underlying medical status, the determinant of inpatient versus outpatient location for their surgeries is based on the complexity of the surgery and the capability of the facility. Dexter and colleagues[2] have proposed that if facility leaders decide what level of surgical complexity can be handled, the ASA Relative Value Guide can aid in determining what procedures qualify. In the example in that work, the proposed facility would have 23-h observation capacity, so the recommendation was that cases that had ASA Relative Value Guide base units of 7 or less, with an anticipated zero or one night stay, were acceptable for the proposed facility.

Good cooperation among anesthesiologists, surgeons, and referring physicians has enabled many more patients to safely undergo surgeries on an ambulatory basis. Attentive screening of the borderline patient can greatly assist in identifying the increasing numbers who can benefit from the ambulatory environment without undue risk, as well as separating those who still require the backup safety net of an inpatient facility.

1. Sabers C, Plevak DJ, Schroeder DR, Warner DO: The diagnosis of obstructive sleep apnea as a risk factor for unanticipated admissions in outpatient surgery. Anesth Analg 2003;96:1328.
2. Dexter F, Macario A, Penning DH: Development of an appropriate list of surgical procedures of a specified maximum anesthetic complexity to be performed at a new ambulatory surgery facility. Anesth Analg 2002;95:78.

mg (0.1 mg/kg in children), granisetron 0.01–0.04 mg/kg, and dolasetron 12.5 mg (0.035 mg/kg in children) are also extremely effective in preventing PONV and in treating established PONV. It should be noted that unlike ondansetron, which is usually effective immediately, dolasetron requires 15 min for onset. An orally disintegrating tablet (ODT) preparation of ondansetron (8 mg) may be useful for treatment and prophylaxis against postdischarge nausea and vomiting. Metoclopramide, 0.15 mg/kg intravenously, is somewhat less effective but is a good alternative to 5-HT_3 antagonists. 5-HT_3 antagonists are not associated with the acute extrapyra-

Table 48–1. Risk factors for postoperative nausea and vomiting.

Patient factors
  Young age
  Female gender, particularly if menstruating on day of
    surgery of in first trimester of pregnancy
  Large body habitus
  History of prior postoperative emesis
  History of motion sickness
Anesthetic techniques
  General anesthesia
  Drugs
    Opioids
    Volatile agents
    ? Neostigmine
Surgical procedures
  Strabismus surgery
  Ear surgery
  Laparoscopy
  Orchiopexy
  Ovum retrieval
  Tonsillectomy
Postoperative factors
  Postoperative pain
  Hypotension

---

midal (dystonic) manifestations and dysphoric reactions that may be encountered with metoclopramide or phenothiazine-type antiemetics. Transdermal scopolamine is effective but can be associated with troublesome side effects in some patients, such as exacerbating glaucoma, urinary retention, and difficulty in visual accommodation. Dexamethasone, 4–10 mg (0.10 mg/kg in children), when combined with another antiemetic is particularly effective for refractory nausea and vomiting. Moreover, it appears to be effective for up to 24 h and thus may be useful for postdischarge nausea and vomiting. Intravenous droperidol 0.625–1.25 mg (0.05–0.075 mg/kg in children), when given intraoperatively, significantly decreases the likelihood of PONV postoperative nausea without significantly prolonging emergence and can effectively treat it. Unfortunately, droperidol now carries a 2001 Food and Drug Administration (FDA) "black box" warning indicating that it can prolong the QT interval and has been associated with fatal cardiac arrhythmias. Because the latter appears to be exceedingly rare and is associated with very high doses (> 25 mg), the FDA warning generated considerable controversy and many clinicians no longer use the drug. Nonpharmacological prophylaxis against PONV includes ensuring adequate hydration (20 mL/kg) after fasting and stimulation of the P6 acupuncture point (wrist). The latter may include application of pressure, electrical current, or injections.

Controversy exists regarding routine prophylaxis for PONV in all patients. Clearly patients with multiple risk factors should receive prophylaxis. Additionally, use of two or more agents is more effective than single agent prophylaxis. Outcome studies and satisfaction surveys suggest little or no difference between routine prophylaxis and treat-as-needed strategies.

Shivering & Hypothermia

Shivering can occur in the PACU as a result of intraoperative hypothermia or the effects of anesthetic agents. It is also common in the immediate postpartum period. The most important cause of hypothermia is a redistribution of heat from the body core to the peripheral compartments (see Chapter 6). A cold ambient temperature in the operating room, prolonged exposure of a large wound, and the use of large amounts of unwarmed intravenous fluids or high flows of unhumidified gases can also be contributory. Nearly all anesthetics, particularly volatile agents, decrease the normal vasoconstrictive response to hypothermia. Although anesthetic agents also decrease the shivering threshold, shivering is commonly observed during or after emergence from general anesthesia. Shivering in such instances represents the body's effort to increase heat production and raise body temperature and may be associated with intense vasoconstriction. Emergence from even brief general anesthesia is sometimes also associated with shivering. Although the shivering can be part of nonspecific neurological signs (posturing, clonus, or Babinski's sign) that are sometimes observed during emergence, it is most often due to hypothermia and is most commonly associated with volatile anesthetics. Regardless of the mechanism, its incidence appears related to duration of surgery and the use of high concentrations of a volatile agent. The shivering occasionally can be intense enough to cause hyperthermia (38–39°C) and a significant metabolic acidosis, both of which promptly resolve when the shivering stops. Both spinal and epidural anesthesia also lower the shivering threshold and vasoconstrictive response to hypothermia; shivering may also be encountered in the recovery room following regional anesthesia. Other causes of shivering should be excluded, such as sepsis, drug allergy, or a transfusion reaction.

Hypothermia should be treated with a forced-air warming device, or (less satisfactorily) with warming lights or heating blankets, to raise body temperature to normal. Intense shivering causes precipitous rises in oxygen consumption, CO_2 production, and cardiac output. These physiological effects are often poorly tolerated by patients with preexisting cardiac or pulmonary impairment. Hypothermia has been associated with an increased incidence of myocardial ischemia, arrhythmias, increased transfusion requirements, and increased duration of muscle relaxant effects. Small intravenous doses of meperidine, 10–50 mg, can dramatically reduce or even stop shivering. Intubated and mechanically ventilated patients can also be sedated and given a muscle relaxant until normothermia is reestablished and the effects of anesthesia have dissipated.

Discharge Criteria

A. PACU

All patients must be evaluated by an anesthesiologist prior to discharge from the PACU unless strict discharge criteria are adopted. Criteria for discharging patients from the PACU are established by the department of anesthesiology and the hospital's medical staff. They may allow PACU nurses to determine when patients may be transferred without the presence of a physician provided all criteria have been met. Criteria can vary according to whether the patient is going to be discharged to an intensive care unit, a regular ward, the outpatient department (phase 2 recovery), or directly home.

Before discharge, patients should have been observed for respiratory depression for at least 20–30 min after the last dose of parenteral narcotic. Other minimum discharge criteria for patients recovering from general anesthesia usually include the following:

(1) Easy arousability

(2) Full orientation

(3) The ability to maintain and protect the airway

(4) Stable vital signs for at least 15–30 min

(5) The ability to call for help if necessary

(6) No obvious surgical complications (such as active bleeding).

Controlling postoperative pain, controlling nausea and vomiting, and reestablishing normothermia prior to discharge are also highly desirable. Scoring systems are widely used. Most assess SpO_2 (or color), consciousness, circulation, respiration, and motor activity (Table 48–2). The majority of patients can meet discharge criteria within 60 min in the PACU. Patients to be transferred to other intensive care facilities need not meet all requirements.

In addition to the above criteria, patients receiving regional anesthesia should also show signs of resolution of both sensory and motor blockade. Complete resolu-

Table 48–2. Postanesthetic Aldrete recovery score.[1,2]

Original Criteria	Modified Criteria	Point Value
Color	**Oxygenation**	
Pink	$SpO_2 > 92\%$ on room air	2
Pale or dusky	$SpO_2 > 90\%$ on oxygen	1
Cyanotic	$SpO_2 < 90\%$ on oxygen	0
Respiration		
Can breathe deeply and cough	Breathes deeply and coughs freely	2
Shallow but adequate exchange	Dyspneic, shallow or limited breathing	1
Apnea or obstruction	Apnea	0
Circulation		
Blood pressure within 20% of normal	Blood pressure ± 20 mm Hg of normal	2
Blood pressure within 20–50% of normal	Blood pressure ± 20–50 mm Hg of normal	1
Blood pressure deviating > 50% from normal	Blood pressure more than ± 50 mm Hg of normal	0
Consciousness		
Awake, alert, and oriented	Fully awake	2
Arousable but readily drifts back to sleep	Arousable on calling	1
No response	Not responsive	0
Activity		
Moves all extremities	Same	2
Moves two extremities	Same	1
No movement	Same	0

[1]Based on Aldrete JA, Kronlik D: A postanesthetic recovery score. Anesth Analg 1970;49:924 and Aldrete JA: The post-anesthesia recovery score revisited. J Clin Anesth 1995;7:89.
[2]Ideally, the patient should be discharged when the total score is 10 but a minimum of 9 is required.

tion of the block is generally desirable to avoid inadvertent injuries due to motor weakness or sensory deficits; some medical centers have nursing protocols that allow earlier discharge to appropriately staffed areas. Documenting resolution of the block is also critically important. Failure of a spinal or epidural block to resolve after 6 h raises the possibility of spinal cord or epidural hematoma, which should be excluded by radiological imaging.

In some centers, outpatients who meet the above discharge criteria when they come out of the operating room may be "fast-tracked" and taken directly to the phase 2 recovery area. Similarly, inpatients who meet the same criteria may be transferred directly from the operating room to their ward.

B. Outpatients

In addition to emergence and awakening, recovery from anesthesia following outpatient procedures includes two additional stages: home readiness (phase 2 recovery) and complete psychomotor recovery. A scoring system has been developed to help assess home readiness discharge (Table 48–3). Recovery of proprioception, sympathetic

Table 48–3. Postanesthesia discharge scoring system (PADS).[1,2]

Criteria	Points
Vital signs	
Within 20% of preoperative baseline	2
Within 20–40% of preoperative baseline	1
> 40% of preoperative baseline	0
Activity level	
Steady gait, no dizziness, at preoperative level	2
Requires assistance	1
Unable to ambulate	0
Nausea and vomiting	
Minimal, treated with oral medication	2
Moderate, treated with parenteral medication	1
Continues after repeated medication	0
Pain: minimal or none, acceptable to patient, controlled with oral medication	
Yes	2
No	1
Surgical bleeding	
Minimal: no dressing change required	2
Moderate: up to two dressing changes	1
Severe: three or more dressing changes	0

[1]Based on Marshall SI, Chung F: Discharge criteria and complications after ambulatory surgery. Anesth Analg 1999;88:508.
[2]Score ≥ 9 is required for discharge.

tone, bladder function, and motor strength are additional criteria following regional anesthesia. For example, intact proprioception of the big toe, minimal orthostatic changes, and normal plantar flexion of the foot are important signals of recovery following spinal anesthesia. Urination before discharge and drinking or eating before discharge are generally no longer required; exceptions include patients with a history of urinary retention and diabetics.

All outpatients must be discharged home in the company of a responsible adult who will stay with them overnight. Patients must be provided with written postoperative instructions on how to obtain emergency help and to perform routine follow-up care. The assessment of home readiness is the responsibility of the physician, preferably an anesthesiologist, who is familiar with the patient. The authority to discharge a patient home can be delegated to a nurse if preapproved discharge criteria are rigorously applied.

Home readiness does not imply that the patient has the ability to make important decisions, to drive, or to return to work. These activities require complete psychomotor recovery, which is often not achieved until 24–72 h postoperatively. All outpatient centers must use some system of postoperative follow-up involving the use of patient questionnaires or preferably phone contacts the day after discharge.

MANAGEMENT OF COMPLICATIONS

RESPIRATORY COMPLICATIONS

Respiratory problems are the most frequently encountered serious complications in the PACU. The overwhelming majority are related to airway obstruction, hypoventilation, or hypoxemia. Because hypoxemia is the final common pathway to serious morbidity and mortality, routine monitoring of pulse oximetry in the PACU leads to earlier recognition of these complications and fewer adverse outcomes.

Airway Obstruction

Airway obstruction in unconscious patients is most commonly due to the tongue falling back against the posterior pharynx (see Chapter 5). Other causes include laryngospasm; glottic edema; secretions, vomitus, or blood in the airway; or external pressure on the trachea (most commonly from a neck hematoma). Partial airway obstruction usually presents as sonorous respiration. Total obstruction causes cessation of airflow, an absence of breath sounds, and marked paradoxic (rocking) movement of the chest. The abdomen and chest should normally rise together during inspiration; however, with airway obstruction, the chest descends as the abdomen rises during each inspiration (paradoxic chest movement). Patients with airway obstruction should receive supplemental oxygen while corrective measures are undertaken. A combined jaw-thrust and head-tilt maneuver pulls the tongue forward and opens the airway. Insertion of an oral or nasal airway also often alleviates the problem. Nasal airways may be better tolerated than oral airways by patients during emergence and may decrease the likelihood of trauma to the teeth when the patient bites down.

If the above maneuvers fail, laryngospasm should be considered. Laryngospasm is usually characterized by high-pitched crowing noises but may be silent, with complete glottic closure. Spasm of the vocal cords is more apt to occur following airway trauma, or repeated instrumentation, or stimulation from secretions or blood in the airway. The jaw-thrust maneuver, particularly when combined with gentle positive airway pressure via a tight-fitting face mask, usually breaks laryngospasm. Insertion of an oral or nasal airway is also helpful in ensuring a patent airway down to the level of the vocal cords. Any secretions or blood in the hypopharynx should be suctioned to prevent recurrence. Refractory laryngospasm should be treated aggressively with a small dose of succinylcholine (10–20 mg) and temporary positive-pressure ventilation with 100% oxygen to prevent severe hypoxemia or negative pressure pulmonary edema. Endotracheal intubation may occasionally be necessary to reestablish ventilation; cricothyrotomy or transtracheal jet ventilation is indicated if intubation is unsuccessful in such instances.

Glottic edema following airway instrumentation is an important cause of airway obstruction in infants and young children. Intravenous corticosteroids (dexamethasone, 0.5 mg/kg) or aerosolized racemic epinephrine (0.5 mL of a 2.25% solution with 3 mL of normal saline) may be useful in such cases. Postoperative wound hematomas following head and neck, thyroid, and carotid procedures can quickly compromise the airway; opening the wound immediately relieves tracheal compression. Rarely, gauze packing may be unintentionally left in the hypopharynx following oral surgery and can cause immediate or delayed complete airway obstruction.

Hypoventilation

Hypoventilation, which is generally defined as a $PaCO_2$ greater than 45 mm Hg, is a common occurrence following general anesthesia. In most instances, the hypoventilation is mild, and many cases are overlooked. Significant hypoventilation is usually clinically apparent only when the $PaCO_2$ is greater than 60 mm Hg or arterial blood pH is less than 7.25. Signs are varied and include excessive or

prolonged somnolence, airway obstruction, slow respiratory rate, tachypnea with shallow breathing, or labored breathing. Mild to moderate respiratory acidosis causes tachycardia and hypertension or cardiac irritability (via sympathetic stimulation), but a more severe acidosis produces circulatory depression (see Chapter 30). If significant hypoventilation is suspected, arterial blood gas measurements should be obtained to assess its severity and guide further management.

Hypoventilation in the PACU is most commonly due to the residual depressant effects of anesthetic agents on respiratory drive. Opioid-induced respiratory depression characteristically produces a slow respiratory rate, often with large tidal volumes. Excessive sedation is also often present, but the patient may be responsive and able to increase breathing on command. Biphasic or recurring patterns of respiratory depression have been reported with all opioids. Proposed mechanisms include variations in the intensity of stimulation during recovery and delayed release of the opioid from peripheral compartments such as skeletal muscle (or possibly the lungs with fentanyl) as the patient rewarms or begins to move. Secretion of intravenously administered opioids into gastric fluid followed by reabsorption has also been described but appears to be an unlikely explanation because of high hepatic extraction for most opioids.

Inadequate reversal, overdose, hypothermia, pharmacological interactions (such as with "mycin" antibiotics or magnesium therapy), altered pharmacokinetics (due to hypothermia, altered volumes of distribution, renal or hepatic dysfunction), or metabolic factors (such as hypokalemia or respiratory acidosis) can be responsible for residual muscle paralysis in the PACU. Regardless of the cause, discoordinated breathing movements with shallow tidal volumes and tachypnea are usually apparent. The diagnosis can be made with a nerve stimulator in unconscious patients; awake patients can be asked to lift their head. The ability to sustain a head-lift for 5 s may be the most sensitive test for assessing the adequacy of reversal.

Splinting due to incisional pain and diaphragmatic dysfunction following upper abdominal or thoracic surgery, abdominal distention, or tight abdominal dressings are other factors that can contribute to hypoventilation. Increased CO_2 production from shivering, hyperthermia, or sepsis can also increase $PaCO_2$ even in normal patients recovering from general anesthesia. Marked hypoventilation and respiratory acidosis can result when these factors are superimposed on an impaired ventilatory reserve due to underlying pulmonary, neuromuscular, or neurological disease.

TREATMENT

Treatment should generally be directed at the underlying cause, but marked hypoventilation always requires controlled ventilation until contributory factors are identified and corrected. Obtundation, circulatory depression, and severe acidosis (arterial blood pH < 7.15) are indications for immediate endotracheal intubation. Antagonism of opioid-induced depression with naloxone is a two-edged sword; the abrupt increase in alveolar ventilation is usually also associated with sudden pain and sympathetic discharge. The latter can precipitate a hypertensive crisis, pulmonary edema, and myocardial ischemia or infarction. If naloxone is used to increase respiration, titration with small increments (0.04 mg in adults) may avoid complications by allowing partial reversal of the respiratory depression without significant reversal of the analgesia. Following naloxone, patients should be watched carefully for recurrence of opioid-induced respiratory depression (renarcotization), as naloxone has a shorter duration than most opioids. Alternatively, doxapram, 60–100 mg, followed by 1–2 mg/min intravenously, may be used; doxapram does not reverse the analgesia, but can cause hypertension and tachycardia. If residual muscle paralysis is present, additional cholinesterase inhibitor may be given. Residual paralysis in spite of a full dose of a cholinesterase inhibitor necessitates controlled ventilation until spontaneous recovery occurs. Judicious opioid analgesia (intravenous or intraspinal), epidural anesthesia, or intercostal nerve blocks are often beneficial in alleviating splinting following upper abdominal or thoracic procedures.

Hypoxemia

Mild hypoxemia is common in patients recovering from anesthesia unless supplemental oxygen is given during emergence. Mild to moderate hypoxemia (PaO_2 50–60 mm Hg) in young healthy patients may be well tolerated initially, but with increasing duration or severity the initial sympathetic stimulation often seen is replaced with progressive acidosis and circulatory depression. Obvious cyanosis may be absent if the hemoglobin concentration is reduced. Clinically, hypoxemia may also be suspected from restlessness, tachycardia, or cardiac irritability (ventricular or atrial). Obtundation, bradycardia, hypotension, and cardiac arrest are late signs. The routine use of a pulse oximeter in the PACU facilitates early detection. Arterial blood gas measurements should be performed to confirm the diagnosis and guide therapy.

Hypoxemia in the PACU is usually caused by hypoventilation, increased right-to-left intrapulmonary shunting, or both. A decrease in cardiac output or an increase in oxygen consumption (as with shivering) will accentuate the hypoxemia. Diffusion hypoxia (see Chapter 7) is an uncommon cause of hypoxemia when recovering patients are given supplemental oxygen. Hypoxemia due to pure hypoventilation is also unusual in patients receiving supplemental oxygen unless marked hypercapnia or a concomitant increase in intrapulmonary shunting is present. Increased intrapulmonary shunting from a decreased functional residual capacity (FRC) relative to closing capacity is the most common cause of hypoxemia following general anesthesia. The greatest reductions in FRC occur following upper abdominal and thoracic surgery. The loss of lung volume is often attributed to microatelectasis, as visible atelectasis is often not evident on a chest film. A semiupright position helps maintain FRC.

Marked right-to-left intrapulmonary shunting ($\dot{Q}s/\dot{Q}t$ > 15%) is usually associated with radiographically discernible findings such as pulmonary atelectasis, parenchymal infiltrates, or a large pneumothorax. Causes include prolonged intraoperative hypoventilation with low tidal volumes, unintentional endobronchial intubation, lobar collapse from bronchial obstruction by secretions or blood, pulmonary aspiration, or pulmonary edema. Postoperative pulmonary edema most often presents as wheezing within the first 60 min after surgery; it may be due to left ventricular failure (cardiogenic), the acute respiratory distress syndrome (ARDS), or the sudden relief of prolonged airway obstruction. In contrast to wheezing associated with pulmonary edema, wheezing due to primary obstructive lung disease, which also often results in large increases in intrapulmonary shunting, is not associated with auscultatory crackles, edema fluid in the airway, or infiltrates on the chest film. The possibility of a postoperative pneumothorax should always be considered following central line placement, intercostal blocks, rib fractures, neck dissections, tracheostomy, nephrectomies, or other retroperitoneal or intraabdominal procedures (including laparoscopy), particularly when the diaphragm might be penetrated. Patients with subpleural blebs or large bullae can also develop pneumothorax during positive-pressure ventilation.

TREATMENT

Oxygen therapy with or without positive airway pressure is the cornerstone of treatment. Routine administration of 30–60% oxygen is usually enough to prevent hypoxemia with even moderate hypoventilation and hypercapnia. Patients with underlying pulmonary or cardiac disease may require higher concentrations of oxygen; oxygen therapy should be guided by SpO_2 or arterial blood gas measurements. Oxygen concentration must be closely controlled in patients with chronic CO_2 retention to avoid precipitating acute respiratory failure. Patients with severe or persistent hypoxemia should be given 100% oxygen via a nonrebreathing mask or an endotracheal tube until the cause is established and other therapies are instituted; controlled or assisted mechanical ventilation may also be necessary. The chest film (preferably an upright film) is invaluable in assessing lung volume and heart size and demonstrating a pneumothorax or pulmonary infiltrates. Infiltrates may initially be absent immediately following aspiration.

Additional treatment should be directed at the underlying cause. A chest tube should be inserted for any symptomatic pneumothorax or one that is greater than 15–20%. Bronchospasm should be treated with aerosolized bronchodilators and perhaps intravenous aminophylline. Diuretics should be given for circulatory fluid overload. Cardiac function should be optimized. Persistent hypoxemia in spite of 50% oxygen generally is an indication for positive end-expiratory pressure (PEEP) or CPAP. Bronchoscopy is often useful in reexpanding lobar atelectasis caused by bronchial plugs or particulate aspiration.

CIRCULATORY COMPLICATIONS

The most common circulatory disturbances in the PACU are hypotension, hypertension, and arrhythmias. The possibility that the circulatory abnormality is secondary to an underlying respiratory disturbance should always be considered before any other intervention.

Hypotension

Hypotension is usually due to decreased venous return to the heart, left ventricular dysfunction, or, less commonly, excessive arterial vasodilatation. Hypovolemia is by far the most common cause of hypotension in the PACU. Absolute hypovolemia can result from inadequate intraoperative fluid replacement, continuing fluid sequestration by tissues ("third-spacing") or wound drainage, or postoperative bleeding. Venoconstriction during hypothermia may mask the hypovolemia until the patient's temperature begins to rise again; subsequent venodilatation results in delayed hypotension. Relative hypovolemia is responsible for the hypotension associated with spinal or epidural anesthesia, venodilators, and α-adrenergic blockade; the increase in venous capacitance reduces venous return in spite of a previously normal intravascular volume in such instances. Hypotension associated with sepsis and allergic reactions is usually the result of both hypovolemia and vasodilatation. Hypotension following a tension pneumothorax or cardiac tamponade is the result of impaired cardiac filling.

Left ventricular dysfunction in previously healthy persons is unusual unless it is associated with severe metabolic disturbances (hypoxemia, acidosis, or sepsis). Hypotension due to ventricular dysfunction is primarily encountered in patients with underlying coronary artery or valvular heart disease, and is usually precipitated by fluid overload, myocardial ischemia, acute increases in afterload, or dysrhythmias.

TREATMENT

Mild hypotension during recovery from anesthesia is common and usually reflects the decrease in sympathetic tone normally associated with sleep or residual effects of anesthetic agents; it typically does not require treatment. Significant hypotension is usually defined as a 20–30% reduction of blood pressure below the patient's baseline level and indicates a serious derangement requiring treatment. Treatment depends on the ability to assess intravascular volume. An increase in blood pressure following a fluid bolus (250–500 mL crystalloid or 100–250 mL colloid) generally confirms hypovolemia. With severe hypotension, a vasopressor or inotrope (dopamine or epinephrine) may be necessary to increase arterial blood pressure until the intravascular volume deficit is at least partially corrected. Signs of cardiac dysfunction should be sought in elderly patients and patients with known heart disease. Failure of a patient to promptly respond to treatment mandates invasive hemodynamic monitoring; manipulations of cardiac preload, contractility, and afterload are often necessary. The presence of a tension pneumothorax, as suggested by hypotension with unilaterally decreased breath sounds, hyperresonance, and tracheal deviation, is an indication for immediate pleural aspiration even before radiographic confirmation. Similarly, hypotension due to cardiac tamponade, usually following chest trauma or thoracic surgery, often necessitates immediate pericardiocentesis or reexploration.

Hypertension

Postoperative hypertension is common in the PACU and typically occurs within the first 30 min after admission. Noxious stimulation from incisional pain, endotracheal intubation, or bladder distention is usually responsible. Postoperative hypertension may also reflect sympathetic activation, which may be part of the neuroendocrine response to surgery or secondary to hypoxemia, hypercapnia, or metabolic acidosis. Patients with a history of systemic hypertension are likely to develop hypertension in the PACU even in the absence of an identifiable cause. The degree of preoperative control over blood pressure bears an inverse relationship to the incidence of postoperative hypertension in such patients. Fluid overload or intracranial hypertension can also occasionally present as postoperative hypertension.

TREATMENT

Mild hypertension generally does not require treatment, but a reversible cause should be sought. Marked hypertension can precipitate postoperative bleeding, myocardial ischemia, heart failure, or intracranial hemorrhage. The decision about what degree of hypertension should be treated must be individualized. In general, elevations in blood pressure greater than 20–30% of the patient's normal baseline or those associated with adverse effects (such as myocardial ischemia, heart failure, or bleeding) should be treated. Mild to moderate elevations can be treated with an intravenous β-adrenergic blocker such as labetalol, esmolol, or propranolol; the calcium channel blocker nicardipine; or nitroglycerin paste. Sublingual nifedipine and hydralazine are also effective but frequently cause reflex tachycardia and have been associated with myocardial ischemia and infarction. Marked hypertension in patients with limited cardiac reserve requires direct intraarterial pressure monitoring and should be treated with an intravenous infusion of nitroprusside, nitroglycerin, nicardipine, or fenoldopam. The end point for treatment should be consistent with the patient's own normal blood pressure.

Arrhythmias

The role of respiratory disturbances, particularly hypoxemia, hypercarbia, and acidosis, in promoting cardiac arrhythmias cannot be overemphasized. Residual effects from anesthetic agents, increased sympathetic nervous system activity, other metabolic abnormalities, and preexisting cardiac or pulmonary disease also predispose patients to arrhythmias in the PACU.

Bradycardia often represents the residual effects of a cholinesterase inhibitor (neostigmine), a potent synthetic opioid (sufentanil), or β-adrenergic blockers (propranolol). Tachycardia may represent the effect of an anticholinergic agent (atropine), a vagolytic drug (pancuronium or meperidine), a β-agonist (albuterol), reflex tachycardia (hydralazine), in addition to more common causes such as pain, fever, hypovolemia, and anemia. Moreover, anesthetic-induced depression of baroreceptor function makes heart rate an unreliable monitor of intravascular volume in the PACU.

Premature atrial and ventricular beats usually represent hypokalemia, hypomagnesemia, increased sympathetic tone, or, less commonly, myocardial ischemia. The latter can be diagnosed with a 12-lead ECG. Supraventricular tachyarrhythmias including paroxysmal supraventricular tachycardia, atrial flutter, and atrial fibrillation are typically encountered in patients with a history of these arrhythmias, and are more commonly encountered following thoracic surgery. The management of arrhythmias is discussed in Chapters 19 and 47.

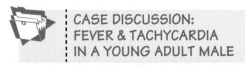

CASE DISCUSSION: FEVER & TACHYCARDIA IN A YOUNG ADULT MALE

A 19-year-old man sustains a closed fracture of the femur in a motor vehicle accident. He is placed in traction for 3 days prior to surgery. During that time, a persistent low-grade fever (37.5–38.7°C orally), mild hypertension (150–170/70–90 mm Hg), and tachycardia (100–126 beats/min) are noted. His hematocrit remains between 30% and 32.5%. Broad-spectrum antibiotic coverage is initiated. He is scheduled for open reduction and internal fixation of the fracture. When the patient is brought into the operating room, vital signs are as follows: blood pressure 162/95 mm Hg, pulse 150 beats/min, respirations 20 breaths/min, and oral temperature 38.1°C. He is sweating and appears anxious in spite of intramuscular premedication with meperidine, 75 mg, and promethazine, 25 mg. On close examination, he is noted to have a slightly enlarged thyroid gland.

Should the surgical team proceed with the operation?

The proposed operation is elective; therefore, significant abnormalities should be diagnosed and properly treated preoperatively, if possible, to make the patient optimally ready for surgery. If the patient had an open fracture, the risk of infection would clearly mandate immediate operation. Even with a closed femoral fracture, needless cancellations or delays should be avoided because nonoperative treatment entails the risks of prolonged bed rest (with traction), including atelectasis, pneumonia, deep venous thrombosis, and potentially lethal pulmonary thromboembolism. In deciding whether to proceed with the surgery, the anesthesiologist must ask the following questions:

(1) What are the most likely causes of the abnormalities based on the clinical presentation?

(2) What, if any, additional investigations or consultations might be helpful?

(3) How would these or other commonly associated abnormalities affect anesthetic management?

(4) Are the potential anesthetic interactions serious enough to delay surgery until a suspected cause is conclusively excluded? The tachycardia of 150 beats/min and the low-grade fever therefore require further evaluation prior to surgery.

What are the likely causes of the tachycardia and fever in this patient?

These two abnormalities may reflect one process or separate entities (Tables 48–4 and 48–5). Moreover, although multiple factors can often be simultaneously identified, their relative contribution is usually not readily apparent. Fever commonly follows major trauma; contributory fac-

Table 48–4. Perioperative causes of tachycardia.

Anxiety
Pain
Fever (see Table 48–5)
Respiratory
Hypoxemia
Hypercapnia
Circulatory
Hypotension
Anemia
Hypovolemia
Congestive heart failure
Cardiac tamponade
Tension pneumothorax
Thromboembolism
Drug-induced
Antimuscarinic agents
β-Adrenergic agonists
Vasodilators
Allergy
Drug withdrawal
Metabolic disorders
Hypoglycemia
Thyrotoxicosis
Pheochromocytoma
Adrenal (addisonian) crisis
Carcinoid syndrome
Acute porphyria

tors can include the inflammatory reaction to the tissue trauma, superimposed infection (most commonly wound, pulmonary, or urinary), antibiotic therapy (drug reaction), or thrombophlebitis. Infection must be seriously considered in this patient because of the risk of bacteria seeding and infecting the metal fixation device placed during surgery. Although tachycardia is commonly associated with a low-grade fever, it is usually not of this magnitude in a 19-year-old patient. Moderate to severe pain, anxiety, hypovolemia, or anemia may be other contributory factors. Pulmonary fat embolism should also be considered in any patient with long bone fracture, particularly when hypoxemia, tachypnea, or mental status changes are present. Lastly, the possibly enlarged thyroid gland, sweating, and anxious appearance together with both fever and tachycardia suggest thyrotoxicosis.

What (if any) additional measures may be helpful in evaluating the fever and tachycardia?

Arterial blood gas measurements and a chest film would be helpful in excluding fat embolism. A repeat hematocrit or hemoglobin concentration measurement would exclude worsening anemia; significant tachycardia may be expected when the hematocrit is below 25–27% (hemoglobin < 8 g/dL) in most patients. The response to an intravenous fluid challenge with 250–500 mL of a colloid solution may be helpful; a decrease in heart rate after the fluid bolus is strongly suggestive of hypovolemia. Similarly, response of the heart rate to sedation and additional opioid analgesia can be helpful in excluding anxiety and pain, respectively, as causes. Although a tentative diagnosis of hyperthyroidism can be made based on clinical grounds, confirmation requires measurement of serum thyroid hormones; the latter usually requires 24–48 h in most hospitals. Signs of infection—such as increased inflammation or purulence in a wound, purulent sputum, an infiltrate on the chest film, pyuria, or leukocytosis with premature white cells on a blood smear (shift to the left)—should prompt cultures and a delay of surgery until the results are obtained and correct antibiotic coverage is confirmed.

The patient is transferred to the PACU for further evaluation. A 12-lead ECG confirms sinus tachycardia of 150 beats/min. A chest film is normal. Arterial blood gas measurements on room air are normal (pH 7.44, $Paco_2$ 41 mm Hg, Pao_2 87 mm Hg, HCO_3^- 27 mEq/L). The hemoglobin concentration is found to be 11 g/dL. Blood for thyroid function tests is sent to the laboratory. The

Table 48–5. Perioperative causes of fever.

Infections
Immunologically mediated processes
  Drug reactions
  Blood reactions
  Tissue destruction (rejection)
  Connective tissue disorders
  Granulomatous disorders
Tissue damage
  Trauma
  Infarction
  Thrombosis
Neoplastic disorders
Metabolic disorders
  Thyroid storm (thyroid crisis)
  Adrenal (addisonian) crisis
  Pheochromocytoma
  Malignant hyperthermia
  Neuroleptic malignant syndrome
  Acute gout
  Acute porphyria

patient is sedated intravenously with midazolam, 2 mg, and fentanyl, 50 μg, and is given 500 mL of 5% albumin. He appears relaxed and pain free, but the heart rate decreases only to 144 beats/min. The decision is made to proceed with surgery using continuous lumbar epidural anesthesia with 2% lidocaine. Esmolol, 100 mg, is administered slowly until his pulse decreases to 120 beats/min, and a continuous esmolol infusion is administered at a rate of 300 μg/kg/h.

The procedure is completed in 3 1/2 hours. Although the patient did not complain of any pain during the procedure and was given only minimal additional sedation (midazolam, 2 mg), he is delirious upon admission to the PACU. The esmolol infusion is proceeding at a rate of 500 μg/kg/min. He has also received propranolol, 24 mg intravenously. Estimated blood loss was 500 mL, and fluid replacement consisted of 2 units of packed red blood cells, 1000 mL of hetastarch, and 9000 mL of lactated Ringer's injection. Vital signs are as follows: blood pressure 105/40 mm Hg, pulse 124 beats/min, respirations 30 breaths/min, and rectal temperature 38.8°C. Arterial blood gas measurements are reported as follows: pH 7.37, $Paco_2$ 37 mm Hg, Pao_2 91 mm Hg, HCO_3^- 22 mEq/L.

What is the most likely diagnosis?

The patient is now obviously in a hypermetabolic state manifested by excessive adrenergic activity, fever, markedly increased fluid requirements, and a worsening mental status. The absence of major metabolic acidosis and lack of exposure to a known triggering agent exclude malignant hyperthermia (see Chapter 44). Other possibilities include a transfusion reaction, sepsis, or an undiagnosed pheochromocytoma. The sequence of events makes the first two unlikely, and the decreasing prominence of hypertension (now replaced with relative hypotension) and increasing fever make the latter unlikely as well. The clinical presentation now strongly suggests thyroid storm.

Emergency consultation is obtained with an endocrinologist, who concurs with the diagnosis of thyroid storm. How is thyroid storm managed?

Thyroid storm (crisis) is a medical emergency that carries a 10–50% mortality rate. It is usually encountered in patients with poorly controlled or undiagnosed Graves disease. Precipitating factors include (1) the stress of surgery and anesthesia, (2) labor and delivery, (3) severe infection, and, rarely, (4) thyroiditis 1–2 weeks following administration of radioactive iodine. Manifestations usually include mental status changes (irritability, delirium, or coma), fever, tachycardia, and hypotension. Both atrial and ventricular arrhythmias are common, particularly atrial fibrillation. Congestive heart failure develops in 25% of patients. Hypertension that often precedes hypotension, heat intolerance with profuse sweating, nausea and vomiting, and diarrhea may be prominent initially. Hypokalemia is present in up to 50% of patients. Levels of thyroid hormones are high in plasma but correlate poorly with the severity of the crisis. The sudden exacerbation of thyrotoxicosis may represent a rapid shift of the hormone from the protein-bound to the free state or increased responsiveness to thyroid hormones at the cellular level.

Treatment is directed toward reversing the crisis as well as its complications. Large doses of corticosteroids (dexamethasone intravenously, 10 mg followed by 2 mg every 6 h) inhibit the synthesis, release, and peripheral conversion of thyroxine (T_4) to triiodothyronine (T_3). Corticosteroids also prevent relative adrenal insufficiency secondary to the hypermetabolic state. Propylthiouracil, 600 mg, followed by 200 mg every 2 h, is used to inhibit synthesis of thyroid hormone. Although methimazole inhibits thyroid hormone production and has a longer half-life, propylthiouracil is preferred because it also inhibits peripheral conversion of T_4. Intravenous preparations are not available for either agent, so they must be administered orally or via nasogastric tube. Iodide is given to inhibit release of thyroid hormones from the gland. The iodide may be given intravenously as sodium iodide, 1 g over 24 h, or enterally as potassium iodide, 100–200 mg every 8 h; the X-ray contrast agent sodium ipodate 1 g/d can alternatively be used. Propranolol not only antagonizes the peripheral effects of the thyrotoxicosis but may also inhibit peripheral conversion of T_4. Combined β_1- and β_2-blockade is preferable to selective β_1-antagonism (esmolol or metoprolol) because excessive β_2-receptor activity is responsible for the metabolic effects. β_2-Receptor blockade also reduces muscle blood flow and may decrease heat production. Supportive measures include surface cooling (cooling blanket), acetaminophen (aspirin is not recommended because it may displace thyroid hormone from plasma carrier proteins), and generous intravenous fluid replacement. Vasopressors are often necessary to support arterial blood pressure. Digoxin is indicated in patients with atrial fibrilla-

tion to control the ventricular rate (see Chapter 19) and those with congestive heart failure. A pulmonary artery catheter greatly facilitates management in patients with signs of congestive heart failure or persistent hypotension by allowing measurements of cardiac output and indices of ventricular filling pressures. β-Adrenergic blockade is contraindicated in patients with low cardiac output.

Propranolol, dexamethasone, propylthiouracil, and sodium iodide are given; the patient is admitted to the ICU, where treatment is continued. Over the next 3 days, his mental status markedly improves. The T_3 and total thyroxine levels on the day of surgery were both elevated to 250 ng/dL and 18.5 mg/dL, respectively. He was discharged home 6 days later on a regimen of propranolol and propylthiouracil with a blood pressure of 124/80 mm Hg, a pulse of 92 beats/min, and an oral temperature of 37.3°C.

SUGGESTED READING

Aldrete JA: The post-anesthesia recovery score revisited. J Clin Anesth 1995;7:89.

American Society of Anesthesiologists Task Force on Postanesthetic Care: Practice guidelines for postanesthetic care. Anesthesiology 2002;96:742.

Chung F: Recovery pattern and home readiness after ambulatory surgery. Anesth Analg 1995;80:896.

Chung F, Mezei G: Adverse outcomes in ambulatory anesthesia. Can J Anaesth 1999;46:R18.

Cohen MM, O'Brian-Pallas LL, Copplestone C, et al: Nursing work load associated with adverse events in the postanesthesia care unit. Anesthesiology 1999;91:1882.

Dexter F, Tinker JH: Analysis of strategies to decrease postanesthesia care costs. Anesthesiology 1995;82:941.

Gan TJ, Meyer T, Apfel CC, et al: Consensus Guidelines for managing postoperative nausea and vomiting. Anesth Analg 2003;97:62.

Hines R, Barash PG, Watrous G, O'Connor T: Complications occurring in the postanesthesia care unit: a survey. Anesth Analg 1992;74:503.

Kovac AL: Prevention and treatment of postoperative nausea and vomiting. Drugs 2000;59:213.

Marshall SI, Chung F: Discharge criteria and complications after ambulatory surgery. Anesth Analg 1999;88:508.

McGrath B, Chung F: Postoperative recovery and discharge. Anesth Clin North Am 2003;21:367.

Mulroy MF, McDonald SB: Regional anesthesia for outpatient surgery. Anesth Clin North Am 2003;21:289.

Pavlin DJ, Rapp SE, Polissar NL, et al: Factors affecting discharge times in adult outpatients. Anesth Analg 1998;87:816.

Rose DK, Cohen MM, DeBoer DP: Cardiovascular events in the postanesthesia care unit: contribution of risk factors. Anesthesiology 1996;84:772.

Stadler M, Bardiau F, Seidel L, et al: Difference in risk factors for postoperative nausea and vomiting. Anesthesiology 2003;98:46.

Witte J De, Sessler DI: Perioperative shivering. Anesthesiology 2002;96:467.

Wu CL, Berenholtz SM, Pronovost PJ, Fleisher LA: Systematic review and analysis of postdischarge symptoms after outpatient surgery. Anesthesiology 2002;96:994.

Critical Care

KEY CONCEPTS

 Brain death criteria can be applied only in the absence of hypothermia, hypotension, metabolic or endocrine abnormalities, neuromuscular blocking agents, or drugs known to depress brain function.

 Neonates' risk of retinopathy of prematurity (ROP) increases with low birth weight and complexity of comorbidities (eg, sepsis). In contrast to pulmonary toxicity, ROP correlates better with arterial than with alveolar O_2 tension.

 Pressure control ventilation (PCV) is similar to pressure support ventilation in that peak airway pressure is controlled but is different in that a mandatory rate and inspiratory time are selected. As with pressure support, gas flow ceases when the pressure level is reached; however, the ventilator does not cycle to expiration until the preset inspiration time has elapsed.

 The disadvantage of PCV is that tidal volume is not guaranteed.

 When compared with oral intubation for extended periods of time in the intensive care unit, nasal intubation may be more comfortable for the patient, more secure (fewer instances of accidental extubation), and less likely to cause laryngeal damage. Nasal intubation, however, has significant adverse events associated with its use.

 When left in place for more than 2–3 weeks, both oral and nasal translaryngeal tracheal tubes (TTs)

predispose patients to subglottic stenosis. If longer periods of mechanical ventilation are necessary, the TT should generally be replaced by a cuffed tracheostomy tube.

 The major effect of positive end-expiratory pressure (PEEP) on the lungs is to increase functional residual capacity.

 A higher incidence of pulmonary barotrauma is observed when excessive PEEP or continuous positive airway pressure is added, particularly at levels greater than 20 cm H_2O.

 Maneuvers that produce sustained maximum lung inflation such as the use of an incentive spirometer can be helpful in inducing cough as well as preventing atelectasis and preserving normal lung volume.

 In patients with acute respiratory distress syndrome, a V_T of > 10 mL/kg is associated with increased mortality.

 Early elective tracheal intubation is advisable when there are obvious signs of heat injury to the airway.

 Because of concern that intermittent hemodialysis associated with hypotension may perpetuate renal injury, continuous renal replacement

(continued on next page)

(continued from previous page)

therapy is increasingly used in critically ill patients with acute renal failure who do not tolerate the hemodynamic effects of intermittent hemodialysis.

 Advanced age (> 70 years), corticosteroid therapy, chemotherapy, prolonged use of invasive devices, respiratory failure, renal failure, head trauma, and burns are established risk factors for nosocomial infections.

 Systemic venodilation and transudation of fluid into tissues result in a relative hypovolemia in patients with sepsis.

 In contrast to nonstressed patients, who require about 0.5 g/kg/d of protein, critically ill patients generally require 1.0–1.5 g/kg/d.

 The gastrointestinal tract is the route of choice for nutritional support when its functional integrity is intact.

 Abrupt withdrawal of total parenteral nutrition (TPN) can precipitate hypoglycemia due to high circulating insulin levels, but this is not a common problem if the patient is not overfed; in this case, 10% glucose can be temporarily substituted for the TPN and gradually decreased.

Critical care medicine—also referred to as intensive care medicine—deals with potentially life-threatening illnesses. Anesthesiologists have played a major role in the development of this multidisciplinary subspecialty. Expertise in airway management, mechanical ventilation, administering potent fast-acting drugs, fluid resuscitation, and monitoring techniques gives the anesthesiologist the technical skills required. Moreover, the emphasis in anesthesia on physiology, pathophysiology, and pharmacology as well as the ability to make a rapid diagnosis and treat acute physiological derangements provides an excellent foundation for evaluating and treating patients who are critically ill. The critical care practitioner (intensivist) also requires a broad base of knowledge that crosses the subspecialties of internal medicine, surgery, pediatrics, neurology, and emergency medicine. Unlike traditional training in these subspecialties, which tends to emphasize single organ systems, intensive care training also provides experience in treating patients with systemic inflammatory response syndrome (SIRS) and multiple organ dysfunction syndrome (MODS). The American Boards of Anesthesiology, Internal Medicine, Pediatrics, and Surgery recognize these requirements and now require specialized training for certification in critical care medicine. Clinicians who have such certification are increasingly recognized by multinational corporations and organizations as making important contributions to the outcomes of hospitalized patients.

The purpose of this chapter is only to provide a survey of critical care medicine. Many items have already been covered in other chapters. Only important topics not previously discussed will be presented.

ECONOMIC, ETHICAL, & LEGAL ISSUES IN CRITICAL CARE COST

Critical care is very expensive. Intensive care unit (ICU) beds constitute only 8–10% of all beds in most hospitals yet account for over 20% of hospital expenditures. One percent of the U.S. gross national product is used to provide care in ICUs. To justify this cost, clear benefits in terms of reductions in morbidity or mortality should be readily demonstrable. Unfortunately, supporting studies are few and often flawed by the use of historical controls. Disease severity, reversibility, previous health status, and age are major determinants of outcome. A method of reliably predicting which patients benefit most from intensive care is needed. Several scoring systems based on the severity of physiological derangements and preexisting health have been proposed, such as the Acute Physiology and Chronic Health Evaluation (APACHE) and Therapeutic Intervention Scoring System (TISS), but none is entirely satisfactory. Survival is generally inversely related to the severity of illness and number of organ systems affected. The Society of Critical Care Medicine in the United States has established Project Impact, a system that allows ICUs to compare their outcomes and the care they provide against a national and international network of ICUs.

Carl C. Hug, Jr, MD, PhD

WHEN IS ENOUGH, ENOUGH? WITHDRAWING CARDIOPULMONARY SUPPORT IN CRITICALLY ILL ICU PATIENTS

There is ... a time to be born, and a time to die.
Ecclesiastes 3.2

My experiences over the past 30 years as a cardiothoracic anesthesiologist and an attending physician in the cardiothoracic and vascular surgical ICUs have allowed me to be a first-hand witness to the marvels of medicine, but they have also caused me to focus attention on the limitations of those marvels in patients near the end of life because of the severity of their disease and/or aging with its progressive loss of reserves. In Hippocrates' words, they become "overwhelmed by their disease."

In the United States, death, the last event in normal life, is a taboo subject for many, and most people avoid preparing for it until late in their own lives, and some not even then. Many attend to last wills and testaments, estate planning, and death taxes, but less than 15% of the adult population is prepared to make decisions about aggressive life-supporting measures. Yet surveys consistently show a strong preference for a dignified, comfortable, and peaceful death at home and a strong wish to avoid dying in a hospital, particularly in an ICU.

The quandary about what to do is particularly acute for the surgical patient who is seeking relief from symptoms, improved functionality, and a better quality of life, but who ends up with a bad outcome requiring ongoing life-supporting measures with little prospect of achieving the goals of the operation.

A substantial number of physicians are not prepared to work through such difficult situations in a humane, nonthreatening, nonadversarial manner or to deal with anger, despair, and other emotions of family members and friends whose expectations have not been met. Professional organizations, medical schools, and residency training programs are just beginning to provide education and guidelines for handling these challenges. Good communication skills are the essential foundation. Communications with the family, friends, and all caregivers have to be timely, consistent (one physician spokesman has advantages), accurate, clear to laypersons, advisory without being dictatorial, focused on what is best for the patient, and aligned with the patient's wishes. A gradual stepwise approach taken over several days allows the family members and friends time to digest the information and to get beyond their normal, initial reactions to the bad news.

The issues to be addressed include, but are not limited to, the following:

1. An accurate summation of the patient's condition in lay terms. (Verify that the message has been understood by asking a family spokesperson to restate it in his or her own words.)

2. The best estimates of survival and recovery to a quality of life satisfactory to the patient. (Recognize that medicine is the science of uncertainty and the art of probabilities and that outcome predictions are never 0% or 100%.)

3. A presentation of realistic options with the benefits, risks, and burdens of each. (Integration of restorative and palliative treatment should be considered early.)

4. A recognition of overall trends (not the transient up-and-down daily variations) in the patient's course. (Distinguish between the effects of inter-

ventions on physiology [eg, increased blood pressure and cardiac output] and their effects on outcome. Failure or limited responses to drugs and other interventions are indications that there are few or no reserves on which the patient can draw.)

5. Discernment of what is in store for the patient in terms of pain, discomfort, and suffering if survival in a debilitated state occurs and the demands of rehabilitation cannot be met.

What signals indicate that it is time to shift the emphasis from aggressive cardiopulmonary support to aggressive comfort care and withdrawal of ongoing resuscitative measures?

1. When an intervention is required that has been rejected by the patient in an advance directive, which ideally should have been reaffirmed preoperatively.

2. When there is a progressive decline in multiple organ systems despite ongoing resuscitation measures. Some physicians view each organ system in isolation and believe that its function is recoverable. However, the simultaneous failure of three or more organ systems predicts death in 30 days or less.[1]

3. When there is overwhelming sepsis indicating breakdown of the gastrointestinal barrier to enteral flora.

4. When it is clear that physical deconditioning resulting from continuous confinement to bed and loss of muscle mass has progressed to the point at which the patient is no longer able to cooperate with rehabilitation, to regain independent function, and to be weaned from mechanical ventilation and the ultimate maximum degree of recovery falls below the minimally acceptable level defined by the patient preoperatively.

5. Severe central nervous system injury (eg, bilateral cortical and/or brain stem infarctions) portends survival of less than 1 year in the absence of other morbidities. With other morbidities and physical deconditioning, the patient is likely to die much sooner and in a state dependent on significant degrees of support.

How should the withdrawal of life-supporting interventions be approached?

1. I review the patient's status and outlook daily with the surrogate and family members and suggest the transition from aggressive life support to aggressive comfort care.

2. I then discuss the options to be considered and offer the choice of any one of the following at this time or a stepwise progression over a period of days:

   a. Do not resuscitate (DNR) status.
   b. No advancement of therapy beyond what is currently ongoing.
   c. Selective withdrawal of therapeutic measures.
   d. Complete withdrawal of all organ-supporting measures, including tracheal extubation, replacement fluids, and nutrition. (An intravenous cannula is left in place for administration of analgesics and sedatives.)

3. I explain exactly what will and will not be done for each option. I go to the patient's bedside intermittently during the withdrawal process to demonstrate my continuing concern and to verify that analgesic and hypnotic drugs are being titrated to need appropriately.

It is important for everyone to understand that (1) morphine-type drugs relieve and prevent dyspnea and (2) patients at the end of life do not experience hunger or thirst as long as moisture of the oropharyngeal membranes is maintained.

Finally, it is important to recognize that two ethical principles are in play. The first is the principle of double effect. All medical therapies and interventions have potential benefits as well as burdens and risks. If the doses of morphine or sedative drug necessary to relieve pain and agitation are high and result in unintended side effects, we accept them, even if the result is death. This is not active euthanasia! The second principle is that withdrawal of medical therapies and interventions is not different from withholding them in respect to the patient's autonomy. There is a broad religious consensus that heroic measures are not mandated to support a heartbeat at the end of life. Withdrawal of such support is not passive euthanasia! It is not artificially prolonging the natural death event.

1. Knaus WA, Wagner DP: Multiple system organ failure: Epidemiology and prognosis. Crit Care Clin 1989;5:221.

ETHICAL & LEGAL ISSUES

The high cost and economic constraints increasingly applied by governments and third-party payers, together with an increased awareness of ethical issues and legal precedents, have changed the practice of critical care medicine. Until recently, nearly all patients in the United States—even those who were clearly terminally ill—received maximal treatment (often contrary to the patient's or family's wishes) for fear of the possible legal repercussions of withholding treatment. "Heroic" measures such as cardiopulmonary resuscitation, mechanical ventilation, and infusion of inotropic and vasoactive drugs were continued until the patient died.

Decisions about when to initiate or terminate treatment can be difficult. Generally, any treatment that can reasonably be expected to reverse illness or restore health is justified, whereas withholding that treatment requires specific ethical justification. Conversely, if treatment will definitely not reverse a disease process or restore health, then the decision to initiate such treatment may not be justified and may be unethical. These complex decisions must involve the patient (or guardian) and the family and must be consistent with hospital policies and state and federal law.

Fortunately, the legal guidelines that can be used by the practitioner in arriving at these decisions are available in nearly all states; although laws vary from state to state, they tend to be similar. The greatest problems are related to withholding treatment and discontinuing artificial life-support systems. Competent patients (ie, individuals who have the capacity to understand and make medical decisions) have the right to refuse treatment and the right to have life-support machines or devices turned off when they so request. Most states allow competent individuals to prepare an advanced directive, usually either a "living will" or a "durable power of attorney for health care," to prevent needless prolongation of life if they become incompetent (eg, irreversible coma). Withholding treatment or discontinuing life support from incompetent minors and adults requires permission of the spouse, guardian, next of kin, or an individual to whom the patient has given power of attorney for health care. In some cases, clarification from the courts may be necessary. "Do not resuscitate" (DNR) or "Allow Natural Death" (AND) orders have been upheld by the courts in cases in which resuscitation clearly offers no hope of curing or reversing the disease process responsible for imminent death.

Artificial support of ventilation and the circulation complicates legal definitions of death. Until recently, most states required only a determination by a physician that irreversible cessation of ventilatory and circulatory function had occurred. All states have added the concept of brain death to that definition. However, some states recognize religious exemptions. In New Jersey, for example, physicians cannot declare brain death "if it would violate the personal religious beliefs of the individual." In addition, although brain death can be established in a pregnant woman, the issue of whether life support can be withdrawn remains subject to both ethical and legal debate. A number of cases of women having given birth posthumously to a viable baby weeks or months after declaration of brain death have now been reported both in the United States and internationally. These cases involve issues of maternal rights, "fetal rights," and paternal rights and have yet to be resolved.

Brain Death

Brain death is defined as irreversible cessation of all brain function. Spinal cord function below C1 may still be present. Establishing brain death gives relief from unjustifiable hope, prolonged anxiety, and financial burdens on families and society. It also allows more efficient utilization of medical resources and potentially allows the harvesting of organs for transplantation.

Brain death criteria can be applied only in the absence of hypothermia, hypotension, metabolic or endocrine abnormalities, neuromuscular blocking agents (NMBAs), or drugs known to depress brain function. A toxicology screen is necessary if sufficient time since admission (at least 3 days) has not elapsed to exclude a drug effect. Moreover, the patient should be observed long enough to establish with reasonable certainty the irreversible nature of the injury. **Generally accepted clinical criteria for brain death include the following:**

(1) Coma

(2) Absent motor activity, including decerebrate and decorticate posturing (spinal cord reflexes may be preserved in some patients)

(3) Absent brain stem reflexes, including the pupillary, corneal, vestibuloocular (caloric), and gag (and/or cough) reflexes

(4) Absence of ventilatory effort with the arterial CO_2 tension 60 mm Hg or 20 mm Hg above the pretest level.

Repeating the examination (not less than 2 h apart) is optional. The number of physician observers varies by state (Florida requires two), as does the level of expertise (Virginia requires a neurologist or neurosurgeon). The apnea test should be reserved for last because of its detrimental effects on intracranial pressure (ICP). Confirmatory tests that may be helpful but are not required include an isoelectric electroencephalogram, absent brain stem auditory evoked potentials, and absence of cerebral perfusion as documented by angiographic, transcranial Doppler, or radioisotopic studies.

Table 49–1. Classification of hypoxias.[1]

Hypoxia	Pathophysiologic Category	Clinical Example
Hypoxic hypoxia	$\downarrow P_{Barom}$ or $\downarrow F_{IO_2}$ (< 0.21)	Altitude, O_2 equipment error
	Alveolar hypoventilation	Drug overdose, COPD exacerbation
	Pulmonary diffusion defect	Emphysema, pulmonary fibrosis
	Pulmonary $\dot{V}/\dot{Q}$ mismatch	Asthma, pulmonary emboli
	$R \rightarrow L$ shunt	Atelectasis, cyanotic congenital heart disease
Circulatory hypoxia	Reduced cardiac output	Congestive heart failure, myocardial infarction, dehydration
Hemic hypoxia	Reduced hemoglobin content	Anemias
	Reduced hemoglobin function	Carboxyhemoglobinemia, methemoglobinemia
Demand hypoxia	$\uparrow$ Oxygen consumption	Fever, seizures
Histotoxic hypoxia	Inability of cells to utilize oxygen	Cyanide toxicity

[1]P_{Barom}, barometric pressure; COPD, chronic obstructive pulmonary disease; $\dot{V}/\dot{Q}$, ventilation/perfusion; $R \rightarrow L$, right to left.

■ RESPIRATORY CARE

Respiratory care (also called respiratory therapy) refers both to the delivery of pulmonary therapy and diagnostic tests and to the allied health profession that has evolved since the 1950s to become an integral part of cardiopulmonary diagnostics and critical care. Respiratory therapists' scope of practice encompasses medical gas therapy, delivery of aerosolized medications, airway management, mechanical ventilation, positive airway pressure therapy, critical care monitoring, cardiopulmonary rehabilitation, and the application of various techniques collectively termed chest physical therapy. The latter includes administering bland and therapeutic aerosols, clearing pulmonary secretions, reexpansion of atelectatic lung, and preserving normal lung function postoperatively or during illness. Diagnostic services may include pulmonary function testing, arterial blood gas analysis, electrocardiography testing, and evaluation of sleep-disordered breathing. The majority of respiratory care procedures are based on clinical practice guidelines known as CPGs, 50 of which have been developed by the American Association for Respiratory Care using best practice/evidence-based medicine criteria.

MEDICAL GAS THERAPY

The therapeutic medical gases include supplemental ambient or hyperbaric oxygen, helium–oxygen mixtures, and nitric oxide. Oxygen is medically indicated for both pulmonary and nonpulmonary disorders. Oxygen is made available in high-pressure cylinders, via pipeline systems, from oxygen concentrators, as well as in liquid form. Heliox is occasionally used to treat the increased work of breathing (WOB) due to upper airway obstructing lesions. Nitric oxide is administered for its dilating effect on the pulmonary vasculature.

The primary goal of oxygen therapy is to prevent or correct hypoxemia and/or tissue hypoxia. Table 49–1 identifies classic categories of hypoxia. Oxygen therapy alone may not correct either hypoxemia or hypoxia. Continuous positive airway pressure (CPAP) or positive end-expiratory pressure (PEEP) may be required to recruit collapsed alveoli. Patients with profound hypercapnia may require ventilatory assistance. High concentrations of oxygen may be indicated for conditions requiring removal of entrapped gas (eg, nitrogen) from body cavities or vessels. The short-term application of high concentrations of oxygen is relatively free of complications.

Supplemental oxygen is indicated for adults, children, and infants (older than 1 month) when PaO_2 is less than 60 mm Hg (7.98 kPa) or SaO_2 or SpO_2 is less than 90% while at rest breathing room air. In neonates, therapy is recommended if PaO_2 is less than 50 mm Hg (6.7 kPa) or SaO_2 is less than 88% (or capillary PO_2 is less than 40 mm Hg [5.33 kPa]). Therapy may be required for patients when clinicians suspect hypoxia based on a review of cardiopulmonary problems or on physical examination. Patients with myocardial infarction, cardiogenic pulmonary edema, acute lung injury (ALI), acute respiratory distress syndrome (ARDS), pulmonary fibrosis, cyanide poisoning, or carbon monoxide inhalation all require supplemental oxygen. Supplemental oxygen is given during the perioperative period because general anesthesia commonly causes a decrease in PaO_2 secondary to increased pulmonary ventilation/perfusion mismatching and decreased functional residual capacity (FRC). Supplemental oxygen should be provided before procedures such as tracheal suctioning or bronchoscopy, which commonly cause arterial desaturation. There is evidence that supplemental oxygen is effective in prolonging survival of patients with chronic obstructive pulmonary disease (COPD) whose resting PaO_2 is lower than 60 mm Hg at sea level. Supplemental oxygen therapy also appears to have a mild beneficial effect on the mean pulmonary arterial pressure and subjective indices of patients' dyspnea.

AMBIENT OXYGEN THERAPY EQUIPMENT

Classifying Oxygen Therapy Equipment

Oxygen given alone or in a gas (mixed with air, helium, or nitric oxide) can be administered as a partial supplement to patients' tidal or minute volume or as the entire source of the inspired volume. This approach provides the basis for classifying devices or systems according to their ability to provide adequate flow levels and a range of fraction of inspired oxygen (FIO_2). Other considerations in selecting therapy include patient compliance, the presence and type of artificial airway, and the need for humidification or an aerosol delivery system.

A. LOW-FLOW OR VARIABLE-PERFORMANCE EQUIPMENT

Oxygen (usually 100%) is supplied at a fixed flow that is only a portion of inspired gas. Such devices are usually intended for patients with stable breathing patterns. As ventilatory demands change, variable amounts of room air will dilute the oxygen flow. Low-flow systems are adequate for patients with

- Minute ventilation less than ~8–10 L/min
- Breathing frequencies less than ~20 breaths/min
- Tidal volumes (VT) less than ~0.8 L
- Normal inspiratory flow (10–30 L/min).

B. HIGH-FLOW OR FIXED-PERFORMANCE EQUIPMENT

Inspired gas at a preset FIO_2 is supplied continuously at high flow or by providing a sufficiently large reservoir of premixed gas. Ideally, the delivered FIO_2 is not affected by variations in ventilatory level or breathing pattern. Profoundly dyspneic and hypoxemic patients may need flows of 100% oxygen in excess of 100 L/min. High-flow systems are indicated for patients who require

- Consistent FIO_2 and/or
- Large inspiratory flows of gas (> 40 L/min).

1. Variable-Performance Equipment (Table 49–2)

Nasal Cannulas

The nasal cannula is available as either a blind-ended soft plastic tube with an over-the-ear head-elastic or dual-flow with under-the-chin lariat adjustment. Sizing is available for adults, children, and infants. Cannulas are connected to flowmeters with small-bore tubing and may be used with a bubble humidifier. The nasal cannula can be rapidly and comfortably placed on most patients. The tension of attachment should be firm yet comfortable enough to avoid pressure sores on the ears, cheeks, and nose. Patients on long-term oxygen therapy most commonly use a nasal cannula. The appliance is usually well tolerated, allows speech and eating/drinking, and is nonclaustrophobic. Cannulas can be combined with spectacle frames for convenience or to improve acceptance by improving cosmesis. Oxygen-conserving cannulas equipped with inlet reservoirs are available for patients receiving long-term oxygen. Since oxygen flows continuously, approximately 80% of the gas is wasted during expiration. This concept has resulted in the use of valved reservoir devices to allow storage of incoming oxygen until inspiration occurs.

Table 49–2. Oxygen delivery devices and systems.

Device/System	Oxygen Flow Rate (L/min)	FIO_2 Range
Nasal cannula	1	0.21–0.24
	2	0.23–0.28
	3	0.27–0.34
	4	0.31–0.38
	5–6	0.32–0.44
Simple masks	5–6	0.30–0.45
	7–8	0.40–0.60
Masks with reservoirs	5	0.35–0.50
Partial rebreathing mask-bag	7	0.35–0.75
	15	0.65–1.00
Nonrebreathing mask-bag	7–15	0.40–1.00
Venturi masks and jet nebulizers	4–6 (total flow = 15)	0.24
	4–6 (total flow = 45)	0.28
	8–10 (total flow = 45)	0.35
	8–10 (total flow = 33)	0.40
	8–12 (total flow = 33)	0.50

The actual FIO_2 delivered to adults with nasal cannulas is determined by oxygen flow, nasopharyngeal volume, and the patient's inspiratory flow (which depends both on VT and inspiratory time). Oxygen from the cannula can fill the nasopharynx during exhalation, yet with inspiration, oxygen and entrained air are drawn into the trachea. The inspired percent oxygen increases by approximately 1–2% (above 21%) per liter of oxygen flow with quiet breathing in adults. Cannulas can be expected to provide inspired oxygen concentrations up to 30–35% with normal breathing and oxygen flows of 3–4 L/min. However, levels of 40–50% can be attained with oxygen flows of greater than 10 L/min for short periods. Usually flows greater than 5 L/min are poorly tolerated because of the discomfort of gas jetting into the nasal cavity and because of drying and crusting of the nasal mucosa.

Data from "normal-breathing subjects" may not be accurate for acutely ill tachypneic patients. Increasing VT and short inspiratory time will dilute the small flow of oxygen. Different levels of mouth-only versus nasal-only breathing patterns and varied inspiratory flow can vary FIO_2 by up to 40%. In clinical practice, flow should be titrated according to vital signs and pulse oximetric and arterial blood gas measurements. Some patients with COPD tend to hypoventilate with even modest oxygen flows, yet are hypoxemic on room air. They may do well with the cannula at flows of less than 1–2 L/min.

Pediatric-sized nasal cannulas are available, and their clinical use has become increasingly common. Some special cannulas allow babies to nurse and subject them to less trauma of the face and nose than oxygen masks. Because of the inherently reduced minute ventilation of infants, flow requirements to the cannula must be proportionately reduced. This generally requires a pressure-compensated flowmeter accurate to deliver oxygen flows in the less than 1–3 L/min range. Hypopharyngeal oxygen sampling from infants breathing with cannulas has demonstrated mean FIO_2s of 0.35, 0.45, 0.6, and 0.68 with flows of 0.25, 0.5, 0.75, and 1.0 L/min, respectively.

Nasal Mask

The nasal mask is a hybrid of the nasal cannula and a face mask. It can be applied to the face by either an over-the-ear lariat or a headband strap. The lower edge of the mask's flanges rests on the upper lip, surrounding the external nose. Nasal masks have been shown to provide supplemental oxygen equivalent to the nasal cannula under low-flow conditions for adult patients. The primary advantage of the nasal mask appears to be patient comfort. Sores can develop around the external nares of long-term nasal cannula wearers. Oxygen is not "jetted" into the nasal cavity as with the cannula. The

nasal mask should be considered if it improves patient comfort and compliance.

Nonreservoir Oxygen Mask

The "simple," or nonreservoir, oxygen-free mask is a disposable lightweight plastic device that covers both nose and mouth. Masks are fastened to the patient's face by adjustment of an elastic headband; some manufacturers provide a malleable metal nose-bridge adjustment device. The face seal is rarely free of "inboard" leaking; therefore, patients receive a mixture of pure oxygen and secondarily entrained room air. This varies depending on size of leak, oxygen flow, and breathing pattern. Some brands of the simple mask connect tubing to a standard tapered fitting; others have a small room air–entrainment hole at the connection.

The body of the mask functions as a reservoir for both oxygen and expired carbon dioxide. A minimum oxygen flow of approximately 5 L/min is applied to the mask to avoid rebreathing and excessive respiratory work. Wearing any mask appliance for long periods of time is uncomfortable. Speech is muffled and drinking and eating are difficult.

The amount of oxygen enrichment of the inspired air depends on mask volume, pattern of ventilation, and the oxygen flow to the mask. It is difficult to predict delivered FIO_2 at specific flows. During normal breathing, it is reasonable to expect an FIO_2 of 0.3–0.6 with flows of 5–10 L/min, respectively. Oxygen levels can be higher with small VT or slow breathing rates. With higher flows and ideal conditions, FIO_2 may approach 0.7 or 0.8.

The nonreservoir mask may be best suited for patients who require higher levels of oxygen than cannulas provide, yet need oxygen therapy for fairly short periods of time. Examples would include medical transport or interim therapy in the postanesthesia care unit or emergency department. It is not the device of choice for patients with severe respiratory disease who are profoundly hypoxemic, tachypneic, or unable to protect their airway from aspiration.

Reservoir Masks

Incorporating some type of gas reservoir is a logical adaptation to the simple mask. Two types of reservoir mask are commonly used: the partial rebreathing mask and the nonrebreathing mask. Both are disposable, lightweight, transparent plastic under-the-chin reservoirs. The difference between the two relates to use of valves on the mask and between the mask and the bag reservoir. Mask reservoirs commonly hold approximately 600 mL or less. The term "partial rebreather" refers to "part" of the patient's expired VT

refilling the bag. Usually that gas is largely dead space that should not result in significant rebreathing of carbon dioxide.

The nonrebreather uses the same basic system as the partial rebreather but incorporates flap-type valves between the bag and mask and on at least one of the mask's exhalation ports. Inboard leaking is common, and room air will enter during brisk inspiratory flows, even when the bag contains gas. The lack of a good facial seal system and a relatively small reservoir can affect delivered oxygen concentration. The key factor to successful application of the masks is to use sufficient flow of oxygen, so the reservoir bag is at least partially full during inspiration. Typical minimum flows of oxygen are 10–15 L/min. Well-fitting partial rebreathing masks provide a range of FIO_2 from 0.35 to 0.60 with oxygen flows up to 10 L/min. With inlet flows of 15 L/min or more and ideal breathing conditions, FIO_2 may approach 1.0. Either style of mask is indicated for patients suspected of significant hypoxemia, with relatively normal spontaneous minute ventilation. Such patients may include victims of trauma, myocardial infarction, or carbon monoxide exposure. Profoundly dyspneic patients with gasping respiration may be better suited with a fixed-performance, high-flow oxygen system.

2. Fixed-Performance (High-Flow) Equipment

Anesthesia Bag or Bag-Mask-Valve Systems

The basic design follows that of the nonrebreathing reservoir mask but with more "capable" components. Self-inflating bags consist of a football-sized bladder, usually with an oxygen inlet reservoir. Anesthesia bags are 1-, 2-, or 3-L non–self-inflating reservoirs with a tailpiece gas inlet. Masks are designed to provide a comfortable leak-free seal for manual ventilation. The inspiratory/expiratory valve systems may vary. The flow to the reservoir should be kept high so that the bags do not deflate substantially. When using an anesthesia bag, operators may frequently have to adjust the oxygen flow and exhaust valve spring tension to respond to changing breathing patterns or demands.

The most common system for disposable and permanent self-inflating resuscitation bags uses a unidirectional gas flow. Although these devices offer the potential for a constant FIO_2 greater than 0.9, tailpiece inlet valves will not open for a spontaneously breathing patient. Opening the valves requires negative pressure bag recoil after compression. If this situation is not recognized, clinicians might be misled into thinking the patient is receiving a specific concentration of oxygen when the contrary is true.

There are limits to the ability of each system to maintain its fixed-performance characteristics. Delivered FIO_2 can equal or approach 1.0 with either anesthesia or self-inflating bags. Spontaneously breathing patients are allowed to breathe only the contents of the system if the mask seal is tight and the reservoir is adequately maintained. Operators must adjust gas flow to the bag to accommodate for any changes in ventilation demand; observation of patient and reservoir provides that information.

A primary concern for clinicians using mask-bag systems is aspiration. Failure to maintain an adequate oxygen supply in the reservoir and inlet flow is another concern. The spring-loaded valve of anesthesia bags must be adjusted properly to prevent overdistention of the bag. Self-inflating bags do not look different when oxygen flow to the unit is inadequate, and they will entrain room air into the bag, thus lowering the delivered FIO_2.

Air-Entrainment Venturi Masks

The gas delivery approach with air-entrainment masks is somewhat different than with an oxygen reservoir. The goal is to create an open system with high flow about the nose and mouth, with a fixed FIO_2. Masks are known as "Venturi" or "Venti-" masks, or high-airflow with oxygen-entrainment (HAFOE) systems. Oxygen is directed by small-bore tubing to a mixing jet; the final oxygen concentration depends on the ratio of air drawn in through entrainment ports. Manufacturers have developed both fixed and adjustable entrainment selections over an FIO_2 range. Most provide instructions for the operator to set a minimum flow of oxygen. Table 49–3 identifies total flow at various inlet flows and FIO_2.

Table 49–3. Air-entrainment mask input flow versus total flow at varying FIO_2.[1]

FIO_2	Inlet Oxygen Flow (Minimum)	Total Flow (L/min)
0.24	4	97
0.28	6	68
0.3	6	54
0.35	8	45
0.40	12	50
0.50	12	33
0.70	12	19
0.80	12	16
1.0	12	12

[1]FIO_2, fraction of inspired oxygen.

Despite the high-flow concept, FIO_2 can vary up to 6% per setting. The air-entrainment masks are a logical choice for patients whose hypoxemia cannot be controlled on lower FIO_2 devices such as the cannula. Patients with COPD who tend to hypoventilate with a moderate FIO_2 are candidates for the Venturi mask. Clinicians providing oxygen therapy by HAFOE therapy should be aware of the previously mentioned problems involving the mask itself. FIO_2 can increase if the entrainment ports are obstructed by the patient's hands, bed sheets, or water condensate. Clinicians should encourage the patient and caregivers to keep the mask on the face continuously. Interruption of oxygen is a serious problem in unstable patients with hypoxemia and or hypercarbia.

Direct analysis of the FIO_2 during air-entrainment mask breathing is possible but difficult to perform accurately. Correlating blood gases with some index of inspiratory flow demand, such as breathing rate, should allow clinicians to know when to suspect that the patient's demands may not be met by the mask's flow. If that occurs, then inlet oxygen flows may need to be increased or an alternate device selected.

Air-Entrainment Nebulizers

Large-volume, high-output or "all-purpose" nebulizers have been used in respiratory care for many years to provide bland mist therapy with some control of the FIO_2. These units are commonly placed on patients following extubation for their aerosol-producing properties. Like the entrainment masks, nebulizers use a pneumatic jet and an adjustable orifice to vary entrained air for various FIO_2 levels at fixed setting points or are continuously adjustable from 0.24 to 1.0. Many commercial devices have an inlet orifice diameter that maximally allows only 15 L/min when the source pressure is 50 psi. This means that on the 100% setting (no air entrainment) output flow is only 15 L/min. Only patients breathing at slow rates and small VT will receive 100% oxygen. This problem has been addressed by the development of high-flow, high-FIO_2 nebulizers. For more common applications that use an FIO_2 of 0.3–0.5, room air is entrained, reducing the FIO_2 and increasing the total flow output to 40–50 L/min.

Knowledge of the air/oxygen ratio and the input flow rate of oxygen allows the total outflow to be calculated. Nebulizer systems can be applied to the patient with many different devices, including aerosol, tracheostomy dome/collar, face tent, and T-piece adapter. These appliances can all be attached via large-bore tubing to the nebulizer. This open system freely vents inspiratory and expiratory gases around the patient's face or out a distal port of a Briggs adapter. Unfortunately, the lack of any valves allows patients to secondarily entrain room air. It is common practice to use either a reservoir bag before

the T or a reservoir tube on the distal side of the T to provide a larger volume of gas than that coming from the nebulizer. The major concern of those applying air-entrainment aerosol therapy with controlled oxygen concentration is that the system provide adequate flow. Clinicians should observe the mist like a tracer to determine adequacy of flow. If a T-piece is used and if the visible mist (exiting the distal port) disappears during inspiration, the flow is inadequate.

Another concern in clinical practice is that excess water in the tubing collects and can obstruct gas flow completely or can offer increased resistance to flow. The latter may increase the FIO_2 above the desired setting. Another complication is bronchospasm in some patients as the sterile water aerosol can be irritating. In such circumstances, a heated (nonaerosol) humidification system should be substituted.

High-Flow Air–Oxygen Systems

Dual air–oxygen flowmeters, air–oxygen blenders, and Down's or Caradyne Whisperflow generators are commonly used for oxygen administration as well as freestanding CPAP and "add-on" ventilator systems. These systems contrast to the air-entrainment nebulizer, as their total output flows do not diminish at FIO_2 greater than 0.4. With these high-flow systems, the total flow to the patient can be independently set (versus FIO_2) to meet or exceed patient needs. This can be done using a large reservoir bag or constant flows in the range of 50 to more than 100 L/min. Clinicians can use a variety of appliances with any of these systems, including aerosol masks, face tents, or well-fitted nonrebreathing system masks with blenders. Face-sealing mask systems can also be constructed but require a reservoir bag with a safety valve to allow breathing if the blender fails. The high flows of gas require use of heated humidifiers of the type commonly used on mechanical ventilators. Humidification offers an advantage for patients with hyperreactive airways. Because of the high flows, such systems are used to apply CPAP for spontaneously breathing patients.

Oxygen Hoods

Although many of the devices previously described have pediatric-sized options, such as cannulas and masks, many young infants and neonates will not tolerate facial appliances. Oxygen hoods cover only the head, allowing access to the infant's lower body while still permitting use of a standard incubator or radiant warmer. The hood is ideal for relatively short-term oxygen therapy for newborns and inactive infants. However, for mobile infants requiring longer term therapy, for example, the nasal cannula, face mask, or full-bed enclosure affords greater mobility.

Normally, oxygen and air are premixed by an air–oxygen blending device and passed through a heated humidifier. Nebulizers should be avoided as the gas source. Most pneumatic jet-type nebulizers create noise levels (> 65 dB) that may cause newborn hearing loss, and cold gas can induce an increase in oxygen consumption. Hoods come in different sizes to accommodate a variety of infants. Some are simple Plexiglas boxes; others have elaborate systems for sealing the neck opening. There is no attempt to completely seal the system, as a constant flow of gas is needed to remove carbon dioxide (minimum flow > 7 L/min). Hood inlet flows of 10–15 L/min are adequate for a majority of patients.

Helium–Oxygen Therapy

Helium–oxygen (heliox) mixtures have a notable, yet limited clinical role. Other than its uses in industry and deep-sea diving, there are a number of medical applications for heliox. Helium is premixed with oxygen in several standard blends. The most popular mixtures are the 80%/20% and 70%/30% helium–oxygen, which have densities that are 1.805 and 1.586 times less dense, respectively, compared with pure oxygen. They are available in large-sized compressed gas cylinders.

In anesthetic practice, pressures needed to ventilate patients with small-diameter tracheal tubes (TTs) can be substantially reduced (halved) when the 80%/20% mixture is used. Patients with acute distress from upper airway–obstructing lesions such as subglottic edema, foreign bodies, and tracheal tumors may obtain relief until more definitive care can be delivered. The evidence is less convincing in treating lower airway obstruction in COPD and acute asthma. Helium mixtures may also be used as the driving gas for small-volume nebulizers for bronchodilator therapy in asthma. However, with 80%/20% heliox flow, the nebulizer needs to be increased to 11 L/min versus the usual 6–8 L/min with oxygen. Patients' WOB can be reduced when heliox is delivered via the mechanical ventilator (noninvasive or via an artificial airway). Nonintubated patients commonly receive heliox therapy via mask with reservoir bag.

Hyperbaric Oxygen

Hyperbaric oxygen therapy uses a pressurized chamber to expose the patient to oxygen tensions exceeding ambient barometric pressure (usually > 760 mm Hg). With a one-person (monoplace) hyperbaric chamber, 100% oxygen is usually used to pressurize the chamber. Larger multiplace chambers allow for the simultaneous treatment of multiple patients and for the presence of medical personnel in the chamber with patients. Multiplace chambers use air to pressurize the chamber, whereas patients receive 100% oxygen by mask, hood, or TT. Commonly established indications for hyperbaric oxygen include decompression sickness, gas embolism, gas gangrene, carbon monoxide poisoning, and treatment of certain wounds.

3. Hazards of Oxygen Therapy

Oxygen therapy can result in both respiratory and non-respiratory toxicity. Important factors include patient susceptibility, the FIO_2, and duration of therapy.

Hypoventilation

This complication is primarily seen in patients with COPD who have chronic CO_2 retention. These patients may have an altered respiratory drive that becomes at least partly dependent on the maintenance of relative hypoxemia. Alternatively, oxygen-mediated release of hypoxic vasoconstriction can result in greater blood flow to areas of high ventilation/perfusion (V̇/Q̇) (see Chapter 23). Elevation of arterial oxygen tension to "normal" can therefore cause severe hypoventilation in these patients. Stable, spontaneously breathing patients with profound hypercarbia ($PaCO_2$ > 80 mm Hg) who are being supported with supplemental oxygen should not have supplemental oxygen discontinued, even for short intervals.

Absorption Atelectasis

High concentrations of oxygen can cause pulmonary atelectasis in areas of low V̇/Q̇ ratios. When nitrogen is "washed out" of the lungs, the lowered gas tension in pulmonary capillary blood results in increased uptake of alveolar gas leading to absorption atelectasis. If the area remains perfused but nonventilated, the resultant intrapulmonary shunt can lead to progressive widening of the alveolar-to-arterial (A–a) gradient.

Pulmonary Toxicity

Prolonged high concentrations of oxygen are known to damage the lungs. Toxicity is dependent both on the partial pressure of oxygen in the inspired gas and the duration of exposure. Alveolar rather than arterial oxygen tension is most important in the development of oxygen toxicity. Although 100% oxygen for up to 10–20 h is generally considered safe (at sea level), concentrations greater than 50–60% for longer periods may lead to toxicity and are undesirable.

Molecular oxygen (O_2) is unusual in that each atom has unpaired electrons in its outer (2P) shell. This gives the molecule the paramagnetic property that allows precise measurements of oxygen concentration. Notably, internal rearrangement of these electrons or their interaction with other atoms (iron) or molecules (xanthine) can produce potentially toxic chemical species. Oxygen toxicity is thought to be due to intracellular generation of highly reactive O_2 metabolites (free radicals) such as superoxide and activated hydroxyl ions, singlet O_2, and hydrogen peroxide. A high concentration of O_2 increases the likelihood of generating toxic species. These metabolites are cytotoxic because they readily react with cellular DNA, sulfhydryl proteins, and lipids. Two cellular enzymes, superoxide dismutase and catalase, provide some protection by sequentially converting superoxide first to hydrogen peroxide and then to water. Additional protection may be provided by antioxidants and free radical scavengers such as glutathione peroxidase, ascorbic acid (vitamin C), α-tocopherol (vitamin E), acetylcysteine, and possibly mannitol; however, clinical evidence supporting the use of these agents in preventing pulmonary toxicity is lacking.

Oxygen-mediated injury of the alveolar–capillary membrane produces a syndrome that is pathologically and clinically indistinguishable from ARDS. Pulmonary capillary permeability increases and the membrane thickens as type I alveolar cells decrease and type II cells proliferate. Tracheobronchitis may also be present initially in some patients. Pulmonary O_2 toxicity in newborn infants is manifested as bronchopulmonary dysplasia.

Retinopathy of Prematurity

Retinopathy of prematurity (ROP), formerly termed retrolental fibroplasia, is a neovascular retinal disorder that develops in 84% of premature survivors born at less than 28 weeks' gestation. Typically, ROP resolves in approximately 80% of these cases without visual loss from retinal detachments or scars. ROP reached epidemic proportions in the 1940s–1950s with unmonitored high (> 0.5 FIO_2) oxygen administration via an incubator. Oxygen therapy promotes disorganized vascular proliferation and fibrosis as well as retinal detachment and can result in blindness. Neonates' risk of ROP increases with low birth weight and complexity of comorbidities (eg, sepsis). In contrast to pulmonary toxicity, ROP correlates better with arterial than with alveolar O_2 tension. The recommended arterial concentrations for premature infants receiving oxygen are 50–80 mm Hg (6.6–10.6 kPa). If an infant requires arterial O_2 saturations of 96%–99% for cardiopulmonary reasons, fear about causing worse ROP is not a reason to withhold the oxygen.

Hyperbaric Oxygen Toxicity

The high inspired O_2 tensions associated with hyperbaric O_2 therapy greatly accelerate O_2 toxicity. The risk and expected degree of toxicity are directly related

Table 49–4. Guidelines suggesting the need for mechanical ventilation.

Respiratory gas tensions	Direct indices
	Arterial oxygen tension < 50 mm Hg on room air, or arterial CO_2 tension > 50 mm Hg in the absence of metabolic alkalosis
	Derived indices
	PaO_2/FIO_2 ratio < 300 mm Hg
	$PA–aO_2$ gradient > 350 mm Hg
	VD/VT > 0.6
Clinical indices	Respiratory rate > 35 breaths/min
Mechanical indices	Tidal volume < 5 mL/kg
	Vital capacity < 15 mL/kg
	Maximum inspiratory force < –25 cm H_2O (ie, –15 cm H_2O)

to the pressures used as well as the duration of exposure. Prolonged exposure to O_2 partial pressures in excess of 0.5 atmospheres absolute (ATA) can cause pulmonary O_2 toxicity. This may present initially with retrosternal burning, cough, and chest tightness and will result in progressive impairment of pulmonary function with continued exposure. Patients exposed to O_2 at 2 ATA or greater are also at risk for central nervous system toxicity. Behavior changes, nausea, vertigo, and/or muscular twitching may or may not precede frank convulsions.

Fire Hazard

Oxygen vigorously supports combustion. Its potential for causing fires and explosions is discussed in Chapter 2.

MECHANICAL VENTILATION

Despite early intervention and aggressive respiratory care, patients in an ICU will often require mechanical ventilation. Mechanical ventilation replaces or supplements normal ventilation by the pulmonary system. In most instances, the problem is primarily that of impaired CO_2 elimination (ventilatory failure). In other instances, mechanical ventilation may be used as an adjunct (usually to positive-pressure therapy; see below) in the treatment of hypoxemia (hypoxemic pulmonary failure). The decision to initiate mechanical ventilation is a clinical one, but certain parameters have been suggested as guidelines (Table 49–4).

Of the two available techniques, positive-pressure ventilation and negative-pressure ventilation, the former has much wider applications and is almost universally used. Although negative-pressure ventilation does not require tracheal intubation, it cannot overcome substantial increases in airway resistance or decreases in pulmonary compliance, and it also limits access to the patient.

During positive-pressure ventilation, lung inflation is achieved by periodically applying positive pressure to the upper airway through a tight-fitting mask (noninvasive mechanical ventilation) or through a tracheal or tracheostomy tube. Increased airway resistance and decreased lung compliance can be overcome by manipulating inspiratory gas flow and pressure. The major disadvantages of positive-pressure ventilation are altered ventilation-to-perfusion relationships, potentially adverse circulatory effects, and risk of pulmonary barotrauma and volutrauma. Positive-pressure ventilation increases physiological dead space because gas flow is preferentially directed to the more compliant, nondependent areas of the lungs, whereas blood flow (which is affected by gravity) favors dependent areas. Reductions in cardiac output are primarily due to decreased venous return to the heart because of the elevated intrathoracic pressure. Barotrauma is closely related to repetitive high peak inflation pressures and underlying lung disease, whereas volutrauma is related to the repetitive collapse and reexpansion of normal or diseased lung.

1. Positive-Pressure Ventilators

Positive-pressure ventilators periodically create a pressure gradient between the machine circuit and alveoli that results in inspiratory gas flow. Exhalation occurs passively. Ventilators and their control mechanisms can be powered pneumatically (by a pressurized gas source), electrically, or by both mechanisms. Gas flow is either derived directly from the pressurized gas source or produced by the action of a rotary or linear piston. This gas flow then either goes directly to the patient (single-circuit system) or, as commonly occurs with operating room ventilators, compresses a reservoir bag or bellows that is part of the patient circuit (double-circuit system).

All ventilators have four phases: inspiration, the changeover from inspiration to expiration, expiration, and the changeover from expiration to inspiration (see Chapter 4). Manipulation of these phases determines V_T, ventilatory rate, inspiratory time, inspiratory gas flow, and expiratory time.

Classification of Ventilators

The complexity of modern ventilators defies simple classification. Incorporation of microprocessor technology into the newest generation of ventilators has further complicated this task. Nonetheless, ventilators are most commonly classified according to their inspiratory phase characteristics and their method of cycling from inspiration to expiration.

A. INSPIRATORY CHARACTERISTICS

Most modern ventilators behave like flow generators. Constant flow generators deliver a constant inspiratory gas flow regardless of airway circuit pressure. Constant flow is produced by the use of either a solenoid (on–off) valve with a high-pressure gas source (5–50 psi) or via a gas injector (Venturi) with a lower-pressure source. Machines with high-pressure gas sources allow inspiratory gas flow to remain constant in spite of large changes in airway resistance or pulmonary compliance. The performance of ventilators with gas injectors varies more with airway pressure. Nonconstant flow generators consistently vary inspiratory flow with each inspiratory cycle (such as by a rotary piston); a sine wave pattern is most common.

Constant-pressure generators maintain airway pressure constant throughout inspiration and irrespective of inspiratory gas flow. Gas flow ceases when airway pressure equals the set inspiratory pressure. Pressure generators typically operate at low gas pressures (just above peak inspiratory pressure).

B. CYCLING (CHANGEOVER FROM INSPIRATION TO EXPIRATION)

Time-cycled ventilators cycle to the expiratory phase once a predetermined interval elapses from the start of inspiration. V_T is the product of the set inspiratory time and inspiratory flow rate. Time-cycled ventilators are commonly used for neonates and in the operating room.

Volume-cycled ventilators terminate inspiration when a preselected volume is delivered. Many adult ventilators are volume cycled but also have secondary limits on inspiratory pressure to guard against pulmonary barotrauma. If inspiratory pressure exceeds the pressure limit, the machine cycles into expiration even if the selected volume has not been delivered. In reality, properly functioning volume-cycled ventilators still do not deliver the set volume to the patient. A percentage of the set V_T is always lost due to expansion of the breathing circuit during inspiration. Circuit compliance is usually about 3–5 mL/cm H_2O; thus, if a pressure of 30 cm H_2O is generated during inspiration, 90–150 mL of the set V_T is lost to the circuit. Loss of V_T to the breathing circuit is therefore inversely related to lung compliance. For accurate measurement of the exhaled V_T, the spirometer must be placed at the TT rather than the exhalation valve of the ventilator.

Pressure-cycled ventilators cycle into the expiratory phase when airway pressure reaches a predetermined

Table 49–5. Ventilatory modes.[1]

Mode	I to E Cycling				E to I Cycling		Allows Spontaneous Ventilation	Weaning Mode
	Volume	Time	Pressure	Flow	Time	Pressure		
CMV	+				+			
AC	+				+	+		
IMV	+				+		+	+
SIMV	+				+	+	+	+
PSV				+		+	+	+
PCV			+		+			
MMV							+	
PC-IRV			+		+			
APRV		+			+		+	
HFJV		+			+		+	

[1]CMV, controlled mechanical ventilation; AC, assist-control ventilation; IMV, intermittent mandatory ventilation; SIMV, synchronized intermittent mandatory ventilation; PSV, pressure support ventilation; PCV, pressure control ventilation; MMV, mandatory minute ventilation; IRV, inverse I:E ratio ventilation; APRV, airway pressure release ventilation; HFJV, high-frequency jet ventilation.

level. VT and inspiratory time vary, being related to airway resistance and pulmonary and circuit compliance. A significant leak in the patient circuit can prevent the necessary rise in circuit pressure and machine cycling. Conversely, an acute increase in airway resistance, or decrease in pulmonary compliance, or circuit compliance (kink) causes premature cycling and decreases the delivered VT. Pressure-cycled ventilators are generally most useful for short-term use only (transport).

Flow-cycled ventilators have pressure and flow sensors that allow the ventilator to monitor inspiratory flow at a preselected fixed inspiratory pressure; when this flow reaches a predetermined level (usually 25% of the initial peak mechanical inspiratory flow rate), the ventilator cycles from inspiration into expiration (see the section on Pressure Support/Pressure Control Ventilation).

C. MICROPROCESSOR-CONTROLLED VENTILATORS

These versatile machines can be set to function in any one of a variety of inspiratory flow and cycling patterns. The microprocessor allows closed-loop control over the ventilator's performance characteristics. Microprocessor-controlled ventilators include the Puritan-Bennett 7200 and 840, Siemens Servo 300, Respironics Espirit and Hamilton Veolar ventilators, and the ventilators on the Ohmeda 7600 and the Drager 6000 anesthesia machines.

Ventilatory Modes

Ventilatory mode is defined by the method by which the ventilator cycles from expiration to inspiration as well as whether the patient is able to breathe spontaneously (Table 49–5 and Figure 49–1). Most modern ventilators are capable of more than one ventilatory mode, and some (microprocessor-controlled ventilators) can combine modes simultaneously.

A. CONTROLLED MECHANICAL VENTILATION (CMV)

In this mode, the ventilator cycles from expiration to inspiration after a fixed time interval. The interval determines the ventilatory rate. Settings on this mode provide a fixed VT and fixed rate (and, therefore, minute ventilation) regardless of patient effort, because the patient cannot breathe spontaneously. Settings to limit inspiratory pressure guard against pulmonary barotrauma. Controlled ventilation is best reserved for patients capable of little or no ventilatory effort. Awake patients with active ventilatory effort require sedation or muscle paralysis.

B. ASSIST-CONTROL (AC) VENTILATION

By incorporating a pressure sensor in the breathing circuit, the patient's inspiratory effort can be used to trigger inspiration. A sensitivity control allows selection of the inspiratory effort required. The ventilator can be set for a fixed ventilatory rate, but each patient effort of sufficient magnitude will trigger the set VT. If sponta-

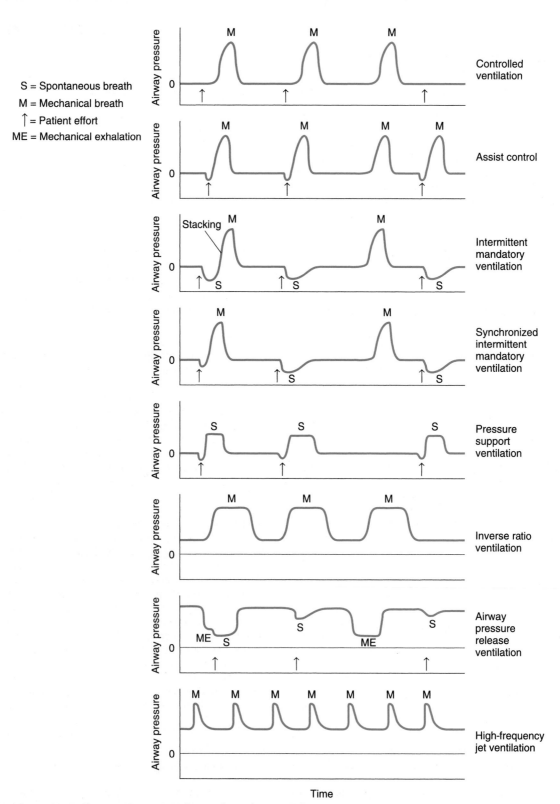

Figure 49–1. Airway pressure waveforms of ventilatory modes.

S = Spontaneous breath
M = Mechanical breath
↑ = Patient effort
ME = Mechanical exhalation

Controlled ventilation

Assist control

Intermittent mandatory ventilation

Synchronized intermittent mandatory ventilation

Pressure support ventilation

Inverse ratio ventilation

Airway pressure release ventilation

High-frequency jet ventilation

neous inspiratory efforts are not detected, the machine functions as if in the control mode.

C. INTERMITTENT MANDATORY VENTILATION (IMV)

IMV allows spontaneous ventilation while the patient is on the ventilator. A selected number of mechanical breaths (with fixed VT) is given to supplement spontaneous breathing. At high mandatory rates (10–12 breaths/min), IMV essentially provides all of the patient's ventilation; at low rates (1–2 breaths/min), it provides minimal mechanical ventilation and allows the patient to breathe relatively independently. The VT and frequency of spontaneous breaths are determined by the patient's ventilatory drive and muscle strength. The IMV rate can be adjusted to maintain a desired minute ventilation. IMV has found greatest use as a weaning technique.

Synchronized intermittent mandatory ventilation (SIMV) times the mechanical breath, whenever possible, to coincide with the beginning of a spontaneous effort. Proper synchronization prevents superimposing (stacking) a mechanical breath in the middle of a spontaneous breath, resulting in a very large VT. As with CMV and AC, settings to limit inspiratory pressure guard against pulmonary barotrauma. The advantages of SIMV include patient comfort, and if used for weaning, the machine breaths provide a backup if the patient becomes fatigued. However, if the rate is too low (4 breaths/min), the backup may be too low, particularly for weak patients who may not be able to overcome the added WOB superimposed by the ventilator during spontaneous breaths.

IMV circuits provide a continuous supply of gas flow for spontaneous ventilation between mechanical breaths. Modern ventilators incorporate SIMV into their design, but older models must be modified by a parallel circuit, a continuous flow system, or a demand flow valve. Regardless of the system, proper functioning of one-way valves and sufficient gas flow are necessary to prevent an increase in the patient's WOB, particularly when PEEP is also used.

D. MANDATORY MINUTE VENTILATION (MMV)

The patient is able to breathe spontaneously and receives mechanical breaths also, while the machine monitors the exhaled minute ventilation. In this mode, the machine then continuously adjusts the number of mechanical breaths so that the sum of spontaneous plus mechanical breaths multiplied by the VT equals the desired set minute ventilation. The role of this mode in weaning remains to be defined.

E. PRESSURE SUPPORT VENTILATION (PSV)

Pressure support ventilation was designed to augment the VT of spontaneously breathing patients and overcome any increased inspiratory resistance from the TT,

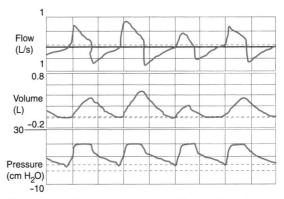

Figure 49–2. Pressure support ventilation. The patient initiates a breath; the machine is set to deliver 15 cm H$_2$O pressure (above 5 cm H$_2$O of continuous positive airway pressure [CPAP]). When flow ceases, the machine cycles into the expiratory mode.

breathing circuit (tubing, connectors, and humidifier), and ventilator (pneumatic circuitry and valves). Microprocessor-controlled machines have this mode, which delivers sufficient gas flow with every inspiratory effort to maintain a predetermined positive pressure throughout inspiration. When inspiratory flow decreases to a predetermined level, the ventilator's feedback (servo) loop cycles the machine into the expiratory phase, and airway pressure returns to baseline (Figure 49–2). The only setting in this mode is inspiratory pressure. The patient determines the respiratory rate and VT varies according to inspiratory gas flow, lung mechanics, and the patient's own inspiratory effort. Low levels of PSV (5–10 cm H$_2$O) are usually sufficient to overcome any added resistance imposed by the breathing apparatus. Higher levels (10–40 cm H$_2$O) can function as a standalone ventilatory mode if the patient has sufficient spontaneous ventilatory drive and stable lung mechanics. The principal advantages of PSV are its ability to augment spontaneous VT, decrease the WOB, and increase patient comfort. However, if the patient fatigues or lung mechanics change, VT may be inadequate, and there is no backup rate if the patient's intrinsic respiratory rate decreases or the patient becomes apneic. Pressure support is often used in conjunction with IMV (Figure 49–3). The IMV machine breaths provide backup, and a low level of pressure support is used to offset the WOB superimposed by the breathing circuit and machine.

F. PRESSURE CONTROL VENTILATION (PCV)

 Pressure control ventilation (PCV) is similar to pressure support ventilation in that peak airway pressure is controlled but is different in that a

Figure 49–3. Intermittent mechanical ventilation with pressure support. M = machine breath → set tidal volume (VT) delivered. S = spontaneous breath, 15 cm of pressure support over 5 cm of PEEP. VT depends on patient effort and lung mechanics.V̇, flow; Paw, partial airway pressure; PEEP, positive end-expiratory pressure.

mandatory rate and inspiratory time are selected. As with pressure support, gas flow ceases when the pressure level is reached; however, the ventilator does not cycle to expiration until the preset inspiration time has elapsed. PCV may be used in both the AC and IMV modes. In AC, all breaths (either machine initiated or patient initiated) are time cycled and pressure limited. In IMV, machine-initiated breaths are time cycled and pressure limited. The patient may breathe spontaneously between the set rate, and the VT of the spontaneous breaths is determined by the patient's pulmonary muscle strength. The advantage of PCV is that by limiting inspiratory pressure, the risks of barotrauma and volutrauma may be decreased. Also, by extending inspiratory time, better mixing and recruitment of collapsed or flooded alveoli may be achieved, provided adequate PEEP levels are used. The disadvantage of PCV is that VT is not guaranteed. Any change in compliance or resistance will affect the delivered VT. This is a major issue in patients with ALI because if the compliance changes without augmenting the pressure, adequate VT may not be attained. PCV has been used on patients with ALI or ARDS, often with a prolonged inspiratory time or inverse I:E ratio ventilation (IRV) (see below) in an effort to recruit collapsed and flooded alveoli. The disadvantage of using IRV with PCV is that the patient needs to be heavily sedated or paralyzed to tolerate this particular ventilatory mode.

With PCV, pressure and inspiratory time are preset, whereas airflow and volume are variable and dependent on the patient's resistance and compliance. With volume ventilation, on the other hand, inspiratory time is also preset but flow and VT are also preset, and in this circumstance the inspiratory pressure can be very high.

G. Inverse I:E Ratio Ventilation

IRV reverses the normal inspiratory to expiratory time ratio of 1:3 or greater to a ratio of greater than 1:1. This may be achieved by adding an end-inspiratory pause, by decreasing peak inspiratory flow during volume-cycled ventilation (CMV), or by setting an inspiratory time such that inspiration is longer than expiration during PCV (PC-IRV). Intrinsic PEEP may be produced during IRV and is caused by air trapping or incomplete emptying of the lung to the baseline pressure prior to the initiation of the next breath. This air trapping increases FRC until a new equilibrium is reached. This mode does not allow spontaneous breathing and requires heavy sedation or neuromuscular blockade. IRV with PEEP is effective for improving oxygenation in patients with decreased FRC. Oxygenation is generally directly proportional to mean airway pressure.

H. Airway Pressure Release Ventilation (APRV)

APRV or bilevel ventilation is a mode in which a high PEEP level is used, during which the patient is allowed to breath spontaneously. Intermittently, the PEEP level decreases to help augment the elimination of CO_2 (Figure 49–4). The inspiratory and expiratory times, high and low PEEP levels, and spontaneous respiratory activity determine minute ventilation. Initial settings include a minimum PEEP of 10–12 cm H_2O and a release level of 5–10 cm H_2O. Advantages of APRV appear to be less circulatory depression and pulmonary barotrauma as well as less need for sedation. This technique appears to be an attractive alternative to PC-IRV for overcoming problems with high peak inspiratory pressures in patients with reduced lung compliance.

I. High-Frequency Ventilation (HFV)

Three forms of HFV are available. High-frequency positive-pressure ventilation (HFPPV) involves delivering a small "conventional" VT at a rate of 60–120 breaths/min. High-frequency jet ventilation (HFJV) utilizes a small cannula at or in the airway through which a pulsed jet of high-pressure gas is delivered at a set frequency of 120–600 times/min (2–10 Hz). The jet of gas may entrain air (Bernoulli effect), which may augment VT. High-frequency oscillation (HFO) employs a driver (usually a piston) that creates to-and-fro gas movement in the airway at rates of 180–3000 times/min (3–50 Hz).

Figure 49–4. Airway pressure release ventilation.

These forms of ventilation all produce V_T at or below anatomic dead space. The exact mechanism of gas exchange is unclear but is probably a combination of effects, including convective ventilation, asymmetrical velocity profiles, Taylor dispersion, pendelluft, molecular diffusion, and cardiogenic mixing. HFJV has found widest use in the operating room. It may be used for laryngeal, tracheal, and bronchial procedures and can be extremely useful in emergency management of the airway when tracheal intubation and conventional positive-pressure ventilation are unsuccessful (see Chapter 5). In the ICU, HFJV may be useful in managing some patients with bronchopleural and tracheoesophageal fistulas when conventional ventilation has failed. Occasionally, HFJV or HFO is used in patients with ARDS to try to improve oxygenation. Inadequate heating and humidification of inspired gases during prolonged HFV, however, can be a problem. Initial settings for HFJV in the operating room are typically a rate of 120–240 breaths/min, an inspiratory time of 33%, and a drive pressure of 15–30 psi. Mean airway pressure should be measured in the trachea at least 5 cm below the injector to avoid an artifactual error from gas entrainment. Carbon dioxide elimination is generally directly proportional to drive pressure, whereas oxygenation is directly proportional to mean airway pressure. An intrinsic PEEP effect is seen during HFJV at high drive pressures and inspiratory times greater than 40%.

J. Differential Lung Ventilation (DLV)

This technique, also referred to as independent lung ventilation (ILV), may be used in patients with severe unilateral lung disease or those with bronchopleural fistula. Use of conventional positive-pressure ventilation and PEEP in such instances can aggravate ventilation/perfusion mismatching or, in patients with fistula, result in inadequate ventilation of the unaffected lung. In patients with restrictive disease of one lung, overdistention of the normal lung can lead to worsening hypoxemia or barotrauma. After separation of the lungs with a double-lumen bronchial tube, differential positive-pressure ventilation with two ventilators is applied to each lung independently. When two ventilators are used, the timing of mechanical breaths is usually synchronized, with one ventilator, the "master," setting the rate for the "slave" ventilator.

2. Care of Patients Requiring Mechanical Ventilation

Tracheal Intubation

Tracheal intubation for mechanical ventilation is most commonly undertaken in ICU patients to manage pulmonary failure. Both nasal and oral (translaryngeal) tracheal intubation appear to be relatively safe for at least 2–3 weeks. When compared with oral intubation for extended periods of time in the ICU, nasal intubation may be more comfortable for the patient, more secure (fewer instances of accidental extubation), and less likely to cause laryngeal damage. Nasal intubation, however, has significant adverse events associated with its use, including significant nasal bleeding, transient bacteremia, submucosal dissection of the nasopharynx or oropharynx, and sinusitis or otitis media (from obstruction of the auditory tubes).

Intubation can often be carried out without the use of sedation or muscle paralysis in agonal and unconscious patients. Topical anesthesia of the airway or sedation, however, is helpful in patients who still have active airway reflexes. More vigorous and uncooperative patients require varying degrees of sedation; administration of an NMBA also greatly facilitates orotracheal intubation. Small doses of relatively short-acting agents are generally used; popular agents include midazolam, etomidate, propofol, and methohexital. Succinylcholine or a nondepolarizing NMBA (mivacuronium or rocuronium) can be used for paralysis after a hypnotic is given.

The time of tracheal intubation and initiation of mechanical ventilation is often a period of great hemodynamic instability. Hypertension or hypotension and bradycardia or tachycardia may be encountered. Responsible factors include activation of autonomic reflexes from stimulation of the airway, myocardial depression and vasodilation from sedative-hypnotic agents, straining by the patient, withdrawal of intense sympathetic activity, and reduced venous return due to positive pressure in the airways. Careful monitoring is therefore required during and immediately following intubation.

When left in place for more than 2–3 weeks, both oral and nasal translaryngeal TTs predispose patients to subglottic stenosis. If longer periods of mechanical ventilation are necessary, the TT should generally be replaced by a cuffed tracheostomy tube. If it is anticipated that a TT will be required for more than 2–3 weeks, and in some institutions for more than 1 week, a tracheostomy is performed within the first few days of intubation.

Initial Ventilator Settings

Depending on the type of pulmonary failure, mechanical ventilation is used to provide either partial or full ventilatory support. For full ventilatory support, CMV, AC, or PCV is generally employed with a respiratory rate of 10–12 breaths/min and a V_T of 8–10 mL/kg; lower V_T (6–8 mL/kg) may be necessary to avoid high peak inflation pressures (> 35–40 cm H_2O) and pulmonary barotrauma and volutrauma. High airway pressures that overdistend alveoli (transalveolar pressure > 35 cm H_2O) have been shown experimentally to promote lung injury. Likewise, VT greater than 10 mL has been associated with increased mortality in patients with ARDS. Partial ventilatory support is usually provided by low SIMV settings (< 8 breaths/min), either with or without pressure support. Lower mean airway pressures (< 20–30 cm H_2O) can help preserve cardiac output and may be less likely to alter normal ventilation/perfusion relationships.

Patients breathing spontaneously on SIMV must overcome the additional resistances of the TT, demand valves, and breathing circuit of the ventilator. These imposed resistances increase the WOB. Small TTs (< 7.0–7.5 mm i.d.) should therefore be avoided whenever possible. The simultaneous use of pressure support 5–15 cm H_2O during SIMV can compensate for TT and circuit resistance.

The addition of 5–8 cm H_2O of PEEP during positive-pressure ventilation preserves FRC and gas exchange. This "physiological" PEEP is purported to compensate for the loss of a similar amount of intrinsic PEEP (and decrease in FRC) in patients following tracheal intubation. Periodic large VT (sigh breaths) is not necessary when physiological PEEP (approximately 5 cm H_2O) and a VT of 6–10 mL/kg are used.

Sedation & Paralysis

Heavy sedation or paralysis may be necessary in patients who become agitated and "fight" the ventilator. Repetitive coughing ("bucking") and straining can have adverse hemodynamic effects, can interfere with gas exchange, and may predispose to pulmonary barotrauma and self-inflicted injury. Sedation with or without paralysis may also be desirable when patients continue to be tachypneic despite high mechanical respiratory rates (> 16–18 breaths/min).

Commonly used sedatives include opioids (morphine or fentanyl), benzodiazepines (diazepam, midazolam, or lorazepam), propofol, and dexmedetomidine. These agents may be used alone or in combination and are most effectively administered by continuous infusion. Nondepolarizing NMBAs are used for paralysis (along with an adequte dose of sedative medication) when all other means to ventilate the patient have failed.

Monitoring

Patients on mechanical ventilation require continuous monitoring for adverse hemodynamic and pulmonary effects resulting from positive pressure in the airways. Continuous electrocardiographic, pulse oximetry, and direct intraarterial pressure monitoring are extremely useful. The latter also allows frequent sampling of arterial blood for respiratory gas analysis. Careful recording of fluid intake and output is necessary to assess fluid balance accurately. An indwelling urinary catheter is very helpful. Central venous and/or pulmonary artery pressure monitoring are indicated in hemodynamically unstable patients and those with a low urinary output. Daily chest radiographs are commonly obtained to assess TT and central line positions, look for evidence of pulmonary barotrauma, help evaluate fluid balance, and monitor the progression of pulmonary disease.

Airway pressures (baseline, peak, and mean), inhaled and exhaled VT (mechanical and spontaneous), and fractional concentration of oxygen should be closely monitored. Monitoring these parameters not only allows optimal adjustment of ventilator settings but helps detect problems with the TT, breathing circuit, and ventilator. Inadequate periodic suctioning of airway secretions and the presence of large mucus plugs are often manifested as increasing peak inflation pressures and decreasing exhaled VT. Moreover, an abrupt increase in peak inflation pressure together with sudden hypotension strongly suggests a pneumothorax.

3. Discontinuing Mechanical Ventilation

The ease of weaning (or liberating) a patient from a ventilator is generally inversely related to the duration of the mechanical ventilation. The process that necessitated mechanical ventilation must be reversed or under control before weaning is attempted. Complicating factors should also be adequately treated, including bronchospasm, heart failure, infection, malnutrition, metabolic acidosis or alkalosis, anemia, increased CO_2 production due to high carbohydrate loads, altered mental status, and sleep deprivation. Underlying lung disease and pulmonary muscle wasting from prolonged disuse are often major factors that complicate weaning.

Weaning from mechanical ventilation may be considered when patients no longer meet general criteria for mechanical ventilation (see Table 49–4). Additional mechanical indices have also been suggested (Table 49–6). Clinical signs of improvement should be supported by laboratory and radiographic findings. The most useful weaning parameters are arterial blood gas tensions, respiratory rate, and rapid shallow breathing

Table 49–6. Mechanical criteria for weaning/extubation.

Criterion	Measurement
Inspiratory pressure	<−25 cm H_2O
Tidal volume	> 5 mL/kg
Vital capacity	> 10 mL/kg
Minute ventilation	< 10 mL
Rapid shallow breathing index	< 100

index (RSBI). Intact airway reflexes and a cooperative patient are also mandatory prior to completion of the weaning process unless the patient has a cuffed tracheostomy tube. Similarly, adequate oxygenation (arterial hemoglobin saturation > 90%) on 40–50% O_2 with less than 5 cm H_2O of PEEP is imperative prior to extubation. When the patient is weaned from the ventilator and extubation is planned, the RSBI is frequently used to help predict who can be successfully weaned from mechanical ventilation and extubated. With the patient breathing spontaneously on a T-piece, the VT and respiratory rate (f) are measured:

$$RSBI = \frac{f(breaths/min)}{V_T(L)}$$

Patients with an RSBI less than 100 can be successfully extubated. Those with an RSBI greater than 120 should remain on some degree of mechanical ventilation.

The most common techniques to wean a patient from the ventilator include SIMV, pressure support, or periods of spontaneous breathing alone on a T-piece or on low levels of CPAP. Mandatory minute ventilation has also been suggested as an ideal weaning technique, but experience with it is more limited.

Weaning with SIMV

With SIMV the number of mechanical breaths is progressively decreased (by 1–2 breaths/min) as long as the arterial CO_2 tension and respiratory rate remain acceptable (generally < 45–50 mm Hg and < 30 breaths/min, respectively). If pressure support is concomitantly used, it should generally be reduced to 5–8 cm H_2O. In patients with acid–base disturbances or chronic CO_2 retention, arterial blood pH (> 7.35) is more useful than CO_2 tension. Blood gas measurements can be checked after a minimum of 15–30 min at each setting. When an IMV of 2–4 breaths is reached, mechanical ventilation is discontinued if arterial oxygenation remains acceptable.

Weaning with PSV

Weaning with PSV alone is accomplished by gradually decreasing the pressure support level by 2–3 cm H_2O while VT, arterial blood gas tensions, and respiratory rate are monitored (using the same criteria as for IMV). The goal is to try to ensure a VT of 4–6 mL/kg and an f of less than 30 with acceptable PaO_2 and $PaCO_2$. When a pressure support level of 5–8 cm H_2O is reached, the patient is considered weaned.

Weaning with a T-Piece or CPAP

T-piece trials allow observation while the patient breathes spontaneously without any mechanical breaths.

The T-piece attaches directly to the TT or tracheostomy tube and has corrugated tubing on the other two limbs. A humidified oxygen–air mixture flows into the proximal limb and exits from the distal limb. Sufficient gas flow must be given in the proximal limb to prevent the mist from being completely drawn back at the distal limb during inspiration; this ensures that the patient is receiving the desired oxygen concentration. The patient is observed closely during this period; obvious signs of fatigue, chest retractions, tachypnea, marked tachycardia, arrhythmias, or hypertension or hypotension should terminate the trial. If the patient appears to tolerate the trial period and the RSBI is less than 100, mechanical ventilation can be discontinued permanently. If the patient can also protect and clear the airway, the TT can be removed.

If the patient has been intubated for a prolonged period or has severe underlying lung disease, sequential T-piece trials may be necessary: periodic trials of 10–30 min are initiated and progressively increased by 5–10 min or longer per trial as long as the patient appears comfortable and maintains acceptable arterial blood gases.

Many patients develop progressive atelectasis during prolonged T-piece trials. This may reflect the absence of a normal "physiological" PEEP when the larynx is bypassed by a TT. If this is a concern, spontaneous breathing trials on low levels (5 cm H_2O) of CPAP can be tried. The CPAP helps maintain FRC and prevent atelectasis.

POSITIVE AIRWAY PRESSURE THERAPY

Positive airway pressure therapy can be used in patients breathing spontaneously as well as those mechanically ventilated. The principal indication for positive airway pressure therapy is a symptomatic decrease in FRC, resulting in absolute or relative hypoxemia. By increasing transpulmonary distending pressure, positive airway pressure therapy can increase FRC, improve (increase) lung compliance, and reverse ventilation/perfusion mismatching. The latter is reflected in a decrease in venous admixture and an improvement in arterial O_2 tension.

Positive End-Expiratory Pressure

Application of positive pressure during expiration as an adjunct to a mechanically delivered breath is referred to as PEEP. The ventilator's PEEP valve provides a pressure threshold that allows expiratory flow to occur only when airway pressure equals or exceeds the selected PEEP level. This threshold usually is provided by a pressurized expiratory valve or diaphragm.

Continuous Positive Airway Pressure

Application of a positive-pressure threshold during both inspiration and expiration with spontaneous breathing is

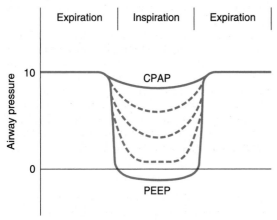

Figure 49–5. Airway pressure during positive end-expiratory pressure (PEEP) and continuous positive airway pressure (CPAP). Note that by increasing inspiratory gas flows, PEEP progressively becomes CPAP.

referred to as CPAP. Constant levels of pressure can be attained only if a high-flow (inspiratory) gas source is provided. When the patient does not have an artificial airway, tightly fitting full-face masks, nasal masks, nasal "pillows" (ADAM circuit), or nasal prongs (neonatal) can be used. Because of the risks of gastric distention and regurgitation, CPAP masks should be used only on alert patients with intact airway reflexes and with CPAP levels less than 15 cm H_2O (less than lower esophageal sphincter pressure in normal persons). Expiratory pressures above 15 cm H_2O require an artificial airway.

CPAP versus PEEP

The distinction between PEEP and CPAP is often blurred in the clinical setting because patients may breathe with a combination of mechanical and spontaneous breaths. Therefore, the two terms are often used interchangeably. In the strictest sense, "pure" PEEP is provided as a ventilator-cycled breath. In contrast, a "pure" CPAP system provides only sufficient continuous or "on-demand" gas flows (60–90 L/min) to prevent inspiratory airway pressure from falling perceptibly below the expiratory level during spontaneous breaths (Figure 49–5). Thus, compared with PEEP, CPAP breathing provides less support but with reduced mean airway pressure. Some ventilators with demand valve–based CPAP systems may not be adequately responsive and result in increased inspiratory WOB. This situation can be corrected by adding low levels of (inspiratory) PSV if in a volume-targeted mode or changing to a pressure-targeted mode. In clinical practice, controlled ventilation, PSV, and CPAP/PEEP support can be

delivered by most modern ICU ventilators. Manufacturers have also developed specific devices to deliver bilevel inspiratory positive airway pressure [IPAP] with expiratory positive airway pressure [EPAP] in either a spontaneous or time-cycled fashion. The term "bilevel positive airway pressure (BiPAP)" has become a commonly used phrase, adding to the confusion of airway pressure terminology.

Pulmonary Effects of PEEP & CPAP

The major effect of PEEP on the lungs is to increase FRC. In patients with decreased lung volume, both PEEP and CPAP increase FRC and tidal ventilation above closing capacity, improve lung compliance, and correct ventilation/perfusion abnormalities. The resulting decrease in intrapulmonary shunting improves arterial oxygenation. Their principal mechanism of action appears to be stabilization and expansion of partially collapsed alveoli. Recruitment (reexpansion) of collapsed alveoli occurs at PEEP or CPAP levels above the inflection point, defined as the pressure level on a pressure–volume curve at which collapsed alveoli are recruited (open); with small changes in pressure there are large changes in volume (Figure 49–6). Although neither PEEP nor CPAP decreases total extravascular lung water, studies suggest that they do redistribute extravascular lung water from the interstitial space between alveoli and endothelial cells toward peribronchial and perihilar areas. Both effects can potentially improve arterial oxygenation.

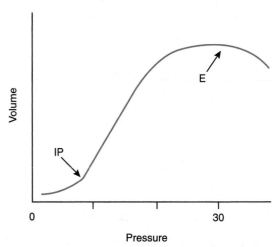

Figure 49–6. Pressure–volume curve for pulmonary system (eg, lung, thoracic). Inflection point (IP) above which the majority of alveoli are recruited. E, result of excessive pressure when alveoli are overdistended and pulmonary compliance decreases.

Excessive PEEP or CPAP, however, can overdistend alveoli (and bronchi), increasing dead space ventilation and reducing lung compliance; both effects can significantly increase the WOB. By compressing alveolar capillaries, overdistention of normal alveoli can also increase pulmonary vascular resistance and right ventricular afterload.

A higher incidence of pulmonary barotrauma is observed when excessive PEEP or CPAP is added, particularly at levels greater than 20 cm H_2O. Disruption of alveoli allows air to track interstitially along bronchi into the mediastinum (pneumomediastinum). From the mediastinum, air can then rupture into the pleural space (pneumothorax) or the pericardium (pneumopericardium) or can dissect along tissue planes subcutaneously (subcutaneous emphysema) or into the abdomen (pneumoperitoneum or pneumoretroperitoneum). Failure of an air leak to seal results in a bronchopleural fistula. Barotrauma may be more closely associated with the higher peak inspiratory pressures that result with increasing level of PEEP or CPAP. Other factors that may increase the risk of barotrauma include underlying lung disease, a high rate of mechanical breaths such that there is stacking of breaths so that intrinsic PEEP develops, large V_T (> 10–15 mL/kg), and young age.

Adverse Nonpulmonary Effects of PEEP & CPAP

These adverse effects are primarily circulatory and are related to transmission of the elevated airway pressure to the contents of the chest. Fortunately, transmission is directly related to lung compliance; thus, patients with decreased lung compliance (most patients requiring PEEP) are least affected.

Progressive reductions in cardiac output are often seen as mean airway pressure and, secondarily, mean intrathoracic pressure rise. The principal mechanism appears to be a progressive decrease in venous return to the heart. Other mechanisms may include leftward displacement of the interventricular septum (interfering with left ventricular filling) because of the increase in pulmonary vascular resistance (increased right ventricular afterload) from overdistention of alveoli, leading to an increase in right ventricular volume. Left ventricular compliance may therefore be reduced; when this occurs, the same preload requires a higher filling pressure. Intravenous fluid administration usually at least partially offsets the effects of CPAP and PEEP on cardiac output. Circulatory depression is most often associated with end-expiratory pressures greater than 15 cm H_2O.

PEEP-induced elevations in central venous pressure and reductions in cardiac output decrease both renal and hepatic blood flow. Circulating levels of antidiuretic hormone and angiotensin are usually elevated. Urinary output, glomerular filtration, and free water clearance decrease.

The increases in central venous pressure also aggravate intracranial hypertension. Increased end-expiratory pressures, because they decrease venous return, may also be manifested as an increase in ICP in patients whose ventricular compliance is decreased. Therefore, in patients on mechanical ventilation for ALI and with evidence of raised ICP, the level of PEEP must be carefully chosen to balance oxygenation requirements against effects on the ICP.

Optimum Use of PEEP & CPAP

The goal of positive-pressure therapy is ultimately to increase oxygen delivery to tissues, while avoiding the adverse sequelae of high (> 0.5) FIO_2. The latter is optimally accomplished only if adequate cardiac output and a hemoglobin concentration greater than 8–10 g/dL are maintained as well. Ideally, mixed venous oxygen tensions or the arteriovenous oxygen content difference should be followed. The salutary effect of PEEP (or CPAP) on arterial oxygen tension must be balanced against any detrimental effect on cardiac output. PEEP or CPAP levels exceeding 15 cm H_2O usually require pulmonary artery pressure monitoring to properly assess circulatory function and allow measurement of mixed venous oxygen tension and calculation of the venous admixture. Volume infusion or inotropic support may be necessary and should be guided by hemodynamic measurements.

At optimal PEEP the maximum beneficial effects of PEEP overshadow any detrimental effects. Practically, PEEP is usually added in increments of 3–5 cm H_2O until the desired therapeutic end point is reached. The most commonly suggested end point is an arterial oxygen saturation of hemoglobin of greater than 88–90% on a nontoxic inspired oxygen concentration (≤ 50%). Many clinicians favor reducing the inspired oxygen concentration to 50% or less because of the potentially adverse effect of higher oxygen concentrations on the lung. Alternatively, PEEP may be titrated to the mixed venous artery oxygen saturation ($S\bar{v}O_2$ > 50–60%). Monitoring lung compliance and dead space has also been suggested.

OTHER RESPIRATORY CARE TECHNIQUES

Several other respiratory care techniques preserve or improve pulmonary function. They include administering aerosolized water or bronchodilators and clearing pulmonary secretions.

An aerosol mist is a gas or gas mixture containing a suspension of liquid particles. Aerosolized water may be administered to loosen inspissated secretions and facilitate their removal from the tracheobronchial tree.

Aerosol mists are also used to administer bronchodilators, mucolytic agents, or vasoconstrictors, although metered-dose inhalers are preferred for administration of bronchodilators. A normal cough requires an adequate inspiratory capacity, an intact glottis, and adequate muscle strength (abdominal muscles and diaphragm). Aerosol mist therapy with or without bronchodilators may induce cough as well as loosen secretions. Additional effective measures include chest percussion or vibration therapy and postural drainage of the various lung lobes.

Maneuvers that produce sustained maximum lung inflation such as the use of an incentive spirometer can be helpful in inducing cough as well as preventing atelectasis and preserving normal lung volume. Patients should be instructed to inhale approximately 15–20 mL/kg and to hold it for 2–3 s before exhalation.

When thick and copious secretions are associated with obvious atelectasis and hypoxemia, more aggressive measures may be indicated. These include suctioning via a nasopharyngeal catheter or flexible bronchoscope or through a TT. When atelectasis is not associated with retention of secretions, a brief period of CPAP by mask or positive-pressure ventilation through a TT is often very effective.

RESPIRATORY FAILURE

Respiratory failure may be defined as impairment of normal gas exchange severe enough to require acute therapeutic intervention. Definitions based on arterial blood gases (see Table 49–1) may not apply to patients with chronic pulmonary diseases; dyspnea and progressive respiratory acidosis must also be present in patients with chronic CO_2 retention. Arterial blood gases typically follow one of several patterns in patients with respiratory failure (Figure 49–7). At one extreme, the derangement primarily affects oxygen transfer from the alveoli into blood, giving rise to hypoxemia (hypoxic respiratory failure); unless severe ventilation/perfusion mismatching is present, CO_2 elimination in these instances is typically normal or even enhanced. At the other extreme, the disorder primarily affects CO_2 elimination (pure ventilatory failure), resulting in hypercapnia; mismatching of ventilation to perfusion is typically absent or minimal. Hypoxemia, however, can occur with pure ventilatory failure when arterial CO_2 tension reaches 75–80 mm Hg in patients breathing room air (see the alveolar gas equation in Chapter 22). Most patients with respiratory failure display a pattern between these extremes.

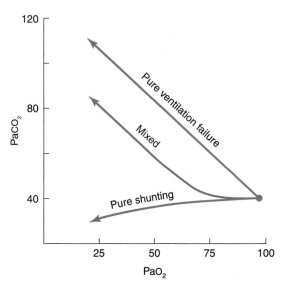

Figure 49–7. Arterial gas tension (room air) patterns during acute respiratory failure.

Treatment

Regardless of the disorder, the treatment of respiratory failure is primarily supportive while the reversible components of underlying disease are being treated. Hypoxemia is treated with oxygen therapy and positive airway pressure (if FRC is decreased), whereas hypercarbia (ventilatory failure) is treated with mechanical ventilation. Other general measures may include using aerosolized bronchodilators, intravenous antibiotics, and diuretics for fluid overload as well as ensuring optimal cardiac function and adequate nutritional support. Some patients may benefit from aminophylline infusions, which can improve diaphragmatic function.

PULMONARY EDEMA

Pathophysiology

Pulmonary edema results from transudation of fluid, first from pulmonary capillaries into interstitial spaces and then from the interstitial spaces into alveoli. Fluid within the interstitial space and alveoli is collectively referred to as extravascular lung water. The movement of water across the pulmonary capillaries is similar to what occurs in other capillary beds and can be expressed by the Starling equation:

$$Q = K \times [(Pc' - Pi) - \sigma(\pi c' - \pi i)]$$

where Q is net flow across the capillary; Pc′ and Pi are capillary and interstitial hydrostatic pressures, respectively; πc′ and πi are capillary and interstitial oncotic pressures, respectively; K is a filtration coefficient related to effective capillary surface area per mass of tissue; and σ is a reflection coefficient that expresses the permeability of the capillary endothelium to albumin. A σ with a value of 1 implies that the endothelium is completely impermeable to albumin, whereas a value of 0 indicates free passage of albumin and other particles/molecules. The pulmonary endothelium normally is partially permeable to albumin, such that interstitial albumin concentration is approximately one-half that of plasma; therefore, πi must be about 14 mm Hg (one-half that of plasma). Pulmonary capillary hydrostatic pressure is dependent on vertical height in the lung (gravity) and normally varies from 0 to 15 mm Hg (average, 7 mm Hg). Because Pi is thought to be normally about –4 to –8 mm Hg, the forces favoring transudation of fluid (Pc′, Pi, and πi) are usually almost balanced by the forces favoring reabsorption (πc′). The net amount of fluid that normally moves out of pulmonary capillaries is small (about 10–20 mL/h in adults) and is rapidly removed by pulmonary lymphatics, which return it into the central venous system.

The alveolar epithelial membrane is usually permeable to water and gases but is impermeable to albumin (and other proteins). A net movement of water from the interstitium into alveoli occurs only when the normally negative Pi becomes positive (relative to atmospheric pressure). Fortunately, because of the lung's unique ultrastructure and its capacity to increase lymph flow, the pulmonary interstitium usually accommodates large increases in capillary transudation before Pi becomes positive. When this reserve capacity is exceeded, pulmonary edema develops.

Pulmonary edema is often divided into four stages:

Stage I: Only interstitial pulmonary edema is present. Patients often become tachypneic as pulmonary compliance begins to decrease. The chest radiograph reveals increased interstitial markings and peribronchial cuffing.

Stage II: Fluid fills the interstitium and begins to fill the alveoli, being initially confined to the angles between adjacent septa (crescentic filling). Gas exchange may remain relatively preserved.

Stage III: Alveolar flooding occurs such that many alveoli are completely flooded and no longer contain air. Flooding is most prominent in dependent areas of the lungs. Blood flow through the capillaries of flooded alveoli results in a large increase in intrapulmonary shunting. Hypoxemia and hypocapnia (due to dyspnea and hyperventilation) are characteristic.

Stage IV: Marked alveolar flooding spills over into the airways as froth. Gas exchange is severely compromised due to both shunting and airway obstruction. Progressive hypercapnia and severe hypoxemia follow.

Causes of Pulmonary Edema

Pulmonary edema usually results from either an increase in the net hydrostatic pressure across the capillaries (hemodynamic or cardiogenic pulmonary edema) or an increase in the permeability of the alveolar–capillary membrane (increased permeability edema or noncardiogenic pulmonary edema). The distinction can often be based on the pulmonary artery occlusion pressure (PAOP), which if greater than 18 mm Hg indicates that hydrostatic pressure is involved in forcing fluid across the capillaries into the interstitium and alveoli. The protein content of the edema fluid can also help differentiate the two. Fluid due to hemodynamic edema has a low protein content, whereas fluid due to permeability edema has a high protein content.

Less common causes of edema include prolonged severe airway obstruction, sudden reexpansion of a collapsed lung, high altitude, pulmonary lymphatic obstruction, and severe head injury, although the same mechanisms (ie, changes in hemodynamic parameters or capillary permeability) also account for these diagnoses. Pulmonary edema associated with airway obstruction may result from an increase in the transmural pressure across pulmonary capillaries associated with a markedly negative interstitial hydrostatic pressure. Neurogenic pulmonary edema appears to be related to a marked increase in sympathetic tone, which causes severe pulmonary hypertension. The latter can disrupt the alveolar–capillary membrane.

1. Increased Transmural Pressure Pulmonary Edema (Cardiogenic Pulmonary Edema)

Significant elevations in Pc′ can increase extravascular lung water and result in pulmonary edema. As can be seen from the Starling equation, a decrease in πc′ may accentuate the effects of any increase in Pc′. Two major mechanisms increase Pc′, namely pulmonary venous hypertension and a markedly increased pulmonary blood flow. Any elevation of pulmonary venous pressure is transmitted passively backward to the pulmonary capillaries and secondarily increases Pc′. Pulmonary venous hypertension usually results from left ventricular failure, mitral stenosis, or left atrial obstruction. Increases in pulmonary blood flow that exceed the capacity of the pulmonary vasculature will also raise Pc′. Marked increases in pulmonary blood flow can be the result of large left-to-right cardiac or peripheral shunts, hypervolemia (fluid overload), severe anemia, or exercise.

Treatment

Management of cardiogenic pulmonary edema involves decreasing the pressure in the pulmonary capillaries.

Generally, this includes measures to improve ventricular function, correct fluid overload with diuretics, or reduce pulmonary blood flow. Pharmacological treatments include morphine, diuretics, vasodilators such as nitrates, preload-reducing agents such as recombinant brain natriuretic peptide (nesiritide) or angiotensin-converting enzyme (ACE) inhibitors (although these decrease both preload and afterload), and inotropes such as dobutamine. Vasodilators, particularly nitrates, have proved extremely useful. By reducing preload, pulmonary congestion is relieved; by reducing afterload, cardiac output may be improved. ACE inhibitors are preferred for patients with pulmonary edema who are also hypertensive. Positive airway pressure therapy is also a useful adjunct for improving oxygenation.

2. Increased Permeability Pulmonary Edema (Noncardiogenic Pulmonary Edema): ALI & ARDS

Extravascular lung water increases in increased permeability pulmonary edema due to enhanced permeability or disruption of the capillary–alveolar membrane. The protective effect of plasma oncotic pressure is lost as increased amounts of albumin "leak" into the pulmonary interstitium; normal—or even low—capillary hydrostatic pressures are unopposed and result in transudation of fluid into the lungs. Permeability edema is seen with ALI (P:F ratio $\leq$ 300 [P = PaO_2 and F = FIO_2]) and is often associated with sepsis, trauma, and pulmonary aspiration; when severe (P:F ratio < 200), it is referred to as ARDS.

Pathophysiology

ALI and ARDS represent the pulmonary manifestation of SIRS. Central to the pathophysiology of ALI and ARDS is severe injury of the capillary–alveolar membrane. Regardless of the type of injury, the lung responds to the ensuing inflammatory response in a similar fashion. The inflammatory response includes the release of large amounts of cytokines and other secondary mediators and activation of the complement, coagulation, fibrinolytic, and kinin cascades. Initial mediators include tumor necrosis factor (TNF), interleukins 1 and 6 (IL-1 and IL-6), platelet-activating factor, as well as various prostaglandins and leukotrienes. Activation of neutrophils and macrophages in the lung exposes the pulmonary parenchyma to oxygen-derived free radicals and proteases. The released mediators increase pulmonary capillary permeability, induce pulmonary vasoconstriction, and alter vascular reactivity such that hypoxic pulmonary vasoconstriction is abolished. Destruction of alveolar epithelial cells (types I and II) is prominent. Alveolar flooding, together with a decrease in surfactant production (due to loss of type II pneumocytes), results in collapse. The exudative phase of ARDS may rapidly resolve or persist for a varying period; it is often followed by a fibrotic phase (fibrosing alveolitis), which in some cases leads to permanent scarring.

Clinical Manifestations

The diagnosis of ALI and ARDS requires the exclusion of significant underlying left ventricular dysfunction (PAOP < 18 mm Hg) combined with a P:F ratio of < 300 and 200, respectively, and the presence of diffuse infiltrates on chest radiograph. The lung is often affected in a nonhomogeneous pattern, although dependent areas tend to be most affected.

ALI and ARDS are most commonly seen in the setting of sepsis and trauma. Patients present with severe dyspnea and labored respirations. Hypoxemia due to intrapulmonary shunting is a universal finding. Although dead space ventilation is increased, arterial CO_2 tension is typically decreased because of a marked increase in minute ventilation. Ventilatory failure may be seen initially in severe cases or may eventually develop due to respiratory muscle fatigue or marked destruction of the capillary–alveolar membrane. Pulmonary hypertension and low or normal left ventricular filling pressures are characteristic hemodynamic findings.

Treatment

In addition to intensive respiratory care, treatment should also be directed at reversible processes such as sepsis or hypotension. Hypoxemia is treated with oxygen therapy. Milder cases may be treated with a CPAP mask, but most patients require intubation and at least some degree of mechanical ventilatory support. **High peak inflation pressures (> 35 cm H_2O) and high VT (> 8–10 mL/kg), however, should also be avoided because overdistention of alveoli (high Paw or high VT) can induce iatrogenic lung injury, as can high FIO_2 (> 0.5).** The latter has not been conclusively demonstrated in humans, but in patients with ARDS, a VT of > 10 mL/kg is associated with increased mortality.

If possible, the FIO_2 should be maintained at $\leq$ 0.5, primarily by increasing PEEP above the inflection point (Figure 49–7). Other maneuvers to improve oxygenation include the use of inhaled nitric oxide, inhaled prostacyclin or prostaglandin E_1 (PGE_1), and ventilation in the prone position. These three techniques improve oxygenation in a majority of patients with ALI but are not risk free and have not been associated with an improvement in survival. Steroids early in ARDS are associated with an increased mortality but are often used (day 4–10) during the fibroproliferative phase of ARDS.

Morbidity and mortality from ARDS are usually due to the precipitating cause or to complications rather than the respiratory failure itself. Among the most common serious complications are sepsis, renal failure, and gastrointestinal (GI) hemorrhage. Nosocomial pneumonia is particularly common in patients with a protracted course. Nosocomial pneumonia is often difficult to diagnose; antibiotics are generally indicated when there is a high index of suspicion (fever, purulent secretions, leukocytosis, and change in chest radiograph). Protected specimen brushings and bronchoalveolar lavage sampling via a flexible bronchoscope may be useful in selected patients. Colonization by gram-negative organisms, breach of mucocutaneous barriers by various catheters, malnutrition, and altered host immunity contribute to a high incidence of infection. Renal failure is usually due to volume depletion, sepsis, or nephrotoxins and substantially increases the mortality rate (to > 60%). Prophylaxis for GI hemorrhage with sucralfate, antacids, H_2 blockers, or proton pump inhibitors is recommended.

DROWNING & NEAR-DROWNING

Drowning, with or without aspiration of water, is death while submerged in water. Near-drowning, with or without aspiration, is to suffocate while submerged and to survive at least temporarily. Both drowning and near-drowning can occur whether or not inhalation (aspiration) of water occurs. If water does not enter the airways, the patient primarily suffers from asphyxia; however, if the patient inhales water, marked intrapulmonary shunting also takes place. Survival depends on the intensity and duration of the hypoxia and water temperature.

Pathophysiology

Ninety percent of drowning patients aspirate fresh water, seawater, brackish water, or other fluids. Although the amount of liquid aspirated is generally small, marked ventilation/perfusion mismatching can result from fluids in the airways and alveoli, reflex bronchospasm, and loss of pulmonary surfactant. Aspiration of gastric contents can also complicate drowning before or after loss of consciousness or during resuscitation.

The hypotonic water aspirated following fresh water drowning is rapidly absorbed by the pulmonary circulation; water cannot usually be recovered from the airways. If a significant amount is absorbed (> 800 mL in a 70-kg adult), transient hemodilution, hyponatremia, and even hemolysis may occur. In contrast, aspiration of salt water, which is hypertonic, draws out water from the pulmonary circulation into the alveoli, flooding them. Hemoconcentration and hypernatremia can occur following saltwater drowning but are uncommon.

Hypermagnesemia and hypercalcemia have also been reported following near-drowning in salt water.

Patients who suffer from cold water drowning lose consciousness when body temperature decreases below 32°C. Ventricular fibrillation occurs at about 28–30°C, but the hypothermia has a protective effect on the brain and may improve outcome providing resuscitation measures are successful.

Clinical Manifestations

Nearly all patients with a significant near-drowning episode have hypoxemia, hypercarbia, and metabolic acidosis. Patients may also suffer from other injuries, such as spine fractures following diving accidents. Neurological impairment is generally related to duration of submersion and severity of asphyxia. Cerebral edema complicates prolonged asphyxia. ALI and ARDS develop in a significant number of patients following resuscitation.

Treatment

Initial treatment of near-drowning is directed at restoring ventilation, perfusion, oxygenation, and acid–base balance as quickly as possible. Immediate measures include clearing and establishing an airway, administering oxygen, and initiating cardiopulmonary resuscitation. In-line stabilization of the cervical spine is necessary while intubating patients who suffer from near-drowning following a dive. Although salt water can often be drained out of the lungs by gravity, this practice should not delay institution of cardiopulmonary resuscitation; abdominal thrusts may promote aspiration of gastric contents. Resuscitation efforts are always continued until the patient is fully assessed and under treatment in a hospital, particularly following cold water drowning. Complete recovery is possible in such instances even after prolonged periods of asphyxia. Management includes tracheal intubation, positive-pressure ventilation, and PEEP. Bronchospasm should be treated with bronchodilators, electrolyte abnormalities corrected, and ALI and ARDS treated as discussed above. If the patient is hypothermic, rewarming should be undertaken over a few hours.

SMOKE INHALATION

Smoke inhalation is the leading cause of death from fires. Affected persons may or may not have sustained a burn. Burn victims who suffer from smoke inhalation have a mortality rate significantly higher than other burn patients. Any exposure to smoke in a fire requires a presumptive diagnosis of smoke inhalation until proved otherwise. A history of loss of consciousness or disorientation or a burn acquired in a closed space is suggestive.

Pathophysiology

The consequences of smoke inhalation are complex because they can involve three types of injuries: heat injury to the airways, exposure to toxic gases, and a chemical burn with deposition of carbonaceous particulates into the lower airways. The pulmonary response to smoke inhalation is equally complex and depends on the duration of the exposure, composition of the material that burned, and presence of any underlying lung disease. Combustion of many synthetic materials produces highly toxic gases such as carbon monoxide, hydrogen cyanide, hydrogen sulfide, hydrogen chloride, ammonia, chlorine, benzene, and aldehydes. When these gases react with water in the airways, they can produce hydrochloric, acetic, formic, and sulfuric acids. Carbon monoxide and cyanide poisoning are common.

Pathological correlates of smoke inhalation include direct mucosal injury resulting in edema, inflammation, and sloughing. Loss of ciliary activity impairs the clearance of mucus and bacteria. Manifestations of ALI and ARDS typically occur 2–3 days after the injury and appear to be more related to the delayed development of SIRS rather than the acute smoke inhalation itself.

Clinical Manifestations

Patients may initially have few if any symptoms of smoke inhalation. Suggestive physical findings include facial or intraoral burns, singed nasal hairs, cough, carbonaceous sputum, and wheezing. The diagnosis can usually be made with flexible bronchoscopy of the upper airway and the tracheobronchial tree. Bronchoscopy reveals erythema, edema, mucosal ulcerations, and carbonaceous deposits. Arterial blood gases may initially be normal or reveal only mild hypoxemia and metabolic acidosis due to carbon monoxide. The chest radiograph is often also initially normal.

Heat injury to the airways is usually confined to supraglottic structures, unless there was prolonged exposure to steam. Progressive hoarseness and stridor are ominous signs of impending airway obstruction, which may develop over 12–18 h. Fluid resuscitation of the patient frequently aggravates the edema.

Carbon monoxide poisoning is usually defined as greater than 15% carboxyhemoglobin in the blood. The diagnosis is made by cooximetric measurements of blood. Carbon monoxide has 200–300 times the affinity of oxygen for hemoglobin. When a carbon monoxide molecule combines with hemoglobin to form carboxyhemoglobin, it decreases the affinity of the other binding sites for oxygen, shifting the hemoglobin dissociation curve to the right. The net result is a marked reduction in the oxygen-carrying capacity of blood.

Moreover, the rate of dissociation for carbon monoxide from hemoglobin is slow with a half-life of approximately 2–4 h. Clinical manifestations are due to tissue hypoxia from impaired oxygen delivery. Levels greater than 20–40% carboxyhemoglobin are associated with neurological impairment, nausea, fatigue, disorientation, and shock. Lower levels may also produce significant symptoms because carbon monoxide also binds cytochrome c and myoglobin. Compensatory mechanisms include increased cardiac output and peripheral vasodilation.

Cyanide toxicity may occur in patients exposed to fumes from fires that contain synthetic materials, particularly those containing polyurethane. The cyanide, which may be inhaled or absorbed through mucosal surfaces and skin, binds the cytochrome system of enzymes and inhibits cellular production of adenosine triphosphate (ATP). Patients present with neurological impairment and lactic acidosis; they typically have arrhythmias, a high cardiac output, and marked vasodilation.

A chemical burn of the respiratory mucosa follows inhalation of large amounts of carbonaceous material, particularly when combined with toxic fumes. Inflammation of the airways results in bronchorrhea and wheezing. Bronchial edema and sloughing of the mucosa lead to obstruction of the lower airways and atelectasis. Progressive ventilation/perfusion mismatching can lead to marked hypoxemia over the course of 24–48 h. Development of SIRS can lead to ALI or ARDS.

Treatment

Fiberoptic bronchoscopy usually establishes the diagnosis of an inhalation injury. Bronchoscopy is usually carried out with a TT over the bronchoscope so that intubation can readily be accomplished if edema threatens the patency of the airway. Early elective tracheal intubation is advisable when there are obvious signs of heat injury to the airway. Patients with hoarseness and stridor require immediate intubation; emergency cricothyrotomy or tracheostomy is necessary if oral or nasal intubation is unsuccessful.

The presence of clinically significant carbon monoxide or cyanide poisoning, as evidenced by obtundation or coma, also requires prompt tracheal intubation and a high inspired oxygen concentration. The diagnosis of carbon monoxide poisoning requires cooximetry measurements because pulse oximeters cannot reliably differentiate between carboxyhemoglobin and oxyhemoglobin. The half-life of carboxyhemoglobin is reduced to 1 h with 100% oxygen; some clinicians advocate hyperbaric oxygen therapy if the patient does not respond to 100% oxygen. The diagnosis of cyanide poisoning is more difficult to make because reliable measurements of cyanide levels are not readily available (normally < 0.1 mg/L). The enzyme rhodanase normally converts cyanide to thiocyanate, which is subsequently eliminated by the kidneys. Treatment for severe cyanide toxicity consists of administering sodium nitrite 300 mg intravenously as a 3% solution over 3–5 min, followed by sodium thiosulfate 12.5 g intravenously in the form of a 25% solution over 1–2 min. Sodium nitrite converts hemoglobin to methemoglobin, which has a higher affinity for cyanide than cytochrome oxidase; the cyanide, which is slowly released from cyanomethemoglobin, is converted by rhodanase to the less toxic thiocyanate.

Marked hypoxemia due to intrapulmonary shunting should be managed with tracheal intubation, oxygen therapy, bronchodilators, positive-pressure ventilation, and PEEP. Corticosteroids are ineffective and increase the rate of infections. As with other forms of ALI, nosocomial infectious pneumonias are common.

■ ACUTE MYOCARDIAL INFARCTION

Acute myocardial infarction (AMI) is a serious complication of ischemic heart disease, with an overall mortality rate of 25%. More than one half of deaths are estimated to occur within the first hour and are usually due to arrhythmias (ventricular fibrillation). With recent advances in interventional cardiology, the hospital mortality rate has been reduced to less than 10–15%. Pump (ventricular) failure is now the leading cause of death in hospitalized patients.

Most myocardial infarctions occur in patients with more than one severely narrowed (> 75%) coronary artery. A transmural infarction occurs in an area distal to a complete occlusion. The occlusion is nearly always due to thrombosis at a stenotic atheromatous plaque. Coronary emboli or severe spasm is less commonly the cause. The size and location of the infarct depend on the distribution of the obstructed vessel and whether collateral vessels have formed. Anterior, apical, and septal infarcts of the left ventricle are usually due to thrombosis in the left anterior descending circulation; lateral and posterior left ventricular infarcts result from occlusions in the left circumflex system, whereas right ventricular and posterior-inferior left ventricular infarcts result from thrombosis in the right coronary artery. In contrast, subendocardial (nontransmural, or "non–Q wave") infarctions usually occur in the setting of a sustained and severe increased myocardial demand in patients with severe stenosis but can also be due to coronary thrombosis.

Following even brief episodes of severe ischemia, prolonged myocardial dysfunction with only a slow and gradual return of contractile function can be observed. This phenomenon of "stunning" is often thought to occur in areas adjacent to infarcted myocardium and can contribute to ventricular dysfunction following AMI. Relief of the ischemia in these areas can restore contractile function. When this phenomenon is observed in the setting of severe chronic ischemia, the myocardium in these noninfarcted but poorly contractile areas is often said to have been "hibernating." Stunning and hibernation are commonly observed in the settings of ischemic cardiac arrest during cardiopulmonary bypass and following myocardial revascularization, respectively.

The immediate treatment of AMI is the administration of oxygen (4–6 L/min), aspirin (160–325 mg), nitroglycerin (sublingual or spray), and morphine (2–4 mg intravenously every 5 min) until the pain is relieved. Remember the acronym: MONA (morphine, oxygen, nitroglycerin, and aspirin) greets all patients. Because the prognosis following AMI is generally inversely proportionate to the extent of necrosis, the current emphasis in management of an evolving myocardial infarction is reperfusion. Based on local resources and timing, angiography with angioplasty and/or a stent with coronary artery bypass surgery backup may be preferred. Alternately, front-loaded alteplase or streptokinase, anistreplase [anisoylated plasminogen streptokinase activator complex (APSAC)], reteplase, or tenecteplase will improve survival. The greatest benefit is if treatment is given within the first hour, but benefit can be seen if treatment is given within 12 h of the AMI.

Patients with ST-segment depression or dynamic T-wave changes (non–Q wave infarction; unstable angina) benefit from antithrombin (heparin) and antiplatelet (aspirin) therapy. All patients without contraindications should receive β-blockers. Other medications such as ACE inhibitors, calcium channel blockers, statins, and so on are indicated based on comorbid conditions. Patients who have recurrent angina should be given nitrates. If angina persists or if there is a contraindication to β-blockers, calcium channel blockers should be administered.

Intraaortic balloon counterpulsation is usually reserved for hemodynamically compromised patients with refractory ischemia. Temporary pacing following AMI is indicated for Mobitz type II and complete heart block, a new bifascicular block, and bradycardia with hypotension. Stable monomorphic ventricular tachycardia, if treated medically and if the patient's ejection fraction is normal, is best managed with procainamide or sotalol. If the ejection fraction is poor, amiodarone at 150 mg intravenous bolus over 10 min is administered. If ventricular tachycardia is polymorphic and the QT interval is normal, abnormal electrolytes should be corrected, ischemia treated, and β-blockers (amiodarone, procainamide, or sotalol can also be given) administered. If the QT interval is prolonged, then in addition to correcting electrolytes, magnesium, overdrive pacing, isoproterenol, phenytoin, or lidocaine is recommended. Lidocaine is the second-tier choice for all four of these indications. Patients with a stable narrow complex supraventricular tachycardia should be treated with amiodarone. Patients with paroxysmal supraventricular tachycardia, whose ejection fraction is preserved, should be treated with a calcium channel blocker, a β-blocker, digoxin, or DC cardioversion. If the ejection fraction is less than 40%, DC cardioversion should be avoided in deference to digoxin, amiodarone, or diltiazem.

Patients with ectopic or multifocal atrial tachycardia should not receive DC cardioversion; instead they should be treated with calcium channel blockers, a β-blocker, or amiodarone. If the ejection fraction is less than 40%, diltiazem could also be considered in addition to amiodarone.

Table 49–7. Reversible causes of azotemia.

Prerenal
Decreased renal perfusion pressure
Hypovolemia
Decreased cardiac output
Hypotension
Increased renal vascular resistance
Neural
Humoral
Pharmacological
Thromboembolic
Postrenal
Urethral obstruction
Bladder outlet obstruction
Prostatic
Bladder tumor
Cystitis
Neurogenic bladder
Bilateral ureteral obstruction
Intrinsic
Calculi
Tumor
Blood clots
Papillary necrosis
Extrinsic
Abdominal or pelvic tumor
Retroperitoneal fibrosis
Inadvertent ureteral ligation

■ RENAL FAILURE

Acute renal failure (ARF) is a rapid deterioration in renal function that is not immediately reversible by altering extrarenal factors, such as blood pressure, intravascular volume, cardiac output, or urinary flow. The hallmark of renal failure is azotemia and frequently oliguria. However, not all patients with acute azotemia have acute renal failure. Likewise, > 500 mL of urine per day does not imply that renal function is normal. Basing the diagnosis of ARF on creatinine levels or an increase in blood urea nitrogen (BUN) is also problematic because creatinine clearance is not always a good measure of glomerular filtration rate.

Typically, ARF is diagnosed by documenting an increase in BUN and plasma creatinine over 24–72 h. In 50% of patients, ARF is secondary to ischemia; in 35% of patients, ARF is due to nephrotoxic causes; and in the remaining 15%, patients have acute tubular interstitial nephritis or acute glomerular nephritis.

Azotemia may be classified as prerenal, renal, and postrenal. Moreover, the diagnosis of ARF (renal azotemia) is one of exclusion; thus, prerenal and postrenal causes must always be excluded.

PRERENAL AZOTEMIA

Prerenal azotemia occurs as a result of hypoperfusion of the kidneys; if untreated, it progresses to ARF. Renal hypoperfusion is most commonly the result of a decrease in arterial perfusion pressure, a marked increase in venous pressure, or renal vasoconstriction (Table 49–7). Decreased perfusion pressure is usually associated with the release of norepinephrine, angiotensin II, arginine vasopressin (AVP, also called antidiuretic hormone), and endothelin. These hormones constrict cutaneous muscle and splanchnic vasculature and promote salt and water retention. The synthesis of vasodilating prostaglandins (prostacyclin and PGE_2) and nitric oxide in the kidneys and the intrarenal action of angiotensin II help maintain glomerular filtration. Use of cyclooxygenase inhibitors or angiotensin-converting enzyme inhibitors in the setting of marked prerenal azotemia can precipitate ARF. The diagnosis of prerenal azotemia is usually suspected from the clinical setting and confirmed by urinary laboratory indices (Table 49–8). Treatment of prerenal azotemia is directed at correcting intravascular volume deficits, improving cardiac function, restoring a normal blood pressure, and reversing increases in renal vascular resistance. The hepatorenal syndrome is discussed in Chapter 35.

Table 49–8. Urinary indices in azotemia.

Index	Prerenal	Renal	Postrenal
Specific gravity	> 1.018	< 0.012	Variable
Osmolality (mmol/kg)	> 500	< 350	Variable
Urine/plasma urea nitrogen ratio	> 8	< 3	Variable
Urine/plasma creatinine ratio	> 40	< 20	Variable
Urine/sodium (mEq/L)	< 10	> 40	Variable
Fractional excretion of sodium (%)	< 1	> 3	Variable
Renal failure index	< 1	> 1	Variable

POSTRENAL AZOTEMIA

Azotemia due to urinary tract obstruction is referred to as postrenal azotemia. Obstruction of urinary flow from both kidneys is usually necessary for azotemia and oliguria/anuria in these conditions. Complete obstruction eventually develops into ARF, whereas prolonged partial obstruction leads to chronic renal impairment. Rapid diagnosis and relief of acute obstruction usually restore normal renal function. Obstruction may be suggested by a physical examination (distended bladder) or a plain radiograph of the abdomen (revealing bilateral renal calculi) but is confirmed by demonstrating dilation of the urinary tract proximal to the site of obstruction. Renal ultrasonography or computed tomography are most commonly used. Treatment depends on the site of obstruction. Obstruction at the bladder outlet can be relieved with catheterization of the bladder or suprapubic cystostomy, whereas ureteral obstruction requires nephrostomy or ureteral stents.

REVERSIBLE AZOTEMIA VERSUS ACUTE RENAL FAILURE

The ability to differentiate prerenal and postrenal azotemia from ARF (renal azotemia) is critical. Exclusion of postrenal azotemia requires visualization of the urinary tract, whereas exclusion of prerenal azotemia depends on the response to treatments aimed at improving renal perfusion. The latter may be facilitated by analysis of urinary composition (see Table 49–8); urinary composition in postrenal azotemia is variable and depends on the duration and severity of obstruction. In prerenal azotemia, tubular concentrating ability is preserved and reflected by a low urinary sodium concentration and high urine/serum creatinine ratio. Calculation of the fractional excretion of filtered sodium ($FENa^+$) may also be extremely useful in the setting of oliguria:

$$FENa^+ = \frac{\text{Urine sodium/serum sodium}}{\text{Urine creatinine/serum creatinine}} \times 100\%$$

$FENa^+$ is less than 1% in oliguric patients with prerenal azotemia but typically exceeds 3% in patients with oliguric ARF. Values of 1–3% may be present in patients with nonoliguric ARF. The renal failure index, which is the urinary sodium concentration divided by the urine/plasma creatinine ratio, is the most sensitive index for diagnosing renal failure. The use of diuretics increases urinary sodium excretion and invalidates indices that rely on urinary sodium concentration as a measure of tubular function. Moreover, intrinsic renal diseases that primarily affect renal vasculature or glomeruli may not affect tubular function and therefore are associated with indices that are similar to prerenal azotemia. Measurement of a 3-h creatinine clearance test can be used to estimate the residual glomerular filtration rate, but several factors must be taken into account. For there to be a good correlation, the increasing serum creatinine must have plateaued.

Etiology of ARF

Causes of ARF are listed in Table 49–9. Up to 50% of cases follow major trauma or surgery; in the majority of instances, ischemia and nephrotoxins are responsible. ARF associated with ischemia and nephrotoxins is generally referred to as acute tubular necrosis. The latter term, however, is inaccurate because intrinsic renal diseases, such as glomerulonephritis and interstitial nephritis, can cause renal failure without tubular necrosis. Moreover, many patients who develop ischemic or nephrotoxic renal failure do not have tubular necrosis on pathological examination. Aminoglycosides, amphotericin B, radiographic contrast dyes, cyclosporine, and cisplatin are the most commonly implicated exogenous nephrotoxins. Amphotericin B, contrast dyes, and cyclosporine also appear to produce direct intrarenal vasoconstriction. Hemoglobin and myoglobin are potent nephrotoxins when they are released during intravascular hemolysis and rhabdomyolysis, respectively. Cyclooxygenase inhibitors, particularly nonste-

Table 49–9. Causes of acute renal failure.

Renal ischemia (50%)
Hypotension
Hypovolemia
Impaired cardiac output
Nephrotoxins (35%)
Endogenous pigments
Hemoglobulin (hemolysis)
Myoglobin (rhabdomyolysis from crush injury and burns)
Radiographic contrast agents
Drugs
Antibiotics (aminoglycosides, amphotericin)
Nonsteroidal antiinflammatory drugs
Chemotherapeutic agents (cisplatin, methotrexate)
Tubular crystals
Uric acid
Oxalate
Sulfonamides
Heavy metal poisoning
Organic solvents
Myeloma protein
Intrinsic renal disease (15%)
Glomerular disease
Interstitial nephritis

roidal antiinflammatory drugs (NSAIDs), may play an important role in at least some patients. Inhibition of prostaglandin synthesis by the latter group of agents decreases prostaglandin-mediated renal vasodilation, allowing unopposed renal vasoconstriction. Other factors predisposing to ARF include preexisting renal impairment, advanced age, atherosclerotic vascular disease, diabetes, and dehydration.

Pathogenesis of ARF

The sensitivity of the kidneys to injury may be explained by their very high metabolic rate and ability to concentrate potentially toxic substances. The pathogenesis of ARF is complex and probably has both a vascular and a tubular basis. Afferent arteriolar constriction, decreased glomerular permeability, direct epithelial cell injury, and tubular obstruction from intraluminal debris or edema can all decrease glomerular filtration. A backleak of filtered solutes through damaged portions of renal tubules may allow reabsorption of creatinine, urea, and other nitrogenous wastes.

Renal ischemia or hypoxia is the likely triggering event in many instances. An imbalance between ATP production and demand in epithelial cells leads to altered ion transport, cellular swelling, altered metabolism of phospholipids, and accumulation of intracellular calcium. Free radical–mediated cell injury can also occur during reperfusion and reoxygenation.

Oliguric versus Nonoliguric ARF

ARF is often classified as oliguric (urinary volume < 400 mL/d), anuric (urinary volume < 100 mL/d), or nonoliguric (urinary volume > 400 mL/d). Nonoliguric ARF accounts for up to 50% of all cases. Patients with nonoliguric ARF typically have urinary sodium concentrations lower than oliguric patients. Moreover, they also appear to have a lower complication rate and to require shorter hospitalizations. Nonoliguric ARF may therefore represent less severe renal injury. In some instances, it may be possible to convert oliguric ARF into nonoliguric ARF by administering mannitol, furosemide, or "renal" doses of dopamine (1–2 μg/kg/min). The resulting increase in urinary output may be therapeutic by preventing tubular obstruction. Mannitol may also decrease cellular swelling and has a free radical scavenging action. Alternatively, the response to diuretic therapy may help identify patients with decreased degrees of renal impairment. However, in recent retrospective studies indicating increased mortality in patients with ARF who receive diuretics, the routine use of diuretics in ARF has been questioned.

Treatment of ARF

ARF accounts for approximately 15% of ICU admissions. Despite the advances in critical care medicine over the past several years, the mortality of ARF remains at approximately 50%. Management of ARF is primarily supportive. Diuretics and mannitol may be used to maintain urinary output in nonoliguric patients. Prospective studies of diuretic use in ARF are lacking. Dopamine has not been shown to be effective in ARF. ARF due to glomerulonephritis or vasculitis may respond to glucocorticoids. Standard treatment for oliguric and anuric patients, who do not increase their urinary output following diuretics, includes restriction of fluid, sodium, potassium, and phosphorus. Daily weight measurements help guide fluid therapy. Fluid intake should generally equal 500 mL plus urinary output. Sodium and potassium intake is limited to 1 mEq/kg/d, whereas protein intake is less than 0.7 g/kg per day and consists mainly of high biological value protein. Hyponatremia can be treated with water restriction. Hyperkalemia may require administration of an ion-exchange resin (sodium polystyrene), glucose and insulin, calcium gluconate, or sodium bicarbonate. Sodium bicarbonate therapy may also be necessary for metabolic acidosis when the serum bicarbonate falls below 15 mEq/L. Hyperphosphatemia requires dietary phosphate restriction and phosphate-binding antacid (aluminum hydroxide). The dosages of renally excreted drugs should be adjusted to the estimated glomerular filtration rate or measured creatinine clearance to prevent accumulation.

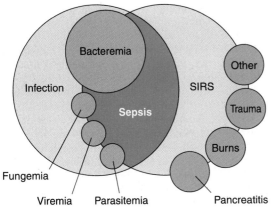

Figure 49–8. The relationship among infection, sepsis, and the systemic inflammatory response system (SIRS). (Modified from the American College of Chest Physicians/Society of Critical Care Medicine Consensus Conference: Definitions for sepsis and organ failure and guidelines for the use of innovative therapies in sepsis. Crit Care Med 1992;20:864.)

Dialysis may be employed to treat or prevent uremic complications (see Table 32–4). A double-lumen catheter placed in the internal jugular, subclavian, or femoral vein is usually used. The high morbidity and mortality rates associated with ARF favor early dialysis, but supporting studies are controversial. Dialysis does not appear to hasten recovery but may in fact aggravate renal injury if hypotension occurs or too much fluid is removed.

Because of concern that intermittent hemodialysis associated with hypotension may perpetuate renal injury, continuous renal replacement therapy (CRRT) (continuous venovenous hemofiltration [CVVHF] and continuous venovenous hemodialysis [CVVHD], which removes fluid and solutes at a slow controlled rate) is increasingly used in critically ill patients with ARF who do not tolerate the hemodynamic effects of intermittent hemodialysis. The main problem associated with CRRT is the expense, as the membrane is prone to clot formation and, therefore, must be periodically replaced. Despite this limitation, many experts believe CRRT is the best way to manage ICU patients with ARF. CRRT is being used not only for ARF (oliguria and uremia) but also to treat metabolic acidosis, fluid overload, and hyperkalemia per se.

Another change in the management of ARF is that whereas protein had been withheld or limited to less than 0.4–0.6 g/kg per day, most nephrologists now believe that nutrition supplementation should not be withheld, and 1.0–1.5 g/kg per day of protein can be given, particularly for patients on CRRT.

■ SEPSIS & SEPTIC SHOCK

The systemic inflammatory response to infection, termed sepsis, is not unique to severe infections because similar manifestations may be encountered with noninfectious illnesses (Figure 49–8). Moreover, it does not necessarily indicate the presence of bacteremia. The use of the term SIRS has been suggested by the Society of Critical Care Medicine (SCCM), European Society of Intensive Care Medicine (ESICM), American College of Chest Physicians (ACCP), American Thoracic Society (ATS), and Surgical Infection Society (SIS) (Table 49–10). The SCCM/ESICM/ACCP/ATS/SIS conference introduced the concept of predisposition, insult infection, response, organ dysfunction (PIRO) to classify sepsis. Severe sepsis exists when the response is associated with organ dysfunction. The term MODS has been suggested to describe progressive dysfunction of two or more organs that is associated with sepsis. Septic shock is defined as acute circulatory failure—systolic blood pressure < 90 mm Hg, mean arterial pressure < 60 mm Hg, or a 40 mm Hg reduction in systolic blood pressure from baseline despite adequate volume resuscitation—in a patient with sepsis.

PATHOPHYSIOLOGY OF SIRS

A mild systemic inflammatory response to any bodily insult may normally have some salutatory effects. However, a marked or prolonged response, such as that associated with severe infections, is often deleterious and can result in widespread organ dysfunction. Although gram-negative organisms account for a majority of infection-related SIRS, many other infectious agents are capable of inducing the same syndrome. These organisms either elaborate toxins or stimulate release of substances that trigger this response. The most commonly recognized initiators are the lipopolysaccharides (LPSs), which are released by gram-negative bacteria. LPS is composed of an O polysaccharide, a core, and lipid A. The O polysaccharide distinguishes between different types of gram-negative bacteria, whereas lipid A, an endotoxin, is responsible for the compound's toxicity. The resulting response to endotoxin involves a complex interaction between macrophages/monocytes, neutrophils, lymphocytes, platelets, and endothelial cells that can affect nearly every organ.

The central mechanism in initiating SIRS appears to be the abnormal secretion of cytokines. These low-molecular-weight peptides and glycoproteins function as intercellular mediators and normally regulate many biological processes, including local and systemic immune

Table 49–10. Diagnostic criteria for sepsis.[1–3]

Infection,[4] documented or suspected, and some of the following
General variables
    Fever (core temperature > 38.3°C)
    Hypothermia (core temperature < 36°C)
    Heart rate > 90/min or > 2 SD above the normal value for age
    Tachypnea
    Altered mental status
    Significant edema or positive fluid balance (> 20 mL/kg
      over 24 h)
    Hyperglycemia (plasma glucose > 120 mg/dL or 7.7 mmol/L)
      in the absence of diabetes
Inflammatory variables
    Leukocytosis (WBC count > 12,000/μL)
    Leukopenia (WBC count < 4000/μL)
    Normal WBC count with > 10% immature forms
    Plasma C-reactive protein > 2 SD above the normal value
    Plasma procalcitonin > 2 SD above the normal value
Hemodynamic variables
    Arterial hypotension[5] (SBP < 90 mm Hg, MAP < 70, or an
      SBP decrease > 40 mm Hg in adults or < 2 SD below nor-
      mal value for age)
    $S\bar{v}O_2 > 70\%$[5]
    Cardiac index[5] > 3.5 L/min per m^2
Organ dysfunction variables
    Arterial hypoxemia ($PaO_2/FIO_2 < 300$)
    Acute oliguria (urine output < 0.5 mL/kg per h or 45 mmol/L
      for at least 2 h)
    Creatinine increase > 0.5 mg/dL
    Coagulation abnormalities (INR > 1.5 or aPTT > 60 s)
    Ileus (absent bowel sounds)
    Thrombocytopenia (platelet count < 100,000/μL)
    Hyperbilirubinemia (plasma total bilirubin > 4 mg/dL or 70
      mmol/L)
Tissue perfusion variables
    Hyperlactatemia (> 1 mmol/L)
    Decreased capillary refill or mottling

---

[1]Reprinted, with permission, from Levy MM, Fink MP, Marshall JC, et al: 2001 SCCM/ESICM/ACCP/ATS/SIS International Sepsis Definitions Conference. Crit Care Med 2003;31:1250.
[2]WBC, white blood cell; SBP, systolic blood pressure; MAP, mean arterial blood pressure; $S\bar{v}O_2$, mixed venous oxygen saturation; INR, international normalized ratio; aPTT, activated partial thromboplastin time.
[3]Diagnostic criteria for sepsis in the pediatric population are signs and symptoms of inflammation plus infection with hyper- or hypothermia (rectal temperature > 38.4°C or < 35°C), tachycardia (may be absent in hypothermia patients), and at least one of the following indications of altered organ function: altered mental status, hypoxemia, increased serum lactate level, or bounding pulses.
[4]Infection defined as a pathological process induced by a microorganism.
[5]$S\bar{v}O_2$ sat > 70% (normally, 75–80%) and cardiac index 3.5–5.5 are normal in children; therefore, neither should be used as a sign of sepsis in newborns or children.

responses, inflammation, wound healing, and hematopoiesis. The most important cytokines released during SIRS are IL-6, adrenomedullin, soluble (s)CD$_{14}$, sELAM-1, MIP-1α, extracellular phospholipase A$_2$, and C-reactive protein. The resulting inflammatory response involves release of potentially harmful phospholipids, attraction of neutrophils, and activation of the complement, kinin, and coagulation cascades.

Increased phospholipase A$_2$ levels release arachidonic acid from cell membrane phospholipids. Cyclooxygenase converts arachidonic acid to thromboxane and prostaglandins, whereas lipoxygenase converts arachidonic acid into leukotrienes (slow-reacting substances of anaphylaxis). Increased phospholipase A$_2$ and acetyltransferase activities result in the formation of another potent proinflammatory compound, platelet-activating factor (PAF). Attraction and activation of neutrophils release a variety of proteases and free radical compounds that damage vascular endothelium. Activation of monocytes causes them to express increased amounts of tissue factor, which in turn can activate both the intrinsic and extrinsic coagulation cascades.

INFECTIONS IN THE ICU

Infections are a leading cause of death in ICUs. Serious infections may be acquired outside the hospital (community acquired) or subsequent to admission for an unrelated illness (nosocomial). The term "nosocomial infection" describes hospital-acquired infections that develop at least 48 h following admission. The reported incidence of nosocomial infections in ICU patients ranges between 10% and 50%. Strains of bacteria resistant to commonly used antibiotics are often responsible. Host immunity plays an important role in determining not only the course of an infection but also the types of organisms that can cause infection. Thus, organisms that normally do not cause serious infections in immunocompetent patients can produce life-threatening infections in those who are immunocompromised (Table 49–11).

Critically ill patients frequently have demonstrable abnormal host defenses, including defective chemotaxis and phagocytosis, altered helper:suppressor T lymphocyte ratios, and impaired humoral immunity. Other host factors include age, drug therapy, integrity of mucosal and skin barriers, and underlying disease. Thus, advanced age (> 70 years), corticosteroid therapy, chemotherapy, prolonged use of invasive devices, respiratory failure, renal failure, head trauma, and burns are established risk factors for nosocomial infections. Patients with burns involving greater than 40% of body surface area have significantly increased mortality from infections. Use of topi-

Table 49-11. Conditions associated with immunocompromise.

Hereditary disorders
    Defects in phagocytosis
    Defects in antibody-mediated (B-cell) immunity
    Defects in cell-mediated (T-cell) immunity
    Defects in complement
    Combined defects
Acquired disorders
    Neutropenia
    Splenectomy
    Acquired immunodeficiency syndrome (AIDS)
    Bone marrow transplantation
    Immunosuppressive therapy
        Organ transplantation
        Autoimmune disorders
    Cytotoxic chemotherapy
    Glucocorticoid therapy
    Radiation therapy
    Malignancies
        Multiple myeloma
        Leukemias
        Lymphomas
    Multiple transfusions

---

cal antibiotics such as sodium mafenide, silver sulfadiazine, and nystatin delays but does not prevent wound infections. Early removal of the necrotic eschar followed by skin grafting and wound closure appears to reverse immunological defects and reduce infections.

Most nosocomial infections arise from the endogenous bacterial flora. Furthermore, many critically ill patients eventually become colonized with resistant bacterial strains. The urinary tract accounts for up to 35–40% of nosocomial infections. Urinary infections are usually due to gram-negative organisms and are associated with the use of indwelling catheters or urinary obstruction. Wound infections are the second most common cause, accounting for up to 25–30%, with pneumonia accounting for another 20–25%. Intravascular catheter-related infections are responsible for 5–10% of ICU infections.

Nosocomial pneumonias are usually caused by gram-negative organisms and are the leading cause of death in many ICUs. GI bacterial overgrowth with translocation into the portal circulation and retrograde colonization of the upper airway from the GI tract followed by aspiration are possible mechanisms for entry for these bacteria. Preservation of gastric acidity inhibits overgrowth of gram-negative organisms in the stomach and their migration into the oropharynx. Tracheal intubation does not appear to provide effective protection because patients commonly aspirate gastric fluid containing bacteria in spite of a properly functioning TT cuff; nebulizers and humidifiers can also be sources of infection. Selective decontamination of the gut with nonabsorbable antibiotics may reduce the incidence of infection but does not change outcome.

Wounds are common sources of sepsis in postoperative and trauma patients; limited antibiotic prophylaxis appears to decrease the incidence of postoperative infections in some groups of patients. Although more commonly seen in postoperative patients, intraabdominal infections due to perforated ulcer, diverticulitis, appendicitis, and acalculous cholecystitis can also develop in critically ill nonsurgical patients. Intravascular catheter-related infections are most commonly due to *Staphylococcus epidermidis, Staphylococcus aureus,* streptococci, *Candida* species, and gram-negative rods. Bacterial sinusitis may be an unrecognized source of sepsis in nasally intubated patients. The diagnosis is suspected from purulent drainage and confirmed by radiographs and cultures.

SEPTIC SHOCK

The SCCM/ESICM/ACCP/ATS/SIS Consensus Conference defines **septic shock** as sepsis associated with hypotension (systolic blood pressure < 90 mm Hg, mean arterial pressure < 60 mm Hg, or systemic blood pressure < 40 mm Hg from baseline) despite adequate fluid resuscitation. Septic shock is usually characterized by inadequate tissue perfusion and widespread cellular dysfunction. In contrast to other forms of shock (hypovolemic, cardiogenic, neurogenic, or anaphylactic), cellular dysfunction in septic shock is not necessarily related to the hypoperfusion. Instead, there may be a metabolic block at the cellular level that contributes to impaired cellular oxidation.

Pathophysiology

A severe or protracted SIRS can result in septic shock. Septic shock is most commonly due to gram-negative infections arising from the genitourinary tract or from the lungs in hospitalized patients, but identical presentations are also seen with other pathogens. Bacteremia is usually present but may be absent. Increased nitric oxide levels may be responsible for the vasodilation. The hypotension is also due to a decreased circulating intravascular volume resulting from a diffuse capillary leak. Many patients also manifest evidence of myocardial depression. Activation of platelets and the coagulation cascade can lead to the formation of fibrin-platelet aggregates, which further compromise tissue blood flow. Hypoxemia resulting from ARDS accentuates tissue hypoxia. The release of vasoactive substances, formation of microthrombi in the pulmonary circulation, or both together increase pulmonary vascular resistance.

HEMODYNAMIC SUBSETS

The circulation in patients with septic shock is often described as either hyperdynamic or hypodynamic. In reality, both represent the same process, but their expression depends on preexisting cardiac function and intravascular volume and where the patient is on the spectrum of response. Systemic venodilation and transudation of fluid into tissues result in relative hypovolemia in patients with sepsis.

Hyperdynamic septic shock is characterized by normal or elevated cardiac output and profound vasodilation (low systemic vascular resistance). Decreased myocardial contractility is often demonstrable even in hyperdynamic patients. Mixed venous oxygen saturation is characteristically high in the absence of hypoxemia and likely reflects the high cardiac output and the cellular metabolic defect in oxygen utilization.

Hypodynamic septic shock, usually seen later in the course of shock, is characterized by decreased cardiac output with low or normal systemic vascular resistance. It is more likely to be seen in severely hypovolemic patients and those with underlying cardiac disease. Myocardial depression is a prominent feature. Mixed venous oxygen saturation may be low in these patients. Pulmonary hypertension is also often prominent in septic shock. Elevation of pulmonary vascular resistance widens the normal pulmonary artery diastolic-to-wedge pressure gradient; large gradients have been associated with a higher mortality rate. The increase in pulmonary vascular resistance may contribute to right ventricular dysfunction.

Clinical Manifestations

Manifestations of septic shock appear to be primarily related to host response rather than the infective agent. Septic shock classically presents with an abrupt onset of chills, fever, nausea (and often vomiting), decreased mental status, tachypnea, hypotension, and tachycardia. The patient may appear flushed and feel

Table 49–12. Initial antibiotic therapy for life-threatening infectious disease syndromes.[1,2]

Syndrome	Pathogens	Initial Empiric Regimens
Cryptogenic sepsis *without* identifiable local infection Community acquired		
Immunocompetent	*Staphylococcus aureus* *Neisseria meningitidis* Group A streptococci	Ceftriaxone or cefotaxime (levofloxicin or gatifloxicin[3]) *plus* vancomycin (*if* MRSA in community acquired infections or has long-term CVC)
A child or elderly adult, or immunocompromised	Same as above *plus* *Streptococcus pneumoniae* (including PRP) *Salmonella* *Listeria*	Ceftriaxone or cefotaxime *plus* ampicillin (vancomycin[3])
Nosocomial	*S. aureus* (including MRSA) Enterococcus (possible VRE) *Pseudomonas aeruginosa* and other resistant gram-negative bacilli	Cefepime, carbapenem, or antipseudomonal penicillin (aztreonam[3]) *plus* ciprofloxacin or tobramycin plus vancomycin (*if* risk MRSA/MRCNS) plus drug for VRE *only* if known culture-positive
Granulocytopenic fever	Same as above	Cefepime or carbapenem *Add* vancomycin (*if* cellulitis, CVC sepsis, septic shock, or known MRSA positive) Ciprofloxacin *plus* vancomycin[3]
Acute bacterial endocarditis Native valve	*S. aureus* Group A streptococci Gram-negative bacilli Enterococcus	Penicillin *plus* nafcillin (vancomycin[3]) plus gentamicin
Prosthetic valve	Same as above *plus* coagulase-negative *Staphylococcus* MRSA Nosocomial gram-negative bacilli *Candida*	Vancomycin *plus* gentamicin

(continued)

Table 49–12. Initial antibiotic therapy for life-threatening infectious disease syndromes.[1,2] (continued)

Syndrome	Pathogens	Initial Empiric Regimens
Susptected IV line sepsis	Same as above	Vancomycin *plus* ciprofloxacin or gentamicin
Presumed bacterial pneumonia		
Community acquired	S. pneumoniae S. aureus Oral anaerobes Enteric gram-negative bacilli Legionella Chlamydia pneumoniae	Ceftriaxone or cefotaxime *plus* azithromycin Levofloxicin or gatifloxicin[3]

Nosocomial or severe
    community acquired
    requiring ICU care
	Same as above *plus*
	P. aeruginosa
	MRSA
		Cefepime or piperacillin-tazobactam or carba-
		  penem (aztreonam[3]) *plus* ciprofloxacin, *plus*
		  vancomycin (*if* risk MRSA)

Sinusitis		
Community acquired	S. pneumoniae Haemophilus influenzae S. aureus	Cefotaxime or ceftriaxone Levofloxicin or gatifloxicin[3] *Add* vancomyucin (if risk MRSA)
Nosocomial	S. aureus (including MRSA) Gram-negative bacilli Fungi	Same as nosocomial pneumonia
Presumed bacterial meningitis		

Community acquired	S. pneumoniae
	H. influenzae type B
	Neisseria meningitidis
	Listeria monocytogenes
		Ceftriaxone, cefotaxime or cefepime *and*
		  vancomycin, *add* rifampin (if also giving
		  corticosteroids)

Nosocomial	Enteric gram-negative bacilli
	P. aeruginosa
	S. aureus (including MRSA) coagulase-
	  negative Staphylococcus
		Cefepime or piperacillin-tazobactam *plus* cipro-
		  floxacin *plus* vancomycin

Intraabdominal infections		

Cholangitis	Enteric gram-negative bacilli
	Enterococci
	Clostridium
		Ciprofloxacin or gentamicin *plus* ampicillin
		  (vancomycin[3])
		Third-generation cephalosporin *plus* ampillicin
		  (vancomycin)
		Carbapenem
		Aztreonam *plus* vancomycin[3]

Secondary peritonitis or
    intraabdominal abscess,
    granulocytopenic typhlitis
	Same as above *plus*
	Bacteroides fragilis
	Other anaerobes
		Metronidazole or clindamycin, *plus* gentamicin
		  or ciprofloxacin *plus* ampicillin (vancomycin[3])
		Ampicillin-sulbactam *and* gentamicin
		Piperacillin-tazobactam *and* gentamicin
		Carbapenem

Spontaneous bacterial peritonitis	Gram-negative bacilli S. pneumoniae	Ceftriaxone or cefotaxime Ciprofloxacin *and* vancomycin[3] Levofloxicin or gatifloxicin[3]
Urosepsis[4]		
Community acquired	Enteric gram-negative bacilli Enterococcus	Ciprofloxacin *and* ampicillin (vancomycin[3]) Gentamicin (tobramycin) *and* ampicillin (vancomycin[3])
Nosocomial	Same as above *plus* P. aeruginosa VRE	Same Carbapenem Give quinupristin or linezolid *only* for docu- mented VRE

(continued)

Table 49–12. Initial antibiotic therapy for life-threatening infectious disease syndromes.[1,2] (continued)

Syndrome	Pathogens	Initial Empiric Regimens
Skin and soft tissue		
Uncomplicated, without granulocytopenia	S. aureus β-Hemolytic streptococci	Nafcillin *with* or *without* penicillin (vancomycin[3]) Vancomycin[3] Ceftriaxone or cefotaxime (children)
Granulocytopenia	S. aureus Gram-negative bacilli, including P. aeruginosa	Cefepime or ticarcillin-clavulate or piperacillin-tazobactam *and* ciprofloxacin or tobramycin *plus* vancomycin
Necrotizing fasciitis	Gram-negative bacilli Clostridia and B. fragilis S. aureus Group A streptococci Vibrio vulnificans	Same as secondary peritonitis Doxycycline Ceftriaxone or cefotaxime
Streptococcal toxic shock syndrome with necrotizing cellulitis	Toxigenic Group A streptococci	Penicillin (vancomycin) *plus* clindamycin
Enteric infection		
Bacterial pathogens	Salmonella Shigella Campylobacter Enteropathogenic Escherichia coli Vibrio	Ciprofloxacin *orally* Ceftriaxone or cefotaxime IV
Antibiotic-associated colitis	C. difficile	Metronidazole (mild or moderately severe) Vancomycin (severe), *also* give IV metronidazole (if ileus)
Toxic shock syndrome	S. aureus Group A streptococci	Nafcillin *and* clindamycin Penicillin G *and* clindamycin
Malaria		
Non-*falciparum* species	Plasmodium vivax Plasmodium malariae Plasmodium ovale	Chloroquine, followed by primaquine[5]
Falciparum	Plasmodium falciparum[6]	Quinine orally (Quinine IV) *plus* doxycycline or clindamycin Atrovaquone-proguanil Mefloquine[7] Artesunate *plus* mefloquine
Rickettsial infections	Ricketssia rickettsii Ricketssia typi Ricketssia prowazeki Ricketssia akari Coxiella burnetii Ehrlichia chaffeensis and Ehrlichia phagocytophilia	Doxycycline Chloramphenicol

[1]Reproduced, with permission, from Maki D: Management of life threatening infections in the ICU. In: *Critical Care Medicine: Perioperative Management.* Murray MJ, Coursin DB, Pearl R, Pough D (editors). Lippincott, Williams & Wilkins, 2002.

[2]MRSA, methicillin-resistant *Staphylococcus aureus*; CVC, central venous catheter; PRP, penicillin-resistant pneumococcus; VRE, vancomycin-resistant enterococci; MRCNS, methicillin-resistant coagulase-negative *Staphylococcus.*

[3]For serious penicillin hypersensitivity.

[4]Gram stain of the urine will show organisms and allow determination, with >98% reliability, whether a drug regimen is needed for gram-negative bacilli alone, for gram-positive cocci alone, or both.

[5]Check for glucose 6-phosphate dehydrogenase deficiency before giving primaquine.

[6]Assume all *falciparum* infections are caused by chloroquine-resistant strain.

[7]Mefloquine resistance is growing.

warm (hyperdynamic) or pale with cool and often cyanotic extremities (hypodynamic); in the latter case, a high index of suspicion is required. In old, debilitated patients and in infants, the diagnosis often is less obvious and hypothermia may be seen.

Leukocytosis with a leftward shift to premature cell forms is typical, but leukopenia can be seen with overwhelming sepsis and is an ominous sign. Progressive metabolic acidosis (usually lactic acidosis) is typically partially compensated by a concomitant respiratory alkalosis. Elevated lactate levels reflect both increased production resulting from poor tissue perfusion and decreased uptake by the liver and kidneys. Hypoxemia may herald the onset of ARDS. Oliguria is most commonly due to the combination of hypovolemia, hypotension, and a systemic inflammatory insult and often progresses to ARF. Elevations in serum aminotransferases and bilirubin are due to hepatic dysfunction. Insulin resistance is uniformly present and produces hyperglycemia. Thrombocytopenia is common and is often an early sign of sepsis. Laboratory evidence of disseminated intravascular coagulation (DIC) is often present but is rarely associated with a bleeding diathesis. The latter responds only to control of the sepsis. Gastric mucosal stress ulceration is common. Respiratory and renal failure are the leading causes of death.

Neutropenic patients (absolute neutrophil count 500/μL) may develop macular or papular lesions that can ulcerate and become gangrenous (ecthyma gangrenosum). These lesions are commonly associated with *Pseudomonas* septicemia but can be caused by other organisms. Perirectal abscesses can develop very quickly in neutropenic patients with few external signs; patients may complain only of perirectal pain.

Treatment

Septic shock is a medical emergency that requires immediate and aggressive intervention. Treatment is threefold: (1) control and eradication of the infection by appropriate and timely intravenous antibiotics (Table 49–12), drainage of abscesses, debridement of necrotic tissues, and removal of infected foreign bodies; (2) maintenance of adequate perfusion with intravenous fluids and inotropic and vasopressor agents; and (3) supportive treatment of complications such as ARDS, ARF, GI bleeding, and DIC.

Antibiotic treatment must be initiated before pathogens are identified but after adequate cultures are obtained (usually of blood, urine, wounds, and sputum). Combination therapy with two or more antibiotics is generally indicated until pathogens are known. In most instances, the combination of a penicillin/β-lactamase inhibitor or third-generation cephalosporin with an aminoglycoside is adequate. Additional diagnostic studies may be indicated (eg, thoracentesis, paracentesis, lumbar puncture, or computed tomographic scans). Debridement and drainage of infections and abscesses should be undertaken expeditiously.

Empiric antibiotic therapy in immunocompromised patients should be based on pathogens that are generally associated with the immune defect (Table 49–13). Vancomycin is added if intravascular catheter-related infection is suspected. Clindamycin or metronidazole should be given to neutropenic patients if a rectal abscess is suspected. Many clinicians initiate amphotericin B, fluconazole, or caspofungin therapy for a presumed fungal infection or when an immunocompromised patient continues to experience fever after 96 h of antibiotic therapy. Granulocyte colony-stimulating factor or granulocyte–macrophage colony-stimulating factor may be used to shorten the period of neutropenia; granulocyte transfusion may occasionally be used in refractory gram-negative bacteremia. Diffuse interstitial infiltrates on a chest radiograph may suggest unusual bacterial, parasitic, or viral pathogens; many clinicians initiate empiric therapy with trimethoprim-sulfamethoxazole and erythromycin in such instances. Nodular infiltrates on a radiograph suggest a fungal pneumonia and may warrant antifungal therapy. Antiviral therapy should be considered in septic patients who are more than 1 month post–bone marrow or solid organ transplantation.

Tissue oxygenation and perfusion are maintained with oxygen therapy, intravenous fluids, inotropes, vasopressors and packed red blood cell transfusions to keep hemoglobin levels > 8–10 g/dL. Marked "third spacing" is characteristic of septic shock. An inotrope should be used if intravenous fluids fail to quickly restore adequate perfusion. Colloid solutions more rapidly restore intravascular volume compared with crystalloid solutions but otherwise offer no proven additional benefit. **Inotropic therapy is generally initiated if 1–3 L of intravenous fluids do not correct the hypotension.** Hematocrit should probably be maintained at or above 24–30% to enhance oxygen delivery. Pulmonary artery catheterization greatly facilitates management in such instances because it allows measurement of PAOP and cardiac output. Most clinicians generally select dopamine as the initial inotrope; others may use dobutamine because it more effectively increases cardiac output and oxygen delivery (Table 49–14). Some studies suggest that patient mortality may be lower if oxygen delivery can be increased. When either dopamine or dobutamine is ineffective in increasing blood pressure and cardiac output, epinephrine (2–18 μg/min) is the agent of choice. In patients with refractory hypotension, norepinephrine, vasopressin, or both are administered with a good improvement in blood pressure but without evidence that it affects outcome. Severe acidosis may decrease the efficacy of inotropes and should therefore generally be corrected (pH > 7.20) with bicarbonate therapy in patients with refractory hypotension.

Table 49–13. Infections associated with altered host immunity.[1]

Host Defect	Pathogens Encountered at the Site of Infection			
	Bloodstream or Disseminated	*Pulmonary*	*Central Nervous System*	*Gastrointestinal*
Hypogammaglobulinemia	*Streptococcus pneumoniae* *Haemophilus influenzae* *Neisseria meningitidis*	*S. pneumoniae* *H. influenzae* *Branhamella catarrhalis*	*S. pneumoniae* *H. influenzae*	*Giardia lamblia*
Splenectomy	Same as above plus *Bartonella*, *Plasmodium*, *Babesia*	As above	As above	
Cell-mediated immunity	*Listeria monocytogenes* *Salmonella* *Mycobacterium tuberculosis* *Coccidioides immitis* *Histoplasma capsulatum* *Cryptococcus neoformans* Cytomegalovirus Varicella-zoster virus Herpes simplex virus	*Legionella* *Nocardia* *Mycobacteria* *C. immitis* *H. capsulatum* *Pneumocystis carinii* Cytomegalovirus	*Listeria* *M. tuberculosis* *C. neoformans* *Toxoplasma gondii* Herpes simplex virus Cytomegalovirus	*Salmonella* *Campylobacter* *Candida* *Cryptosporidium* *Entamoeba histolytica* *Strongyloides stercoralis* Cytomegalovirus Herpes simplex virus

Tumorous obstruction	Cholangitis
	  Gram-negative bacilli
	  Enterococcus
	  Clostridium
	Urosepsis
	  Gram-negative bacilli
	  Enterococcus
	  Candida
	Pneumonia
	  Staphylococcus
	  S. aureus
	  Oral anaerobes
		S. pneumoniae
		S. aureus
		Oral anaerobes
				Gram-negative bacilli
				Enterococci
				Clostridium
				Bacteroides fragilis

Granulocytopenia	Gram-negative bacilli:
	  Pseudomonas aeruginosa
	  Staphylococci
	  Fusarium spp.
	  Candida spp.
		Gram-negative
		Staphylococci
		Aspergillus
			Aspergillus
			Candida
				Candida
				Clostridium difficile
				Other clostridia
				Herpes simplex virus

Reactivation of latent infections	*H. capsulatum* *C. immitis* *Plasmodium*	*M. tuberculosis*	*M. tuberculosis* *H. capsulatum* *C. immitis* *Toxoplasma gondii*	*S. stercoralis*
Central venous catheter	*Staphylococcus epidermidis* *S. aureus* *Corynebacterium*, group *JK* *Mycobacterium* *Bacillus* *Candida* *Fusarium* *Trichosporon*			

[1]Reproduced, with permission, from Maki D: Management of life threatening infections in the ICU. In: *Critical Care Medicine: Perioperative Management.* Murray MJ, Coursin DB, Pearl R, Prough D (editors). Lippincott, Williams & Wilkins, 2002.

Table 49–14. Effects of inotropes and vasopressors in septic patients.

Agent	Blood Pressure	Cardiac Output	Oxygen Delivery
Dopamine	↑↑	↑	↑
Dobutamine	0 or ↑	↑↑	↑↑
Norepinephrine	↑↑	0	0
Epinephrine	↑↑↑	↑↑↑	↑↑↑
Vasopressin	↑↑	0	0

Even in the absence of arterial hypotension, "renal" doses of dopamine may help maintain urinary output but have not been shown to improve outcome. The use of corticosteroids, naloxone, opsonins (fibronectin), and monoclonal antibodies directed against lipopolysaccharide in septic shock has been disappointing, but inhibitors of the coagulation cascade show promise. One such agent, activated protein C, drotrecogin alfa, has been approved by the U.S. Food and Drug Administration for use during sepsis. Because of the expense of this agent and questions about long-term outcome, many ICUs have criteria for when it can be administered to patients that are derived from the original study results (Table 49–15).

■ GASTROINTESTINAL HEMORRHAGE

Acute GI hemorrhage is a common reason for admission to the ICU. Advanced age (> 60 years), comorbid conditions, hypotension, marked blood loss (> 5 units), and recurrent hemorrhage (rebleeding) after 72 h increase mortality. Management consists of simultaneous and rapid evaluation and identification of the site of bleeding and stabilization. Although volume resuscitation is similar, the clinician must attempt to differentiate between upper GI and lower GI bleeding. A history of hematemesis indicates bleeding proximal to the ligament of Treitz. Melena often indicates bleeding proximal to the cecum. Hematochezia (bright red blood from the rectum) indicates either very brisk upper GI bleeding or more commonly lower GI bleeding. The former is likely to be associated with hypotension. The presence of maroon stools usually localizes the bleeding to the area between the distal small bowel and the right colon.

At least two large-bore (14–16 gauge) intravenous cannulas should be placed, and blood should be sent for laboratory analysis (including hematocrit, hemoglobin, platelet count, prothrombin time, and activated partial thromboplastin time). The patient should also be typed and crossed for at least 4–6 units. Fluid resuscitation guidelines are discussed in Chapter 29. Serial hematocrits are useful but may not accurately reflect true blood loss. Intraarterial blood pressure monitoring is very helpful. Central venous cannulation is useful for both venous access and pressure measurements. Placement of a nasogastric tube may help identify an upper GI source if bright red blood or "coffee grounds"–appearing material can be aspirated; inability to aspirate blood, however, does not rule out an upper GI source.

Upper GI Bleeding

Lavage through a nasogastric tube can help assess the rate of bleeding and facilitate esophagogastroduodenos-

Table 49–15. Adult drotrecogin alfa guidelines.

Note: Do not prescribe if more than 48 h has passed since patient first met criteria below.
Positive cultures or suspected infection that is being treated.
At least **three** of the following four criteria of systemic inflammatory response syndrome:
 Core temperature > 38°C or < 36°C
 Heart rate > 80 beats/min
 Respiratory rate > 20 breaths/min or a $Paco_2$ < 32 mm Hg
 White cell count > 12,000/mm^3 or < 4000/mm^3
At least one organ or system dysfunction presumed due to sepsis.
None of the following contraindications exist:
 Prior adverse reaction or hypersensitivity
 Known active bleeding at any site
 Recent surgery (within 12 h)
 Closed head injury, intracranial or spinal surgery, or stroke within 3 months
 Documented intracranial mass lesion, cerebral herniation, or intracranial neoplasm
 Recent or planned epidural catheter (within 2 h)
 APACHE II score less than 25
The following conditions may increase the risk from drotrecogin but the risk-to-benefit assessment may be acceptable:
 Recent gastrointestinal bleeding (within 6 weeks)
 Thrombocytopenia (< 30 × 10^9/L) or an international normalized ratio < 3
 Recent use of IIb/IIIa glycoprotein inhibitors or thrombolytics **or** full anticoagulation with any type heparin or warfarin
 Chronic severe hepatic disease
 Known bleeding disorders
 Pregnancy
 Intracranial arteriovenous malformation or aneurysm
 Single organ failure
 Surgery within 30 days

copy (EGD). EGD should be performed whenever possible to diagnose the cause of bleeding. Failure to visualize the source by endoscopy because of brisk bleeding requires arteriography. Both EGD and arteriography can also be used therapeutically to stop the bleeding. The most common causes of upper GI bleeding, in decreasing order of frequency, are duodenal ulcer, gastric ulcer, erosive gastritis, and esophageal varices. Erosive gastritis may be due to stress, alcohol, aspirin, NSAIDs, and possibly corticosteroids. Less common causes include angiodysplasia, erosive esophagitis, Mallory–Weiss tear, gastric tumor, and aortoenteric fistula.

Bleeding from peptic ulcers (gastric or duodenal) can be coagulated via EGD. Surgery is generally indicated for severe hemorrhage (> 5 U) and recurrent bleeding. H_2-receptor blockers are ineffective in stopping the bleeding but may reduce the likelihood of rebleeding. Selective arteriography of the bleeding vessel allows localized infusion of vasopressin (0.15–0.20 U/min) or arterial embolization.

The most effective treatment for erosive gastritis is prevention. Proton pump inhibitors, H_2-receptor blockers, antacids, and sucralfate are all effective for prevention. Many gastroenterologists advocate the routine administration of a proton pump inhibitor. Once bleeding has occurred, there is generally no specific therapy.

Endoscopic therapy, either with bipolar electrocoagulation or heater probes, is the most effective nonsurgical treatment that reduces blood transfusions, rebleeding, hospital stay, and the need for urgent surgery. Intravenous vasopressin infusions (0.3–0.8 U/min) are generally not as effective; concomitant infusion of nitroglycerin can help reduce portal pressure and may reduce the incidence of cardiac complications. Intravenous propranolol can also lower portal venous pressure and may reduce variceal bleeding. Balloon tamponade (Sengstaken–Blakemore, Minnesota, or Linton tubes) may be used as adjunctive therapy but usually require elective tracheal intubation to protect the airway against aspiration.

Lower GI Bleeding

Common causes of lower GI bleeding include diverticulosis, angiodysplasia, neoplasms, inflammatory bowel disease, ischemic colitis, infectious colitis, and anorectal disease (hemorrhoids, fissure, or fistula). Rectal examination, anoscopy, and sigmoidoscopy can usually diagnose very distal lesions. As with EGD, colonoscopy usually allows definitive diagnosis and is often useful therapeutically. A technetium-99–labeled red blood scan can be used to identify the source of bleeding when colonoscopy cannot be carried out because of inadequate preparation.

Cauterization of the site of bleeding is often possible via colonoscopy. When colonoscopy is unavailable or not possible because of brisk bleeding, selective arteriography can be used to identify the source, which is either embolized or infused with vasopressin. Surgical treatment is reserved for severe or recurrent hemorrhage.

■ NUTRITIONAL SUPPORT

The importance of maintaining adequate nutrition in critically ill patients cannot be overemphasized. Severe malnutrition causes widespread organ dysfunction and increases perioperative morbidity and mortality rates. Nutritional repletion may improve wound healing, restore immune competence, and reduce morbidity and mortality rates in critically ill patients.

OVERVIEW OF NUTRITION

Maintenance of normal body mass, composition, structure, and function requires the periodic intake of water, energy substrates, and specific nutrients. Nutrients that cannot be synthesized from other nutrients are characterized as "essential." Remarkably, relatively few essential nutrients are required to form the thousands of compounds that make up the body. Known essential nutrients include 8–10 amino acids, 2 fatty acids, 13 vitamins, and approximately 16 minerals.

Energy is normally derived from dietary or endogenous carbohydrates, fats, and protein. Metabolic breakdown of these substrates yields the ATP required for normal cellular function. Dietary fats and carbohydrates normally supply most of the body's energy requirements. Dietary proteins provide amino acids for protein synthesis; however, when their supply exceeds both essential and nonessential amino acid requirements, they also function as energy substrates. The metabolic pathways of carbohydrate, fat, and amino acid substrates overlap such that some interconversions can occur through metabolic intermediates (see Figure 34–3). Excess amino acids can therefore be converted to carbohydrate or fatty acid precursors. Excess carbohydrates are stored as glycogen in the liver and skeletal muscle. When glycogen stores are saturated (200–400 g in adults), excess carbohydrate is converted to fatty acids stored as triglycerides primarily in fat cells.

Normal Energy Requirements

Total energy requirements vary widely and depend on the basal metabolic rate (BMR), specific dynamic action (energy required for digestion of meals), and a person's activity level. BMR is energy expenditure measured in the morning immediately after awakening, 12 h after the last meal, and in a state of thermal neutrality. Clinically, basal energy expenditure (BEE) in kilocalories can be estimated by the Harris–Benedict equation, using weight in kilograms, height in centimeters, and age in years:

$$\text{Males: BEE} = 66 + (13.7 \times \text{weight [kg]}) + (5 \times \text{height [cm]}) - (6.8 \times \text{age})$$

$$\text{Females: BEE} = 655 + (9.6 \times \text{weight [kg]}) + (1.8 \times \text{height [cm]}) - (4.7 \times \text{age})$$

BEE is increased by temperature (13% per °C), and degree of stress (see below).

Organ-Specific Substrate Utilization

Variations in the ability to store glycogen and triglycerides, enzyme pathways, and membrane transport mechanisms result in differing substrate utilizations between organs. Neurons, red cells, and cells of the renal medulla normally utilize only glucose. The liver, heart, skeletal muscle, and renal cortex preferentially rely on fatty acid metabolism for energy.

Starvation

The physiology of starvation is such that the protein content of essential tissues is spared. As blood glucose concentration begins to fall during fasting, insulin secretion decreases, whereas glucagon increases. Hepatic and, to a lesser extent, renal glycogenolysis and gluconeogenesis are enhanced. Because glycogen supplies are depleted within 24 h, gluconeogenesis becomes increasingly important. The liver primarily uses deaminated amino acids (alanine and glutamine) as precursors for glucose synthesis. Only neural tissue, renal medullary cells, and erythrocytes continue to utilize glucose, in effect sparing tissue proteins. Lipolysis in adipose tissue is enhanced, so that fats become the principal energy source. Glycerol from the triglycerides enters the glycolytic pathway and fatty acids are broken down to acetyl-coenzyme A (CoA). Excess acetyl-CoA results in the formation of ketone bodies (ketosis). Some fatty acids can contribute to gluconeogenesis. If starvation is prolonged, the brain, kidneys, and muscle also begin to utilize ketone bodies efficiently.

NUTRITION IN CRITICAL ILLNESS

Perioperative critical illnesses are usually characterized by tissue injury, a neuroendocrine stress response, and cachexia. The response to injury involves increases in the secretion of catecholamines, cortisol, glucagon, thyroxine, angiotensin, aldosterone, growth hormone, ACTH, antidiuretic hormone, and thyroid-stimulating hormone. Insulin secretion is at least initially decreased

but may subsequently rise due to increasing levels of growth hormone.

Catecholamines, glucagon, and perhaps growth hormone promote glycogenolysis, whereas glucagon and possibly cortisol induce gluconeogenesis. Hyperglycemia is characteristic and reflects increased hepatic production as well as decreased utilization by peripheral tissues. Moreover, decreased tolerance to glucose loads occurs, apparently as a result of both decreased insulin secretion and peripheral resistance to its actions. Both effects are probably due to increased catecholamine secretion, which also enhances lipolysis. Both protein synthesis and breakdown are increased, but the latter exceeds the former, so that there is a net loss of tissue protein. During sepsis, muscle utilization of fat and carbohydrate is impaired, resulting in increased protein breakdown. Moreover, cells appear to rely more on branched-chain amino acids. Circulating levels of glutamine are decreased. Glutamine is the most prevalent free amino acid in the body. It is an important intermediate in a large number of metabolic pathways. Moreover, rapidly proliferating cells, such as those of the immune system and the GI tract, utilize this amino acid as an energy source.

Administration of glucose during acute illnesses fails to suppress protein breakdown. An adequate intake of calories and proteins can decrease but not prevent protein catabolism in a stressed patient.

Nutritional Assessment of Patients

Evaluation of nutritional status is central to nutritional support of critically ill patients. With the subjective global assessment, a clinician takes a history to detect weight loss, dietary habits, and symptoms of hypoproteinemia (edema) and examines the patient for evidence of loss of skeletal mass or fat stores, edema, or jaundice. The patient is then classified as being normally nourished or mildly or severely malnourished. Alternatively, anthropometric measurements, cutaneous hypersensitivity tests, and laboratory determinations can be used to classify a patient's degree of malnutrition. Patients requiring close assessment include those with less than 80% acceptable body weight or weight loss exceeding 10% in the preceding 6 months, those with serum albumin < 3 g/dL or serum transferrin < 150 mg/dL, those with skin anergy, and those with low total lymphocyte counts (< 1200 cells/μL).

Comparison of body weight to acceptable body weight criteria and measurement of skinfolds are generally indicative of body fat stores. Midarm muscle circumference measurements and the urinary creatinine excretion to height index reflect skeletal protein muscle mass. Serum albumin and transferrin measurements generally indicate protein synthetic ability, although the serum albumin is a better marker of severity of illness.

Prealbumin, because of its shorter half-life, is therefore monitored to try to help assess adequacy of anabolism.

Calculating Energy Requirements

Caloric requirements are usually derived by means of the Harris–Benedict equation (see above). Some clinicians multiply the BMR by a stress factor according to the degree of tissue injury and severity of illness:

$$Stress\ factor = 1–1.25\ for\ mild\ starvation$$
$$= 1.25–1.5\ for\ moderate\ to\ severe\ illness$$
$$= 1.5–1.75\ for\ severe\ illness$$

Most nutritionists, however, give critically ill patients only 20–30 kcal/kg per day because such patients have impaired cellular metabolism—glucose and fatty acids are not completely oxidized. Instead, metabolic intermediates are transported from the cells back to the liver where they are recycled (substrate cycling), increasing metabolic rate even further.

Calculating Energy Expenditure

The resting energy expenditure (REE [not truly basal as the patient is stressed]) can be calculated using indirect calorimetry. This technique relies on measuring oxygen consumption and carbon dioxide production, according to the following formula:

$$REE = (3.94 \times \dot{V}o_2) + (1.11 \times \dot{V}co_2)$$

This calculation is not accurate during gluconeogenesis and lipogenesis.

The respiratory quotient (RQ), $\dot{V}o_2/\dot{V}co_2$, may indicate the primary fuel utilized: An RQ of 1 reflects glucose utilization; a quotient of 0.7 reflects lipid oxidation. Values above 1 reflect lipogenesis.

Calculating Protein Requirements

In contrast to nonstressed patients, who require about 0.5 g/kg/d of protein, critically ill patients generally require 1.0–1.5 g/kg/d. Increasing protein intake to > 1.5 g/kg/d increases anabolism and catabolism such that there is no increase in net protein balance.

ENTERAL NUTRITION

The GI tract is the route of choice for nutritional support when its functional integrity is intact. Enteral feedings can be used to provide complete or supplemental nutrition. Enteral nutrition is simpler, cheaper, less complicated, and associated with fewer complications than parenteral nutrition. Moreover, enteral nutrition appears to better preserve GI structure and function than the parenteral route; studies also suggest that early (1–3 days) enteral nutrition may blunt the hypermetabolic response to improve the host response to infection.

Enteral feedings are most often given as a continuous infusion through a small-bore nasogastric or nasoduodenal tube, gastrostomy, or feeding jejunostomy tube. Therapy is usually initiated at a rate of 25 mL/h and is increased slowly over the course of a few days until the desired caloric and protein goals are reached. Most enteral formulas contain polymeric mixtures of proteins, fats, and carbohydrates. Numerous preparations are available. Selection is based on osmolality and fat content. Some formulas are composed of elemental low-residue formulas. Elemental formulas are indicated in patients with short bowel syndrome, GI fistula, and inflammatory bowel disease and those who have been NPO (nil per os) for weeks; they are readily absorbed and have low residues. Medium-chain triglycerides (MCTs) are composed of 8–10 carbon-chain fatty acids that do not require bile salts or pancreatic enzymes for absorption; MCT oils are indicated for patients with pancreatic insufficiency and cholestasis.

Diarrhea is one of the most common problems with enteral feedings and is usually related to either hyperosmolarity of the solution or lactose intolerance. Gastric distention is another complication that increases the risk of regurgitation and pulmonary aspiration; duodenal or jejunostomy tubes should decrease its incidence. Progressive abdominal distention or large gastric residual volumes are indicative of ileus and should prompt discontinuation of enteral feedings.

PARENTERAL NUTRITION

Total parenteral nutrition (TPN) is indicated if the GI tract cannot be used or if absorption is inadequate. TPN formulas utilize hyperosmolar solutions of amino acids, glucose, and lipids mixed together. The hypertonic nature of these solutions requires central venous access. Electrolytes, trace elements, and a multivitamin preparation are added. Parenteral glucose solutions provide only 3.4 kcal/g (compared with 4 kcal/g for dry carbohydrate) because their glucose concentration is expressed as the monohydrate. Fats are given in the form of a fat emulsion that can be infused separately if not mixed with the glucose–amino acid solution. Fat emulsions are available as either 10% (1.1 kcal/mL) or 20% (2 kcal/mL). Failure to give fat at least once a week may result in essential fatty acid deficiency, which is manifested as dermatitis, alopecia, hepatomegaly (fatty liver), and defective immunity. To infuse an adequate amount of calories in the least volume, fat is often given on a daily basis.

Table 49–16. Complications of total parenteral nutrition.

Catheter-related
  Pneumothorax
  Hemothorax
  Chylothorax
  Hydrothorax
  Air embolism
  Cardiac tamponade
  Thrombosis
    Subclavian vein
    Vena cava
    Pulmonary thromboembolism
  Catheter sepsis
Metabolic
  Azotemia
  Hepatic dysfunction
  Cholestasis
  Hyperglycemia
    Hyperosmolar coma
    Diabetic ketoacidosis
  Excessive CO_2 production
  Hypoglycemia (due to interruption of infusion)
  Metabolic acidosis or alkalosis
  Hypernatremia
  Hyperkalemia
  Hypokalemia
  Hypocalcemia
  Hypophosphatemia
  Hyperlipidemia
  Pancreatitis
  Fat embolism syndrome
  Anemia
    Iron
    Folate
    B_{12}
    ? Copper
  Vitamin D deficiency
  Vitamin K deficiency
  Essential fatty acid deficiency
  Hypervitaminosis A
  Hypervitaminosis D

The amount of amino acids given is determined by estimated protein requirements (see above), whereas glucose and fat are given to the desired caloric requirements (see above). Fat calories generally should account for 30–40% of the desired caloric requirements. Excessive reliance on glucose exacerbates problems with hyperglycemia and increases CO_2 production. The latter may be a problem in weaning patients with a compromised pulmonary reserve from mechanical ventilation.

Complications of TPN are either metabolic or related to central venous access (Table 49–16). Over-feeding with excess amounts of glucose can increase energy requirements and production of carbon dioxide; the respiratory quotient can exceed 1 because of lipogenesis. Overfeeding can lead to reversible cholestatic jaundice. Mild elevations of serum transaminases and alkaline phosphatase may reflect fatty infiltration of the liver resulting from overfeeding.

TPN can be modified for patients with significant hepatic or renal impairment. Altering the amino acid load may be beneficial in patients with hepatic encephalopathy. Plasma amino acid concentrations tend to be altered in these patients: phenylalanine and methionine are usually elevated, whereas branched-chain amino acids (leucine, isoleucine, and valine) are reduced. Amino acid formulations for patients with liver disease (HepatAmine) are therefore rich in branched-chain amino acids but low in aromatic amino acids. Patients with hepatic encephalopathy can be tried on Hepat-Amine, which is continued if there is evidence of improvement in the mental status.

Protein content is no longer reduced in patients with ARF. With the availability of CRRT, it is better to feed these patients adequate amounts of protein (1.0–1.5 g of protein/kg/d). Total TPN volume, acid–base balance, and potassium content must be altered based on patient assessment.

Monitoring Patients on TPN

Initiation of TPN requires close metabolic monitoring. The most common problem is hyperglycemia. A gradual increase in the infusion rate decreases the severity of hyperglycemia and allows sufficient time for enhanced endogenous insulin secretion. Stressed patients often require the addition of insulin to the TPN solution. Abrupt withdrawal of TPN can precipitate hypoglycemia due to high circulating insulin levels, but this is not a common problem if the patient is not overfed; in this case, 10% glucose can be temporarily substituted for the TPN and gradually decreased. Serum glucose measurements should generally be measured every 4 h until they stabilize. Other measurements (serum electrolytes, BUN, creatinine) are obtained daily. Calcium, phosphate, and magnesium concentrations and liver tests (including prealbumin) can be checked weekly. The complete blood cell count (including a differential count) should also be monitored. Lipid clearance can be checked by measuring a serum triglyceride level if there is any evidence of lipemia or concern about pancreatitis or if patients have a history of abnormal lipoprotein concentrations. Twenty-four-hour nitrogen balance studies are sometimes used in checking the efficacy of nutritional support:

$$\text{Nitrogen balance} = \text{input} - \text{output},$$
$$\text{Nitrogen output} = (\text{UNN} \times 1.2 \times \text{urinary volume}) + 2\,\text{g}$$

where UUN = urinary urea nitrogen concentration (g/L). The 2 g in the above equation represents fecal and integumentary nitrogen losses. UUN is multiplied by 1.2, as urea nitrogen represents only 80% of urinary nitrogen losses. Ideally, TPN should result in a positive nitrogen balance, but this is rarely, if ever, achieved in critically ill patients.

Anesthetic Management of Patients Receiving TPN

Patients who are receiving TPN often require surgical procedures. They require careful preoperative evaluation because of the large number of potentially serious complications that can be associated with TPN (Table 49–16). Metabolic abnormalities are relatively common and should generally be corrected preoperatively. Hypophosphatemia is a serious and often unrecognized complication that can contribute to postoperative muscle weakness and respiratory failure.

When TPN infusions are suddenly stopped or decreased perioperatively, hypoglycemia may develop. Frequent measurements of blood glucose concentration are therefore required in such instances during general anesthesia. On the other hand, if the TPN solution is continued unchanged, excessive hyperglycemia resulting in hyperosmolar nonketotic coma or ketoacidosis (in diabetics) is also possible. The neuroendocrine stress response to surgery frequently aggravates glucose intolerance. Some clinicians routinely reduce the rate of the TPN infusion, whereas others substitute a 10% dextrose solution; however, with the current practice of not overfeeding patients, it is often safe to discontinue TPN completely. **Regardless of whether the TPN infusion is continued, reduced, replaced with 10% dextrose, or stopped, subsequent therapy should be based on blood glucose measurements.** Blood glucose concentration should generally be maintained between 100 and 150 mg/dL. Lastly, to decrease the likelihood of catheter sepsis, the integrity of the TPN infusion-catheter system generally should not be violated with drug injections. Separate infusions should be used for injection of anesthetic agents and administration of other perioperative fluids and blood.

PERIPHERAL PARENTERAL NUTRITION

When a 3–4% amino acid solution is added to a 5–10% dextrose solution, the resulting solution is still hypertonic but can generally be infused through a peripheral vein without irritation. Simultaneous infusion of a 1% fat emulsion through the same intravenous catheter further reduces the concentration and provides additional calories. Volume constraints limit caloric intake with peripheral parenteral nutrition to a maximum of 800–1200 kcal/d, which is satisfactory in a majority of patients.

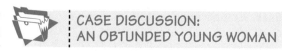

CASE DISCUSSION: AN OBTUNDED YOUNG WOMAN

A 23-year-old woman is admitted to the hospital obtunded with slow respirations (7 breaths/min). Blood pressure is 90/60 mm Hg and the pulse is 90 beats/min. She was found at home in bed with empty bottles of diazepam, acetaminophen with codeine, and fluoxetine lying next to her.

How is the diagnosis of a drug overdose made?

The presumptive diagnosis of a drug overdose usually must be made from the history, circumstantial evidence, and any witnesses. Signs and symptoms may not be helpful. Confirmation of a suspected drug overdose or poison ingestion usually requires delayed laboratory testing for the suspected agent in body fluids. Intentional overdoses (self-poisoning) are the most common mechanism and typically occur in young adults who are depressed. Ingestion of multiple drugs is common. Benzodiazepines, antidepressants, aspirin, acetaminophen, and alcohol are the most commonly ingested agents.

Accidental overdoses frequently occur in intravenous drug abusers. Commonly abused substances include opioids, stimulants (cocaine and amphetamine), and hallucinogens (phencyclidine [PCP]). Younger children occasionally accidentally ingest caustic household alkali (eg, drain cleaner), acids, and hydrocarbons (eg, petroleum products). Organophosphate poisoning (parathion and malathion) usually occurs in adults following agricultural exposure. Overdoses and poisoning less commonly occur as an attempted homicide.

What are appropriate steps in managing this patient?

Regardless of the type of drug or poison ingested, the principles of initial supportive care are the same. Airway patency and adequate ventilation and oxygenation must be established. Unless otherwise indicated, oxygen therapy (100%) should probably be administered. Hypoventilation and obtunded airway reflexes require tracheal intubation and mechanical ventilation. Many clinicians routinely administer naloxone (up to 2 mg), dextrose 50% (50 mL), and thiamine (100 mg) intravenously to all obtunded or comatose patients until a diagnosis is established; this may help exclude or treat opioid overdose, hypoglyce-

mia, and Wernicke–Korsakoff syndrome, respectively. The dextrose can be omitted if a glucose determination can be obtained by a fingerstick. In this case, intubation should be performed prior to naloxone because the respiratory depression is likely due to both the codeine and the diazepam.

Blood, urine, and gastric fluid specimens should be obtained and sent for drug screening. Blood is also sent for routine hematological and chemistry studies (including liver function). Urine is usually obtained by bladder catheterization, and gastric fluid can be aspirated from a nasogastric tube; the latter should be placed after intubation to avoid pulmonary aspiration. Alternatively, emesis material may be tested for drugs in conscious persons.

Hypotension should generally be treated with intravenous fluids unless the patient is obviously in pulmonary edema; an inotrope may be necessary in some instances. Seizure activity may be the result of hypoxia or a pharmacological action of a drug (tricyclic antidepressants) or poison. Seizure activity is unlikely in this patient because she ingested diazepam, a commonly used anticonvulsant.

Should flumazenil be administered?

Flumazenil should generally not be administered to patients who overdose on both a benzodiazepine and an antidepressant and those who have a history of seizures. Reversal of the benzodiazepine's anticonvulsant action can precipitate seizure activity in such instances. Moreover, as is the case with naloxone and opioids, the half-life of flumazenil is shorter than that of benzodiazepines. Thus, it is often preferable to ventilate the patient until the benzodiazepine effect dissipates, the patient regains consciousness, and the respiratory depression resolves.

Should any other antidotes be given?

Because the patient also ingested an unknown quantity of acetaminophen (paracetamol) administration of N-acetylcysteine (NAC; Mucomyst) should be considered. Acetaminophen toxicity is due to depletion of hepatic glutathione, resulting in the accumulation of toxic metabolic intermediates. Hepatic toxicity is usually associated with ingestion of more than 140 mg/kg of acetaminophen. NAC prevents hepatic damage by acting as a sulfhydryl donor and restoring hepatic glutathione levels. If the patient is suspected of having ingested a toxic dose of acetaminophen, an initial dosage of NAC (140

mg/kg orally or by nasogastric tube) should be administered even before plasma acetaminophen levels are obtained; additional doses are given according to the measured plasma level. If the patient cannot tolerate oral or gastric administration of NAC, if the patient is pregnant, or if the risk of hepatotoxicity is high, NAC should be given intravenously.

What measures might limit drug toxicity?

Toxicity might be reduced by decreasing drug absorption or enhancing elimination. GI absorption of an ingested substance can be reduced by emptying stomach contents and administering activated charcoal. Both methods can be effective up to 12 h following an ingestion. If the patient is intubated, the stomach is lavaged carefully to avoid pulmonary aspiration. Emesis may be induced in conscious patients with syrup of ipecac 30 mL (15 mL in a child). Gastric lavage and induced emesis are generally contraindicated for patients who ingest caustic substances or hydrocarbons because of a high risk of aspiration and worsening mucosal injury.

Activated charcoal 1–2 g/kg is administered orally or by nasogastric tube with a diluent. The charcoal irreversibly binds most drugs and poisons in the gut, allowing them to be eliminated in stools. In fact, charcoal can create a negative diffusion gradient between the gut and the circulation, allowing the drug or poison to be effectively removed from the body.

Alkalinization of the serum with sodium bicarbonate for tricyclic antidepressant overdose is beneficial because, by increasing pH, protein binding is enhanced; the sodium decreases sodium channel inhibition, and if seizures occur the alkalinization prevents acidosis-induced cardiotoxicity.

What other methods can enhance drug elimination?

The easiest method of increasing drug elimination is forced diuresis. Unfortunately, this method is of limited use for drugs that are highly protein bound or have large volumes of distribution. Mannitol or furosemide with saline may be used. Concomitant administration of alkali (sodium bicarbonate) enhances the elimination of weakly acidic drugs such as salicylates and barbiturates; alkalization of the urine traps the ionized form of these drugs in the renal tubules and enhances urinary elimination. Hemodialysis generally has a limited role in this type of setting; it is *usually reserved for patients with severe toxicity who continue to deteriorate despite aggressive supportive therapy.*

SUGGESTED READING

American Heart Association: Guidelines 2000 for Cardiopulmonary Resuscitation and Emergency Cardiovascular Care. Circulation (Suppl) 2000;102:I86.

Levy MM, Fink MP, Marshall JC, et al: 2001 SCCM/ESICM/ACCP/ATS/SIS International Sepsis Definitions Conference. Crit Care Med 2003;31:1250.

Murray MJ, Coursin DB, Pearl RG, Prough DS: *Critical Care Medicine. Perioperative Medicine.* Lippincott, Williams & Wilkins, 2002.

Noble DW: Acute renal failure and diuretics: Propensity, equipoise, and the need for a clinical trial. Crit Care Med 2004;32:1794.

Parillo JE, Dellinger RP (editors): *Critical Care Medicine. Principles of Diagnosis and Management.* W.B. Saunders, 2001.

Silvester W, Bellomo R, Cole L: Epidemiology, management, and outcome of severe acute renal failure of critical illness in Australia. Crit Care Med 2001;29:1910.

Star RA: Treatment of acute renal failure. Kidney Int 1998;54:1817.

Ward JJ: Medical gas therapy. In: *Respiratory Care: A Guide to Clinical Practice,* 4th ed. Burton GG, Hodgkin JE, Ward JJ (editors). Lippincott-Raven, 1997.

Index

NOTE: A *t* following a page number indicates tabular material and *f* following a page number indicates a figure.

Peripheral nerve

Nerve root

Trigeminal
- Ophthalmic branch
- Maxillary branch
- Mandibular branch

Anterior cutaneous nerve of neck

Supraclavicular nerves

Axillary nerve

Medial cutaneous nerve of arm
Lateral cutaneous nerve of arm

Medial cutaneous nerve of forearm

Lateral cutaneous nerve of forearm

Radial

Median

Ulnar
Lateral femoral cutaneous
Obturator
Medial femoral cutaneous
Anterior femoral cutaneous

Lateral cutaneous nerve of calf

Saphenous

Superficial peroneal

Sural

Lateral and medial plantar

Deep peroneal

Post. Mid. Ant
Lateral thoracic rami
Anterior thoracic rami

C3
C4
C5
T2
T3
T4
T5
T6
T7
T8
T9
T10
T11
T12
T2
T1
C6
L1
L1
L2
C8
C7
L3
L4 L5
C6
S1

X = Iliohypogastric
† = Ilioinguinal
* = Genitofemoral
█ Dorsal nerve of penis
▓ Perineal